Dr. D'Amato

C0-AVD-979

Dr. D'Amato

Clinical Pediatric Gastroenterology

Clinical Pediatric Gastroenterology

Steven M. Altschuler, M.D.
Physician-in-Chief
Children's Hospital of Philadelphia

Chair, Department of Pediatrics
University of Pennsylvania School of Medicine
Philadelphia, Pennsylvania

Chris A. Liacouras, M.D.
Director of Pediatric Endoscopy
Children's Hospital of Philadelphia

Assistant Professor of Pediatrics
University of Pennsylvania School of Medicine
Philadelphia, Pennsylvania

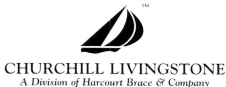

CHURCHILL LIVINGSTONE
A Division of Harcourt Brace & Company
Philadelphia London Toronto Montreal Sydney Tokyo

CHURCHILL LIVINGSTONE
A Division of Harcourt Brace & Company

The Curtis Center
Independence Square West
Philadelphia, Pennsylvania 19106

Library of Congress Cataloging-in-Publication Data

Clinical pediatric gastroenterology / [edited by] Steven M.
  Altschuler, Christopher A. Liacouras.

    p.   cm.

   ISBN 0-443-05542-4

   1. Pediatric gastroenterology.   2. Liver—Diseases.
I. Altschuler, Steven. II. Liacouras, Christopher A.
   [DNLM: 1. Gastrointestinal Diseases—in infancy & childhood.
2. Liver Diseases—in infancy & childhood. 3. Pancreatic Diseases—
in infancy & childhood. 4. Biliary Tract Diseases—in infancy &
childhood. WS 310 P37127 1998]

RJ446.P34 1998 618.92′33—dc21

DNLM/DLC   97-47601

CLINICAL PEDIATRIC GASTROENTEROLOGY   ISBN 0-443-05542-4

Printed in the United States of America

Last digit is the print number: 9   8   7   6   5   4   3   2   1

PREFACE

The growth of managed care is forcing pediatric providers to reconstruct and integrate the health care delivery system with a focus away from specialty-dominated care and toward a primary care model. With this development in mind, *Clinical Pediatric Gastroenterology* has been designed to provide the primary care physician with the essential information necessary to diagnose and manage gastrointestinal and nutritional problems of childhood. Equally important, it also provides the criteria for referral of patients with more complicated diagnostic or therapeutic problems to specialty centers. Thus, this text is intended to facilitate care of pediatric patients with gastrointestinal and nutritional problems by providing a basis for primary care providers and specialists to cooperate and integrate care.

The contributing authors have been selected because of expertise based on their clinical experience, a track record of successful interactions with referring primary care providers, and their appreciation of the monumental changes occurring in health care. They have all written concise, practical, and easy to read chapters that facilitate access to and interpretation of up-to-date clinical information on a wide variety of pediatric gastrointestinal and nutritional issues. During the editorial process, care has been taken to ensure that each chapter conforms to a standard format. We hope that the reader will use the text to help determine for an individual patient the most appropriate level of care in the most appropriate setting at the most appropriate time.

As editors, we would like to thank all contributing authors for their hard work and interest in this project. Their commitment to excellence in patient care and education is readily apparent.

STEVEN M. ALTSCHULER, M.D.
CHRIS A. LIACOURAS, M.D.

CONTRIBUTORS

STEVEN M. ALTSCHULER, M.D.

Chair, Department of Pediatrics, University of Pennsylvania School of Medicine; Physician-in-Chief, Children's Hospital of Philadelphia, Philadelphia, Pennsylvania
Irritable Bowel Syndrome

LINDA ARNOLD, M.D.

Senior Fellow, Gastroenterology and Nutrition, Department of Pediatrics, University of Pennsylvania School of Medicine; Division of Gastroenterology and Nutrition, Children's Hospital of Philadelphia, Philadelphia, Pennsylvania
Foreign Bodies and Caustic Ingestions

MARK BAGARAZZI, M.D.

Assistant Professor, Department of Pediatrics, Allegheny University of the Health Sciences MCP Hahnemann School of Medicine; Attending Physician, Division of Immunology, St. Christopher's Hospital for Children, Philadelphia, Pennsylvania
Parasites

ROBERT N. BALDASSANO, M.D.

Assistant Professor, Department of Pediatrics, University of Pennsylvania School of Medicine; Director, Inflammatory Bowel Disease Center, Division of Gastroenterology and Nutrition, Children's Hospital of Philadelphia, Philadelphia, Pennsylvania
Diarrhea; Portal Hypertension

JAY BARTH, M.D.

Assistant Professor, Department of Pediatrics, Mount Sinai School of Medicine; Assistant Attending Physician, Department of Pediatric Gastroenterology and Nutrition, Mount Sinai Medical Center, New York, New York
Lactose Intolerance

LOUIS BELL, M.D.

Associate Professor of Pediatrics, University of Pennsylvania School of Medicine; Attending Physician, Division of Emergency Medicine and Section of Infectious Disease, Children's Hospital of Philadelphia, Philadelphia, Pennsylvania
Parasites

RICHARD D. BELLAH, M.D.

Associate Professor, Departments of Radiology and Pediatrics, University of Pennsylvania School of Medicine; Director, Division of Ultrasound, Department of Radiology, Children's Hospital of Philadelphia, Philadelphia, Pennsylvania
Abdominal Ultrasound

JULIA A. BILODEAU, M.S.N., R.N., C.P.N.P.

Advanced Practice Nurse, Division of Gastroenterology and Nutrition, Children's Hospital of Philadelphia, Philadelphia, Pennsylvania
Parenteral Nutrition and Care of Central Venous Lines

JOHN T. BOYLE, M.D.

Associate Professor, Department of Pediatrics, Case Western Reserve University School of Medicine; Chief, Division of Gastroenterology and Nutrition, Rainbow Babies and Children's Hospital, Cleveland, Ohio
Achalasia

DELMA L. BROUSSARD, M.D.

Assistant Professor, Department of Pediatrics, University of Pennsylvania School of Medicine, Philadelphia, Pennsylvania
Dysphagia; Manometry; Pseudo-obstruction

KURT A. BROWN, M.D.

Assistant Professor, Department of Pediatrics, University of Pennsylvania School of Medicine; Attending Physician, Division of Gastroenterology and Nutrition, Children's Hospital of Philadelphia, Philadelphia, Pennsylvania
Eosinophilic Enteritis; Pancreatitis

EMIL CHUANG, M.D.

Assistant Professor, Division of Gastroenterology and Nutrition, Duke University School of Medicine, Durham, North Carolina
Alpha-1-Antitrypsin Deficiency

WILLIAM J. COCHRAN, M.D.

Clinical Associate Professor, Department of Pediatrics, Pennsylvania State University College of Medicine, Hershey; Associate, Department of Pediatric Gastroenterology and Nutrition, Geisinger Medical Center, Danville, Pennsylvania
Diarrhea; Portal Hypertension

ROBERT M. COHN, M.D.

Associate Professor, Department of Pediatrics, University of Pennsylvania School of Medicine; Deputy Director, Clinical Laboratories, and Senior Physician, Division of Metabolism, Children's Hospital of Philadelphia, Philadelphia, Pennsylvania
Laboratory Testing: Metabolic Testing

ANDREW M. DAVIDOFF, M.D.

Surgical Fellow, University of Pennsylvania School of Medicine; Chief Resident of Surgery, Department of Surgery, Children's Hospital of Philadelphia, Philadelphia, Pennsylvania
Laparoscopy

KATHERINE MACRAE DELL, M.D.

Fellow, Division of Nephrology, Department of Pediatrics, Children's Hospital of Philadelphia, Philadelphia, Pennsylvania
Hemolytic Uremic Syndrome

PATRICIA A. DERUSSO, M.D.

Section on Human Iron Metabolism, Cell Biology and Metabolism Branch, National Institute of Child Health and Human Development, Bethesda, Maryland
Iron Overload Conditions

CARLO DI LORENZO, M.D.

Associate Professor, Department of Pediatrics, Children's Hospital of Pittsburgh, Pittsburgh, Pennsylvania
Hirschsprung's Disease

KAREN D. FAIRCHILD, M.D.

Assistant Professor, Department of Pediatrics, University of Maryland School of Medicine; Attending Physician, University of Maryland Hospital, Baltimore, Maryland
Necrotizing Enterocolitis

KENNETH E. FELLOWS, M.D.

Professor, Department of Radiology, University of Pennsylvania School of Medicine; Radiologist-in-Chief, Department of Radiology, Children's Hospital of Philadelphia, Philadelphia, Pennsylvania
Angiography and Interventional Procedures; Vascular Disorders of the Liver

DAVID A. FERENCI, M.D.

Clinical Instructor, Department of Pediatrics, University of Minnesota; Consultant, Department of Pediatric Gastroenterology, Children's Healthcare, Minneapolis, Minnesota
Celiac Disease

FRANCIS M. GIARDIELLO, M.D.

Associate Professor, Department of Medicine, Johns Hopkins University School of Medicine, Baltimore, Maryland
Polyps

JAMES B. GIBSON, M.D., Ph.D.

Assistant Professor, Section of Genetics, Department of Pediatrics, University of Arkansas College of Medicine for Medical Sciences; Attending Physician, Medical Genetics, Arkansas Children's Hospital and University Hospital UAMS, Little Rock, Arkansas
Galactosemia

JANE M. GOULD, M.D.

Clinical Assistant Professor, Department of Pediatrics, University of Pennsylvania School of Medicine; Assistant Physician, Primary Care, Children's Hospital of Philadelphia, Philadelphia, Pennsylvania
Pancreatitis

RICHARD J. GRAND, M.D.

Professor, Departments of Pediatrics, Gastroenterology, and Nutrition, Tufts University School of Medicine; Chief, Division of Pediatric Gastroenterology and Nutrition, New England Medical Center, Boston, Massachusetts
Wilson's Disease

BARBARA A. HABER, M.D.

Assistant Professor of Pediatrics, Department of Pediatrics, University of Pennsylvania School of Medicine; Division of Gastroenterology and Nutrition, Children's Hospital of Philadelphia, Philadelphia, Pennsylvania
Hepatomegaly; Tyrosinemia

M. PATRICIA HARTY, M.D.

Assistant Professor, Department of Radiology, University of Pennsylvania School of Medicine; Radiologist, Department of Radiology, Children's Hospital of Philadelphia, Philadelphia, Pennsylvania
Plain Abdominal Radiography

JANICE B. HEIKENEN, M.D.

Department of Pediatrics, Division of Gastroenterology, Medical College of Wisconsin and Children's Hospital of Wisconsin, Milwaukee, Wisconsin
Congenital Anomalies of the Pancreas and Biliary Tract

SYDNEY HEYMAN, M.D.

Professor, Division of Nuclear Medicine, Department of Radiology, University of Pennsylvania School of Medicine; Director, Division of Nuclear Medicine, Children's Radiology Associates, Philadelphia, Pennsylvania
Nuclear Medicine

MARK A. HOFFMAN, M.S., M.D.

Assistant Professor, Department of Surgery, Uniformed Services University of the Health Sciences, Bethesda, Maryland; Attending Surgeon, General Surgery Service, Walter Reed Army Medical Center, Washington, District of Columbia
Congenital Anomalies of the Intestine

CELESTE M. HOLLANDS, M.D.

Resident, Department of Surgery, Children's Surgical Associates, Children's Hospital of Philadelphia, Philadelphia, Pennsylvania
Congenital Anomalies of the Intestine

ANNE M. HUBBARD, M.D.

Associate Professor, Department of Radiology, University of Pennsylvania School of Medicine; Director, Body Magnetic Resonance Imaging, Department of Radiology, Children's Hospital of Philadelphia, Philadelphia, Pennsylvania
Magnetic Resonance Imaging

JEFFREY S. HYAMS, M.D.

Professor and Vice-Chairman, Department of Pediatrics, University of Connecticut School of Medicine, Farmington; Head, Division of Digestive Diseases, Connecticut Children's Medical Center, Hartford, Connecticut
Inflammatory Bowel Disease

MARK J. INTEGLIA, M.D.

Fellow in Pediatric Gastroenterology, Tufts University School of Medicine and Floating Hospital for Children at New England Medical Center, Boston, Massachusetts
Wilson's Disease

DIANE S. JAKOBOWSKI, M.S.W., C.R.N.P.

Interim Administrator, Multi Organ Transplant Program, University of Pennsylvania Health System, Philadelphia, Pennsylvania
Management of Ostomies

WENDY JESHION, M.D.

Senior Gastroenterology and Nutrition Fellow, University of Pennsylvania School of Medicine; Division of Gastroenterology and Nutrition, Children's Hospital of Philadelphia, Philadelphia, Pennsylvania
Clostridium difficile

HELEN A. JOHN, M.D.

Senior Gastroenterology/Nutrition Fellow, Division of Pediatric Gastroenterology and Nutrition, University of Pennsylvania School of Medicine and Children's Hospital of Philadelphia, Philadelphia, Pennsylvania
Cystic Fibrosis–Related Gastrointestinal and Liver Disease; Gastrointestinal and Hepatobiliary Disease in the Acquired Immunodeficiency Syndrome

MAUREEN M. JONAS, M.D.

Assistant Professor, Department of Pediatrics, Harvard Medical School; Associate, Division of Gastroenterology and Nutrition, Children's Hospital, Boston, Massachusetts
Biliary Atresia

HOWARD A. KADER, M.D.

Fellow, Gastroenterology and Nutrition, University of Pennsylvania School of Medicine; Division of Gastroenterology and Nutrition, Children's Hospital of Philadelphia, Philadelphia, Pennsylvania
Abdominal Pain

BERNARD S. KAPLAN, M.B., B.Ch.

Professor, Department of Pediatrics, University of Pennsylvania School of Medicine; Director, Division of Nephrology, Children's Hospital of Philadelphia, Philadelphia, Pennsylvania
Hemolytic Uremic Syndrome

PAIGE KAPLAN, M.D.

Professor, Division of Pediatrics, University of Pennsylvania School of Medicine; Senior Physician, Departments of Metabolism and Genetics, Children's Hospital of Philadelphia, Philadelphia, Pennsylvania
Gaucher's Disease and Niemann-Pick Disease

GREGORY F. KEENAN, M.D.

Assistant Professor, Departments of Pediatrics and Medicine, University of Pennsylvania School of Medicine; Acting Section Chief, Section of Rheumatology, Children's Hospital of Philadelphia, Philadelphia, Pennsylvania
Henoch-Schönlein Purpura

JANICE A. KELLY, M.D.

Clinical Assistant Professor of Pediatrics, Private Practice, Bryn Mawr, Pennsylvania
Uncommon Intestinal Diseases: Mallory Weiss Tear

SANDRA S. KRAMER, M.D.

Professor, Department of Radiology, University of Pennsylvania School of Medicine; Associate Radiologist-in-Chief, Department of Radiology, Children's Hospital of Philadelphia, Philadelphia, Pennsylvania
Abdominal Computed Tomography

CHRIS A. LIACOURAS, M.D.

Assistant Professor, Department of Pediatrics, University of Pennsylvania School of Medicine; Director of Pediatric Endoscopy, Children's Hospital of Philadelphia, Philadelphia, Pennsylvania
Abdominal Masses; Abdominal Pain; Clostridium difficile; Foreign Bodies and Caustic Ingestions; Helicobacter pylori in Pediatrics; Laboratory Testing: Pancreatic Function Tests; Percutaneous Enteral Access and Care of Gastrostomy Tubes; Splenomegaly; Uncommon Intestinal Diseases: Shwachman's Syndrome; Upper Endoscopy

KAREN LIQUORNIK, M.D.

Fellow, Department of Gastroenterology and Nutrition, Children's Hospital of Philadelphia, Philadelphia, Pennsylvania
Helicobacter pylori in Pediatrics; Upper Endoscopy

FREDERICK R. LONG, M.D.

Chief, Body CT and MRI, Children's Radiological Institute, Columbus Children's Hospital, Columbus, Ohio
Contrast Studies

ERIC S. MALLER, M.D.

Assistant Professor, Department of Pediatrics, University of Pennsylvania School of Medicine; Attending Physician and Medical Director, Liver Transplant Program, Division of Pediatrics, Department of Gastroenterology and Nutrition, Children's Hospital of Philadelphia, Philadelphia, Pennsylvania
Chronic Autoimmune Hepatitis; Jaundice; Liver Function Tests; Liver Transplantation

JOHN M. MARIS, M.D.

Assistant Professor, Department of Pediatrics, University of Pennsylvania School of Medicine; Assistant Physician, Division of Oncology, Children's Hospital of Philadelphia, Philadelphia, Pennsylvania
Hepatoblastoma and Hepatocellular Carcinoma

MARIA R. MASCARENHAS, M.D.

Assistant Professor, Department of Pediatrics, University of Pennsylvania School of Medicine; Director, Nutrition Support Service, Department of Gastroenterology and Nutrition, Children's Hospital of Philadelphia, Philadelphia, Pennsylvania
Failure to Thrive and Malabsorption; Parenteral Nutrition and Care of Central Venous Lines

ALICE T. MAZUR, M.S., R.N.

Nurse Practitioner, Division of Metabolism, Department of Pediatrics, Children's Hospital of Philadelphia, Philadelphia, Pennsylvania
Gaucher's Disease and Niemann-Pick Disease

KARAN MCBRIDE, M.D.

Senior Fellow and Research Fellow, Division of Gastroenterology and Nutrition, Children's Hospital of Philadelphia, Philadelphia, Pennsylvania
Chronic Autoimmune Hepatitis; Liver Transplantation

RANDOLPH MCCONNIE, M.D.

Clinical Instructor in Pediatrics, University of Minnesota School of Medicine; Clinical-Private Practice, Minneapolis, Minnesota
Peptic Ulcer Disease

KARIN L. MCGOWAN, Ph.D.

Associate Professor, Department of Pediatrics and Microbiology, University of Pennsylvania School of Medicine; Director, Clinical Microbiology Laboratory, Department of Pediatrics, Children's Hospital of Philadelphia, Philadelphia, Pennsylvania
Gastrointestinal Microbiology Testing

JAMES S. MEYER, M.D.

Assistant Professor, Department of Radiology, University of Pennsylvania School of Medicine; Staff Radiologist, Department of Radiology, Children's Hospital of Philadelphia, Philadelphia, Pennsylvania
Magnetic Resonance Imaging; Plain Abdominal Radiography

KEVIN E. C. MEYERS, M.B., B.Ch.

Fellow, Division of Nephrology, Department of Pediatrics, Children's Hospital of Philadelphia, Philadelphia, Pennsylvania
Hemolytic Uremic Syndrome

JEFFREY E. MING, M.D., Ph.D.

Fellow, Divisions of Metabolism and Human Genetics, Children's Hospital of Philadelphia, Philadelphia, Pennsylvania
Gaucher's Disease and Niemann-Pick Disease

MUNIR MOBASSALEH, M.D.

Associate Professor, Department of Pediatric Gastroenterology and Nutrition, Tufts University School of Medicine, Boston, Massachusetts
Bacterial Infections

ANDREW E. MULBERG, M.D., F.A.A.P.

Assistant Professor and Director, Gastroenterology Fellowships, Division of Pediatric Gastroenterology, Department of Pediatrics, University of Pennsylvania School of Medicine; Attending Physician, Division of Gastroenterology and Nutrition, Children's Hospital of Philadelphia, Philadelphia, Pennsylvania
Cystic Fibrosis–Related Gastrointestinal and Liver Disease; Gastrointestinal and Hepatobiliary Disease in the Acquired Immunodeficiency Syndrome; Protein-Losing Enteropathy

KAREN F. MURRAY, M.D.

Fellow, Departments of Gastroenterology and Nutrition, Children's Hospital, Boston, Massachusetts
Biliary Atresia

MICHAEL N. NEEDLE, M.D.

Assistant Professor, Department of Pediatrics, University of Pennsylvania School of Medicine; Attending Physician, Division of Oncology, Children's Hospital of Philadelphia, Philadelphia, Pennsylvania
Cancer of the Gastrointestinal Tract

JOHN J. NICOTRA, M.D.

Clinical Instructor, Department of Radiology, University of Pennsylvania School of Medicine; Assistant Attending Radiologist, Department of Radiology, Children's Hospital of Philadelphia, Philadelphia, Pennsylvania
Abdominal Computed Tomography

MICHAEL J. PALMIERI, Ph.D.

Scientific Director, Metabolic Diagnostic Laboratory, Children's Hospital of Philadelphia, Philadelphia, Pennsylvania
Laboratory Testing: Metabolic Testing

SUSAN N. PECK, M.S.N., R.N., C.P.N.P.

Clinical Nurse Specialist, Division of Gastroenterology and Nutrition, Children's Hospital of Philadelphia, Philadelphia, Pennsylvania
Percutaneous Enteral Access and Care of Gastrostomy Tubes

DAVID A. PICCOLI, M.D.

Acting Division Chief and Director, Clinical Service, Division of Gastroenterology and Nutrition, Children's Hospital of Philadelphia, Philadelphia, Pennsylvania
Breath Testing; Hepatic Fibrosis; Viral Hepatitis

RANDI G. PLESKOW, M.D.

Assistant Professor of Pediatrics, Gastroenterology, and Nutrition, Department of Pediatrics, Tufts University School of Medicine; Pediatric Gastroenterologist, Division of Gastroenterology and Nutrition, Floating Hospital for Children at New England Medical Center, Boston, Massachusetts
Wilson's Disease

RICHARD A. POLIN, M.D.

Professor, Department of Pediatrics, Division of Neonatology, University of Pennsylvania School of Medicine; Senior Physician, Department of Pediatrics, Division of Neonatology, Children's Hospital of Philadelphia, Philadelphia, Pennsylvania
Necrotizing Enterocolitis

CATHY POON, Pharm.D.

Assistant Professor of Clinical Pharmacy, Department of Pharmacy Practice and Pharmacy Administration, Philadelphia College of Pharmacy and Science; Adjunct Assistant Professor of Pediatrics in Pharmacy, Department of Pediatrics, School of Medicine and Adjunct Assistant Professor, Science and Role Development Division, School of Nursing, University of Pennsylvania, Philadelphia, Pennsylvania; Pediatric Clinical Specialist, Department of Pharmacy, Children's Regional Hospital—Cooper Hospital/University Medical Center, Camden, New Jersey
Parenteral Nutrition and Care of Central Venous Lines

JYOTI P. RAMAKRISHNA, M.D.

Associate, Department of Pediatrics, Duke University School of Medicine; Divisions of Hepatology and Nutrition, Duke Children's Hospital, Durham, North Carolina
Liver Failure

ELIZABETH B. RAND, M.D.

Assistant Professor, Department of Pediatrics, University of Pennsylvania School of Medicine; Assistant Physician, Division of Gastroenterology and Nutrition, Children's Hospital of Philadelphia, Philadelphia, Pennsylvania
Alagille Syndrome; Percutaneous Liver Biopsy

DOUGLAS C. B. REDD, M.D.

Assistant Professor, Departments of Radiology and Surgery, University of Pennsylvania School of Medicine; Interventional Radiologist, Department of Radiology, Children's Hospital of Philadelphia, Philadelphia, Pennsylvania
Angiography and Interventional Procedures; Percutaneous Enteral Access and Care of Gastrostomy Tubes; Vascular Disorders of the Liver

EVE A. ROBERTS, M.D., F.R.C.P.C.

Associate Professor of Paediatrics, Medicine, and Pharmacology, University of Toronto Faculty of Medicine; Attending Physician, Division of Gastroenterology and Nutrition, Hospital for Sick Children, Toronto, Ontario, Canada
Drug Hepatitis

LOUISE SCHNAUFER, M.D.

Professor, Division of Pediatric Surgery, Department of Surgery, University of Pennsylvania School of Medicine; Senior Surgeon, Division of Pediatric General and Thoracic Surgery, Children's Hospital of Philadelphia, Philadelphia, Pennsylvania
Management of Ostomies

EDISIO SEMEAO, M.D.

Fellow, Division of Gastroenterology, Department of Pediatrics, University of Pennsylvania School of Medicine; Fellow, Division of Gastroenterology and Nutrition, Children's Hospital of Philadelphia, Philadelphia, Pennsylvania
Irritable Bowel Syndrome

TIMOTHY SENTONGO, M.D.

Second Year Gastroenterology and Nutrition Fellow, Division of Gastroenterology and Nutrition, Children's Hospital of Philadelphia, Philadelphia, Pennsylvania
Uncommon Intestinal Diseases: Shwachman's Syndrome

STEPHEN E. SHAFFER, M.D.

Clinical Assistant Professor, Department of Pediatrics, Jefferson Medical College of Thomas Jefferson University, Philadelphia, Pennsylvania; Pediatric Gastroenterologist, Division of Gastroenterology, duPont Hospital for Children, Wilmington, Delaware
Esophageal pH Monitoring; Gastroesophageal Reflux

RAANAN SHAMIR, M.D.

Lecturer, Divisions of Gastroenterology and Nutrition, Schneider Children's Medical Center of Israel; Attending Physician, Tel-Aviv University Sackler School of Medicine, Tel-Aviv, Israel
Malnutrition; Short Bowel Syndrome

HAROHALLI SHASHIDHAR, M.D.

Senior Fellow in Pediatric Gastroenterology and Nutrition, Department of Pediatrics, Floating Hospital for Children at New England Medical Center, Boston, Massachusetts
Bacterial Infections

EDWIN SIMPSER, M.D.

Assistant Professor, Department of Pediatrics, New York University School of Medicine, New York; Chief, Division of Pediatric Nutrition, North Shore University Hospital–New York University School of Medicine, Manhasset, New York
Gastrointestinal Allergy

AZAM SOROUSH, M.D.

Fellow, Division of Gastroenterology and Clinical Nutrition, Department of Pediatrics, University of Pennsylvania School of Medicine; Clinical Instructor, Division of Pediatrics, Department of Gastroenterology and Nutrition, Children's Hospital of Philadelphia, Philadelphia, Pennsylvania
Protein-Losing Enteropathy

ROBERT H. SQUIRES, JR., M.D.

Associate Professor, Division of Gastroenterology and Nutrition, Department of Pediatrics, University of Texas Southwestern Medical Center at Dallas Southwestern Medical School, Dallas, Texas
Colonoscopy; Gastrointestinal Bleeding

PERRY W. STAFFORD, M.D.

Assistant Professor, Division of Pediatric Surgery, Department of Surgery, University of Pennsylvania School of Medicine; Attending Pediatric Surgeon, Children's Hospital of Philadelphia, Philadelphia, Pennsylvania
Laparoscopy

VIRGINIA A. STALLINGS, M.D.

Associate Professor, Department of Pediatrics, University of Pennsylvania School of Medicine; Chief, Nutrition Section, Division of Gastroenterology and Nutrition, Children's Hospital of Philadelphia, Philadelphia, Pennsylvania
Bone Densitometry; Resting Energy Expenditure

ANDREW M. TERSHAKOVEC, M.D.

Assistant Professor, Department of Pediatrics, University of Pennsylvania School of Medicine; Associate Physician, Division of Gastroenterology and Nutrition, Children's Hospital of Philadelphia, Philadelphia, Pennsylvania
Vitamin Deficiency

WILLIAM R. TREEM, M.D.

Professor, Department of Pediatrics, Duke University School of Medicine; Chief, Divisions of Gastroenterology, Hepatology, and Nutrition, Duke Children's Hospital, Durham, North Carolina
Liver Failure; Sucrase-Isomaltase Deficiency

JOHN TUNG, M.D.

Clinical Instructor of Pediatrics, University of Pennsylvania School of Medicine; Division of Gastroenterology, Children's Hospital of Philadelphia, Philadelphia, Pennsylvania
Splenomegaly

MENNO VERHAVE, M.D.

Assistant Professor, Department of Pediatrics, Tufts University School of Medicine; Division of Pediatric Gastroenterology and Nutrition, New England Medical Center, Boston, Massachusetts
Lactose Intolerance

RITU VERMA, M.D.

Clinical Instructor, University of Pennsylvania School of Medicine; Attending Physician, Division of Gastroenterology and Nutrition, Children's Hospital of Philadelphia, Philadelphia, Pennsylvania
Vomiting

DROR WASSERMAN, M.D.

Fellow, Division of Gastroenterology and Nutrition, and Clinical Instructor, Department of Pediatrics, Children's Hospital of Philadelphia, Philadelphia, Pennsylvania
Ascites

WILLIAM J. WENNER, M.D.

Assistant Professor, Department of Pediatrics, University of Pennsylvania School of Medicine; Associate Physician, Division of Gastroenterology and Nutrition, Children's Hospital of Philadelphia, Philadelphia, Pennsylvania
Constipation and Encopresis; Uncommon Intestinal Diseases: Bacterial Overgrowth of the Intestine; Uncommon Intestinal Diseases: Rectal Prolapse; Viral Hepatitis

STEVEN L. WERLIN, M.D.

Professor, Department of Pediatrics, Medical College of Wisconsin; Director, Division of Gastroenterology, Department of Pediatric Gastroenterology and Nutrition, Children's Hospital of Wisconsin, Milwaukee, Wisconsin
Congenital Anomalies of the Pancreas and Biliary Tract

STEVEN M. WILLI, M.D.

Assistant Professor, Division of Endocrinology, Department of Pediatrics, Medical University of South Carolina College of Medicine; Clinical Associate Physician, General Clinical Research Center, Medical University of South Carolina Children's Hospital, Charlestown, South Carolina
Glycogen Storage Diseases

MICHAEL WILSCHANSKI, M.B.B.S.

Department of Pediatrics, Hebrew University; Consultant, Department of Pediatric Gastroenterology, Shaare Zedek Medical Center, Jerusalem, Israel
Malnutrition; Short Bowel Syndrome

DONNA ZEITER, M.D.

Assistant Professor, Department of Pediatrics, University of Connecticut School of Medicine, Farmington; Attending Physician, Departments of Pediatric Digestive Diseases and Nutrition, Connecticut Children's Medical Center, Hartford, Connecticut
Laboratory Testing: Intestinal Testing; Peritonitis; Uncommon Intestinal Diseases: Bezoars

BABETTE ZEMEL, Ph.D.

Clinical Assistant Professor, Division of Gastroenterology and Nutrition, Department of Pediatrics, Children's Hospital of Philadelphia, Philadelphia, Pennsylvania
Anthropometric Assessment of Nutritional Status

CONTENTS

SECTION III
DISEASES OF THE LIVER, PANCREAS, AND GALLBLADDER

SECTION IV
USE AND INTERPRETATION OF DIAGNOSTIC TESTS

1

ABDOMINAL MASSES

CHRIS A. LIACOURAS

Often abdominal masses in children are found by an unsuspected parent or by a physician, during a routine physical examination. In pediatrics, most abdominal masses have no specific signs or symptoms but usually require urgent attention. When evaluating a pediatric abdominal mass, an organized approach is paramount in determining its etiology. Table 1-1 provides the differential diagnosis of abdominal masses arranged anatomically by location. This approach allows the physician to consider the cause of an abdominal mass as it pertains to a specific abdominal organ.

HISTORY

The age of the patient is often a helpful clue as to the cause of the abdominal mass. While most abdominal masses diagnosed during the first 3 months of life are benign, the likelihood of malignancy increases with age. In the newborn, most masses are retroperitoneal, with more than one-half originating in the kidney, and less than 20% arising in the intestine (Table 1-2). The most common renal mass in newborns is hydronephrosis, which can arise from extrinsic compression (vascular) or chronic vesicoureteral reflux. Bilateral hydronephrosis in males is often secondary to posterior urethral valves. Other causes of renal masses include polycystic kidney disease, multicystic dysplastic kidney disease, and renal vein thrombosis. With regard to neonatal tumors, mesoblastic nephroma is the most common neonatal renal tumor, while nephroblastomatosis is a rare lesion characterized by small localized nodules and may be a precursor

to Wilms tumor. Other common causes of neonatal abdominal masses include adrenal hemorrhage, congenital anomalies, and teratoma.

In preschool-age children, approximately 20% of abdominal masses arise from the gastrointestinal tract, while 5% originate from the liver or biliary tree. Wilms tumor and neuroblastoma typically occur in young children, while ovarian disorders present in adolescence. Important historical questions include the frequency and quality of bowel movements (constipation, intussusception), use of medications, history of abdominal trauma (pancreatic pseudocyst), history of weight loss (tumor, intestinal abscess from Crohn's disease), presence of jaundice (liver/biliary disease), hematuria, or dysuria (renal disease), intercourse (pregnancy), and fever (abscess). In infants, a full bladder is often mistaken for an abdominal mass, while in neonates a palpable liver edge can be normal and is often appreciated. Severe constipation in older children and adolescents can present as a large, hard mass extending from the pubis past the umbilicus. Finally, gastric distention should be considered in all children who present with a tympanitic epigastric mass.

PHYSICAL EXAMINATION

The abdomen of a normal infant and child should be completely soft and nontender. As a child grows, increased abdominal wall musculature may give greater resistance on examination, but the abdomen should continue to be soft to deep palpation. When evaluating an

TABLE 1-1. Etiology of Abdominal Masses by Location

Right upper quadrant	Periumbilical
Liver	Intestine
Hepatomegaly	Omental/mesenteric cyst
Hepatitis	Intestinal duplication
Vascular anomaly	Obstruction
Tumor	Midgut volvulus
Gallbladder	Lympangioma
Hydrops	Constipation
Cholecystitis	Gaseous distention
Gallstones	Ascites
Biliary tree	**Right lower quadrant**
Obstruction	Intestine
Choledochal cyst	Abscess (appendix, Crohn's
Intestine	disease)
Duodenal atresia	Intussuception
Pyloric stenosis	Meckel's duplication cyst
Duplication	Phlegmon
Duodenal hematoma	Lymphoma
Left upper quadrant	Inguinal hernia
Spleen	Ovary/testis
Splenomegaly	Torsion
Cyst	Cyst
Tumor	Ectopic pregnancy
Epigastric	Teratoma (dermoid)
Stomach	Tumor
Gastric bezoar	Undescended testis
Gastric volvulus	**Left lower quadrant**
Duplication	Ovary/testis (see Right lower
Tumor	quadrant)
Pancreas	Intestine
Pseudocyst	Constipation
Pancreatitis	Sigmoid volvulus
Duplication	**Hypogastrium**
Right/left mid-abdomen	Uterus
Kidney	Hydrometrocolpos
Hydronephrosis	Pregnancy
Wilms tumor	Congenital anomaly
Neuroblastoma	Bladder
Cystic kidney disease	Obstruction
Congenital anomaly	Posterior urethral valves
Adrenal	
Pheochromocytoma	
Tumor	
Hemorrhage	

TABLE 1-2. Common Abdominal Masses in the Newborn

Renal vein thrombosis	Pyloric stenosis
Hydronephrosis	Nephroblastomatosis
Adrenal hemorrhage	Mesoblastic nephroma
Cystic kidney disease	Posterior urethral valves

abdominal mass, the examiner should note its size, mobility, tenderness, firmness, and border edge. Auscultation and percussion have become a lost science; however, these diagnostic techniques can be extremely useful in determining the etiology of an abdominal mass. Solid masses (liver and spleen) and tumors typically resonate a dull sound, while hollow organs (gaseous intestine and stomach) provide a high pitch on percussion. Ascites is associated with shifting dullness. With regard to auscultation, a vascular tumor may provide a bruit and borborygmi can be heard in various intestinal disorders. A palpable liver edge does not always indicate pathology. In infants and children with right sided pulmonary disease, the liver edge may extend below the ribs. Whenever the liver edge is palpable, auscultation of the liver span should be attempted to determine whether hepatomegaly is present. By contrast, a palpable spleen almost certainly marks the presence of a disease process. Palpable tumors are frequently hard and immobile, and teratomas are generally large, extending across the midline, with cystic and calcium components. Most important is the location of the mass (Table 1-1).

DIAGNOSTIC STUDIES

Routine blood work, including a complete blood count (CBC) and chemistry panel, are useful tests, as the CBC can indicate anemia or hemolysis, while an abnormal chemistry panel can indicate renal disease (blood-urea nitrogen [BUN], creatinine), liver disease (alanine aminotransferase [ALT], aspartate aminotransferase [AST], alkaline phosphate), gallbladder disease (bilirubin, gamma-glutamyltransferase [GGTP], pancreatic disease (amylase), or intestinal disease (hypoalbuminemia).

Abdominal ultrasound is the most useful pediatric diagnostic test for the evaluation of abdominal masses because the paucity of fat in children enhances its diagnostic detail. Ultrasonography is readily available and easily obtained at most institutions, requires little preparation, usually identifies the involved organ, and can differentiate solid from cystic masses. If a diagnosis cannot be made, ultrasound can provide clues as to the next most logical diagnostic study. The disadvantage of ultrasound is its operator variability and its limitations when bowel gas obscures underlying abdominal tissues.

Computed tomography (CT) provides the best anatomic detail of all studies commonly in use and can provide more detail when there is overlying gas or bone. Other useful radiologic tests include plain abdominal radiographs (presence of calcifications, extension into the chest), magnetic resonance imaging (MRI) (vascular lesions of liver, major vessels, and tumors), radio-isotope hepato-iminodiacetic acid (HIDA) scan (liver, gallbladder) and intravenous urography (Wilms tumor, cystic kidney disease). Intestinal contrast studies (upper GI, barium enema) and intestinal endoscopy can be of bene-fit when the mass involves the intestine. Occasionally, laparoscopy can be useful for direct intraperitoneal visu-alization and biopsy of abdominal masses.

REFERRAL

Except for the diagnosis of constipation, the presence of an abdominal mass requires immediate attention. For all masses in children, diagnostic studies should be per-formed expeditiously at a center capable of diagnosing pediatric disorders. Once the abnormality is identified, the appropriate pediatric subspecialist should be con-sulted.

EMERGENCIES

Of all the diseases listed in Table 1-1, patients who pres-ent with an abdominal mass and with either signs or symptoms of intestinal obstruction, including severe, colicky abdominal pain, bilious vomiting, and increase in heart rate (intussusception, volvulus, gastric torsion, toxic megacolon), should be hospitalized as soon as possi-ble (Table 1-3). Other emergencies include ovarian tor-sion, ectopic pregnancy, biliary obstruction (stone, hy-drops), and pancreatitis (pseudocyst). Initial diagnostic studies should include an abdominal ultrasound and plain abdominal radiographs, as well as a surgical consul-tation. The remaining causes of abdominal masses re-quire urgent care and timely evaluation.

TABLE 1-3. Abdominal Masses That Require Immediate Hospitalization

Intussusception	Biliary obstruction (stone, hydrops)
Midgut/sigmoid volvulus	Pancreatic pseudocyst
Gastric torsion/bezoar	Ectopic pregnancy
Toxic megacolon	Incarcerated inguinal hernia
Ovarian torsion	

REFERENCES

1. Taylor LA, Ross AJ III. Abdominal masses. In: Walker WA, Durie PR, Hamilton JR et al. Eds. Pediatric Gastrointestinal Disease. Philadelphia: BC Decker, 1991:132–145

2. Healey PJ, Hight DW. Abdominal masses. In: Wyllie R, Hyams JS, Eds. Pediatric Gastrointestinal Disease. Philadel-phia: WB Saunders, 1993:281–292

3. Schwartz MW. Abdominal masses. In: Schwartz MW, Curry TA, Charney EB, Ludwig S, Eds. Principles and Practice of Clinical Pediatrics. Chicago: Year Book, 1987:139–143

4. Swischuk LE, Hayden CK Jr. Abdominal masses in children. Pediatr Clin North Am 1985;32:1281–1298

5. Mahaffey SM, Rychman RC, Martin LW. Clinical aspects of abdominal masses in children. Semin Roentgenol 1988;23:161–174

6. Merten DF, Kirks DR. Diagnostic imaging of pediatric abdom-inal masses. Pediatr Clin North Am 1985;32:1397–1426

7. Hartman GE, Schochat SJ. Abdominal mass lesions in the newborn: diagnosis and treatment. Clin Perinatol 1989;16:123–135

2

ABDOMINAL PAIN

HOWARD A. KADER
CHRIS A. LIACOURAS

Evaluating abdominal pain in infants, children, and sometimes adolescents is very difficult even to those experienced in treating children. Clinical experience along with a high index of suspicion in the appropriate age group is essential in determining the diagnosis and etiology of abdominal pain in most children.[1] Often minimal historic information regarding the patient's pain is available; most symptoms are usually derived from the patient's actions and any associated symptoms described by the caregiver. By contrast, specific details may be offered by the child when prompted; thus, it is always useful to involve the patient in the history and physical examination, whenever possible.

Abdominal pain can be classified as acute or chronic (emergent or nonemergent) functional or secondary to a pathologic disease process. Functional disorders consist of variations from the norm but without evidence of proven tissue-related organic disease. Pathologic disorders are caused by an underlying disease that precipitates the patient's symptoms. Identifying infants, children, and adolescents with acute, emergent pathology is of the utmost importance to permit appropriate intervention in a timely manner. Acute (emergent), unremitting abdominal pain that occurs suddenly and has no prior history is considered a medical emergency and children should be immediately evaluated by a physician (Table 2-1). Chronic abdominal pain relates to symptoms continuing for 3 or more months.[2] Chronic functional abdominal pain is commonly associated with irritable bowel syndrome and often entails intermittent obstipation or diarrhea, gas pains, somatization, increased flatulence; in the

past it was often referred to as recurrent abdominal pain of childhood.[2–4]

PATHOPHYSIOLOGY

Abdominal pain occurs from one of three afferent pain pathways: visceral, somatic, or referred. Visceral pain is poorly localized and dull and is usually induced by the distention of hollow organs lined with smooth muscle, by capsular stretching, or by vascular ischemia. Somatic pain is perceived as sharp, acute, severe pain that arises from receptors lining the peritoneum and abdominal wall. Referred pain emanates from visceral pain that is referred to a somatic location.

ACUTE ABDOMEN

The single most important factor in the evaluation of abdominal pain is to determine whether a medical emergency exists.[5,6] The symptoms of intestinal inflammation, perforation, hemorrhage, and obstruction can be very similar, especially in young children. Because the risk of congenital anomalies is greater in children as compared to adults, disorders such as malrotation, volvulus, hypertrophic pyloric stenosis, and intestinal duplication should be entertained in any patient with an acute abdomen. In general, appendicitis continues to be the most common cause of an acute abdomen; however, the diag-

TABLE 2-1. Causes of Acute Emergent Abdominal Pain

Gastrointestinal	Nongastrointestinal
Pancreatitis	Pyelonephritis
Cholelithiasis/cholecystitis	Renal calculi
Malrotation with volvulus	Ureteropelvic junction obstruction
Intussusception	
Appendicitis	Ovarian torsion or rupture of ovarian cyst
Crohn's disease	
Ulcerative colitis	Tubo-ovarian abscess
Henloch-Schönlein purpura	Psoas abscess
Hemolytic uremic syndrome	Ectopic pregnancy
Porphyria	
Intestinal adhesions	
Strangulated hernia	
Mesenteric vasculitis	

nosis of appendicitis in pediatrics can be quite difficult, especially in preschool-age children.[7] The first symptom of appendicitis is periumbilical pain associated with nausea, vomiting, and sometimes fever. Subsequently, the "classic" symptom of right lower quadrant pain occurs. Unfortunately, the vast majority of infants and toddlers with appendicitis present instead with extreme irritability, inconsolable crying, and vomiting without an exact location of pain. Symptoms of intestinal obstruction (bilious vomiting, electrolyte disturbances, borborygmi, ileus) or gastrointestinal (GI) bleeding, as well as physical signs such as abdominal guarding and rebound tenderness, should alert the physician to an acute abdomen. Appropriate diagnostic tests and surgical consultation should then be performed.

CLINICAL PRESENTATION

Abdominal pain can present alone or in combination with other findings. Usually, the characteristics of the pain often lead to a diagnosis.[8] A detailed history is essential in determining a diagnosis.[9] Several important questions about the patient's abdominal pain should be asked, including the acuity or chronicity of the pain; the characteristics of the pain (constant or intermittent, dull ache or sharp cramps); the site and radiation of the pain; its relationship to movement, stress, foods, and medication; and those factors that exacerbate or relieve the pain. Questions should be asked regarding the association of the abdominal pain with other GI and constitutional symptoms, such as fever, headache, cough, emesis, heartburn, diarrhea, constipation, rectal bleeding, dysuria, menses, vaginal discharge, growth failure, weight loss, rashes, anemia, or arthritis. A child who can communicate often provides helpful information when asked to point to the location of the pain with one finger.

Whenever a patient or parent comments that the pain awakens the child from sleep, concerns for organic disease are high. The location of the pain is extremely useful (Table 2-2). Apley's rule states that the further the location of the pain from the umbilicus, the greater the likelihood of an underlying organic disorder.[2,10] In one prospective study of 377 patients from a major children's

TABLE 2-2. Etiology of Abdominal Pain Based on Location

Right upper quadrant	Left upper quadrant
Cholecystitis/cholangitis	Pneumonia
Peptic ulcer disease	Splenic infarction/ hemorrhage/trauma
Pneumonia (right lower lobe)	Gastritis/peptic ulcer disease
Gallstones	Esophagitis
Pelvic inflammatory disease (Fitz-Hugh-Curtis)	
Peritonitis	
Gastritis	
Epigastric	
Pancreatitis	
Gastroesophageal reflux/esophagitis	
Gastritis (*Helicobacter pylori*)	
Peptic ulcer disease	
Esophageal stricture/foreign body	
Right mid- or lower quadrant	Left mid- or lower quadrant
Appendicitis	Pyelonephritis
Mesenteric adenitis	Ureteropelvic junction obstruction
Meckel's diverticulitis	
Pyelonephritis	Ovarian torsion/cyst
Renal calculi	Tubo-ovarian abscess
Ureteropelvic junction obstruction	Renal calculi
Ovarian torsion/cyst/abscess	
Inflammatory bowel disease (Crohn's disease)	
Pelvic inflammatory disease	
Periumbilical	
Gastroenteritis	
Intussusception	
Irritable bowel syndrome	
Inflammatory bowel disease	
Functional abdominal pain	
Peritonitis	
Constipation	
Lactose intolerance	
Hypogastric	
Constipation	
Cystitis/bladder anomalies	
Irritable bowel syndrome	
Inflammatory bowel disease	
Sigmoid volvulus	
Pelvic inflammatory disease	

emergency department, the diagnosis most often associated with the complaint of abdominal pain was abdominal pain of unknown etiology, followed by gastroenteritis, appendicitis, constipation, urinary tract infection, viral illness, streptococcal pharyngitis, pharyngitis, pneumonia, and otitis media.[11] Appendicitis in this study occurred in only 8% of patients.

FUNCTIONAL ABDOMINAL PAIN

Functional abdominal pain typically begins between 4 and 14 years of age, with girls more often affected than boys by a ratio of 1.5 : 1.[2,12] This pain is periumbilical in location, is associated with an altered bowel pattern, and almost never awakens the child from sleep; however, it can be quite severe and can affect normal activity.[3,13] Some authorities use the term recurrent abdominal pain interchangeably with functional abdominal pain.[14] Strictly defined, functional abdominal pain is the most common etiology of nonorganic abdominal pain.[2] Many investigators now believe that functional abdominal pain is related to irritable bowel syndrome[15] (see Ch. 31). While the etiology of functional abdominal pain is unknown, the current theory is that it is due to either altered GI motility or hypersensitivity to general visceral afferent pain/stretch sensors and the patient responds to the stimulus with pain.[16] Other possible factors include external environmental stressors (physical or psychosocial), specific foods, previous GI infection, or genetic predisposition. The main detriment of recurrent abdominal pain is the effect on the patient's social life as school, friends, family, and extracurricular activities are affected. Depending on the outcome, the symptoms of functional abdominal pain may reinforce the behavior. Generally, functional abdominal pain resolves completely in 30% to 50% of patients by 2 to 12 weeks after diagnosis.[17,18]

PHYSICAL EXAMINATION

A properly performed physical examination is essential for any child who presents with abdominal pain. In general, the same examination you would perform on an adolescent or adults should be performed on younger children. An attempt should be made to localize the pain, identify abdominal masses, evaluate the liver and spleen, inspect the perianal area, and perform a rectal examination with Hemoccult testing. A proper abdominal exam should include (1) looking at the abdomen for distention or irregularities; (2) listening to the abdomen for the presence and quality of bowel sounds; (3) palpate the abdomen in all four quadrants for masses, organomegaly, tenderness, involuntary guarding, and rebound tenderness; and (4) percussing the abdomen for tenderness,

dullness (shifting), resonance, or tympany. Obviously, a kinder, gentle approach should be used when examining children; however, the thought that an unpleasant examination should not be performed should not be immediately dismissed, as several key elements may be missed, leading to an inaccurate or delayed diagnosis. Rebound tenderness is a reliable finding with regard to an acute abdomen; however, it is often difficult to elicit this response in young children. Completion of a growth chart is imperative, preferably with older plots as well.

DIAGNOSTIC EVALUATION

Laboratory evaluation of abdominal pain can be limited or extensive, depending on the history and physical examination. In general, initial laboratory evaluation includes a complete blood count (CBC) with differential, electrolytes, blood-urea nitrogen (BUN), creatinine, amylase, lipase, and if warranted, liver function tests (LFTs), sedimentation rate, or C-reactive protein. If the patient is anemic, has an anion gap acidosis, elevated lipase or erythrocyte sedimentation rate (ESR), low albumin, or abnormal LFTs further investigation should be pursued. Anemia should alert the physician either to GI bleeding or to chronic disease with malabsorption or malnutrition. An elevated sedimentation rate may indicate intestinal or hepatic inflammation, while hypoalbuminemia also suggests malabsorption. Stool evaluation in the correct clinical setting should include a smear for white blood count (WBC), culture for bacteria and viruses (including *Clostridium difficile* and rotavirus), along with ova and parasite cultures ×3.

Radiologic studies should also be considered, especially in children who present with acute abdominal pain. Initial radiographic evaluation should include an acute obstructive series with supine and upright abdominal radiographs. Whenever intestinal obstruction or an acute abdomen is present either a barium enema (intussusception, sigmoid volvulus), an abdominal ultrasound (appendicitis, cholelithiasis, choledochocyst, intussusception, renal calculi, ureteropelvic junction obstruction, ovarian cyst, tubo-ovarian abscess, abscess, ascites), or an upper GI series (obstruction, inflammatory bowel disease) should be performed. Diagnostic endoscopy should be performed whenever GI bleeding is present or when the above tests do not lead to a diagnosis.

TREATMENT AND MANAGEMENT

Initiation of treatment depends on the patient's diagnosis. The interpretation, treatment, and management of these diseases are discussed in succeeding chapters.

REFERENCES

1. Mason JD. The evaluation of acute abdominal pain in children. Emerg Med Clin North Am 1996;14:615–627

2. Apley J. The Child With Abdominal Pains. London: Blackwell Scientific, 1975

3. Faull C, Nicol AR. Abdominal pain in six year olds: an epidemiological study in a new town. Child Psychol Psychiatry 1986;27:251–260

4. Bury RG. A study of 111 children with recurrent abdominal pain in childhood. Aust Pediat J 1987;23:117–119

5. Davenport M. Acute abdominal pain in children. BMJ 1996;313:498–501

6. Rosenberg NM. Emergency versus casual pediatric emergency medicine. Pediatr Emerg Care 1995;11:255–258

7. Hatch EI. The acute abdomen in children. Pediatr Clin North Am 1985;32:1151–1164

8. Hardikar W, Feekery C, Smith A et al. *Helicobacter pylori* and recurrent abdominal pain in children. Pediatr Gastroenterol Nutr 1996;22:148–152

9. Pearigen PD. Unusual causes of abdominal pain. Emerg Med Clin North Am 1996;14:593–613

10. Wright JE. Left sided abdominal pain in childhood. Aust NZ Surg 1994;64:703–704

11. Reynolds SL, Jaffe DM. Diagnosing abdominal pain in a pediatric emergency department. Emerg Care 1992;8:126–128

12. Stone RT, Barbero GT. Recurrent abdominal pain in childhood. Pediatrics 1970;45:732–738

13. Apley J, Naish N. Recurrent abdominal pains: a field survey of 1000 school children. Arch Dis Child 1958;33:165–170

14. Hyams JS. Recurrent abdominal pain in children: commentary. Curr Opin Pediat 1995;7:529–532

15. Hyams JS, Treem WR, Justinich CJ et al. Characterization of symptoms in children with recurrent abdominal pain: resemblance to irritable bowel syndrome. J Pediatr Gastroenterol Nutri 1995;20:209–214

16. Boyle JT. Abdominal pain. In: Walker WA, Durie PR, Watkins JB, Eds. Pediatric Gastrointestinal Disease: Pathophysiology, Diagnosis, Management. Vol. 1. 2nd Ed. Philadelphia: Mosby, 1996:205–226

17. Ho K. Noncardiac chest pain and abdominal pain. Ann Emerg Med 1996;27:457–460

18. Stein MT Zeltzer L. Recurrent abdominal pain. Dev Behav Pediatr 1995;16:277–281

3

DIARRHEA

ROBERT N. BALDASSANO
WILLIAM J. COCHRAN

Diarrheal disease is a significant problem that affects 500 million children worldwide.[1] The estimated number of children who die each year from diarrhea ranges from 5 to 18 million.[2] Although the mortality rate is not as high in the United States as in underdeveloped countries, there are still about 300 U.S. deaths from diarrhea each year.[3] In the United States, there are approximately 220,000 admissions annually for diarrhea, accounting for 10% of all young children who are hospitalized.[4] As this is so common a problem, it is important for all health care workers who care for children to know how to evaluate and manage diarrheal illness.

PATHOPHYSIOLOGY

Diarrhea is present when there is an increase in the frequency, volume, or liquidity of the bowel movement relative to the usual habit of each individual. Often urgency, perianal discomfort, or incontinence is present. When making the diagnosis of diarrhea, one must also be familiar with the great variability of stool patterns among normal infants. Typically, children excrete 5 to 10 g/kg day,[5] while healthy adults excrete 100 to 200 g/day. Diarrhea results when there is a disturbance in the normal intestinal fluid and electrolyte transport. The most common causes of diarrhea in the infant are excessive fluid and nonabsorbable carbohydrate intake, invasion of the intestinal barrier by microorganisms, inflammatory processes, and drugs.[6]

TYPES OF DIARRHEA

Osmotic Diarrhea

Osmotic diarrhea is caused either by ingesting solutes that cannot be digested or absorbed or by diseases that prevent the patient from absorbing solutes that are normally absorbed. The accumulation of these nonabsorbable solutes in the intestine results in an increase in the intraluminal osmotic pressure, which retards water and electrolyte absorption. Therefore, if the ingestion of solute is discontinued, the diarrheal condition will improve. Stool analysis is also helpful in determining the presence of an osmotic diarrhea.

In osmotic diarrhea, a solute will make up the principal part of the osmolality of the stool; this differs from nonosmotic conditions in which Na, K, Cl, and HCO_3 are the principal components. The stool osmolality should be isosmotic with the serum, approximately 280 mOsm. The following formula for nonosmotic diarrhea can be represented by

$$2 \times ([Na^+] + [K^+]) \approx 280 \text{ mOsm}$$

However, in osmotic diarrhea, the formula is as follows:

$$2 \times ([Na^+] + [K^+]) < 280 \text{ mOsm}.$$

The most common example of a disorder that affects absorption of a particular food is lactose intolerance. This disorder is a functional deficiency of the enzyme lactase from the brush border of the small intestine. Lactose cannot be broken down and is therefore unable to be absorbed. Thus, undigested lactose draws water into the intestine, resulting in diarrhea.

An example of a disorder that would affect absorption of a specific substance is Crohn's disease of the terminal ileum. In this disease, the terminal ileum does not appropriately reabsorb bile salts, resulting in a decrease in the bile salt pool, which will interfere with the normal absorption of fats. In celiac disease, malabsorption of many different food groups results from destruction of the epithelial lining of the entire small intestine. By damaging the villi, there is a loss in the absorptive surface area, as well as a loss of many brush-border enzymes. The extent of intestinal damage determines the severity of malabsorption.

The causes of osmotic diarrhea generally involve malabsorption of a solute in the small intestine, but the colon can also be the site of osmotic diarrhea. Since the colon has less absorptive capacity than the small intestine, conditions that affect the colon usually produce mild symptoms. An example is microscopic or collagenous colitis. In these disorders, malabsorption results from lymphocytic infiltration of the lamina propria or from a thickening of collagen bands underlying the muscularis mucosa, respectively.

Finally, motility disorders must be included, as rapid intestinal transit time causes inadequate digestion, promoting nonabsorbed solutes. Examples are irritable bowel syndrome, hyperthyroidism, and pseudo-obstruction.[6]

Secretory Diarrhea

The gastrointestinal (GI) tract absorbs large amounts of water and electrolytes. Na^+ is the electrolyte most responsible for water absorption. The epithelial cells located on the villi are the cells responsible for absorption of fluid, while the cells located in the crypts are responsible for secretion. Absorption of fluid secondary to Na^+ transport is accomplished by different transport (pump) mechanisms. These include the electrogenic Na^+ pump and the neutral Na^+ pump. There are two types of electrogenic Na^+ pumps. One is a recently described Na^+ channel, and the other is a pump that requires both Na^+ and d-glucose, d-galactose, or a number of l-amino acids. Neutral Na^+ transport involves several transport proteins resulting in NaCl absorption. This transport mechanism is responsible for many diarrheal states because it is inhibited by second messengers (cyclic adenosine monophosphate [cAMP], cyclic guanosine monophosphate [cGMP], Ca^{2+}, and diacylglycerol).[7]

Active secretion occurs in the crypts by Cl^- transport. Chloride transport increases with greater concentration of many of the second messengers. Therefore, substances that increase the concentration of second messengers will result in decreased absorption of NaCl and increased secretion of Cl^-, resulting in diarrhea. In treating cholera, with the knowledge that there is an increase in cAMP, one can use the Na^+-coupled glucose transport pump (cAMP-independent pump) to maximize absorption. By understanding this phenomenon of coupled transport, oral rehydration solutions have been developed for the management of diarrhea.[6]

CLINICAL ASPECTS

When taking the history, several key questions need to be considered. What is the age of the child? The child's age is important, as many illnesses typically present at certain ages. Also, young children are at greater risk of significant dehydration from acute diarrhea. Thus, during the initial clinical assessment the physician must determine the degree of dehydration. The most accurate way is to compare present weight with a recent past weight. This usually is impossible because a recent weight is not often available. Signs and symptoms of dehydration (Table 3-1) during the initial evaluation are helpful in determining the degree of dehydration and appropriate therapy.

Is the diarrhea chronic or self-limited? Self-limited diarrhea usually indicates infection. One must ask if there has been recent travel to areas endemic with giardiasis, amebiasis, or *Campylobacter*. Chronic diarrhea may indicate the presence of an immunologic disorder such as irritable bowel disease (IBD) or celiac disease.

Is the diarrhea associated with an inflammatory syndrome? Inflammatory disorders typically cause extraintestinal symptoms, such as fever, arthritis, anemia, leukocytosis, and/or blood or mucus in the stool. Patients with noninflammatory disorders generally have milder symptoms and would not have mucus in the stool.

TABLE 3-1. Degrees of Dehydration

Degree	Description
Mild, 5% (50 ml/kg)	10–15% increase in pulse rate Decreased tears Concentrated urine Slightly dry appearance of skin and mucous membranes
Moderate, 10% (100 ml/kg)	Depressed fontanelle Sunken eyeballs Decreased turgor Coolness, acrocyanoses, mottling of skin Weak rapid pulse rate Normal blood pressure
Severe, 15%	Shock

Does the diarrhea originate in the large or small intestine? Small intestine pathology usually results in a large volume of diarrhea and may also result in malabsorption of particular nutrients. Large bowel pathology usually results in smaller volume (1 to 2 L/day) of diarrhea, unless there is a secretory element to the diarrhea. Inflammation of the large intestine is more likely to present with gross blood and mucus in the stool, along with symptoms of fecal urgency and tenesmus.

Does the patient have other medical problems that may predispose to diarrhea? Infectious causes of diarrhea are common in patients who have acquired immunodeficiency syndrome (AIDS) and other immunodeficiencies. Previous surgeries can create a predisposition to bacterial overgrowth, or the removal of the ileocecal valve can result in bile salt–induced diarrhea. Neurologic disorders may result in abnormal intestinal motility. Cystic fibrosis can lead to fat malabsorption. A family history can also be helpful in considering certain genetic disorders in children who present with chronic diarrhea.

PHYSICAL EXAMINATION

Careful physical examination will determine initial management and can often point to the diagnosis. For acute diarrhea, the degree of dehydration (Table 3-1) should be determined immediately. A key part of the physical examination is determination of height, weight, and head circumference. Previous measurements are mandatory for proper evaluation of a patient. Monitoring the growth of the child is essential, since healthy thriving children will have a different differential diagnosis than the poorly growing ill child. Does the patient have scleral icterus, finger clubbing, skin rash or peripheral edema? On abdominal examination, one must evaluate bowel sounds, abdominal tenderness and distention, and determine whether there are any abdominal masses or the presence of organomegaly. A rectal examination is very important when evaluating the possibility of perianal disease, such as rectal tags, fissures, hemorrhoids, fistulas, abnormal sphincter tone, and rectal tenderness.[6]

DIFFERENTIAL DIAGNOSIS OF ACUTE DIARRHEA

Acute diarrhea is most commonly associated with an infectious agent. Causes of acute, and at times chronic, gastroenteritis include viruses, bacteria, and parasites.

Viral Pathogens

Rotavirus, Norwalk agent, adenovirus, and other enteroviruses generally cause an acute enteritis. Generally, a short incubation period of 2 to 5 days is followed by inflammation of the intestinal lamina propria and varying degrees of villous and microvillous shortening. Soon afterward, the viral particles are excreted causing symptoms such as vomiting, diarrhea, fever, and abdominal cramping. These symptoms usually subside within 7 days. However, in infants, viruses can cause chronic diarrhea for up to 2 months secondary to severe villous flattening and a delay in mucosal healing (postinfectious gastroenteritis).

Bacterial Pathogens

Enteric bacterial pathogens promote diarrhea through three mechanisms: direct mucosal invasion, toxin production, or adherence to the intestinal epithelium. Patients with bacterial gastroenteritis often present with fever, abdominal pain, and blood or mucus in the stool. Again, the diarrhea is typically self-limited and resolves within 10 days. However, several pathogens, including *Salmonella*, *Shigella*, *Yersinia enterocolitica*, *Campylobacter jejuni*, *Aeromonas hydrophila*, and *Plesiomonas*, *Shigelloides*, can cause persistent diarrhea. *Clostridium difficile* produces a toxin that can cause pseudomembranous colitis and, while typically associated with antibiotic administration,[8] it can occur spontaneously. Stool cultures should be obtained in all children who present with persistent diarrhea, with specific requests for the above mentioned pathogens and *C. difficile* toxin. A fresh stool specimen, on ice, is necessary to measure the *C. difficile* toxin. (For in-depth discussion, see Chs. 18 and 20.)

Several parasites can initiate diarrhea. *Giardia lamblia* thrives in freshwater streams and well water. A *Giardia* infection can cause abdominal distention, diarrhea and, at times, failure to thrive. *Giardia* is easily passed from child to child through the fecal-oral route; it can be particularly troublesome in day care centers and schools. Another parasite, *Entamoeba histolytica*, produces a severe colitis; however, it is generally acquired only by travel to underdeveloped countries. When parasites are suspected, stool specimens should be collected for ova and parasites. In order to obtain the best results, specimen bottles containing a parasite preservative should be used, and three separate stool specimens should be collected to provide maximum yield. In the face of high suspicion, a duodenal intubation is necessary because as many as 50% of stools from patients proved to have giardiasis do not contain the parasite.[9] The antibiotics for the common infections are listed on Table 3-2.[8] (For detailed discussion, see Ch. 35.)

TREATMENT OF ACUTE DIARRHEA

The management of acute diarrhea can be divided into two phases. During the first, normal fluid and electrolyte status must be restored and maintained. This can be ac-

TABLE 3-2. Antibiotic Treatment for Infectious Gastroenteritis

Organism	Therapy	Comments
Salmonella	Third-generation cephalosporin	Treat only invasive disease or those at risk of invasive disease
Shigella	Trimethoprim-sulfamethoxazole	Increasing resistance to trimethoprim-sulfamethoxazole
Yersinia	Unknown	
Aeromonas	Unknown	
Pleisiomonas	Trimethoprim-sulfamethoxazole	
Campylobacter	Erythromycin	
Clostridium difficile	Metronidazole	Alternate therapy—vancomycin
Enterohemorrhagic Escherichia coli	Unknown	
Enterotoxigen Escherichia coli	Trimethoprim-sulfamethoxazole	
Giardia	Furoxone/Flagyl	
Entamoeba	Flagyl	

complished with oral rehydration solutions or intravenous fluids. During the second phase, formula and food are reintroduced.[10]

Regardless of the cause of acute diarrhea, the initial treatment is supportive. For most children, this therapy can be accomplished with oral rehydration solutions. Children who are severely dehydrated (greater than 10%) should be rehydrated intravenously. Understanding that a solution containing both sodium and glucose will maximize water absorption by using the electrogenic Na$^+$ pump (see section on Secretory Diarrhea), oral rehydration solutions have been developed. The most widely used solution worldwide is the World Health Organization (WHO) oral rehydration solution. In the United States, commercially prepared solutions are available (Table 3-3). Parents can make a rehydration solution by adding $\frac{1}{2}$ teaspoon salt and 3 tablespoons sugar to one quart of water. However, this is usually not recommended because this solution lacks potassium, and parents often make errors when preparing the solution.[10]

The American Academy of Pediatrics recommends giving the rehydration solution used to correct the deficit over 6 hours and should contain 75 to 90 mEq sodium per liter. After correcting the deficit (determined by the degree of dehydration), a lower concentration of sodium (40 to 60 mEq sodium per liter) is required for maintenance hydration. Care must be taken not to recommend common household beverages that are low in sodium and high in carbohydrates. Many cases of hyponatremia have been reported that led to seizure after an infant was given clear liquid as therapy for dehydration.

The physician should give specific guidelines for oral intake to the family. The general recommendations for fluid maintenance in children are as follows[11]:

For the first 10 kg of body weight, administer 100 ml/kg/day.

For children weighing 10 to 20 kg, give an additional 50 ml/kg/day for each kilogram over 10 kg.

For children weighing more than 20 kg, give the previous amount plus an additional 20 ml/kg/day for each kilogram over 20 kg.

Knowing both the maintenance and deficit fluid necessary to correct the dehydration, recommendations for therapy can be given. For example, if a 10-kg infant presents with 5% dehydration, the family should be in-

TABLE 3-3. Oral Rehydration Solutions

Solution	Carbohydrate (g/L)	Sodium (mEq/L)	Potassium (mEq/L)	Base (mEq/L)
Recommended				
World Health	20 (glucose)	90	20	30
Pedialyte RS	25 (glucose)	75	20	30
Pedialyte	25 (glucose)	45	20	30
Infalyte	30 (rice syrup)	50	25	30
Common household beverages (not recommended)				
Jell-O water ($\frac{1}{2}$ strength)	80	6–17	0	0
Apple juice	100–150	2	20	0
Cola	50–150	2	0.1	13
Gatorade	45	20	3	3
Tea	0	0	0	0

structed to give 500 ml (50 ml/kg) fluid for the deficit fraction plus 40 ml/h for the maintenance fraction. This would result in a fluid rate of approximately 125 ml/hr for 6 hours. Therefore, the family should be instructed to give 2 tablespoons (30 ml), solution containing 75 to 90 mEq sodium per liter every 15 minutes for the first 6 hours; the solution should then be changed to contain 40 to 60 mEq of sodium per liter and given at a rate of at least 40 ml (1⅓ tablespoons) per hour. The infant should not be given a full bottle, as a thirsty infant may drink rapidly and vomiting may result. The parents must also replace ongoing stool losses at about 10 ml/kg for each diarrheal stool.[10]

It is very important to continue feeding children with mild dehydration and to begin feeding as soon as possible after rehydration for children with moderate to severe dehydration. Many studies have shown that fasting results in villus atrophy leading to a decrease in absorptive surface area.[12] Also, fasting will result in starvation stools. The infant should continue breast feeding or full-strength formula feedings. Clinical trials have compared the use of lactose-containing versus lactose-free diets during diarrheal illnesses and have shown that infants tolerated the lactose-containing formula as well as the lactose-free formula.[10] Therefore, the infant's formula should not change during the time of the illness. Older children should be given foods low in fats and simple sugars. The traditional BRAT diet is good, and children should eat frequently.

DIFFERENTIAL DIAGNOSIS OF CHRONIC DIARRHEA

The etiology of chronic diarrhea can range from benign, self-limited diseases to a life-threatening organic illness (Table 3-4). The differential diagnosis in the child who shows failure to thrive is quite different than that of a healthy, well-nourished child. The remaining discussion concentrates on the diagnosis and treatment of the common causes of chronic diarrhea in childhood. When an uncommon cause of diarrhea is suspected, referral to a pediatric gastroenterologist is indicated.[10]

Postinfectious Gastroenteritis

In most children, enteric viral infections are acute and uncomplicated. However, in infants, several viruses can cause a severe enteritis resulting in prolonged intestinal mucosal damage for up to 2 months. Since the intestinal brush border is destroyed, acquired carbohydrate intolerance and malabsorption can occur. During this illness, carbohydrates, proteins, fats, and fluid may all be inadequately absorbed, leading to significant weight loss and dehydration. Clinically, children initially present with

TABLE 3-4. Etiology of Chronic Diarrhea

Common causes
Infectious
    Bacterial (*Salmonella, Shigella, Campylobacter, Yersinia, Aeromonas, Plesiomonas*)
    Parasitic (*Giardia, Cryptosporidium, Entamoeba*)
    Clostridium difficile
    Viral (rotavirus, adenovirus, Norwalk agent)
Drug-induced diarrhea
    Antibiotics
    Laxative abuse
    Chemotherapy
Dietary causes
    Intolerance to specific foods
    Sorbitol
    Formulas
    Malnutrition
Primary or secondary lactose intolerance
Encopresis
Irritable bowel syndrome
Milk-protein/soy allergy
Nonspecific diarrhea of infancy
Inflammatory bowel disease
Celiac disease
Anatomic abnormalities
    Malrotation, short-bowel syndrome

Uncommon causes
Congenital carbohydrate malabsorption
Congenital villous atrophy
Endocrine disorders
    Hyperthyroidism
    Congenital adrenal hyperplasia
    Diabetes
Eosinophilic gastroenteritis
Familial polyposis
Hemolytic-uremic syndrome
Henoch-Schönlein purpura
Hirschprung's enterocolitis
Immune system defects
Intestinal pseudo-obstruction
Necrotizing enterocolitis
Pancreatic disorders/fat malabsorption
    Cystic fibrosis
    Shwachman's disease
    Chronic pancreatitis, pancreatic insufficiency

(Adapted from Baldassano and Liacouras,[6] with permission.)

fever and diarrhea, followed by intractable watery diarrhea. These patients usually respond to elemental formulas such as Alimentum, Progestimil, and Nutramigen. Elemental formulas are lactose free, contain hydrolyzed amino acids, and have medium-chain triglycerides, all of which improve absorption across damaged intestinal epithelium. While these formulas provide excellent nutrition, infants typically produce four to five loose green stools per day; therefore, these infants should have their weight monitored very closely, as the number or consistency of the stools will not always provide an accurate assessment of the child's illness. Acute weight loss or dehydration will necessitate hospitalization. Severe cases may require continuous nasogastric feeding or parenteral hyperalimentation. In these instances, a small bowel biopsy can help define the severity of the lesion. Postinfectious gastroenteritis may resolve in as short as 2 weeks, or it may last as long as several months.[6]

Dietary Causes

Adverse GI symptoms to foods have been described for hundreds of years. While *food allergy* is defined as a pathologic immune-mediated process that occurs in response to an offending antigen, a *food intolerance* describes an abnormal physiologic response to an ingested food or food additive.[14] A variety of foods contain pharmacologically active substances that can produce an extensive array of GI symptoms. Most commonly, foods cause diarrhea, abdominal pain, and vomiting. Other symptoms include anaphylaxis, skin rash, and bronchospasm. A number of inciting agents, such as sulfites, aflatoxins, tricothecenes, and other food additives, can be found in a variety of foods (Table 3-5). If a food intolerance is suspected, that food should be withdrawn from the child's diet.[6]

Lactose Intolerance

Lactose intolerance is frequently the cause of chronic diarrhea in pediatric cases. There are several forms of lactose intolerance, which include congenital lactase deficiency, acquired lactase deficiency secondary to a mucosal abnormality of the small intestine, and, most commonly, late-onset lactose intolerance. Symptoms can be quite severe ranging from abdominal distention, flatulence, and bloating to vomiting and/or explosive, watery diarrhea. (For further details, see Ch. 32.)

Milk-Protein Allergy

Strictly speaking, milk-protein allergy (MPA) is a pathologic immune reaction induced by milk-protein antigens. The incidence of true MPA in children ranges from 1%

TABLE 3-5. Foods That Cause Gastrointestinal Adverse Reactions

Cabbage	Carrots	Celery
Chocolate	Licorice	Fava beans
Peppers	Radishes	Rhubarb
Soybeans	Turnips	Mushrooms
Watercress	Tea	Potatoes
Chick peas	Spinach	Sorrel

(Adapted from Fadal,[13] with permission.)

to 7%.[14] Furthermore, up to 50% of children with MPA can have a concomitant soy-protein allergy.[15] Finally, maternally ingested antigens, which pass into human breast milk, can also cause a milk/soy-protein allergy.[16] The allergy resolves once the antigen is removed from the mother's diet.

Commonly, MPA is overdiagnosed. Many times infants with colic, loose stools, and gastroesophageal reflux disease are falsely classified as having an allergy to milk. This misdiagnosis leads to increased parental expense and concern and to an unwarranted restricted diet. Therefore, physicians need to develop an organized method to diagnose MPA.

Clinically, infants with MPA present with heme-positive or bloody diarrhea and poor growth. Other associations include urticaria, wheezing, and skin rash. When considering the diagnosis of MPA, abnormal laboratory tests such as a blood count with a peripheral eosinophilia, a decreased hemoglobin, a decreased serum albumin or total protein, or more classically the presence of eosinophils in the stool can help confirm the diagnosis. The true diagnosis relies on the classic Goldman challenge test.[17] (For further details, see Ch. 15.)

Drug-Induced Diarrhea

Diarrhea can often be a significant side effect of many pharmacologic agents. Drugs can cause diarrhea by increasing GI motility, through direct mucosal injury, by altering intestinal microflora, or by decreasing intraluminal digestion and absorption. Antibiotics have long been known to cause diarrhea in infants and children. Antibiotics can alter bowel flora and cause loose watery stools. Furthermore, they can cause pseudomembranous colitis (see the section Infections). Penicillins and cephalosporins have been shown to cause diarrhea through direct competition for absorption. Also, erythromycin can affect intestinal motility. Therefore, a change in antibiotic therapy can be helpful in eliminating the diarrhea.

While antibiotics typically produce most of the GI side effects in children, several other agents deserve mention. In today's society, laxative abuse should be considered for all patients, particularly adolescent girls who present with unexplained chronic diarrhea. Bethanechol, cisapride, and metoclopramide are frequently used in children with gastroesophageal reflux disease and, at times, can cause a significant diarrhea. Finally, mucositis and enteritis can follow radiation therapy and chemotherapy.[6]

Inflammatory Bowel Disease

IBD includes two disorders: Crohn's disease and ulcerative colitis. Clinically, the presentation of IBD is quite variable and depends on the severity of the inflamed bowel, the site of the diseased bowel, and the chronicity of the disease. Most commonly, children present with growth failure, diarrhea, abdominal pain, stool mixed with mucus or blood, or weight loss; however, the presentation can often be extremely subtle.[18] When considering the diagnosis of IBD, a careful history and a review of the child's height, weight, and weight for height curves may distinguish chronic from acute disease. On physical examination, patients may present with arthritis, arthralgias, mouth sores, erythema nodosum, or perianal disease. Furthermore, an elevated sedimentation rate, a low hemoglobin, a decreased albumin, or guaiac-positive stools can aid in the diagnosis. It is not uncommon for the sedimentation rate to be normal in Crohn's disease, especially when there is only small bowel involvement. While radiologic studies such as an upper GI series or a barium enema can confirm the location of the disease, a flexible colonoscopy should be performed in order to obtain direct visual and histologic information regarding the disease process. Treatment depends on the location and severity of the inflamed bowel and should be determined by a pediatric gastroenterologist. (For further details, see Ch. 30.)

Celiac Disease

Celiac disease, also known as gluten-sensitive enteropathy, is a disease of the proximal small intestine characterized by severe intestinal mucosal damage. The damage occurs secondary to an allergic response to the antigen, gluten. Celiac disease leads to diarrhea, malabsorption, and poor growth. Furthermore, vitamin deficiencies, iron-deficiency anemia, heme-positive stools, and acquired lactose intolerance frequently develop. Celiac disease can present anytime after gluten is introduced into the diet, from 6 months to adulthood. Most commonly, affected persons are of European ethnic origin; specifically, Irish, English, and Australian descendants. The incidence of celiac disease varies, depending on geographic location and nationality. In Ireland, celiac disease occurs in 1 of every 600 births, while in North America, its incidence approaches 1 in every 6,000 births.

While specific laboratory testing such as a d-xylose test, antiendomysial antibody, and/or antigliadin antibody screen may provide clues to the diagnosis, Celiac disease can only be diagnosed by intestinal biopsy. All too often, physicians falsely diagnose the disease without biopsy confirmation, and this can lead to an unwarranted, severely restricted lifetime diet. Moreover, a small percentage of patients with celiac disease develop lymphoma later in life, making accurate diagnosis essential. Therefore, if celiac disease is suspected, we recommend formal histologic diagnosis. The diagnosis requires three biopsies: an abnormal biopsy on a standard diet, a normal biopsy on a gluten-free diet, followed by another abnormal biopsy after gluten is reintroduced into the diet. Referral to a pediatric gastroenterologist is indicated.[6] (For further details, see Ch. 19.)

Fat Malabsorption/Pancreatic Disorders

Steatorrhea, or fatty stools, can be caused by pancreatic dysfunction, bile salt abnormalities, bacterial overgrowth, small intestine mucosal disease, or an abnormality of the terminal ileum. Clinically, patients who present with one of the above disorders pass large, greasy, foul-smelling stools. Children with fat malabsorption present with poor growth, fat-soluble vitamin deficiency, and increased fat in their stools. The causes of pancreatic dysfunction include cystic fibrosis, Shwachman's syndrome,[19] pancreatitis, surgical manipulation,[22] and pancreatic insufficiency of unknown etiology. Bacterial overgrowth causes bile salt deconjugation and should be considered in patients who have had recent surgery. Bile salt malabsorption typically promotes a watery diarrhea.

Fat malabsorption should be considered in all children who exhibit poor growth and bulky, foul-smelling diarrhea. Outpatient testing should include a 3-day calorie count, a 72-hour stool fecal fat collection, and serum amylase, lipase, and sweat tests. Referral to a pediatric gastroenterologist is also indicated.

Encopresis

Encopresis or "soiling" is the involuntary passage of loose stool.[21] In the toddler or older child, encopresis often presents as diarrhea and is almost always caused by severe constipation. Encopresis and constipation are very common in children.[22] Therefore, any apparently healthy child who has a history of uncontrollable diarrhea should be evaluated for constipation/encopresis. A digital rectal examination usually proves the diagnosis; however, a normal exam does not always dispel the diagnosis. If constipation is being strongly considered, an abdominal radiograph can help provide the correct diagnosis. Therapy relies on an initial, aggressive bowel cleansing using Fleet enemas, followed by maintenance therapy using Kondremul, a mineral oil preparation, at 2 to 3 tablespoonfuls twice or three times daily. (For further details, see Ch. 22.)

Irritable Bowel Syndrome

Intermittent diarrhea, abdominal discomfort, flatulence, and occasional constipation are characteristic symptoms of irritable bowel syndrome (IBS). Typically, the child's history may include the rapid onset of abdominal cramping followed by a loose bowel movement with resolution of symptoms. These episodes can be related to various environmental or emotional stressors. Furthermore, children with IBS can present with diarrhea alternating with periods of constipation. A careful history and physical examination is needed to exclude more serious illness. While there is no pathognomonic diagnostic test that proves IBS, occasionally an abdominal radiograph demonstrating constipation can help confirm the diagnosis.

Current therapy consists of a high-fiber diet, fiber supplements, and behavioral modification. Fiber not only regulates bowel motility but also acts as a bulking agent in stool production. Foods such as raw vegetables, nuts, and bran cereals provide a high degree of fiber. Citrucel, a fiber supplement, can also be added. Finally, relaxation techniques and counseling can help to improve the GI symptomatology. (For further details, see Ch. 31.)

Idiopathic or Nonspecific Chronic Diarrhea

Chronic nonspecific diarrhea, or "toddler's diarrhea," is an unexplained, persistent diarrhea that typically occurs in young children aged 1 to 3 years. Although these children have diarrhea, they are active and appear healthy, and they continue to grow and develop normally. Clinically, infants with nonspecific diarrhea pass 5 to 10 loose watery stools each day.[23] The stools often appear to contain undigested food particles, and the diarrhea may be cyclical in nature. In other words, there may be weeks of normal stooling followed by weeks of diarrhea. Nonspecific diarrhea may last a few weeks or several years; however, symptoms generally resolve by 4 years of age.

While most cases of nonspecific diarrhea have no definable cause, occasionally an inciting agent contributes to the diarrhea. Sorbitol, a nonabsorbable carbohydrate, can produce an osmotic diarrhea. Sorbitol is present in many foods, especially sugar-free products, candy, and pear juice (Table 3-6). Occasionally, excessive fluid intake and a poor diet can also contribute to nonspecific diarrhea. Often, toddlers prefer an unbalanced diet

TABLE 3-6. Sorbitol Content of Various Foods and Drugs

Food	Sorbitol Content
Natural foods	
Pears	≤4.6 g/100 g dry weight
Prunes	≤2.4 g/100 g dry weight
Plums	≤15.8 g/100 g dry weight
Sweet cherries	≤12.6 g/100 g dry weight
Fruit juices	
Apple juice	0.3–0.9 g/dl
Pear juice	0.4–0.9 g/dl
Dietetic foods	
Sugar-free gum	1.3–2.2 g/piece
Diabetic jams	≤57 g/100 g

(Adapted from Greenberger,[24] with permission.)

which consists of low-residue, high-carbohydrate, low-fat foods. More to the point, young children may drink up to 40 ounces of clear liquids each day. This particular combination may give rise to loose, frequent stools. When this history is identified, we recommend that a high-fat diet be instituted along with a reduction in clear fluid intake to 12 to 15 ounces/day.[6]

Other Causes

Apart from the previously discussed disorders, there are many other less common causes of diarrhea in children (Table 3-4). Children who exhibit chronic diarrhea without a clear etiology should be referred to a pediatric gastroenterologist.

MANAGEMENT OF CHRONIC DIARRHEA

Since the differential diagnosis of chronic diarrhea is quite extensive, every pediatrician needs to develop an organized consistent laboratory approach, in order to determine its etiology. We recommend that a differential diagnosis be defined for each patient followed by the selection of appropriate laboratory and diagnostic tests that will help confirm the diagnosis.

The causes of chronic diarrhea can be categorized by age and symptoms. With regard to the differential diagnosis, we pay particular attention to the common causes of diarrhea, that is, infections, dietary changes, and drug effects. Second, we review the child's growth curve, since gradual weight loss and an abnormally low weight for height indicates chronic disease. Next, we assess the patient's age and we determine whether blood is present in the stools. Using these criteria, a workable differential can be developed. Afterward, laboratory testing can help to identify the specific diagnosis.

LABORATORY EVALUATION

The initial workup can be accomplished in most pediatric offices. On the basis of these findings an intelligent decision can be made as to what type of diagnostic evaluation is warranted. The first set of tests would include measurement of height and weight, complete blood count (CBC) with differential, sedimentation rate, electrolytes with liver function tests, stool guaiac, stool culture, stool for ova and parasite, and stool for *C. difficile* toxin. Evaluation of the stool specimen is absolutely necessary. Everyone's definition of diarrhea is different, and the description of the stool given by the parent may be much different from that of the physicians. Having the parent bring a sample in a diaper to the office permits determination of the stool weight, color, consistency, and presence of blood or mucus. Where cells are present, determination of whether the cells are neutrophils or eosinophils is performed next, especially for infants in whom a milk/soy allergic gastroenteritis is suspended. When performing the rectal examination the index finger should be used in any child with a normal anus and who weighs more than 4 kg. The child should be placed in the left lateral recumbent position with knees flexed facing away from the physician. If the child is having loose stools, a lubricated 8 to 10 Fr feeding tube can be inserted into the rectum and then aspirated with a 20-ml syringe. Depending on the results of the workup, the next set of tests may be performed or referral to a pediatric gastroenterologist may be necessary. These tests include a sweat test, 72-hour fecal fat, hydrogen breath test, and d-xylose.

A sweat test can be performed in hospitals that perform them frequently. False positive results must be considered if the total amount of sweat is low (less than 100 mg). Low amount of sweat could be secondary to evaporation and would result in a falsely high concentration of NaCl. Also, the amount of chloride in the sweat test may be falsely low in children with cystic fibrosis in the face of significant edema.

A 72-hour stool fecal fat test requires patient cooperation but when properly carried out is the most definitive test for steatorrhea. The patient is placed on a diet high in long-chain fats (2 g/kg) for 3 days. A careful diet history is necessary to determine fat intake. All stools passed within a 72-hour period must be collected and immediately frozen to prevent bacterial breakdown of the fat. Fat malabsorption is determined if greater than 7% of the dietary fat is excreted in the stool. False-negative results can be secondary to poor stool collection, inadequate dietary intake of fat, or not freezing the stool immediately.

D-xylose absorption test is a very useful study to estimate the surface area of the small intestinal mucosa. The principle of the test is that d-xylose absorption is independent of bile salts, pancreatic secretions and intestinal mucosal disaccharidases. The dose of $14.5/m^2$ is given orally, and the serum level of d-xylose is determined at 1 hour after ingestion (normal greater than 36 mg/dl). Any disorder that results in villous atrophy will have an abnormal result. Abnormal results usually require a small bowel biopsy to determine the diagnosis. At this time, referral to a pediatric gastroenterologist is usually necessary. (For further details, see Ch. 79.)

Hydrogen (lactose) breath test works on the principle that H_2 gas is produced by bacterial fermentation of carbohydrate (lactose), then absorbed, and excreted in the breath. The usual carbohydrate use is lactose. If there is adequate lactase in the small intestine, lactose will be completely absorbed, and no lactose will enter the colon. Thus, colonic bacteria will be unable to ferment the lac-

tose and no H_2 gas will be produced. False negatives can result if a child is on antibiotics obliterating the colonic bacteria or if the child does not have H_2-producing bacteria in the colon. (For further details, see Ch. 76.)

Endoscopy has become one of the most useful diagnostic procedures in pediatric gastroenterology. It permits direct visualization of the mucosa of the colon, esophagus, stomach, duodenum, and hepatobiliary tract in infants and children. It has dramatically improved our understanding of the diseases that affect these parts of the GI tract. In the hands of a skilled pediatric endoscopist, these studies not only enhance diagnostic accuracy but can be performed safely.[8] (For further details, see Ch. 72.)

REFERENCES

1. Hirschhorn N. The treatment of acute diarrhea in children. An historical and physiological perspective. Am J Clin Nutr 1980;33:637–663

2. Elliot KM, Knight J, Eds. Acute Diarrhea in Childhood. Ciba Foundation Symposium No. 42. Amsterdam: Elsevier/Excerpta Medica, 1976:341

3. Kilgore PE, Holman RC, Clarke MJ. Trends of diarrheal disease-associated mortality in US children, 1968 through 1991. JAMA 1995;274:1148

4. Glass RI, Lew JF, Gangarosa RE. Estimates of morbidity and mortality rates for diarrheal disease in American children. J Pediatr 1991;118:527

5. Anderson DH. Celiac syndrome. I. Determination of fat in feces; reliability of two chemical methods and microscopic estimate; excretion of feces and of fecal fat in normal children. Am J Dis Child 1945;69:141–151

6. Baldassano RN, Liacouras CA: Chronic diarrhea: a practical approach to the pediatrician. In: Schwartz MW, Ed. Difficult Diagnoses in Pediatrics. Pediatric Clin North Am 1991;38:667–686

7. Rood RP, Donowitz M. Regulation of small intestinal Na$^+$ absorption by protein kinases: implication for therapy of diarrheal diseases. Viewpoints Dig Dis 1990;22:1–5

8. Christie DL, Ament ME. Ampicillin-associated colitis. J Pediatr 1975;87:657

9. Ament ME, Rubin CE. Relation of giardiasis to abnormal intestinal structure and function in gastrointestinal immunodeficiency syndromes. Gastroenterology 1972;62:216

10. Limbos MP, Lieberman JM. Management of acute diarrhea in children. Contemp Pediatr 1995;12:68–88

11. Cochran Wj, Klish WJ. Treating acute gastroenteritis in infants. Drug Protocol 1987;2:88–93

12. Butzner JD, Gall DG. Refeeding enhances intestinal repair during acute enteritis in infant rabbits subjected to protrin-energy malnutrition. Pediatrics 1986;109:277

13. Fadal RG. Introduction to food allergy and other adverse reactions to foods. Res Staff Physician 1988;34:23–33

14. Gerrard JW, Mackenzie JWA, Goluboff N et al. Cow's milk

allergy: prevalence and manifestations in an unselected series of newborns. Acta Paediatr 1973;234:1–21

15. Shibaski M, Suzuki S, Tajima S et al. Allergenicity of major components of soybean. Int Arch Allergy Appl Immunol 1980;61:441–448

16. Machtinger S, Moss R. Cow's milk allergy in breast fed infants: the role of allergen and maternal secretory IgA antibody. J Allergy Clin Immunol 1986;77:341–347

17. Goldman AS, Anderson DW, Sellers WA et al. Milk Allergy I. Oral challenge with milk and isolated milk proteins in allergic children. Pediatrics 1963;32:425–443

18. Motil K, Grand R. Ulcerative colitis and Crohn's disease in children. Pediatr Rev 1987;9:109

19. Aggett PJ, Cavanagh NPC, Matthew DJ et al. Shwachman's syndrome. A review of 21 cases. Arch Dis Child 1980;55: 331–347

20. Poley JR, Hofmann AF. Role of fat malabsorption in pathogenesis of steatorrhea in ileal resection. Fat digestion after two sequential test meals with and without cholestyramine. Gastroenterology 1976;71:38–44

21. Hatch TF. Encopresis and constipation in children. Pediax Clin North Am 1980;35:257–280

22. Levine MD. Children with encopresis: a descriptive analysis. Pediatrics 1975;56:412–416

23. Davidson M, Wasserman R. The irritable colon of childhood (chronic non-specific diarrhea syndrome). J Pediatr 1966; 69:1027–1038

24. Greenberger NJ: Diagnostic approach to the patient with a chronic diarrheal disorder. Disease a Month 1990;36:131–79

4

DYSPHAGIA

DELMA L. BROUSSARD

Swallowing is a finely coordinated process involving multiple muscle groups of the oropharynx and esophagus, which are controlled by both the central nervous system (CNS) and the enteric nervous system.[1,2] There are three phases of swallowing: oral, pharyngeal, and esophageal. After mastication and mixing of food with saliva, the oral phase of deglutition involves the voluntary movement of a bolus posteriorly by the tongue, toward the oropharynx. Once in the oropharnyx, the bolus activates sensory receptors that initiate the involuntary pharyngeal phase of swallowing. Simultaneous with the entry of the bolus into the pharynx, the soft palate is elevated against the posterior wall, preventing regurgitation into the nasopharyngeal area. Additionally, respirations temporarily stop, and the epiglottis is lowered backward over the larynx to further protect the airway. During the pharyngeal phase, food is transported across the relaxed upper esophageal sphincter (UES) and into the esophagus, where the esophageal phase begins. Relaxation of the UES starts as a swallow is initiated and is maintained until the bolus passes into the esophagus. The lower esophageal sphincter (LES) relaxation occurs almost simultaneous with the UES relaxation to enable liquids to enter the stomach without difficulty before the peristaltic wave reaches the LES.

CLINICAL SYMPTOMS OF DYSPHAGIA

Dysphagia is a broad term for subjective or objective swallowing difficulty that includes food sticking and gagging with feeds. Odynophagia is the complaint of pain with swallowing. The discomfort associated with dysphagia is commonly perceived to be proximal to the actual site of obstruction, although this sensation is occasionally referred distally. Dysphagia may be specifically described by older children and adolescents, however infants and young children are more likely to present with other symptoms that may be associated with swallowing dysfunction[3] (Table 4-1). For example, in infants and small children, heartburn or esophagitis may present as irritability or food refusal,[4] which can ultimately result in failure to thrive.

TABLE 4-1. Symptoms Sometimes Associated With Dysphagia

Aspiration
    Cough, choke, gag
    Recurrent pneumonia
    Bronchospasm

Nasopharyngeal regurgitation (sneezing)

Oral regurgitation (drooling, if severe—unable to handle own secretions)

Abnormalities of voice
    "Wet" voice—due to laryngeal soiling from dysfunctional swallowing
    Hoarse voice—due to laryngeal inflammation
    "Nasal" voice—due to velopharyngeal insufficiency and nasopharyngeal air escape

Swallowing behavior
    Posturing of head and neck during swallowing
    Rapid or slow intake; multiple swallows; pocketing of food in cheeks

(Modified from Orenstein,[3] with permission.)

Difficulty in the initiation of swallowing, such as a poor sucking reflex, suggests an abnormality of the oral or cricopharyngeal phases of swallowing. Coughing, gagging, choking, nasopharyngeal regurgitation, or cyanosis with feeding may be associated with an oropharyngeal disorder interfering in the transfer of food from the mouth to the upper esophagus. Regurgitation of food from the stomach or esophagus to the mouth is a common manifestation of functional and structural esophageal disorders. Recurrent pneumonia, bronchospasm, or a change in voice quality may be the presenting symptoms of chronic aspiration either from direct aspiration or following regurgitation of food from the esophagus or the stomach. In older children and adolescents, studies have reported that noncardiac chest pain is most often associated with esophageal disorders.[5,6] It is not uncommon, however, for patients to have difficulty distinguishing between dysphagia and odynophagia.[7] Odynophagia is commonly associated with severe esophageal inflammation.

DIFFERENTIAL DIAGNOSIS

Conditions resulting in dysphagia may be broadly divided into structural and functional disorders (Table 4-2). Dysphagia that is greater with solids than with liquids suggests a fixed esophageal narrowing, whereas dysphagia that is equal for both solids and liquids suggests a motility

TABLE 4-2. Differential Diagnosis of Dysphagia

Structural causes

Anatomic abnormalities of the oropharynx
    Cleft lip or palate
    Macroglossia
    Lingual ankyloglossia
    Pierre-Robin malformation
    Cleft larynx
    Retropharyngeal mass or abscess

Anatomic abnormalities of the esophagus
    Tracheoesophageal fistula
    Congenital esophageal stenosis resulting from tracheobronchial remnants
    Esophageal stricture, web, or ring
    Esophageal mass or tumor
    Foreign body
    Vascular rings and dysphagia lusorum
    Paraesophageal hernia
    Esophageal diverticula

Functional causes

Disorders affecting neuromuscular coordination of swallowing
    Cerebral palsy
    Bulbar atresia or palsy
    Brain stem glioma
    Arnold-Chiari malformation
    Myelomeningocele
    Familial dysautonomia
    Tardive dyskinesia
    Nitrazepam-induced dysphagia
    Postdiphtheric and polio paralysis
    Möbius' syndrome (cranial nerve abnormalities)
    Myasthenia gravis
    Infant botulism
    Congenital myotonic dystrophy
    Oculopharyngeal dystrophy
    Muscular dystrophies and myopathies
    Cricopharyngeal achalasia
    Polymyositis/dermatomyositis
    Rheumatoid arthritis

Disorders affecting esophageal peristalsis
    Achalasia
    Chagas disease
    Diffuse esophageal spasm
    Pseudoobstruction
    Scleroderma
    Mixed connective tissue disease
    Systemic lupus erythematosus
    Polymyositis/dermatomyositis
    Rheumatoid arthritis

Mucosal infections and inflammatory disorders causing dysphagia
    Candida pharyngitis or esophagitis
    Peptic esophagitis
    Herpes simplex esophagitis
    Human immunodeficiency virus infection
    Cytomegalovirus esophagitis
    Medication-induced esophagitis
    Crohn's disease
    Behçet's disease
    Chronic graft-versus-host disease

Other miscellaneous disorders associated with swallowing difficulties
    Foreign body
    Globus pharyngeus
    Epidermolysis bullosa dystrophica
    Central nervous system trauma
    Toxin: tetanus, lead poisoning, rabies
    Metabolic: hyperthyroid, hypothyroid

(Adapted from Rudolph,[43] with permission.)

disorder. Many of the conditions associated with disordered swallowing that present in infancy are a result of anatomic congenital anomalies. Esophageal narrowing may occur as a result of a congenital or acquired stenosis, a web, tumor, or an extrinsic compression of the esophagus.[8] The most common congenital esophageal anomaly is esophageal atresia associated with tracheal esophageal fistula. In utero, the lung bud divides in two, becoming the trachea ventrally and the esophagus dorsally. Any changes in this developmental process results in anomalies of either the esophagus or trachea, or both, frequently with an esophageal fistula. Primary repair of the esophageal atresia restores continuity but often progresses to stricture formation. Additionally, surgical repair does not ensure normal esophageal motility. Manometric studies of the esophagus following repair of esophageal atresia reveal disordered motility in almost all subjects.[9–11] Complications of esophageal atresia also include recurrent pneumonia as a result of an incompetent LES with gastroesophageal reflux and aspiration.[11]

Other structural lesions resulting in dysphagia include vascular malformations, such as an aberrant right subclavian artery, which passes behind the esophagus, consequently compressing it.[12] Other vascular abnormalities include a double aortic arch which may compress both the trachea and esophagus forming a complete vascular ring. Acquired anatomic defects from caustic ingestions or prior surgical trauma may also result in dysphagia.

FUNCTIONAL DISORDERS OF THE UPPER ESOPHAGUS

The cricopharyngeal muscle, which largely controls the UES, must relax completely and allow the anterior and superior movement of the larynx to ensure safe delivery of a bolus into the esophagus. Decreased cricopharyngeal pressures may be observed in myoneuronal conditions such as amylotrophic lateral sclerosis, myasthenia gravis, oculopharyngeal muscular dystrophy, dystrophia myotonica, and polymyositis[13] due to decreases in the tonic closure of the UES. Cricopharyngeal achalasia (dysfunction) is also associated with CNS lesions such as Arnold-Chiari malformation.[14] Before surgical decompression of an Arnold–Chiari malformation, incomplete relaxation of the UES or pharyngo-UES incoordination has been observed.

Symptoms of congenital cricopharyngeal dysfunction appear shortly after birth or during the neonatal period.[15] Pooling of saliva at the back of the pharynx, repeated aspirations, and choking are common presenting symptoms for these disorders.[16] Cricopharyngeal incoordination has been described as a transient condition in the newborn period.[16,17] The diagnosis can be made

radiographically using cinefluoroscopy. The clinical course is variable. Some infants progressively improve and become symptom free, while others experience fatal aspiration.[18,19]

A delay in cricopharyngeal relaxation results in a bolus being pushed from the pharynx before the UES is opened. A delay in cricopharyngeal opening of more than one-third of second has been associated with pulmonary aspiration.[20] Delayed cricopharyngeal opening has been observed in patients with Riley-Day syndrome,[20] as well as with nitrazepam administration.[21] The normal cricopharyngeal relaxation that preceeds pharyngeal contraction returns after discontinuation of nitrazepam. Cinefluoroscopy shows abnormal relaxation of the UES and the slow passage of barium.[15,16,18,22] Manometry has confirmed the incomplete UES relaxation in some patients, in addition to showing abnormal esophageal manometry.[15]

Treatment of cricopharyngeal dysphagia is directed toward the primary problem, although most cases will be idiopathic in children. Both cricopharyngeal achalasia and incoordination have been treated with dilation[16] or cricopharyngeal myotomy[23] in children. A more conservative approach using nutrition and positioning has also been effective in the management of some children.[15] Therefore, it is recommended that management of these disorders include "aggressive" nutritional support[24] with dilation in the patients with significant complications,[16] reserving surgery as a last resort.[24]

FUNCTIONAL DISORDERS OF THE ESOPHAGUS

Many systemic conditions affect the control or function of the oropharyngeal and esophageal muscles and are consequently associated with dysphagia (Table 4-2). Neurologic diseases or conditions may affect the neuromuscular coordination of swallowing through either the motor neurons of the bulbar tract or the brain stem region controlling the swallowing muscles.[25] Diseases of the neuromuscular junction such as myasthenia gravis and infant botulism frequently present with swallowing difficulty due to proximal esophageal weakness.

Esophageal achalasia is a primary motor disorder associated with swallowing difficulty. Most of the cases in the United States are idiopathic; however Chagas disease can mimic achalasia following ganglion destruction. The precise pathophysiology of esophageal achalasia is unclear, but it is hypothesized that postganglionic inhibitory neurons are reduced, absent, or impaired in the proximal dilated portion of the esophagus.[26] Achalasia disease is a rare disorder in adults, and even rarer in children under 15 years of age.[27] In general, the most common complaints are vomiting and dysphagia. The regur-

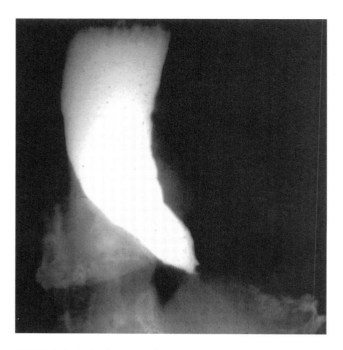

FIGURE 4-1. Barium esophagram demonstrating a dilated esophagus and the classic "beak" at the gastroesophageal junction in a patient with achalasia. (Courtesy of Dr. Steven M. Altschuler, MD, University of Pennsylvania School of Medicine, Philadelphia, PA.)

gitated food is often undigested because it has not mixed with gastric secretions. Patients also report that food gets stuck in the middle of the chest.[28]

A plain chest radiograph suggests esophageal achalasia if there is an air-fluid level in the esophagus or a widened mediastinum. Barium swallow demonstrates aperistalsis of the esophagus and a dilated esophageal body with distal narrowing at the esophageal junction (Fig. 4-1). The diagnosis is confirmed by manometry, which characteristically shows (1) aperistalsis of the esophagus with simultaneous contractions, (2) an increased LES pressure, and (3) incomplete relaxation of the esophagus with swallowing.[29]

The goal of therapy for achalasia is to reduce LES pressure and thereby relieve the distal esophageal obstruction. The most common procedure is pneumatic dilation of the esophagus, which applies direct pressure to the LES muscle in order to tear the muscle fibers. This procedure has a variable response rate, and it is not uncommon for patients to have multiple dilations. Those patients who fail pneumatic dilation may be candidates for surgical[30] or laparoscopic[31–33] myotomy. Nurko,[34] summarized the outcomes of the more common treatment modalities (e.g., dilation and surgical myotomy) in children. Pharmacologic agents such as isosorbide dinitrate and nifedipine have also been shown to decrease

LES pressures in adults[35,36] and children[37] with achalasia; however, the role of pharmacologic therapy as a primary treatment remains unclear.

Abnormal esophageal motor function has been reported in children with muscular dystrophy,[38] mixed connective tissue disease, and scleroderma.[39] Similar to the adult population, Flick and colleagues[39] reported symptoms of esophageal dysfunction in 73% of 17 patients with progressive systemic sclerosis and mixed connective tissue disease. The most frequent complaints were regurgitation and heartburn. Manometric studies demonstrated decreased LES pressure, low amplitude, and simultaneous contractions within the esophageal body. Children with progressive muscular dystrophy also showed decreased upper esophageal body amplitudes when compared to controls; however, no specific esophageal symptoms were reported despite the manometric abnormality.

DIAGNOSTIC EVALUATION

Initial evaluation of swallowing disorders begins with a thorough history to determine whether a birth or past medical history would predispose the patient to neurologic injury. Feeding problems are not an uncommon presentation of neurologic conditions. After a careful history and examination of the head and neck and nervous system, it is helpful to observe the feeding of the child, if this is not contraindicated by complaints of cyanosis or apnea. The initial evaluation of dysphagia should include a radiographic contrast study to look for structural abnormalities. Cinefluoroscopy during a barium swallow permits direct evaluation of the swallowing mechanism of the oropharynx and esophagus, in addition to laryngeal aspiration or nasopharyngeal regurgitation.[40,41] In some clinical situations, variations in the consistency of barium can be used to determine the best consistency to normalize swallowing function.

Although abnormal oropharyngeal and esophageal activities can be demonstrated with fluoroscopy, esophageal manometry is used to describe patterns of motility. (For a discussion of manometry, see Ch. 74.) There is good correlation, however, between manometric and radiologic findings of oropharyngeal[22] and esophageal[42] disorders. Endoscopy is reserved for histologic or structural evaluation (e.g., stricture confirmation or mass evaluation), as well as endoscopic procedures of the esophagus.

Therapy for dysphagia is directed toward the primary disorder when a definitive therapy is available. Otherwise supportive care is given with the primary emphasis on nutrition. Changes in food texture or positioning of the head and neck can prevent airway aspiration in some patients. Alternatively, dysphagia may be so severe as to require enteral feeds through a gastrostomy or a gastrointestinal feeding tube, in order to deliver adequate nutrition. In extreme cases of aspiration of saliva into the respiratory tract, more radical surgery may need to be considered.

REFERENCES

1. Kahrilas P. Pharyngeal structure and function. Dysphagia 1993;8:303–307

2. Dodds W. The physiology of swallowing. Dysphagia 1989; 3:171–178

3. Orenstein SR. Dysphagia and vomiting. In: Wyllie R, Hyams JS, Eds. Pediatric Gastrointestinal Disease. Philadelphia: Harcourt Brace Jovanovich, 1993:135–149

4. Dellert SF, Hyams JS, Treem WR, Geertsma MA. Feeding resistance and gastroesophageal reflux in infancy. J Pediatr Gastroenterol Nutr 1993;17:66–71

5. Glassman MS, Medow MS, Berezin S, Newman LJ. Spectrum of esophageal disorders in children with chest pain. Dig Dis Sci 1992;37:663–666

6. Berezin S, Medow MS, Glassman MS, Newman LJ. Esophageal chest pain in children with asthma. J Pediatr Gastroenterol Nutr 1991;12:52–55

7. Decktor DL, Allen ML, Robinson M. Esophageal motility, heartburn, and gastroesophageal reflux: variations in clinical presentation of esophageal dysphagia. Dysphagia 1990;5: 211–215

8. Enterline H, Thompson J. Congenital defects, rings, and webs. In: Enterline H, Thompson J, Eds. Pathology of the Esophagus. New York: Springer-Verlag, 1984:23–41

9. Werlin SL, Dodds WJ, Hogan WJ et al. Esophageal function in esophageal atresia. Dig Dis Sci 1981;26:796–800

10. Orringer MB, Kirsh MM, Sloan H. Long term esophageal function following repair of esophageal atresia. Ann Surg 1977;186:436–443

11. Whitington PF, Shermeta DW, Seto DS et al. Role of lower esophageal sphincter incompetence in recurrent pneumonia after repair of esophageal atresia. J Pediatr 1977;91:550–554

12. Orenstein SR. Manometric demonstration of aberrant right subclavian artery associated with dysphagia. J Pediatr 1984; 3:634–636

13. Vantrappen G, Hellmans J. Diseases of the Esophagus. New York: Springer-Verlag, 1974:399

14. Putnam PE, Orenstein SR, Pang D et al. Cricopharyngeal dysfunction associated with Chiari malformations. Pediatrics 1992;89:871–876

15. Reichert TJ, Bluestone CD, Seiber WK et al. Congenital cricopharyngeal achalasia. Ann Otol 1977;86:603–610

16. Dinari G, Danzinger Y, Mimouni M et al. Cricopharyngeal dysfunction in childhood: treatment by dilatations. J Pediatr Gastroenterol Nutr 1987;6:212–216

17. Frank MM, Gatewood OM. Transient pharyngeal incoordination in the newborn. Am J Dis Child 1966;111:178–181

18. Utian HL, Thomas R. Cricopharyngeal incoordination in infancy. Pediatrics 1969;43:402–406

19. Benson PF. Transient dysphagia due to muscular incoordination. Proc R Soc Med 1962;55:237–240

20. Kilman WJ, Goyal RK. Disorders of pharyngeal and upper esophageal sphincter motor function. Arch Intern Med 1976;136:592–601

21. Wyllie E, Wyllie R, Rothner AD, Erenberg G. The mechanism of nitrazepam induced-drooling and aspiration. N Engl J Med 1986;314:35–38

22. Hurwitz AL, Nelson JA, Haddad JK. Oropharyngeal dysphagia: manometric and cine esophagraphic findings. Dig Dis 1975;20:313–323

23. Bishop HC. Cricopharyngeal achalasia in childhood. J Pediatr Surg 1974;9:775–778

24. Fisher SE, Painter M, Milmoe G. Swallowing disorders in infancy. Pediatr Clin North Am 1981;28:845–853

25. Fischer RA, Ellison GW, Thayer WR et al. Esophageal motility in neuromuscular disorders. Ann Intern Med 1965;63: 229–248

26. Holloway RH, Dodds WJ, Helm JF et al. Integrity of cholinergic innervation to the lower esophageal sphincter in achalasia. Gastroenterology 1986;90:924–929

27. Berquist WE, Byrne WJ, Ament ME et al. Achalasia: diagnosis, management, and clinical course in 16 children. Pediatrics 1983;71:798–805

28. Boyle JT, Cohen S, Watkins J. Successful treatment of achalasia in childhood by pneumatic dilatation. J Pediatr 1981; 99:35–40

29. Cohen S. Motor disorders of the esophagus, review. N Engl J Med 1979;301:184–192

30. Lemmer JH, Coran AG, Wesley JR et al. Achalasia in children: treatment by anterior esophageal myotomy (modified Heller operation). J Pediatr Surg 1985;20:333–338

31. Swanstrom LL, Pennings J. Laparoscopic esophagomyotomy for achalasia. Surg Endosc 1995;9(3):286–290

32. Anselmino M, Hinder RA, Filipi CJ, Wilson P. Laparoscopic Heller cardiomyotomy and thoracoscopic esophageal long myotomy for the treatment of primary esophageal motor disorders. Surg Laparosc Endosc 1993;3:437–441

33. Pellegrini C, Wetter LA, Patti M et al. Thoracoscopic esophagomyotomy. Initial experience with a new approach for the treatment of achalasia. Ann Surg 1992;216:291–296

34. Nurko S. Motor disorders of the esophagus. In: Walker WA, Durie PR, Hamilton JR, Walker-Smith JA, Watkins JB, Eds. Pediatric Gastrointestinal Disease. Philadelphia: BC Decker, 1991:399

35. Gelfond M, Rosen P, Gilat R. Isosorbide dinitrate and nifedipine treatment of achalasia: a clinical, manometric and radionuclide evaluation. Gastroenterology 1982;83:963–969

36. Hongo M, Traub M, McAllister RG, McCallum RW. Effects of nifedipine on esophageal motor function in humans: correlation with plasma nifedipine concentration. Gastroenterology 1984;86:8–12

37. Maksimak M, Perlmutter DH, Winter HS. The use of nifedipine in the treatment of achalasia in children. J Pediatr Gastroenterol Nutr 1986;5:883–886

38. Staiano A, Del Giudice E, Romano A et al. Upper gastrointestinal tract motility in children with progressive muscular dystrophy. J Pediatr 1992;121:720–724

39. Flick JA, Boyle JT, Tuchman DN et al. Esophageal motor abnormalities in childrenn and adolescents with scleroderma and mixed connective tissue disease. Pediatrics 1988;82: 107–111

40. Ott DJ, Gelfand DW, Wu WC. Radiological evaluation of dysphagia. JAMA 1986;256:2718–2721

41. Jones B, Donner MW. Examination of the patient with dysphagia. Radiology 1988;167:319–326

42. Hewson EG, Ott DJ, Dalton CB et al. Manometry and radiology. Gastroenterology 1990;98:626–632

43. Rudolph CD. Feeding disorders in infants and children. J Pediatr 1994;125:S120

5

FOREIGN BODIES AND CAUSTIC INGESTIONS

L I N D A   A R N O L D
C H R I S   A .   L I A C O U R A S

FOREIGN BODIES

Foreign body ingestions, although generally benign, remain a common cause of morbidity and mortality in the United States, with up to 1,500 deaths per year attributable to complications from objects lodged in the upper gastrointestinal (GI) tract.[1,2] Eighty percent of foreign body ingestions occur in the pediatric age group.[1,3] While Binder and Angerson[4] found that children ingesting foreign bodies have a tendency toward developmental delay or a high-risk social situation, most series report foreign body ingestions in developmentally normal children in the care of their parents.[2,5] A slightly increased incidence in males has been reported by some investigators, and up to 10% of patients will have a history of previous ingestion. While up to one-half of foreign body ingestions may be witnessed, a history of ingestion is frequently not available. Coins are the items most frequently ingested,[1,2,5–10] followed by food, toy parts, and jewelry. Sharp objects comprise 10% of foreign bodies.

Clinical Symptoms

Symptoms of foreign body ingestion include gagging, vomiting, choking, odynophagia, or a sticking sensation in the chest.[4] Neck, throat, and chest pain may also occur. Dysphagia may be a late symptom, and mild to moderate respiratory distress may result from the mass effect of an esophageal foreign body impinging on the trachea.[10] It is important to remember that the location of discomfort may not correlate with the anatomic location of the foreign body and that mucosal lacerations secondary to a foreign body ingestion may produce similar symptoms.[11] By contrast, 40% of children with documented foreign bodies may be asymptomatic.[4,9] Additionally, up to 25% of foreign bodies may not be seen radiographically.[10] Whenever history or symptoms are suggestive of a foreign body ingestion, further investigation is warranted regardless of radiographic findings.

Passage of Foreign Body

As many as 80% to 90% of ingested foreign bodies will pass spontaneously, with an average transit time of 4 to 7 days.[1,2,5,11] Among foreign bodies documented to be in the stomach, up to 99% will pass within 5 days.[9] Impaction and delays in transit are most common at sites of anatomic narrowing, specifically, the cricopharyngeus, the lower esophageal sphincter, the pylorus, the ligament of Treitz, and the ileocecal valve.[2,10] Children with esophageal pathology such as a congenital narrowing, esophagitis, or abnormal motility may have an increased risk of esophageal impaction (and an increased probability of recurrence).[7,9]

Rules for Passage

Most investigators report that objects greater than 2 cm in diameter and longer than 5 cm are less likely to pass beyond the pylorus.[1,2,11] Elongated objects can also "hang up" or perforate the duodenal sweep.[11] Foreign bodies of these dimensions should be removed endoscopically. Otherwise, the decision to remove an object endoscopically should be based on the size, shape, and location of the object along with the risk of perforation or obstruction and the patient's clinical symptoms.

Methods of Removal

Although some investigators have described the use of the Foley catheter to remove esophageal foreign bodies, flexible endoscopy with general anesthesia is the preferred method in children, as it offers airway protection and permits visual evaluation of the esophagus, stomach, and duodenum.

Complications

Complications of foreign body ingestion include esophageal perforation, airway obstruction or aspiration, esophageal or intestinal perforation, and tracheoesophageal or esophagoaortic fistula formation.[5,9] The most commonly reported fatality from ingested foreign bodies results when a hot dog lodges in a toddler's esophagus and impinges on the trachea, resulting in airway obstruction.[10]

Specific Types of Foreign Bodies

COINS

Most foreign bodies are directly accessible to children. It is not surprising that coins, and pennies in particular, account for the majority of esophageal foreign bodies. The most common coin to lodge in the esophagus is a quarter. Recent surveys of practicing pediatricians indicate that most asymptomatic patients do not receive radiographs following coin ingestion.[5,9] This practice persists despite recommendations by most investigators that all children with a suspected coin ingestion receive radiographs to document location.[6–8] This recommendation arises from the knowledge that coins that lodge in the esophagus may damage the surrounding mucosa resulting in possible tracheal compression with airway obstruction or erosion into the mediastinum.[6,7] Although symptomatic patients are more likely to have esophageal lodgement, different series have reported that 7% to 44% of children with esophageal coins may be asymptomatic.[6–8] Esophageal foreign bodies can begin to ulcerate into the esophageal wall within 24 hours.

Choking or coughing is frequently reported at the time of ingestion. On presentation, children may complain of localized throat or chest pain, increased salivation with or without drooling, and vomiting, or dysphagia.[7,8,12,13] Radiographs including both the cervical esophagus and the stomach should be obtained. A coin lodged in the esophagus will generally appear en face in the anteroposterior projection while tracheal coins will appear en face in the lateral view. Ros and Cetta[9] propose the use of metal detectors to verify coin ingestion and identify possible lodgement when radiographs are either not available or undesirable. This method does not allow for distinction between esophageal and tracheal coins or between coins at the gastroesophageal junction and those in the stomach.

Connors et al.[6] reviewed the records of 73 patients with esophageal coins. In that series, more than 70% of coins were located in the proximal esophagus, 7% in the mid-esophagus, and 20% in the distal esophagus. The median age for children with proximal or mid-esophageal coins was 28 months and the median time of endoscopic removal was 15.5 hours. The median age for children with coins lodged in the distal esophagus was 57 months, and 60% of these coins passed within 5 hours.[6] Schunk et al.[7] prospectively studied 52 consecutive patients with a history of coin ingestion. In this study 9% of patients showed no coin on radiography and 40% demonstrated a coin in the stomach or intestine. Of those with esophageal coins, 63% were located at the thoracic inlet, 10% at the aortic arch, and 20% at the gastroesophageal junction.[7]

Serious complications following coin ingestion are generally associated with prolonged impactions.[7] Recently, the composition of the penny was changed in 1982 from 45% copper to 47.5% zinc with copper plating. Zinc is a more corrosive material than copper. Canadian dimes are also highly corrosive.

When a child presents with a history of a coin ingestion, radiographs should be obtained. Endoscopic removal of the coin, with airway protection, should be performed on all symptomatic patients and in all patients with upper or mid-esophageal coins. Children with coins in the distal esophagus may be observed for up to 24 hours, at which time endoscopic removal should be attempted if the coin has not passed. Most coins that have lodged in the stomach will pass through the remainder of the GI tract without difficulty. Four weeks should be allowed for gastric coins to pass, with weekly radiographs if passage of the coin in the stool is not documented. However, if after 4 weeks the coin has remained in the stomach, or if the patient develops upper intestinal symptoms, endoscopic removal is required. An abdominal radiograph should always be performed immediately prior to endoscopy.

FOOD AND MEAT

Meat and bone impaction are the most common esophageal foreign bodies seen in adults.[1] The classic presentation is that of the "café coronary," typified by the diner who has meat impacted at the level of the cervical esophagus, placing pressure on the anterior aspect of the trachea, and resulting in sudden onset of airway obstruction.

In children, meat impactions are rare in the absence of congenital or acquired defects of the esophagus, such as esophageal atresia, strictures, webs, rings, achalasia, or other motor disorders.[2,11] Steak and hot dogs are most commonly implicated, with food boluses lodging above the mechanically obstructing lesion, most often in the distal esophagus.[2,11]

When a child presents with a positive history and is symptomatic, no radiographs are needed to confirm the diagnosis of meat impaction, although plain films may be useful in checking for bone fragments. Concerning symptoms include discomfort, increased salivation, respiratory distress, or the inability to handle secretions; all the above symptoms are indications for immediate endoscopic removal of the impaction.[1,2,11] Following removal of the obstructing mass, the endoscopist should look for signs of esophageal injury and for underlying lesions.[1]

If the child is comfortable and is handling secretions well, the physician may safely observe the child and wait for spontaneous passage up to 24 hours.[1,2] If passage has not occurred, the impaction should be removed endoscopically, a task that will be more difficult after fragmentation. Several authors have advocated the use of intravenous glucagon for distal esophageal food impactions. Glucagon decreases lower esophageal sphincter tone and smooth muscle spasm and is relatively safe, with side effects including nausea and retching. Glucagon therapy has been reported to have a 30% to 50% success rate, has no effect on esophageal motor function or relaxation of distal strictures or esophageal rings (frequently implicated in meat impaction), and has been reported to cause aspiration.[1]

Papain- or gas-forming agents should not be used. Likewise, impacted food should never be pushed through the esophagus blindly using a catheter or endoscope. All these techniques increase the risk of perforation.

SHARP OBJECTS

While sharp objects account for only 10% of foreign body ingestions, they are responsible for most gastrointestinal complications. In a review of multiple series, Webb[1] reports rates of perforations ranging from 15% to 35%; the ileocecal valve is the most frequent site of perforation. Bones, pins, and toothpicks are the most common culprits; nails and razors have also been implicated. Given the high morbidity and mortality associated with toothpick and bone ingestion in particular, immediate endoscopic or surgical removal is often safer than observation.

When a child presents with a history or symptoms consistent with the ingestion of a sharp foreign body, radiographs should be obtained to document position. Lateral neck films may show cervical esophageal bone fragments that are not visible in the anteroposterior projection.[12] Esophageal sharp objects should be removed immediately, as esophageal perforation can result in hemorrhage, sepsis, or mediastinitis. The occurrence of upper GI bleeding in a patient with a history of sharp foreign body ingestion should alert the clinician to the possibility of a fistula between the esophagus and surrounding vasculature.[11] Objects longer than 5 cm and greater than 2 cm in diameter are unlikely to pass the pylorus.[1,2]

If the object has passed beyond the pylorus, the patient should receive daily radiographs and be monitored closely for symptoms such as fever, GI bleeding, and abdominal pain. A high roughage diet has been suggested but laxatives should not be used. The bowel exhibits a "mural withdrawal reflux," whereby the muscle wall reflexively dilates in response to mucosal contact with a sharp object. The resulting axial flow generally leaves the sharp end trailing.[1,11] By the time a sharp object reaches the transverse colon, it is generally surrounded by fecal material and passes through the remainder of the colon safely.[1] Surgical removal is indicated if a patient becomes symptomatic or if the object becomes localized to a specific segment intestine through serial radiographs.

BATTERIES

It is estimated that 500 to 850 button batteries are ingested each year in the United States. Two deaths from battery ingestion have been reported.[14] Litovitz presented a series of 125 battery ingestions reported to the National Battery Ingestion Hotline between August 1982 and June 1983.[15] Seventy percent of battery ingestions occur in children between the ages of 6 and 12. Nearly one-half of the batteries were found loose or discarded, while one-third had been removed from a product before ingestion. Of special note, 33.9% of ingested batteries came from hearing aids (often the child's own).

Optimal management following button battery ingestion requires a radiograph to locate the battery. Batteries lodged in the esophagus should be removed immediately, and the esophagus should be inspected for signs of injury. When endoscopic removal proves unsuccessful, the battery is often advanced into the stomach, from which it will often pass spontaneously. When a battery is allowed to remain lodged in the esophagus, local tissue damage may result from a combination of pressure necrosis, direct corrosive action, and low-voltage burns.[16]

Corrosion of the ingested battery results in leakage of the alkaline contents. Animal studies have demonstrated mucosal necrosis within 1 hour, with ulceration occurring within as early as 2 hours; burns have been reported by 4 hours and perforation within 6 hours. When the cells lodge in the esophagus, tracheoesophageal fistulas, stricture formation, and erosion can occur. In cases of esophageal lodgement, a barium swallow should be performed at 24 to 36 hours and again at 10 to 14 days, looking for strictures and late fistula formation. In the stomach, mucosal erosions, gastritis, and minor GI bleeding are less frequently seen.[16]

In the series conducted by Litovitz,[15] 90% of gastric button batteries passed spontaneously. Seventy percent passed within 48 hours with a range of 12 hours to 14 days. Ipecac treatment uniformly failed to expel ingested batteries though some recommend metoclopramide for cells beyond the esophagus. While batteries larger than 23 mm should be removed if they remain in the stomach for more than 48 hours, small batteries (e.g., watch, hearing aid) may be allowed to pass spontaneously. Patients should be monitored closely for anorexia, fever, abdominal pain, vomiting, and tarry stools.[14,16] If after 3 or 4 days the battery has not passed, endoscopy should be performed.

Concerns have been raised about possible mercury toxicity following button battery ingestion. Mercanic oxide is poorly absorbed from the GI tract. Even with corrosion or rupture, serum mercury levels are only minimally elevated; the risk of toxicity is low.

CAUSTIC INGESTIONS

Pathophysiology

Ingestions cause liquefactive necrosis and can rapidly penetrate the layers of the GI tract. Various degrees of caustic ingestion involvement can occur, including first-degree burns defined by superficial involvement of the mucosa, second-degree burns defined by transmural mucosal involvement, and third-degree burns, representing full-thickness injury, often leading to peritonitis or mediastinitis.[17] GI perforation may begin within hours or days of the event. Peri-intestinal inflammation with pain may be noted in patients with second- or third-degree burns, even without perforation. In patients with severe mucosal lesions, a superbacterial infection may occur. Upon healing, scarring and stricture formation may develop and ulcerations may be visualized for several months after the initial ingestion.

Clinical Symptoms

Symptoms typically begin from the moment of ingestion. Children experience immediate mouth or chest pain, coughing, crying, drooling, mouth burns, and dysphagia. Whenever a caustic ingestion occurs, the Poison Control Center should be notified, and the patient should be immediately seen by a physician. If possible, the caustic agent should be identified by the caretaker, and the container should accompany the child to the physician's office. The physician should conduct a thorough examination of the patient's oropharynx and should discuss any immediate therapies with the Poison Control Center.

Symptoms of airway obstruction should be immedi-

ately addressed. However, GI symptoms may not always correlate with the degree of GI involvement. Esophageal and gastric burns have been reported to occur despite lack of burns in the mouth and oropharynx.[18] Aspiration may complicate caustic ingestions and can be documented by clinical examination, pulse oximetry, and chest radiography. Patients who have full-thickness mucosal burns are usually acutely ill, febrile, and tachycardic.

Complications

Aspiration pneumonia, peritonitis, mediastinitis, and sepsis may occur following a caustic ingestion. GI complications include perforation, stricture, or fistula formation. Mortality generally ranges from 2% to 10%, but in severe cases the figure can approach 100%. Morbidity includes esophageal or gastric strictures requiring enteral tube feeding, dilation, and, in rare cases, surgical revision.

Alkali Ingestions

Caustic injury to the GI tract frequently occurs in the pediatric population. Lye ingestions are the most common agents encountered and contribute to most oropharyngeal, esophageal, and gastric lesions. When swallowed, lye can cause a variety of mucosal lesions, ranging from a few oral burns to deep, perforating, circular erosions of the esophagus. Lye is often present in routine household cleaners (e.g., Liquid-Plumber and Drano); the main ingredient is usually sodium hydroxide. The extent of tissue injury is often unrelated to the amount of the ingested agent. Major mucosal lesions and perforation has been reported to occur following licking a bottle cap or using an unwashed spoon.[19,20]

Acid Ingestion

Acid ingestion occurs less frequently than alkali ingestion. While acids can cause mucosal burns and destruction, they typically only cause superficial mucosal damage and are less likely to cause perforation. The stomach is most commonly affected by acid ingestion; however, acids may cause esophageal disease.

Treatment

Vomiting should never be induced because of the risk of potentiating injury to the esophagus and causing aspiration pneumonia. All children suspected of a caustic ingestion should be admitted to a hospital for observation. The patient's vital signs should be stabilized and respiratory compromise addressed. Upper endoscopy should be performed in all patients within 48 hours; it is impossible to determine the extent of esophageal or gastric mucosal disease on the basis of the clinical findings visualized in the oropharynx. The stomach and duodenum should be also be evaluated endoscopically, as burns are commonly noted in the gastric antrum, pylorus, and duodenal bulb. General anesthesia should be used to aviod all risk of aspiration. While many endoscopists perform endoscopy with the first 12 hours of ingestion,[21] some endoscopists prefer to wait 48 hours in order to visualize late-forming ulcers and fibrin deposits.

If there is no evidence of mucosal burn, the patient can be discharged after tolerating a normal diet. Patients with first-degree burns are observed in the hospital for 48 to 96 hours. Within 48 hours, a liquid or soft diet is generally tolerated, and the patient may be discharged. Patients with second- or third-degree esophageal or gastric burns may require prolonged hospitalization. Broad-spectrum antibiotics are recommended by many gastroenterlogists to prevent bacterial superinfection, which could contribute to stricture formation. Steroids are also commonly administered to patients with severe mucosal burns in a dose of 1 to 2 mg Solu-Medrol (methylprednisolone) per day, in order to reduce edema, inflammation, and fibrosis.[22] Enteral feeding by nasogastric, gastrostomy, or jejunostomy tube may be required if a significant stricture forms.

Referral

All patients who present with a caustic ingestion should be taken seriously. Immediate examination and communication with the local Poison Control Center is mandatory. In all but a select number of cases, patients will require observation in the hospital and evaluation by a gastroenterologist.

REFERENCES

1. Webb WA. Management of foreign bodies of the upper gastrointestinal tract. Gastroenterology 1988;94:204–216

2. Gryboski JD. Traumatic injury of the esophagus. In: Walker WA, Durie PR, Hamilton JR, Walker-Smith JA, Watkins JB, Eds. Pediatric Gastrointestinal Disease. 2nd Ed. St. Louis: Mosby-Year Book, 1996:430–451

3. O'Neill JA, Holcomb GW, Neslett WW. Management of tracheobronchial and esophageal foreign bodies in children. J Pediatr Surg 1983;18:475–479

4. Binder L, Anderson WA. Pediatric gastrointestinal foreign body ingestions. Ann Emerg Med 1984;13:61–66

5. Paul RI, Christoffel KK, et al. Foreign body ingestions in children: risk of complication varies with site of initial health care contact. Pediatrics 1993;91:121–127

6. Connors GP, Chamberlain JM, Ochsenschlager DW. Symptoms and spontaneous passage of esophageal coins. Arch Pediatr Adolesc Med 1995;149:36–39

7. Schunk JE, Cornel H, Bolte R. Pediatric coin ingestions: a prospective study of coin location and symptoms. Am J Dis Child 1989;143:546–548

8. Hodge D, Tecklenburg F, Fleisher G: Coin ingestion: does every child need a radiograph? Ann Emerg Med 1985;14:105–108

9. Ros SP, Cetta F. Metal detectors: an alternative approach to the evaluation of coin ingestions in children. Pediatr Emerg Care 1992;8:134–136

10. Friedman EM. Caustic ingestions and foreign bodies in the aerodigestive tract of children. Pediatr Clin North Am 1986;36:1403–1410

11. Hamilton JR, Polter DE. Gastrointestinal foreign bodies. In: Sleisenger MH, Fordtran JS, Eds. Gastrointestinal Disease. 5th Ed. Philadelphia: WB Saunders, 1993:286–292

12. Caravati EM, Bennett DL, McElwee NE. Pediatric coin ingestion: a prospective study on the utility of routine roentgenograms. Am J Dis Child 1989;143:549–551

13. Nandi P, Ong GB. Foreign body in the oesophagus: review of 2394 cases. Br J Surg 1978;65:5–9

14. Kutirutzm TL. Battery ingestions: product accessibility and clinical cource. Pediatrics 1985;5:469–476

15. Litovitz TL. Battery ingestions: product accessibility and clinical course. Pediatrics 1985;75:469–476

16. Studley JG, Linehan IP, Ogilvie AL, Dowling BL. Swallowed button batteries: is there a consensus on management? Gut 1990;31:867–870

17. Gryboski JD. Traumatic injury of the esophagus. In: Walker WA, Durie PR, Hamilton JR, Walker-Smith JA, Watkins JB, Eds. Pediatric Gastrointestinal Disease. Philadelphia: BC Decker, 1991:377–379

18. Sellers SL, Spence RA. Chemical burns of the esophagus. J Laryngol Otol 1987;101:1211–1213

19. Leape L, Ashcraft KW, Scrapilli DG, Holder TM. Hazard to health—liquid lyei. N Engl J Med 1971;284:478–480

20. Habener SA. Letter to the editor. N Engl J Med 1971;284:143

21. Sugawa C, Mullins RJ, Lucas CE, Leibold WC. The value of early endoscopy following caustic ingestion. Surg Gynecol Obstet 1981;143:553–556

22. Postlethwait RW. Chemical burns of the esophagus. Surg Clin North Am 1987;63:915–924

6

GASTROINTESTINAL BLEEDING

ROBERT H. SQUIRES, JR.

The presence of visible blood in stool or emesis is frightening to the child, family, and, at times, the physician. While patients with obvious gastrointestinal (GI) bleeding will quickly seek medical attention, those with occult intestinal blood loss are problematic. Iron-deficiency anemia or guaiac-positive stools may be the only evidence of intestinal bleeding. Therefore, a prioritized diagnostic and therapeutic approach to the child with suspected intestinal blood loss is critical to avoid a delay in diagnosis for the seriously ill child and unnecessary tests in the stable patient.[1–5]

CLINICAL WORKUP

General Assessment

For the ill-appearing child, simultaneous initiation of resuscitative, diagnostic, and therapeutic measures is required. A well-appearing child is evaluated with a patient and by focused selection of diagnostic tests or therapeutic trials. For example, a child with hypovolemic shock as a consequence of a ruptured esophageal varix, duodenal ulcer, or Meckel's diverticulum commands a different diagnostic and management strategy than does the otherwise healthy child with blood-streaked stools and suspected milk-protein–induced colitis, anal fissure, or juvenile polyp.

The patient may appear ill as a result of the underlying condition associated with GI blood loss (e.g., inflammatory bowel disease, infectious diarrhea) or as a consequence of a hemodynamically significant hemorrhage. The latter is identified by careful assessment of the child's general appearance and vital signs. Blood pressure, obtained with an appropriate size cuff, and heart rate are the most sensitive measures of significant blood loss, regardless of the hematocrit. In the cooperative patient, evidence of postural hypotension may be the first sign of decreased vascular volume. A decrease in the systolic blood pressure of more than 15 mm Hg, together with an increase in heart rate when the patient stands from a recumbent position, reflects significant vascular compensation for blood or fluid loss. Important physical findings include pallor of the skin and mucous membranes and prolonged capillary refill (greater than 2 seconds) to indicate poor peripheral perfusion.

Hematemesis defines blood in emesis and suggests a recent or ongoing hemorrhage proximal to the ligament of Treitz. Blood denatured by gastric fluids appears as black flecks, often described as "coffee grounds." *Hematochezia* represents bright red or maroon-colored blood in the stool from a source localized to the colon, unless the patient sustained a brisk, hemodynamically significant upper intestinal hemorrhage. Streaks of bright red blood limited to the exterior of the stool occur with an anal fissure or perianal streptococcal infection, but when mixed with stool, a more proximal lesion is suggested (e.g., polyp, colitis). *Melena* describes a black, tarry stool, associated with bleeding proximal to the ileocecal valve. Rarely, melena results from bleeding in the right colon if colonic transit is sufficiently delayed to allow bacteria to denature the hemoglobin.

Factitious hematochezia or melena is seen with certain artificial food colorings, foods, medications, and swallowed blood (Table 6-1). Commercial dye No. 2 and No. 3 red, found in some breakfast cereals and fruit

TABLE 6-1. Causes of Factitious Intestinal Bleeding

Hematemesis
    Commercial dyes No. 2 and No. 3 (Frankenberry stool)
    Swallowed maternal blood at delivery or breast feeding
    Bleeding from the nose, mouth, or pharynx
    Swallowed nonhuman blood

Melena
    Iron preparations
    Licorice
    Blueberries
    Spinach
    Beets
    Bismuth (e.g., Pepto-Bismol)
    Lead
    Charcoal
    Dirt
    Swallowed nonhuman blood

Hematochezia
    Menstruation
    Commercial dyes No. 2 and No. 3
    Ampicillin
    Hematuria

drinks, can give stool or emesis a bloody appearance (e.g., Frankenberry stool).[6] Black stool is associated with the ingestion of iron preparations, licorice, blueberries, bismuth, lead, dirt, and charcoal. Blood swallowed from lesions in the mouth or nose or, in the case of a neonate, during delivery or breast feeding, can be regurgitated and resemble an upper intestinal hemorrhage. Swallowed nonhuman blood or a self-inflicted oral mucosal lesion is considered if Munchausen syndrome by proxy is suspected.

Tests to verify blood in the stool are based on either leukodyes, fluorescent antibodies to porphyrin, or antihemoglobin antibodies (Table 6-2). Leukodyes (e.g., guaiac, orthotolidine) use the peroxidase-like activity found in hemoglobin to induce an oxidative reaction with the reagent to produce a blue color. The sensitivity

TABLE 6-2. Tests for Occult Blood

Guaiac or other leukodye
    Hemoccult
    Hemoccult II
    Hemoccult II Sensa
    Gastroccult

Fluorescent antibody to porphyrin
    HemoQuant

Antihemoglobin antibody
    Heme/detect
    FECA-EIA
    Heme Select

TABLE 6-3. Substances That Interfere With Fecal Occult Blood Tests

False-positive
    Meat (rare or well done)
    Horseradish
    Turnips
    Ferrous sulfate (stool pH <6.0)
    Tomatoes
    Fresh red cherries
False-negative
    Vitamin C
    Storage of specimen >4 days

of the tests varies significantly.[7,8] Unfortunately, peroxidase activity is also found in animal blood, myoglobin, iron preparations, and certain plants (e.g., horseradish, turnips, tomatoes, fresh red cherries). Ingestion of these and other items can lead to a false-positive result[9,10] (Table 6-3).

Consumption of vitamin C, even the amounts found in standard multivitamins, and storage of the specimen longer than 4 days may produce false-negative results.[11,12] Gastroccult (SmithKline Diagnostics, Philadelphia, PA) appears to be the most reliable method for the evaluation of occult blood in gastric juice.[13] The HemoQuant stool test (SmithKline Diagnostics) is a quantitative fluorometric technique used to assay porphyrin and is more specific than leukodyes for detecting blood in the stool.[14] Ingestion of red meat appears to be the only interfering substance for the HemoQuant test. The most specific, but expensive, tests use antihemoglobin antibodies and are usually performed in a reference laboratory.[15] Highly sensitive and specific tests for occult blood in the stool were developed to screen adults for colon cancer. However, the sensitivity of leukodye-based tests is sufficient for pediatric patients.

Few laboratory studies are necessary to evaluate a patient with intestinal bleeding. In addition to the hemoglobin and hematocrit, a low mean corpuscular volume may indicate chronic blood loss. Thrombocytopenia occurs in patients with hypersplenism, hemolytic uremic syndrome, necrotizing enterocolitis, or sepsis. Evidence of a coagulopathy as a cause or consequence of the hemorrhage is detected by measurement of the prothrombin time and partial thromboplastin time. If Munchausen syndrome by proxy is suspected blood, stool or emesis is usually "laced" by the conspirator with blood other than the child's. In this setting, blood in stool or emesis can be examined for blood type or nucleated red blood cells not seen with human blood.

Upper Intestinal Bleeding

HISTORY

Important clues to the diagnosis are obtained with a careful history, physical examination, and knowledge of the

TABLE 6-4. Causes of Acute Upper Intestinal Bleeding

Site	Common	Uncommon
Esophagus		
	Esophagitis	Esophagitis
	Acid reflux[b]	Viral (herpes,
	Pill induced	cytomegalovirus)
	Mallory-Weiss tear	Allergic[b]
		Fungal
		Caustic ingestion
		Varices[a]
		Dieulafoy's disease[a]
		Aortoesophageal fistula[a]
		Foreign body
		Duplication cyst
Stomach		
	Gastritis	Gastritis
	Prolapse	Crohn's disease
	gastropathy[b]	Portal hypertension
	Aspirin	Ulcer
	NSAIDs	Zollinger-Ellison
	H. pylori	syndrome
	Stress	Elevated intracranial
	ulcer/gastritis	pressure
		Dieulafoy's disease[a]
		Duplication cyst
		Leiomyoma
		Varices[a]
		Vascular malformations
Duodenum		
	Ulcer	Dieulafoy's disease
	H. pylori	Duplication cyst
	Duodenitis	Foreign body
	Crohn's disease	Varices
		Lymphoid hyperplasia
		Vascular malformations
		Hemobilia
Other		
	Swallowed blood[b]	Swallowed blood +
	During delivery	Munchausen by proxy
	Breast milk	Coagulopathy
	Nasopharynx	
	Oral pharynx	

[a] Always or often associated with hemodynamically significant bleeding.
[b] Never associated with hemodynamically significant bleeding.

potential causes of upper intestinal bleeding in infants and children (Table 6-4). The age and clinical condition of the patient will help prioritize the differential diagnosis.

Hemodynamically significant hemorrhage in a neonate is usually caused by a gastric or duodenal ulcer. Physiologic stress associated with fetal distress, perinatal asphyxia, sepsis, or a recent surgical procedure may precede the bleeding episode, although it can also occur in an apparently healthy, term infant.[16] Medications associated with gastric mucosal injury include tolazoline (pulmonary hypertension), indomethacin (patent ductus arteriosus), or dexamethasone (stimulate lung maturity).[17,18] If the newborn is clinically well and bleeding is not significant, it is proper to rule out swallowed maternal blood, which can occur either at delivery (e.g., melena neonatorum) or during breast feeding.[19]

In older infants and children, a sudden unexpected hemodynamically significant hemorrhage can occur with intestinal varices, Dieulafoy's disease, intestinal vascular malformations, hemobilia, or gastric ulceration secondary to physiologic stress (e.g., sepsis, shock, surgery) or ingestion of standard doses of aspirin or other nonsteroidal anti-inflammatory drugs (NSAIDs).[20–23] Occasionally, paroxysmal retching or coughing creates a rent in the mucosa along the gastroesophageal junction (Mallory-Weiss tear), which results in bleeding of varying severity.[24] More commonly, the amount of blood seen after a vomiting episode is small and is neither life-threatening nor hemodynamically significant. In these cases, bleeding is attributed to superficial mucosal injury from physical trauma to the stomach as it prolapses through the gastroesophageal junction (prolapse gastropathy).[25] Evidence of pruritus or jaundice suggests the presence of chronic liver disease, portal hypertension, and varices. Portal vein thrombosis may occur as a consequence of omphalitis or umbilical vein catheterization in the newborn, with subsequent development of extrahepatic portal hypertension later in childhood.[26] A careful and direct history of prescription and nonprescription medications can identify drugs, such as aspirin and other NSAIDs (e.g., indomethacin, ibuprofen, naproxen, tolmetin, sulindac) associated with mucosal erosion, ulceration, and bleeding.[27,28] Abdominal trauma (e.g., bicycle handle bar injury, automobile accident, blunt abdominal injury) may fracture intrahepatic blood vessels. Blood may then flow freely through the intrahepatic bile ducts into the small intestine, a condition known as hemobilia.[29] Recurrent episodes of upper intestinal bleeding without a readily identifiable source occurs with Dieulafoy's disease or other vascular malformations and with hemobilia.[23]

Fortunately, most patients with hematemesis do not have a clinically significant hemorrhage. In these patients, a history of dysphagia, odynophagia, nighttime cough, or water brash may suggest esophagitis (infectious, acid-related, eosinophilic), caustic ingestion, or an esophageal foreign body. Nausea, intermittent vomiting, and epigastric abdominal pain, especially if pain awakens the patient from sleep, are symptoms that suggest peptic ulcer disease, gastritis, or esophagitis.[30] Recent epistaxis or facial trauma may result in swallowed blood. GI blood loss is uncommon in patients with a coagulopathy, unless there is also a mucosal lesion (e.g., esophagitis, gastritis, ulcer).[31]

PHYSICAL EXAMINATION

A careful systematic physical examination will often provide clues to the diagnosis. The anterior nares should be inspected for evidence of recent bleeding or injury. Blood in the hypopharynx suggests bleeding from adenoidal or tonsillar tissue. The buccal mucosa should be examined, particularly at the level of the second and third molars, for evidence of trauma. Facial petechiae are seen after intense coughing or retching. Not all patients with liver disease are jaundiced. Hepatosplenomegaly can be missed unless the abdominal examination begins at the level of the pelvic rim and then gradually advances to the costal margin. Splenomegaly may be the only sign of portal hypertension. Other signs of liver disease and portal hypertension include prominent abdominal vessels, excoriations of the skin as a consequence of pruritus, clubbing of the digits, and telangiectasia. The finding of cutaneous hemangiomas may suggest the presence of other hemangiomas within the upper intestine. Blood originating from the lungs (hemoptysis) that is swallowed and regurgitated is uncommon in children but should be considered if lung disease is present (e.g., tuberculosis, pulmonary hemosiderosis).

Lower Intestinal Bleeding

HISTORY

Blood in the stool may result from a lesion anywhere from the mouth to the anus. Melena or guaiac-positive stools may provide the only evidence of bleeding proximal to the ligament of Treitz. Those lesions not reviewed in the prior section are presented in Table 6-5.

Hemodynamically significant rectal bleeding is uncommon, although it can occur with necrotizing enterocolitis, Hirschsprung's disease, vascular malformations, and Meckel's diverticulum.[32,33] Necrotizing enterocolitis presents in premature infants but has been reported in otherwise healthy-appearing newborns.[34–36] Delayed passage of meconium or severe constipation in infancy is associated with Hirschsprung's disease.[37] If the infant appears well and presents with a blood-streaked stool, a feeding and stool history may suggest milk-protein (cow, soy or human) intolerance or an anal fissure.[38,39] Infectious enterocolitis is uncommon during the perinatal period, but can present with a paucity of systemic symptoms.[40]

In the older child, as in the infant, the most common cause of rectal bleeding is a rectal fissure that occurs as a consequence of a recent gastroenteritis or passing of a large firm stool. Infectious enterocolitis is more common in the older child, who will likely experience symptoms of fever, vomiting, diarrhea, and tenesmus. An encounter with potentially undercooked meat (e.g., on a picnic, during travel) or a cluster of patients with bloody diarrhea suggests an infectious cause.[41] *Clostridium difficile*–

TABLE 6-5. Causes of Lower Intestinal Bleeding

Common	Uncommon
Infant	
Anal fissure	Vascular lesions
Milk-protein intolerance	Hirschsprung's enterocolitis
Necrotizing enterocolitis	Coagulopathy
Swallowed maternal blood	Intestinal duplication
	Meckel's diverticulum
	Intussuception
	Infectious enterocolitis
Older child	
Anal fissure	Inflammatory bowel disease
Intussusception	(<4 years of age)
Infectious enterocolitis	Vascular malformations
Salmonella	Intestinal duplication
Shigella	Henoch-Schönlein purpura
Campylobacter	Coagulopathy
Escherichia coli O157	Typhlitis
Yersinia enterocolitica	Infectious diarrhea
Clostridium difficile toxin	Cytomegalovirus
Inflammatory bowel disease	Amebiasis
(>4 years of age)	Hemorrhoids
Meckel's diverticulum	Colonic or rectal varicies
Nodular lymphoid hyperplasia	Ulceration at surgical
Perianal streptococcal cellulitis	anastamosis
	Solitary ulcer of the rectum
	Sexual abuse
	Rectal trauma

associated enterocolitis is considered if the child has received antibiotics within 1 month of presentation.[42] Abdominal distention, vomiting, and colicky abdominal pain in association with listlessness and apathy suggest intussusception.[43] Hematochezia and intense cramping abdominal pain may precede the characteristic rash on the buttocks and lower extremities seen with Henoch-Schönlein purpura.[44] Although clinical manifestations of inflammatory bowel disease (IBD) are protean, a history of vague or severe abdominal discomfort, anorexia, and weight loss accompanied by hematochezia or guaiac-positive stools make its consideration essential.[45,46] A history of vascular insufficiency to the bowel (e.g., actual or suspected necrotizing enterocolitis, Stevens-Johnson syndrome) can lead to a stricture of the involved segment, which may not be clinically evident until years after the event.[47,48] Hematochezia or occult blood in the stool from mucosal erosions near the stricture may be the only signs of previous injury to the intestine. Also, mucosal ulcerations can occur at the anastomotic site of bowel removed for any cause.[49] Inflammatory or juvenile polyps are common between ages 4 and 10 and can present with either streaks of blood on the stool or with a frightening amount of painless rectal bleeding that is not hemodynamically significant.[50] However, a family history of intestinal polyps or colon cancer in young relatives suggests a more serious familial polyp syndrome (e.g., Gardner's syndrome, Peutz-Jeghers syndrome).[51] A history of travel or exposure to areas endemic for parasitic infestation or infectious diseases may prompt an investigation for hookworm, strongyloidiasis, ascariasis, tuberculosis, or amebiasis. Questions regarding the ingestion of food containing red dye are asked whenever the substance in the stool is thought not to be blood.

PHYSICAL EXAMINATION

An anal fissure can be difficult to detect and requires the anal opening to be gently, but completely exposed. Intense perianal erythema likely represents cellulitis caused by group A beta-hemolytic streptococcus.[52] Skin tags or a perianal fistula may be the only manifestation of Crohn's disease.[53] Hemorrhoids are uncommon in children without portal hypertension.[54] Henoch-Schönlein purpura is characterized by a petechial or purpuric rash on the buttocks or posterior aspect of the lower extremities. A right lower quadrant mass in the infant or toddler with hematochezia suggests intussusception; in the older patient, Crohn's disease would be more likely. Pigmented freckles on the lips, buccal mucosa, hard-palate, or ventral surface of the fingers suggests Peutz-Jeghers syndrome.

Syndromes and Associations

Intestinal bleeding is associated with a variety of syndromes or clinical conditions (Table 6-6). Blue rubber bleb nevus syndrome, hereditary hemorrhagic telangiectasia (Osler-Weber-Rendu disease), and Klippel-Trenaunay syndrome are associated with intestinal blood loss from mucosal vascular malformations.[55–59] Disorders associated with cyclic neutropenia, such as Hermansky-Pudlak syndrome and glycogen storage disease type 1b may develop an inflammatory bowel disease similar to Crohn's disease.[60,61] Connective tissue disorders, especially Ehlers-Danlos syndrome type IV (ecchymotic) and pseudoxanthoma elasticum, are associated with intestinal bleeding as a consequence of fragile vascular epithelia.[62] Rectal bleeding noted in patients with epidermolysis bullosa can result from esophageal and rectal strictures, anal fissures, and friable perianal skin.[63] Hirschsprung's disease, Meckel's diverticulum, and pyloric stenosis occur more frequently in patients with trisomy 21.[64] Hemangioma, telangiectasis, venous ectasia, and inflammatory bowel disease have been described in patients with Turner's syndrome.[65,66]

DIAGNOSIS

Radiography

A plain-film radiograph of the abdomen will identify pneumatosis (e.g., necrotizing enterocolitis), toxic megacolon (e.g., Hirschsprung's disease, ulcerative colitis),

TABLE 6-6. Conditions Associated With Intestinal Bleeding

Condition	Intestinal Lesion
Turner's syndrome	Venous ectasia Inflammatory bowel disease
Epidermolysis bullosa	Anal fissure Colonic stricture
Down's syndrome	Hirschsprung's disease Meckel's diverticulum Pyloric stenosis
Ehlers-Danlos syndrome	Fragile vascular walls
Hermansky-Pudlak syndrome	Inflammatory bowel disease Platelet dysfunction
Blue rubber bleb nevus syndrome	Vascular malformations
Hereditary hemorrhagic telangiectasia (Osler-Weber-Rendu disease)	Vascular malformations Epistaxis
Klippel-Trenaunay syndrome	Vascular malformation
Pseudoxanthoma elasticum	Fragile vascular walls
Glycogen storage disease, type 1b	Inflammatory bowel disease

gastric bezoar, or pneumoperitoneum. A contrast study of the stomach and small intestine or colon can demonstrate mucosal, submucosal, and structural abnormalities, which include varices, nodularity of the gastric antrum, gastric tumor, malrotation, stricture, and thickening of the bowel wall as seen with Crohn's disease. As contrast material can interfere with other studies, such as endoscopy and radionucleotide scans, prioritization and timing of studies is essential for successful identification of the bleeding source.

Apt-Downey Test

The Apt-Downey test is a reliable method to determine whether red cells are of fetal or maternal origin.[19] A sample of red blood from emesis or stool is diluted with water and centrifuged to separate the particulate material. The supernatant is mixed with 0.25 N (1%) sodium hydroxide (5 : 1). A pink color is produced if the hemoglobin is fetal in origin or yellow-brown if adult. The test requires a sufficient quantity of bright red blood as denatured blood (e.g., "coffee-ground" emesis, melena) will be read falsely as adult.

Nasogastric Lavage

Nasogastric lavage to evaluate the presence of blood in the stomach has limited efficacy.[67,68] Blood may not be retrieved following gastric lavage despite the presence of a gastric lesion. Likewise, the presence of blood in the gastric fluid does not isolate bleeding to the stomach, as it can be swallowed from the nasopharynx, lungs, esophagus, or refluxed from the duodenum proximal to the ligament of Treitz. Normal saline at room temperature should be the only fluid used to lavage the stomach. Chilled or "iced" saline does not stop bleeding but can cause central hypothermia, particularly in the infant or young child.

Esophagogastroduodenoscopy

Esophagogastroduodenoscopy (EGD) is a safe and reliable tool, when performed by an endoscopist experienced with children and their diseases, and is performed using intravenous sedation or general anesthesia.[69,70] Upper GI endoscopy will identify mucosal abnormalities of the esophagus, stomach, and duodenum. However, not all patients with hematemesis require endoscopy. Sound clinical judgment is needed to determine whether findings at endoscopy will either change patient management or require specific therapy (e.g., sclerotherapy, thermo- or electrocoagulation).

As seen through the endoscope, the normal esophagus has a delicate mucosal surface with easily identifiable submucosal vessels. The distal 1 to 2 cm appears slightly erythematous but is related to the normal confluence of vessels at the gastroesophageal junction. Esophagitis from acid reflux has a range of endoscopic findings that include obscuration of submucosal vessels and friable mucosa with or without ulcerations.[71] However, the mucosa may appear normal; only a biopsy will identify histologic abnormalities consistent with acid reflux (e.g., thickened basal cell layer, elongated rete pegs, mucosal eosinophilia). Esophageal inflammation and injury may result from viral or fungal infection.[72,73] Patients with herpes esophagitis have a diffuse ulcerative esophagitis with intensely friable mucosa. By contrast, cytomegalovirus (CMV) is more likely to cause single or multiple discrete aphthous ulcerations. A thick cottage cheese-like exudate is seen with fungal esophagitis. Two ulcerations opposed to one another ("kissing ulcers") are characteristic of pill esophagitis or of prolonged entrapment of a foreign body such as a coin.[74] Crohn's disease rarely involves the esophagus but should be considered if aphthoid ulcerations are seen at endoscopy and granuloma is found on histologic sections.[75] Esophageal varices are easily identified, unless endoscopy is performed immediately following a bleeding episode when, in some cases, the vessels may be collapsed.

Within the stomach, ulcerations are most commonly found in the antrum or along the lesser curvature. Antral modularity, a result of lymphoid hyperplasia, is associated with *Helicobacter pylori* infection in children.[76] Aphthoid ulcerations are seen with Crohn's disease. Vascular lesions occur anywhere within the stomach. Dieulafoy's lesion, a rare cause of massive hemorrhage due to rupture of a large tortuous submucosal artery, is often hidden in the fundus or cardiac portion of the stomach.[23] Gastric varices are usually clustered around the gastroesophageal junction. Visualization of a Mallory-Weiss tear requires careful examination of the gastric side of the gastroesophageal junction. Multiple submucosal hemorrhages are seen in the fundus of patients with prolapse gastropathy.

While duodenal ulcerations occur most often within the bulb just distal to the pylorus, they can be found in the second or third portion of the duodenum. Blood can be seen flowing from the ampulla of Vater in patients with hemobilia.

On rare occasions, visualization of the entire small bowel is necessary. New, but expensive, fiberoptic instruments are available to evaluate the small intestine.[77] Small bowel enteroscopy is often coupled with surgical exploration.

Flexible Sigmoidoscopy

Flexible sigmoidoscopy identifies mucosal disease of the rectosigmoid and distal descending colon.[78] In most cases, minimal or no sedation is required to complete the procedure. However, careful patient monitoring will ensure patient safety and comfort. Flexible sigmoidoscopy is useful to assess hematochezia. Finding evidence of colitis or a polyp may abrogate the need for complete colonoscopy. In addition, a polyp can be removed if proper electrocautery equipment is available. A normal flexible sigmoidoscopy with biopsy and persistent hematochezia suggests a more proximal lesion.

Colonoscopy

Colonoscopy is indicated to evaluate patients with an unexplained iron-deficiency anemia and guaiac-positive stools, IBD, and persistent hematochezia unexplained by flexible sigmoidoscopy.[79,80] It is generally not indicated for acute infectious diarrhea, for evidence of toxic megacolon, or in a patient with neutropenia. Protocols to cleanse the colon prior to the procedure are available.[81] Intravenous sedation or general anesthesia is required if the procedure extends beyond the rectosigmoid. Ideally, evaluation should include intubation of the terminal ileum.[82]

Normal colonic mucosa appears pristine with visible submucosal vessels. Erythema, friability, modularity, and ulcerations are nonspecific signs of colonic inflammation. Mucosal biopsies are obtained, even with normal-appearing mucosa, as granuloma, eosinophils, or a mixed cellular infiltrate to suggest acute or chronic colitis can be found.

Meckel's Scan with Technetium-99m Pertechnetate

The use of Meckel's scan with technetium-99m pertechnetate will localize within the mucous cells of functional gastric mucosa and identify ectopic gastric mucosa found within a Meckel's diverticulum or an intestinal duplication cyst.[83,84] Active bleeding is not required for a scan to be positive. The scan may be enhanced by administration of an H_2-receptor antagonist or pentagastrin prior to the scan.[85,86] False-positive results occur with ureteral obstruction, arteriovenous malformation, hemangioma, or an inflammatory mass such as that seen in Crohn's disease.[87] A false-negative scan should not delay surgical exploration if clinical suspicion of a bleeding Meckel's diverticulum is high.

Bleeding Scan With Technetium-99m–Labeled Red Cells

Intermittent small volume intestinal bleeding that eludes endoscopic detection is evaluated with a bleeding scan although identification of a suspected lesion is rarely achieved.[88,89] An aliquot of the patient's blood is removed, labeled with technetium-99m and then injected into the patient while under a gamma counter. Images are taken over the abdomen every 5 minutes for the first hour to detect extravasation of the tagged red cells into the intestinal lumen. As technetium-tagged red cells remain the circulation for up to 5 days, intermittent bleeding can be assessed. A bleeding rate of 0.1 to 0.3 ml/min or 500 ml/day is necessary for a positive scan. If active bleeding is not identified during the initial imaging phase, additional images are taken at regular intervals for up to 24 hours. If extravasation of tagged red cells is detected, more frequent images are obtained to confirm and better localize the source of bleeding. Unfortunately, intestinal peristalsis propels extravasated blood distally and limits the test's ability to precisely identify the location of the hemorrhage. Angiography or endoscopy is needed to confirm the precise location of the bleeding site.

Angiography

Ongoing hemorrhage at a rate of 0.5 ml/min or greater is needed for angiography to identify the bleeding source accurately.[90,91] Once the patient is hemodynamically stable, has established urine output, and is properly sedated, the experienced angiographer systematically evaluates branches of the celiac axis, superior and inferior mesenteric arteries. Arterial injection of iodinated contrast material is followed by rapid sequence exposures to include the arterial and venous phase of the injection. A bleeding mucosal lesion is identified by extravasation of contrast into the intestinal lumen. An arteriovenous malformation is identified by an early venous return. A vascular "blush" identifies a vascular lesion (e.g., tumor, hemangioma, telangiectasia). If a bleeding site is identified, the catheter may be used therapeutically to embolize the lesion or to selectively infuse petressin. Also, if surgery is necessary, methylene blue can be injected to make the bleeding site visible to the surgeon.

MANAGEMENT

Shock and Resuscitation

A common mistake is to underestimate the amount of blood loss in a hemorrhaging patient. Any child who presents with blood in emesis or stool should be considered a potential emergency. If hypotension, orthostatic changes in pulse or blood pressure, tachycardia, an altered level of consciousness, or prolonged capillary refill are present, the patient should be observed in an intensive care unit (ICU), where prompt, aggressive treatment can be life-saving. One, but preferably two, large-bore intravenous catheters must be promptly placed to permit rapid infusion of extracellular-like fluids and blood products. A multilumen central venous catheter also provides acceptable venous access. Provide supplemental oxygen to maximize the oxygen-carrying capacity of available red cells. Initial blood work should include a complete blood count, serum electrolyte concentrations, liver and renal function tests, coagulation studies, and a cross-match for blood. At least one blood volume of packed red blood cells or whole blood should be available for immediate use. After intravenous access is secure, extracellular-like fluid in aliquots of 15 to 20 ml/kg or more are infused to maintain perfusion, until blood is available. Fresh frozen plasma is used to correct coagulation abnormalities, and platelet transfusions are given if the platelet count is less than 50,000. Central venous pressure and urine output are closely monitored to guide resuscitation efforts. Early involvement of members of the gastroenterology, radiology, critical care, and surgery teams will strengthen the coordinated effort to diagnose and manage the patient.

Ideally, investigation of the cause and location of the hemorrhage begins after adequate resuscitation. Occasionally, bleeding is torrential and aggressive diagnostic and therapeutic measures must proceed in an unstable patient.

Nonvariceal Upper Intestinal Bleeding

If the bleeding episode is not hemodynamically significant, did not require a blood transfusion, and has ceased clinically, and if a mucosal erosion or ulcer is suspected, empiric acid-reduction therapy may be considered without diagnostic endoscopy (see Ch. 36). Patients with a history compatible with an acute self-limited bleeding episode (e.g., pyloric stenosis, recent ingestion of a NSAID, prolapse gastropathy) with rapid clearance of the nasogastric aspirate may also be managed conservatively. Endoscopy for upper intestinal bleeding is indicated for active, persistent, or recurrent bleeding, for assessment of a hemodynamically significant hemorrhage (e.g., anemia requiring transfusion, hypotension, shock), or to distinguish between variceal and nonvariceal bleeding.

If endoscopy is performed, the endoscopist should be prepared to "intervene" at the time of the procedure to stop or abate the hemorrhage. Indications for endoscopic therapeutic hemostasis include active bleeding from a visible vessel within an ulcer crater, or under an adherent clot, and the presence of a nonbleeding visible vessel. If the suspected lesion has a nonbleeding adherent clot or has a clean base, therapeutic intervention could be withheld.

The three commonly used methods of endoscopic hemostasis for nonvariceal bleeding are bipolar electrocoagulation (BICAP, Circon-American ACMI, Stamford, CT), heater probe (Olympus Corp., Lake Success, NY), and injection sclerosis.[92–94] Each of these methods requires washing excess fluid and blood from the ulcer crater to provide optimal visualization of the vessel to be treated. The BICAP and heater probe rely on the generation of heat to coagulate the surrounding tissue. Injection sclerosis uses epinephrine, absolute alcohol, or sclerosing agents (e.g., polidocanol, tetradecyl) to achieve hemostasis by a combination of vessel constriction and tissue pressure that results from the injection of fluid into the interstitial space. The method chosen usually depends on the equipment and experience available at each institution.

Potential complications following therapeutic endoscopy include perforation or precipitation of uncontrolled bleeding. The BICAP and heater probe are designed to limit the area of tissue injury and minimize the risk of perforation; however, extensive experience of their use in children is not available. Complications from injection sclerotherapy are comparable to other methods (see Ch. 51).

Variceal Bleeding

Patients with variceal bleeding are managed initially in the intensive care unit.[95–99] Although replacement of blood and blood products is critical, overly aggressive transfusion therapy may increase portal pressure and precipitate recurrent variceal bleeding. Therefore, the hematocrit should be maintained at close to 30 g/dl. Fortunately, most episodes of variceal bleeding in children stop spontaneously with supportive care. If bleeding continues, a number of treatment regimens are available for

TABLE 6-7. Acute Management of Variceal Hemorrhage

Supportive care
    Monitor in intensive care unit
    Fluid resuscitation
    Maintain hematocrit about 30 g/dl
    Administer platelets if <50,000
    Correct coagulopathy
Pharmacologic
    Vasopressin
    Somatostatin
    Octreotide
Endoscopic
    Sclerotherapy
    Band ligation
    Thrombin injection
Mechanical
    Segstaken-Blakemore
Surgical
    Portosystemic shunt
    Esophageal transection
    Liver transplantation

acute management (Table 6-7). Data from controlled trials that support different treatment methods in children are limited. Attentive but conservative management of the pediatric patient often yields acceptable outcomes and avoids complications associated with invasive management.

Pharmacologic management of acute variceal bleeding is intended to reduce portal pressure with minimal systemic side effects.[100–102] Vasopressin, somatostatin, and octreotide decrease splanchnic arterial blood flow, followed by a decrease in portal blood flow and pressure. Dose schedules are derived from adult studies and clinical experience, as there are no placebo-controlled trials in children. Vasopressin (0.2 to 0.4 U/1.73 m^2/min) has been used in children, although its efficacy has never been critically evaluated. Complications associated with vasopressin include hypertension, bradycardia, dysrhythmias, venous thrombosis, and tissue injury if the peripheral infusion extravasates into the subcutaneous tissue. Somatostatin and its analogue, octreotide, are as effective as vasopressin in interrupting a bleeding episode and have fewer side effects.[103,104]

Two methods used to control variceal bleeding endoscopically are sclerotherapy and endoscopic variceal ligation (EVL).[105–107] Sclerotherapy involves the endoscopic injection of a chemical irritant (e.g., ethanolamine, tetradecyl sulfate) into a varix or the paravariceal tissue. The sclerosant will initiate an intense inflammatory response that results in fibrosis and obscuration of the varix. Sclerotherapy does not require special equipment and can be performed with a small-caliber endoscope. EVL requires an adult-size endoscope equipped with a clip-on hollow cylinder at the tip, which allows a varix to be sectioned into the device. Once the varix is entrapped within the cylinder, an elastic band is released from the device to act as a tourniquet around the varix. After each ligation, the endoscope must be removed and the apparatus reloaded with another band. Up to a dozen band ligations are performed with each treatment, which requires frequent removal and replacement of the endoscope. To facilitate frequent esophageal intubations, an overtube can be passed into the esophagus, through which the endoscope can be passed. The overtube protects the epiglottis and hypopharyngeal tissue from injury due to accidental discharge of the band. Both methods are equally effective in treating esophageal varices. The decision to use either sclerotherapy or EVL will depend on the size of the patient, equipment availability, and experience of the endoscopist.

Clinically significant complications follow endoscopic sclerosis in up to 20% of patients. Chest pain, likely due to esophageal spasm or chemical mediastinitis, will occur in 25% to 50% of patients. Low-grade fever, generally unrelated to bacteremia, is present in up to 50% of patients. Esophageal ulceration occurs in virtually all patients within 48 hours of the injection, thereby increasing the likelihood of rebleeding. Esophageal stricture or perforation are rare complications, occurring in 2% to 3% of patients. Although chest radiographic abnormalities such as symptomatic plural effusions are noted frequently, acute respiratory failure is rare. Bacteremia occurs at a frequency sufficient to require patients at risk of bacterial endocarditis to receive prophylactic antibiotics. Paralysis as a result of spinal cord necrosis has been reported. Thrombosis of intra-abdominal vessels (e.g., portal and splenic vein) has been described, although the etiology remains unclear. Finally, acute pericarditis and cardiac dysrhythmias may occur.

EVL has virtually no systemic complications. However, chest pain, recurrent esophageal bleeding, ulceration, and stricture may occur with EVL. Esophageal perforation and death are reported with placement of the overtube. Technical difficulties limit the use of EVL to adolescents and larger children (see Ch. 51).

Emergent surgical intervention is associated with high morbidity and mortality and should be reserved for the most desperate cases.[108] Surgical techniques used in children include esophageal transection, portosystemic shunt, and liver transplantation.

Lower Intestinal Bleeding

Flexible sigmoidoscopy, early in the evaluation of the patient with rectal bleeding, will identify distal colitis or a colonic polyp. If sigmoidoscopy fails to identify a source of bleeding, and the blood loss is hemodynamically sig-

nificant or ongoing, a Meckel's scan may diagnose a Meckel's diverticulum or intestinal duplication. Gastric lavage may demonstrate evidence of upper intestinal bleeding. If the diagnosis remains elusive, a full colonoscopy to the terminal ileum will identify inflammatory bowel disease or vascular malformation. Biopsies should be obtained even if the mucosa appears normal. If bleeding persists, upper endoscopy to detect an ulcer or vascular malformation is considered. Selective angiography or small bowel enteroscopy is reserved for patients with persistent, clinically significant symptoms despite standard efforts to identify the source of bleeding. Surgical laparotomy can be life-saving for patients with an ongoing intestinal hemorrhage.

OCCULT OR CHRONIC INTESTINAL BLEEDING

When the source of intestinal blood loss is not obvious, a careful reassessment of the patient's history and physical examination is needed to uncover additional clues to the diagnosis.[109] Any of the causes for upper or lower intestinal bleeding may be associated with chronic or occult blood loss. It is important to ensure that the patient is passing blood and that the blood is coming from the intestinal tract. Upper endoscopy and colonoscopy along with mucosal biopsy to look for eosinophilia, chronic inflammation, and granuloma formation can provide important information. If these studies are negative, a Meckel's scan may identify a Meckel's diverticulum or intestinal duplication. A tagged red cell study or angiography can be undertaken, depending on the estimated rate of bleeding. If the intestinal hemorrhage is substantial and persists despite efforts to identify the source, surgically assisted small bowel enteroscopy may be necessary.

REFERENCES

1. Hyams JS, Leichtner AM, Schwartz AN. Medical progress: recent advances in diagnosis and treatment of gastrointestinal hemorrhage in infants and children. J Pediatr 1985; 106:1–9

2. Laine L. Rolling review: upper gastrointestinal bleeding. Aliment Pharmacol Ther 1993;7:207–232

3. Olson AD, Hillemeier AC. Gastrointestinal Hemorrhage. In: Wyllie R, Hyams JS, Eds. Pediatric Gastrointestinal Disease: Pathophysiology, Diagnosis, Management. Philadelphia: WB Saunders, 1993:251–270

4. Perrault JF, Berry R. Gastrointestinal bleeding. In: Walker WA, Durie PR, Hamilton JR, Walker-Smith JA, Watkins JB, Eds. Pediatric Gastrointestinal Disease. 2nd Ed. St. Louis: CV Mosby, 1996:323–342

5. Vinton NE. Gastrointestinal bleeding in infancy and childhood. Gastroenterol Clin North Am 1994;23:93–122

6. Payne JV. Benign red pigmentation of stool resulting from food coloring in a new breakfast cereal (the Frankenberry stool). Pediatrics 1996;33:33

7. Allison JE, Tekawa IS, Ransom LJ, Adrian AL. A comparison of fecal occult-blood tests for colorectal-cancer screening. N Engl J Med 1996;334:115–159

8. Ransohoff DF, Lang CA. Improving the fecal occult-blood test. N Engl J Med 1996;334:189–190

9. Lifton LJ, Kreiser J. False-positive stool occult blood tests caused by iron preparations. Gastroenterology 1982;83:860–863

10. Ostrow JD, Mulvaney CA, Hansell JR, Rhodes RS. Sensitivity and reproducibility of chemical tests for fecal occult blood with an emphasis on false-positive reactions. Dig Dis 1973;18:930–940

11. Stroehlein JR, Fairbanks VF, Go VLW et al. Hemoccult stool tests: false-negative results due to storage of specimens. Mayo Clin Proc 1976;51:548–552

12. Jaffe RM, Kasten B, Young DS, MacLowry JD. False-negative stool occult blood tests caused by ingestion of ascorbic acid (vitamin C). Ann Intern Med 1975;83:824–826

13. Rosenthal P, Thompson J, Singh M. Detection of occult blood in gastric juice. J Clin Gastroenterol 1984;6:119

14. Ahlquist DA, McGill DB, Schwartz S et al. Fecal blood levels in health and disease. A study using HemoQuant. N Engl J Med 1985;312:1422

15. Frommer JJ, Kupparis A, Brown MK. Improved screening for colorectal cancer by immunological detection of occult blood. BMJ 1988;296:1092

16. Man DWK. Massive upper gastrointestinal bleeding from hemorrhagic gastritis in the newborn. Aust NZ J Surg 1986;56:871

17. Butt W, Auldist A, McDougall P. Duodenal ulceration: a complication of tolazaline therapy. Aust Pediatr J 1986;22:221

18. O'Neil EA, Chivals WJ, O'Shea MD. Dexamethasone treatment during ventilator dependency: possible life threatening gastrointestinal complications. Arch Dis Child 1992;67:10

19. Apt L, Downey W. Melena neonatorum; the swallowed blood syndrome, a simple test for the differentiation of adult and fetal hemoglobin in bloody stools. J Pediatr 1955;47:6–12

20. Cook DJ, Reeve BK, Guyatt GH et al. Stress ulcer prophylaxis in critically ill patients. JAMA 1996;275:306–314

21. Lacroix J, Infante-Rivard C, Gauthier M et al. Upper gastrointestinal tract bleeding acquired in a pediatric intensive care unit: prophylaxis trial with cimetidine. J Pediatr 1986;108:1015–1018

22. Ross AJ, Siegel KR, Bell W et al. Massive gastrointestinal hemorrhage in children with posterior fossa tumors. J Pediatr Surg 1987;22:633–636

23. Pointer R, Schwab G, Konigsrainer A, Dietze O. Endoscopic treatment of Dieulafoy's disease. Gastroenterology 1988;94:563–566

24. Cannon RA, Lee G, Cox KL. Gastrointestinal hemorrhage due to Mallory-Weiss syndrome in an infant. J Pediatr Gastroenterol Nutr 1985;4:323

25. Laine L, Weinstein WM. Subepithelial hemorrhages and erosions of human stomach. Dig Dis Sci 1988;33:490–503

26. Cohen J, Edelman RR, Chopra S. Portal vein thrombosis: a review. Am J Med 1992;92:173–182

27. Bergman GF, Philippidis P, Naiman JL. Severe gastrointestinal hemorrhage and anemia after therapeutic doses of aspirin in normal children. J Pediatr 1976;88:501–503

28. Fries JF, Williams CA, Bloch DA, Michel BA. Nonsteroidal anti-inflammatory drug-associated gastropathy: incidence and risk factor models. Am J Med 1991;91:213–222

29. Lackgren G, Olsen LL, Wassen C. Hemobilia in childhood. J Pediatr Surg 1988;23:105–108

30. Laine L, Peterson WL. Bleeding peptic ulcer. N Engl J Med 1994;331:717–727

31. Jaffin BW, Bliss CM, Lamont JT. Significance of occult gastrointestinal bleeding during anticoagulation therapy. Am J Med 1987;83:269–273

32. St-Vil D, Brandt ML, Panic S et al. Meckel's diverticulum in children: a 20-year review. J Pediatr Surg 1991;26:1289–1292

33. Trugeon DK, Barnett JL. Meckel's diverticulum. Am J Gastroenterol 1990;85:777–781

34. Nowicki P. Intestinal ischemia and necrotizing enterocolitis. J Pediatr 1990;117:S14–S19

35. Wiswell TE, Robertson CF, Jones TA, Tuttle DJ. Necrotizing enterocolitis in full-term infants. Am J Dis Child 1988;142:532–553

36. West KW, Rescorla FJ, Grosfeld JL, Vane DW. Pneumatosis intestinalis in children beyond the neonatal period. J Pediatr Surg 1989;24:818–822

37. Lifschitz CH, Bloss R. Persistence of colitis in Hirschsprung's disease. J Pediatr Gastroenterol Nutr 1985;4:291–293

38. Bishop JM, Hill DJ, Hosking CS. Natural history of cow milk allergy: clinical outcome. J Pediatr 1990;116:862–867

39. Machida HM, Catto Smith AG, Gall DG et al. Allergic colitis in infancy: clinical and pathologic aspects. J Pediatr Gastroenterol Nutr 1994;19:22–26

40. Raucher HS, Eichenfield AH, Hodes HL. Treatment of *Salmonella* gastroenteritis in infants. The significance of bacteremia. Clin Pediatr 1983;22:601–604

41. Belongia EA, MacDonald KL, Parham GL et al. An outbreak of *Escherichia coli* O157:H7 colitis associated with consumption of precooked meat patties. J Infect Dis 1991;164:338–343

42. Kelly CP, Pothoulakis C, Lamont JT. *Clostridium difficile* colitis. N Engl J Med 1994;330:257–262

43. Bruce J, Huh YS, Cooney DR et al. Intussusception: evolution of current management. J Pediatr Gastroenterol Nutr 1987;6:663–674

44. Tomomasa T, Hsu JY, Itoh K, Kuroume T. Endoscopic findings in pediatric patients with Henoch-Schönlein purpura and gastrointestinal symptoms. J Pediatr Gastroenterol Nutr 1987;6:725–729

45. Gryboski JD. Crohn's disease in children 10 years old and younger: comparison with ulcerative colitis. J Pediatr Gastroenterol Nutr 1994;18:174–182

46. Grand RJ, Ramakrishna J, Calenda KA. Inflammatory bowel disease in the pediatric patient. Gastroenterol Clin North Am 1995;24:613–632

47. Nanjundiah P, Lifschitz CH, Gopalakrishna GS et al. Intestinal strictures presenting with gastrointestinal blood loss. J Pediatr Surg 1989;24:174–176

48. Edell DS, Davidson JJ, Muelenar AA, Majure M. Unusual manifestation of Stevens-Johnson syndrome involving the respiratory and gastrointestinal tract. Pediatrics 1992;89:429–432

49. Sondheimer JM, Sokol RJ, Narkewicz MR, Tyson RW. Anastomotic ulceration: a late complication of ileocolonic anastomosis. J Pediatr. 1995;127:225–30

50. Cynamon HA, Milov DE, Andres JM. Diagnosis and management of colonic polyps in children. J Pediatr 1989;114:593–596

51. Foulkes WD. A tale of four syndromes: familial adenomatous polyposis, Gardner syndrome, attenuated APC, and Turcot syndrome. Q J Med 1995;88:853–863

52. Kokx NP, Comstock JA, Facklam RR. Streptococcal perianal disease in children. Pediatrics 1987;80:659–663

53. Markowitz J, Grancher K, Rosa J et al. Highly destructive perianal disease in children with Crohn's disease. J Pediatr Gastroenterol Nutr 1995;21:149–153

54. Johansen K, Bardin J, Orloff MJ. Massive bleeding from hemorrhoidal varices in portal hypertension. JAMA 1980;244:2084–2085

55. Moodley M, Ramdial P. Blue rubber bleb nevus syndrome: case report and review of the literature. Pediatrics 1993;92:160–162

56. Azizkhan RG. Life-threatening hematochezia from a rectosigmoid vascular malformation in Klippel-Trenaunay syndrome: long-term palliation using an argon laser. J Pediatr Surg 1991;26:1125–1128

57. Reilly PJ, Nostrant TT. Clinical manifestations of hereditary hemorrhagic telangiectasia. Am J Gastroenterol 1984;79:363–367

58. Cynamon HA, Milov DE, Andres JM. Multiple telangiectases of the colon in childhood. J Pediatr 1988;112:928–930

59. Perry WH. Clinical spectrum of hereditary hemorrhagic telangiectasis (Osler-Weber-Rendu disease). Am J Med 1987;82:989–997

60. Roe TF, Thomas DW, Gilsanz V et al. Inflammatory bowel disease in glycogen storage disease type 1b. J Pediatr 1986;109:55–59

61. Garay SM, Gardella JE, Fazzini EP, Goldring RM. Hermansky-Pudlak syndrome. Pulmonary manifestations of a ceroid storage disorder. Am J Med 1979;66:737–747

62. Nardone DA, Reuler JB, Girard DE. Gastrointestinal complications of Ehlers-Danlos syndrome. N Engl J Med 1979;300:863

63. Ergun GA, Lin AN, Dannenberg AJ, Carter DM. Gastrointestinal manifestations of epidermolysis bullosa, a study of 101 patients. Medicine (Baltimore) 1992;71:121–127

64. Knox G, E., Ten Bensel RW. Gastrointestinal malformations in Down's syndrome. Minn Med 1972;12:542–544

65. Burge DM, Middleton AW, Kamath R, Fasher BJ. Intestinal haemorrhage in Turner's syndrome. Arch Dis Child 1981;56:557–569

66. Weinrieb IJ, Fineman RM, Spiro HM. Turner syndrome and inflammatory bowel disease. N Engl J Med 1976;294:1221–1222

67. Cuellar RE, Gavaler JS, Alexander JA et al. Gastrointestinal tract hemorrhage: the value of a nasogastric aspirate. Arch Intern Med 1990;150:1381–1384

68. Basuk PM, Isenberg JI. Gastric lavage in patients with gastrointestinal hemorrhage: yea or nay? Arch Intern Med 1990;150:1379–1380

69. Ament ME, Berquist WE, Vargas J, Perisic V. Fiberoptic upper intestinal endoscopy in infants and children. Pediatr Clin North Am 1988;35:141–155

70. Squires RH, Morriss R, Schluterman S et al. Efficacy, safety, and cost of intravenous sedation versus general anesthesia in children undergoing endoscopic procedures. Gastrointest Endosc 1995;41:99–104

71. Black DD, Haggitt RC, Orenstein SR, Whitington PF. Esophagitis in infants. Morphometric histological diagnosis and correlation with measures of gastroesophageal reflux. Gastroenterology 1990;98:1408–1414

72. Ashenburg C, Rothstein FC, Dahms BB. Herpes esophagitis in the immunocompetent child. J Pediatr 1986;108:584–587

73. Baehr PH, McDonald GB. Esophageal infections: risk factors, presentation, diagnosis, and treatment. Gastroenterology 1994;106:509–532

74. Webb WA. Management of foreign bodies of the upper gastrointestinal tract: update. Gastrointest Endosc 1995;41:39–51

75. Mashako MNL, Cezard JP, Navarro J et al. Crohn's disease lesions in the upper gastrointestinal tract: correlation between clinical, radiological, endoscopic, and histological features in adolescents and children. J Pediatr Gastroenterol Nutr 1989;8:442–446

76. Bujanover Y, Konikoff F, Baratz M. Nodular gastritis and Helicobacter pylori. J Pediatr Gastroenterol Nutr 1990;11:41–44

77. Morrissey JF, Reichelderfer M. Gastrointestinal endoscopy. N Engl J Med 1991;325:1142–1149

78. Cucciara s, Guandalini S, Staiano A et al. Sigmoidoscopy, colonoscopy, and radiology in the evaluation of children with rectal bleeding. J Pediatr Gastroenterol Nutr 1983;2:667–671

79. Steffen RM, Wyllie R, Sivak M et al. Colonoscopy in the pediatric patient. J Pediatr 1989;115:507–513

80. Kawamitsu T, Nagashima K, Tsuchiya H et al. Pediatric total colonoscopy. J Pediatr Surg 1989;24:371–374

81. Vanner SJ, MacDonald PH, Paterson WG et al. A randomized prospective trial comparing oral sodium phosphate with standard polyethylene glycol-based lavage solution (Golytely) in the preparation of patients for colonoscopy. Am J Gastroenterol 1990;85:422–427

82. Zwas FR, Bonheim NA, Berken CA, Gray S. Diagnostic

yield of routine ileoscopy. Am J Gastroenterol 1995;990:1441–1443

83. Kong MS, Huang SC, Tzen KY, Lin JN. Repeated technetium-99m pertechnetate scanning for children with obscure gastrointestinal bleeding. J Pediatr Gastroenterol Nutr 1994;18:284–287

84. Wilson JP, Wenzel WW, Campbell JB. Technetium scans in the detection of gastrointestinal hemorrhage: preoperative diagnosis of enteric duplication in an infant. JAMA 1977;237:265–266

85. Treves S, Grand RJ, Eraklis AJ. Pentagastrin stimulation of technetium-99m uptake by ectopic mucose in a Meckel's diverticulum. Radiology 1978;128:711

86. Petrokubi RJ, Baum S, Rohrer GV. Cimetidine administration resulting in improved pertechnetate imaging of Meckel's diverticulum. Clin Nucl Med 1978;3:385–388

87. Rodgers BM, Youssef S. 'False positive' scan for Meckel diverticulum. J Pediatr 1975;87:239–240

88. Bentley DE, Richardson JD. The role of tagged red blood cell imaging in the localization of gastrointestinal bleeding. Arch Surg 1991;126:821–824

89. Majd M. Radionuclide imaging in pediatrics. Pediatr Clin North Am 1985;32:1573–1579

90. Athanasoulis CA. Therapeutic applications of angiography. N Engl J Med 1980;302:1117–1124

91. Afshani E, Berger PE. Gastrointestinal tract angiography in infants and children. J Pediatr Gastroenterol Nutr 1986;5:173–186

92. Cook DJ, Guyatt GH, Salena BJ, Laine LA. Endoscopic therapy for acute nonvariceal upper gastrointestinal hemorrhage: a meta-analysis. Gastroenterology 1992;102:139–148

93. Laine L. Multipolar electrocoagulation in the treatment of active upper gastrointestinal tract hemorrhage, a prospective controlled trial. N Engl J Med 1987;316:1613–1617

94. Raigopal C, Palmer KR. Endoscopic injection sclerosis: effective treatment for bleeding peptic ulcer. Gut 1991;32:727–729

95. Crass RA, Keeffe EB, Pinson CW. Management of variceal hemorrhage in the potential liver transplant candidate. Am J Surg 1989;157:476–478

96. Terblanche J, Burroughs AK, Hobbs KEF. Controversies in the management of bleeding esophageal varices. N Engl J Med 1989;320:1393–1398, 1469–1475

97. Cello JP, Crass RA, Grendell JH, Trunkey DD. Management of the patient with hemorrhaging esophageal varices. JAMA 1986;256:1480–1484

98. D'Amico G, Pagliaro L, Bosch J. The treatment of portal hypertension: a meta-analytic review. Hepatology 1995;22:332–354

99. Grose RD, Hayes PC. Review article: the pathophysiology and pharmacological treatment of portal hypertension. Aliment Pharmacol Ther 1992;6:521–540

100. Burroughs AK. Somatostatin and octreotide for variceal bleeding. J Hepatol 1991;13:1–4

101. Tuggle DW, Bennett KG, Scott J, Tunell WP. Intravenous vasopressin and gastrointestinal hemorrhage in children. J Pediatr Surg 1988;23:627–629

102. Grace ND. Management of portal hypertension. Gastroenterologist 1993;1:39–58

103. Sung JJY, Chung SCS, Lai C et al. Octreotide infusion or emergency sclerotherapy for variceal haemorrhage. Lancet 1993;342:637–641

104. Valenzuela JE, Schubert T, Fogel MR et al. A multicenter, randomized, double-blind trial of somatostatin in the management of acute hemorrhage from esophageal varices. Hepatology 1989;6:958–961

105. Stringer MD, Howard ER, Mowat AP. Endoscopic sclerotherapy in the management of esophageal varices in 61 children with biliary atresia. J Pediatr Surg 1989;24:438–442

106. Laine L, Cook D. Endoscopic ligation compared with sclerotherapy for treatment of esophageal variceal bleeding. Ann Intren Med 1995;123:280–287

107. Fox VL, Carr-Locke DL, Connors PJ, Leichtner AM. Endoscopic ligation of esophageal varices in children. J Pediatr Gastroenterol Nutr 1995;20:202–208

108. Maksoud JG, Goncalves MEP, Porta G et al. The endoscopic and surgical management of portal hypertension in children: analysis of 123 cases. J Pediatr Surg 1991;26:178–181

109. Perrault J, Fleming R, Dozois RR. Surreptitious use of salicylates: a cause of chronic recurrent gastroduodenal ulcers. Mayo Clin Proc 1988;63:337–342

7

HEPATOMEGALY

BARBARA A. HABER

The clinician who finds hepatomegaly on physical examination must first determine the significance of the finding. Hepatomegaly is the clinical perception of liver enlargement that is influenced by relationships between the liver and adjacent structures and by the anatomic variation from person to person. A myriad of factors alter the perception of liver size, including pneumothorax, perihepatic abscess, retroperitoneal mass, chronic obstructive lung disease, pectus excavatum, narrowed costal angles, flared costal margins, and Reidel's lobe (a tongue-like downward projection of the right liver lobe). In other words, a palpable liver is not necessarily an enlarged liver.

To determine whether a liver is enlarged, it is important to establish the expected liver size. The normal adult liver extends from the right fifth intercostal space in the midclavicular line to the right costal margin and descends below the costal margin with inspiration. Posteriorly, liver dullness is usually present on percussion below the ninth rib. Size correlates with age as does the palpable margin below the rib cage. The liver of infants is relatively large constituting 5% of body weight. From birth to adulthood, the liver normally increases in mass by at least 10-fold. In 1926, Zamkin studied 2,100 normal infants and children by palpation. He found palpable livers in 100% of infants less than 1 year of age and in 50% of children aged 10 to 12 years. These numbers may be higher than that found for many clinicians; however, they do highlight the difference between the pediatric liver examination and the adult exam.

LIVER EXAMINATION

An accurate examination of the liver is the most important way to establish the significance of a liver that is perceived to be large. The physical examination of the liver must include size (midclavicular span), shape (symmetric or asymmetric), consistency (soft, firm, stony-hard), surface morphology (smooth, irregular, or nodular), edge (sharp, rounded), tenderness, rubs, and bruits. Each of these qualities provides information about the underlying pathology.

Liver Size

The size of the liver is most accurately determined by percussion of the upper border and either percussion or palpation of the lower border in the midclavicular line. Its size should be recorded and compared to norms for age. The span of the liver varies with age. Table 7-1 was compiled by Naveh and Berant, who reviewed the literature. With inspiration, the liver moves down 1 to 3 cm; at expiration, it is acceptable to palpate the liver 1 cm below the costal margin throughout childhood and 2 cm in infancy. These data would suggest proceeding with an evaluation for liver spans exceeding 7 cm in patients less than 2 years old.

Shape

Asymmetry would suggest space-occupying lesions such as tumor, abscess, and cysts. However, proximal bile duct obstruction, radiation injury, or lobular infarction may also produce asymmetry as a result of hypertrophy of one lobe and atrophy of another. The liver should not cross the midline.

TABLE 7-1. Normative Values for Liver Span

Age	Span (cm)
Birth	5.6–5.9
2 mo	5
1 yr	6
2 yr	6.5
3 yr	7
4 yr	7.5
5 yr	8
12 yr	9

Firmness

A firm texture suggests infiltration, fibrosis, or congestion.

Surface Nodularity

Nodularity is found with liver cirrhosis or neoplasms.

Tenderness

A diffusely tender liver occurs when the capsule is distended, as found with acute parenchymal inflammation or congestion. Focal tenderness is more suggestive of an abscess, an infected cyst, or an infarcted focal lesion.

Rubs

A rub is the sound of the liver moving against the abdominal or chest wall. This occurs when there is inflammation of the liver capsule and is usually associated with trauma (including liver biopsy), infection (gonococcemia), and malignancy.

Bruit

A bruit is heard when there is increased hepatic arterial flow. This can occur with vascular lesions (e.g., arteriovenous fistula, hemangiomas) and liver tumors.

PATHOPHYSIOLOGY

Hepatomegaly may be a manifestation of either intrinsic liver disease or systemic illness. A firm foundation in the structure of the liver is essential to understanding how the liver enlarges.

Mature Liver Morphology

The liver is a highly vascular organ with a total liver blood flow approximating 20% to 25% of cardiac output in the adult. Portal blood from the intestines delivers approximately 70% of the blood flow to the liver. The remainder of the blood supply is derived from the systemic circulation through the hepatic artery. There is mixing of portal and systemic blood within the sinusoids. All the blood eventually drains from the liver through the hepatic veins to the inferior vena cava. Hepatocytes are arranged in a labyrinth of interconnecting plates of 20 to 25 cells in length within the acini. The plates are one cell thick; portal blood flows through the sinusoids across several sides of the hepatocyte from the periphery of the acinus toward the central vein. These plates are arranged like spokes on a wheel emanating from a central vein. The periphery is punctuated by portal triads, each composed of a hepatic artery, a portal vein, and bile ducts. Lining the sinusoids are antacids and Kupffer cells (fixed tissue macrophages).

By number, the liver is composed of 60% hepatocytes, approximately 17% to 20% endotholelial cells and close to the same proportion of Kupffer cells, 3% to 5% are bile duct cells. The remaining cell types constitute less than 1% and include cells such as Ito cells and oval cells.

Immature Liver Morphology

The liver does not establish mature morphology until 1 and 2 years of age. Before birth and early in development, hepatocytes are poorly organized, and the cells have limited contact with one another. During development, the hepatocytes develop a more linear array, and biliary structures, which initially are solid, develop a lumen. At birth, many of the liver cords are still two cells thick. This configuration generally resolves by 2 years of age. Hematopoietic elements are prominent in the first few postpartum weeks and then disappear.

Hepatomegaly results when the relative proportion for any cellular component or compartment. For example, hepatomegaly results when the number or size of hepatocytes increase or results when the sinusoidal space increases. Hepatomegaly can also occur through infiltration by foreign cells.

MECHANISMS OF HEPATOMEGALY

The mechanisms involved in the sudden or gradual onset of liver enlargement are varied and complex.

Congestion

The sinusoidal and vascular spaces account for 15% of the liver volume. These spaces expand with increased venous pressure as with right heart failure, atrial tachycardia, constrictive pericarditis, thrombosis of the hepatic veins, or veno-occlusive disease.

Inflammation

An inflammatory response to hepatocellular destruction causing Kupffer cell lysis occurs with infectious hepatitis and toxin response. Infections also elicit an inflammatory response, such as bacteremia, viral hepatitis, Epstein-Barr virus (EBV), syphilis, leptospirosis, histoplasmosis, brucellosis, toxoplasmosis, tuberculosis, ascariasis, amebiasis, amebic abscess, and pyogenic abscess.

Infiltration

Infiltration occurs with invasion by foreign cells and endogenous tumorous cells, including leukemic, lymphomatous and lymphocytic infiltrates, hepatoma, hepatic cell carcinoma, infantile choriocarcinoma, hepatoblastoma, hemangioma, hemangioendothelioma, Hodgkin's disease, neuroblastoma, Wilms' tumor, gonadal tumors, histiocytosis X, and Letterer-Siwe disease.

Storage/Fat Accumulation

Storage occurs when there is either an inborn error of metabolism or an acquired block to a metabolic pathway. Each of these processes can lead to the accumulation of by-products within the hepatic parenchyma or Kupffer cells. Fat accumulates in malnutrition, hydrocarbon ingestion, corticosteroids and tetracycline.

Proliferation of Liver Cells

Proliferation of hepatocytes occurs with tumors such as hepatoma and hepatoblastoma.

Hematopoietic Element Proliferation

Erythropoietic tissue can normally be found within the hepatic sinusoids during the first weeks of life. In erythroblastosis fetalis, the islands of blood-forming elements are enlarged, producing a large liver. Other hemolytic anemias can also lead to hepatomegaly in infancy due to expansion of blood-forming elements such as sickle cell disease.

Kupffer Cell Proliferation

Kupffer cells which act as phagocytes within the liver proliferate in sepsis, acute hepatitis, and toxic injury.

Ito Cell Hypertrophy

Ito cells respond to excessive ingestion of vitamin A by proliferating and storing the vitamin. The space of Disse becomes obliterated, and the cells deposit collagen, resulting in progressive hepatic fibrosis.

Proliferation of Multiple Cell Types

Proliferation of multiple cell types can occur with congenital hepatic fibrosis, biliary obstruction such as in biliary atresia and infectious hepatitis.

Space-Occupying Lesions

Congenital cysts, especially choledochal cyst, *Echinococcus* cyst, traumatic cyst, and inflammatory cyst, can all result in an enlarged liver.

CLINICAL PRESENTATION

Nutritional History

Nutritional history is important in establishing the possibility of steatosis. Factors such as a short period of starvation or excessive vitamin A can lead to liver enlargement.

Medications

Medications can lead to steatosis (phenobarbital, Dilantin, corticosteroids), peliosis hepatitis (androgens) or cancer (androgens, chemotherapy).

Age of Onset

Age of onset can be an important clue to etiology. In the newborn, congenital cysts, perinatal infections, and erythroblastosis fetalis are some of the diseases to be considered, while in the older infant cystic fibrosis, metabolic diseases, histiocytic syndromes, and tumors become more common. In the school-age child and adolescent, autoimmune hepatitis, liver disease with inflammatory bowel disease, Wilson's disease, and alcoholic hepatitis should be considered.

Travel

Travel to foreign countries or certain areas of the United States may raise the possibility of infections that cause liver enlargement, such as schistosomiasis, amebiasis, nematodes, leptospirosis, malaria, or tuberculosis. The most systematic approach to developing an appropriate differential involves defining the problem by age and associated findings (Tables 7-2 and 7-3).

PHYSICAL EXAMINATION

A thorough history and physical examination can often provide important information to help arrive at an appropriate differential.

TABLE 7-2. Diagnosis of Hepatomegaly

Hepatomegaly with aggressive cirrhosis	Hepatomegaly with hypoglycemia	Hepatomegaly with neuromuscular problems
Tyrosinemia type 1	Glycogen storage disease type I, II, III	Fulminant or relapsing
Glycogen storage disease type IV	Hereditary fructose intolerance	Organic acidemias
Idiopathic congenital cirrhosis	Hereditary fructose 1–6 diphosphatase deficiency	Urea cycle defects
Neonatal hemochromatosis	Islet cell lesions (infant of diabetic mother)	Progressive CNS deterioration
Hepatomegaly with moderately aggressive cirrhosis	Erythroblastosis	Niemann-Pick
Wilson's disease	Beckwith's syndrome	Gangliosidosis (GM1)
Galactosemia	Galactosemia	Mucopolysaccharidosis type 1 Hurler
Hereditary fructose intolerance	Cirrhosis	Gaucher type II
Alpha-1 antitrypsin deficiency	Hypopituitarism	Glycogen storage disease type VIII
Thalassemia major	Hepatosplenomegaly	Metachromatic leukodystrophy
Wolman's disease	Gangliosidosis (GM1)	Myopathic presentation
Biliary atresia	Niemann-Pick disease type A	Glycogen storage disease type II
	Sandhoff's	
	Gaucher's (infantile)	
	Hurler's	
	Marotasux-Lamy	
	I-Cell	
	Galactosemia	
	Glycogen storage disease type I	
	Cirrhosis with portal hypertension	

Physical Findings

JAUNDICE

Conjugated hyperbilirubinemia and jaundice characterize acute and chronic hepatitis and extrahepatic obstruction. This is an unusual finding in infiltrative processes or chronic congestive syndromes. Jaundice prior to pruritus typifies intrahepatic disease, and pruritus prior to jaundice suggests extrahepatic obstruction.

FEVER

Fever is a common but variable finding and therefore is not a major diagnostic tool.

SPLENOMEGALY

Acute splenomegaly suggests viral infection, hepatic or portal vein thrombosis, infection, or malignant dissemination. Chronic enlargement of the spleen suggests chronic liver disease and portal hypertension or a storage disorder.

ASCITES

Ascites is a manifestation of chronic liver disease, hepatic venous obstruction, or peritoneal inflammation. It is rarely associated with acute viral or toxic hepatitis.

NEUROLOGIC DISEASE

A variety of neurologic manifestations are found in association with liver disease and can help tailor the evaluation. The associated neurologic findings and underlying pathology include microcephaly (congenital infections), hydrocephalus (congenital syphilis or tumor), tremors, dystonia or dysarthria (Wilson's disease, lipid storage diseases), iritis (hepatitis with inflammatory bowel disease), Kayser-Fleisher rings (Wilson's disease), cataracts (Wilson's disease, galactosemia), and papilledema (hypervitaminosis A).

RENAL DISEASE

Renal cysts are associated with congenital hepatic fibrosis.

Laboratory Evaluation

Baseline laboratory tests are used for the initial evaluation and routine monitoring of liver disease. These tests include complete blood count (CBC), erythrocyte sedimentation rate, liver function tests, clotting studies, albumin, and total protein. Some laboratory tests can help refine the differential. An AST/ALT elevated above 1,000 implies acute viral, autoimmune, drug, or ischemic injury. An elevated alkaline phosphatase (ALP) or GGT suggest obstruction or infiltrative disorder.

TABLE 7-3. Diagnosis of Hepatomegaly and Associated Clinical Findings

Illness in infancy with hepatic
  dysfunction
  Infection
  Alpha-1-antitrypsin deficiency
  Tyrosinemia type 1
  Galactosemia
  Hereditary fructose intolerance
  Wolman's disease
  Zellweger syndrome
  Urea-cycle defects
  Cystic fibrosis
  Neimenn-Pick disease
  Beckwith-Wiedermann syndrome
  Methylmalonic acidemia
  Infantile sialidosis
  Biliary atresia
  Maternal diabetes
  Congestive heart failure
  Hemolytic anemia
  Isoimmunization disorders
  Hemorrhage into the liver
  Inspissated bile syndrome
  Hemangioma of the liver
  Metastatic neuroblastoma
  Neonatal iron storage disease

Appearance in childhood with illness
  Visceral larva migrens (toxocariasis)
  Hemolytic anemia
  Hand-Schüller-Christian disease
  Chediak-Higashi syndrome
  Chronic granulomatous disease
  Metastatic tumors
  Alpha-1-antitrypsin deficiency
  Cystic fibrosis
  Wilson's disease
  Glycogen storage disease type IV
  Tyrosinemia type 1

Illness in infancy with systemic findings
  Neuroblastoma
  Beta-thalassemia
  Mucopolysaccharidoses
  Histiocytosis X (Letlener-Siwe disease)
  Sickle cell disease
  Glycogen storage disease types I, II, III,
    IV, V
  Hereditary fructose intolerance
  Generalized gangliosidosis
  Fucosidosis
  Gaucher's disease
  Neimann-Pick disease
  Farber's disease
  Wolman's disease
  Crigler-Najlar
  Mannosidosis
  Familial intrahepatic cholestasis
  Albers-Schomberg syndrome
  Mucolipidosis I and II
  Aase's syndrome
  Klippel-Trenaunay-Weber syndrome
  Carnitine deficiency
  Familial erythrophagocytic
    tymphohistiocytosis
  Lysinuric protein intolerance
  Multiple sulfatase deficiency

Appearance at any age and generally ill-
  appearing
  Sepsis
  Starvation
  Infection
  Drug/toxin
  Leukemia and lymphoma
  Cystic fibrosis
  CHF or restrictive pericarditis
  Tangier's disease
  Budd-Chiari syndrome
  Veno-occlusive disease
  Diabetes mellitus
  Autoimmune chronic active hepatitis
  Juvenile rheumatoid arthritis
  Wilson's disease
  Systemic lupus erythematosus
  Alpha-1-antitrypsin
  Hyperlipoproteinemia types IV and V
    (after first decade of life)
  Hypervitaminosis A
  Primary sclerosing cholangitis
  Histiocytic proliferation syndromes

Hepatomegaly in the older infant and
  child without apparent illness
  Congenital hepatic fibrosis
  Cholesterol ester storage disease
  Glycogen storage disease type I, VI, IX
  Iron deficiency
  Hepatoblastoma
  Congenital lipoproteinemia
  Homocystinuria
  Moore-Federmann syndrome
  Autoimmune chronic active hepatitis
  Acquired immunodeficiency syndrome

Albumin and prothrombin time (PT)/partial thromboplastin time (PTT) reflect hepatocellular synthetic function. Late-stage liver disease may occur with normal serum enzymes but with abnormal albumin and clotting studies. Parenteral vitamin K administration is a valuable tool to distinguish extrahepatic obstruction from intrahepatic injury.

Ultrasound is always useful in determining the anatomy and texture of the liver. If a vascular process is suspected, a Doppler study should be requested, which can help determine flow to the liver through the portal vein and hepatic artery, as well as the flow of blood leaving the liver through the hepatic veins into the inferior vena cava. Scintigraphy can be helpful to assess the uptake and excretory capacity of the liver cells. Liver biopsy is performed in patients with chronic disease (greater than 3 months) or in patients in whom liver tissue may provide an etiology. Liver biopsies can be performed percutaneously or operatively, depending on the accessibility of the lesion and the risk of the procedure. ERCP or cholangiogram is used to define lesions of the biliary system.

REFERRAL PATTERN

The finding of liver enlargement in infancy and childhood almost always requires an extensive evaluation in order to distinguish benign self-limited processes from serious life-threatening conditions. Very rarely does an infant or young child have a self-limited illness with transient hepatomegaly for which mere observation is appropriate. Therefore, almost all patients with significantly elevated liver function tests and all patients with any other associated finding, such as fever, weight loss, splenomegaly, or jaundice, should undergo diagnostic evaluation.

Emergency referrals are made for suspected liver failure, tumors, metabolic liver disease, and infections that may benefit from the rapid intervention. The best parameters to follow for liver failure are the liver's synthetic capacity and transaminases. Transfer of care to a medical center should be made emergently for any patient with coagulopathy (PT greater than 14), significantly elevated transaminases, decreased albumin or total protein and bilirubin greater than 20 mg/dl. If hepatitis presents with altered mental status, again the transfer should be rapid and consultation with a gastroenterologist should be made immediately. If hepatitis presents with altered mental status, the transfer should be rapid and consultation with a gastroenterologist immediate. The changes in mentation may be due to liver failure or an underlying metabolic problem. Infection may be suspected if there is a fever, liver tenderness, travel history, or a septic picture based on blood tests.

CONCLUSION

Hepatomegaly is associated with a vast number of diseases, many of which are serious. A careful history and physical examination are the most important initial steps the clinician must take in order to develop an appropriate differential and appropriate testing.

REFERENCES

1. Czaja AJ. Axioms on hepatomegaly. Hosp Med 1980;60: 43–57
2. Walker WA, Mathis RK. Hepatomegaly: an approach to differential diagnosis. Pediatr Clin North Am 1975;22:929–942
3. Lawson EE, Grand RJ, Neff RK, Cohen LF. Clinical estimation of liver span in infants and children. Am J Dis Child 1978;132:474–476
4. Reiff MI, Osborn LM. Clinical estimation of liver size in newborn infants. Pediatrics 1983;71:46–48
5. Naveh Y, Berant M. Assessment of liver size in normal infants and children. J Pediatr Gastroenterol Nutr 1984;3:346–348

8

JAUNDICE

ERIC S. MALLER

Jaundice is defined as the presence of a yellow or yellow-green hue to the skin, sclerae, and mucous membranes due to elevation of bilirubin in serum. Jaundice usually becomes apparent at total serum bilirubin levels of 5 mg/dl but may be apparent at lower levels, particularly if searched for on examination as scleral discoloration. Jaundice in the newborn is a common problem for the general pediatrician and is the primary focus of this chapter. Jaundice in the older infant, school-age child, or adolescent is much less common and will be discussed only briefly.

The first task in the diagnostic evaluation is to ascertain whether the jaundice is due to conjugated (direct) or unconjugated (indirect) hyperbilirubinemia. Most infants will have an unconjugated hyperbilirubinemia, usually of a benign and physiologic nature. By contrast, the presence of elevated direct serum bilirubin (operationally defined as a direct bilirubin fraction greater than or equal to 2 mg/dl or accounting for greater than or equal to 15% of the total serum bilirubin) is never "physiologic" and implies a cholestatic and therefore a pathologic state.[1-4] The first 90 days of postnatal life are a particularly important period as an upper limit of time in which to diagnose and initiate definitive surgical therapy, should the infant have extrahepatic biliary atresia. Surgical correction attempted for biliary atresia beyond 90 days of post-natal life is associated with decreased success and a significantly poorer prognosis than surgery carried out earlier than 90 days of age.

Measurement of serum direct bilirubin has traditionally been performed by dye (van den Bergh) methods. This method has been replaced increasingly in many clinical laboratories by measurements of conjugated, un-conjugated, and delta-bilirubin, a fraction of conjugated bilirubin covalently bound to albumin. Although direct and conjugated bilirubin measurements are often used interchangeably, direct bilirubin values are, strictly speaking, approximated more accurately by the sum of the measured values of conjugated and delta-bilirubin. Therefore, the definition of cholestasis (the interruption of normal bile flow anywhere along the pathway from the hepatocyte to the delivery of bile into the duodenum) described above may need to be modified such that values of conjugated bilirubin (as opposed to direct bilirubin) below 2 mg/dl may also define a cholestatic state.

UNCONJUGATED HYPERBILIRUBINEMIA

Unconjugated jaundice in the newborn is common, occurring in up to 50% of full-term newborns and in a higher percentage of premature infants. The vast majority have so-called physiologic jaundice, due in part to delayed or inefficient conjugation of bilirubin. Other causes of unconjugated jaundice in the newborn are listed in Table 8-1. The older child with unconjugated jaundice usually has a hemolytic disorder or has Gilbert syndrome, a disorder of decreased bilirubin conjugation and possibly other aspects of hepatic bilirubin clearance.

DEVELOPMENT OF BILE FLOW AND NEONATAL CHOLESTASIS

Unfortunately, many of the processes responsible for the efficient generation of bile flow in the newborn and young infant are immature during early life. The liver of

TABLE 8-1. Causes of Unconjugated Hyperbilirubinemia

Physiologic jaundice (usually less than 14 days of age)

Breast feeding–associated jaundice

Hemolytic anemia due to red cell enzyme or membrane structural defect: (glucose-6-phosphate dehydrogenase [G6PD] deficiency, pyruvate kinase deficiency, hereditary spherocytosis, elliptocytosis)

Hemolysis due to Rh or ABO blood group incompatibility

Extravascular increased bilirubin load due to cephalohematoma or bruising after traumatic birth, swallowed maternal blood, or infant bleeding from neonatal clotting disorders

Sepsis

Endocrinopathy: congenital hypothyroidism and infants of diabetic mothers

Familial benign unconjugated hyperbilirubinemia (Lucey-Driscoll syndrome)

Defect in hepatic conjugation of bilirubin (Crigler-Najjar I and II)

Upper GI tract obstruction (e.g., pyloric stenosis, duodenal atresia, web, or stenosis)

---

the newborn and young infant may have little reserve when insulted by a variety of agents and may consequently demonstrate clinically significant cholestasis.

Terminology

Neonatal cholestasis, neonatal direct or conjugated hyperbilirubinemia, and neonatal hepatitis are terms used interchangeably to refer to the pathologic condition of cholestasis of the newborn liver caused by a large and diverse group of disorders (Table 8-2). The term *neonatal obstructive jaundice* has also been used to describe the cholestatic state in the newborn, despite the fact that the vast majority of disorders causing neonatal cholestasis are not truly anatomically obstructive in nature. *Idiopathic neonatal hepatitis* is also used by many to describe a specific diagnosis in the cholestatic newborn in which extensive investigation has failed to reveal as a cause any of the known disorders that lead to neonatal conjugated hyperbilirubinemia. The percentage of newborns with these generic and nonspecific diagnoses has, however, been steadily decreasing over time as new specific disorders that lead to neonatal liver disease are uncovered and their pathophysiology elucidated. The most recent example of such disorders is the recognition of the inherited disorders of bile acid synthesis due to single enzyme defects that may present during the newborn period with neonatal hepatitis.[5,6]

The neonate with cholestasis may be affected with any one of many complex differential diagnostic possibilities. It is critical that the clinican rapidly distinguish among the various disorders that are potentially responsible for the cholestatic state, since the outcome of treatment may well depend on the rapidity of diagnosis and initiation of appropriate medical or surgical therapy. This is a challenging task, because many of the disorders causing neonatal cholestasis are individually rare; some may require sophisticated assays not readily available to the practicing neonatologist or general pediatrician in the community.

EPIDEMIOLOGY AND CLINICAL PRESENTATION

Although many conditions may cause cholestasis in the newborn, their presentation is usually clinically similar. The findings usually include jaundice and hepatomegaly, together with other manifestations of decreased bile flow, such as dark urine and hypopigmented or frankly acholic stool. Splenomegaly may be apparent at presentation in as many as 50% of cases. It is more likely to be seen in cases of congenital infection or disorders resulting in early cirrhosis and portal hypertension, such as biliary atresia. The infant may rarely present with hypoglycemia due to compromised hepatic glycogen reserve, impaired gluconeogenesis, or (rarely) panhypopituitarism, including congenital growth hormone and cortisol deficiency. The infant with early severe liver disease and decreased hepatic parenchymal synthetic function together with malabsorption of fat-soluble vitamins including vitamin K due to cholestasis may present with life-threatening bleeding from the gastrointestinal (GI) tract or in the central nervous system (CNS). Infants presenting later with decreased hepatic synthesis of albumin and sodium retention may have ascites and peripheral edema.

Biochemical features usually include evidence of hepatocellular injury with elevated serum aminotransferases (ALT, AST). Cholestasis (impairment of bile flow) is evidenced by increased serum values of serum alkaline phosphatase, 5'-nucleotidase, and most specifically, gamma-glutamyltransferase (GGT) and serum bile acids. Serum lipids, especially cholesterol, may be elevated as well, particularly in bile duct paucity disorders, such as arteriohepatic dysplasia (Alagille syndrome). Some of these patients may experience severe itching (pruritus).

Jaundice with increased conjugated bilirubin may be present in the first few days of life. It is only rarely present immediately after birth, except in cases of complete biliary obstruction (other than biliary atresia). It is important to remember that conjugated (i.e., pathologic) hyperbilirubinemia, particularly that due to biliary atresia, may evolve after an initial physiologic and apparently benign unconjugated elevation in bilirubin. The initial presentation of benign physiologic jaundice can be falsely reassuring. A jaundiced infant with cholestatic

TABLE 8-2. Differential Diagnosis of Neonatal Conjugated Hyperbilirubinemia

Extrahepatic disorders

Biliary atresia

Extrahepatic biliary hypoplasia

Choledochal cyst

Congenital bile duct stricture

Spontaneous perforation of the bile duct

Common bile duct gallstones/"sludge"

Anomalies of the pancreaticobiliary junction (e.g., choledochocele)

Neoplasia

Intrahepatic disorders

Idiopathic
  Idiopathic neonatal hepatitis
  Recurrent intrahepatic cholestasis
    Familial benign recurrent cholestasis
    Hereditary cholestasis with lymphedema (Aagenaes syndrome)
  Persistent intrahepatic cholestasis
    Arteriohepatic dysplasia (Alagille syndrome)
    Byler's disease (severe intrahepatic cholestasis with progressive hepatocellular disease)
    Cholestasis in North American Indians (? microfilament dysfunction)
    Nonsyndromic paucity of intrahepatic ducts
    Sclerosing cholangitis
    Trihydroxycoprostanic acidemia (defective bile acid metabolism)
    Zellweger syndrome (cerebrohepatorenal syndrome)
    Transient intrahepatic cholestasis
    Inspissated bile syndrome

Anatomic disorders
  Congenital hepatic fibrosis with polycystic kidney and liver disease
  Cystic dilation of the intrahepatic biliary tree (Caroli disease)

Hepatitis
  Infectious causes
  Toxoplasmosis
  Syphilis
  Congenital rubella
  Cytomegalovirus (CMV)
  Herpes simplex virus (HSV)
  Varicella zoster virus (VZV)
  Hepatitis B virus (HBV)
  Hepatitis C virus (HCV)
  Human immunodeficiency virus (HIV)
  Tuberculosis
  Listeriosis
  Echovirus (types 11, 14, 19)
  Coxsackie virus

Parvovirus B19
Reovirus 3 ?
Toxins/drugs
  Parenteral nutrition–induced cholestasis
  Gram-negative sepsis with possible endotoxemia (e.g., urinary tract infection, necrotizing enterocolitis)
  Medicines (e.g., trimethoprim-sulfamethoxazole, anticonvulsants)
Metabolic disorders
  Disorders of carbohydrate metabolism
    Galactosemia
    Glycogenosis IV
    Hereditary fructose intolerance
  Disorders of lipid metabolism
    Gaucher disease
    Niemann-Pick disease (type C)
    Wolman disease (cholesterol ester storage)
  Disorders of amino acid metabolism
    Tyrosinemia
  Disorders of bile acid metabolism
    3-β-hydroxysteroid dehydrogenase/isomerase deficiency
    δ-4-3-oxosteroid 5β-reductase deficiency
  Disorders of the electron transport chain
    Cytochrome c oxidase deficiency
    Other mitochondrial enzymopathies
  Metabolic disorders in which the pathophysiology is uncharacterized
    α-1-antitrypsin deficiency
    Arginase deficiency
    Cystic fibrosis
    Familial erythrophagocytic lymphohistiocytosis
    Hypopituitarism
    Hypocortisolism
    Infantile copper overload
    Multiple acyl-CoA dehydrogenase deficiency (glutaric aciduria type II)
    Neonatal iron-storage disease
Chromosomal/syndromic abnormalities
  Trisomy 17, 18, or 21
  Turner syndrome
  Donohue syndrome (leprechaunism)
  Polysplenic syndrome (heterotaxy)
Systemic disease
  Post-shock or post-asphyxia
  Congestive heart failure
  Hypoplastic left heart syndrome
  Generalized hemangiomatosis
Miscellaneous
  Histiocytosis X
  Intestinal obstruction
  Neonatal lupus erythematosus

TABLE 8-3. Causes of Neonatal Cholestasis for Which the Outcome May Be Adversely Affected by Delayed Diagnosis and Treatment

Disorder	Consequence of Delayed Diagnosis	Therapy
Biliary atresia	Worse prognosis/need for liver transplantation	Kasai portoenterostomy
Choledochal cyst	Secondary biliary cirrhosis	Operative resection
Congenital syphilis	Osteomyelitis, death	Penicillin
Disorders of bile acid synthesis	Hepatic failure, death	Oral bile acid therapy
Galactosemia	CNS damage, gram-negative sepsis	Dietary galactose elimination
Hereditary fructose intolerance	Shock, death	Fructose (and sucrose) elimination from the diet
Hypopituitarism	Hypoglycemia, shock	IV glucose infusion, hormone replacement
Sepsis, urinary tract infection	Meningitis, death	Antibiotics

liver disease may then present on subsequent follow-up at 2 to 6 weeks after birth. Therefore, even if earlier determinations have suggested a benign noncholestatic cause of the jaundice, any infant jaundiced beyond 2 weeks of age should have a serum direct or conjugated bilirubin determination together with serum aminotransferase levels performed.

DIFFERENTIAL DIAGNOSIS

The more routine clinical, laboratory and radiographic assessments used to initially evaluate the infant with cholestatic liver disease usually do not provide a specific diagnosis. Individual test results are rarely diagnostic. Consequently, an extensive and complex laboratory investigation is essential to attempt to differentiate among those disorders which may be fatal or have a poorer prognosis if diagnosis and treatment are delayed (Table 8-3). As many as 60% to 70% of patients with neonatal cholestasis will have either extrahepatic biliary atresia or will have idiopathic neonatal hepatitis. Alpha-1-antitrypsin deficiency follows in incidence, approximately 8% of patients. The actual percentage mix of diagnoses appears to vary in several series, probably in part due to referral patterns.[7,8]

SELECTED CLINICAL DISORDERS THAT CAN CAUSE NEONATAL CHOLESTASIS EXTRAHEPATIC BILIARY DISEASE

Extrahepatic Biliary Atresia

Biliary atresia is the most common disorder causing neonatal cholestasis. Diagnosis and treatment need to be carried out rapidly to achieve a satisfactory outcome. If operated on before 2 months of age, bile flow may be reestablished in up to 90% of patients.[9] The success rate

decreases to below 20% if the patient is more than 90 days old at operation.[10,11]

Biliary atresia may be associated with the polysplenia syndrome and anomalies such as preduodenal portal vein, interrupted inferior vena cava, congenital cyanotic heart disease, and intestinal malrotation. These patients may represent a distinct subgroup who have a poorer prognosis.[12–14] In biliary atresia, it appears that an inflammatory process leading to scarring of the intra- and extrahepatic biliary ducts develops over time. We have observed the progression of this process on sequential liver biopsies. There are also isolated reports of infants who developed biliary atresia documented on reoperation when jaundice failed to resolve after an initial exploration showed an apparently normal biliary tree.[15,16]

The etiology of biliary atresia remains unknown. Several viral agents have been implicated, including some that have been shown to cause hepatobiliary injury in animals. However, none of these associations has been proven to be causal.[17–22]

When a hepatobiliary scintiscan (DISIDA scan) cannot demonstrate excretion of tracer from the biliary tree into the small bowel and a needle liver biopsy demonstrates interlobular bile duct proliferation, biliary atresia must be ruled out by exploratory laparotomy and intraoperative cholangiogram. If no definitive extrahepatic biliary ducts can be demonstrated on cholangiogram or dissection, a hepatoportoenterostomy is performed. The surgeon dissects and excises the fibrotic remnants of the extrahepatic bile ducts up to the hilum of the liver and its junction with the hepatic parenchyma. Then a jejunojejunostomy (Roux-en-Y anastomosis) is constructed, and the free limb is brought up to and sutured to the exposed small biliary branches present at the resection line in the hilum. This operation is called a Kasai procedure.

Before the advent of the Kasai procedure, mortality was virtually 100% by 2 years of age in unoperated patients. Rates of achieving long-term good bile flow postoperatively vary widely from 80% in Japanese series to

25% to 40% in Western series. Approximately 36% to 56% of patients lived to age 5 years during the preliver transplantation era, but many children maintain an only partially stable clinical state with many complications of chronic liver disease and cirrhosis. Episodes of bacterial cholangitis may accelerate the progression of chronic liver failure in the post-Kasai patient. Approximately 57% to 80% of children post-Kasai procedure will ultimately require liver transplantation at some time.[23] However, the Kasai procedure may allow continued growth and development to a size and weight that allow a greater pool of potential donor organs for subsequent liver transplant. Some patients may avoid liver transplant indefinitely.

Choledochal Cyst and Anomalies of the Pancreaticobiliary Junction

Choledochal cysts are rare, accounting for only approximately 2% of 731 referred cases of neonatal conjugated hyperbilirubinemia in a large regional pediatric hepatology service in England.[24] There is a markedly higher incidence in the Far East, and a female to male incidence ratio has been estimated at 2–5:1.[25,26] The cyst produces biliary obstruction in almost 50% of cases. Diagnosis is made by nuclear medicine scan or, more commonly, by ultrasound and rarely by ERCP, the test of choice to demonstrate a choledochocele, a localized dilation of the terminal common bile duct at the ampulla of Vater as it enters the duodenum. Unlike biliary atresia, which may be associated with cystic collections of bile at or near the hepatic hilum and which may be difficult to distinguish from a choledochal cyst by ultrasound, choledochal cyst may be associated with dilation of the intrahepatic bile ducts due to obstruction of the common duct. (Dilation of the intrahepatic ducts never occurs with biliary atresia, probably due to the inflammation which also involves the intrahepatic ducts and thus prevents their dilation, even with complete extrahepatic obstruction.) Prompt surgical excision is the therapy of choice for a choledochal cyst. Resection relieves the ongoing obstruction to bile flow and also prevents the long-term risk of cholangiocarcinoma associated with retained abnormal cyst epithelium.

Other Extrahepatic Causes of Neonatal Cholestasis

Disorders of the extrahepatic biliary tree other than biliary atresia are relatively rare as a cause of neonatal cholestasis. They include spontaneous perforation of the bile duct, neoplasms, and cholelithiasis, congenital bile duct stenosis, or extrahepatic biliary hypoplasia (sometimes associated with an intrahepatic bile duct paucity such as Alagille syndrome, also known as arteriohepatic dysplasia). Cholelithiasis in infancy, though relatively rare, is usually related to biliary stasis and the formation of "sludge" or frank stones. It occurs in the setting of other systemic disorders such as cystic fibrosis or a hemolytic disorder. Parenteral nutrition, even over a few weeks, may cause biliary "sludge" or actual stones to form.[27] The ill premature infant who has respiratory distress and is treated with frequent diuretics such as furosemide for fluid overload and unable to take any enteral feedings that would otherwise stimulate the enterohepatic circulation is at special risk. An operative cholangiogram has been reported to "flush out" sludge and reestablish bile flow without further therapy.[28]

INTRAHEPATIC DISORDERS

Idiopathic Neonatal Hepatitis

Idiopathic neonatal hepatitis accounts for 30% to 40% of all infants presenting with neonatal cholestasis. It is a diagnosis of exclusion when known causes of neonatal cholestasis have been excluded. The liver biopsy shows multinucleated giant cells. However, other disorders including biliary atresia may demonstrate this finding on liver biopsy. Bile duct proliferation, which implies extrahepatic biliary obstruction, is conspicuously absent. The major physical findings include jaundice and hepatomegaly with variable splenomegaly. If present, other findings, such as purpura, microcephaly, rash, cataract, microcephaly, and cardiac murmur, should suggest other etiologies, most importantly congenital infection. The prognosis, once thought to be almost universally good, is now recognized as only fair. In various series,[29–33] an average of approximately 74% (range 60% to 94%) recover without persistent liver disease, 7% (range 2% to 22%) have chronic liver disease, and 20% (range 5% to 31%) die of progressive liver disease. These infants likely represent a heterogeneous population without specific known mechanisms of injury and likely include several disorders whose pathophysiology and natural history have not been delineated.

PERSISTENT INTRAHEPATIC CHOLESTASIS DISORDERS

Arteriohepatic Dysplasia (Alagille Syndrome)

Alagille syndrome, or arteriohepatic dysplasia, is a chronic cholestatic disorder (described in more detail in Ch. 4) characterized by paucity of the interlobular bile ducts (defined as fewer than 0.5 duct on average per portal triad). These features are associated with some or all of the following findings: extrahepatic biliary hypoplasia, pulmonary outflow tract abnormalities ranging from valvar or peripheral pulmonic stenosis most commonly, and rarely to severe right-sided congenital cardiac disease. Other associated anomalies include butterfly or cleft vertebrae, a variety of ocular findings, bone abnormalities, hypogonadism, developmental delay, and a characteristic cholestatic facies. This facies includes a prominent forehead, moderate hypertelorism with deep-set eyes, a small pointed chin, and a saddle or straight nose that, in profile, may be in the same plane as the forehead. These features usually become more prominent as the child ages but may be present at birth.[34] Others have suggested that these facies may be less specific and can result from any condition of chronic cholestasis of early onset in children.[35] The extrahepatic biliary tree is patent but often hypoplastic.

The importance of recognizing the possibility of arteriohepatic dysplasia in the newborn or young infant with cholestasis lies in distinguishing it from extrahepatic biliary atresia and avoiding operative intervention, if possible. Alagille syndrome appears to be inherited as an autosomal dominant, though with quite variable penetrance and clinical severity. Misdiagnosis has implications not only for the individual patient, but also for genetic counseling with regard to occurrence in future offspring as well.[34,36]

Nonsyndromic Paucity of Interlobular Bile Ducts

Paucity of the interlobular bile ducts is seen without the features of arteriohepatic dysplasia (Alagille syndrome). There may or may not be an associated diagnosed primary disease. Prognosis of bile duct paucity in an associated disease (e.g., alpha-1-antitrypsin deficiency) is generally that of the associated disease.

Other Idiopathic Intrahepatic Disorders

Byler's disease was first reported in an Amish kindred of the same name in which there was neonatal cholestasis with progressive cholestatic liver disease leading to biliary cirrhosis, chronic liver failure, and death.[37] Despite pronounced jaundice, pruritus, and elevations of serum bile acids and alkaline phosphatase, serum GGT as well as 5'-nucleotidase and cholesterol, normally markedly elevated in other severe cholestatic disorders, were all normal or near normal.[38] Recently, it has been observed in patients with inborn errors of bile acid synthesis that normal GGT as well as cholelithiasis is common, interestingly, both features of the clinical presentation of Byler's disease.[39]

Several disorders of peroxisomes associated with neonatal cholestasis have been described, the most important of which is the cerebrohepatorenal or Zellweger syndrome. This syndrome is characterized by absent peroxisomes and structurally abnormal mitochondria

seen on electron microscopy of liver specimens. Consequently, there is abnormal beta-oxidation of fatty acids with bile acid precursors present with abnormal side chain structure. Hepatomegaly and cholestasis are usually present at birth together with profound hypotonia, a characteristic facies consisting of prominent forehead, triangular mouth, low-set abnormal ears, widely open metopic suture, and hypertelorism with upslanting palpebral fissures. Psychomotor retardation with cerebral dysgenesis and pigmentary retinopathy, as well as cortical glomerular cysts of the kidney seen on ultrasound, is also found.[40]

HEPATOCELLULAR DISORDERS

Perinatal Infectious Hepatitides

Intrauterine infections are commonly associated with a picture of neonatal cholestasis.

Cytomegalovirus

Cytomegalovirus (CMV) infection of the newborn may be acquired transplacentally, at delivery, or infection may occur in the postnatal period, but only 5% to 10% of infected patients show clinical symptoms.[41] Hepatomegaly in 75% to 90% and a direct hyperbilirubinemia in 60% are the most consistent abnormal findings in neonatal CMV infection.[42] Other findings in severely affected infants include thrombocytopenia, hemolytic anemia, cataracts, microcephaly, intracranial calcifications, chorioretinitis, and ultimately psychomotor retardation. Liver biopsy findings include a giant cell hepatitis frequently with the occurrence of intranuclear viral inclusions in bile duct epithelial cells, but less commonly in hepatocytes. Most neonates recover completely, although progression to hepatic failure or presinusoidal portal hypertension has been noted.[43]

The CMV infection is diagnosed by viral isolation or rapid antigen detection in secretions or from tissue, such as liver biopsy specimens and detection of elevated IgM antibodies in infant serum.

Toxoplasmosis

Toxoplasma gondii is a protozoan intracellular parasite passed to the fetus in utero after it is acquired by the mother in infected cat feces or from ingestion of inadequately cooked meat, especially lamb or pork, hence the importance of eliciting this exposure in the maternal prenatal history. Only 10% of patients with congenital toxoplasmosis have serious disease as newborns, usually with CNS and hepatic involvement; 40% of all affected infants have cholestasis and 60% have hepatosplenomegaly. Other clinical findings consist of purpura, microcephaly, chorioretinitis, intracranial calcification, meningoencephalitis, and psychomotor retardation. Liver biopsy may show areas of necrosis with a generalized hepatitis. Diagnosis may be made by demonstration of the parasite in liver tissue with specific fluorescent antibody staining. More commonly, it is made by Wright stain of CSF or inferred by elevated IgM titer in infant serum.[42]

Rubella

Congenital rubella hepatitis may be present in 20% of infected neonates,[42] and a history of a rubella-like illness in pregnancy should suggest the diagnosis. Clinically, the infected neonate may have hepatosplenomegaly (in up to 60%), thrombocytopenia, congenital cardiac disease, deafness, and low birth weight. Biopsy findings may include giant cells, focal areas of necrosis, and severe cholestasis with extramedullary hematopoiesis. Bile duct proliferation may be present as well, erroneously suggesting extrahepatic obstruction.[44] Diagnosis is usually established by elevated IgM antibody in the affected infant's serum. The virus can be isolated from nasopharyngeal, urine, spinal fluid, and liver cultures. Infants with hepatitis confined to the neonatal period usually recover from the liver involvement without the development of chronic liver disease. The incidence and importance of congenital rubella have fortunately decreased during the last two decades due to widespread maternal immunization against the disease.

Herpes Simplex Virus

Neonates may manifest symptoms of disseminated herpes infection including liver involvement. The average time of onset is 6 days of age. An eruption consisting of vesicular, purpuric, or necrotic lesions is present on the skin or oropharyngeal mucosa of the affected infant, and hepatosplenomegaly and jaundice are noted several days later. Infection may take a fulminant course with massive hepatic necrosis in which the liver may no longer be palpable, associated with gastrointestinal bleeding, coagulopathy, encephalitis, and seizures. Infection is usually acquired from an unrecognized maternal genital lesion, usually due to herpes simplex virus type 2 (HSV 2). Liver biopsy shows a giant cell hepatitis with acidophilic hepatocyte intranuclear viral inclusions. Treatment initiated promptly with intravenous acyclovir may be life-saving.

Syphilis

Although recently considered rare, congenital infection with the spirochete *Treponema pallidum* has had a resurgence with the general rise in other sexually transmitted diseases, including human immunodeficiency virus (HIV). There is a spectrum of clinical severity in neonatal infection, though severe infections characterized

by prematurity, apnea, hepatosplenomegaly, hydrops fetalis, rash, hemolytic anemia, and cutaneous hemorrhage, may carry a poor prognosis for the neonate if unrecognized and left untreated. A mortality rate of up to 40% has been reported.[45] Cholestasis may appear within the first 24 hours of life, or findings may develop over days to weeks. Liver biopsy shows centrilobular mononuclear inflammation and a characteristic dissecting fibrosis. Diagnosis is by serology or demonstration of organisms in skin or mucosal lesions. Treatment is with parenteral penicillin.

Hepatitis B Virus

Vertical transmission of hepatitis B from mother to infant occurs when the mother has acquired the infection in the third trimester or if the mother, especially if she is e-antigen positive, is a chronic carrier of the virus. Most of the infected infants are asymptomatic, with acute icteric hepatitis developing in less than 5% of perinatally infected infants.[46] Fulminant hepatic failure may rarely develop in the newborn.[47]

OTHER PERINATAL INFECTIONS OF THE LIVER

The enteroviruses, coxsackie B and echovirus, may produce acute hepatitis with cholestasis in the first few weeks of life. Infection with coxsackie B is usually more serious with mortality rates as high as 30% to 50% with hepatitis, myocarditis, and meningoencephalitis. Echovirus infection is usually mild, although there are reports, including nursery outbreaks, of fatal fulminant liver failure. Treatment of fulminant cases has generally been supportive with poor outcome, but successful liver transplantation in an affected 2-week-old infant without recurrence of infection in the graft was reported.[48]

Vertical transmission of hepatitis C virus has now been documented, although it appears to occur more uncommonly than hepatitis B virus, especially without concomitant HIV infection. Not enough data are yet available to determine how often this virus might cause hepatitis in the infected newborn. Perinatal HIV infection has been reported in at least one case in association with perinatal liver disease.[49] Perinatal varicella infection is another rare cause of neonatal cholestasis and hepatitis.

METABOLIC DISEASES

Alpha-1-Antitrypsin Deficiency

Alpha-1-antitrypsin deficiency is the most common inherited metabolic cause of neonatal cholestasis, present in about 10% of patients (Table 8-3) (for further discussion, see Ch. 10). The expression of alpha-1-antitrypsin, a protease inhibitor, is controlled by more than 30 different alleles with the protease inhibitor phenotype, or Pi type, of the patient's protein named alphabetically by its mobility on an electrophoresis gel. The most common allele, M, appears in normal concentrations in serum and has normal function. The slowest moving allele, Z, when present in a homozygous individual (i.e., Pi ZZ phenotype) is associated with serum protease inhibitor activity of only 10% to 15% of normal levels present in a Pi MM individual. Jaundice in homozygous ZZ-deficient infants typically has its onset in the first 8 weeks of life, but only approximately 10% of Pi ZZ individuals will demonstrate prolonged neonatal cholestasis. Up to 60% will have abnormal aminotransferases at 6 months of age; in 75% jaundice will resolve, in those who are affected, within 7 months. Progression to fulminant liver failure in the early perinatal period is encountered rarely.

Liver biopsy in alpha-1-antitrypsin may show features that overlap with biliary atresia or idiopathic neonatal hepatitis. In Pi ZZ patients, the biopsy usually shows periodic acid-Schiff (PAS) positive staining material in the cytoplasm of hepatocytes, which is resistant to digestion by the enzyme diastase, although this finding may rarely be absent early on. This highlights the need for prompt and accurate protease inhibitor (Pi) typing information prior to consideration of operative cholangiogram to exclude extrahepatic obstruction. Currently, the only curative therapy for the minority who develop acute or chronic liver failure is liver replacement.

Other Metabolic Disorders Presenting With Neonatal Cholestasis

A variety of other inherited metabolic diseases may present during the newborn or early perinatal period with cholestatic liver disease. Cystic fibrosis rarely presents during the newborn period with neonatal cholestasis. Glycogen storage disease type IV, a deficiency of the brancher enzyme in the synthesis of glycogen, may present in the older infant and results in growth failure and hypotonia, with hepatosplenomegaly and usually cirrhosis in early childhood. Liver transplantation is the only definitive therapy and has been successfully carried out in a number of cases. Hereditary fructose intolerance is a rare inborn error of carbohydrate metabolism that presents with hyperchloremia, hypokalemia, hypophosphatemia, lactic acidosis, hypoglycemia, and liver decompensation when the patient is exposed to fructose or to the fructose-containing disaccharide sucrose. Diagnosis is by determination of deficient enzyme activity in hepatic tissue. Treatment involves removing fructose and sucrose from the diet and results in dramatic improvement in the patient's clinical status and clinical liver disease.

Galactosemia, a rare disorder most commonly due to deficiency of the enzyme galactose-1-phosphate uridyl transferase, is characterized in the newborn by cholestatic liver disease, hepatomegaly, emesis, hypoglycemia, and growth failure. This disorder must be rapidly excluded by testing the urine for reducing sugars by the Clinitest, which will be positive even while the urine dipstick test (a glucose oxidase assay sensitive only specifically to glucose) is negative. Importantly, the patient must be taking feedings, either breast milk or formula, which contain lactose (a disaccharide made up of galactose and glucose). The diagnosis is confirmed by direct assay of the enzymatic activity in red blood cells, assuming the patient has not recently received a red cell transfusion that may give a false-positive result. Rapid diagnosis and treatment with a diet that excludes lactose are essential because of the rapid development of irreversible CNS or liver damage and acidosis. In addition, infants with this disorder who are untreated have a higher than average risk of developing gram-negative sepsis, which in itself may be fatal.[50] Tyrosinemia may also present with a neonatal hepatitis picture, sometimes fulminant. (This disorder is described in greater detail in Ch. 60.)

The most recently described inherited disorders associated with neonatal cholestatic liver disease are the inborn errors of bile acid synthesis. These disorders may have been responsible for some of the cases previously described as idiopathic neonatal hepatitis and for many of such cases that appeared to have a familial incidence with severe liver disease during the newborn period, with poor prognosis. The technique of fast-atom bombardment (FAB) mass spectrometry (MS), available at only a few specialized centers in the United States and Europe, can be done on microliter amounts of urine and can serve as a fast and relatively cheap screening method. In affected infants, this assay reveals the presence of large amounts of bile acid precursors excreted in the urine. Samples suspicious for a bile acid disorder then need to be confirmed by more sophisticated and labor intensive methods. Oral bile acid therapy has been successful in a small number of patients.

DIAGNOSTIC GOALS AND CLINICAL AND LABORATORY EVALUATION

In light of the comments above, there are three goals of the diagnostic evaluation of the newborn or young infant with cholestasis. First, rapidly exclude life-threatening disorders such as bacterial sepsis or disorders such as galactosemia, which may predispose to gram-negative sepsis or cause ongoing damage to the liver or CNS the longer it is left untreated. Second, exclude those patients with a disorder amenable to surgical therapy such as choledochal cyst, bile duct stricture or perforation, or biliary atresia. Finally, avoid surgical exploration, if possible, in those infants for whom the cause of cholestasis is intrahepatic in nature (bile duct paucity disorders such as Alagille syndrome). The overall approach to the infant with neonatal cholestasis is outlined in Table 8-4.

CLINICAL FEATURES

The information from the clinical history will rarely provide the definitive clues to the cause of the neonatal cholestasis. Some important exceptions include a history of unexplained febrile illness in the mother during pregnancy that may suggest a congenital infection of the infant. There may be a history of specific exposure to raw meat or soiled cat litter, which can harbor the protozoan *Toxoplasma gondii*. Maternal and infant titers for the so-called TORCH infections including toxoplasmosis, herpes simplex, rubella, cytomegalovirus, and syphilis should be obtained, even in uncomplicated pregnancies. Syphilis is the key congenital infection to exclude, since this disorder can be treated with penicillin. A history of intravenous drug abuse in either parent should be sought. Testing for hepatitis B virus should be done on mother's blood and, if positive for hepatitis B surface antigen, on the infant's serum as well. Since vertical transmission of hepatitis C virus has been documented, this is a potential cause of newborn liver disease. Antibody testing of the infant for hepatitis C may be unrevealing in the newborn period, so that testing for hepatitis C should be done on the mother's serum, or testing for hepatitis C RNA in serum by polymerase chain reaction (PCR) may be done on infant or maternal serum. Testing for infection with human immunodeficiency virus (HIV) should be considered in otherwise undiagnosed cases as well. Neonatal lupus causing intrahepatic cholestasis has been reported[51,52] so a history of lupus in the mother may be relevant as well.

It may be helpful to elicit any history of cholestasis in the newborn or later childhood period of the infant's siblings or offspring of the parents' close relatives. Such a positive family history may indicate an inherited metabolic disorder. These disorders include cystic fibrosis, the cerebrohepatorenal syndrome of Zellweger, hereditary fructose intolerance, galactosemia, tyrosinemia, or alpha-1-antitrypsin deficiency, all autosomal recessive disorders, and several of which are discussed in more detail elsewhere in this textbook. Alagille syndrome (arteriohepatic dysplasia) (for further discussion, see Ch. 4) is probably inherited as an autosomal dominant disorder. This disorder may account for recurrent cases of neonatal cholestasis among several siblings or close relatives in some instances. Tyrosinemia (due to abnormal tyrosine degradation) and Zellweger syndrome (due to absence of the subcellular organelle, the peroxisome) may be

TABLE 8-4. Diagnostic Evaluation of the Infant With Cholestasis

History and physical examination

General screening of clinical status and liver function
  Complete blood count, peripheral blood smear, reticulocyte count; maternal and infant blood types and Coombs' test on infant's blood, where indicated
  Liver enzymes—aspartate (AST) and alanine (ALT) aminotransferases, alkaline phosphatase, and gamma-glutamyltransferase (GGT)
  Liver synthetic function—total protein, albumin; prothrombin (PT) and partial thromboplastin (PTT) times
  Serum bile acids
  Stool pigment

Blood
  Serology: cytomegalovirus, herpes, rubella
  Toxoplasmosis, syphilis, HIV
  Hepatitis B and C markers (mother and infant)
  Alpha-1-antitrypsin level with protease inhibitor (Pi) typing
  Thyroxine and thyroid stimulating hormone
  Plasma amino acids
  Blood culture
  Serum iron, total iron-binding capacity and ferritin
  Serum for maternal and infant serology for lupus erythematosus

Urine
  Urine culture
  Urinalysis
  Urine-reducing substance (Clinitest)
  Urine for organic acids
  Urine for FAB-MS screen for bile acid intermediates

Cerebrospinal fluid (CSF)
  CSF culture
  CSF Gram stain
  CSF cell count

Sweat chloride concentration

Intestinal fluids
  Stool for viral isolation, if indicated
  24-hour duodenal intubation fluid sample

Radiologic evaluation
  Ultrasound, with Doppler vascular flow assessment
  Hepatobiliary scintigraphy (DISIDA scan)
  Operative cholangiogram—if operated on to rule out extrahepatic obstruction

Liver biopsy
  Percutaneous or operative wedge sample

screened for by analysis of plasma and urine for amino acids and urine for organic acids. (Both disorders are discussed in greater detail in Ch. 60.) Hereditary fructose intolerance and galactosemia may be screened for by testing the urine for reducing substances by Clinitest, assuming the patient is ingesting the potential offending sugar in the diet at the time of the urine screening.

The infant's history may include a history of persistent vomiting or misdiagnosed severe "reflux" and could suggest a metabolic disorder such as galactosemia or hereditary fructose intolerance. A history of total parenteral nutrition (TPN) use for at least 2 weeks or exposure to certain drugs, such as trimethoprim-sulfamethoxazole or anticonvulsants, and a variety of other drugs may suggest a toxic cholestatic jaundice.

On physical examination, microcephaly, chorioretinitis, and petechiae should suggest a congenital infection. The presence of a pulmonary outflow murmur and typical facies should raise the possibility of arteriohepatic dysplasia. Totally depigmented (acholic) stools may suggest extrahepatic obstruction. However, the infant's stools may be pigmented, and hepatomegaly may rarely be absent, even in the presence of total extrahepatic obstruction.

Therefore, the history and physical examination will only rarely differentiate intrahepatic causes from extrahepatic causes that require operative intervention. Only with the combination of findings on history and physical examination, together with extensive laboratory and radiographic testing, can we reliably distinguish between intra- and extrahepatic causes of the cholestasis. An attempt has been made to differentiate intrahepatic and extrahepatic causes of cholestasis based on four major clinical findings: stool color 10 days after admission, birth weight, age in days at onset of acholic stools, and several clinical features of liver involvement[1]; however, these features are unable to distinguish intrahepatic from extrahepatic causes with certainty.

LABORATORY TESTS

As noted in Table 8-4, initial laboratory tests are designed to assess the overall degree of inflammation and cholestasis by obtaining serum for aminotransferases (ALT and AST) and serum fractionated bilirubin and gamma-glutamyltransferase (GGT). Overall liver synthetic function is measured by serum albumin concentration and prothrombin and partial thromboplastin times and especially to alert the clinician to an imminent risk of bleeding.

More specialized tests are required to rule out the metabolic and infectious causes as detailed in Table 8-4. The maximal value of obtaining plasma amino acid levels is in the early detection of tyrosinemia. However, significant liver disease of any cause will yield elevations of methionine, tyrosine, and phenylalanine, confounding the diagnosis without more specific testing of certain urinary metabolites by mass spectrometry. As mentioned above, Clinitests of the urine in patients with galactosemia or hereditary fructose intolerance will only be instructive if the patient is actually ingesting the offending sugars at the time of assay of the urine. False-positive sweat tests have been noted in a variety of conditions, including failure to thrive, cortisol deficiency states, and hypopituitarism, the latter two of which can, in their own

right, cause neonatal cholestasis. Some advocate the 24-hour aspiration of duodenal contents by direct nasoduodenal tube to assess adequacy of bile flow. Normal feedings continue to stimulate bile flow. Some have suggested that if no pigment is discernible or no bilirubin is assayable in the specimen, extrahepatic obstruction is suggested with 90% certainty.[53] In summary, no single biochemical test can exclude extrahepatic obstruction with certainty despite the proposal and subsequent abandonment of several candidates such as lipoprotein X, bile acids, and GGT.

RADIOLOGIC EVALUATION

Liver Ultrasound

On presentation of the infant with neonatal cholestasis, one of the first and most valuable studies that should be ordered is a hepatobiliary ultrasound examination. This study may detect a choledochal cyst, biliary stones or sludge and ascites, which if present early in the infant's course may suggest a perforation of the bile duct and tumors. Although not specific, absence of the gallbladder at least suggests biliary atresia, but its presence does not rule out atresia. Bile duct dilation suggests a cause of extrahepatic obstruction other than biliary atresia, as this disorder is never associated with that finding. Intrahepatic ductal involvement in biliary atresia, also part of the disorder, probably prevents dilation of the ducts despite complete obstruction distally.

Radionuclide Studies

Hepatobiliary scintigraphy, using technetium[99]-labeled derivatives of iminodiacetic acid (IDA), such as disofenin (DISIDA), allows assessment of hepatic blood flow and, most importantly, hepatocyte uptake and biliary excretion. The healthy hepatocyte rapidly takes up the radionuclide, and excretion of the isotope into bile is detected in the small intestine within 1 hour. Poor uptake with normal or delayed excretion into the bowel is seen in hepatitis and other intrahepatic disorders. In infants with biliary atresia, uptake is usually normal, particularly early in the course before significant injury to the liver results from ongoing biliary obstruction. However, there is no evidence of excretion into the gut lumen, despite normal uptake even on delayed images of up to 24 hours. Absence of excretion does not prove the presence of biliary atresia or even of extrahepatic obstruction. This is because intrahepatic causes of severe cholestasis can also cause failure of excretion. Excretion of the tracer into bowel rules out biliary atresia (except in the rare case of delayed development of atresia as noted above) and obviates the need for urgent operative cholangiogram and exploration.

LIVER BIOPSY, OPERATIVE EXPLORATION, AND CHOLANGIOGRAM

We perform percutaneous liver biopsy for almost every patient with neonatal cholestasis, unless extrahepatic obstruction appears certain, as in the case of the visualization of a choledochal cyst on ultrasound. In case of failure to detect excretion on DISIDA scan with a negative laboratory workup and evidence of bile ductular proliferation and often periportal expansion by fibrosis and inflammatory infiltrate, the infant is surgically explored, a wedge liver biopsy is performed and an intraoperative cholangiogram is attempted. In infants older than 1 month of age, liver biopsy provides differentiation of extrahepatic from intrahepatic causes in more than 90% of cases, if more than 5 portal tracts are present.[54]

CONJUGATED HYPERBILIRUBINEMIA IN THE OLDER CHILD

Jaundice with elevated direct bilirubin is uncommon in the older child (Table 8-5). Causes include viral hepatitis due to hepatitis viruses A, B, and C and the hepatitis D virus, which may co-infect or superinfect patients with hepatitis B infection. Most cases of acute viral hepatitis are anicteric. Occasionally, Epstein-Barr virus (EBV) and other viruses causing systemic disease, such as cytomegalovirus (CMV) and varicella, can cause clinical hepatitis. Other causes include autoimmune hepatitis, most common in adolescent girls, and toxic hepatitis due to idiosyncratic reactions to a variety of drugs or the intentional ingestion of hepatotoxic drugs such as acetaminophen in suicide attempts among teenagers and young adults. Metabolic and inherited disorders causing chronic liver disease in older children include alpha-1-antitrypsin deficiency, which more often presents with complications of portal hypertension, such as acute variceal bleeding, rather than jaundice. Cystic fibrosis—associated liver disease may progress to a chronic stage with clinical jaundice in the older child. However, jaundice is rarely, if ever, the presenting sign, unless the patient develops obstructive jaundice from a gallstone or acute cholecystitis, both of which are more common in these patients because of abnormal viscous bile.

Finally, any child above the age of 3 or 4 years who presents with acute or chronic liver disease should be investigated for the possibility of Wilson's disease. This is a potentially treatable disorder with copper chelation therapy. If undiagnosed, this disorder may progress to irreversible chronic liver disease or present with fulminant liver failure no longer amenable to drug therapy and necessitating emergent liver transplantation.

Other disorders of the bile ducts such as sclerosing

TABLE 8-5. Causes of Conjugated Hyperbilirubinemia in the Older Child and Adolescent

Viral hepatitis
    Acute hepatitis A
    Acute or chronic hepatitis B, C, D
    Cytomegalovirus
    Epstein-Barr virus
    Varicella
    Other systemic viral infections
Autoimmune hepatitis
    Type 1 (anti-smooth muscle antibody and/or antinuclear antibody positive)
    Type 2 (anti-liver-kidney microsomal antibody positive)
Biliary tract disorders
    Cholelithiasis
    Cholecystitis
    Sclerosing cholangitis
    Choledochal cyst
    Intrahepatic bile duct dilation in association with congenital hepatic fibrosis
    Bacterial cholangitis
Metabolic/inherited disorders
    Alpha-1-antitrypsin deficiency
    Cystic fibrosis
    Wilson's disease
Toxic hepatitis
    Drugs (e.g., acetaminophen, sulfa drugs, anticonvulsants)
    Toxins
    Chemotherapeutic agents
    Radiation
Vascular disorders
    Budd-Chiari syndrome
    Veno-occlusive disease

cholangitis (with or without associated inflammatory bowel disease) and bile duct malformations such as choledochal cyst or the dilated intrahepatic ducts often associated with congenital hepatic fibrosis and polycystic kidney disease may present with jaundice. These disorders may predispose to bacterial cholangitis due to stasis of bile and poor drainage of the biliary tree. Finally, rare patients with acute hepatic venous outflow obstruction, so-called Budd-Chiari syndrome, or acute or chronic veno-occlusive disease in patients treated with chemotherapy or radiation to the right upper quadrant may present with acute or chronic icteric hepatitis.[55]

REFERRAL PATTERN

Children with unexplained hyperbilirubinemia for greater than 1 week should be referred to a pediatric gastroenterologist. Additionally, any child with jaundice and liver disease coupled with synthetic dysfunction should undergo immediate referral for possible liver failure.

REFERENCES

1. Alagille D. Cholestasis in the first three months of life. Prog Liver Dis 1979;6:471–485

2. Burton EM, Babcock DS, Heubi JE, Gelfand MJ. Neonatal jaundice: clinical and ultrasonographic findings. South Med J 1990;83:294–302

3. Motala C, Ireland JD, Hill ID, Bowie MD. Cholestatic disorders of infancy—etiology and outcome. J Trop Pediatr 1990; 36:218–222

4. Mieli-Vergani G, Howard ER, Mowat AP. Liver disease in infancy: a 20 year perspective. Gut 1991(suppl):S123–128

5. Setchell KDR. Disorders of bile acid synthesis. In: Walker WA, Durie PR, Hamilton JR et al, eds. Pediatric Gastrointestinal Disease: Pathophysiology, Diagnosis, Management. Philadelphia: BC Decker, 1991;992–1013

6. Setchell KDR, Suchy FJ, Welsh MB et al. *Delta*-4,3-oxosteroid 5 *beta*-reductase deficiency described in identical twins with neonatal hepatitis—a new inborn error in bile acid synthesis. J Clin Invest 1988;82:2135–2146

7. Moyer MS, Balistreri WF. Prolonged neonatal obstructive jaundice. In: Walker WA, Durie PR, Hamilton JR et al, eds. Pediatric Gastrointestinal Disease: Pathophysiology, Diagnosis, Management. Philadelphia: BC Decker, 1991; 835–848

8. Mowat AP. Liver Disorders in Childhood, 2nd Ed. New York: Butterworths, 1987;24–71

9. Kasai M. Treatment of biliary atresia with special reference to hepatic portoenterostomy and its modifications. Prog Pediatr Surg 1974;6:5–15

10. Altman RP. The portoenterostomy procedure for biliary atresia: a five year experience. Ann Surg 1987;188:351–362

11. Lilly JR, Altman RP. Hepatic portoenterostomy (the Kasai operation) for biliary atresia. Surgery 1975;78:76–86

12. Silveira TR, Salzano FM, Howard ER, Mowat AP. Congenital structural abnormalities in biliary atresia: evidence for etiopathogenic heterogeneity and therapeutic implications. Acta Paediatr Scand 1991;80:1192–1199

13. Davenport M, Savage M, Mowat AP, Howard ER. Biliary atresia splenic malformation syndrome: an etiologic and prognostic subgroup. Surgery 1993;113:662–668

14. Carmi R, Magee CA, Neill CA, Karrer FM. Extrahepatic biliary atresia and associated anomalies: etiologic heterogeneity suggested by distinctive patterns of associations. Am J Med Genetics 1993;45:683–693

15. McDonald PJ, Stehman FB, Stewart DR. Infantile obstructive cholangiography. Am J Dis Child 1979;133:518–522

16. DeLorimier AA. Surgical management of neonatal jaundice. N Engl J Med 1974;268:1284–1286

17. Morecki R, Glaser JH, Cho S et al. Biliary atresia and reovirus 3 infection. N Engl J Med 1982;307:481–484

18. Morecki R, Glaser JH, Johnson AB, Kress Y. Detection of

19. reovirus type 3 in the porta hepatis of an infant with extrahepatic biliary atresia: ultrastructural and immunocytochemical study. Hepatology 1984;4:1137–1142

19. Riepenhoff-Tarty M, Schaekel K, Clark HF et al. Group A rotaviruses produce extrahepatic biliary obstruction in orally inoculated newborn mice. Pediatr Res 1993;33:394–399

20. Lee CY. Cytomegalovirus as an important cause of neonatal hepatitis in Taiwan. Acta Paediatr Sin 1979;20:271–272

21. Chang M-H, Huang H-H, Huang E-S et al. Polymerase chain reaction to detect human cytomegalovirus in livers of infants with neonatal hepatitis. Gastroenterology 1992;103: 1022–1025

22. Brown WR, Sokol RJ, Levin MJ et al. Lack of correlation with reovirus 3 and extrahepatic biliary atresia or neonatal hepatitis. J Pediatr 1988;113:670–676

23. Maller ES, Piccoli DA. Diagnostic evaluation and care of the child with biliary atresia. In: Hoffman MA, ed. Current Controversies in Biliary Atresia. Austin, TX: RG Landes, 1992;45–61

24. Dick MC, Mowat AP. Hepatitis syndrome in infancy—an epidemiologic survey with 10-year follow-up. Arch Dis Child 1985;60:512–520

25. Howell C, Templeton J, Weiner S et al. Antenatal diagnosis and early surgery for choledochal cyst. J Pediatr Surg 1983; 18:387–393

26. Yamaguchi M. Congenital choledochal cyst. Analysis of 1,433 patients in the Japanese literature. Am J Surg 1980; 140:653–657

27. Enzenauer RW, Montrey JS, Baria PJ, Woods J. Total parenteral cholestasis: a cause of mechanical biliary obstruction. Pediatrics 1985;76:905–908

28. Cooper A, Ross AJ III, O'Neill JA et al. Resolution of intractable cholestasis associated with total parenteral nutrition following biliary irrigation. J Pediatr Surg 1985;20: 772–774

29. Lawson EE, Boggs JD. Long-term follow-up of neonatal hepatitis: safety and value of surgical exploration. Pediatrics 1974; 52:650–655

30. Chang MH, Hsu HC, Lee CY et al. Neonatal hepatitis: a follow-up study. J Pediatr Gastroenterol Nutr 1987;6: 203–207

31. Deutsch J, Smith AL, Danks DM, Campbell PE. Long-term prognosis for babies with neonatal liver disease. Arch Dis Child 1985;60:447–451

32. Danks DM, Campbell PE, Smith AL, Rogers J. Prognosis of babies with neonatal hepatitis. Arch Dis Child 1977;52: 368–372

33. Odievre M, Hadchouel M, Landrieus P et al. Long-term prognosis for infants with intrahepatic cholestasis and patent extrahepatic biliary tract. Arch Dis Child 1981;56:373–376

34. Alagille D, Estrada A, Hadchouel M et al. Syndromic paucity of interlobular ducts (Alagille syndrome or arteriohepatic dysplasia): review of 80 cases. J Pediatr 1987;110:195–200

35. Sokol RJ, Heubi JE, Balistreri WF. Intrahepatic "cholestatic facies": is it specific for Alagille syndrome? J Pediatr 1983; 103:205–208

36. Markowitz J, Daum F, Kahn EI et al. Arteriohepatic dyspla-

sia, I. Pitfalls in diagnosis and management. Hepatology 1983;3:74–76

37. Clayton RJ, Iber FL, Reubner BH, McKusick VA. Byler's disease: fatal familial intrahepatic cholestasis in an Amish kindred. J Pediatr 1965;67:1026–1028

38. Maggiore G, Bernard O, Riely CA et al. Normal gamma glutamyltransferase activity identifies a group of infants with idiopathic cholestasis with poor prognosis. J Pediatr 1987; 111:251–252

39. Setchell KDR, Piccoli DA, O'Connell NC et al. Progressive intrahepatic cholestasis with normal γ glutamyltransferase is highly associated with the 3-hydroxysteroid dehydrogenase/isomerase deficiency, an inborn error in bile acid synthesis—a new category of metabolic disease. Hepatology 1993; 18(4,2):178A

40. Kelley RI. Reviews: the cerebrohepatorenal syndrome of Zellweger. Am J Hum Genet 1983;16L:503–517

41. Reynolds DW, Stagno S, Hosty TS et al. Maternal cytomegalovirus excretion and perinatal infection. N Engl J Med 1973; 289:1–5

42. Felber S, Sinatra F. Systemic disorders associated with neonatal cholestasis. Semin Liver Dis 1987;7:108–118

43. McCracken GH, Shinefeld HR, Cobb R et al. Congenital cytomegalic inclusion disease: a longitudinal study of 20 patients. Am J Dis Child 1969;117:522–539

44. Esterly JR, Slusser RJ, Ruebner BH. Hepatic lesions in the congenital rubella syndrome. J Pediatr 1967;71:676–685

45. Petorius PJ, Roode H. Obstructive jaundice in early infancy. Afr Med J 1974;48:811–815

46. Tong MJ, Thursby MW, Lin J-H et al. Studies on the maternal-infant transmission of hepatitis B virus and HBV infection within families. Prog Med Virol 1981;27:137–147

47. Sinatra F, Shah P, Weissman JY, et al. Perinatal transmitted acute icteric hepatitis B in infants born to hepatitis B surface antigen-positive and anti-hepatics B e-positive carrier mothers. Pediatrics 1982;70:557–559

48. Chuang EC, Maller ES, Hoffman MA et al. Successful treatment of fulminant echovirus 11 infection in a neonate by orthotopic liver transplantation. J Pediatr Gastroenterol Nutr 1993;17:211–214

49. Witzleben CL, Marshall GS, Wenner W et al. HIV as a cause of giant cell hepatitis. Hum Pathol 1988;19:603–605

50. Levy HL, Sepe SJ, Shih VE et al. Sepsis due to *Escherichia coli* in neonates with galactosemia. N Engl J Med 1977;297: 823–825

51. Rosh JR, Silverman ED, Groisman G et al. Intrahepatic cholestasis in neonatal lupus erythematosus. J Pediatr Gastroenterol Nutr 1993;17:310–312

52. Laxer RM, Roberts EA, Gross KR et al. Liver disease in neonatal lupus erythematosus. J Pediatr 1990;116:238–242

53. Greene HL, Helinek GL, Moran R, O'Neill J. A diagnostic approach to prolonged obstructive jaundice by 24-hour collection of duodenal fluid. J Pediatr 1979;95:412–414

54. Brough AJ, Bernstein J. Conjugated hyperbilirubinemia in early infancy: a re-assessment of liver biopsy. Hum Pathol 1974;5:507–516

55. Mews C, Sinatra F. Chronic liver disease in children. Pediatr Rev 1993;14:436–444

9

LIVER FAILURE

JYOTI P. RAMAKRISHNA
WILLIAM R. TREEM

Acute liver failure, also known as fulminant hepatic failure (FHF), constitutes a medical emergency. The major part of this chapter is devoted to dealing with its causes, pathophysiology, diagnosis, and management. Chronic liver disease can lead to cirrhosis and to subsequent liver failure or end-stage liver disease. This is usually a more gradual process and is dealt with toward the end of the chapter. There is considerable overlap in the management strategies for both acute and chronic hepatic failure.

FHF has been defined as the acute onset of coagulopathy and encephalopathy within 8 weeks of the onset of symptoms of liver disease in a patient with no evidence of pre-existing liver disease. Liver failure is considered subfulminant when the interval between the onset of symptoms and encephalopathy is greater than 8 weeks.[1,2] These traditional definitions are useful, as most studies still refer to them.

The primary aims of this chapter are to help the pediatrician recognize the clinical manifestations of liver failure, to arrive at the diagnosis in a timely fashion, to institute appropriate management, to be able to recognize good and bad prognostic factors, and to know when to refer a child to a tertiary care center. It is important to realize that time is of the essence when dealing with a patient with acute hepatic failure, as the patient's condition can deteriorate rapidly, leading to death within a few days of initial presentation. With the best available management in the setting of an intensive care unit (ICU), the mortality of FHF is 60% to 70%. The availability of liver transplantation has brought this figure

down to 20 to 40%.[3] These figures highlight the seriousness of this condition and emphasize the need to provide optimal care.

CAUSES OF ACUTE HEPATIC FAILURE

The causes of FHF, and their frequencies compiled from several studies,[1-6] are listed in Table 9-1. Most of these are based on combined adult and pediatric data.

Hepatitis A

About 0.1% to 0.2% of acute cases of hepatitis A progress to hepatic failure. The prognosis for hepatic failure associated with hepatitis A is better than the prognosis for other causes, with survival approaching 60%.

Hepatitis B

Hepatitis B remains the single largest identifiable cause of FHF, which occurs in 0.5% to 1% of acute cases. Mutations in the hepatitis B surface antigen (HBsAg) region of the virus can lead to HBsAg-negative hepatitis, but this accounts for only a very small percentage of the cryptogenic cases of FHF. Infection with viruses that have precore region mutations that lead to hepatitis B 'e' antigen (HBeAg)-negative disease has a more aggressive

TABLE 9-1. Causes of Acute Hepatic Failure

Source	Percent
Viral	
Hepatitis A	2–8
Hepatitis B	15–40
Hepatitis C	0–3
Hepatitis D	
Hepatitis E	
Other viruses (rare)	
Toxic	
Acetaminophen	18–56
Other drugs/toxins	5–18
Metabolic	5–14
Other	
Cryptogenic	20–40

(Data from references 1–6.)

course and leads to FHF more frequently. HBeAg is thought to be responsible for immunologic tolerance; therefore, in HBeAg-negative cases there is an increase in the host immune response, leading to a greater degree of hepatocyte damage.

Hepatitis C

Hepatitis C is a rare cause of FHF in most series. Earlier, questions had been raised about the diagnostic tests being used, but recent studies using polymerase chain reaction (PCR) on blood and liver tissue have corroborated the fact that this virus is rarely found in cases of FHF. Hepatitis C may be seen more frequently in association with acute liver failure in certain geographic areas, such as Japan and Taiwan. It has been suggested that co-infection or superinfection with hepatitis B in a chronic carrier of hepatitis C is associated with FHF.

Hepatitis D

Hepatitis D, or delta hepatitis, is only infectious if acquired in conjunction with hepatitis B. Co-infection (acquisition at the same time as or soon after), or superinfection (later acquisition in a chronic case), with hepatitis B increases the risk of developing FHF to about 50%. In parts of the world where hepatitis D virus is endemic, it is responsible for a larger percentage of cases of FHF, but in North America it is seen mostly in intravenous drug abusers, and rarely if at all in children.

Hepatitis E

Hepatitis E virus is endemic in some areas of Asia and Africa and has been seen as sporadic cases in the United States and Europe.[5] It rarely causes FHF, except in pregnant women.

Other Causes

Rare viral causes of acute hepatic failure include Epstein-Barr virus, herpes simplex virus (HSV), cytomegalovirus (CMV), and adenovirus. Most of the cases reported have occurred as part of a disseminated infection in immunocompromised hosts; however, there are occasional reports of FHF due to these viruses occurring in immunocompetent patients.

Among the nonviral causes of FHF, acetaminophen toxicity constitutes the major identifiable category.[1–3] It accounts for 10% to 20% of cases of FHF in the United States and closer to 50% in the United Kingdom. It is the commonest cause of FHF in the United Kingdom.

Other drugs that can cause acute liver failure include halothane, isoniazid, carbamazepine, phenytoin, valproate, sulfonamides, and tetracycline. Toxicity from *Amanita* mushrooms can occur, and as few as three medium-size mushrooms could be lethal.

Metabolic causes such as Wilson's disease at initial presentation, galactosemia, hereditary fructose intolerance, tyrosinemia, neonatal hemochromatosis, disorders of fatty acid oxidation, Reye's syndrome, and acute fatty liver of pregnancy, are rare but should be borne in mind.

Miscellaneous causes include hepatic vein thrombosis (Budd-Chiari syndrome), ischemic liver disease and shock, autoimmune hepatitis, hyperthermia, massive malignant infiltration, and primary graft rejection after liver transplant.

Cryptogenic liver failure has been thought to be viral in origin and is also called non-A, non-B, non-C hepatitis. Flavivirus and togavirus-like particles have been seen in some cases; however, in most cases, no viral agent can be identified. Also no potential environmental toxin has been implicated.[1,5] There is a fairly high incidence of aplastic anemia (28%) in these cases, which also suggests a viral etiology.[4]

PATHOPHYSIOLOGY

Biopsies taken at autopsy or at liver transplantation demonstrate massive hepatocyte necrosis. Diffuse hepatic microvesicular steatosis is rarely seen in children and is associated with Reye's syndrome or with some toxic or metabolic insults; also, some metabolic defects can lead to macrovesicular fat deposition. Typical viral inclusions may be seen in CMV and HSV infections. Although helpful in making a diagnosis, biopsy findings do not affect the management, and cannot be used to predict the outcome, limiting the value of liver biopsy.

The loss of functional hepatocytes leads to a series of metabolic derangements. The functions that are affected include gluconeogenesis; bilirubin elimination; ureagenesis; lactate uptake; protein synthesis; synthesis of clotting factors I, II, V, VII, IX, and X; and detoxification of various metabolites. The clinical manifestations of these impairments are jaundice, hypoglycemia, metabolic acidosis, coagulopathy, and encephalopathy.

Coagulopathy

The coagulopathy of hepatic failure has multiple etiologies.[2-4] First, there is decreased hepatic synthesis of fibrinogen and factors II, V, VII, IX, and X. Since the cause is poor synthetic function, the coagulopathy usually cannot be corrected with vitamin K. The prothrombin time and levels of factors V and VII are sensitive indicators that can be used to monitor the course and prognosis of liver failure. Since these tests are based on clotting factors that have a short half-life in the circulation, they represent current hepatic function. The use of plasma supplements within the previous 48 to 72 hours makes these tests difficult to interpret.

Patients with acute liver failure have thrombocytopenia, due to both peripheral consumption of platelets and bone marrow suppression. Gastrointestinal (GI) hemorrhage is frequently seen when the platelet count drops to less than 50,000/mm.[3]

Disseminated intravascular coagulation (DIC) is also a late complication of liver failure, although a marked derangement of the prothrombin time and partial thromboplastin time (PT/PTT) with elevated D-dimers is more likely to be due to sepsis. This further exacerbates the coagulopathy.

Infections

Impaired immune function combined with the performance of multiple invasive procedures places these patients at high risk of infections, and up to 80% develop bacterial infections.[1-4] *Staphylococcus* species, *Streptococcus* species, and gram-negative bacteria are the most common causes. These originate in the skin and in the respiratory and GI tracts. Infections may be partly due to poor clearance of portal venous blood by Kupffer cells in the failing liver. Other contributory factors are complement deficiencies, abnormal opsonization, and impaired neutrophil adherence. Intravenous catheters, urinary catheters, and endotracheal tubes increase the risk of infection, as do H_2-blockers by decreasing the acid in the stomach, which normally acts as a barrier to bacterial and fungal infections in the upper GI tract. About 40% of deaths in acute liver failure are due to sepsis, and ongoing infections can preclude liver transplant.[3] Fungal infections are seen in as many as one-third of patients, mostly secondary to the use of broad-spectrum antibiotics. *Candida albicans* and *Aspergillus* infections are the most commonly isolated organisms. Fever and leukocytosis are frequently absent, and frequent cultures are the only means of diagnosing these infections.

Encephalopathy

Encephalopathy is a hallmark of acute liver failure and is progressive unless the liver failure is reversed. Early agitation, erratic behavior, and hyperkinesia rapidly give way to somnolence and coma within a period of hours to days. Hepatic encephalopathy is thought to be secondary to the accumulation of inhibitory neurotransmitters, such as gamma-aminobutyric acid (GABA), and other neurotoxic metabolites.[2,7] Although the ammonia levels often correspond with the degree of encephalopathy, the accumulation of ammonia is not the sole cause; however it probably plays a contributory role in the development of mental status changes. Indirect evidence has shown elevated levels of benzodiazepine receptor ligands in the brain and cerebrospinal fluid of animal models. In animal and human studies, elevated brain concentrations of benzodiazepines have been reported, and the benzodiazepine receptor antagonist flumazenil has been shown to ameliorate hepatic encephalopathy.[7-9] Since all the implicated metabolites are produced in the intestinal tract by gut flora, the treatment of hepatic encephalopathy involves restricting protein in the diet, antibiotics to clear the gut of bacteria, and the administration of lactulose to alter gut pH and induce diarrhea. The altered pH level creates an unfavorable environment for the gut flora, hence diminishing their production of nitrogenous metabolites. The staging of hepatic encephalopathy is given in Table 9-2. Cerebral edema is a frequent occurrence in cases of fulminant hepatic failure and is the commonest cause of death in most series.[1-5] Eighty percent of patients in stage IV coma have cerebral edema. This is probably due to increased permeability of the blood-brain barrier due a direct toxic effect of circulating metabolites; inhibition of the Na-K ATPase has also been demonstrated. Both events lead to movement of fluid into the intracellular compartment. There is usually an iatrogenic component of fluid overload because of the need for volume support and blood products. Edema can also be secondary to hypoglycemia or ischemia from hypotension and poor perfusion. Intracranial pressure monitoring is recommended once a patient is in stage III

TABLE 9-2. Stages of Hepatic Encephalopathy

Stage	Description
I	Slow mentation, confusion, inability to concentrate, changes in mood, personal and sleep habits
II	Drowsiness, inappropriate behavior, disorientation; gross motor incoordination
III	Stuporous but arousable; unable to obey commands; marked confusion, slurred speech; hyperreflexia
IV	Deep coma, not arousable; may respond to deep pain by decerebrate or decorticate posturing

(Data from Treem[2] and Kirsh et al.[3])

coma; every effort must be made to prevent or treat cerebral edema.

Multiorgan Failure

Renal failure is a common occurrence in FHF. It is more common in acetaminophen ingestion due to direct nephrotoxicity. In acute hepatic failure, renal involvement is due to either the hepatorenal syndrome, acute tubular necrosis, or intravascular volume depletion.[1-4] Hepatorenal syndrome is an unexplained functional renal impairment. It is the commonest cause of renal failure in FHF. The diagnosis and management of renal failure require central venous pressure monitoring. Moreover, the development of renal failure in FHF carries a poor prognosis. Cardiovascular changes include vasodilation and hypotension, which may be refractory to fluid administration and inotropic agents. This is hypothesized to be due to circulating endotoxin or mediators such as serotonin, renin, aldosterone, and prostaglandins.[10] Pulmonary edema is also seen in FHF, probably secondary to increased vascular permeability. Although there is insufficient time for varices and splenomegaly to develop, portal hypertension is often present. Metabolic acidosis is due to anaerobic metabolism in the tissues as a result of poor perfusion. Lactic acid accumulates in the circulation and is inadequately cleared by the liver.

CLINICAL PRESENTATION

Although jaundice is a common presenting complaint, it is important to remember that clinical jaundice may not be evident in the initial stages of acute hepatic failure. Patients may present with bleeding due to coagulopathy manifesting as easy brusing, excessive bleeding from injuries, or epistaxis. Other nonspecific presenting symptoms include personality changes, mood swings, and bizarre or violent behavior. The GI tract is the commonest site of bleeding, which is usually related to a low platelet count (less than 50,000/mm^3). The acute onset of a prolonged PT (more then 16 to 18 seconds) should suggest FHF.

PHYSICAL EXAMINATION

A thorough physical examination and a high index of suspicion are the key factors in making an early diagnosis of acute hepatic failure. In a child who is old enough to talk, orientation to time, place, and person must be determined. Agitation, confusion, and slow mentation are early signs of encephalopathy. Parents may report recent poor school performance, deterioration of handwriting or other fine motor skills, and lack of concentration.

The vital signs may reveal a low-grade fever that may be due to viral hepatitis, but it may also be due to a secondary infection, a common complication. Peripheral vasodilation can cause hypotension due to poor hepatic elimination of vasoactive substances. Tachycardia with pallor and cold, clammy extremities may be due to significant bleeding and hypovolemia. Bradycardia and systemic hypertension are indicative of cerebral edema.

Scleral icterus may or may not be present. Easy bruising is seen with coagulopathy. Peripheral edema and ascites suggest a more longstanding process, as do clubbing and cutaneous spider angiomas. Fetor hepaticus is a musty odor due to circulating mercaptans that may not always be detectable in children with fulminant hepatic failure, although it is considered a diagnostic feature in adults.

Although a shrunken liver may be detected as a reduced area of hepatic dullness on percussion, this finding may be difficult to appreciate. In acute liver failure, splenomegaly is usually not a feature. Rectal examination can yield guaiac-positive or tarry stools in a patient who has not yet shown clinically evident bleeding.

Central nervous system examination may detect increased muscle tone, brisk reflexes, and sluggish pupillary responses in the presence of cerebral edema. Tremor and asterixis (hepatic flap) should be elicited. All patients presenting with bizarre or violent behavior of acute onset must be suspected to have hepatic encephalopathy as a possible cause.

DIAGNOSIS

The diagnosis of acute liver failure is based on findings of coagulopathy and of an encephalopathy in association with the recent onset of liver disease. Corroborative, confirmatory, and basic diagnostic laboratory tests are listed in Table 9-3. These are important not only in arriving at a diagnosis, but also as a guideline for initiating management.

INITIAL MANAGEMENT

The goal of initial management is to establish quickly the diagnosis and to stabilize and support the patient, with a view to ensuring the best possible outcome.[1-4,6,10] The findings from the history, physical examination, and initial laboratory tests are sufficient to establish the diagnosis, determine the level of concern, and guide the decisions regarding hospitalization and referral to a tertiary care center at the appropriate time. The bilirubin and liver enzymes tell us about the existence of liver disease and the degree of hepatocyte necrosis, but a prolonged PT suggests liver synthetic dysfunction and hepatic de-

TABLE 9-3. Laboratory Evaluation for Suspected Fulminant Hepatic Failure

Test	Description
Hematology	CBC with platelets and differential count,[a] PT/PTT,[a] factor V (with or without factor VII) level
Biochemistry	Serum bilirubin,[a] AST,[a] ALT,[a] alkaline phosphatase,[a] GGT, total protein and albumin,[a] ammonia[a]; blood glucose[a]; BUN, creatinine,[a] electrolytes[a]
Serology/ microbiology	Anti-HAV Ab(IgM) HepBsAg, anti-HBcAb(IgM) Anti-HCV Ab—second-generation assay RIBA CMV titers—IgG and IgM Blood and urine cultures, if febrile
Other	Acetaminophen level, toxicologic screen of blood and urine Serum copper and ceruloplasmin Blood type Urinalysis, urine electrolytes, serum, and urine osmolarity

Abbreviations: Anti-HAV Ab, antihepatitis A virus antibody titer; HepBsAg, hepatitis B surface antigen; Anti-HBcAb, antihepatitis B core antibody; Anti-HCV Ab (RIBA), antihepatitis C virus antibody by radioimmunoblot assay; CBC, complete blood count; CMV, cytomegalovirus; AST, aspartate aminotransferase; ALT, alanine aminotransferase; GGT, gamma-glutamyl transferase; BUN, blood-urea nitrogen; PT/PTT, prothrombin time/partial thromboplastin time.

[a] Laboratory tests that should be sent as "stat."

compensation. The ammonia level in children usually corresponds to the degree of encephalopathy, although an occasional patient may be encephalopathic with a normal ammonia level or appear normal with an elevated blood ammonia level. Hypoglycemia must be looked for and corrected and renal function continuously monitored.

Office Setting

If the patient is seen in the office setting with suspected acute-onset liver disease, all studies must be performed as quickly as possible (Table 9-3) and the results reviewed before the patient leaves the office. Prolonged PT, elevated ammonia level, or deranged renal function tests warrant hospitalization. Also, any possibility of drug- or toxin-induced hepatic damage must be assessed. If these issues are satisfactorily dealt with, and it is determined that the patient has acute hepatitis with no evidence of liver failure, the patient may go home on a high-carbohydrate, protein-restricted diet. Prolonged periods of fasting should be avoided and bed rest advised, with a return visit arranged within 24 to 48 hours. Parents should be cautioned to watch for deepending jaundice, aberrant behavior, lethargy, drowsiness, or confusion and for decreased urine output or bleeding from any site. They must be given a phone number at which a physician can be reached at any time, should the need arise. Return visits should be frequent initially, with careful evaluation of mental status, thorough general physical examination, and repetition of selected laboratory tests.

Hospitalization

Hospitalization is advisable for all children with liver disease who have nausea and vomiting, who are therefore at risk of hypoglycemia and volume depletion. Also, all children with deep jaundice, a prolonged PT, elevated serum ammonia level, or signs of encephalopathy however mild, should be admitted to the hospital. Hospital care consists of restricting protein intake to 1 g/kg/day and a high-carbohydrate intake. This can be done by mouth, through a nasogastric tube, or intravenously. In most patients who are hospitalized, the oral route cannot be relied on due to markedly diminished intake. Bolus feedings through a nasogastric tube may be appropriate, but intravenous access should be obtained for all hospitalized patients. If the patient is maintained on intravenous fluids, the dextrose content should be 10% or more. Blood glucose levels should be monitored frequently. Careful monitoring of intake and output is essential, and it is often necessary to pass a urinary catheter for accurate documentation. Tests that must be done twice a day initially include complete blood count (CBC), PT/PTT, with platelets, ammonia, blood urea nitrogen (BUN), creatinine, electrolytes, alamine aminotransferase (ALT), aspartate aminotransferase (AST), and bilirubin. Frequent assessments of mental status must be made. Parenteral vitamin K (5 to 10 mg/dose) daily for 3 days should be given, although it may not correct the PT. Plasma and blood products should be restricted to cases with active bleeding, or when invasive procedures are planned. Intravenous ranitidine (6 mg/kg/day) or an equivalent H_2-receptor antagonist should be started as prophylaxis against gastrointestinal bleeding. Surveillance cultures of blood, urine, and other possible sites should be obtained, and broad-spectrum antibiotics started if there is any suspicion of infection. Urinary electrolytes and osmolarity are useful in the management of renal failure associated with FHF. Urinary electrolytes should be obtained before administration of diuretics.

Referral

It is wise to refer patients early to a liver transplant center, keeping in mind that deterioration can occur within hours and that the mortality rate even with the best of treatment is 60% to 70%. Any patient with a bilirubin of 15 mg/dl or greater, a PT of greater then 16 to 18 seconds (4 seconds more than the control) or signs of encephalopathy, no matter how stable he or she appears, belongs in an ICU at a center equipped to perform pediatric liver transplants. While arrangements to transfer the patient are being made, the above management measures must be initiated. In addition, bleeding warrants administration of blood or fresh frozen plasma as indicated. Platelets should be transfused to maintain the platelet count at greater than 50,000/mm^3, as this lowers the chances of GI bleeding. As far as possible, all blood products should be CMV negative until the CMV status of the patient is known. This is done in anticipation of possible liver transplantation and subsequent immunosuppression, when a recently acquired CMV infection can endanger the graft.

Encephalopathic patients can be started on lactulose with or without neomycin to reduce the gut bacterial load and decrease the absorption of introgenous substances. These are given by mouth or by nasogastric tube. In all cases characterized by agitation or seizures, it is important to remember that *benzodiazepines and barbiturates must be avoided* as they can worsen encephalopathy. Narcotics and phenytoin are the preferred therapeutic options. Patients already in stage III encephalopathy need to be treated for cerebral edema with fluid restriction, head elevation, and endotracheal intubation, to protect the airway and ensure adequate ventilation. Noxious stimuli should be avoided in patients with suspected cerebral edema, as such stimuli cause swings in intracranial pressure. Hence, when possible, patients should be transported to a referral center before the development of stage III encephalopathy. Hyperventilation to keep the PCO$_2$ at less than 25 mm Hg may be of limited value. Intravenous mannitol 0.25 to 0.5 g/kg/dose can be used as required, keeping serum osmolarity at approximately 320 mosm/L. Once these patients are transferred to a suitable ICU, the need for intracranial pressure monitoring can be determined. The goal of such monitoring is to maintain a cerebral perfusion pressure (mean arterial pressure -- intracranial pressure) of at least 50 mm Hg.

In many cases, with supportive treatment and monitoring, the patient will start to recover with improved mental status and normalization of the PT and serum ammonia, in conjunction with falling liver enzymes. Such patients may be advanced to oral feedings as specified above and then discharged home with close follow-up management and parent education regarding diet and signs of deterioration. It must be remembered that falling levels of liver enzymes in conjunction with a rising PT or bilirubin, or both, may in fact be an ominous sign signifying massive hepatocyte necrosis.

PROGNOSIS

The etiology of hepatic failure is important in predicting the outcome. Patients with acetaminophen toxicity do well if given adequate supportive care, whereas patients with hepatotoxicity due to other drugs have a poor prognosis.[1-6,10,11] Among the viral causes, hepatitis A carries the best prognosis and non-A, non-B, non-C or cryptogenic hepatitis the worst.

A variety of other factors are of prognostic value. Patients aged 10 to 40 years do better than the very young or very old. Jaundice occurring more than 7 days before encephalopathy is considered a bad prognostic sign. Patients with stage III or IV encephalopathy also carry a poor prognosis. In acetaminophen toxicity, a blood pH level of less than 7.3, serum creatinine of greater than 3.4 mg/dl, and a PT of more than 100 seconds are indicators of a poor outcome. In other causes of liver failure, a PT of more than 50 seconds and serum bilirubin of greater than 17.5 mg/dl are associated with a poor prognosis.

It is important to be aware of these prognostic indicators in order to make decisions regarding immediate management and the optimum time to list these patients for liver transplantation.

LIVER TRANSPLANTATION

In the pediatric population, 11% to 13% of all liver transplants are performed for the indication of fulminant hepatic failure.[2-6,10,11] The 1-year survival after transplantation is 55% to 75% in various series of children with FHF, as compared to an almost 90% survival rate in all liver transplant recipients. Therefore, it is crucial, for any case of FHF, to weigh the expected outcome against the possible outcome after transplantation. For example, in patients with acetaminophen toxicity who have none of the above indicators of a poor prognosis, the survival rate is 80% with good medical management. Conversely, patients with non-A, non-B or cryptogenic FHF have a poor prognosis and should be considered for transplant as soon as acute hepatic failure is diagnosed.

The perfect time to perform liver transplantation is when the patient's liver has failed irreversibly, but the other organ systems are capable of complete recovery. In reality, such circumstances are rarely found, and the decision is not an easy one to make. Of the patients listed for transplant, some will die waiting for an organ, and others will be precluded from surgery due to sepsis, cerebral edema, or multiorgan failure. Therefore, it is recommended that patients be listed as soon as the diagnosis is made. In the event of spontaneous recovery, the patient can be removed from the list.

Contraindications to transplantation include (1) a disease course known to have an equal or better outcome than that associated with transplantation by using available alternative therapy; (2) impairment of other organ systems (either patients who have pre-existing cardiac, renal, neurologic, or other disease, or those with involvement of these organs secondary to liver failure); (3) a questionable neurologic outcome due to cerebral edema and stage III or IV encephalopathy; (4) the presence of systemic infection; and (5) processes such as malignancy or viral disease that have a high possibility of recurrence in the donor organ. Acute or fulminant viral hepatitis is not a contraindication, whereas chronic active hepatitis B or human immunodeficiency virus (HIV) positivity is considered a contraindication by most transplant centers.

At most centers, cadaveric liver transplants are performed. Only a few offer living-related donor transplants, since in these cases there is an added risk to the donor. Size-matched livers are preferable, although recently the techniques for reduced size grafts have improved and many centers are reporting comparable survival rates.

OTHER TREATMENT METHODS

Auxiliary liver transplantation, where in the donor liver or a part of it is placed in the abdomen without removal of the patient's own liver, has been performed on occasion when the original liver was thought to be capable of regeneration. Once the liver began to function again, the donor liver was removed.[10,11]

A number of hepatic support systems have been tried.[1,2,4,10] These include dialysis, plasmapheresis, and charcoal hemoperfusion. Although they are useful to correct fluid and electrolyte problems, these support systems have not significantly improved hepatic encephalopathy or overall patient survival. There are case reports that document some success with filtering blood through devices lined with isolated human or porcine hepatocytes. Other experimental therapies include the use of acetylcysteine and prostaglandin E_1 (PGE_1), but these have not shown a benefit when studied in randomized controlled trials. Alternatives to liver transplantation that are currently being investigated are hepatocyte transplantation, extracorporeal pig liver perfusion, and xenotransplantation.[1,10]

CHRONIC LIVER FAILURE

All the conditions that lead to cirrhosis can eventually present with chronic liver failure[12] (Table 9-4). Long-standing or end-stage liver disease is associated with certain problems not seen in acute cases of liver failure. The significant problems are discussed below.

Portal hypertension can result in bleeding from esophageal and gastric varices, the development of ascites, and the consequences of hypersplenism. Variceal bleeding is often a life-threatening event, as a large amount of blood can be lost in a short period of time.

TABLE 9-4. Causes of Chronic Liver Failure in Children

Viral
  Hepatitis B
  Hepatitis C
  Cytomegalovirus (CMV)
  Herpes simplex virus (HSV)
  Epstein-Barr virus (EBV)
  Echovirus
  Rubella
Metabolic
  Alpha-1-antitrypsin deficiency
  Tyrosinemia
  Hereditary fructose intolerance
  Galactosemia
  Cystic fibrosis
  Wilson's disease
Biliary ducts
  Biliary atresia
  Alagille's syndrome
  Nonsyndromic paucity of intrahepatic bile
Miscellaneous
  Total parenteral nutrition
  Autoimmune hepatitis
  Sclerosing cholangitis
  Neonatal hemochromatosis
  Zellweger's syndrome
  Indian childhood cirrhosis

(Data from Treem[2] and Whitington.[4])

Bleeding into the GI tract can precipitate encephalopathy and liver failure in a patient with previously compensated cirrhosis. Chronic blood loss can also occur from the congestive gastropathy and enteropathy seen in patients with portal hypertension. In the presence of ascites, spontaneous bacterial peritonitis can occur. Gram-negative enteric bacteria account for the 60% to 80% of cases, although staphylococcal and streptococcal species (especially *Streptococcus pneumoniae*) have been isolated. The diagnosis is made by abdominal paracentesis and analysis and culture of the ascitic fluid. Even with appropriate antibiotic therapy, bacterial peritonitis carries a high mortality rate. Hypersplenism can lead to a reduced platelet count, which, in addition to the coagulopathy of liver disease, can increase the risk of bleeding. Anemia and a reduction in the white blood cell count are also associated with hypersplenism.

Malnutrition and growth failure are commonly seen in children with chronic liver disease. This condition can be due to poor caloric intake secondary to anorexia, suboptimal absorption of nutrients (fat and the fat-soluble vitamins A, D, E, and K) due to a low level of intraluminal bile acids, and excessive losses due to diarrhea and steatorrhea. High replacement doses of fat-soluble vitamins are commonly required to achieve adequate blood levels, so that the complications of vitamin deficiency (e.g., nightblindness, xerophthalmia, rickets, irreversible neurologic damage, bleeding) can be avoided. Poor growth and a low serum albumin in spite of adequate caloric and protein intake are signs of hepatic decompensation; these patients should be listed for liver transplantation.

Pulmonary changes include the development of arteriovenous shunts, which can lead to dyspnea and cyanosis. Cardiovascular changes are seen with alteration in the systemic and pulmonary vascular resistance, leading to hyperdynamic circulation. Skin changes found in chronic liver disease include palmar erythema and spider angiomata. Digital clubbing is also a feature of longstanding liver disease.

Other presenting signs and symptoms, as well as the management of end-stage liver disease, are much the same for liver failure due to either a chronic process or an acute insult. (For a discussion of the management of acute GI bleeding from esophageal varices, see Ch. 51). As compared to patients with FHF, patients with chronic liver disease have poorer reserves of liver and other organ function and are likely to be malnourished. The decision to list these patients for transplantation is an easier one to make, as there is little chance of spontaneous recovery. If transplanted before the onset of stage III encephalopathy or multiorgan failure, the outcome is better than in fulminant hepatic failure.[11]

REFERENCES

1. Lidofsky SD. Fulminant hepatic failure. Crit Care Clin 1995; 11:415–430
2. Treem WR. Hepatic failure. In: Walker WA, Durie PR, Hamilton RJ, Walker-Smith JA, Watkins JB, Eds. Pediatric Gastrointestinal Disease. 2nd Ed. St. Louis: Mosby-Year Book, 1996:343–393
3. Kirsh BM, Lam N, Layden TJ, Wiley TE. Diagnosis and management of fulminant hepatic failure. Compr Ther 1995; 21:166–171
4. Whitington PF. Fulminant hepatic failure in children. In: Suchy FJ, Ed. Liver Disease in Children. St. Louis: Mosby-Year Book, 1994:180–213
5. Pappas SC. Fulminant viral hepatitis. Gastroenterol Clin North Am 1995;24:161–173
6. Attilasoy E, Berk PD. Fulminant hepatic failure: pathophysiology, treatment, and survival. Annu Rev Med 1995;46: 181–191
7. Jones EA, Yurdayin C, Basile AS. The GABA hypothesis—state of the art. Adv Exp Med Biol 1994;368:89–101
8. Basile AS, Pannell L, Jaouni T et al. Brain concentrations of benzodiazepines are elevated in an animal model of hepatic encephalopathy. Proc Natl Acad Sci USA 1990;87: 5263–5267
9. Basile AS, Hughes RD, Harrison PM et al. Elevated brain concentrations of 1,4-benzodiazepines in fulminant hepatic failure. N Engl J Med 1991;325:473–478
10. Hoofnagle JH, Carithers RL Jr, Shapiro C, Ascher N. Fulminant hepatic failure: summary of a workshop. Hepatology 1995;21:240–252
11. Whitington PF, Alonso EM, Piper JB. Pediatric liver transplantation. Semin Liver Dis 1994;14:303–317
12. Hardy SC, Kleinman RE. Cirrhosis and chronic liver failure. In: Suchy FJ, Ed. Liver Disease in Children. St. Louis: Mosby-Year Book, 1994:214–248

10

FAILURE TO THRIVE AND MALABSORPTION

MARIA R. MASCARENHAS

Failure to thrive is the term used to describe poor growth in infants and children. This can be due to a lack of weight gain as well as weight loss. Early recognition of failure to thrive is important to prevent malnutrition and its complications. From a gastrointestinal (GI) point of view, failure to thrive requires a search for possible malabsorption. However, it must be remembered that non-GI causes of failure to thrive also exist (Table 10-1).

Other descriptive terms for failure to thrive include decreasing growth percentiles, diminished weight for height ratio, and nutritional dwarfism. Data exist for the average increase in weight and height (length) with increasing age (Table 10-2). Because children are frequently seen for routine checkups, these values may be used as a guideline for determining adequacy of weight and height (length) increases. Because failure to thrive is often secondary to GI malabsorption or maldigestion, these disease processes are described below.

The diagnosis of failure to thrive is made on the basis of any one of the following signs: (1) decrease in weight, height, or head circumference percentiles over time; (2) decreased weight for height (if no serial plots are available); or (3) decreased mid-arm circumference-to-head circumference ratio.

MALABSORPTION AND MALDIGESTION

Malabsorption is the abnormal absorption of nutrients from the diet. Once eaten, food must be digested, absorbed, and transported from the villi on the intestinal mucosal surface into the bloodstream before the body is able to use it. Maldigestion is the abnormal digestion of food before it is absorbed. In addition, several other factors are required for normal digestion including the production of adequate amounts of bile and pancreatic juice, an intact GI mucosal surface, and sufficient intestinal length. Abnormal motility can predispose the patient to bacterial overgrowth, which can cause secondary malabsorption. Therefore, normal functioning of the GI tract and allied organs is required for normal digestion and absorption.

Malabsorption of protein, carbohydrate and fat can occur alone or in combination depending on the etiology of malabsorption (Table 10-3). Protein malabsorption usually occurs with fat and carbohydrate malabsorption in conditions characterized by intestinal inflammation and mucosal damage. Protein-losing enteropathy occurs when protein is the predominant nutrient malabsorbed (i.e., intestinal lymphangiectasia or from increased venous pressure in the intestine due to right-sided heart failure).

Carbohydrate malabsorption is common and occurs with the ingestion of poorly absorbed sugars (e.g., sorbitol) or disorders of mucosal (e.g., celiac disease) or intraluminal phases of digestion (e.g., pancreatic insufficiency). Transient mucosal injury can result from viral gastroenteritis or before treatment of a *Giardia* infestation or celiac disease. Intestinal recovery can be variable and depends on the age of the patient, the underlying disease state, and the patient's nutritional status.

The absorption of fat is a complex process requiring

TABLE 10-1. Differential Diagnosis of Failure to Thrive by Organ System

Gastrointestinal
　　Inflammatory bowel disease, celiac disease, postviral enteropathy, chronic liver disease, cystic fibrosis
Genetic syndromes
　　Cornelia De Lange, Turner's syndromes, etc.
Malignancies
　　Lymphoma, leukemia, brain tumor
Immunologic disorders
　　SCIDS, DiGeorge's syndrome
Infections
　　Tuberculosis, HIV, congenital CMV
Rheumatologic disorders
　　JRA, RA, SLE
Renal disease
　　Chronic renal failure, RTA, cystic kidney disease
Pulmonary disease
　　Cystic fibrosis, BPD, bronchiectasis
Endocrine disorders
　　Growth hormone deficiency, thyroid deficiency
Cardiac disorders
　　Congenital heart disease, chronic heart failure
Neurologic disorders
　　Cerebral palsy
Psychosocial
　　Child neglect, mental illness in caretaker, poverty

TABLE 10-2. Average Increases in Weight and Height in Healthy Infants and Children

Age	Weight Gain[a]	Height Gain (cm/yr)
0–3 mo	25–30 g/day	23–28
3–6 mo	20 g/day	23–28
6–12 mo	12 g/day	23–28
12–18 mo	8 g/day	7.5–13
18–24 mo	6 g/day	7.5–13
2–7 yr	38 g/mo	5–13
7–9 yr	56–62 g/mo	5–6.5
9–11 yr	67–77 g/mo	5–6.5
11–13 yr	85–110 g/mo	5–6.5

[a] Based on growth velocity of the 50th percentile weight for age from the National Center for Health Statistics growth charts.

TABLE 10-3. Classification of Malabsorption

Carbohydrate malabsorption
Monosaccharide
　　Congenital glucose-galactose deficiency
　　Fructose intolerance
　　Sorbitol intolerance
Disaccharide
　　Lactase deficiency
　　　　Congenital
　　　　Acquired (post-enteritis syndrome)
　　Sucrase-isomaltase deficiency
Polysaccharide
　　Amylase deficiency
　　　　Congenital (cystic fibrosis)
　　　　Acquired (chronic, recurrent pancreatitis)
Fat malabsorption
Bile salt deficiency
　　Cholestasis
　　Resection of terminal ileum
　　Primary bile salt malabsorption
Exocrine pancreatic insufficiency
　　Cystic fibrosis
　　Shwachman's syndrome
　　Chronic pancreatitis
Intestinal lymphangiectasia
Abetalipoproteinemia
Congenital lipase deficiency
Inadequate surface area
　　Celiac disease
　　Flat villous lesion
Protein malabsorption
Exocrine pancreatic insufficiency (cystic fibrosis)
Protein-losing enteropathy
　　Intestinal lymphangiectasia
　　Congenital heart failure
　　Malignancy
　　Severe mucosal injury (i.e., IBD)
Inadequate surface area
　　Celiac disease
　　Flat villous lesion
　　Postviral enteropathy

three phases: (1) intraluminal digestion, (2) mucosal absorption, (3) and proper intestinal transport. Abnormalities in intraluminal digestion result from abnormal bile or pancreatic secretion and affect lipolysis and micellar formation (i.e., cystic fibrosis, recurrent pancreatitis, Shwachman's syndrome, liver disease, and ileal resection [decreased intraluminal bile salt concentration]). Bacterial overgrowth promotes maldigestion secondary to deconjugation of bile acids that reduces intraluminal bile acid concentration. Mucosal damage from any etiology promotes fat malabsorption secondary to poor uptake (i.e., postviral enteropathy). Abnormalities of fat transport also result in malabsorption (i.e., intestinal lymphangiectasia, abetalipoproteinemia).

ETIOLOGY

The causes of failure to thrive are varied and can be discussed by organ system or by pathophysiology (Table 10-1 and 10-4). The best way to think about this condition is to decide whether organic disease is present or whether psychosocial factors play a role.[1] The latter, also called nonorganic failure to thrive, psychosocial failure to thrive, or emotional deprivation syndrome, may be due to psychosocial disturbances in the caretaker, poor feeding technique, errors in formula preparation, poor maternal infant interaction and bonding, unusual food fads of the caretaker, child neglect, or abuse. In some patients with chronic illness, psychosocial factors may occur secondarily illustrating the fact that organic and nonorganic causes of failure to thrive can coexist in the same patient.[2]

Organic Failure to Thrive

The causes of organic failure to thrive can be divided into four major categories: decreased caloric intake, inadequate luminal digestion, inadequate intestinal absorption or increased intestinal losses, and increased caloric requirements. Decreased caloric intake may be secondary to anorexia or, more importantly, poor appetite secondary to GI disease, such as seen in gastroesophageal reflux, gastritis, duodenitis, or esophageal or gastric dysmotility causing either difficulty with the suck-and-swallow mechanism or delayed gastric emptying.

Inadequate luminal digestion may be due to either bile salt deficiency or pancreatic insufficiency. Inade-

quate absorptive uptake with increased losses is seen with disaccharide deficiency, inadequate length of intestine (i.e., short gut), and any disease that causes mucosal damage (i.e., Crohn's disease). Increased caloric requirements may be seen with chronic disease and endocrine abnormalities.

CLINICAL PRESENTATION

History

A detailed history can point to the diagnosis in the majority of patients. Both parents and all caretakers may need to be interviewed. Questions need to be asked about the presence of vomiting, diarrhea, gastroesophageal reflux (GER), and anorexia. Details about bowel movements may suggest fat malabsorption (e.g., foul-smelling or floating bowel movements) or carbohydrate malabsorption (i.e., frequent, watery diarrhea causing perianal irritation or increased flatus and abdominal distention).

It is very important to obtain previous growth data (baby book) or, if unavailable, to inquire about changes in clothing or shoe size. A quick 24-hour diet recall can give an estimate of caloric intake, amount, quality, preparation, and eating habits of the family. One may need to inquire into the feeding beliefs and practices of the parents. Poor growth has been attributed to poor caloric intake and to quality of food because of the parent's fear of obesity, hypercholesterolemia, or religious or cultural beliefs.[3,4] When conducting a review of systems, it is important to ask about chronic diseases (i.e., lung disease, heart failure). It is also important to inquire about a history of previous abdominal surgery that may suggest short bowel syndrome. Details about site of resection are important, since the area of resection affects the type of nutrient deficiency (Table 10-5).

Birth history may be significant, as 10% to 40% of patients with failure to thrive have a birth weight of less than 2.5 kg.[5-7] About 50% to 70% of patients with failure to thrive will have developmental delay.[8] Finally, the family history of chronic illness should be investigated, especially for hereditary diseases, familial patterns of growth, and age of menarche in female members of the family.

Physical Examination

Physical examination of an infant or child with failure to thrive should always include an accurate measurement of weight and height/length using age-appropriate equipment.[9] For children younger than 24–36 months of age, head circumference should be measured as well. All current and previous growth points should be plotted. Arm anthropometry can be performed by trained dietitians and compared with known standards (see Ch. 11). How-

TABLE 10-4. Etiology of Failure to Thrive

Organic
Decreased caloric intake
  Decreased oral intake
  Anorexia
  Gastroesophageal reflux (GER)
  Vomiting (brain tumor)
  Inability to suck or swallow (cerebral palsy)
Inadequate luminal digestion
  Bile salt deficiency (cholestasis, terminal ileal surgery)
  Pancreatic insufficiency (cystic fibrosis)
Inadequate absorptive uptake with increased losses
  Abnormal mucosa (celiac disease, IBD)
  Enzyme deficiency (glucose-galactose, sucrase-isomaltase, lactase—congenital/acquired)
  Inadequate length of intestine (short bowel syndrome)
Increased caloric requirements
  Thyrotoxicosis
  Chronic disease (BPD, heart failure, IBD, cancer, immunodeficiency)

Nonorganic

TABLE 10-5. Sites of Absorption of Ingested Nutrients

Duodenum
    Calcium
    Magnesium
    Iron
    Monosaccharide (glucose and xylose)
    Disaccharides

Jejunum
    Protein
    Fat
    Fat-soluble vitamins A, D, and E
    Water-soluble vitamins (thiamin, riboflavin, pyridoxine, folic
      acid, ascorbic acid)

Ileum
    Bile salts
    Vitamin B_{12}

Colon
    Fluid
    Electrolytes

ever a mid-arm circumference-to-head circumference ratio can be obtained easily. A value of less than 0.27 is suggestive of severe malnutrition (normal = greater than 0.3).[10] Careful observation of the child and his or her interaction with the parent or caretaker can be invaluable. One may even need to observe the child feeding. Failure of the child to make eye contact could suggest psychosocial dysfunction. Irritability during feeding can occur with chronic pain, celiac disease, and chronic inflammation. Physical signs of malnutrition can be visualized in a child's hair texture, mouth, and eyes. The child's nails should be examined for koilonychia, clubbing, and Beau's lines. The abdomen should be examined for distention, previous abdominal scars, hepatosplenomegaly, and increased bowel sounds. Evidence of perianal disease suggests inflammatory bowel disease.

A rectal examination will help in the determination of stool consistency and heme positivity. Blood in stool is usually associated with intestinal protein loss.

Growth Charts

Plotting growth points on age- and sex-appropriate growth charts is invaluable in the assessment of a patient with failure to thrive. While charts for normal children between birth and 18 years of age have been available for many years, new charts (birth to 36 months) for following premature infants are available.[11,12] Growth-velocity charts can also be used to follow patients with failure to thrive.[13,14]

While most children with failure to thrive fall below the fifth percentile, it is preferable when diagnosing this condition to look at changes in growth percentiles over

time (crossing percentiles). A child who started at the 90th percentile and has not gained weight over a 3-year period (25th percentile) has failure to thrive.

It is well known that between 6 to 18 months of age, children can normally change their growth percentiles and from then on grow along these new lower percentiles. Children with failure to thrive usually will drop in weight percentile, before a change in height and head circumference occurs. In general, head circumference is the last growth parameter to be affected in a child with failure to thrive. If both height and weight decrease, this suggests that the child has been having problems for at least 2 to 3 months. Figures 10-1 to 10-3 demonstrate growth patterns seen in health and two intestinal diseases.[15]

A child growing consistently below the fifth percentile may have constitutional short stature. These children tend to have a normal or slightly enlarged head circumference, with weight and height slightly below, but following, the fifth percentile curve. Bone age is usually delayed when compared to height age or chronological age. In familial short stature, bone age is equal to chronologic age, but height age is retarded. Parental height can be used to predict a patient's final height. In growth hormone deficiency, weight gain continues with normal weight velocity, but height gain and height velocity are delayed. Bone age is significantly more delayed than patient's height age (also seen in hypothyroidism).

Patients with organic failure to thrive will have normal growth parameters initially. If one looks back in time, the point of growth faltering can be correlated with the onset of the disease process. Patient's with chronic illness can have a bone age equal to, or slightly less than, height age. It is known that small-for-gestational age (SGA) neonates probably will remain small throughout their lives. Their height, weight, and head circumference will always be small. This pattern is seen in congenital cytomegalovirus (CMV) infections, perinatal asphyxia, and prematurity.

Another method in evaluating failure to thrive is to look at weight and height velocity. A decrease in weight velocity greater than 3 standard deviations (SD) from the mean requires a workup, but a decrease of less than 2 SD suggests a need for close observation. The third percentile usually correlates with 2 SD below the mean. Anthropometry (triceps skinfold and mid-arm circumference measurements) can also be used to diagnose failure to thrive. Age- and sex-appropriate charts are available.[9]

Differential Diagnosis

The differential diagnosis of failure to thrive can be multifactorial. As mentioned earlier, some patients may have organic as well as nonorganic causes for this condition.

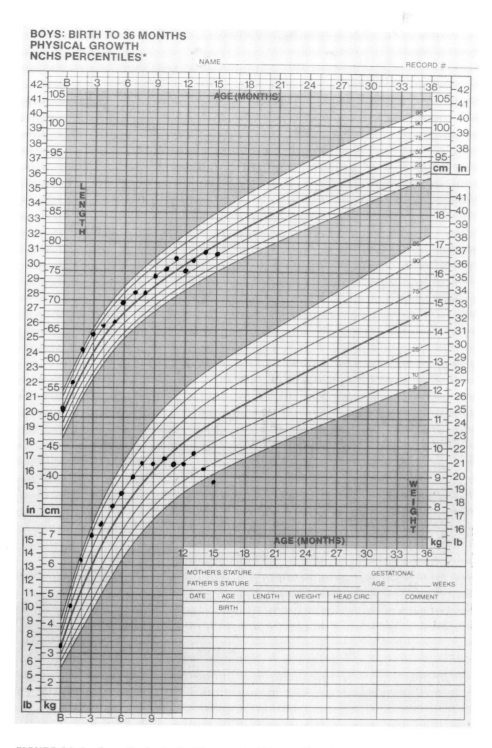

BOYS: BIRTH TO 36 MONTHS
PHYSICAL GROWTH
NCHS PERCENTILES*

FIGURE 10-1. Growth chart of a 15-month-old boy with celiac disease. (Data printed on chart are from the Fels Longitudinal study, Wright State University School of Medicine, Yellow Springs, OH. © 1982 Ross Laboratories.)

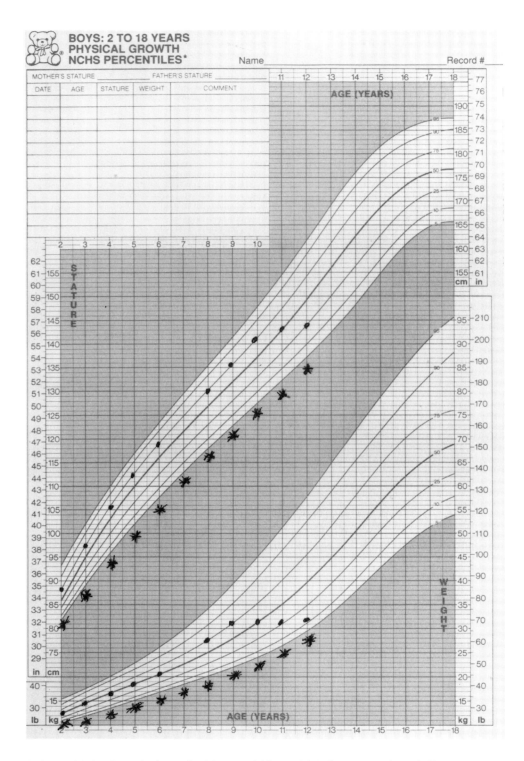

FIGURE 10-2. Growth chart of a 12-year-old boy with inflammatory bowel disease (●) and genetic short stature (*). (Data printed on chart are from the National Center for Health Statistics (NCHS), Hyattsville, MD. © 1982 Ross Laboratories.)

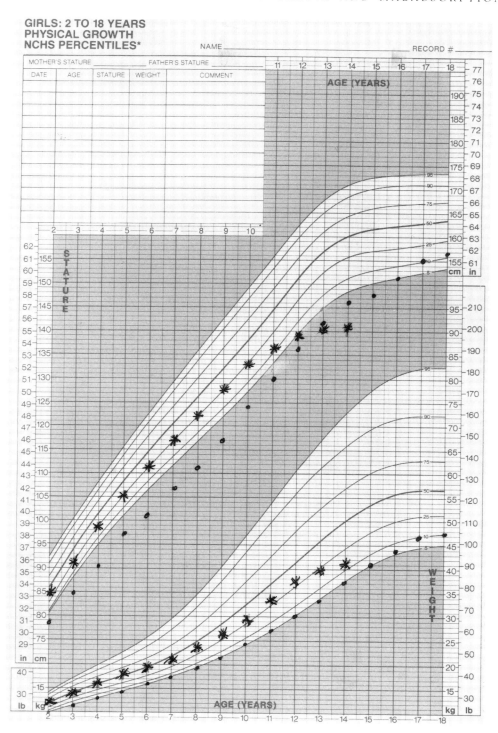

FIGURE 10-3. Growth chart of an 18-year-old girl with constitutional delay (●) and a 14-year-old with growth hormone deficiency (*). (© 1982 Ross Laboratories.)

A good history and physical examination can narrow the list of possible diagnoses. While interviewing the patient, it is a good idea to decide whether he or she has organic or nonorganic failure to thrive and, if malabsorption is present, to attempt to determine the form of malabsorption (Table 10-3). A disease-specific evaluation can then be embarked upon without putting the child through unnecessary testing. Alternatively, one can develop a list of differential diagnoses on the basis of age (Table 10-6).

TABLE 10-6. Age-Based Differential Diagnosis of Failure to Thrive

Early Infancy (0–6 mo)	Late Infancy (6–12 mo)	Children (1–13 yr)	Adolescent (13–18 yr)
Esophagitis	Celiac disuse	Celiac disease	IBD
GER	GER	IBD	HIV infection
Improper formula preparation	SBS	Cystic fibrosis	Malignancy
RTA	RTA	Cerebral palsy	Eating disorder
Cystic fibrosis	BPD	Malignancy	Chronic infection
Cerebral palsy	Cystic fibrosis	Immunodeficiency	Immunodeficiency
SBS	Cerebral palsy	GI allergies	Cystic fibrosis
BPD	GI allergies	HIV infection	Cerebral palsy
HIV infection	Postviral enteritis	Postviral enteritis	Celiac disease
Heart failure	HIV infection	Chronic infection	
Pyloric stenosis	Heart failure	Chronic renal failure	
GI allergies	Chronic infection	Chronic UTI	
Postviral enteritis	Chronic renal failure	Psychosocial	
Chronic infection	Chronic UTI		
Chronic renal failure	Psychosocial		
Chronic UTI			
Psychosocial			

Abbreviations: GER, gastroesophageal reflux; RTA, renal tubular acidosis; SBS, short bowel syndrome; BPD, bronchopulmonary dysplasia; HIV, human immunodeficiency virus; UTI, urinary tract infection; IBD, inflammatory bowel disease.

Diagnostic Testing

Diagnostic testing is invaluable for determining the etiology of failure to thrive in those patients in whom an organic etiology is suspected (Table 10-7). In some patients with nonorganic failure to thrive, some simple screening tests can help make the diagnosis of failure to thrive (Table 10-8) (for details on individual tests, see the section on diagnostic testing).

MANAGEMENT

Management of failure to thrive depends on the cause of the disease. Nutritional rehabilitation is an integral part of therapy. In some children, caloric intake of 120% to 150% of the recommended daily allowance (RDA) may be required to achieve adequate growth. Disease-specific therapy should be instituted with correction (if possible) of the underlying condition. Often, one must treat the underlying problem and at the same time provide additional calories for "catch-up" growth. Specific nutrient abnormalities also need to be corrected (see Table 10-9 for the principles of treatment of malabsorptive disorders).

In those patients with carbohydrate malabsorption, removal of the offending agent from the diet (e.g., glucose, galactose, and/or lactose) should result in improved symptomatology. Patients with sorbitol intolerance must decrease the amount of sorbitol in their diet. Supplemental enzymes may be required in children with primary or secondary lactose intolerance (lactase) and sucrase-isomaltase deficiency (sucrase-isomaltase). Patients with polysaccharide intolerance will need to avoid starch and use pancreatic enzymes. Some patients benefit from receiving rice- or corn-based glucose polymers, which are well tolerated, have low osmolality, and are well absorbed. Patients with bacterial overgrowth may benefit from ingesting yogurt with active cultures, as the bacteria are able to survive the acid pH level of the stomach and are active in the intestine.

Patients with fat malabsorption have symptomatic improvement when prescribed a low-fat diet. Supplementation with medium-chain triglycerides (MCT) may be required to improve their caloric intake. Fat-soluble vitamin (A, D, E, and K) deficiencies should be corrected. Patients with exocrine pancreatic insufficiency require pancreatic enzyme supplementation. Acid blockade with H_2-blocker therapy has been reported to improve pancreatic enzyme activity.[16] Protein and calorie supplements may also be required. Younger children may be given a formula rich in MCT oil to improve fat absorption. Older children may ingest MCT oil or carbohydrate supplements to improve caloric intake. Patients with intestinal lymphangiectasia require MCT supplements, fat-soluble vitamin therapy, and a low-fat diet.[17]

TABLE 10-7. Diagnostic Testing for Failure to Thrive

1. Diet record (3 day)
2. Stool tests: stool for white blood cells and eosinophils
    Stool for ova and parasites
    Stool for *Clostridium difficile* toxin
3. Blood tests: complete blood count
    Serum electrolytes
4. Specific tests for malabsorption
    a. Carbohydrate malabsorption
        Stool pH and reducing substances
        Stool electrolytes, bicarbonate, and osmolality
        Lactose and other breath H_2 tests
        Xylose absorption test
        Small bowel biopsy for pathology and enzyme analysis
    b. Fat malabsorption
        PT/PTT
        Serum carotene/25-hydroxyvitamin D/vitamin E level
        Fecal smear for fat (qualitative)
        72-hour fecal fat collection (quantitative)
        Bentiromide absorption test
        Pancreatic stimulation test
        Small bowel biopsy
    c. Protein malabsorption
        Serum total protein and albumin level
        Stool hemoccults
        Urinalysis
        24-hour stool alpha-1-antitrypsin clearance
        Small bowel biopsy
5. Miscellaneous tests
    Urinalysis
    Sweat test
    Serum folate and vitamin B_{12} levels
    Thyroid function tests
    Resting energy expenditure
    Bone age
    HIV testing

TABLE 10-8. Diagnostic Testing: Cost-Effective Approach

1. Diet record (3 day)
2. Stool examination
    Hemoccult
    Clinitest
    White blood tests and eosinophils
    Fat smear
    Ova and parasites
3. Complete blood count
4. Serum electrolytes, liver function and kidney function tests, cholesterol, triglycerides, calcium, phosphorus, total protein, albumin
5. Sweat test
6. Lactose breath test
7. Xylose absorption test
8. Serum vitamin E level
9. Urinalysis and culture

TABLE 10-9. Treatment of Malabsorption

Carbohydrate intolerance
    Remove offending carbohydrate from the diet
    Replacement enzyme therapy
Fat malabsorption
    Low-fat diet
    Correct fat-soluble enzyme deficiencies
    Supplemental fat-soluble vitamins
    Medium-chain tryglyceride supplementation
    Pancreatic enzyme replacement
    Calorie supplements
Protein malabsorption
    Protein and calorie supplements
    Treat underlying disease
    Correct any coexisting nutritional abnormalities

In general, patients with protein malabsorption require treatment of the underlying condition in addition to protein and calorie supplements. Patients with specific GI disorders require disease-specific therapy. Patients who have celiac disease demand a gluten-free diet; they also need to be put on a lactose-free diet until mucosal healing has occurred.[18] Patients with inflammatory bowel disease need aminosalicylates, immunosuppressive therapy, a high-calorie–high-protein diet, and multivitamin supplementation.[19] Patients with short bowel syndrome require antibiotics for bacterial overgrowth, medium-chain triglyceride containing supplements if they have had extensive ileal resection, and high-protein and high-calorie diets enterally or parenterally.[20] *Giardia* infestation is treated with metronidazole and other antiparasite medications. Acrodermatitis enteropathica requires zinc supplementation.[21] Patients with ileal resection and vitamin B_{12} malabsorption will need parenteral vitamin B_{12} therapy. Some patients with decreased caloric intake and/or increased caloric requirements will require caloric supplements (oral, through a tube, or by parenteral nutrition).

REFERENCES

1. Sills RH. Failure to thrive: the role of clinical and laboratory evaluation. Am J Dis Child 1978;132:967–969
2. Homer C, Ludwig S. Categorization of the etiology of failure to thrive. Am J Dis Child 1981;135:848–851
3. Pugliese MT, Weyman-Daum M, Moses N et al. Parenteral health beliefs as a cause of non-organic failure to thrive. Pediatrics 1978;80:175–182
4. Pugliese MT, Lifshitz F, Grad G et al. Fear of obesity: a cause of short stature and delayed puberty. N Engl J Med 1983; 309:513–518
5. Mitchell W, Gorrell R, Greenberg R. Failure to thrive: a study in a primary care setting. Pediatrics 1980;65:971–977

6. Oates RK, Yu J. Children with non-organic failure to thrive: A community problem. Med J Aust 1971;2:199–203

7. Shaheen E, Alexander D, Truskowsky M et al. Failure to thrive: a retrospective profile. Clin Pediatr 1986;7:255–261

8. Berwick DM. Non-organic failure to thrive. Pediatr Rev 1980;1:265–270

9. Lohman TG, Roche AF, Martorell R. Anthropometric Standardization Reference Manual. Champaign, IL: Human Kinetics Books, 1988

10. Sasanow SR, Georgieff MK, Pereira GR. Mid arm circumference and midarm/head circumference ratios: standard curves for anthropometric assessment of neonatal nutritional status. J Pediatr 1986;109:311–315

11. The Infant Health and Development Program. Enhancing the outcomes of low-birth-weight, premature infants. JAMA 1990;263:3035–3042

12. Casey PH, Kraemer HC, Bernbaum J et al. Growth status and growth rates of a varied sample of low birth weight, preterm infants: a longitudinal cohort from birth to three years of age. J Pediatr 1991;119:599–605

13. Tanner JM, Davies PSW. Clinical longitudinal standards for height and height velocity for North American children. J Pediatr 1985;107:317–329

14. Roche AF, Himes JH. Incremental growth charts. Am J Clin North Am 1980;33:2041–2052

15. Cohen P, Rosenfeld RG. Disorders of growth. In: MacAnarney XX, Kreipe XX, Orr XX, Comerci XX, Eds. Textbook of Adolescent Medicine. Philadelphia: WB Saunders, 1992: 56:494–508

16. Durie PR et al. Effect of cimetidine and sodium bicarbonate on pancreatic replacement therapy in cystic fibrosis. Gut 1980;21:778–786

17. Tift WL, Lloyd JK. Intestinal lymphangiectasia: long-term results with MCT diet. Arch Dis Child 1975;50:269–276

18. Barr DGD, Shmerling DH, Brader A. Catchup growth in malnutrition, studies in coeliac disease after institution of gluten-free diet. Paediatr Res 1972;6:521–527

19. Hofley PM, Piccoli DA. Inflammatory bowel disease in children. Med Clin North Am 1994;78:1281–1302

20. Treem WR. Short bowel syndrome. In: Wyllie R, Hyams JS, Eds. Pediatric Gastrointestinal Disease: Pathophysiology, Diagnosis, Management. Philadelphia: WB Saunders, 1993: 573–603

21. Hambidge KM, Walravens PA: Disorders of mineral metabolism. Clin Gastroenterol 1982;11(1):87–117

11

MALNUTRITION

RAANAN SHAMIR
MICHAEL WILSCHANSKI

DEFINITION

The term *malnutrition* refers to either underfeeding or overfeeding and is associated with a patient who is underweight or overweight, respectively. This chapter discusses malnutrition caused by underfeeding. This form of malnutrition is a major health hazard in the developing world. During 1975 to 1990, the total prevalence of underweight children (i.e., the percentage below 2 standard deviations (SD) from the mean with regard to weight for age, ages zero to 5 years) in developing countries was estimated to be approximately 34%.[1] Insufficient nutrient intake and recurrent infections are the main causes of malnutrition. Children may present with malnutrition in the form of kwashiorkor (protein-deficient, energy-sufficient), marasmus (protein- and energy-deficient) or a combination of marasmus and kwashiorkor. In general, malnutrition is referred to as protein-energy malnutrition (PEM).

In Western societies, primary PEM is hardly seen.[2] However, malnutrition secondary to acute and chronic disease states is commonly seen, with a 25% to 60% prevalence of malnutrition in hospitalized pediatric patients.[3-5] Inadequate caloric intake (Fig. 11-1), inadequate absorption and assimilation, failure of utilization, or increased metabolic needs are the basis for this type of malnutrition.

CLINICAL WORKUP

Diagnosing Malnutrition

The first step in the diagnosis of PEM is taking an adequate history. Anorexia is common in sick children and is characteristic of a wide range of disease states, such as anorexia nervosa,[6] congestive heart failure due to congenital heart disease or cardiomyopathy,[7,8] inflammatory bowel disease (IBD) due to abdominal pain and discomfort,[9] and in patients with malignancies as a result of chemotherapy.[10] Anorexia is only one of the causes that contribute to reduced food intake. In many disease states, laboratory and imaging testing require that patients remain nothing per os (NPO), which can be a major cause of reduced food intake in hospitalized patients. In addition, keeping patients NPO is commonly used as a treatment modality. As early as 1948, studies comparing fasting to the continued use of a formula during acute gastroenteritis demonstrated a beneficial effect of formulas in nutrient retention.[11] Nevertheless bowel rest is still a common practice in the management of acute gastroenteritis, despite the guidelines published by the American Academy of Pediatrics in 1996. In this situation as well as in other disease states (i.e., IBD,[12] where bowel rest is a common practice), decreased food intake aggravates a fragile balance between increased energy and protein needs and excessive nutrient loss. A list of common diseases causing malnutrition is given in Table 11-1.

Clues to the existence of PEM are provided when other causes of diminished food intake exist. Causes of diminished food intake include hypotonicity, hypertonicity, an abnormal swallowing mechanism, an altered level of consciousness, regurgitation, or vomiting. Questions that are appropriate when evaluating infants and children include the type of milk used for feeding, the precise way in which the formula is diluted, intake of formula, and changes in eating patterns. The number of meals, snacks, and their content should also be evaluated, and questions should be asked about specific foods. Deficient food intake should not be missed during history taking. In adolescence, it is important to find out about

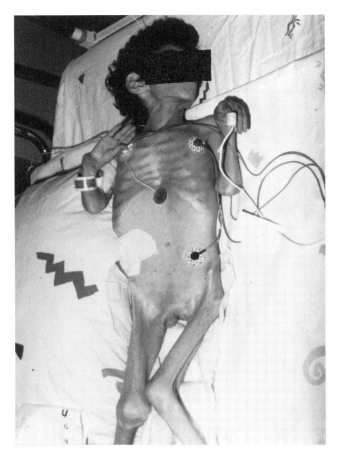

FIGURE 11-1. A 13-year-old patient with cerebral palsy who is suffering from severe chronic malnutrition.

special diets, the number and content of meals and snacks, skipping meals, avoidance of specific foods, and physical activity. Questions should be asked about recent weight loss and whether this weight loss was voluntary.

Nutritional assessment that is crucial for making the diagnosis of PEM is discussed in Chapter 80. The physical examination can be useful in determining specific causes for increased energy needs. Common abnormal physical findings associated with increased needs include burns, trauma, closed-head injury, fever, and sepsis. Increased nutrient loss (e.g., diarrhea, intestinal mucosal inflammation, burns) should also be considered.

It is well known that inadequate food intake leads to weight loss and growth retardation. However, classifications of malnutrition were based solely on weight and age. The classification published by Gomez et al.[13] did not use international criteria and defined severe malnutrition (third-degree) as weight for age (current weight divided by weight at the 50th percentile for the patient's age) less than the 60th percentile. First- and second-degree malnutrition were defined as the 75th to 90th percentile of weight for age and as the 60th to 75th percentile of weight for age, respectively.

Acute PEM affects weight, while chronic PEM affects both weight and height. Therefore, in order to diagnose PEM, age and weight are not sufficient. In addition to recording age and weight, length (before 2 years of age) or height (after 2 years of age) should be measured; subsequently, two indexes should be calculated: (1) weight for height, and (2) height for age. Weight for height provides the current nutritional status of the patient, while deficient height for age provides evidence for chronic malnutrition. In order to plot the weight and height on the growth chart, the World Health Organization (WHO) has recommended to use the growth charts based on the National Center for Health Statistics (NCHS) data.[14] These charts can be used worldwide, as healthy children have similar growth potential regardless of ethnic background, and weight and height relate to each other similarly in all age groups. The use of growth charts provides a practical method for establishing the presence and degree of PEM.

For nutritional assessment, the current accepted classification is based on the Waterlow criteria for malnutrition,[15] which defines wasting as a deficient weight

TABLE 11-1. Diseases Commonly Associated With Malnutrition

Anorexia nervosa

Burns

Cancer

Cardiac
    Surgery
    Congenital heart disease

Central nervous system
    Cerebral palsy
    Neuromuscular disorders

Infectious diseases (chronic)

Gastrointestinal diseases
    Celiac disease
    Cystic fibrosis
    Inflammatory bowel disease
    Intestinal pseudo-obstruction
    Intractable diarrhea
    Milk-protein enteropathy
    Pancreatitis
    Short bowel syndrome

Immunodeficiencies (including AIDS)

Intrauterine growth retardation

Liver disease—chronic

Metabolic disorders

Pulmonary disease

Renal disease—chronic

Transplantation

Trauma

for height, and stunting as a deficient height for age (Table 11-2). According to these criteria, patients may be classified as adequately nourished, as having acute PEM (wasted but not stunted), or as having acute and chronic PEM (wasting and stunting). Patients who are stunted but not wasted may or may not be suffering from nutritional short stature. The degree of wasting carries implications for treatment and for the risk of refeeding, discussed later in this chapter. For adolescents, body mass index (BMI) may be used for the diagnosis of PEM.[16] A BMI (weight/height^2) below 15 at ages 11 to 13 and BMI below 16.5 at ages 14 to 17 suggests a diagnosis of PEM in both males and females.

Other anthropometric measurements, such as mid-arm circumference (MAC), used to assess skeletal protein mass, and skinfold measurements, used to assess fat mass, are useful in following patients with PEM but are not used routinely for diagnosis (for more information on these tests refer to Ch. 80). Laboratory testing can also support the diagnosis of PEM. Table 11-3 summarizes the spectrum of initial laboratory tests to be considered in children with PEM.

Clinical Presentation of Malnutrition

The child with severe PEM can present solely with signs of malnutrition or with a combined picture of the primary disease and malnutrition (Table 11-1). Three presentations of malnutrition can be diagnosed based on clinical findings: kwashiorkor, marasmic-kwashiorkor, and marasmus. In all three entities, a deficiency of protein and energy is present, therefore, the term protein calorie malnutrition has been given to the full spectrum of clinical presentations. Kwashiorkor occurs when protein deficiency dominates the presentation, while marasmus is considered when energy deficiency is primarily present. Marasmic-kwashiorkor is a combination of both.

TABLE 11-2. Classification of Acute (Wasting) and Chronic (Stunting) PEM

Weight/Height^a		Height/Age^b	
%	Description	%	Description
90–110	Normal weight	>95	Normal height
80–90	Mild wasting	90–95	Mild stunting
70–80	Moderate wasting	85–90	Moderate stunting
<70	Severe wasting	<85	Severe stunting

^{a} First, ideal weight for height should be calculated. On the growth chart, find where actual height intersects with the 50th percentile and drop a line to the intersection with the 50th percentile in weight. This is the ideal body weight for actual height. Weight/Height is calculated by dividing the current weight by the ideal weight for height.

^{b} Current height divided by ideal height for age (50th percentile).

(Data from Waterlow.[15])

TABLE 11-3. Laboratory Tests in Severe PEM^a

Assessment of visceral protein stores
  Albumin/transferin/prealbumin
Electrolytes
  Sodium, potassium, chloride, bicarbonate
Minerals
  Calcium, phosphorus, magnesium, zinc
Renal function
  Blood urea nitrogen, creatinine
Liver enzymes
  Alanine aminotransferase, aspartate aminotransferase, alkaline phosphatase
Other tests
  Complete blood count
  Glucose
  Cholesterol
  Triglycerides
  Vitamins A, E, and D (25-OH)
  Prothrombin time

^{a} Since infections are common in malnourished children, appropriate cultures are mandatory. Chest film and electrocardiogram are also part of the routine.

KWASHIORKOR

Kwashiorkor was first described in Africa as a disease that occurs in an older sibling after the next child is born. In North America, cases of kwashiorkor were described when children were fed calorie-sufficient but protein-deficient formulas.[17–21] Kwashiorkor is common after the age of 18 months and occurs when a child receives a diet rich in carbohydrates but lacking protein. Children with kwashiorkor commonly present with edema, hypoproteinemia, fatty liver, and mental status changes, including apathy and anorexia. Cutaneous manifestations include fine, brittle hair, dry skin or skin with areas of hypopigmentation, and erythematous lesions that may progress into widespread erosions with a flaky paint appearance particularly over the limbs and buttocks.[22] Children who suffer from kwashiorkor have depleted protein stores, with reduced muscle mass. Weight loss may not be appreciated due to the presence of edema.

MARASMUS

Marasmus develops as a consequence of partial starvation and occurs predominantly in the first year of life. It is caused by the body's physiologic adaptation to starvation, and is the result of deficient energy, protein, vitamins, and minerals. Severe weight reduction, stunting, muscle wasting, depleted subcutaneous fat, and dry wrinkled skin are common. The marasmic child is usually apathetic but is aware of his or her surroundings. The lack of facial subcutaneous fat commonly gives the child the appearance of an old man. Hypothermia, bradycardia, bradypnea, and hypotension appear late in the course of starvation and carry high risk of mortality if not treated promptly. Marasmic children differ from children with kwashiorkor, as they lack hepatomegaly and edema. These findings can be present in marasmic-kwashiorkor.

PHYSICAL FINDINGS OF NUTRIENT DEFICIENCY

A thorough evaluation should include the evaluation of specific clinical signs and symptoms of nutrient deficiencies (e.g., nightblindness, xerophthalmia, Bitot's spots, keratomalacia in vitamin A deficiency). Serum testing for specific nutrients are often not helpful as they may show either low or normal levels. One should keep in mind that normal values do not rule out depleted body stores and low levels of carrier proteins can give rise to low serum levels despite adequate stores. In the presence of steatorrhea, fat-soluble vitamin deficiencies should be evaluated. Although uncommon, malnutrition can be a primary cause of pancreatic insufficiency.

In severe PEM, laboratory testing often reveals a low hemoglobin due to reduced red cell mass and reduced hematopoiesis. Hypoproteinemia and hypoalbuminemia are present in edematous children (kwashiorkor, marasmic kwashiorkor), while hypoglycemia is common in marasmic children when fasted for a few hours. Hypoglycemia can also occur as secondary to refeeding syndrome. During starvation, the intracellular concentration of sodium increases, while intracellular concentrations of potassium and magnesium are decreased. In addition, there is increased urinary loss of potassium, magnesium, zinc, calcium, and phosphorus. These chemical abnormalities can occur even when serum levels are initially within the normal range.

MANAGEMENT OF THE CHILD WITH PEM

Children with PEM may suffer from dehydration.[23,24] Before attempting to correct the nutritional deficiencies, the patient should be rehydrated and serum chemistries corrected.

Refeeding Syndrome

The complications of feeding severely malnourished patients, termed refeeding syndrome, have been known since World War II and result from metabolic and physiologic alterations caused by the administration of calories and nutrients to a system that has adapted to starvation.[24] These complications may be caused by the administration of intravenous glucose,[25,26] total parenteral nutrition,[27,28] or enteral nutrition.[29] Treatment of the malnourished child can only be understood in the setting of expected complications.

1. *Fluid intolerance*: Refeeding can cause extracellular water retention due to carbohydrate administration.[24,30] Fluid retention is also aggravated by sodium intake.[24]

2. *Cardiopulmonary complications*: Malnutrition causes a reduction in left ventricular mass, cardiac output, and respiratory tissue.[31–34] Refeeding increases extracellular fluid, cardiac output,[32] minute ventilation, oxygen consumption, and carbon dioxide production.[35] Thus, congestive heart failure and respiratory distress can complicate the treatment of malnourished children, especially when severe anemia is present.

3. *Hypophosphatemia*: A common and life-threatening complication of the refeeding syndrome is hypophosphatemia.[25–29] A malnourished child responds to glucose administration with insulin release. The result is a shift of phosphorus from the extracellular to the intercellular spaces, increasing the intracellular phosphorus requirements for ATP production and phosphorylated intermediates in the glycolytic pathway. The clinical signs of severe hypophosphatemia include congestive heart failure, dysrhythmia, hypotension, respiratory failure, muscle weakness, paresthesias, confusion, coma, convulsions, rhabdomyolysis, hemolytic anemia, and decreased immunocompetence. Deaths due to hypophosphatemia have been documented secondary to suboptimal supplementation of phosphorus.[27]

4. *Hypokalemia*: A common complication of refeeding is hypokalemia, the result of elevated plasma insulin levels, rapid glucose infusion, and increased intracellular potassium that occurs following the recovery of lean body mass.[16,24] Diarrhea and vomiting are other possible causes of hypokalemia. Signs of hypokalemia include skeletal muscle weakness, decreased peristalsis, ileus, decreased ability of the kidney to concentrate urine, and various electrocardiographic (ECG) abnormalities (T-wave changes, U waves, and ST-segment depression).

5. *Glucose metabolism*: Hypoglycemia may be part of the initial presentation of the malnourished child or it may develop in the early stages of refeeding. Hyperglycemia is also seen during refeeding and is caused by glucose administration exceeding the body's ability to maintain normoglycemia.[36] Sepsis and stress (e.g., surgery, trauma) are other causes of hyperglycemia due to increased levels of circulating glucagon and cortisol.

6. *Hypomagnesemia*: Magnesium is an important component of the intracellular space, as it serves as a cofactor in many enzymatic systems. During repletion, serum levels tend to be low despite adequate renal conservation.[37] Signs of magnesium deficiency include anorexia, nausea, vomiting, irritability, depression, tremors, convulsions, tetany, paresthesias, and ECG changes. Since magnesium depletion interferes with parathyroid hormone (PTH) synthesis and release,[38]

hypomagnesemia and hypocalcemia often coexist, and signs of deficiency may reflect both deficiencies.

7. *Hypocalcemia*: Hypocalcemia usually resolves with the normalization of magnesium serum levels. In the presence of hypoalbuminemia, true ionized serum calcium levels need to be determined, either by correcting serum levels for the degree of hypoalbuminemia or by directly measuring ionized calcium.

In light of all possible complications, feeding of the malnourished child should be provided cautiously. After fluid resuscitation, feeding should be started, preferably using the enteral route. When establishing feeds, it is safe to start with a previously tolerated regimen or with 25 to 50 kcal/kg (current weight). This is followed by gradually increasing energy and protein intake.[23,39,40] Serum electrolytes, glucose, potassium, calcium, phosphorus, and magnesium should be monitored daily. To achieve catch-up growth, 2 to 3 g/kg of protein and 150 to 200 kcal/kg may be needed. Catch-up growth calculations are based on ideal body weight, as defined in Table 12-2. Growth is the best indicator for appropriate management and is the best guide for the tapering of nutrition supplementation (when the patient approaches ideal body weight). Whenever possible, feeds should be provided ad libitum and tube supplementation provided only if necessary. In many disease states, nutritional supplementation should continue for a prolonged period. If nasogastric feedings is used for more than a few weeks, insertion of gastrostomy tube should be considered.[41]

SEVERE PEM AND DISEASE

This section focuses on IBD as a model for disease in which malnutrition is common. It should be kept in mind that in IBD as well as in other disease commonly associated with malnutrition (Table 11-1), failure to diagnose or treat the malnutrition results in growth failure, increased incidence of infection, increased incidence of perioperative complications, and increased morbidity and mortality.[8,9,12,42,43]

Inflammatory Bowel Disease: a Model for Diseases Commonly Associated With Malnutrition

IBD refers to chronic inflammatory conditions of the intestine, mainly Crohn's disease and ulcerative colitis (see Ch. 30).

Malnutrition is a major issue in IBD. Several mechanisms underline malnutrition in IBD:

1. *Decreased food intake*: Inadequate caloric intake is thought to be common in children with IBD and growth retardation.[43] The decreased intake is caused by anorexia, nausea, vomiting, impaired taste sensation, dietary restrictions imposed by the physician, and dietary restrictions imposed by the patient for fear of abdominal pain and diarrhea.[12,23]

2. *Malabsorption*: There are multiple causes for malabsorption in patients with IBD secondary to a loss of intestinal absorptive surface due to inflammation of the small bowel mucosa or resection of small bowel segments (Crohn's disease). Figure 11-2 provides a schematic presentation of causes and consequences of malabsorption in IBD.

3. *Increased nutrient loss*: Excessive loss of nutrients is well documented in IBD. Protein-losing enteropathy is usually present in active IBD. Blood loss, fistula drainage, and liver disease contribute to the hypoproteinemia. Protein loss from inflamed mucosa may be extensive and in Crohn's disease is highly correlated with disease activity.[44] In addition, blood loss causes iron depletion, and diarrhea causes electrolyte loss (potassium, magnesium, and zinc).[45] Zinc loss is correlated with the volume of the diarrhea. Zinc depletion occurs with steatorrhea, as do losses of other divalent cations (e.g., calcium, magnesium, copper), and fat soluble vitamins.[44]

4. *Increased energy requirements*: Inflammation has not been shown to cause chronic malnutrition due to increased energy needs in IBD.[12] Infections and fever may contribute to increased energy needs.[9]

5. *Drug-nutrient interactions*: Corticosteroids suppress intestinal calcium absorption.[44] The risk of calcium deficiency is exacerbated when milk products are avoided in order to achieve low lactose intake. Sulfasalazine is a competitive inhibitor of folate absorption that necessitates monitoring folic acid blood levels.

At diagnosis, 85% of pediatric patients with Crohn's disease and 65% of those with ulcerative colitis have weight loss.[9] Similarly, in adults, 80% of Crohn's disease patients and 60% of ulcerative colitis patients may develop weight loss.[12,46,47] In children, growth failure complicates the clinical picture and is present in 10% to 40% of children with IBD.[48] In addition, height velocity may be reduced in 88% of patients with Crohn's disease.[49] Malnutrition is the main cause of the growth failure seen in IBD. Nutritional rehabilitation has been shown to restore normal growth in these children.[50,51] Hypoalbuminemia is common in IBD and can be found in as many as 60% of patients with Crohn's disease and in 35% of patients with ulcerative colitis. Nutritional anemias (iron deficiency, vitamin B_{12} deficiency, folic acid deficiency) are also common in children with IBD and can be found in 75% of children with Crohn's disease and in 60% of children with ulcerative colitis. Iron defi-

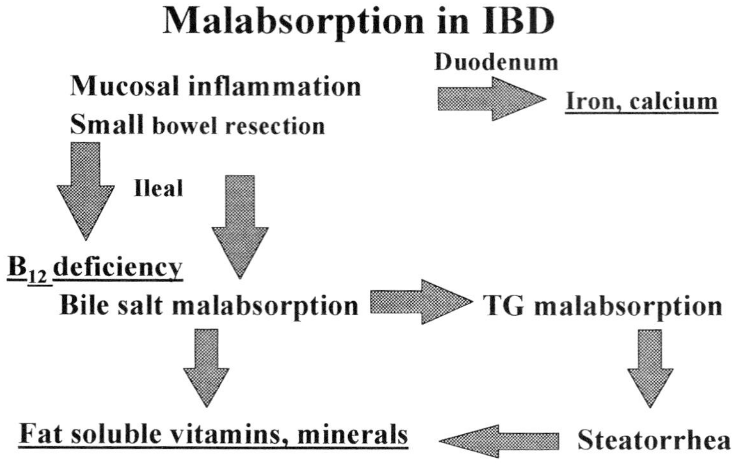

Malabsorption in IBD

Mucosal inflammation
Small bowel resection

Duodenum
→ **Iron, calcium**

Ileal

B$_{12}$ deficiency
Bile salt malabsorption ⇒ **TG malabsorption**

Fat soluble vitamins, minerals ⇐ **Steatorrhea**

FIGURE 11-2. Schematic presentation of causes for malabsorption in inflammatory bowel disease.

ciency may be present due to intestinal blood loss, poor dietary intake, or decreased absorption. Patients with severe terminal ileum disease or resection are at risk of vitamin B$_{12}$ deficiency. Vitamin B$_{12}$ deficiency may also occur in the presence of bacterial overgrowth. Folate deficiency occurs in patients with IBD due to decreased absorption (Crohn's disease) or to increased utilization in chronic inflammation, or with the use of sulfasalazine.[52] In addition to hypoalbuminemia and anemia, multiple deficiencies have been reported in IBD, including zinc, calcium, magnesium, water-soluble vitamins (vitamins C and B$_6$, niacin, and biotin), and fat-soluble vitamins (vitamins E, A, D, and K).

Adequate nutrition with restoration of weight gain and catch-up growth is the cornerstone of the nutritional therapy. In addition, enteral nutrition or parenteral nutrition is likely to facilitate remission in 60% to 80% of patients with acute exacerbation of Crohn's disease.[53] Parenteral nutrition, elemental diets, oligopeptide diets, and polymeric diets have been described as useful in inducing remission in Crohn's disease.[9,12,54] It was recently suggested that supplementary enteral feeds may have a role in maintaining remission in pediatric Crohn's disease.[55] Enteral nutrition is the preferred route of nutrition supplementation, and the use of parenteral nutrition is reserved for patients who cannot tolerate or fail to improve on enteral feeds.[53]

CONCLUSION

Malnutrition is an important manifestation of both acute and chronic disease. The prevalence of malnutrition in hospitalized pediatric patients is 25% to 60%. IBD, in which nutritional therapy restores catch-up growth and facilitates remission, is one example for the important role of malnutrition in the pathophysiology, clinical presentation, and treatment of the pediatric patient.

REFERENCES

1. United Nations. Second report on the world nutrition situation. Lavenham, Suffolk, England: Vol. 1. Lavenham Press, 1992

2. Owen G, Lippman G. Nutritional status of infants and young children USA. Pediatr Clin North Am 1977;24:211–277

3. Merritt RJ, Suskind RM. Nutritional survey of hospitalized pediatric patients. Am J Clin Nutr 1979;32:1320–1325

4. Cooper A, Jakobowski D, Spiker J et al. Nutritional assessment. J Pediatr Surg 1981;16:554–560

5. Hendricks KM, Duggan C, Gallagher L, et al. Malnutrition in hospitalized pediatric patients. Current prevalence. Arch Pediatr Adolesc Med 1995;149:1118–1122

6. Lucas AR, Huse DM. Behavioural disorders affecting food intake: anorexia nervosa and bulimia nervosa. In: Shils ME, Olson JA, Shike M, Eds. Modern Nutrition in Health and Disease. Philadelphia: Lea & Febiger; 1994:977–983

7. Rosenthal A. Nutritional considerations in the prognosis and treatment of children with congenital heart disease. In: Suskind RM, Lewinter S, Eds. Textbook of Pediatric Nutrition. New York: Raven Press, 1993:383–391

8. Cameron JW, Rosenthal A, Olson AD. Malnutrition in hospitalized children with congenital heart disease. Arch Pediatr Adolesc Med 1995;149:1098–1102

9. Seidman E, LeLeiko N, Ament M et al. Nutritional issues in pediatric inflammatory bowel disease. J Pediatr Gastroenterol Nutr 1991;12:424–438

10. Shils ME. Nutrition and diet in cancer management. In: Shils ME, Olson JA, Shike M, Eds. Modern Nutrition in Health and Disease. Philadelphia: Lea & Febiger, 1994: 1317–1348

11. Chung AW, Viscorova B. The effect of early feeding versus early oral starvation on the course of infantile diarrhea. J Pediatr 1948;33:14–22

12. Lewis JD, Fisher RL. Nutrition support in inflammatory bowel disease. Med Clin North Am 1994;78:1443–1456

13. Gomez F, Galvan RR, Frenk S et al. Mortality in second and third degree malnutrition. J Trop Pediatr 1956;2:77–83

14. Hamill PVV, Drizd TA, Johnson CL et al. Physical growth: National Center for Health Statistics percentiles. Am J Clin Nutr 1979;32:607–629

15. Waterlow JC. Note on the assessment and classification of protein-energy malnutrition in children. Lancet 1973;2:87–89

16. Torun B, Chew F. Protein-energy malnutrition. In: Shils ME, Olson JA, Shike M, Eds. Modern Nutrition in Health and Disease. Philadelphia: Lea & Febiger, 1994:950–976

17. Latham MC. The dermatoses of kwashiorkor in young children. Semin Dermatol 1991;10:270–272

18. Chase HP, Kumar V, Caldwell RT, O'Brien D. Kwashiorkor in the United States. Pediatrics 1980;66:972–976

19. Sinatra FR, Merritt RJ. Iatrogenic kwashiorkor in infants. Am J Dis Child 1981;135:21–23

20. Taitz LS, Finberg L. Kwashiorkor in the Bronx. Am J Dis Child 1966;112:76–78

21. John TJ, Blazovich J, Lightner ES et al. Kwashiorkor not associated with poverty. J Pediatr 1977;90:730–735

22. Lozoff B, Fanaroff AA. Kwashiorkor in Cleveland. Am J Dis Child 1975;129:710–711

23. Suskind D, Murthy KK, Suskind RM. The malnourished child: an overview. In: Suskind RM, Lewinter-Suskind L, Eds. The Malnourished Child. New York: Raven Press, 1990:1–22

24. Solomon SM, Kirby DF. The refeeding syndrome: a review. J Parent Enteral Nutr 1990;14:90–97

25. Gundersen K, Bradley RF, Marble A. Serum phosphorus and potassium levels after intravenous administration of glucose. N Engl J Med 1954;250:547–554

26. Hessov I, Jensen NG, Rasmusen A. Prevention of hypophosphatemia during postoperative routine glucose administration. Acta Chir Scand 1980;146:109–114

27. Weinsier RL, Krumdieck CL. Death resulting from overzealous total parenteral nutrition: The refeeding syndrome revisited. Am J Clin Nutr 1981;34:393–399

28. Silvis SE, Paragas PD Jr. Paresthesias, weakness, seizures and hypophosphatemia in patients receiving hyperalimentation. Gastroenterology 1972;62:513–520

29. Maier-Dobersberger T, Lochs H. Enteral supplementation of phosphate does not prevent hypophosphatemia during refeeding of cachectic patients. J Parent Enteral Nutr 1994;18:182–184

30. Bloom WL. Carbohydrates and water balance. Am J Clin Nutr 1967;20:157–162

31. Keys A, Henschel A, Taylor HL. The size and function of the human heart at rest in semi-starvation and in the subsequent rehabilitation. Am J Physiol 1947;50:153–169

32. Heymsfield SB, Bethel RA, Ansley JD et al. Cardiac abnormalities in cachectic patients before and during nutritional repletion. Am Heart J 1978;95:584–594

33. Murciano D, Rigaud D, Pingleton S et al. Diaphragmatic function in severely malnourished patients with anorexia nervosa. Effects of renutrition. Am J Respir Crit Care Med 1994;150:1569–1574

34. Arora N, Rochester D. Effect of general nutritional and muscular status on the human diaphragm. Am Rev Respir Dis suppl. 1977;115:84A

35. Heymsfield SB, Casper K. Continuous nasoenteric feeding: bioenergetic and metabolic response during recovery from semistarvation. Am J Clin Nutr 1988;47:900–910

36. Wolfe RR. Carbohydrate metabolism and requirements. In: Rombeau JL, Caldwell MD, Eds. Clinical Nutrition: Parenteral Nutrition. 2nd Ed. Philadelphia: WB Saunders, 1993:113–131

37. Freeman J, Wittine M, Stegink L, Mason ED. Effects of magnesium infusions on magnesium and nitrogen balance during parenteral nutrition. Can J Surg 1982;25:570–574

38. Anast CS, Mohs JM, Kaplan SL, Burns TW. Evidence for parathyroid failure in magnesium deficiency. Science 1972;177:606–608

39. Hendricks KM, Walker WA. Protein-calorie malnutrition: nutrition management. In: Hendricks KM, Walker WA, Eds. Manual of Pediatric Nutrition. Philadelphia: BC Decker, 1990:260–264

40. Burton BT, Foster WR. Nutrition in disease. In: Burton BT, Foster WR, Eds. Human Nutrition. New York: McGraw-Hill, 1988:277–300

41. Hohenbrink K, Nicol JJ. Enteral nutrition support. In: Gottschlich MM, Matarese LE, Shronts EP, Eds. Nutrition Support Dietetics. Core Curriculum. 1993:182–185

42. Chandra RK. Nutrition immunity and infection: present knowledge and future directions. Lancet 1983;1:688–691

43. Hofley PM, Piccoli DA. Inflammatory bowel disease in children. Med Clin North Am 1994;78:1281–1302

44. Sitrin MD. Nutrition support in inflammatory bowel disease. NCP 1992;7:53–60

45. Rosenberg IH, Bengoa JM, Sitrin MD. Nutritional aspects of inflammatory bowel disease. Annu Rev Nutr 1985;5:463–484

46. Silk DBA, Payne-James J. Inflammatory bowel disease: nutritional implications and treatment. Proc Nutr Soc 1989;48:355–361

47. Driscoll RH, Rosenberg IH. Total parenteral nutrition in inflammatory bowel disease. Med Clin North Am 1978;62:185–201

48. Motil KJ, Grand RJ. Nutritional management of inflammatory bowel disease. Pediatr Clin North Am 1985;32:447–469

49. Kanof ME, Lake AM, Bayless TM. Decreased height velocity in children and adolescents before the diagnosis of Crohn's disease. Gastroenterology 1988;95:1523–1527

50. Aiges H, Markowitz J, Rosa J, Daum F. Home nocturnal supplemental nasogastric feedings in growth-retarded adolescents with Crohn's disease. Gastroenterology 1989;97:905–910

51. Kirschner BS, Klish JR, Kalman SS et al. Reversal of growth retardation in Crohn's disease with therapy emphasizing oral nutritional restitution. Gastroenterology 1981;80:10–15

52. Afonso JJ, Rombeau JL. Parenteral nutrition for patients with inflammatory bowel disease. In: Rombeau JL, Caldwell MD, Eds. Clinical Nutrition: Parenteral Nutrition. 2nd Ed. Philadelphia: WB Saunders, 1993:427–441

53. American Society for Parenteral and Enteral Nutrition Board of Directors. Guidelines for the use of parenteral and enteral nutrition in adults and pediatric patients. J Parenteral Enteral Nutr suppl. 1993;17:1SA–52SA

54. Griffiths AM, Ohlsson A, Sherman PM, Sutherland LR. Meta-analysis of enteral nutrition: a primary treatment of active Crohn's disease. Gastroenterology 1995;108:1056–1067

55. Wilschanski M, Sherman P, Pencharz P et al. Supplementary enteral nutrition maintains remission in paediatric Crohn's disease. Gut 1996;38:543–548

12

SPLENOMEGALY

JOHN TUNG
CHRIS A. LIACOURAS

The spleen sits retroperitoneally in the left hypochondriac region in the abdomen between the fundus of the stomach and the diaphragm. It is approximately 12 cm in length, 7 cm in breadth, 3 to 4 cm in thickness, and weighs 170 g in adulthood. In infants, the spleen weighs about 20 g. Four ligaments maintain the spleen in its position: splenophrenic, splenorenal, splenocolic, and gastrosplenic. The gastrosplenic ligament vascular carries the gastrosplenic vessels. The spleen lies on an oblique long axis, parallel to the tenth rib in the mid-axillary line, completely covered by the ninth and eleventh ribs. This makes the spleen susceptible to rupture in rib fractures.

The spleen has functions in erythropoiesis and in immune regulation. The functional units of the spleen can be divided into the red and white pulp. The red pulp consists of blood-filled sinuses and reticuloendothelial cells. The white pulp consists of periarterial collections of lymphocytes and monocytes that resemble germinal centers of the lymphatic system. Most of these cells enter the pulp cords, placing them in direct contact with a meshwork of mononuclear phagocytic cells and triggering host defense. Blood leaves the cords through small membranous slits of 1- to 5-μm width, reaching the sinuses. Approximately 10% of blood bypasses this filtering mechanism, to enter the venous circulation directly. The narrow slits in the pulp cords act to clear abnormal cells, such as spherocytes, antibody-coated platelets, and abnormal erythrocytes. In the fetus, the spleen is a hematopoietic tissue until the end of the second trimester.

SPLENOMEGALY

The spleen is normally palpable in 30% of newborns and in 15% of infants before 6 months age. Subsequently, a palpable spleen greater than 1 cm below the left costal margin signifies splenomegaly. The finding of splenomegaly is usually a coincidental finding during routine physical examination. In most cases, the finding of splenomegaly is pathologic. The causes of splenomegaly can be conveniently grouped into several categories: (1) infections; (2) disorders of immunoregulation; (3) disorders of splenic blood flow; (4) diseases associated with abnormal erythrocytes; (5) infiltrative diseases of the spleen; and (6) miscellaneous diseases. Table 12-1 depicts a clinically useful way of classifying splenomegaly.

CAUSES OF SPLENOMEGALY

Newborn Period

Sepsis is the most likely cause of splenomegaly in the newborn. Infection can be acquired in utero or perinatally. Perinatal infections may be associated with prolonged rupture of membranes. There is an increased risk with maternal fever, urinary tract infections, and vaginal colonization with group B streptococcus, *Escherichia coli*, *Neisseria gonorrhoeae*, *Listeria*, *Chlamydia*, *Candida*, and herpes simplex virus. Congenital infections (TORCH) are those acquired in utero and may be associated with other malformations.

TABLE 12-1. Causes of Splenomegaly in Children

Infections
    Viral disease
        Epstein-Barr virus
        Cytomegalovirus
    Bacterial disease
        Septicemia
    Others
        Malaria
        Toxoplasmosis
Neoplasms
    Leukemia
    Hodgkin's disease
Storage disorders
    Niemann-Pick
    Gaucher's disease
Hemolytic disease
    Hemolytic anemia
        Early sickle cell
        Hereditary spherocytosis
        Thalassemia
    Extramedullary hematopoiesis
Autoimmune
    Systemic lupus erythematosus
    Rheumatoid arthritis
Secondary to portal hypertension
    Liver disease causing portal hypertension
        Congenital hepatic fibrosis
        Biliary atresia
    Vascular disorders
        Cavernous transformation of the portal vessels
    Portal/splenic vein thrombosis
    Budd-Chiari syndrome
Congestive heart disease

Infections

Up to 60% of patients with infectious mononucleosis have detectable splenomegaly as determined by ultrasonographic criteria.[1] The most common cause of infectious mononucleosis is Epstein-Barr virus, a member of the herpesvirus family that affects the B lymphocytes. A blood smear reveals atypical lymphocytes which are activated T lymphocytes that respond to infected B lymphocytes. The enlarged spleen is vulnerable to trauma; rupture has been reported in 0.1% to 0.5% of patients.[2] In these patients, splenic rupture is usually associated with trauma, although it can occur spontaneously.[3] It would be prudent to caution against all contact sports until the spleen normalizes. Other infectious causes of transient splenomegaly include parvovirus, group A streptococcus, adenovirus, coxsackievirus, and rubella virus.[4] Rare infections include chronic Q fever due to *Coxiella burnetti*[5] and cat-scratch fever.[6] Outside the United States, splenomegaly is caused by hepatosplenic schistosomiasis, tuberculosis, human immunodeficiency virus (HIV), and malaria.

Portal Hypertension

Portal hypertension is an important cause of splenomegaly in childhood (for further details, see Ch. 51).

Cavernous Transformation of the Portal Vein

Neovascularization and the appearance of numerous tortuous blood vessels at the liver base without a main portal vein is termed cavernous transformation. Although the cause of cavernous transformation is often unknown, a small population of children who had umbilical vein catheters as neonates may present later in life with portal vein thrombosis (PVT). Other causes of PVT include protein C and S deficiency estrogen supplementation, smoking, hyperviscosity pylephlebitis, and complications of liver transplantation. Following the thrombotic event, new vessels enlarge to bypass the thrombotic site, creating the transformation. Patients with cavernous transformation almost always develop portal hypertension, resulting in splenomegaly. Because esophageal variceal bleeding is a major complication of portal hypertension, physicians should always attempt to determine the cause of splenomegaly. There is no specific treatment for cavernous transformation other than supportive care and therapy for esophageal varices; however, in many patients, new collateral vessels may form around the transformation, bypassing the obstruction and decompressing the portal hypertension.

Budd-Chiari Syndrome

Budd-Chiari syndrome is caused by an obstruction of the inferior vena cava or hepatic veins producing congestive hepatomegaly, gross ascites, and splenomegaly. The obstruction may be due to a variety of causes, such as those seen in PVT. Other causes include congenital webs, irradiation, chemotherapy, or extraluminal compression by tumor or lymph nodes. Treatment is by bypassing the obstruction by transjugular intrahepatic shunt portacaval (TIPS) or by liver transplantation.

Congenital Heart Disease

Congestive splenomegaly can occur secondary to congenital heart disease. Heart disease causes elevated pressure in the vena cava, which is transmitted to the portal and splenic veins.[7]

Bone Marrow Transplantation

Veno-occlusive disease occurs 1 to 3 weeks after bone marrow transplantation. Patients can develop ascites, hepatosplenomegaly, and elevated liver enzyme levels. Chronic graft-versus-host disease and rejection often leads to liver dysfunction, portal hypertension, and splenomegaly. Lymphoproliferative disease is a complication that occurs after organ transplantation and develops when immunosuppression causes a premalignant or malignant proliferation of lymphocytes with concurrent Epstein-Barr virus (EBV) infection.

Malignancy

The spleen is almost always enlarged and is one of the first signs of many childhood malignancies.

Hemolytic Disorders

Chronic hemolytic anemias secondary to diseases that create abnormal hemoglobin and autoimmune hemolytic anemia may produce splenomegaly. In a male child with a history of jaundice, abdominal pain, splenomegaly, and a family history of anemia, hereditary spherocytosis should be strongly considered. Children in the early stages of sickle cell disease often have splenomegaly, even though these patients later become functionally asplenic, as splenic infarcts cause the spleen to involute. Idiopathic thrombocytopenic purpura (ITP) is an immune-mediated disease characterized by thrombocytopenia, purpura, or petechiae; bone marrow aspiration shows megakarocytes in normal or increased numbers.

Gaucher's Disease

Gaucher's disease is caused by defective acid beta-glucosidase activity resulting in cerebroside (glucosylceramide) accumulation in the reticuloendothelial cells of the liver, spleen and bones. It is the most prevalent genetic disease of Ashkenazi Jews. This lysosomal storage disease commonly presents with bleeding associated with thrombocytopenia and splenomegaly. Gaucher's disease and Niemann-Pick syndrome should always be considered in any asymptomatic child who has a significantly enlarged spleen[8,9] (see Ch. 52).

Niemann-Pick Disease

Niemann-Pick disease is an autosomal recessive disorder resulting from a defect of cholesterol esterification leading to accumulation of sphingomyelin in the reticuloendothelial cells of the brain, liver, and spleen. These children have the classic cherry-red maculae[10] (see Ch. 52).

Cholesteryl Ester Storage Disease

Cholesteryl ester storage disease is a rare lysosomal storage disease manifested by excessive storage of cholesteryl esters by macrophages. These patients have massive splenomegaly.[11]

Autoimmune Disorders

While disease such as rheumatoid arthritis, systemic lupus erythematosus, sarcoidosis, and amyloidosis are not commonly seen in children, in adults these diseases have been associated with splenomegaly.

Extracorporeal Membrane Oxygenation and Hemodialysis

Extracorporeal membrane oxygenation (ECMO) is used in neonates who present with diaphragmatic hernias and meconium aspiration syndrome.[12] Hemodialysis is accepted therapy for renal failure. Both treatments may cause splenomegaly.[13] A possible explanation for the condition is splenic sequestration of abnormal blood cells and platelets that undergo mechanical shearing in the respective mechanical circuits.

Idiopathic Splenomegaly

The traditional teaching is that a palpable spleen is always abnormal. However, a few case reports describe a number of patients in whom multiple investigations failed to show any abnormalities despite the clear demonstration of splenomegaly but who are otherwise physically healthy.[14,15]

SPLENIC RUPTURE

An enlarged spleen is always at risk of rupture, even by even minor trauma. A palpable spleen is an unprotected organ and minor falls or injury to the left flank can cause injury to the splenic capsule. The spleen and liver are the two intrabdominal organs most commonly injured by blunt trauma. Children with splenic injury present with diffuse abdominal pain, left upper quadrant pain, or pain referred to the left shoulder due to subphrenic blood accumulation. However, a ruptured spleen can also be present in the absence of any tenderness. Since no supportive connective tissue or muscular walls can regulate blood flow in the spleen, splenic rupture can be associated with very rapid blood loss or death. Therefore, physicians must always be observant for signs and symptoms or hemorrhage in patients with possible splenic trauma. Spontaneous splenic rupture has been described in the literature and can be caused by infectious mononucleosis, sepsis, congenital afibrinogenemia, pregnancy, angiosarcoma of the spleen, peliosis of the spleen, acute *Plasmodium vivax* infection, abscesses of the spleen, and hydatid disease.

PHYSICAL EXAMINATION

The examiner should stand on the patient's right side, placing the left hand beneath the patient's left costovertebral angle pushing the spleen anteriorly. Since the spleen enlarges in the direction toward the right lower quadrant, the examination is conducted with the palmar surface of the right hand feeling for the notched anterior surface, palpating from the right lower quadrant, inching toward the left costal margin, and moving only when the patient expires. A common error is to start palpating at the expected splenic site at the left costal margin; however, in the case of a very enlarged spleen, the notched anterior surface may be below the point at which palpation begins.

Another maneuver used is to roll the patient on his right side. Using the left hand, the examiner pushes on the left lateral wall of the lower rib cage aiding gravity to bring the spleen downward while palpating upward with the right hand. It is sometimes difficult to differentiate an enlarged spleen from an enlarged kidney; however, the kidney is slightly mobile, while the spleen is fixed. Occasionally, a palpable spleen may be normal and only felt secondary to displacement. Whenever a spleen is palpated, its size should be determined through percussion as diseases that cause the left diaphragm or stomach to be pushed inferiorly may cause the spleen to migrate below the rib cage. Serial measurements of the spleen are useful in splenomegaly. Traditionally, measurements are made perpendicular from the left costal margin in the direction of spleen enlargement.

DIAGNOSIS

The finding of splenomegaly is almost always made by physical examination. Often, laboratory studies show a depression of all blood components (hemoglobin, white cells and platelets) secondary to sequestration. Rarely, other diagnostic modalities, such as abdominal ultrasound or computed tomography (CT) scan will prompt an investigation for the cause of splenomegaly. Every patient with splenomegaly should undergo an abdominal ultrasound for evaluation of possible portal hypertension and vascular abnormalities of the hepatosplenic circulation, liver disease and infection (EBV, cytomegalovirus [CMV]), and metabolic disease and trauma.

In anyone suspected of splenic injury, a careful history and low threshold for imaging (ultrasound, CT scan) studies is the key to avoiding a misdiagnosis. These tests may even have to be repeated multiple times during the evaluation.[16] In the absence of positive CT findings in a patient with possible splenic trauma, one needs to be aware of late-onset hemorrhage due to delayed rupture of the spleen.[17–19] Surgical consultation should be obtained.

TREATMENT

Management of splenomegaly depends on the etiology (see Chapters on specific diseases). Management of blunt splenic trauma includes observation in an intensive care setting with aggressive supportive care and monitoring. Every effort is made to preserve the spleen. Occasionally a liver-to-spleen radionuclide study or splenorrhaphy are required. If an operation is necessary, every effort is made to preserve a portion of the spleen as splenectomy has been associated with increased risks of infection with capsular organisms such as *Streptococcus pneumoniae*, *Neisseria meningitidis*, *Escherichia coli*, and *Haemophilus influenzae*. Mortality from sepsis in these asplenic patients varies from 50% to 80%. Asplenic patients should receive prophylactic pneumococcal vaccination and prophylatic antibiotics and should be monitored closely by their primary physician.

CONCLUSION

In children, the presence of splenomegaly should always be considered abnormal. While transient infections, such as EBV or CMV, may promote an enlarged spleen, the cause of splenomegaly should always be determined, as severe complications can occur even in asymptomatic patients.

REFERENCES

1. Dommerby H, Stangerup SE, Stangerup M, Hancke S. Hepatosplenomegaly in infectious mononucleosis, assessed by ultrasonic scanning. J Laryngol Otol 1986;100:573–579
2. Safran D, Bloom GP. Spontaneous splenic rupture following infectious mononucleosis. Am Surg 1990;56:601–605
3. MacGowan JR, Mahendra P, Ager S, Marcus RE. Thrombocytopenia and spontaneous rupture of the spleen associated with infectious mononucleosis. Clin Lab Haematol 1995;17: 93–94
4. Currie JM, Adamson DJ, Brown T, Dawson AA. The fifth cause of splenomegaly?—Parvovirus B19. Clin Lab Haematol 1992;14:327–330
5. Laufer D, Lew PD, Oberhansli I et al. Chronic Q fever endocarditis with massive splenomegaly in childhood. J Pediatr 1986;108:535–539

6. Greenbaum B, Nelson P, Marchildon M, Donaldson M. Hemolytic anemia and hepatosplenomegaly associated with cat-scratch fever. J Pediatr 1986;108:428–430

7. Bennett MR, Shiu MF. Ebstein's anomaly associated with splenomegaly and reversible hypersplenism. Br Heart J 1991; 65:223–224

8. Sibille A, Eng CM, Kim SJ et al. Phenotype/genotype correlations in Gaucher disease type I: clinical and therapeutic implications. Am J Hum Genet 1993;52:1094–1101

9. Pastores GM, Sibille AR, Grabowski GA. Enzyme therapy in Gaucher disease type 1: dosage efficacy and adverse effects in 33 patients treated for 6 to 24 months. Blood 1993;82: 408–416

10. Omarini LP, Frank-Burkhardt SE, Seemayer TA et al. Niemann-Pick disease type C: nodular splenomegaly. Abdom Imag 1995;20:157–160

11. Shawker T, Guzzetta P, Comly M et al. Cholesterol ester storage disease: a patient with massive splenomegaly and splenic abscess. Am J Gastroenterol 1988;83:687–692

12. Hamano K, Hiraoka H, Kouchi Y et al. Klippel-Trenaunay syndrome associated with splenomegaly: report of a case. Surg Today 1995;25:272–274

13. Platts MM, Anastassiades E, Sheriff S et al. Spleen size in chronic renal failure. BMJ 1984;289:1415–1418

14. Arkles LB, Gill GD, Molan MP. A palpable spleen is not necessarily enlarged or pathological. Med J Aust 1986;145: 15–17

15. Hesdorffer CS, Macfarlane BJ, Sandler MA et al. True idiopathic splenomegaly—a distinct clinical entity. Scand J Haematol 1986;37:310–315

16. Raptopoulos V. Abdominal trauma. Emphasis on computed tomography. Radiol Clin North Am 1994;32:969–987

17. Velanovich V, Tapper D. Decision analysis in children with blunt splenic trauma: the effects of observation, splenorrhaphy, or splenectomy on quality-adjusted life expectancy. J Pediatr Surg 1993;28:179–185

18. Spencer DD, Ragland JJ. Delayed splenic rupture: an unusual cause of the acute surgical abdomen. J Am Osteopath Assoc 1993;93:249–251

19. Kluger Y, Paul DB, Raves JJ et al. Delayed rupture of the spleen—myths, facts, and their importance: case reports and literature review. J Trauma 1994;36:568–571

13

VITAMIN DEFICIENCY

ANDREW M. TERSHAKOVEC

Vitamins are essential nutrients that must be supplied exogenously (e.g., in the diet, sunlight). The following chapter details the more important fat- and water-soluble vitamin abnormalities that may present clinically. Pathophysiology, clinical presentation, physical findings, diagnosis, treatment, and supplementation are discussed.

VITAMIN A

Vitamin A has important functions in vision, cell differentiation, morphogenesis, and immune function. In addition, vitamin A deficiency is one of the leading causes of blindness and death in the world. However, overt vitamin A deficiency is rare in the Western world due to the wide availability of foods containing vitamin A and food supplementation.

Clinical Presentation

Xerophthalmia, including Bitot's spots (white foamy conjunctival lesions), is generally pathognomonic for vitamin A deficiency. Early conjunctival changes include thickened wrinkled areas of conjunctivae that appear dry.[1] However, as overt vitamin A deficiency is rare in the United States, xerophthalmia may be misdiagnosed as conjunctivitis that is not responsive to antibiotic therapy.[2] It is crucial to avoid misdiagnosing this condition, as the process can proceed to corneal perforation and blindness. In addition to corneal changes, fundoscopic examination of a person with xerophthalmia may show yellow-white dots on the retina.[1]

Nightblindness or some degree of limited night vision due to decreased rhodopsin levels and vitamin A deficiency may have a subtle presentation. Surveys have shown that persons at risk of vitamin A deficiency (e.g., children with cystic fibrosis) may suffer from some degree of nightblindness, yet not objectively complain of a problem.[3] Follicular hyperkeratosis has also been associated with vitamin A deficiency, although it is not specific to this deficiency.

Children with significant malabsorption and steatorrhea are at risk of vitamin A deficiency. Because of their increased need for growth and reduced vitamin A stores, young children seem particularly vulnerable to the development of vitamin A deficiency. Similarly, since the liver is important in the absorption of fats and fat-soluble vitamins, vitamin A deficiency may be exacerbated in persons with significant liver disease.[4]

Vitamin A supplementation has been noted to decrease morbidity and mortality in areas of the world where poor vitamin A status is endemic.[5-8] Supplementation is useful even in children who show no clinical signs of a vitamin A deficiency. In particular, the deleterious effect of low vitamin A levels in children with measles has been described, and the benefit of supplementing children with severe measles has been demonstrated. These observations have been extended to children in the United States, where the severity of a child's measles has been inversely associated with vitamin A levels.[9-11] However, it is not altogether clear whether these low levels are really indicative of low vitamin A stores or a defect in mobilizing the stores of vitamin A.

Diagnosis

Although unusual in the United States, vitamin A deficiency can occur in a child without evidence of malabsorption solely on the basis of dietary inadequacy. How-

TABLE 13-1. Dosage Recommendations for Oral Administration of Vitamin A

Malabsorption syndrome (prophylaxis), short bowel syndrome, liver disease, or cystic fibrosis
    Children <8 years: 5,000–10,000 U/day
    Children >8 years and adults: 10,000–50,000 U/day; adjust dose based on blood levels

Supplementation in measles
    Children <1 year: 100,000 units/day for 2 days
    Children >1 year: 200,000 units/day for 2 days

Severe deficiency with xerophthalmia
    Children 1–8 years: 5,000–10,000 U/kg/day for 5 days or until recovery occurs
    Children >8 years and adults: 500,000 U/day for 3 days, then 50,000 U/day for 14 days, then 10,000–20,000 U/day for 2 months

Deficiency (without corneal changes)
    Children <1 year: 10,000 units/kg/day for 5 days, then 7,500–15,000 U/day for 10 days
    Children 1–8 years: 5,000–10,000 U/kg/day for 5 days, then 17,000–35,000 U/day for 10 days
    Children >8 years and adults: 100,000 U/day for 3 days, then 50,000 U/day for 14 days

(Adapted from Darby,[14] with permission.)

ever, a diet would have to be extremely restricted to cause vitamin A deficiency. In these cases, the physician should always consider the potential for a feeding disorder, significant socioeconomic limitations, abuse, or neglect. In addition, restricted diets superimposed on malabsorption may combine to induce the deficiency.

While conjunctival changes of xerophthalmia are diagnostic of vitamin A deficiency, repeated bouts of vitamin A deficiency may cause permanent changes resembling Bitot's spots, which may not be indicative of a current deficiency.[12] Functional tests of visual adaptation to darkness may also be used for indirect evaluation of vitamin A status.[13] Plasma vitamin A levels are the most practical and available laboratory evaluation of vitamin A status.

Treatment

With conjunctival changes, treatment constitutes medical emergency to prevent loss of vision. Dosage recommendations for oral administration are listed in Table 13-1.[14]

Toxicity

Although it is important to treat rapidly and effectively, the potential for toxicity must be considered. Neurologic changes, vertigo, pseudotumor cerebri, vomiting, diarrhea, erythema, and peeling skin are associated with tox-

icity. Severe overdoses can be fatal. In addition, relatively low doses (>10,000 IU/day) may be teratogenic, so the potential for pregnancy must be considered with adolescent girls.[15–17]

Vitamin A deficient children who are on a diet low in vitamin A should be treated therapeutically and given dietary counseling. Diets deficient in vitamin A can be modified relatively easily to provide adequate amounts of vitamin A. Liver, eggs, dairy products, fish, dark green leafy vegetables, and yellow and orange fruits and vegetables are good sources of vitamin A and related compounds.[4]

As low vitamin A levels have been observed in children with severe cases of measles, the American Academy of Pediatrics suggests that vitamin A supplementation be considered in the circumstances listed in Table 13-2.[15] Similarly, vitamin A deficiency should be considered in certain subsections of the U.S. population. For example, a survey of low income children in Iowa demonstrated that 25% had marginal vitamin A status.[18]

VITAMIN D

Clinical Presentation

Vitamin D is produced as a by-product of sun exposure of the skin. Children at risk include those who are dark pigmented or who do not get much skin sun exposure (e.g., chronically ill children and those who cover most of their bodies with clothing [cultural or religious cus-

TABLE 13-2. Potential Indications for Vitamin A Supplementation During Measles

Patients aged 6 months to 2 years hospitalized with measles and its complications (e.g., croup, pneumonia, diarrhea). Limited data are available regarding the safety and need for vitamin A supplementation for infants younger than 6 months of age.

Patients older than 6 months of age with measles who have any of the following risk factors and who are not already receiving vitamin A:
    Immunodeficiency (e.g., HIV infection, congenital immunodeficiencies, immunosuppressive therapy)
    Ophthalmologic evidence of vitamin A deficiency, including night blindness, Bitot's spots (grayish-white deposits on the bulbar conjunctiva adjacent to the cornea), or xerophthalmia
    Impaired intestinal absorption (e.g., biliary obstruction, short bowel syndrome, cystic fibrosis)
    Moderate to severe malnutrition, including that associated with eating disorders
    Recent immigration from area in which high mortality rates from measles have been observed

(Data from American Academy of Pediatrics.[15])

tom]). Children with cerebral palsy of cognitive and motor deficits and those who are receiving anticonvulsant therapy for a seizure disorder commonly have limited sun exposure and altered hepatic vitamin D metabolism induced by the anticonvulsant therapy; they may be receiving a diet deficient in calcium and vitamin D. Since breast milk is normally low in vitamin D, breast-fed infants of vitamin D deficient mothers or of mothers who get limited sun exposure or have dark skin pigmentation are also at risk of vitamin D deficiency.[19] Finally, children with significant malabsorption and steatorrhea exhibit malabsorption of vitamin D and calcium (which binds with the unabsorbed fat to form unabsorbable compounds). In children with significant renal disease and, less commonly, in those with significant liver disease, the role of other bodily organs in the intermediary metabolism of vitamin D, can lead to the production of inadequate levels of the active form of vitamin D.

Physical Findings

The classic signs of rickets include bowing of the legs; widening of the epiphyses of the long bones of the arms, legs (seen as thickened or widened wrists and ankles), and distal aspect of the anterior ribs (rachitic rosary); craniotabes; pigeon breast deformity of the chest; muscle weakness; and bone pain. Affected toddlers may stop walking as a result of discomfort and bone pain. As rickets is a condition affecting growing children, children in rapid growth phases (e.g., infancy and adolescence) are more susceptible. Conversely, children who are not growing as a result of illness or other conditions may not display the florid signs of rickets despite a significant vitamin D deficiency. In addition, limited winter sun exposure can lead to frank rickets in children with borderline vitamin D status, during the winter or early spring, especially in northern climates.

Diagnosis

Serum calcium levels are usually maintained until a severe case of vitamin D deficiency has developed. High parathyroid hormone (PTH) levels (secreted to maintain a normal calcium level) help mobilize bone calcium to maintain serum calcium levels. This activity is clinically presented by the rachitic changes in bone described above and by an elevated alkaline phosphatase level. The high PTH levels increase renal absorption of calcium and losses of phosphorus.

Laboratory Evaluation

The classic laboratory presentation of vitamin D deficiency includes a normal serum calcium, elevated PTH and alkaline phosphatase levels, and low serum phosphorus levels. Of note, in the case of significant malnutrition and resultant decreased growth, alkaline phosphatase levels may be reduced, becoming significantly elevated only when nutrient delivery and growth are re-established. The best measure of vitamin D status is 25-hydroxyvitamin D.[20] Other vitamin D levels (e.g., 1,25 dihydroxyvitamin D) may be normal or even elevated despite clinical vitamin D deficiency.

Other Causes

Vitamin D deficiency must be differentiated from other more unusual causes of rickets. Evaluation of the response to an appropriate dose of vitamin D can be used as a diagnostic test to help differentiate between vitamin D deficiency and the other forms of rickets (vitamin D resistant, vitamin D dependent). Children with vitamin D resistant rickets (due to excessive renal phosphorus losses) have bowing of the lower extremities but not other bony changes or hyperparathyroidism related to vitamin D deficiency. These children tend to have depressed phosphorus levels, as compared to children with vitamin D deficient rickets who have normal PTH levels.

Vitamin D dependent rickets, caused by a defect in the 25-hydroxylation of vitamin D or by a defect in the appropriate utilization of vitamin D, usually presents with the classic changes associated with vitamin D deficiency. These children also have low calcium and phosphorus levels and high PTH levels.

Treatment

Prior to starting vitamin D supplements, hypocalcemic children with vitamin D deficiency should receive calcium supplements until their calcium levels approach normal. Rapid supplementation of vitamin D in hypocalcemic vitamin D deficient children may precipitate dangerously low serum calcium levels. Treatment recommendations for oral administration of vitamin D are listed in Table 13-3.[14]

Supplementation

Oversupplementation can cause hypercalcemia. Care must be taken when using nutritional supplements enriched in vitamin D. For example, a case of hypervitaminosis D related to the prolonged use of premature infant formula has been described.[21] The clinical response and calcium and vitamin D levels should be monitored when treating rickets.

VITAMIN E

Clinical Presentation

Although specific clinical syndromes related to vitamin E deficiency have been well described in animals; the clinical presentation of vitamin E deficiency is less well

TABLE 13-3. Dosage Recommendations for Oral Administration of Vitamin D

Nutritional rickets and osteomalacia
    Children and adults (with normal absorption): 25–125 μg/day (1,000–5,000 units)
    Children with malabsorption: 250–625 μg/day (10,000–25,000 units)
    Adults with malabsorption: 250–7,500 μg/day (10,000–300,000 units)

Vitamin D-dependent rickets
    Children: 75–125 μg/day (3,000–5,000 units); maximum: 1,500 μg/day (60,000 units)
    Adults: 250–1,500 μg/day (10,000–60,000 units)

Vitamin D-resistant rickets
    Children: Initial: 1,000–2,000 μg/day (40,000–80,000 units) with phosphate supplements; daily dosage is increased at 3- to 4-month intervals in 250- to 500-μg (10,000–20,000 unit) increments
    Adults: 250–1,500 μg/day (10,000–60,000 units) with phosphate supplements

Dietary supplementation for specific medical conditions
    Children with cystic fibrosis: 10–20 μg/day (400–800 units)
    Children with malabsorption: 25 μg/day (1,000 units)
    Children with liver disease: 100–200 μg/day (4,000–8,000 units)
    Children with renal failure: 100–1,000 μg/day (4,000–40,000 units)

(From Darby,[14] with permission.)

defined in humans. In premature infants, retinopathy of prematurity and hemolysis have been reported to be related to vitamin E deficiency, but this reported association is controversial.[22,23]

Vitamin E deficiency has also been described in association with a wide variety of syndromes associated with steatorrhea. In pediatrics, one of the most common conditions associated with vitamin E deficiency is cystic fibrosis. Shortened erythrocyte survival has been associated with vitamin E deficiency, presumably related to reduced antioxidant activity and resultant hemolysis. An increase in erythrocyte survival and an improved hemoglobin level after vitamin E supplementation have been observed in vitamin E deficient persons.[24–26]

Children with chronic vitamin E malabsorption may develop neurologic dysfunction. For example, children with abetalipoproteinemia seem to suffer neurologic problems related to vitamin E deficiency.[27] (Children with abetalipoproteinemia become vitamin E deficient because of an inability to form chylomicrons and thus efficiently absorb fat and potentially because of a diminished vitamin E carrying capacity related to hypolipoproteinemia.) The neurologic signs and symptoms may be subtle at first, presenting initially with decreased or absent deep tendon reflexes progressing to spinocerebellar ataxia. Ataxia, decreased vibration and position sense,

ophthalmoplegia, muscle weakness, ptosis, dysarthria, pigmented retinopathy, and decreased vision have all been described.[28] In children with lifelong malabsorption, the initial neurologic changes are usually observed by 18 to 24 months of age and become disabling by 10 years of age. In general, the neurologic changes associated with vitamin E deficiency are very responsive to vitamin E therapy, though treatment in a beta lipoproteinemia may have limited efficacy.

Vitamin E Deficiency Syndrome

Isolated vitamin E deficiency syndrome is a unique inborn error of metabolism, unrelated to any of the other disorders associated with vitamin E deficiency (e.g., malabsorption, hypolipoproteinemia). This disease appears to be inherited as an autosomal recessive trait. The neurologic disorder related to this syndrome does not typically involve the eyes.[28] The presentation may be difficult to differentiate from idiopathic ataxia, movement disorders, or peripheral neuropathy; therefore, any child evaluated for these conditions should have its vitamin E level measured.

Diagnosis

The early clinical presentation of vitamin E deficiency can be subtle, leading to a low threshold for formal evaluation of vitamin E status. In practical terms, serum levels are used to evaluate vitamin E status, although these levels do not always reflect the true vitamin E status. A peroxide hemolysis test can be used as an index of antioxidant potential[25,29] and a serum vitamin E level can be used as a screen for deficiency (a normal level rules out deficiency).

Serum vitamin E levels vary with lipoprotein level.[30–32] Children at risk of vitamin E deficiency commonly have altered serum lipid levels. For example, children with fat malabsorption commonly have low serum lipids, while those with liver disease and cholestasis commonly have elevated lipid levels. The best way to evaluate vitamin E status is to obtain a ratio of serum vitamin E to total serum lipids (mg/g).[31] A vitamin E level lower than 0.6 mg/g total serum lipids is thought to represent a deficient state. If total serum lipid levels are unavailable, serum cholesterol or triglycerides can be used to approximate the adjustment for the serum lipid level.[29,30] Serum cholesterol or triglyceride levels are generally more useful in adjusting serum vitamin E levels in adults than in children.

Treatment

Children with significant steatorrhea should receive prophylactic vitamin E supplementation. The range of prophylactic doses varies significantly, depending on the condition and degree of malabsorption. In general, the recommended dose by the oral or enteral route is as follows: 25 to 50 IU/day for infants, 50 to 100 IU/day for children under 10 years, 100 IU/day for 10- to 18-year-olds, and 200 IU/day for those older than 18 years.[22]

Vitamin E deficient children should receive 50 IU/kg/day (25 to 50 IU/day for neonates and premature infants) of vitamin E by the oral or enteral route. In cases of very significant malabsorption and for persons with abetalipoproteinemia, the dose may be increased to 100 or 200 IU/kg/day, as indicated. Water-miscible forms of vitamin E may also be better absorbed in such cases, with the usual starting dose of the water-miscible form 15 to 25 IU/kg/day. If an adequate response is not achieved through enteral supplementation, parenteral supplementation should be considered (e.g., parenteral multivitamin solution, as used with parenteral nutrition).

Toxicity

Although vitamin E appears to be safe even when using very large doses, toxicity producing a vitamin K related coagulopathy and interference with vitamin K and A absorption have been reported.[32]

VITAMIN K

Clinical Presentation

Vitamin K deficiency presents with a bleeding tendency either in response to cuts, trauma, or surgery or as spontaneous bleeding in severe cases. Cases can also mimic child abuse.[33] Vitamin K is widely distributed in food and is produced by intestinal bacteria. Thus, persons who have generalized malabsorption, fat malabsorption, or altered intestinal bacteria (e.g., children receiving chronic antibiotics) are at risk of vitamin K deficiency.

Hemorrhagic disease of the newborn can present during the first day of life (early onset), during the first week of life (classic), or during the first few weeks of life (late onset).[34] Newborns are relatively deficient in vitamin K, as the placenta does not efficiently deliver vitamin K to the fetus. In addition, the immaturity of the neonate's liver and the lack of bacteria (which normally produce vitamin K) in the newborn's gut contribute to the potential problem.[34,35] Since breast milk is a poor source of vitamin K, breast-fed children who did not receive adequate vitamin K prophylaxis at birth may develop late-onset hemorrhage. Infants with malabsorption, however fed, can be similarly affected. Early-onset hemorrhage is usually associated with maternal drug administration (e.g., anticonvulsants, warfarin). Classic and late-onset cases are predominantly idiopathic.[34]

Older children generally present with vitamin K deficiency secondary to malabsorptive disorders, such as cystic fibrosis, short bowel syndrome, or cholestasis. Disruption of colonic flora and associated vitamin K production due to chronic antibiotic administration generally will not cause a significant coagulopathy without another risk factor for vitamin K deficiency (e.g., inadequate diet or malabsorption). Bleeding associated with the administration of small amounts of heparin (e.g., to keep an intravenous line patent) may unmask a previously subclinical vitamin K deficiency.[36]

Diagnosis

Any child presenting with abnormal or excessive bleeding should be evaluated for vitamin K status. Assays for accurate evaluation of vitamin K levels are not currently available for clinical use.[37] Therefore, indirect measures of coagulation status are used. A prolonged prothrombin time (PT) is consistent with vitamin K deficiency. Normalization of the PT after one or more doses of 2.5 to 5 mg intravenous (IV), intramuscular (IM), or oral (PO) vitamin K is diagnostic. It is important to note, however, that a child may be relatively vitamin K deficient, yet have a normal PT. Since infants with hemorrhagic disease of the newborn may have lower vitamin K levels due to low maternal vitamin K levels, evaluation of coagulation status of the mothers of infants with hemorrhagic disease of the newborn should be considered.

Treatment

Prophylactic intramuscular injections of 1 mg of vitamin K should be given to all newborn infants. The association described between intramuscular vitamin K and childhood leukemia and cancer[38,39] is not consistent with most existing epidemiologic data (e.g., no significant increase in the incidence of childhood leukemia was seen after the 1961 recommendation of the American Academy of Pediatrics to give prophylactic intramuscular vitamin K to all newborns).[40,41] Given the morbidity and mortality of hemorrhagic disease of the newborn, concrete evidence of a risk that outweighs the known risks of hemorrhaging must be demonstrated. Although some centers have demonstrated the relative safety of the use of multiple doses of oral vitamin K supplementation with newborns,[42] others suggest that an increase in the incidence of hemorrhagic disease of the newborn has accompanied the use of oral vitamin K prophylaxis.[34] Similarly, the use of maternal vitamin K supplementation in breast-fed children in place of direct infant supplementation has mixed efficacy.[43,44] Therefore, medical caregivers must very carefully judge the potential risk when making a change from the established practice of intramuscular vitamin K, as well as the added compliance and follow-up issues raised by the use of a multiple dosing oral regimen. For children bleeding from hemorrhagic disease of the newborn, immediate administration of vitamin K, 1 to 2 mg IM or IV is recommended and may be repeated as indicated. Intravenous use is rarely associated with anaphylaxis. Thus, IV administration is for emergencies only.

Prophylaxis

Prophylactic doses for children at risk of the development of vitamin K deficiency (e.g., children with malabsorption or those receiving chronic antibiotics) should be considered. Although it is difficult to be specific with dosing recommendations, infants and children generally receive vitamin K 1 to 5 mg/day to once or twice per week. Prolonged enteral maintenance therapy is usually effective in all but the most extreme cases of malabsorption. In those children at risk of significant bleeding, intramuscular or intravenous administration is indicated (although intramuscular injections may be contraindicated for those who have a coagulopathy). Parenteral doses usually range from 1 to 5 mg.

As vitamin K is well stored in the body, daily supplementation is unnecessary. The dosage schedule can thus be adapted to optimize compliance. Children requiring ongoing vitamin K supplementation should have PT regularly monitored.

VITAMIN B$_{12}$

Gastric parietal cells produce intrinsic factor. Intrinsic factor binds free vitamin B$_{12}$. The vitamin B$_{12}$-intrinsic factor complex is then absorbed in the terminal ileum. Functional or structural abnormalities of the stomach or terminal ileum can prevent adequate absorption of vitamin B$_{12}$. Since pancreatic bicarbonate and trypsin also facilitate this process, pancreatic dysfunction is another factor predisposing to vitamin B$_{12}$ deficiency. Additionally, colonic bacteria ingest vitamin B$_{12}$. Those with small bowel bacterial overgrowth may develop a vitamin B$_{12}$ deficiency. Despite these risk factors, as the body is very efficient in processing vitamin B$_{12}$, it may take years or even decades for persons who malabsorb vitamin B$_{12}$ or who ingest a vitamin B$_{12}$ deficient diet to manifest the clinical signs and symptoms of vitamin B$_{12}$ deficiency.

Clinical Presentation

In most cases, a macrocytic anemia precedes the development of neurologic disease. Folate supplementation may block the development of the anemia, which prevents easy diagnosis until the neurologic signs are evident. The neurologic dysfunction related to vitamin B$_{12}$ deficiency seems to be related to myelination defects and includes paresthesia, especially of the hands and feet, loss of vibratory and position sense, unsteadiness, ataxia, poor memory, confusion, depression, hallucinations, and psychosis.[45] Severe forms may cause long lasting, if not permanent, damage, even after adequate treatment.[46]

A rare autosomal recessive syndrome caused by the inability to secrete intrinsic factor or by the secretion of a functionally limited intrinsic factor has been described (congenital pernicious anemia). Children with this disease usually present at 9 months to 11 years of age after stores of vitamin B$_{12}$ gained in utero are exhausted.[47]

Diagnosis

Vitamin B$_{12}$ is essential to hematopoiesis. Therefore, a deficiency causes a macrocytic anemia. Disrupted DNA synthesis causes megaloblastic (i.e., containing hypersegmented nuclei) white blood cells. In most cases, the megaloblastic anemia precedes the neurologic disease of vitamin B$_{12}$ deficiency; however, in some persons the evaluation of a complete blood count for mean corpuscular volume and hemoglobin level is not an adequate screening test. A serum vitamin B$_{12}$ level is generally an adequate test of vitamin B$_{12}$ status, although signs of clinical deficiency have been reported despite normal serum levels.

Schilling Test

If the etiology of the deficiency is not obvious, the Schilling test is recommended to help identify the defect associated with the deficiency. This involves giving labeled vitamin B$_{12}$ orally with and without intrinsic factor to help differentiate between a deficiency of intrinsic factor and malabsorption.

Treatment

Since vitamin B$_{12}$ is not present in plant foodstuffs, strict vegetarians need to take vitamin B$_{12}$ supplements. In cases of true deficiency, intramuscular or deep subcutaneous administration is recommended. For congenital pernicious anemia, 1,000 μg/day for at least 2 weeks, followed by maintenance doses of 50 μg/month, should be given. For vitamin B$_{12}$ deficiency in older children, 100 μg/day for 10 to 15 days (total dose 1.0 to 1.5 mg), then once or twice weekly, and then 60 μg/month is recommended. For older adolescents and adults, 30 μg/day for 5 to 10 days and 100 to 200 μg/month is recommended.[14]

OTHER WATER-SOLUBLE VITAMINS

True deficiencies of water-soluble vitamins, other than vitamin B$_{12}$, are rare in the developed countries, given the relative abundance of a wide range of foods and

TABLE 13-4. Clinical Signs of Water-Soluble Vitamin Deficiencies

Vitamin	Signs of Clinical Deficiency
Biotin	Dermatitis, anorexia, muscle pain, alopecia
Vitamin B_{12}	Megaloblastic anemia, dementia, peripheral neuropathy, methylmalonic acidemia
Folate	Megaloblastic anemia, pancytopenia, peripheral neuropathy, neural tube defects in offspring
Niacin (pellagra)	Dermatitis, diarrhea, dementia
Pantothenic acid	Depression, hypotension, weakness, abdominal pain
Pyridoxine	Dermatitis, glossitis, cheilosis, peripheral neuritis, irritability, convulsions, anemia
Riboflavin	Photophobia, cheilosis, glossitis, corneal vascularization, poor growth, dyssebacia, angular stomatitis
Thiamine	Beriberi: neuritis, edema, heart failure, anorexia, aphonia; Wernicke-Korsakoff syndrome; infantile beriberi: anorexia, vomiting, pallor, restlessness, insomnia, aphonia or hoarse cry, convulsions, opisthotonos, constipation
Ascorbic acid	Infantile scurvy: fretfulness, pallor, anorexia, localized joint swelling and tenderness, costochondral junction enlargement (scorbutic rosary), skin and mucous membrane hemorrhage, bone, joint, and muscle pain, perifollicular hemorrhages, gingivitis, loose teeth

(Adapted from McLaren[49] and Greer,[50] with permission.)

TABLE 13-5. Conditions Commonly Associated With Deficiencies or Requiring Vitamin Supplementation in Children and Adolescents

Sickle cell anemia (folate)

Chronic hemolytic anemia (folate)

Breast-fed infants (vitamin K, vitamin D)

Breast-fed infants of mothers with nutritional deficiencies (dependent on maternal deficiency)

Infants born to mothers receiving anticonvulsant therapy (vitamin K, vitamin D)

Chronic diarrhea/malabsorption/steatorrhea (fat-soluble vitamins)

Crohn's disease (fat-soluble vitamins, vitamin B_{12})

Short bowel syndrome (fat-soluble vitamins, vitamin B_{12})

Cystic fibrosis (fat-soluble vitamins)

Cholestasis (fat-soluble vitamins)

Terminal ileal resection/disease (fat-soluble vitamins, vitamin B_{12})

Biliary atresia (fat-soluble vitamins)

Abetalipoproteinemia/hypobetalipoproteinemia (fat-soluble vitamins)

Intestinal bacterial overgrowth (fat-soluble vitamins, vitamin B_{12})

Cholestyramine administration (fat-soluble vitamins)

Sulfasalazine administration (folate)

Adolescent girls who may become pregnant (multivitamins, especially folate)

Strict vegetarians (vitamin B_{12})

(Adapted from data in McLaren.[49])

food supplementation. The need for some of these vitamins is increased in some metabolic disorders, whereas certain metabolic disorders may respond to increased vitamin supplementation (e.g., thiamine-responsive maple syrup urine disease, treatment of glutaric acidemia type II with increased riboflavin supplementation). For the child who presents with signs and symptoms of a water-soluble vitamin deficiency (Table 13-4), more than a cursory evaluation should be undertaken to find the true etiology.[48,49] Several medical conditions require increased micronutrient levels of water-soluble vitamins (Table 13-5). For example, small bowel bacterial overgrowth (Table 13-6) may precipitate a deficiency in vitamin B_{12}, while those with sickle cell disease or other chronic hemolytic anemias have increased folate requirements due to the rapid production and turnover of red cells.

TABLE 13-6. Potential Causes of Small Intestine Bacterial Overgrowth

Gastrointestinal dysmotility
  Pseudo-obstruction (idiopathic)
  Scleroderma
  Following bowel or surgery resection
  Medications (e.g., opiates, morphine)

Decreased gastric acid secretion

Blind loop

Loss of ileocecal valve

Intestinal fistula

Structural abnormalities of gastrointestinal tract

Malnutrition

(From Heyman and Perman,[51] with permission.)

REFERENCES

1. Tielsch JM, Sommer A. The epidemiology of vitamin A deficiency and xerophthalmia. Annu Rev Nutr 1984;4: 183–205

2. Duffy TP. Clinical problem-solving. N Engl J Med 1994;330: 994–996

3. Rayner RJ, Tyrrell JC, Hiller EJ et al. Night blindness and conjunctival xerosis caused by vitamin A deficiency in patients with cystic fibrosis. Arch Dis Child 1989;64: 1151–1156

4. Olson JA. Vitamin A, retinoids, and carotenoids. In: Shils ME, Olson JA, Shike M, Eds. Modern Nutrition in Health and Disease. Philadelphia: Lea & Febiger, 1994:287–307

5. Coutsoudis A, Broughton M, Coovadia HM. Vitamin A supplementation reduces measles morbidity in young African children: a randomized, placebo-controlled, double-blind trial. Am J Clin Nutr 1991;54:890–895

6. Hussey GD, Klein M. A randomized, controlled trial of vitamin A in children with severe measles. N Engl J Med 1990; 323:160–164

7. West KP, Kokhrel RP, Katz J et al. Efficacy of vitamin A in reducing preschool child mortality in Nepal. Lancet 1991; 338:67–71

8. Fawzi WW, Herrera MG, Willett WC et al. Dietary vitamin A intake and the risk of mortality among children. Am J Clin Nutr 1994;59:401–408

9. Frieden TR, Sowell AL, Henning KJ et al. Vitamin A levels and severity of measles. Am J Dis Child 1992;146:182–186

10. Butler JC, Havens PL, Sowell AL et al. Measles severity and serum retinol (vitamin A) concentration among children in the United States. Pediatrics 1993;91:1176–1181

11. Arrieta AC, Zaleska M, Stutman HR, Marks MI. Vitamin A levels in children with measles in Long Beach, California. J Pediatr 1992;121:75–78

12. Sommer A. Field Guide to the Detection and Control of Xerophthalmia. Geneva: World Health Organization, 1982

13. Goodman DS. Biosynthesis, absorption and hepatic metabolism of retinol. In: Sporn MB, Roberts AB, Goodman DS, Eds. The Retinoids. New York: Academic Press, 1984;1–39

14. Darby M, Ed. The Children's Hospital of Philadelphia Pharmacy Handbook and Formulary. Alphabetical Listing of Drugs. Hudson, OH: Lexi-Comp, 1995

15. American Academy of Pediatrics. Measles. In: Peter G, Ed. 1997 Red Book: Report of the Committee on Infectious Diseases. 24th ed. Elk Grove Village, IL: American Academy of Pediatrics, 1997;346

16. Oakley GP, Erickson JD. Vitamin A and birth defects (letter). N Engl J Med 1995;333:1414–1415

17. Rothman KJ, Moore LL, Singer MR et al. Teratogenicity of high vitamin A intake. N Engl J Med 1995;333:1369–1373

18. Spannaus-Martin DJ, Tanumihardio S, Cook L, Olson JA. The vitamin A statuses of young children with several ethnic groups in a socioeconomically disadvantaged urban population. FASEB 1994;8:A94

19. Committee on Nutrition of the American Academy of Pediatrics. Vitamin and mineral supplement needs of healthy children in the United States. In: Barness LA, Ed. Pediatric Nutrition Handbook. Elk Grove Village, IL: American Academy of Pediatrics 1993;34–42

20. Holick MF. Vitamin D. In: Shils ME, Olson JA, Shike M, Eds. Modern nutrition in health and disease. Philadelphia: Lea & Febiger, 1994;308–325

21. Nako Y, Fukushima N, Tomomasa T et al. Hypervitaminosis D after prolonged feeding with a premature formula. (letter) Pediatrics 1993;92:862–864

22. Farrell PM, Roberts RJ. Vitamin E. In: Shils ME, Olson JA, Shike M, Eds. Modern nutrition in health and disease. Philadelphia: Lea & Febiger, 1994;326–341

23. Phelps DL. Current perspectives on vitamin E in infant nutrition. Am J Clin Nutr 1987;46:187–191

24. Farrell PM, Machlin LJ. Human health and disease. In: Machlin LJ, Ed. Vitamin E, a Comprehensive Treatise. New York: Marcel Dekker, 1980;520–620

25. Farrell PM, Bieri JG, Fratantoni JF et al. The occurrence and effects of human vitamin E deficiency. A study of patients with cystic fibrosis. J Clin Invest 1977;60:233–241

26. Kelleher J, Miller MG, Littlewood JM et al. The clinical effects of correction of vitamin E depletion in cystic fibrosis. Int J Vitam Nutr Res 1987;57:253–259

27. Scully RE, Mark EJ, McNeely WF, McNeely BU. Case records of the Massachusetts General Hospital, Case 35–1992. N Engl J Med 1992;327:628–635

28. Sokol RJ. Vitamin E deficiency and neurologic disease. Annu Rev Nutr 1988;8:351–373

29. Farrell PM, Levine SL, Murphy MD, Adams AJ. Plasma tocopherol levels and tocopherol-lipid relationships in a normal population of children as compared to healthy adults. Am J Clin Nutr 1978;31:1720–1726

30. Horwitt MK, Harvey CC, Dahm CH, Searcy MT. Relationship between tocopherol and serum lipid levels for determination of nutritional adequacy. Ann NY Acad Sci 1972;203: 223–236

31. Sokol RJ, Heubi JE, Iannaccone ST et al. Vitamin E deficiency with normal serum vitamin E concentrations in children with chronic cholestasis. N Engl J Med 1984;310: 1209–1212

32. Bieri JG, Corash L, Hubbard VS. Medical uses of vitamin E. N Engl J Med 1983;308:1063–1071

33. Wetzel RC, Slater AJ, Dover GJ. Fatal intramuscular bleeding misdiagnosed as suspected nonaccidental injury, case report. Pediatrics 1995;95:771–773

34. Shearer MJ. Vitamin K. Lancet 1995;345:229–234

35. Nelson WE, Behrman RE, Kliegman RM, Arvin AM, Eds. Blood disorders. In: Nelson's Textbook of Pediatrics, 15th ed. Philadelphia: WB Saunders, 1996;499–505

36. Shah MC, Schwarz KB. Hazards of small amounts of heparin, in a patient with subclinical vitamin K deficiency. JPEN J Parent Ent Nutr 1989;13:324–325

37. von Kries R, Greer FR, Suttie JW. Assessment of vitamin K status of the newborn infant. J Pediatr Gastroenterol Nutr 1993;16:231–238

38. Golding J, Paterson M, Kinlen LJ. Factors associated with childhood cancer in a national cohort study. Br J Cancer 1990;52:304–308

39. Golding J, Greenwood R, Birmingham K, Mott M. Childhood cancer, intramuscular vitamin K, and pethidine given during labour. BMJ 1992;305:341–346

40. Vitamin K Ad Hoc Task Force of the American Academy of Pediatrics. Controversies concerning vitamin K and the newborn. Pediatrics 1993;91:1001–1003

41. Draper G, McNinch A. Vitamin K for neonates: the controversy. BMJ 1994;308:867–868

42. Clark FI, James EJ. Twenty-seven years of experience with oral vitamin K1 therapy in neonates. J Pediatr 1995;127:301–304

43. Greer FR, Marshall S, Cherry J, Suttie JW. Vitamin K status of lactating mothers, human milk, and breast-feeding infants. Pediatrics 1991;88:751–756

44. Greer FR, Marshall S, Suttie JW. Maternal vitamin K1 supplements—effects on human milk concentrations and intakes in breast feeding infants. Pediatr Res 1994; 35:312A

45. Herbert V, Das KC. Folic acid and vitamin B_{12}. In: Shils ME, Olson JA, Shike M, Eds. Modern Nutrition in Health and Disease. Philadelphia: Lea & Febiger, 1994;402–425

46. Graham SM, Arvela OM, Wise GA. Long-term neurologic consequences of nutritional vitamin B_{12} deficiency in infants. J Pediatr 1992;121:710–714

47. Megaloblastic anemias. In: Behrman RE, Kliegman RM, Arvin AM, Eds. Nelson's Textbook of Pediatrics, 15th ed. Philadelphia: WB Saunders, 1996;1384–1387

48. Barness LA, Curran JS. Nutritional requirements. In: Behrman RE, Kliegman RM, Arvin AM, Eds. Nelson's Textbook of Pediatrics, 15th ed. Philadelphia: WB Saunders, 1996; 141–151

49. McLaren DS. Clinical manifestations of human vitamin and mineral disorders: a resume. In: Shils ME, Olson JA, Shike M, Eds. Modern Nutrition in Health and Disease. Malvern, PA: Lea & Febiger, 1994;909–923

50. Greer FR. Nutritional needs of the full-term and low-birthweight infant. In: Rudolph AM, Ed. Rudolph's Pediatrics. 19th Ed. Norwalk, CT: Appleton & Lange, 1991;240

51. Heyman MB, Perman JA. Nutrition in bacterial overgrowth syndromes of gastrointestinal tract. In: Grand RJ, Sutphen JL, Dietz WH, Eds. Pediatric Nutrition—Theory and Practice. Boston: Butterworths, 1987;446

14

VOMITING

RITU VERMA

Vomiting involves the forceful expulsion of the contents of the stomach. This unpleasant activity may be a protective reflex, since it promotes rapid expulsion of ingested toxins or relieves pressure in hollow organs distended by distal obstruction. Vomiting is a feature of many disorders. It may be the only presenting symptom of many diseases, including disorders causing increased intracranial pressure, metabolic diseases, and anatomic and mucosal gastrointestinal (GI) abnormalities. It is often preceded by nausea and retching.

Nausea is an epigastric or abdominal sensation accompanied by a variety of autonomic changes, including reduced gastric tone, contractions, secretion, and mucosal blood flow; increased salivation, sweating, pupil diameter, and heart rate; and changed respiratory rhythm.[1] Duodenal gastric reflux may occur during nausea, accompanied by retrograde peristalsis from the small intestine to the antrum or by generalized simultaneous contractions of the antrum and the duodenum.[2,3]

Retching is an involuntary effort to vomit and may be seen as preparatory maneuvers to vomiting. The effort consists of spasmodic contractions of the somatic muscles of the diaphragm and the abdominal wall at the same time the lower esophageal sphincter relaxes. The lower esophageal sphincter is also pulled cephalad by contraction of the striated longitudinal muscles of the upper esophagus and may herniate through the crural hiatus, preventing the increased intra-abdominal pressure from being transmitted to the lower esophageal sphincter.[4] During retching, gastric material is moved into the esophagus by the combination of increased positive intra-abdominal pressure and increased negative intra-

thoracic pressure, but this material may be returned to the stomach by secondary peristalsis.[5]

PATHOPHYSIOLOGY

The response of vomiting is mediated by neural efferents in the vagal, phrenic, and spinal nerves (Fig. 14-1). Input to these nerves is from the brain stem "vomiting center." There is no single anatomic structure identified as the "vomiting center," but the final pathway is through medullary intraneurons in the solitary tract nucleus and a variety of sites in the nearby reticular formation.

DIFFERENTIAL DIAGNOSIS OF VOMITING

Vomiting is a prominent feature of many disorders. The causes may be classified as follows: (1) disorders of various systems in the body, (2) age of the patient, and (3) associated symptoms or signs. Table 14-1 presents a list of disorders associated with vomiting; however, because the differential diagnosis varies with the age of the patient, it is very helpful for the physician treating these patients to follow specific guidelines (Table 14-2). Severe congenital anatomic, genetic, and metabolic disorders are more commonly seen during the neonatal period. Feeding intolerances as new foods are introduced, gastroesophageal reflux, and less severe congenital diseases occur in infancy. Peptic infection and psychogenic causes are more prominent with increasing age.[6]

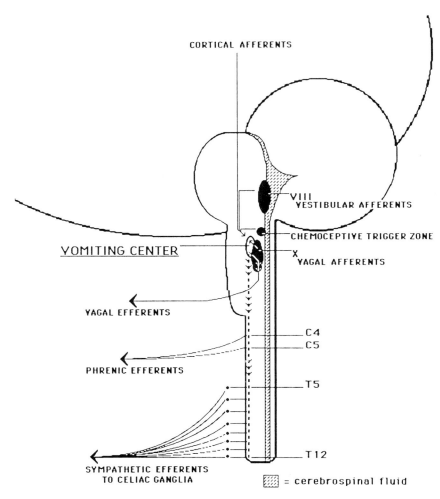

FIGURE 14-1. Neuroanatomy of vomiting. Midsagittal view of a portion of the cerebral cortex, the cerebellum, the pons, the medulla, and the spinal cord. The vomiting center receives input from the cortex, from the vestibular system (via the vestibular nucleus—VIII), from the blood (via the chemoceptive trigger zone—the area postrema), and from the gastrointestinal periphery (via the vagal nuclei—X). Output from the vomiting center through vagal, phrenic, and sympathetic nerves produces the complex stereotypic behavior associated with emesis. (Adapted from Orenstein,[5] with permission.)

ASSOCIATED SIGNS AND SYMPTOMS

Vomiting can have several causes. Often the physician must determine the severity of the illness to prioritize the care. Associated signs and symptoms help streamline the workup of the patient (Table 14-3).

VOMITING SYNDROMES

Regurgitation

Regurgitation is the effortless return of gastric contents to the mouth and not usually associated with nausea or retching. This is characteristic of infant gastroesophageal reflux (GER) (for an in-depth discussion, see Ch. 25).

Cyclical Vomiting Syndrome

Cyclical vomiting syndrome is uncommon and is characterized by recurrent episodes of nausea and vomiting without identifiable organic cause. It is usually a diagnosis of exclusion, managed symptomatically, and of un-

known prognosis. Episodes are usually of rapid onset, often starting during sleep or in the early morning, persisting for hours to days, and separated by symptom-free intervals that can range from several weeks to a year. The episodes may end spontaneously or may produce severe fluid and electrolyte imbalance, requiring fluid management. In most cases, there are few residual complications, and patients suddenly seem better. Each patient has the same pattern to each attack, and often stress or minor intercurrent illness is noted at onset. Headaches of various types are present in up to 25% of patients, as reported in some series.[7] In 62% of cases, there is a familial and personal history of irritable bowel symptoms.[8] A meticulous search for organic diseases that produce recurrent episodes of vomiting should be undertaken. Important in the differential diagnosis are urea cycle defects, organic acid metabolism and gastric and intestinal motility disorders, peptic diseases, central nervous system (CNS) abnormalities (especially seizures), familial dysautonomia, obstructive uropathy, obstructive cholangiopathy, familial pancreatitis, malrotation, duplication, strictures, diverticula of the intestines, adrenal insufficiency, and diabetes mellitus.[6]

TABLE 14-1. Differential Diagnosis of Vomiting

Gastrointestinal

Anatomic
  Oropharynx: cleft palate, macroglossia
  Esophageal: stricture, web, ring, atresia, tracheoesophageal fistula
  Stomach: pyloric stenosis, web, duplication, microgastria
  Intestine: duodenal atresia, malrotation, duplication
  Colon: Hirschsprung's disease, imperforate anus
  Annular pancreas
  Choledochal cyst
Motility
  Achalasia
  Gastroesophageal reflux
  Pseudo-obstruction
Foreign body/bezoar
Obstruction
  Intussusception
  Volvulus
  Incarcerated hernia
Cholecystitis or cholelithiasis
Eosinophilic enteritis
Appendicitis
Necrotizing enterocolitis
Peritonitis
Celiac disease
Peptic ulcer
Trauma
  Duodenal hematoma
  Pancreatitis (pseudocyst)

Neurologic

Intracranial mass lesions
  Tumor
  Cyst
  Subdural hematoma
Cerebral edema
Hydrocephalus
Pseudotumor cerebri
Migraine (head, abdominal)
Seizures

Renal

Obstructive uropathy
  Ureteropelvic junction obstruction
  Hydronephrosis
  Nephrolithiasis
Renal insufficiency
Glomerulonephritis
Renal tubular acidosis

Metabolic

Inborn errors of metabolism
  Galactosemia
  Fructose intolerance
  Hereditary fructose intolerance
  Amino acid or organic acid metabolism
  Urea cycle defects
  Fatty acid oxidation disorders
  Lactic acidosis
  Lysosomal storage diseases
  Peroxisomal disorders

Genetic

Smith-Lemli-Opitz syndrome
Trisomy 21, 13, 18 syndromes
Familial dysautonomia
Prader-Willi syndrome—newborn
Cornelia de Lange's syndrome
Cri-du-chat syndrome

Infectious

Sepsis
Meningitis
Urinary tract infection
Parasites
Giardia
Ascaris
Helicobacter pylori
Otitis media
Bordetella pertussis
Viral
  Gastroenteritis
  Viral hepatitis (A, B, C)

Endocrine

Diabetes
  Diabetic ketoacidosis (DKA)
  Gastroparesis
Adrenal insufficiency

Respiratory

Pneumonia
Sinusitis
Pharyngitis

Immunologic

Milk/soy protein allergy
Cryptosporidium (AIDS)
Graft-versus-host reaction
Chronic granulomatous disease

Other

Pregnancy
Rumination
Bulimia
Psychogenic
"Cyclic vomiting" syndrome
Overfeeding
Medications/drugs/vitamin toxicity
Vascular (superior mesenteric artery syndrome)
Child abuse—chronic subdural
Chronic congestive heart failure

(Adapted from Wyllie R. Pediatric endoscopy. Gastrointest Endosc Clin North Am 1994;4:60–61.)

TABLE 14-2. Differential Diagnosis of Vomiting by Age

Newborn
    Congenital obstructive gastrointestinal malformations
        Atresias or webs of esophagus or intestine
        Meconium ileus or plug; Hirschsprung's disease
    Inborn errors of metabolism

Infant
    Acquired or milder obstructive lesions: pyloric stenosis, mal-
        rotation and volvulus, intussusception
    Metabolic diseases, milder inborn errors of metabolism
    Nutrient intolerances
    Functional disorders: gastroesophageal reflux
    Psychosocial disorders: rumination, injury due to child abuse

Child—most causes from Table 14-1

Adolescent—most childhood causes, plus pregnancy, drugs (of abuse, suicide), eating disorders

(Adapted from Orenstein,[5] with permission.)

Investigations should be targeted toward conditions suggested by the history. Symptomatic treatment, such as intravenous fluids and nasogastric suction, should be instituted as early as possible. Lorazepam, butyrophenones, and benzamides can be helpful on occasion. Propranolol has been used prophylactically in some cases.[9] Family education about the benign nature of the condition and early initiation of appropriate treatment are very important. Psychological evaluation may also be helpful.

Psychogenic Vomiting

Psychogenic vomiting is a syndrome that has no organic cause. Cortical and psychological input may cause nausea and vomiting. This syndrome is usually chronic, associated with stress and with meals. It can be easily suppressed, and relief can be obtained by hospitalization. Vomiting may be self-induced.

Rumination

Rumination is frequent regurgitation of previously ingested food into the mouth. The food is then re-chewed and swallowed or spit out. It is not associated with nausea, retching, or vomiting. Rumination is often seen in mentally retarded children, in cases of child neglect, in neonates during prolonged hospitalization,[10] in children and infants with untreated GER,[11] and in older children (in association with bulimia). Adults and older children may regurgitate by contracting the abdominal muscles.[12] Treatment should include increased personal attention, especially during feeds, and behavior therapy, except in the cases of GER and bulimia. Differentiation from the other causes of vomiting should be pursued; this may entail extensive testing.

Abdominal Migraine

A patient with abdominal migraine may present with abdominal pain that could be epigastric or periumbilical, accompanied by nausea, vomiting, and diarrhea. Other symptoms, such as fever, irritability, and vertigo, may also be associated. In 30% to 40% of patients, headaches are reported as well. These attacks occur suddenly and may last for variable periods; such attacks are consistent in character within the same person. Patients are asymptomatic between attacks. There may be a family history of migraine headaches. Prophylactic propranolol is helpful, and ergotamine may abort an episode.

Superior Mesenteric Artery Syndrome

Superior mesenteric artery syndrome is characterized by extrinsic compression of the duodenum, between the superior mesenteric artery anteriorly and the aorta posteriorly, as the superior mesenteric artery crosses over the duodenum in the root of the mesentery.[13] The compression is usually to the right of the midline, often with proximal dilation. These patients usually experience bilious vomiting and epigastric abdominal pain relieved by vomiting and by placement in the prone or knee-chest position. This is often seen in patients who have undergone significant weight loss, lengthy bed rest, or prior abdominal surgery. Adolescents and young adults are most often affected.

Bulimia

Bulimia is an eating disorder of psychogenic origin, characterized by recurrent episodes of binge eating, followed by purging induced by vomiting, diarrhea, diet, and exercise.[15] This condition is most commonly seen in adolescents and college-age girls.

DIAGNOSTIC STUDIES

Evaluation is based on the associated signs and symptoms of vomiting and the final narrowed-down differential diagnosis. Suggested screening laboratory investigations of prolonged vomiting exhibited by any child would include complete blood count, blood chemistry, urinalysis, urine culture, blood urea nitrogen (BUN) and creatinine, amylase and lipase, stool for occult blood, leukocytes, and parasites. The approach depends on the history and physical examination: (1) radiologic investigations, for example, plain abdominal radiographs, for obstruction; (2) abdominal ultrasound in cases of pyloric stenosis; and (3) an upper GI series to rule out any anatomic abnormalities. Endoscopic evaluation of the upper GI tract is helpful if one is concerned about inflammation as well as obtaining cultures for infections, for example

TABLE 14-3. Differential Diagnosis of Vomiting by Associated Symptoms and Signs

Contents of vomitus
Undigested: achalasia
Blood or "coffee grounds": gastritis, ulcers, esophagitis, varices
Initially without, then with, blood: Mallory Weiss tear
Bile: postampullary obstruction
Clear, large volume: Zollinger-Ellison syndrome
Malodorous, feculent: stasis with bacterial overgrowth, gastrocolic fistula, ischemic injury to gut

Force of vomiting
Projectile: pyloric stenosis and other gastric obstruction, gastroesophageal reflux (occasionally), metabolic disease
Forceless regurgitation: gastroesophageal reflux

Relationship of vomiting to time of day or mealtime
Early morning: high intracranial pressure, pregnancy, gag due to sinusitis
Mealtime: peptic ulcer disease, psychogenic

Relationship of vomiting to particular foods
Cow, soy, gluten: protein intolerance
Other or multiple: allergic enteropathies, eosinophilic gastroenteropathy, metabolic disease (e.g., hereditary fructose intolerance)

Periodicity of vomiting
Paroxysmal, cyclic: carcinoid, pheochromocytoma, porphyria, diencephalic syndrome, epilepsy, familial dysautonomia

Other gastrointestinal symptoms and signs
Nausea: lack of nausea suggests raised intracranial pressure, gut obstruction
Esophageal pain: esophagitis (may be secondary to chronic vomiting)
Dysphagia: esophageal disease
Diarrhea: infectious enteritis, partial luminal obstruction, toxin
Constipation or distention: luminal obstruction, hypercalcemia
Delayed vomiting, succussion splash: gastric outlet obstruction or stasis
Visible peristalsis: luminal obstruction, especially pyloric
Bowel sounds: obstruction versus atony
Abdominal pain or tenderness: may localize diseased organ, define severity
Abdominal mass
   Lesions produced by luminal or vascular obstruction
   Inflamed or neoplastic lesions
   Congenital malformations, pyloric "tumor"

Abdominal scars: postoperative adhesions or stenoses; surgical vagotomy
Jaundice
   Hepatitis, hepatobiliary malformation
   Urinary tract infection or pyloric stenosis in neonate

Neurologic symptoms and signs: metabolic, toxic, central nervous system disease
Headache, vertigo, visual changes (photophobia, scotomata, field outs)
Abnormal tone, seizures
Funduscopic or fontanelle evidence of increased intracranial pressure

Other organ system symptoms and signs
Cardiac (hypotension or hypertension: intestinal ischemia, paroxysmal diseases (see below)
Urinary: pyelonephritis, hydronephrosis, renal calculi, hypertension
Respiratory: pneumonia, otitis, aspiration due to vomiting

Degree of well-being
Well
   Gastroesophageal reflux
   Stimulation of gag reflex
   Rumination, psychosocial, psychogenic, malingering
Acutely ill—often with dehydration, electrolyte abnormalities
   Surgical emergencies (luminal or vascular obstruction)
   Gastroenteritis, hepatitis, pancreatitis, sepsis, meningitis
   Ingestions
   Pain: may help localize diseased organ
   Fever: inflammatory lesions (e.g., appendicitis, peritonitis, pyelonephritis)
Chronically ill—often with malnutrition ("failure to thrive")
   Metabolic disease (especially if abnormalities of tone and development)
   Partial or intermittent obstructions

Epidemiologic information
Epidemics: gastrointestinal infections, toxic exposures
Family history: migraine, peptic ulcer disease, etc.

(Adapted from Orenstein,[5] with permission.)

Helicobacter pylori, duodenal *Giardia,* and gastritis. Manometry of the upper GI tract is helpful in defining primary or secondary motility abnormalities causing vomiting.

THERAPY

Therapy should be directed at the specific cause, if identified. In addition, any complications of vomiting, such as metabolic or nutritional or inflammatory, should be treated. Psychotherapy is often helpful. Antiemetic drugs are useful in patients with persistent vomiting to reduce the metabolic and nutritional consequences. However, the use of these drugs without a clear understanding of the cause of vomiting is not recommended. The use of these agents is contraindicated in most infants and children with vomiting secondary to gastroenteritis, anatomic abnormalities, surgical emergencies, and expanding intracranial lesions. Antiemetic agents are useful for motion sickness, cancer chemotherapy, postoperative nausea and vomiting, cyclical vomiting syndrome, gastroparesis, and other GI motility disorders. Table 14-4

TABLE 14-4. Antiemetic and Antinausea Drugs With Indications and Possible Mechanisms of Action

Chemical Name	Representative Brand Name	Indication	Mechanism
Antihistamines			
Diphenhydramine	Benadryl	Motion sickness, mild chemotherapy-induced vomiting	Most likely labyrinthine suppression, possibly via anticholinergic effect as well as H_1-receptor antagonism in the central pattern generator
Hydroxyzine	Vistaril, Atarax		
Dimenhydrinate	Dramamine		
Promethazine	Phenergan		
Meclizine	Antivert		
Anticholinergics			
Hyoscyamine	Scopolamine	Prophylaxis of motion sickness	Antimuscarinic effect, probably at the level of the labyrinth or central pattern generator
Substituted benzamides			
Metoclopramide	Reglan	Chemotherapy, motility disorders, especially gastroparesis, GER	D_2-receptor blockade at the chemoreceptive trigger zone (CTZ) and enteric nervous system; in high dose, exhibits 5-HT_3 activity enterically
Trimethobenzamide	Tigan	Often used during vomiting associated with acute gastroenteritis—?efficacy.	D_2-receptor blockade
Cisapride	Propulsid	May abort some cases of cyclic vomiting Motility disorders, GER	Enteric acetylcholine release
5-HT_2-Receptor antagonists			
Ondansetron	Zofran	Chemotherapy	5-HT_3-receptor blockade most important at the enteric level, but possibly some effect at the CTZ and central pattern generator
Granisetron	Kytril		
Cannabinoids			
Dronabinol	Marinol	Chemotherapy, but used less and less because of more efficacious drugs and central side effects	Unknown
Nabilone	Cesamet		
Benzodiazepines			
Lorazepam	Ativan	Chemotherapy—especially lorazepam. Preferred because of rapid effect and short duration	These drugs probably act via central GABA inhibition producing sedation and anxiolysis
Diazepam	Valium		
Midazolam	Versed		
Phenothiazines			
Prochlorperazine	Compazine	Chemotherapy, cyclic vomiting, acute gastritis; rarely used in pediatrics because of extrapyramidal side effects	D_2-receptor antagonist at CTZ
Chlorpromazine	Thorazine		
Perphenazine	Trilafon		
Promethazine	Phenergan		
Butyrophenones			
Droperidol	Inapsine	Cyclic vomiting, intractable vomiting from acute gastritis, chemotherapy, postoperative nausea and vomiting	D_2-receptor blockade at the CTZ; central anxiolysis and sedation
Haloperidol	Haldol		
Domperidone	Motilium	Chemotherapy, motility disorders (especially gastroparesis, GER)	D_2-receptor blockade at enteric nervous system
Corticosteroids			
Dexamethasone	Decadron	Mild chemotherapy-induced vomiting or in combination with other antiemetics; emesis resulting from increased intracranial pressure	Unknown, possibly decreased enteric prostaglandin synthesis

(Adapted from Sondheimer,[6] with permission.)

outlines some of the available drugs, as well as indications and possible mechanisms of action.

REFERRAL PATTERN

Chronic vomiting should always be considered abnormal, and an etiology should be sought. Referrals should be made if there is significant weight loss, severe abdominal pain, GI bleeding, evidence of a surgical acute abdomen, or an abnormal neurologic examination.

REFERENCES

1. Lang IM, Sarna SK. Motor and myoelectric activity associated with vomiting, regurgitation, and nausea. In: Wood J, Ed. Motility and Circulation. Vol. 1. In: Schultz SG, Ed. Gastrointestinal System, Section 6. Handbook of Physiology. New York: Oxford University Press, 1989:1179–1198

2. Ingelfinger FJ, Moss RE. The activity of the descending duodenum during nausea. Am J Physiol 1942;136:561–566

3. Thompson BG, Malagelada JR. Vomiting and the small intestine. Dig Dis Sci 1982;27:1121–1125

4. Johnson HD, Laws JW. The cardia in swallowing, eructation, and vomiting. Lancet 1966;2:1268–1273

5. Orenstein SR. Dysphagia and vomiting. In: Wyllie R, Hyams JS, Eds. Pediatric Gastrointestinal Disease: Pathophysiology, Diagnosis, Management. Philadelphia: WB Saunders, 1993: 144

6. Sondheimer JM. Vomiting. In: Walker WA, Durie PR, Hamilton JR et al, Eds. Pediatric Gastrointestinal Disease: Pathophysiology, Diagnosis, and Management. Vol. 1. 2nd Ed. St. Louis: Mosby-Year Book, 1996:200

7. Jernigan SA, Ware LM. Reversible quantitative EEG changes in a case of cyclic vomiting: evidence for migraine equivalent. Dev Med Child Neurol 1991;33:80–85

8. Fleisher DR, Matar M. Review: the cyclic vomiting syndrome: a report of 71 cases and literature review. J Pediatr Gastroenterol Nutr 1993;17:361–369

9. Weitz R. Prophylaxis of cyclic vomiting with propranolol. Drug Intell Clin Pharm 1982;16:161–162

10. Sheagren TG et al. Rumination—a new complication of neonatal intensive care. Pediatrics 1980;66:551–555

11. Herbst J, Friedland GW, Zhoraiske FF. Hiatal hernia and rumination in infants and children, J Pediatr 1971;78: 261–265

12. Amarnath RP, Abell TL, Malagelada JR. The rumination syndrome in adults. Ann Intern Med 1986;105:513–518

13. Fromm S, Cash JM. Superior mesenteric artery syndrome: an approach to the diagnosis and management of upper gastrointestinal obstruction of unknown etiology. South Dakota J Med 1990;43:5–10

14. McLain CJ et al. Gastrointestinal and nutritional aspects of eating disorders. J Am Coll Nutr 1993;12:466–474

15. Liacouras CA. Vomiting. In: Schwartz MW, Ed. The 5 Minute Pediatric Consult. Baltimore: Williams & Wilkins, 1997: 64

15

GASTROINTESTINAL ALLERGY

EDWIN SIMPSER

Adverse reactions to foods are often categorized into two types: allergy or intolerance. It is important to distinguish between these two types of reactions, since the therapeutic approaches vary. Food *intolerance* can result from reactions related to various properties and components of the food products themselves or to deficiencies and abnormalities in the host (e.g., lactose intolerance). Food *allergy* specifically relates to an immunologically mediated reaction secondary to the ingestion of a food product. These reactions can be seen in a number of organs, most commonly the skin, respiratory tract, and the gastrointestinal (GI) tract. GI food allergies are characterized by the onset of GI symptoms related to an immunologically mediated reaction in the GI tract.[1] This chapter focuses on one of the most common GI food allergies in infants and children: cow milk protein and soy protein allergy.

PATHOPHYSIOLOGY

The development of an allergic reaction to a food product is the result of interaction between food allergens, the GI tract, and the immune system.[2] The glycoprotein portion of the food is the usual allergen. In the case of cow milk protein, there are more than 25 known immunogenic proteins. Studies comparing single cow milk proteins as to their ability to elicit an allergic response show that beta-lactoglobulin, the major whey protein, has the highest level of antigenicity. The other major protein component, casein, is next in terms of clinical significance. Human breast milk has also been shown to contain a variety of food proteins including cow milk, egg,

wheat, and peanut.[3] Thus, even exclusively breast-fed infants can be found to have GI manifestations of food allergy. Soy proteins have also been found to be allergenic and, although it has been suggested that soy is less allergenic than cow milk, this is not well documented. It does seem likely, although also not well proven, that soy allergy develops as a secondary event after initial sensitization to cow milk protein.

The development of GI allergic reactions to cow and soy protein is felt to be related to genetic predisposition followed by sensitization (Table 15-1). Although the molecular basis for this genetic predisposition is not well understood, the data presented by Kjellman[4] clearly show a rise in risk of milk protein sensitivity, with the similar history of atopy in families in which one parent, a sibling, or both parents, have atopy.[4]

Sensitization has been shown to occur in utero, although this probably constitutes less than 5% of infant food allergies. More commonly, however, sensitization occurs when genetically predisposed infants are exposed early to antigens, whether it be in infant formula or in maternal breast milk.

The GI tract is quite efficient in its ability to form a barrier to a variety of ingested antigens, as well as other toxins and intestinal pathogens.[5] However, this mucosal barrier is often immature in the newborn infant until approximately 4 months of age, predisposing the child to macromolecular absorption of a variety of antigens. In addition, damage to the intestinal mucosa, such as that induced by an acute gastroenteritis, leads to a break in the mucosal barrier and to possible sensitization to cow milk. It has been hypothesized that exposure to cow

TABLE 15-1. Pathogenesis of GI Allergy

Genetic predisposition

Sensitization
    In utero
    Early exposure

Defective mucosal barrier
    GI immaturity
    Infectious

milk protein during an episode of acute gastroenteritis is a significant contributor to the incidence of food-sensitive enteropathy. Components of this gut mucosal barrier include mucosal epithelial cells; the GI tract's unique mucous layer; normal intestinal peristalsis; gastric acid and pepsin; proteolytic enzymes; as well as the gut immune system, including gut-associated lymphatic tissues, secretory IgA, and cell-mediated immunity. A breakdown in any or some of the components of this intricate system may lead to sensitization and subsequent allergy.

There is significant controversy, especially among allergists and gastroenterologists, as to the specific antibody reactions classified as milk protein allergy. Many allergists classify only IgE antibody-related reactions as true food allergy. However, in addition to IgE-associated reactions, studies have also shown elevated IgG antibodies and immune complexes in infants with cow milk protein allergy. In addition, a number of investigators believe there is also a link between cell-mediated immunity and GI epithelial damage and food allergy. To date, no single immunoglobulin specificity has been demonstrated to be solely responsible for a food allergic reaction.[3] It is possible that the variation in clinical presentation of GI food allergies may in part be related to different immune responses. This lack of immunoglobulin specificity in food allergy makes antibody determination, although of some diagnostic value, secondary to the clinical diagnostic technique.

CLINICAL PRESENTATION

The prevalence of cow milk protein allergy has been estimated to be somewhere between 1% and 8%. Children with underlying problems such as atopic dermatitis may have a much higher incidence of milk protein allergy as well as other food allergies.[6] It would appear that the incidence of primary allergy to soy is significantly less than that to cow milk, probably within the range of 0.5%. However, when soy is used as a substitute for cow milk in children with cow milk protein allergy, there is anywhere from a 15% to 50% incidence of allergic reaction to the soy. One study suggested cross-reactivity of up to 80%.[7]

There are a variety of clinical manifestations of allergy to either cow or soy protein. In addition to the GI disorders listed in Table 15-2, infants and children have been found to have anaphylactoid reactions; acute urticaria and/or angioedema; atopic dermatitis; and respiratory symptoms, including rhinitis, nasal congestion, and wheezing. GI symptoms appear to present most often independent of the skin or respiratory tract, but they are not mutually exclusive. Certainly, anaphylaxis or shock, or both, can be seen in a subset of patients with GI presentations of milk protein allergy.

The two most common presenting manifestations of GI allergy are cow milk–sensitive enteropathy and allergic colitis. Interestingly, these two entities rarely occur together, suggesting different pathogenic pathways.

Enteropathy

Cow milk protein–related enteropathy presents most commonly in children under the age of 2 years, with the salient features being diarrhea and failure to thrive. Some newborn infants will have a more acute form that will present with vomiting as well as diarrhea. Children's appetite may be poor, related to the discomfort caused by the offending allergen and by the malabsorption of nutrients such as carbohydrate, causing gassiness and bloating. The enteropathy is characterized by abnormal small intestinal mucosa, often patchy in nature, with features similar to those of celiac disease (i.e., mucosal atrophy). The abnormalities in small intestinal mucosa are reversed by elimination of cow milk from the diet. Rarely, if ever, do children present after 2 years of age, and in most cases, the symptoms resolve after age 3 and children are able to tolerate cow milk.

An associated disaccharide intolerance accompanies this enteropathy. Thus, children will often present with symptoms of lactose intolerance, making diagnosis somewhat confusing. In general, however, lactose intolerance is uncommon in children under the age of 2 years with-

TABLE 15-2. GI Manifestations of Cow Milk or Soy Protein Allergy

Acute enteropathy (anaphylactoid)
    Vomiting with or without diarrhea
    Edema

Enteropathy (slow onset)
    Vomiting
    Diarrhea
    Failure to thrive
    Malabsorption

Colitis
    Diarrhea
    Bloody stools

? Colic

out some other underlying pathology (e.g., acute gastroenteritis with subsequent mild disaccharidase deficiency). However, any child presenting with chronic symptoms of lactose intolerance (i.e., bloating, gassiness, loose stools) in this age group should be investigated for entities that cause small intestine mucosal damage, including milk protein allergy.

Allergic Colitis

Most patients with allergic colitis have the onset of disease within the first few months of life.[8] Similar to those with enteropathy, most children are tolerant of milk protein by the time they reach the age of 2 or 3 years. Some infants present as early as in the first week of life, suggesting an in utero sensitization.

Infants most often present with rectal bleeding, at times associated with diarrhea. Indeed, milk protein allergy is likely the most common cause of pathologic rectal bleeding in infancy. These infants do not show significant weight loss, nor is the colitis associated in general with vomiting. There may be an associated history of irritability, and a small subset of children may present with a shock-like picture.[9] Most children do not have associated fever, anemia, or other constitutional signs or symptoms. The onset of allergic colitis may be acute, even as short as 24 hours after initial feeding of an antigenic substance, but it is more often insidious, with a considerable interval between the introduction of cow milk and the onset of symptoms.[8] Allergic colitis has been described in babies who are exclusively breast fed. Some of those children will respond to elimination of milk protein from the mother's diet, implicating the transfer of proteins from the mother's diet into the breast milk, thereby sensitizing the infant.

Colic

In addition to the clinical syndromes described above, there has been a controversy as to whether cow milk protein allergy is a cause of infantile colic. A group from Sweden has championed this theory and has published a number of studies supporting this idea. Although it is likely that the symptoms of colic are multifactorial, this group used a double-blind crossover study to show, somewhat convincingly, that whey protein can indeed cause infantile colic.[10]

DIAGNOSIS

In virtually every paper and textbook that discusses the diagnosis of an infant or child with milk protein allergy, the approach is to stress the use of classic diagnostic criteria and "elimination and challenge." In practice, how-

TABLE 15-3. Differential Diagnosis of Colitis in Infancy

Infection (bacterial, amebic)
Hirschsprung's disease
Milk protein allergy
Necrotizing enterocolitis
Inflammatory bowel disease
Eosinophilic gastroenteritis
Hemolytic uremic syndrome

ever, many physicians, be they general practitioners or pediatric gastroenterologists, will often make the diagnosis on the basis of clinical history and a few on any laboratory tests that may have been performed. This approach has its drawbacks, since symptoms associated with milk allergy can be caused by other entities, and an empirical diagnosis may unnecessarily relegate a child to long-term expensive dietary restrictions.

Because the gastroenterologic manifestations of milk protein allergy present somewhat independently, that is, either as colitis or as an enteropathy, the approach to a differential diagnosis can largely be based on these presenting symptoms. Therefore, for the child presenting with the symptoms of enteropathy (i.e., chronic diarrhea and failure to thrive), the differential diagnosis would include milk protein allergy, celiac disease, lactose intolerance, cystic fibrosis, chronic infections (parasites), and other disorders causing malabsorption/maldigestion. The differential diagnosis of the child presenting with bloody diarrhea in infancy is presented in Table 15-3.

Diagnostic Tests

For the child presenting with colitis, one needs to take a careful history that can relate the onset of symptoms to feeding, along with a family history or personal history of allergy, or both. Small amounts of red blood may be secondary to an anal fissure. Unfortunately, no single laboratory or biochemical test is either sensitive or specific enough to be diagnostic of allergic colitis.[8] Many infants will have either peripheral eosinophilia and/or leukocytosis noted on a complete blood count or eosinophils in their stool samples. The fecal eosinophils can be seen on Wright stain, but it may also be seen as pinkish crystals (Charcot-Leyden crystals) on an ova and parasite stain. These findings are highly suggestive, but not diagnostic, of allergic colitis. Given the above-mentioned differential diagnosis, one needs to obtain a stool culture and a stool for ova and parasites to rule out an infectious cause. At times, the clinical presentation of allergic colitis can mimic that of enterocolitis induced by Hirschsprung's disease. Rectal examination may be suggestive of

Hirschsprung's. In order to differentiate those symptoms, radiologic or manometric studies can be diagnostic of Hirschsprung's disease. Some centers will rely on a rectal suction biopsy to help differentiate Hirschsprung's disease from allergic colitis. The rectal biopsy can be diagnostic of Hirschsprung's disease or, if eosinophilia is noted, allergy is the most likely diagnosis. At many pediatric GI centers, endoscopy is thought to be a better approach to making a pathologic diagnosis of allergic colitis because the disease can be focal or "patchy," with the rectosigmoid the area most likely involved. In the study by Odze et al.[9] it was noted that rectal biopsies showed significant variability and that upwards of 40% of patients would not be diagnosed if only a single rectal biopsy was done. Therefore, if rectal biopsy is used to make a histologic diagnosis, as opposed to directed endoscopic biopsies, multiple biopsies need to be taken. The same investigators described that the most salient histologic feature of allergic colitis was the presence of focal eosinophilic infiltration of the mucosa, in particular the lamina propria.

For the child presenting with possible milk protein-induced enteropathy, the diagnosis can be much more difficult. Although stool and blood tests may be helpful, in these patients, very often the diagnosis hinges on a small bowel biopsy, immunologic tests, and the gold standard of elimination and challenge. Often entities such as cystic fibrosis and chronic parasitic infections are ruled out before an intestinal biopsy is undertaken. Serologic studies for celiac disease should be done as well. It is imperative to obtain measurements of IgA antibodies to gliadin as well as IgA antiendomysial antibodies. The latter are much more specific for celiac disease, as opposed to antigliadin IgG antibodies, which are quite nonspecific and can often be seen in children with milk protein allergy. Once some of these other diagnoses have been excluded, one can proceed to specific testing for milk allergy, including small intestinal biopsy, immunologic tests, and elimination and challenge.

Intestinal Biopsy

As in allergic colitis, the intestinal biopsy in milk protein allergy can be "patchy." Abnormal areas can have subtotal mucosal atrophy, often associated with an eosinophilic infiltration of the mucosa and lamina propria. When this eosinophilia is not present, the mucosal pattern may mimic that of celiac disease. The biopsy is quite helpful in differentiating other diagnoses such as lymphangiectasia and microvillus inclusion disease. Also on occasion, endoscopy can be helpful to obtain duodenal juice for analysis of pancreatic enzyme function, as well as to diagnose chronic parasitic infection such as giardiasis. Gastric (antral) and duodenal biopsies are also useful in the diagnosis of eosinophilic gastroenteritis which is discussed elsewhere in this text.

Immunologic/Skin Tests

Skin tests for GI food allergy have been widely used but are not universally accepted. One must be careful to include defined and standardized food antigens in the testing, to avoid nonspecific irritations that are nondiagnostic. Also, children under 3 years of age may have negative skin tests, especially those with delayed reactions. Children who have IgE-mediated responses are the most likely to have a positive skin test.

From the standpoint of immunologic testing, some physicians use total IgE and radioallergosorbent test (RAST) as indicators of food allergy. Unfortunately, RAST testing is fraught with false-positive results, but newer techniques using enzyme-linked immunosorbent assay (ELISA) methodology may be helpful.[11] Although RAST are also probably most useful for immediate reactors, a study by Hill et al.[12] suggests that a small percentage of delayed responders may also have positive RASTS. These tests are generally not useful in young infants because of a significant number of false-positive results.

Elimination and Challenge

Many physicians believe that the gold standard for diagnosis of cow milk allergy is an unequivocal and reproducible reaction to elimination and challenge. Some require a double-blind placebo-controlled challenge. The criteria for the diagnosis were originally established by Goldman et al.[13]: (1) improvement in symptoms after elimination of cow milk, (2) relapse of symptoms after 48 hours of challenge, and (3) a total of three challenges causing relapse. These criteria have proved difficult to use on a routine basis. Multiple challenges are quite difficult to obtain, and some children will relapse at some point beyond 48 hours after exposure. Also, significant observer bias is associated with the challenge; in addition, most physicians are uncomfortable with challenging patients who displayed previous anaphylactic reactions.[3] Powell[14] suggested a modified protocol for elimination and challenge that can be followed for most infants and children. This protocol includes using small amounts of liquid initially to observe for anaphylaxis, followed by increasing doses of the challenge food (cow milk). Most pediatricians and many pediatric gastroenterologists find even this modified approach difficult and use it only for children with the most severe reactions and more often in older children (at least 1 year of age) as an indicator of resolution of the allergy, not as a diagnostic tool during the initial workup.

Given that there is no gold standard laboratory test, the limited clinical use of controlled challenges, and the reluctance of pediatricians to obtain blood work or biopsies for neonates, it is very likely that many pediatricians are making a clinical diagnosis of cow milk protein allergy in children who are not truly allergic. This can have significant implications, especially nutritionally, when parents limit the milk and diary product intake of an older infant and child, often limiting calories and important micronutrients (e.g., calcium) in the process.

TREATMENT

The treatment of milk protein allergy in infancy and childhood requires removal of the offending antigen (cow milk and/or soy) and substitution of a nonantigenic or lower antigenic formula. Although breast milk would be an appropriate substitute for formulas containing cow milk protein, it is often no longer available by the time the diagnosis is made, as the mother has already weaned the child from the breast. In addition, once sensitized, these infants may react to the small quantities of antigens that cross into maternal breast milk.

Hydrolysate formulas have been used for many years for children with milk allergy. These include casein hydrolysate formulas and, more recently, a formula with a whey hydrolysate protein. The casein hydrolysate formulas contain enzymatically degraded proteins with low molecular weight. In general, they are hypoallergenic and, because they also contain glucose polymer and some contain medium chain triglyceride (MCT) they are better absorbed in the child with severe enteropathy. Unfortunately, one of the drawbacks to these hydrolysate formulas is their poor palatability, but with time most infants accept the formula. Recently a small number of studies have suggested the efficacy of the whey hydrolysate formulas for the treatment and prevention of milk protein allergy.[15,16] Physicians should recognize that it may take upward of 2 weeks for clinical improvement (e.g., blood or guaiac-positive stools can persist), even while on these formulas. As long as the infant is thriving and remains clinically stable, further intervention should not be necessary.

A number of infants are extremely sensitive to milk protein and react even to hydrolysate formulas, with such conditions as shock or anaphylaxis. These highly sensitive infants often require treatment with free amino acid–containing formulas. In the past, most of these formulas were designed for adults and, even with modification, were suboptimal for use in infants. A new infant formula with free amino acids has recently shown to be efficacious for children with severe milk protein allergy.[17]

In addition, a subset of infants present with such severe reactions to milk protein that they require intravenous nutrition for a short period to stabilize their nutritional status before attempting a new formula. This is often the child who presents with either severe enteropathy or anaphylaxis and shock related to exposure to milk protein. These infants are best started, when clinically stable, on an amino acid–based formula, progressing slowly to a casein hydrolysate.

Because of the known cross-reactivity between soy protein and cow milk protein,[7] many physicians prefer to use the casein or whey hydrolysate formulas, as opposed to soy formula, as a treatment for milk protein allergy. More than likely, however, although this is not well studied, many children do respond when switched empirically from cow milk formula to soy formula, either by their parents or by their pediatricians, because of presumed intolerance to their milk protein formula.

In those exclusively breast-fed infants who are sensitive to proteins that cross into the maternal breast milk, the initial approach is the removal of all milk protein from the maternal diet. This is not always successful, and some of these patients may require either hydrolysate formulas or even the free amino acid–based formulas.

Prevention

One important facet of milk protein allergy is the prevention of allergy in infants and children at risk, given the genetic predisposition. Thus, if there is a strong family history of atopic disease, or if a sibling has a history of milk protein allergy, preventive measures should be undertaken. Most physicians believe that those children should be exclusively breast fed. If this is not possible, the use of either a soy protein formula or a hydrolysate formula as the initial formula in these infants is recommended. For those infants who have a strong history and who are breast fed, it would seem logical to modify the maternal diet, to remove milk protein.[3] Given the risk of allergy in these infants, avoidance of other allergenic foods is warranted. Thus, the introduction of solid food should wait at least until after 6 months of age in those infants.

Because most milk protein allergy is transient, there is often a question as to when children can be safely rechallenged and tolerate milk protein in their diet. Most investigators recommend waiting until age 18 to 24 months, as most children are no longer allergic at that age. Of course, a subset of infants can tolerate milk protein earlier than this period, and others who will retain their allergy for many years (age 5 or older). Children whose reaction to milk protein in infancy included anaphylaxis and/or shock or angioedema should be challenged in a controlled environment, with very small volumes. More than likely, this should be done in an office setting in which epinephrine is available.

REFERRAL PATTERN

For the infant presenting with classic signs and symptoms of allergic colitis, most pediatricians will make the diagnosis either empirically or using a test such as a complete blood count and stool studies for eosinophils and to rule out enteric infection. Although many physicians switch formulas when a child presents with bloody stools, I consider it worthwhile to at least attempt to make a diagnosis, so that one can make appropriate recommendations for long-term dietary care. If the diagnosis is unclear, or if there is a suspicion of possible Hirschsprung's disease, the child should be referred to a pediatric gastroenterologist for further diagnosis, which will more than likely include either a rectal biopsy or a colonoscopy.

In the child whose symptoms suggest milk protein-related enteropathy, the pediatrician must have a clear understanding of the differential diagnosis and should progress in the evaluation accordingly. Diagnostic tests as outlined above can be obtained initially by the pediatrician. If the diagnosis is uncertain, referral to a pediatric gastroenterologist for further diagnostic testing and a possible small intestinal biopsy will be necessary. Obtaining an appropriate history and performing these evaluations can be time-consuming for a pediatrician in a busy practice. As a result, some physicians are inclined to refer the children at an earlier stage to a pediatric gastroenterologist, who deals with these differential diagnoses on a regular basis. On occasion, infants with milk allergy will have severe reactions (even mimicking sepsis) and require hospitalization. Clearly, a pediatric gastroenterologist should be consulted for those children, as well.

Once the diagnosis of milk protein allergy is confirmed, the child can be followed by the regular pediatrician, including the performance of the milk protein challenge. Those children who remain allergic for an extended period of time, or who in the second year of life begin to refuse the hydrolysate or amino acid–based formulas, should receive counseling on appropriate caloric intake and calcium supplementation. This can be done either by the pediatrician or by a pediatric nutritionist.

REFERENCES

1. Walker JA. Food intolerance in infancy. In: Hamberger R, Ed. Allergology, Immunology, and Gastroenterology. New York: Raven Press, 1989:127–134

2. Sampson HA. Adverse reactions to food. In: Middleton E, Reed CE, Ellis EF, Adkinson NF, Unginger JW, Busse MW, Eds. Allergy: Principles and Practices. St. Louis, MO: CV Mosby, 1991:1661–1686

3. Stern M. Gastrointestinal allergy. In: Walker WA, Dubrie PR, Hamilton JR, Walker-Smith JA, Watkins JB, Eds. Pediatric Gastrointestinal Disease: Pathophysiology, Diagnosis, and Management. Philadelphia: BC Decker, 1991;1: 557–574

4. Kjellman NIM. Atopic disease in seven year old children: incidence and relation to family history. Acta Paediatr 1977; 66:465–471

5. Kerner JA. Formula allergy and intolerance. In: Ament M, Ed. Pediatric Gastroenterology. Part II. Gastroenterol Clin North Am 1995;24:1–25

6. Burkes AW, Mallary SB, Williams LW et al. Atopic dermatitis: clinical relevance of food hypersensitivity reactions. J Pediatr 1981;113:447–451

7. Eastham EJ. Soy protein allergy. In: Hamberger R, ed. Allergology, Immunology, and Gastroenterology. New York: Raven Press, 1989:223–236

8. Goldman HG, Proujansky R. Allergic proctitis and gastroenteritis in children. Clinical and mucosal biopsy features in 53 cases. Am J Surg Pathol 1986;10:75–86

9. Odze RO, Bines J, Lechtner AM et al. Allergic proctocolitis in infants. A perspective clinical-pathologic biopsy study. Hum Pathol 1993;24:668–674

10. Loth EL, Lindberg T. Cow's milk whey protein elicits symptoms of infant colic in colicky formula fed infants: a double blind crossover study. Pediatrics 1989;83:262–266

11. Atkins FM, Metcalfe DD. The diagnosis and treatment of food allergy. Annu Rev Nutr 1984;4:233–255

12. Hill DJ, Firer MA, Shelton MJ et al. Manifestations of milk allergy in infancy: clinical and immunologic findings. J Pediatr 1986;109:270–276

13. Goldman AS, Anderson DW, Sellars WA et al. Milk allergy. I. Oral challenge with milk and isolated milk proteins in allergic children. Pediatrics 1963;32:425–443

14. Powell GK. Milk- and soy-induced enterocolitis of infancy: clinical features and standardization of challenge. J Ped 1978; 93:553–560

15. Vandenplas Y, Malfruit A, Dabb I. Short term prevention of cow's milk protein allergy in infants. Immunol Allergy Pract 1989;11:17–24

16. Meritt RJ, Carter M, Haight M. Whey protein hydrolysate formula for infants with gastrointestinal intolerance to cow milk and soy protein in infant formulas. J Pediatr Gastroenterol Nutr 1990;11:78–82

17. Vanderhoof JA, Kaufman SS, Murray NP et al. Evaluation of neocate in infants with milk protein induced colitis. J Pediatr Gastroenterol Nutr 1995:21:331

16

ACHALASIA

JOHN T. BOYLE

From a functional point of view, the esophagus can be divided into three zones: the upper esophageal sphincter (UES), the esophageal body, and the lower esophageal sphincter (LES).[1] The proximal 40% of the esophagus, including the UES, is striated muscle; the distal 60% is smooth muscle, including the LES. At rest, the esophageal body is quiet and without motor activity, whereas the sphincters maintain a state of contraction that serves as a protective barrier to esophagopharyngeal and gastroesophageal reflux. The act of swallowing triggers an involuntary coordinated motor pattern within the esophagus in which the food bolus is transferred through a relaxed UES into the esophagus and propelled through a relaxed LES by a progressive aboral circular contraction called peristalsis.

Achalasia is the best characterized motility disorder of the esophagus.[2] It is defined by failure of the LES to relax completely with swallowing and by absence of peristalsis in the body of the esophagus. The cardinal symptom of achalasia is dysphagia, or difficulty swallowing (the sensation of food being "stuck"). Dysphagia is produced by the residual gradient between esophagus and stomach that remains during swallowing and the absence of normal progressive aboral esophageal contractions to propel luminal contents toward the stomach.

Achalasia is uncommon at any age, but less than 5% of patients present during childhood or adolescence. The incidence in children is less than 0.1 per 100,000 per year.[3] Most cases are sporadic. Familial occurrences, however, suggest that genetic factors may play a role in the pathogenesis of the disease. Achalasia has also been described as part of several distinct multisystem syndromes suggesting a generalized neuromuscular disorder as the mode of origin.

PATHOPHYSIOLOGY

Esophageal function involves numerous interacting control mechanisms within the central and enteric nervous systems.[1] Extrinsic control for esophageal motor function resides in the brain stem. Innervation of both the striated and smooth muscle segments of the esophagus, including the sphincters, is via the vagus nerve. In humans, swallow-induced peristalsis appears to result primarily from sequencing and activation of postganglionic intramural excitatory cholinergic neurons. Under normal circumstances, the central control mechanism exerts the dominant influence on these neurons for initiation and coordination of peristalsis. Resting tone in the LES is predominantly a property of the muscle itself, although this tone is regulated by a balance between many excitatory and inhibitory influences. The relaxation on swallowing is caused by active inhibition of muscle through nonadrenergic, noncholinergic inhibitory neurons and cessation of tonic neural excitation to the sphincter. It is increasingly evident that nonadrenergic, noncholinergic neurons use nitric oxide as a neurotransmitter.[4]

The cause of achalasia remains unknown. Whatever the underlying cause, the disease leads to damage to the intrinsic and extrinsic innervation of the esophagus. The most consistent neuropathic lesion reported has been degeneration or loss of the esophageal myenteric plexus.[5] Nerve fiber degeneration in both the extra- and intraesophageal portions of the esophagus, as well as neuronal loss in the dorsal motor nucleus of the vagus nerve, has also been reported in some patients.[6] Postganglionic denervation of the LES is believed to be the primary pathophysiologic abnormality. Absence or functional impairment of the inhibitory innervation of the LES is hypothesized to result in the incomplete relaxation of the LES in achalasia. Animal models of achalasia have been established using nitric oxide inhibitors such as N-nitro-L-arginine (L-NNA).[7] The elevated resting LES pressure frequently observed in patients with achalasia suggests that the integrity of the excitatory cholinergic pathway remains intact but is now unopposed by inhibitory influences. The etiology of the esophageal aperistalsis is unclear. Disruption of peristalsis may be an extension of the primary neural defect that causes LES dysfunction. Several cases have been reported of return of peristalsis after forceful disruption of the LES, suggesting that the defect at the LES can result in a secondary reversible derangement of peristalsis.[8]

Most pediatric cases of achalasia occur sporadically in older children, suggesting that it is an acquired disease. One of the important difficulties in identifying the cause of the disease is the long interval between the start of the pathologic process and the onset of symptoms. Goldblum et al.[5] have reported variable myenteric chronic inflammation in deep longitudinal muscle strips obtained at esophagomyotomy in adult patients with achalasia. In most cases, inflammation is patchy, and found within and surrounding myenteric nerves. It is difficult in such cases to determine whether such myenteric inflammation is the primary cause of ganglion cell loss and myenteric nerve injury or a secondary phenomenon. However, in some patients, there is lymphocytic infiltration into ganglion cell cytoplasm (ganglionitis) suggesting that depletion of ganglion cells in selected cases of achalasia could be secondary to inflammatory destruction. An infectious etiology is supported by Chagas disease, in which a parasite, *Trypanosoma cruzi*, causes damage to the myenteric plexus and an esophageal motor pattern similar to idiopathic achalasia. To date, however, a hypothesized neurotropic virus has yet to be identified, although varicella-zoster virus DNA has been identified in the esophageal myenteric plexus in sporadic adult cases.[9] In the absence of a documented infectious etiology, the common pathologic finding of a round cell infiltration of the myenteric plexus has raised speculation regarding an immune-mediated abnormality.

There is also evidence in adults that achalasia may be part of a generalized motility disorder. Motor abnormalities of the stomach, small bowel, gallbladder, and sphincter of Oddi have been described in some patients.[10] Yet, symptomatic motility disorder in the gut below the cardia is almost unknown in achalasia.

Achalasia has been described as part of several distinct multisystem syndromes, suggesting a generalized neuromuscular disorder as the mode of origin. Achalasia may be a harbinger of a generalized familial autonomic and sensorimotor polyneuropathy, termed Allgrove syndrome. Allgrove syndrome was originally described as the association of chronic adrenal insufficiency due to adrenocorticotropic hormone (ACTH) insensitivity, achalasia, and alacrima. Subsequent case reports have described the association of a progressive autonomic and sensorimotor polyneuropathy. Variants of the syndrome with different combinations of the three major abnormalities have been reported. Achalasia has also been associated with Alport's syndrome, Rozycki syndrome (deafness, vitiligo, short stature, muscular weakness), mental retardation, and microcephaly.

The report of sporadic familial occurrence suggests possible genetic predisposition or exposure to a common environmental triggering mechanism.[11] The appearance in both sexes, high incidence of parental consanguinity, and perceived normality of the parents in most familial cases have suggested an autosomal recessive mode of inheritance, with genes fully penetrant in the homozygous patient. However, survey of 1,012 first-degree relatives of 159 patients with achalasia failed to show a single case.[12] Thus, a distinct hereditary childhood disorder is probably very rare.

Other diverse disorders can cause a similar manometric picture of achalasia, including trauma (postsurgical fundoplication) and malignancy (by either direct extension into the LES or the remote effects of a distant tumor).[2]

CLINICAL PRESENTATION

Clinical manifestations of achalasia may include dysphagia (difficulty swallowing), nocturnal regurgitation, and noncardiac chest pain. Dysphagia is the cardinal symptom of achalasia. The disease is characterized by an insidious onset and indolent course, such that the diagnosis can remain elusive for years. Initially, the dysphagia may be episodic and related to size and character of the food bolus. With time, dysphagia slowly worsens and typically occurs for both solids and liquids. The patient may describe the site of obstruction at the suprasternal notch or the xyphoid area. As dysphagia worsens, the patient may develop maneuvers to facilitate eating, including repeated swallowing, eating only small quantities, drinking larger volumes of water, or arching backward with swallows. In severe cases, the esophagus may empty only by filling with food and secretions with gravitational pressure, forcing food through the nonrelaxing LES.

Children commonly regurgitate undigested food, which unlike gastroesophageal reflux is neither sour nor bitter. Regurgitation tends to occur at night because of the recumbent position. Food or secretions are often noticed on the pillow in the morning. Halitosis is a common complaint. Regurgitation can lead to microaspiration or gross aspiration, resulting in night cough or bronchospasm, or even aspiration pneumonia or lung abscess. The initial suggestion of achalasia may come from an upright chest radiograph showing a widened mediastinum caused by a dilated esophagus or by an air-fluid level in the posterior mediastinum. Chest pain may be a predominant symptom when there are spasm-like, high-pressure nonperistaltic contractions in the esophageal body. In such cases, the disease is referred to as vigorous achalasia.

Complications in children include weight loss, failure to thrive, aspiration pneumonia, reactive airway disease, and candida esophagitis. Weight loss is directly related to the severity of dysphagia. In infants and small children, respiratory problems, feeding problems, and poor weight gain may be the predominant symptoms. Adults are at risk of the development of esophageal carcinoma.

DIAGNOSIS

The diagnosis of achalasia is made by barium swallow radiography, esophageal manometry, and upper endoscopy. The characteristic radiograph is of a dilated intrathoracic esophagus with an air-fluid level. The LES tapers to a point, giving the distal esophagus a bird's beak–like appearance that does not open with swallowing. Radiologic criteria for achalasia include aperistalsis of the esophagus and failure of relaxation of the LES segment.

Esophageal manometry is the gold standard for the diagnosis of achalasia. A normal esophageal manometry demonstrates end-expiratory esophageal pressures 1 to 2 mmHg lower than gastric pressure, a resting LES tone of 15 to 25 mmHg, and complete LES relaxation to gastric baseline pressure and peristalsis in the entire body with contraction pressures in excess of 40 mmHg during swallowing. The classic manometric findings for the diagnosis of achalasia include (1) elevated basal end-expiratory esophageal pressure relative to gastric pressure; (2) elevated basal LES pressure (greater than 25 mmHg); (3) impaired relaxation of the LES during swallowing; (4) absence of peristalsis throughout the esophageal body during swallowing; and (5) low-amplitude (20- to 40-mmHg) tertiary esophageal pressure contractions. The resting LES pressure is actually elevated in 60% of achalasia cases. Impaired LES relaxation is the most important diagnostic criterion. Most patients have partial relaxation of the LES. To diagnose achalasia, the residual LES pressure between the esophagus and stomach should exceed 10 mmHg. Early in the course of the disease, intermittent peristalsis or peristaltic contractions in the proximal esophagus may be observed, and LES pressure may be within the normal range (15 to 25 mmHg). Vig-

orous (high-amplitude) simultaneous contractions may also be present early in the disease. Several adult patients with radiologic manifestation of achalasia and esophageal peristalsis have been described as having complete LES relaxation.[13] In such cases, the possibility of scleroderma, CREST syndrome (calcinosis, Reynaud's [phenomenon], esophageal [dysfunction], sclerodactyly, telangiectasia), and pseudo-obstruction must be considered prior to proceeding to pneumatic dilation or surgical therapy.

All patients should undergo endoscopy prior to forceful dilation or surgery. The purpose of endoscopy is to ensure passage of the endoscope through the gastroesophageal junction with minimal resistance, absolutely ruling out an anatomic obstruction. Moderate to marked resistance to passage of the endoscope through the gastroesophageal junction within the context of erosive esophagitis should raise suspicion of caustic ingestion, scleroderma, or reflux esophagitis. Endoscopy performed prior to pneumatic dilation will rule out candida esophagitis, a complication of esophageal food and fluid retention, and a contraindication to forceful dilation of the gastroesophageal junction.

TREATMENT

There is no therapy to restore LES relaxation or peristalsis. The treatment of achalasia is palliative and directed toward the symptomatic relief of the functional obstruction at the lower esophageal sphincter. Management may involve medical therapy, forceful dilation of the LES, or surgical esophagomyotomy. The initial treatment is controversial. No studies have been performed in children to compare the effectiveness of the different therapies.

Pneumatic dilation is the most effective, nonsurgical therapy available for the treatment of achalasia.[14,15] The goal is to weaken the resistance at the gastroesophageal junction by partially ripping the LES muscle. Objective long-term improvement in swallowing, weight gain, and respiratory symptoms clinical outcome has been reported in 60% to 80% of pediatric patients. The initial LES pressure or the diameter of the esophagus does not influence the probability of responding to dilation. Endoscopy is performed before each dilation to rule out candida esophagitis. If gross esophagitis is present, dilation is delayed until successful treatment is accomplished. Pneumatic dilation is a skilled procedure that requires experience. The procedure should only be performed in institutions where there is skilled surgical backup. The technique varies from institution to institution with main areas of difference, including the type of dilator used, inflation parameters, and duration of inflation. Because of limitations of dilator size, the procedure should only be performed in children over 6 years of age. Fluoroscopic guidance should always be used to position the dilating balloon across the diaphragmatic hiatus and to ensure that axial tension does not result in movement of the balloon during inflation. I currently use a Rigiflex achalasia dilator (Microvasive, Watertown, MA)[16] balloon, made of a modified polyethylene and mounted on a flexible catheter, inflated to 7 psi/m^2 for 45 seconds under fluoroscopic guidance, with the patient in the left semirecumbent position under deep conscious sedation or general anesthesia. Following recovery from sedation or anesthesia, a radiologic examination of the esophagus using water-soluble contrast material is obtained to exclude perforation. Fasting is maintained for at least 12 hours in hospital, during which the patient's vital signs are monitored every 4 hours. The patient is refed a regular diet the morning after dilation, with significant improvement in swallowing function if dilation has been successful. Lack of immediate improvement predicts poor outcome. Poor outcomes from treatment with pneumatic dilation include lack of significant objective clinical benefit, short-term benefit with recurrence of dysphagia within 6 months, and major complication, such as perforation. A second dilation using a higher inflation pressure should be undertaken if degree or duration of clinical benefit are a concern. Surgical myotomy should be undertaken if there is poor outcome following two dilations. The frequency of complications following pneumatic dilation appears to be no greater in children than in adults. Figures reported in the literature are within the range of 1% to 10%. Complications include esophageal perforation, tear, hematoma, or hemorrhage. The key to successful management of perforation is early recognition and treatment. Perforation is usually detected on postdilation esophagraphy but should be suspected in any patient in whom fever, prolonged chest pain, or unexplained tachycardia develops within 8 hours of the procedure. Any of the above symptoms should generate repeat esophagraphy, using water-soluble contrast material. Patients with perforation should receive prompt surgical intervention to limit progression of mediastinitis. Surgery usually involves a left posterolateral thoracotomy, closure of the perforation, establishment of adequate drainage, and performance of a surgical esophagomyotomy on the contralateral side. Follow-up studies in adults report outcomes similar to elective esophagomyotomy if emergency surgery is performed within 24 hours of perforation. Fever in the absence of chest pain or radiologic evidence of perforation or aspiration should be treated with bowel rest and broad-spectrum antibiotics for 5 to 7 days.[14] Esophageal hematomas are usually asymptomatic and resolve spontaneously. Bleeding at the gastroesophageal junction is rare and almost never life-threatening. Gastroesophageal reflux disease is uncommon after pneumatic dilation; if it does occur, it will usually respond to antisecretory therapy.[17]

Esophagomyotomy involves partial destruction of the LES by longitudinal incision of the esophageal circular muscle at the gastroesophageal junction (modified Heller myotomy). As with pneumatic dilation, surgical approach and technique vary from institution to institution. Experience of the surgeon is an important factor in surgical outcome. Surgical approach may be through the chest or abdomen, using classic thoracotomy, laparotomy, or laparoscopy.[18–22] The length and depth of the myotomy are important. Too deep a myotomy can lead to perforation of the esophageal mucosa, too short an incision can lead to incomplete sectioning of the LES and persistent dysphagia, and too long an incision on the gastric side can lead to intractable postoperative gastroesophageal reflux. The various modifications of the Heller procedure yield good to excellent outcome, defined as subjective improvement of dysphagia and resolution of achalasia-related complications in 70% to 90% of patients. The major complication of the surgical approach is the development of intractable gastroesophageal reflux, esophagitis, and peptic stricture formation. Many surgeons also perform a partial or loose antireflux fundoplication at surgical myotomy. In some patients with achalasia treated with pneumatic dilation or esophagomyotomy, esophageal peristalsis may return.[8]

Medical therapy has not been well studied for chronic treatment of achalasia in children. Thus, the long-term clinical efficacy of medical therapy such as calcium channel antagonists and nitrates remains unproved.[23] Calcium channel blocking agents interfere with calcium flux across cell membranes and diminish contractions of both vascular and visceral smooth muscle. Nifedipine significantly reduces LES pressure for more than 1 hour and has been useful in the short-term management of achalasia in children.[24] However, the development of drug tolerance, together with concern regarding long-term cardiac side effects, make it unlikely that current calcium channel antagonists will replace pneumatic dilation or esophagomyotomy as the primary treatment of achalasia. Nitrates such as isosorbide dinitrate also decrease LES pressure. In adults, nitrates compare favorably to calcium channel antagonists for objective improvement of postprandial dysphagia; their use has not been studied in children. Experimental approaches to the therapy of achalasia include the use of nitric oxide agonists[25] and local injection of botulinum toxin into the sphincter muscle.

PROGNOSIS

Longitudinal population studies in adults with achalasia suggest that the disease does not influence life expectancy. Such studies are not available for patients with onset of the disease in childhood. Achalasia in children should be viewed as a chronic functional illness that can be treated effectively by pneumatic dilation or Heller esophagomyotomy. Treatment does not cure dysphagia but, combined with maneuvers to facilitate swallowing and expected improvements in medical therapy, should allow relatively normal feeding behavior. Long-term management of the patient must include personal support and an understanding of the potential for recurrent symptoms, complications of therapy, and possible development of neoplasia. The risk of esophageal carcinoma is relatively small.

REFERRAL PATTERN

The primary care physician should suspect a disorder of the esophageal phase of swallowing based on a history of dysphagia, feeding difficulty or feeding aversion behavior, or chronic cough or bronchospasm associated with feeding difficulty or weight loss. Achalasia should also be suspected in any patient with alacrima or chronic adrenal insufficiency due to ACTH insensitivity in whom feeding difficulty or failure to thrive develops despite cortisone replacement therapy.

The primary care physician should initiate the diagnostic evaluation by ordering a barium esophagram. All patients with symptoms on barium esophagraphy suggestive of achalasia should be referred to a pediatric gastroenterologist for esophageal manometry and endoscopy, to verify the diagnosis. Management of achalasia requires ongoing collaboration between the primary care physician, pediatric gastroenterologist, and pediatric surgeon.

REFERENCES

1. Diamant NE. Physiology of esophageal motor function. Gastroenterol Clin North Am 1989;18:179–194
2. Reynolds JC, Parkman HP. Achalasia. Gastroenterol Clin North Am 1989;18:223–255
3. Mayberry JF, Atkinson M. Achalasia and other diseases associated with disorders of gastrointestinal motility. Hepatogastroenterology 1986;33:206–207
4. Mearin F, Mourelle M, Guarner F et al. Absence of nitric oxide synthase in the gastroesophageal junction of patients with achalasia. Gastroenterology 1993;104:A550
5. Goldblum JR, Rice TW, Richter JE. Histologic features in esophagomyotomy specimens from patients with achalasia. Gastroenterology 1996;111:648–654
6. Casella RR, Brown AL, Sayre GB, Ellis FH. Achalasia of the esophagus: pathologic and etiologic considerations. Ann Surg 1964;160:474–486
7. Helm JF, Layman RD, Eckert MD. Effect of chronic administration of Nw-Nitro-L-arginine (LNNA) on the opossum

esophagus and lower esophageal sphincter (LES) resembles achalasia. Gastroenterology 1992;103:1375
8. Cucchiara S, Staiano A, DiLorenzo C et al. Return of peristalsis in a child with esophageal achalasia treated by Heller's myotomy. J Pediatr Gastroenterol Nutr 1986;5:150–152
9. Robertson CS, Martin BA, Atkinson M. Varicella-zoster virus DNA in the esophageal myenteric plexus in achalasia. Gut 1993;34:299–302
10. Mearin F, Papo M, Malagelada JR. Impaired gastric relaxation in patients with achalasia. Gut 1994;36:363–368
11. Westley CR, Herbst JJ, Goldman S, Wiser WC. Infantile achalasia: inherited as an autosomal recessive disorder. J Pediatr 1975;87:243–246
12. Mayberry JF, Atkinson M. A study of swallowing difficulties in first degree relatives of patients with achalasia. Thorax 1985;40:391–393
13. Katz PO, Richter JE, Cowan R, Castell DO. Apparent complete lower esophageal sphincter relaxation in achalasia. Gastroenterology 1986;90:978–983
14. Boyle JT, Cohen S, Watkins JB. Successful treatment of achalasia in childhood by pneumatic dilatation. J Pediatr 1981;99:35–40
15. Berquist WE, Byrne WJ, Ament ME et al. Achalasia: diagnosis, management, and clinical course in 16 children. J Pediatrics 1983;71:798–805
16. Kadakia SC, Wong RK. Graded pneumatic dilatation using Rigiflex achalasia dilators in patients with primary esophageal achalasia. Am J Gastroenterol 1993;88:34–38
17. Azizkhan RG, Tapper D, Eraklis A. Achalasia in childhood: a 20 year experience. J Pediatr Surg 1980;15:452–456
18. Lemmer JH, Coran AG, Wesley JR et al. Achalasia in children: Treatment by anterior esophageal myotomy (modified Heller Operation). J Pediatr Surg 1985;20:333–338
19. Myers NA, Jolley SG, Taylor RT. Achalasia of the cardia in children: a worldwide survey. J Pediatr Surg 1994;29:1375–1379
20. Vane DW, Cosby K, West K, Grosfeld JL. Late results following esophagomyotomy in children with achalasia. J Pediatr Surg 1988;23:515–519
21. Allen KB, Ricketts RR. Surgery for achalasia of the cardia in children: the Dor-Gavriliu procedure. J Pediatr Surg 1992;27:1418–1421
22. Pellegrini C, Wetter LA, Patti M et al. Thoracoscopic esophagomyotomy. Ann Surg 1992;216:291–299
23. Gelfond M, Rozen P, Gilat T. Isosorbide dinitrate and nifedipine treatment of achalasia: a clinical, manometric and radionucleotide evaluation. Gastroenterology 1982;83:963–969
24. Maksimak M, Perlmutter DH, Winter HS. The use of nifedipine for the treatment of achalasia in children. J Pediatr Gastroenterol Nutr 1986;5:883–886
25. Marzio L, Cennamo L, DeLaurentiis MF, Grossi L. Cimetropium bromide reduces esophageal lower sphincter pressure and transit time in patients affected by primary achalasia. Gastroenterology 1993;104:A547
26. Pasricha PJ, Ravich WJ, Hendrix TR et al. Intrasphincteric botulinum toxin for treatment of achalasia. N Engl J Med 1995;322:774–778

17

GASTROINTESTINAL AND HEPATOBILIARY DISEASE IN THE ACQUIRED IMMUNODEFICIENCY SYNDROME

HELEN A. JOHN
ANDREW E. MULBERG

Acquired immunodeficiency syndrome (AIDS)–related gastrointestinal (GI) disease is most easily differentiated and understood by examining the specific and distinct effects of the human immunodeficiency virus (HIV) on individual organ systems. GI disorders are extremely common in persons infected with HIV. Because the GI tract lumina lack a strong physical barrier, infection with HIV accentuates this vulnerability.[1] For example, the effects of HIV infection on the enterocyte lead to malabsorption, while infection of the biliary epithelium results in AIDS cholangiopathy. This chapter discusses specific infections and other processes associated with AIDS and related illnesses.

CLINICAL PRESENTATION

The presentation of GI and hepatobiliary disease in children with AIDS can be variable. The GI sites of involvement include oral and esophagogastric, small bowel and colonic, hepatobiliary, and pancreatic and unusual GI manifestations of AIDS. Nutritional considerations in children with AIDS also play an important pathophysiologic role in the development of severe cachexia and malnutrition.

Mouth and Esophagus

Signs and symptoms of esophagitis, resulting from herpes simplex virus (HSV), *Candida*, and cytomegalovirus (CMV), lead to the presentation of common complaints in children with AIDS, including odynophagia, difficulty swallowing, chest pain, mouth ulcers, or discrete lesions. Other manifestations include oral hairy leukoplakia and lesions secondary to human papillomavirus.[2] Oral candidiasis and hairy oral leukoplakia in adults and recurrent HSV stomatitis in children are indicators of moderately severe disease in the classification of AIDS-related disease.[2] The classification of HIV-associated oral lesions in HIV infection is given in Table 17-1. Treatment options are listed in Table 17-2.

Stomach

A decrease in the acidity of the stomach without a clear pathophysiologic basis commonly develops in adults with AIDS.[3] No data are available in the literature regarding children. While the exact cause is unknown, the mechanism by which the HIV organism specifically causes achlorhydria may result from direct damage to the acid-producing parietal cell. The specific implications of decreased gastric acid relate to the altered bioavailability

TABLE 17-1.　Classification of HIV-Associated Oral Lesions

Lesions strongly associated with HIV infection
　Candidiasis
　Leukoplakia
　Kaposi's sarcoma
　Non-Hodgkin's lymphoma
　Periodontal disease
　　Necrotizing gingivitis
　　Linear gingival erythema
Lesions less commonly associated with HIV infection
　Bacterial infections
　　MAI
　Melanotic hyperpigmentation
　Necrotizing gingivitis
　Salivary gland disease (xerostomia)
　Aphthous ulceration (secondary to HSV type I)
　Viral infections
　　HSV
　　Papillomavirus
　　Varicella-zoster

(Adapted from Kline,[2] with permission.)

of certain drugs, including ketoconazole, and to the development of specific GI infections in patients with AIDS as a result of altered stomach defenses. In addition, the pharmacokinetics of drugs requiring gastric acidity may be altered, which can cause increased morbidity and mortality in these patients.

Of interest is the report of isolated antral narrowing in a 33-year-old man with AIDS who presented with nausea and postprandial vomiting. Radiographs of the upper GI tract showed a 4-cm-long, irregular, narrowed segment in the antrum proximal to the pylorus. Esophagogastroduodenoscopy showed diffuse erythema of spores

TABLE 17-2.　Treatment Options for AIDS-Associated Gastrointestinal Disease: Oral Cavity and Esophagus

Disease	Treatment
Oral candidiasis	Nystatin, clotrimazole troches
Esophageal candidiasis	Ketoconazole, fluconazole, amphotericin B
Oral hairy leukoplakia	Acyclovir
Herpes simplex virus	Acyclovir, foscarnet
Ulcers of unknown etiology	Systemic steroids, intralesional corticosteroid injections
CMV infection of esophagus or stomach	Intravenous gancyclovir, foscarnet

and active antritis. *Cryptosporidium* is more often a common pathogen in the etiology of infectious diarrhea.

Infectious Etiology of Diarrhea

One of the most common presentations of children with AIDS or AIDS-related complex include infectious diarrhea. Multiple etiologies of diarrhea have been described but typically occur secondary to infection. These infections include *Cryptosporidium*, CMV, *Salmonella* (nontyphoidal), *Isospora belli*, *Candida*, *Mycobacterium avium-intracellulare*, *Campylobacter*, *Microsporum* (i.e., *Enterocytozoon bieneusi*), *Giardia lamblia*, *Strongyloides*, *Entamoeba coli*, and *Plesiomonas*. HIV by itself can also be a primary enteric pathogen.[1] Treatment protocols for these infections are presented in Table 17-3.

Noninfectious Etiology of Enteropathy and Other Intestinal Disorders

AIDS ENTEROPATHY

AIDS enteropathy is a specific process that develops as a result of the HIV infection. The clinical syndrome is manifested by nonbloody, watery and non–mucus-containing diarrhea, resulting in weight loss and marked increase in mortality.[1] A correlation of GI symptoms can be made with in situ hybridization using p24, a specific antigen expressed by HIV. Endoscopic examination shows villous atrophy, increased crypt hyperplasia, and increased intraepithelial lymphocytes. These findings are nonspecific and also observed in celiac disease, acute graft-versus-host disease, and intestinal allograft rejection. In children, various GI presentations have been described, including idiopathic villous atrophy and bacterial opportunistic infections.[4]

SURGICAL PROBLEMS AND HIV INFECTION

AIDS-related abdominal pathology has been reported to include perforation secondary to CMV, Kaposi's sarcoma, and lymphoma; intussusception in young adults; obstruction secondary to lymphoma and lymphoid hyperplasia; *Strongyloides* infestation; primary peritonitis secondary to *Cryptococcus* and CMV; terminal ileitis secondary to CMV and MAI; cholecystitis (calculous and acalculous); cholangitis and papillary stenosis; GI bleeding; and appendicitis.[5,6] Such presentations are probably less common in children with AIDS.

Hepatobiliary Disease

One of the more common manifestations of AIDS in children is chronic active hepatitis. The proposed mechanism involves an autoimmune reaction secondary to HIV. Patients present with hepatomegaly and with elevated transaminases and normal alkaline phosphatase

TABLE 17-3. Treatment of Intestinal Disease in HIV Infection

Organism	Drug or Procedure
Cryptosporidium parvum	Paromomycin, octreotide, antimotility agents
Enterocytozoon bieneusi	Trimethoprim-sulfamethoxazole, metronidazole, paromomycin
Isospora belli	Trimethoprim-sulfamethoxazole, trimethoprim
Giardia lamblia	Metronidazole, furazolidone, quinacrine hydrochloride
Entamoeba histolytica	Metronidazole, followed by iodoquinol
Bacterial enteritis (i.e., *Shigella*, *Campylobacter*, and *Salmonella*)	Conventional antibiotics
Pseudomembranous colitis	Vancomycin, metronidazole
Strongyloides stercoralis	Thiabendazole
Blastocystis hominis	Oral metronidazole
Microsporum	Octreotide, albendazole
Secondary intestinal disease	
Cytomegalovirus	Gancyclovir, foscarnet
Mycobacterial infections	Combinations using amikacin, rifampin, ethambutol, clofazimine, ciprofloxacin
Fungal infections (*Candida, Cryptococcus, Coccidioides*)	Fluconazole
Herpes simplex virus type 2	Oral or parenteral acyclovir, foscarnet
CMV infection	Gancyclovir
Venereal disease	Antibiotics, intralesional or systemic steroids for deep anal ulcer
Neoplastic disease	
Kaposi's sarcoma	Chemotherapy, interferon, radiation therapy, laser ablation of symptomatic ulcers
Lymphomas	Combination chemotherapy
Neoplasms (squamous cell carcinomas)	Surgical resection, chemotherapy, laser photocoagulation

levels. Laboratory testing indicates elevated alkaline phosphatase in most cases (87%) and a rise in transaminases in 40% of patients presented by Negra et al.[7] Histopathologic features include giant cell hepatitis, bridging portal fibrosis, piecemeal necrosis, bile duct epithelial destruction, sinusoidal hyperplasia, steatosis, and cholestasis.[8–12]

A recent review of 15 pediatric patients with AIDS (aged 21 to 48 months) who underwent percutaneous liver biopsy demonstrated 13% with chronic hepatopathy, 13% with granulomatous hepatitis, 7% with acute hepatitis, and 53% with a reactive hepatitis.[7] Patients with a hepatic parenchymal infiltrate (especially giant cell transformation) may have associated lymphocytic interstitial pneumonitis.[11] The differential diagnosis of these nonspecific liver abnormalities must always include infectious hepatitis (including A, B, C, D, CMV, herpes and, rarely, *Pneumocystis carinii*), a toxin-mediated hepatitis (e.g., Bactrim, AZT), or AIDS cholangiopathy.

AIDS cholangiopathy is manifested by signs and symptoms of sclerosing cholangitis. Etiologic factors include CMV and *Cryptosporidium*. In adults, a reversible cause of AIDS cholangiopathy has been attributed to successful chemotherapeutic treatment of a disseminated

B-cell non-Hodgkin's lymphoma.[13] Other rare manifestations of hepatobiliary disease in children have included cholecystitis secondary to CMV and *Serratia marcescens*, cat-scratch disease presenting as hepatic granulomas, and adenovirus-associated hepatic necrosis. Another manifestation that has been reported includes peliosis hepatis secondary to rickettsial infection (*Rochalimaea henselae*). Table 17-4 outlines an evaluation for patients with AIDS who present with hepatobiliary abnormalities. Table 17-5 lists eriterin for an HIV-positive child with diarrhea who has had a recent history of travel and patient contact.

Pancreatic Disease

Pancreatic disease is usually indicative of progressive AIDS disease. Acute pancreatitis occurs in 12% of children with AIDS and represents a poor prognostic finding. In a recent histopathologic review of autopsy specimens from children who died of AIDS, the pancreatic histopathology ranged from acute and chronic pancreatitis to nonspecific changes, including edema, fibrosis, inspissated material within acini and ducts, and nodular lymphoplasmacytic infiltrate.[14] The medications used to

TABLE 17-4. Evaluation of Elevated Transaminases and Bilirubin in Children With AIDS

History: recent viral infection, medications

Physical examination: presence of hepatosplenomegaly or jaundice

Hepatitis screen, hepatitis C polymerase chain reaction in neonates: TORCH titers

If above negative, check creatinine phosphokinase, aldolase to rule out HIV myositis

If GGT elevated, do abdominal ultrasound to rule out gallstones and evaluate bile ducts for dilation

If recent change in medication, consider withholding the medication and repeat liver enzymes in 2–3 days

Consider abdominal ultrasound with Doppler if splenomegaly present to evaluate portal vein and direction of blood

If none of the above diagnostic, consider liver biopsy and diagnostic cholangiogram by endoscopic retrograde cholangiopancreatography (ERCP) or percutaneous cholangiogram by gallbladder injection; send tissue for bacterial cultures and for viruses, such as hepatitis virus B or C, CMV, or Epstein-Barr virus; special stains for acid-fast bacteria

treat AIDS are the most common cause of acute pancreatitis in adults. These drugs include 2′, 3′-dideoxyinosine, parenteral or aerosolized pentamidine isethionate, octreotide, and the sulfonamides.[15] In addition, infectious agents can cause pancreatitis. Pancreatic tumors such as Kaposi's sarcoma and Burkitt's and non-Hodgkin's lymphomas have been described in adults; however, to date no pancreatic tumors have been reported.[14]

Whether AIDS-related opportunistic infections lead to chronic pancreatitis and exocrine pancreatic insufficiency is presently unknown. Chronic pancreatitis may have some relationship to the development of chronic diarrhea that plagues many AIDS patients.

TABLE 17-5. HIV-Positive Child With Diarrhea Who Has a History of Recent Travel and Patient Contact

Stool for ova and parasites, *Cryptosporidium*, *Clostridium difficile*, and bacterial culture

If diarrhea persistent, stop feeding to identify secretory versus osmotic diarrhea; send stool for osmolarity, electrolytes along with serum osmolarity; if secretory, send stool for *Vibrio* species and other enteric pathogens (i.e., *Cryptosporidium*)

If stool studies negative, consider upper endoscopy to rule out *Helicobacter pylori*, duodenal fluid for culture and giardiasis; biopsies for disaccharidases and flexible sigmoidoscopy

Nutritional Considerations in AIDS

ETIOLOGY OF NUTRITIONAL DEFICIENCIES IN AIDS

Patients with AIDS develop malnutrition from a variety of etiologies: (1) decreased nutrient intake from anorexia, vomiting, nausea, stomatitis, odynophagia, dysphagia, epigastric pain, dyspepsia, and depression; (2) increased nutrient loss from diarrhea and nonspecific AIDS enteropathy; (3) malabsorption of fat, carbohydrate, vitamin B_{12}, folate, thiamin, zinc, selenium; and (4) increased nutrient requirements secondary to fever, catabolism, sepsis, medications, and neoplasms.

Nutritional assessment of patients with AIDS should include the following paradigm: (1) monitoring dietary intake, body weight, height, head circumference, signs of wasting, and malnutrition; (2) monitoring laboratory parameters, including albumin, total iron binding capacity (TIBC), iron, zinc, and a complete blood count (CBC); (3) adjusting intake and diet to degree of GI function; (4) maintaining adequate caloric intake and minimizing catabolic state, dependent on factors previously discussed.

LABORATORY TESTS

Specific laboratory tests may be helpful in the diagnosis of AIDS-related GI diseases.

1. *CBC with differential*—usually mild to moderate leukocytosis. Occasionally, specific infections, including *Isospora belli* infection, is not associated with leukocytosis. Eosinophilia may be seen in parasitic infections, such as *Strongyloides stercoralis*.
2. *Electrolytes/serum osmolarity*—in chronic diarrhea, patient may have metabolic acidosis with decreased sodium and potassium levels; in osmotic diarrhea, serum osmolarity is less than the osmolarity found in the stools; in secretory diarrhea, the serum osmolarity is equal to stool osmolarity. Secretory diarrhea seen in infections with enterotoxigenic strains of *Escherichia coli* and *Vibrio* species
3. *Blood cultures*—Bacterial isolation, CMV, *Mycobacterium*
4. *Stool studies*—Microscopy to detect parasites, fecal leukocytes, routine stool cultures, stool culture requiring special media (*Aeromonas*, enteropathogenic *Escherichia coli*, *Mycobacterium avium-intracellulare*, *Vibrio* species, *Yersinia enterocolitica*), stool enzyme-linked immunosorbent assay [ELISA] for rotavirus, enteric adenovirus, *Clostridium difficile* toxins A and B, *Giardia lamblia*, acid-fast stains for *Cryptosporidium*, *Cyclospora* species, and *Microsporum* and trichrome staining for *Microsporum* and *Blastocystis hominis*.

TREATMENT

The treatment protocols for all GI diseases reported in AIDS-related infections are delineated in Tables 17-1 to 17-4.

Chronic Active Hepatitis

No definitive treatment modality is available for chronic active hepatitis.

Referral Pattern

Specific referral to a pediatric gastroenterologist may be suggested with the development of organ-specific disease.

REFERENCES

1. Edison SA, Kotler DP. How HIV infection and AIDS affect the gastrointestinal tract. J Crit Illness 1992;7:37–56

2. Kline MW. Oral manifestations of pediatric human immunodeficiency virus infection: a review of the literature. Pediatrics 1996;97:380–388

3. Lake-Bakaar G, Quadros E, Beidass S et al. Gastric secretory failure in patients with the acquired immunodeficiency syndrome (AIDS). Ann Intern Med 1988;109:502–504

4. McLoughlin LC, Nord KS, Joshi VV et al. Severe gastrointestinal involvement in children with the acquired immunodeficiency syndrome. J Pediatr Gastroenterol Nutr 1987;6:517–524

5. Wood BJ, Kumar PN, Cooper C et al. AIDS-associated intussusception in young adults. J Clin Gastroenterol 1995;21:158–162

6. Bharucha S, Brandt LJ. Abdominal surgery and the acquired immunodeficiency syndrome. Pract Gastroenterol 1996;18:22C–22J

7. Negra MD, Queiroz W, Taveras CJR et al. Liver disorders in pediatric AIDS patients. Pediatr AIDS HIV Infect 1993;4:222–226

8. Kahn E, Greco A, Daum R et al. Hepatic pathology in pediatric acquired immunodeficiency syndrome. Hum Pathol 1991;22:1111–1119

9. Duffy LF, Daum F, Kahn E et al. Hepatitis in children with acquired immune deficiency syndrome. Gastroenterology 1986;90:173–181

10. Schneiderman DJ, Arenson DM, Cello JP et al. Hepatic disease in patients with the acquired immune deficiency syndrome (AIDS). Hepatology 1987;7:925–930

11. Jonas MM, Roldan EO, Lyons HJ et al. Histopathologic features of the liver in pediatric acquired immune deficiency syndrome. J Pediatr Gastroenterol Nutr 1989;9:73–81

12. Witzleben CL, Marshall GS, Wenner W et al. HIV as a cause of giant cell hepatitis. Hum Pathol 1988;19:603–605

13. Teare JP, Price DA, Foster GR et al. Reversible AIDS-related sclerosing cholangitis. Hepatology 1995;23:209–211

14. Kahn E, Anderson VM, Greco MA, Magid M. Pancreatic disorders in pediatric acquired immune deficiency syndrome. Hum Pathol 1995;26:765–770

15. Miller TL, Winter HS, Luginbuhi LM et al. Pancreatis in pediatric human immunodeficiency infection. J Pediatr 1992;120:233–237

18

BACTERIAL INFECTIONS

HAROHALLI SHASHIDHAR
MUNIR MOBASSALEH

Diarrheal disease is a leading cause of mortality and morbidity in children younger than 5 years of age, throughout the world. An estimated one billion episodes of diarrhea and four million deaths occur annually in the pediatric age group, with most occurring in the developing world.[1] Children less than 2 years of age have the highest incidence of diarrhea, which peaks at 6 to 11 months of age. In the developing world, the estimated median incidence of acute diarrhea is 2.6 episodes per child per year,[2] with an average case fatality rate of 0.2%.[3] Incidence data from the developed world are limited. A U.S. study estimated that 21 to 37 million episodes of acute diarrhea occur annually in 16.5 million children less than 5 years of age. Approximately 10% of these episodes lead to physician visits, with 220, 000 hospitalizations and approximately 400 deaths.[4]

Acute enteric infections are associated with a higher incidence of complications in children compared to adults. The morbidity from acute bacterial diarrhea results from dehydration and its associated sequelae. However, the main impact of chronic diarrhea is in causing malnutrition that leads to increased mortality. In the developing countries, case fatality rates dramatically increase to 14% in cases of persistent diarrhea.[5] In addition, immunosuppression due to chemotherapy, bone marrow and solid organ transplants, and human immunodeficiency virus (HIV) infections result in further increases in morbidity and mortality. In one multicenter study, bacterial pathogens were identified in 8% of watery diarrheal episodes and in 20% of bloody diarrheal episodes.[6] In the United States, the predominant bacterial pathogens causing diarrheal illness include *Campylobacter*, *Salmonella*, *Escherichia coli* serotype 0157 : H7, and *Shigella*.

Common routes of spread of diarrheal illnesses include fecal-oral and person-to-person transmission and contaminated food and water. The precise mode of spread for various organisms is dependent on the characteristics of the specific organism, which include the required infective inoculum, carriage rate in human and nonhuman hosts, and the ability to survive outside of human hosts.

The mechanisms involved in the pathogenesis of bacterial diarrhea are diverse: (1) secretion of enterotoxins causing increased fluid secretion into the gut lumen; (2) elaboration of cytotoxins causing cell destruction and resulting in inflammatory (dysenteric) diarrhea; (3) direct invasion of intestinal cells with intracellular multiplication and cell-to-cell spread causing mucosal inflammation and decreased absorptive surface; and (4) adhesion to enterocytes resulting in cytoskeletal changes. Some toxins possess both enterotoxic and cytotoxic effects, and certain bacteria cause illness by more than one pathogenic mechanism (Table 18–1). Most toxins are multimeric proteins with A and B subunits. The B subunit is the binding component, while the A subunit mediates the biologic effects of the toxin.[7]

The following discussion on bacterial causes of diarrheal illness in children excludes *Clostridium difficile* infection (for an in-depth discussion, see Ch. 20).

TABLE 18-1. Summary of Bacterial Enteropathogens

Organism	Pathogenic Mechanisms	Clinical Presentation	Risk Factors
Salmonella	Cell invasion Systemic spread Enterotoxins	Dysenteric or watery, profuse stools Fecal leukocytes	Contaminated poultry, beef, and eggs
Shigella	Cell invasion systemic spread Shiga toxin	Dysentery Fecal leukocytes	Poor sanitation; day care centers
Campylobacter jejuni	Colonization and adherence Cytotoxin	Dysenteric or bloody stools Fecal leukocytes	Contaminated poultry, milk, and water; domestic pets
Enterotoxigenic *E. coli*	Colonization Heat-labile and heat-stable enterotoxins	Acute watery diarrhea	Travel to endemic area
Enteropathogenic *E. coli*	Localized adherence Effacing and attaching lesion	Acute or persistent diarrhea	Children in developing countries
Enterohemorrhagic *E. coli*	Attachment Shiga-like toxin	Nonbloody or bloody stools	Undercooked ground beef
Enteroaggregative *E. coli*	Localized or diffuse adherence	Persistent diarrhea	Poor sanitation; infants in developing countries
Enteroinvasive *E. coli*	Cell invasion Systemic spread	Dysentery	Poor sanitation
Yersinia enterocolitica	Cell invasion Systemic spread Enterotoxin	Acute watery or dysenteric stools Pseudoappendicitis syndrome	Contaminated pork, milk, and water
Vibrio cholerae	Adherence Heat-labile enterotoxin	Profuse, watery diarrhea	Endemic areas
Vibrio parahaemolyticus	Cell invasion ?Enterotoxin	Acute watery or dysenteric stools	Contaminated shellfish
Aeromonas, Plesiomonas	Adherence Invasion Cyto- and enterotoxins	Acute, watery or dysenteric stools—chronic	Contaminated aquatic sources

GENERAL PRINCIPLES OF THERAPY

Children are more susceptible to dehydration because they have a higher proportion of total body water composed of extracellular fluid, a larger body surface area relative to weight, and a more severe or prolonged course of illness complicated by vomiting. In the acute setting, correction of fluid and electrolyte deficits assumes priority irrespective of the cause of diarrhea. Oral rehydration therapy (ORT), considered one of the significant medical advances of the twentieth century, has revolutionized diarrheal therapy in the developing world. ORT is based on the physiologic principle that glucose enhances transport of sodium and fluid across the intestinal epithelium. The current recommended composition of oral rehydrating solutions (ORS) is glucose, 2.0% to 2.5% (110–140 mmol/L);

sodium, 75 to 90 mmol/L; potassium, 20 mmol/L; anions, 20% to 30% as base; and the remainder as chloride.[8] Most children with mild to moderate dehydration can be effectively treated with ORS at 50 to 100 ml/kg over a 4-hour period. Severe dehydration, intractable vomiting, and neurologic disturbances are indications for intravenous rehydration with isotonic solution, until hemodynamic stability is achieved. Replacement of ongoing losses is essential and is estimated at 10 ml/kg for each stool and 2 ml/kg for each emesis.[9]

In order to prevent the malnutrition associated with chronic and recurrent diarrhea, early refeeding is essential. Malabsorption is rarely severe enough to preclude early institution of enteral nutrition, which is especially important in younger children in the developing countries. Total parenteral nutrition is occasionally necessary in cases of protracted diarrhea.

PREVENTION

Prevention of diarrheal disease spread should be instituted at the community, family, and individual levels. Food-borne transmission is prevented by improvements in production, processing, and storage of meat and food products. Provision of pasteurized milk, clean drinking water, and monitoring of swimming waters are primary considerations. Prevention of person-to-person spread involves the isolation of infected individuals. Strict hand-washing remains as the single most effective mode of prevention, particularly in day care centers, food establishments, and health care institutions. At the family level, washing of vegetables and safe storage of cooked and processed foods at optimal temperatures are essential for prevention.

BACTERIAL ENTEROPATHOGENS

Salmonella

Salmonella is a gram-negative, flagellated bacillus, currently recognized as a single species, Salmonella choleraesuis. Thus, S. typhi, S. paratyphi, S. typhimurium, and S. enteritidis are different serotypes of the same species.

Salmonella infection has two distinct clinical presentations: typhoidal salmonella causing enteric or typhoid fever and nontyphoidal salmonella, primarily causing gastroenteritis. Typhoid fever, caused by a S. typhi and S. paratyphi, is a global health problem that has a lower incidence in the United States. Most sporadic cases are related to foreign travel, most frequently to Mexico and the Indian subcontinent,[10] and are transmitted by food and water contaminated with the excreta of its only host, humans. Enteric fever is uncommon in children less than 1 year of age.

The incidence of nontyphoidal salmonella, mostly caused by S. enteritides and S. typhimurium, has recently increased in the United States.[11] An estimated 1 to 2 million cases occur annually, with the highest attack rate in infancy. Nontyphoidal salmonella has a variety of animal hosts. Eggs and undercooked poultry are most commonly involved in transmission. Contrary to popular belief, person-to-person transmission through food handlers and health care workers is unusual,[12] except in neonatal and infantile cases of salmonella.

PATHOGENESIS

Gastric acid is the first barrier to salmonella. Hence, antacid therapy, gastric surgery, and reduced gastric acid production in neonates increase the risk of infection. Secretory IgA and mucus also play a role in the defense against bacterial penetration. Salmonella infects the enterocytes and M cells, followed by internalization to sub-mucosal lymphoid tissue and entry into the systemic circulation. Chromosomal genes encode for virulence factors, resulting in enterocyte invasion, survival within the macrophage, and acid resistance.[13] Other virulence factors include plasmid-mediated enterotoxins. Host factors that increase susceptibility include immune suppression, malaria, sickle cell disease, and absent or decreased splenic function.

CLINICAL PRESENTATION

Typhoid fever; gastroenteritis; focal infections of the nervous system, bones, and joints; and a chronic carrier state comprise the clinical spectrum of Salmonella. The different clinical pictures may overlap, and patients with gastroenteritis may have fever and bacteremia, while gastroenteritis may occur in typhoid fever.

Typhoid fever presents with fever and prominent systemic features, including lethargy and headache. Characteristic features include a skin rash (rose spots), relative bradycardia, and splenomegaly. Gastroenteritis presents with abdominal cramps, nausea, and vomiting and has an incubation period of about 6 to 48 hours. Stools can be dysenteric or watery and profuse (cholera-like) lasting 3 to 7 days. Systemic symptoms of fever, chills, headache, and myalgia may occur. The overall mortality of nontyphoidal Salmonella infection is reported to be less than 0.5%.[11]

Complications of nontyphoidal salmonella include pseudoappendicitis syndrome, consisting of fever, severe abdominal pain, and right lower quadrant tenderness. Focal infections, including meningitis, are more common in children, and osteomyelitis and arthritis occur with increased frequency in association with sickle cell disease.[14] Reactive arthritis, which has an association with HLA B27 antigen, may occur after the onset of diarrhea and usually lasts an average of 6 months.[14]

The chronic carrier state, defined as prolonged carriage of Salmonella in stool and urine for greater than 1 year, has an incidence up to 4% in typhoidal infections but occurs less commonly in nontyphoidal salmonella (less than 1%).[12]

DIAGNOSIS

Fecal leukocytes are usually present, and stool cultures of fresh stool specimens establish the diagnosis. Serotyping is based on the agglutination of somatic (O) and flagellar (H) antigens. Positive blood cultures in the first week and stool cultures in the second week confirm the diagnosis of typhoid fever. Serum antibody response usually occurs later in typhoidal Salmonella infection.

TREATMENT

Primary therapy in nontyphoidal illness consists of correction of fluid and electrolyte imbalance. Antimicrobial therapy may be associated with a higher clinical relapse rate.[15] However, patients at increased risk of bacteremia (neonates, those with sickle cell disease, and immunosuppressed persons) and those with focal infections are candidates for antibiotic therapy with ampicillin, trimethoprim-sulfamethoxazole, or third-generation cephalosporins. Amoxicillin and trimethoprim-sulfamethoxazole have been used for 6 weeks in the eradication of chronic carrier states. Cholecystectomy may be necessary in chronic carriers with gallstones. An oral typhoid vaccine is indicated for prophylaxis in persons traveling to endemic areas. The vaccine has not been well studied in children.

Shigella

Shigella is a gram-negative bacillus comprising four species: *S. dysenteriae*, *S. flexneri*, *S. boydii*, and *S. sonnei*. Shigellosis is prevalent worldwide, and the main mode of transmission is fecal-oral person-to-person spread. In the United States, *S. sonnei* is the predominant species, causing shigellosis.[16] The small inoculum dose required (10 to 100 organisms) to cause infection facilitates spread and explains its association with overcrowding, poverty, poor personal hygiene, and sanitation. Children in day care centers are at high risk for shigellosis.[17] Endemic shigellosis is predominant in children less than 10 years of age but is uncommon before 6 months of age.

PATHOGENESIS

Bacterial genes encoding for various pathogenic factors are present on both the chromosomes and plasmids. Virulence determinants include the following[18]: (1) chromosomally encoded superoxide dismutase helps in bacterial survival by inhibition of the bactericidal activity of free O_2 radicles in the gastrointestinal (GI) tract; (2) plasmid-encoded invasiveness and ability to multiply within enterocytes; and (3) chromosomally encoded Shiga toxin produced by *S. dysenteriae* type I, exhibits cytotoxic, enterotoxic and neurotoxic effects and inhibits protein synthesis.

Shiga toxin binds to a cell surface glycolipid receptor globotriaosylceramide (Gb_3). The expression of Gb_3 is lacking in neonatal rabbits and progressively increases with age.[19] The secretory response to the toxin parallels the level of receptor expression and thus may explain the relative resistance of human neonates to shigellosis.

CLINICAL PRESENTATION

Shigella infection presents with generalized constitutional symptoms, including fever, fatigue, malaise, and loss of appetite. Nausea and vomiting are common, and the initial watery diarrhea may progress to bloody dysenteric stools within hours to days. Shigellosis in the United States is usually mild, due to the predominance of *S. sonnei* infection. In the developing countries, shigellosis

tends to be a more severe illness complicated by toxic megacolon and perforation, resulting in increased mortality. The severity of the inflammatory response is dependent on the infective dose and on the presence of underlying malnutrition.

Unique clinical features occasionally occur, including hyponatremia, rectal prolapse in younger children, and protein-losing enteropathy leading to malnutrition and growth failure.[20] Bacteremic spread is rare in *S. sonnei* infections. Other complications include hemolytic uremic syndrome (HUS) (see the discussion below, *Enterohemorrhagic E. coli*), encephalopathy, and seizures. Reactive arthritis and Reiter's syndrome are extraintestinal complications that exhibit strong association with HLA B27 histocompatibility antigen.

DIAGNOSIS

A clinical picture compatible with shigellosis and a stool smear with more than 50 leukocytes per high-powered field is sufficient to make a presumptive diagnosis. DNA probes and polymerase chain reaction (PCR) testing of the various virulence factors are more sensitive and useful in the diagnosis of patients pretreated with antibiotics. Serologic studies are of epidemiologic interest only.

TREATMENT

Primary modality of therapy consists of fluid and electrolyte correction, with particular attention to correction of hyponatremia and hypoglycemia in malnourished children. Seizures are managed as any febrile seizures. Antimicrobial agents (Table 18-2) lower mortality and shorten the duration of illness. First-line antibiotics are trimethoprim-sulfamethoxazole and ampicillin. Third-generation cephalosporins are reserved for resistant strains.

Campylobacter jejuni

Campylobacter jejuni, a small spiral-shaped gram-negative bacterium, is reportedly the most common bacterial cause of diarrhea in the developed world.[20a] This fastidious organism is susceptible to a variety of physical and chemical agents, including atmospheric oxygen. *C. fetus* and *C. coli* cause similar enteric illnesses. The incidence is highest in summer and late fall and follows a bimodal age distribution: children less than 1 year and those aged 15 to 24 years.[21] Most infections occur sporadically or in family clusters. *C. jejuni* is a normal commensal of domestic pets and poultry; at-risk groups include farmers, butchers, and people with pets. Transmission, requiring a low inoculum, spreads through contaminated water, milk, and undercooked poultry.

TABLE 18-2. Antimicrobial Therapy for Selected Bacterial Diarrheal Illnesses

Organism	Antimicrobial Agent	Dosage (mg/kg/dose, max) Frequency, Duration	Remarks
Salmonella	Ampicillin or TMP-SMX or Ceftriaxone or Cefotaxime Chronic carrier state: Amoxicillin	35 (1,000) q4h ×14 days 5/25 (160/800) q12h ×14 days 50 (3,000) q6h ×14 days 15 q8h ×6 wk 75 (2,000) bid ×14 days	Indicated in invasive or focal infection; not indicated for uncomplicated gastroenteritis
Shigella	TMP-SMX or Ampicillin or Ciprofloxacin[a] or Ceftriaxone	5/25 (160/800) q12h ×5 days 20 (500) q6h ×5 days 500 (1,000) q12h ×5 days 50 (1,500) q24h ×5 days	Therapy indicated for most patients with dysentery
Campylobacter jejuni	Erythromycin or Ciprofloxacin[a]	10 (250) q6h ×5–7 days 500 (1,000) q12h ×5–7 days	None needed in mild cases
Enterotoxigenic *Escherichia coli*	TMP-SMX or Ciprofloxacin[a]	5/25 (160/800) q12h ×3–5 days 500 (1,000) q12h ×3–5 days	
Enteroinvasive *E. coli*	Same as in shigellosis		
Enteropathogenic *E. coli*	TMP-SMX	5/25 (160/800) q12h	Antibiotic therapy controversial; no controlled studies
Enterohemorrhagic *E. coli*	?TMP-SMX		Antibiotic therapy not well enough established to be beneficial
Enteroadherent *E. coli*	No data available		
Yersinia enterocolitica	TMP-SMX or Ciprofloxacin[a]	5/25 (160/800) q12h 500 (1,000) q12h	Indicated in invasive/focal disease; duration of optimal therapy not well established
Vibrio cholerae 01	TMP/SMX or tetracycline[b] or doxycycline[b]	5/25 (160/800) q12h ×3 days 10 (250) q6h ×3 days 6 (300) q12h ×3 days	
Vibrio parahaemolyticus	Tetracycline[b] or Cefotaxime	10 (250) q6h 50 (2,000) q6h	Therapy needed only in severe cases
Aeromonas, Plesiomonas	Same as in shigellosis		

Abbreviation: TMP-SMX, trimethoprim-sulfamethoxazole.

[a] Ciprofloxacin has not been approved for patients less than 17 years of age.

[b] Tetracycline is only used in patients more than 9 years of age.

(Modified from Pickering and Matson,[39] with permission.)

PATHOGENESIS

The motility and spiral-shaped structure of *Campylobacter* enable it to move through intestinal mucous.[22] It is unclear whether enterocyte adherence is necessary for infection; however, invasion of both the colon and small intestine results in a histologic picture mimicking idiopathic inflammatory bowel disease. Other pathogenic mechanisms include production of a cytotoxin and a cholera-like enterotoxin.

CLINICAL PRESENTATION

Campylobacter enteritis is clinically indistinguishable from that of *Salmonella* or *Shigella*. A typical feature, however, is a prodromal nonspecific flu-like illness. Abdominal pain can be very severe and may be the sole symptom in 10% of cases.[23] Vomiting and bloody stools are more common in neonates and infants. Most *C. jejuni* infections are self-limited, with milder disease seen in children than in adults. Complications include seizures and Guillain-Barre syndrome due to possible cross-reactivity between peripheral myelin and *Campylobacter* antigens.[24]

DIAGNOSIS

The presumptive diagnosis is based on the presence of fecal leukocytes and erythrocytes in association with a compatible clinical picture. Stool culture confirms the diagnosis. Identification of organisms on dark-field microscopy or stained smear are useful for rapid diagnosis.

Detection of serum antibodies, which peak between 2 to 4 weeks, is useful in retrospective diagnosis of patients presenting with Guillain-Barré syndrome.

TREATMENT

Correction of fluid and electrolyte imbalance is sufficient in most cases of *Campylobacter* infection. Erythromycin is the antibiotic of choice in more severe cases (Table 18-2).

Escherichia coli

Six types of *E. coli* are known to be pathogenic to humans: enterotoxigenic, enterohemorrhagic, enteropathogenic, enteroinvasive, enteroaggregative, and diffuse-adherent. The virulence of *E. coli* depends on the various encoding genes residing on bacterial chromosomes or plasmids specific for the different types of *E. coli*.

ENTEROTOXIGENIC *E. COLI*

Enterotoxigenic *E. coli* (ETEC) is a major cause of diarrheal illness in the developing world. It is the leading cause of "traveler's diarrhea" to endemic areas. ETEC is acquired mainly by contaminated food or water and requires a large inoculum for infection. Children are at an increased risk at the time of weaning, especially in areas of the world with poor sanitation.

Pathogenesis

ETEC diarrhea is mediated by plasmid-encoded enterotoxins that are either heat-stable (ST) or heat-labile (LT). ST causes increased intestinal fluid secretion through activation of guanylate cyclase resulting in increased cyclic/guanosine monophosphate (cGMP), while LT acts through activation of adenylate cyclase, increasing cAMP.[7] In addition, ETEC produces fimbrial attachments called colonization factor antigens (CFA) that mediate enterocyte adherence.

Clinical Presentation

Clinical illness caused by ETEC is characterized by watery, nonbloody, nonmucoid diarrhea, usually without fever or abdominal pain. The incubation period is 14 to 50 hours. The diarrhea can be of varying severity but is usually mild and self-limited, except in malnourished children.

Diagnosis

Specific assays for toxins are not available in clinical laboratories and are rarely necessary. The diagnosis is based on the clinical picture and, if necessary, by stool culture and identification of recognized ETEC serotypes.

Treatment

ETEC infection does not usually require antibiotic therapy. ORT is a safe and effective method for replacing fluid and electrolyte losses. Trimethoprim-sulfamethoxazole reportedly shortens the course and decreases the duration of bacterial fecal shedding.[25]

ENTEROPATHOGENIC *E. COLI*

Enteropathogenic *E. coli* (EPEC) was the first diarrheagenic *E. coli* recognized in newborn nursery outbreaks. It is a frequent cause of diarrhea across the world but is less common in the developed countries, including the United States. Fecal-oral person-to-person spread is the primary mode of transmission. Contamination of food and water is reportedly rare. The increase in day care centers and immunocompromised hosts contributes to the observed increase in incidence in the United States.

Pathogenesis

EPEC is neither invasive nor toxigenic; however, it attaches intimately to intestinal epithelial cells. The plasmid-encoded EPEC adherence factor results in the formation of a bundle-forming pilus responsible for localized adherence. This is followed by activation of the attachment and effacement chromosomal genes, eaeA and eaeB, resulting in binding to intestinal cells and leading to the accumulation of filamentous actin which forms the cupping or "pedestal lesion" on the enterocyte.[26] The precise relationship between these EPEC effects on the cell and the resultant diarrhea remains unclear.

Clinical Presentation

The clinical course is usually mild and self-limited; however, infants may have profuse watery diarrhea associated with vomiting and low-grade fever. EPEC may result in chronic protracted diarrhea in approximately 25% of infected children.[27] Acute EPEC outbreaks in the United States have involved pediatric day care centers, all of which were self-limited. The high mortality rates observed in the developing countries may be related to the protracted illness resulting in severe malnutrition.

Diagnosis

Identification of EPEC serotypes is performed by the agglutination method using polyvalent antisera. DNA probes for virulence factors are more accurate but depend on the availability of fluorescent microscopy and tissue cultures.

Treatment

Correction of fluid and electrolyte imbalance is the mainstay of therapy. The use of bismuth subsalicylate (100 mg/kg/dose) decreases fluid secretion and reduces the duration of diarrhea. Antibiotic use is controversial and is not usually required, except in protracted cases.

ENTEROHEMORRHAGIC E. COLI

The enterohemorrhagic E. coli (EHEC) serotype, 0157 : H7, was first identified as a cause of bloody diarrheal outbreaks linked to a fast food restaurant chain in 1982.[28] Transmission is mostly by undercooked beef and occasionally by contaminated cider or water. Fecal-oral person-to-person contact has also been reported, particularly in day care centers.[29] Sporadic cases peak during the warm season, while outbreaks have no seasonal predilection. Although 0157 : H7 is the main serotype causing diarrheal outbreaks and HUS, many other non-0157 EHEC serotypes have been isolated[29] (for a detailed discussion, see Ch. 27).

Pathogenesis

EHEC secrete cytotoxins similar in structure and biologic effects to Shiga toxin, hence the name Shiga-like toxins (SLT). Two types of SLT are antigenically distinct: SLT1 and SLT2, with SLT1 more similar to Shiga toxin.[26] The diarrhea caused by EHEC has been attributed to both the phage-encoded SLT and the plasmid-encoded adhesion factor.[29]

Clinical Presentation

EHEC infection has an incubation period of 3 to 4 days and results in both bloody and nonbloody diarrhea, which can progress to HUS. Patients present with abdominal pain, vomiting, and diarrhea, which remain nonbloody in most cases. Fever and progression to hemorrhagic colitis can occur by the second or third day, indicating a more severe illness.

Complications of EHEC 0157 : H7 infection include bowel necrosis and perforation, toxic megacolon, GI strictures, and extraintestinal manifestations such as HUS, thrombotic thrombocytopenic purpura, myocardial ischemia, pulmonary edema, hepatitis, and neurologic abnormalities.[30]

HUS is characterized by microangiopathic hemolytic anemia, thrombocytopenia, renal failure, and neurologic manifestations. This syndrome can occur at the end of the diarrheal illness, when stool cultures may be negative. Colonic vascular damage by SLT can facilitate systemic access to toxins and inflammatory mediators, resulting in endothelial glomerular injury and progression to HUS. The renal failure in HUS can be accompanied by hypokalemia secondary to diarrheal losses. Risk factors for the development of HUS include extremes of age, bloody diarrhea, fever, leukocytosis, female gender, mental retardation, and absence of P1 antigen on erythrocytes.[31] The overall incidence of HUS in sporadic EHEC infection is 5% to 10%.[29]

Diagnosis

Stool cultures for serotyping is the standard method of diagnosis. The timing of stool cultures is important as the highest yield is within 1 week of onset of diarrheal symptoms. Detection of antibody to the lipopolysaccharides of 0157 : H7 is helpful in those presenting late in the illness, when stool cultures are negative. Infants shed organisms longer than do older children and adults. Colonoscopy in active EHEC infection indicates patchy hemorrhagic colitis, which is most pronounced in the cecum and right-sided colon.

All patients less than 5 years of age who present with acute bloody diarrhea, especially with fever and leukocytosis, should be monitored for possible progression to HUS. A careful smear analysis for helmet or burr cells, urine microscopy for hematuria, and monitoring of blood-urea nitrogen (BUN), serum creatinine, and complete blood count (CBC) are essential.

Treatment

There is no specific therapy for EHEC diarrhea. Antibiotic use is controversial, and antimotility agents may increase risk of neurologic complications.[31] A child with EHEC infection should be kept out of school or a day care center until a stool culture is negative.

ENTEROINVASIVE E. COLI

Enteroinvasive E. coli (EIEC) causes an illness similar to shigellosis. Both organisms share biochemical properties and virulence mechanisms. Like Shigella, EIEC possesses invasive properties; however, the presence of Shiga toxin is unique to S. dysenteriae.

Clinical Presentation

Clinical features include dysenteric stools with abdominal cramping and tenesmus. Bacteremia does not usually occur. Fecal leukocytes are present, and confirmatory diagnosis is by stool culture.

Treatment

Data regarding antibiotic therapy for EIEC are limited, but indications are similar to those for shigellosis (Table 18-2).

ENTEROAGGREGATIVE AND DIFFUSELY ADHERENT E. COLI

Enteroaggregative E. coli (EaggEc) and diffusely adherent E. coli (DAEC) have specific adherence patterns to Hep-2 cell-line cultures. EaggEc demonstrates a "stacked brick" pattern, while DAEC exhibits a diffusely adherent configuration. None of these two types of E. coli secretes enterotoxins, and both show similarities to EPEC. Recent epidemiologic studies have associated aggregative

E. coli with protracted diarrhea in developing countries.[32]

Pathogenesis

The pathogenesis of infection is by intimate attachment of bacteria to the enterocyte surface, predominantly in the colon.[33] Plasmid-encoded adherence factors enable the bacterium to express a flexible bundle-forming pilus. Diarrhea may be related to the reduction in absorptive capacity, secondary to mucosal damage.

Clinical Presentation

EaggEC predominantly cause persistent diarrheal episodes lasting more than 14 days. This can lead to significant malnutrition in the developing countries.

Treatment

Correction of fluid and electrolyte deficits are primary considerations. However, enteral and parenteral nutritional support are especially important.

Yersinia enterocolitica

Yersinia enterocolitica and *Yersinia pseudotuberculosis* are gram-negative organisms that cause gastroenteritis. *Y. enterocolitica* accounts for 1% to 3% of diarrheal outbreaks in children.[34] Undercooked pork and contaminated milk are important in the spread of disease.

PATHOGENESIS

Bacterial pathogenesis includes enterocyte binding, invasion, localization within lymphoid tissue, and extracellular multiplication. These are mediated by virulence factors that are either chromosomally or plasmid mediated. A heat-stable enterotoxin akin to that of cholera is also produced by *Y. enterocolitica*.

CLINICAL PRESENTATION

Yersinia infection in children predominantly causes enterocolitic symptoms, including abdominal pain, fever, diarrhea, and vomiting. Grossly bloody stools occur in up to 25% of patients.[34] Illness tends to be prolonged for up to 3 weeks.

Pseudoappendicitis syndrome is a characteristic clinical feature that occurs in older children. Associated complications include intestinal perforation, intussusception, peritonitis, and toxic megacolon. Septicemic illness, observed in some cases, is associated with a high fatality rate of up to 50%. Hemochromatosis and other states of iron overload are factors that predispose to severe yersinial infection. Long-term complications include reactive arthritis, Reiter's syndrome, and ankylosing spondylitis. Prolonged inflammation and diffuse ulceration of small bowel and colon with the associated joint involvement may closely mimic idiopathic inflammatory bowel disease.

DIAGNOSIS

Stool culture on selective media may require up to 4 weeks for growth.

TREATMENT

Yersinial infections are self-limited; therefore, antibiotics are not generally required except for patients at high risk of invasive disease, as described for salmonella. Third-generation cephalosporins and trimethoprim-sulfamethoxazole are the antibiotics of choice (Table 18-2).

Vibrio cholerae

Vibrio cholerae is a gram-negative bacillus that causes a profuse, watery diarrhea leading to serious rapid dehydration associated with significant mortality. Worldwide, there are an estimated 5.5 million cases of cholera diarrhea each year, with more than 100,000 resultant deaths.[35] Most cases in the United States occur in travelers to the South American continent. Transmission is by fecal contamination of water and food. Lasting immunity is usual after a natural infection.

PATHOGENESIS

The pilus-mediated adherence of *Vibrio* to the enterocyte is the initial step in pathogenesis. The major virulence factor is the chromosomally encoded cholera toxin,[7] which binds to GM_1 gangliosides and results in increased luminal fluid secretion by the activation of adenylate cyclase, which increases the AMP production.

CLINICAL PRESENTATION

The incubation period is usually 1 to 3 days. In endemic areas, cholera primarily affects nonimmune children aged 2 to 15 years. In nonendemic areas, infection can occur at any age. Risk factors include low gastric acidity and possibly *H. pylori*[36] infection. The clinical picture is characterized by vomiting and profuse watery diarrhea leading to severe rapid dehydration. The stools are rich in sodium, potassium, bicarbonate, and chloride, causing significant electrolyte imbalance and prerenal azotemia. Hypoglycemia can also occur in young children.

DIAGNOSIS

Stool specimens contain large numbers of organisms identified by Gram stain and wet-mount examination, showing the typical comma-shaped organisms with a single polar flagellum and the characteristic mobility. Stool culture and specific serotype identification by polyvalent antiserum agglutination confirm the diagnosis.

TREATMENT

Aggressive rehydration is the primary therapy. The advent of ORS revolutionized the treatment of cholera and dramatically reduced mortality. Intravenous rehydration is indicated for severe dehydration or vomiting. Oral antibiotics can reduce stool volume and shorten the duration of illness (Table 18-2). Chemoprophylaxis of family members of affected patients is not recommended. The currently available cholera vaccine is of limited value in prevention.

Non-Cholera *Vibrio*

Vibrio parahemolyticus is the most common *Vibrio* pathogen isolated in the United States in association with a self-limited gastroenteritis related to ingestion of contaminated shellfish. Treatment is primarily supportive.

Aeromonas and *Plesiomonas*

Aeromonas and *Plesiomonas* are motile gram-negative bacilli that belong to the family Vibrionaceae and are increasingly recognized as enteric pathogens. *Aeromonas* is transmitted through contamination of well water. Contaminated aquatic sources and shell fish play a role in transmission of plesiomonal infections. *A. hydrophila* and *P. shigelloides* are the most commonly isolated species.

PATHOGENESIS

Virulence factors for *Aeromonas* include adherence fimbria, invasiveness, and production of cyto- and enterotoxins.[37] Pathogenic factors for *Plesiomonas* include invasiveness and production of a hemolysin enterotoxin.

CLINICAL PRESENTATION

The highest attack rate involves children less than 3 years of age. Patients present with fever, vomiting, diarrhea, and abdominal pain.[37] The acute diarrhea can be watery or dysenteric; however chronic diarrhea lasting for weeks to months has also been described.

DIAGNOSIS

Stool smear is devoid of leukocytes. *Aeromonas* grows on commonly used culture media, co-infection with other pathogens is common.

TREATMENT

Antibiotics are generally not required in this usually self-limited infection. There are no reliable data on the use of antibiotics in therapy.

Edwardsiella

Edwardsiella is a recently described enteric pathogen that causes an illness similar to that of *Aeromonas* and *Plesiomonas*. In a significant proportion of patients, infection may remain asymptomatic.

Mycobacterium avium-intracellulare

Mycobacterium avium-intracellulare (MAC) is an acid-fast bacillus recently recognized as a pathogen in immunocompromised children.

PATHOGENESIS

MAC invades the Peyer's patches and mesenteric lymph nodes, predominantly of the small intestine.

CLINICAL PRESENTATION

In acquired immunodeficiency syndrome (AIDS), MAC is the most commonly isolated bacterial agent causing systemic symptoms[38] and is associated with chronic diarrhea and abdominal pain. No clinical manifestations are usually seen in immunocompetent patients.

DIAGNOSIS

The diagnosis is made by histologic examination of the GI tissue and by culture of the organism from stools or duodenal aspirates obtained during upper endoscopy.

TREATMENT

Antituberculosis agents in three- or four-drug regimens are employed with limited success. Recently, azithromycin and clarithromycin have shown promise.

Food Poisoning Syndromes

Food poisoning is a syndrome of gastroenteritis occurring within 24 hours of ingestion of an offending agent, usually a bacterially derived preformed toxin. The common causes of food poisoning include the following[16]:

1. *Staphylococcus aureus. S. aureus* causes a toxin-mediated disease 1 to 6 hours after ingestion of contaminated foods, especially processed meat. Severe abdominal cramps, vomiting, and diarrhea are common features that resolve within 24 hours.
2. *Bacillus cereus. B. cereus* causes two distinct syndromes: an emetic syndrome similar to staphylococcal food poisoning and a second syndrome characterized by predominant diarrhea. Poisoning results mostly from ingestion of contaminated cooked rice and symptoms usually resolve within 24 hours.

3. *Clostridium perfringens. C. perfringens* causes a self-limited diarrheal syndrome with abdominal pain and vomiting.

4. *Clostridium botulinum. C. botulinum* causes infant botulism presenting with muscular weakness and paralysis due to toxin-induced neuromuscular junction blockade. Bulbar palsy and cranial nerve involvement are typical complications requiring prolonged intensive supportive therapy. Contaminated honey is a common source of disease transmission.

REFERRAL PATTERNS

Most bacterial diarrheal illnesses can be treated by primary care physicians, except for a few specific clinical situations. Bloody stools, particularly if associated with fever in children younger than 5 years of age, should be closely monitored for possible progression to HUS, which requires referral to a center that has the requisite facilities. Warning signs include fever, leukocytosis, azotemia, or a peripheral blood smear with hemolytic features (helmet/burr cells). In addition, bloody stools in an infant may indicate an acute surgical or medical emergency, including intussusception, volvulus, Hirschsprung's associated enterocolitis, and necrotizing enterocolitis, which require early referral. Another clinical situation in which referral to a specialist is indicated is protracted diarrhea associated with intolerance to reinstitution of enteral feeding indicating continuing malabsorption, which may necessitate parenteral nutrition. Disseminated or complicated infections with *Salmonella*, *Shigella*, or *Yersinia* merit similar consideration for referral to a specialist.

REFERENCES

1. Claeson M, Merson MH. Global progress in the control of diarrheal disease. Pediatr Infect Dis J 1990;9:345–355
2. Bern C, Martines J, de Zoysa I, Glass RI. The magnitude of the global problem of diarrhoeal disease: a ten year update. Bull WHO 1992;70:705–714
3. Institute of Medicine. Committee on Issues and Priorities for New Vaccine Development. New Vaccine Development: Establishing Priorities. Vol II. Diseases of Importance in Developing Countries. Washington, DC: National Academy Press, 1986
4. Glass RI, Lew JF, Gangarosa RE et al. Estimates of morbidity and mortality rates for diarrheal disease in American children. J Pediatr 1991;118:27–33
5. Bhan MK, Arora NH, Ghai KR et al. Major factors in diarrhoea related mortality among rural children. Indian J Med Res 1986;83:9–12
6. Blaser MJ, Wells JG, Feldman R et al. Campylobacter enteri-

7. Acheson DWK. Enterotoxin in acute infective diarrhoea. J Infect 1992;24:225–245
8. American Academy of Pediatrics Committee on Nutrition: Use of oral fluid therapy and post-treatment feeding following enteritis in children in a developed country. Pediatrics 1985;75:358–361
9. Duggan C, Santosham M, Glass R. The management of acute diarrhea in children: oral rehydration, maintenance and nutritional therapy. MMWR 1992,41:RRIG:1–20
10. Ryan CA, Hargrett-Bean NT, Blake PA. *Salmonella typhi* infections in the United States, 1975–1984: increasing role of foreign travel. Rev Infect Dis 1989;11:1–8
11. Centers for Disease Control and Prevention. Outbreak of *Salmonella enteritides* infection associated with consumption of raw shell eggs. MMWR 1992;21:369–372
12. Buchwald DS, Blaser MJ. A review of human salmonellosis. II. Duration of excretion following infection with non-*typhi Salmonella*. Rev Infect Dis 1984;6:345–356
13. Pace J, Hayman MJ, Galan JE. Signal transduction and invasion of epithelial cells by *Salmonella typhimurium*. Cell 1992; 72:505–514
14. Cohen JI, Bartlett JA, Corey GR. Extra-intestinal manifestations of *Salmonella* infections. Medicine (Baltimore) 1987; 66:349–388
15. Nelson JD, Kusmiesz H, Jackson LH, Woodman C. Treatment of *Salmonella* gastroenteritis with ampicillin, amoxicillin or placebo. Pediatrics 1980;65:1125–1130
16. Bishai WR, Sears CL. Food poisoning syndromes. Gastroenterol Clin North Am 1993;22:579–608
17. Centers for Disease Control. Shigellosis in child day care centers. MMWR 1992;41:440–442
18. Hale TL. Genetic basis of virulence in shigella species. Microbiol Rev 1991;55:206–224
19. Mobassaleh M, Donohue-Rolfe A, Jacewicz M et al. Pathogenesis of *Shigella* diarrhea: evidence for a developmentally regulated glycolipid receptor for Shigella toxin involved in the fluid secretory response of small bowel. J Infect Dis 1988; 157:1023–1031
20. Bennish ML, Salam MA, Wahed MA. Enteric protein loss during shigellosis. Am J Gastroenterol 1993;88:53–57
20a. Skirrow MB, Blaser MJ. Campylobacter Jejuni In: Blaser MJ. Smith PD, Greenberg HB, Guerrant RG Eds. Infections of Gastrointestinal Tract. New York, Raven Press, P826:1995
21. Tauxe RV, Hargrett-Bean N, Patton CM et al. *Campylobacter* isolates in the United States, 1982–1986. MMWR 1988;37(SS-2):1–13
22. Walker RI, Caldwell MB, Lee EC et al. Pathophysiology of *Campylobacter enteritis*. Microbiol Rev 1986;50:81–94
23. Wilson PG, Davies JR, Hoskins TW et al. Epidemiology of an outbreak of milk-borne enteritis in a residential school. In: Pearson AD, Skirrow MB, Rowe B, Davies JR, Jones DM, Eds. *Campylobacter* II Proceedings of the Second International Workshop on *Campylobacter* Infections. London: Public Health Laboratory Service, 143, 1983
24. Fujimoto S, Amako K. Guillain-Barre syndrome and *Campylobacter jejuni* infection. Lancet 1990,335:1350

(continued) tis in the United States. A multicenter study. Ann Intern Med 1983;98:360

25. Black RE, Levine MM, Clements ML et al. Treatment of experimentally induced enterotoxigenic *Escherichia coli* with trimethoprim, trimethoprim-sulfamethoxazole or a placebo. Rev Infect Dis 1982;4:540–545

26. Donnenberg MS, Kaper JB. Minireview: enteropathogenic *Escherichia coli*. Infect Immun 1992;60:3953–3961

27. Hill SM, Phillips AD, Walker-Smith JA. Enteropathogenic *Escherichia coli* and life-threatening chronic diarrhea. Gut 1991;32:154–158

28. Riley LW, Remis RS, Helgerson SD et al. Hemorrhagic colitis associated with a rare *Escherichia coli* serotype. N Engl J Med 1983;308:681–685

29. Pickering LK, Obrig TG, Stapleton FB. Hemolytic-uremic syndrome and enterohemorrhagic *Escherichia coli*. Pediatr Infect Dis J 1994;13:459–476

30. Levin M, Walters MDS, Barratt TM. Hemolytic uremic syndrome. In: Arnoff SC, Hughes WT, Kehl S, Speck WT, Wald ER, Eds. Advances in Pediatric Infectious Diseases. Vol. 4. Chicago: Year Book, 51–81, 1989

31. Griffin PM, Tauxe RV. The epidemiology of infections caused by *Escherichia coli* 0157 : H7, other enterohemorrhagic *E. coli*, and the associated hemolytic uremic syndrome. Epidemiol Rev 1991;13:60–98

32. Bhan MK, Raj P, Levine MM et al. Enteroaggregative *Escherichia coli* associated with persistent diarrhea in a cohort of rural children in India. J Infect Dis 1989;159:1061–1064

33. Vial PA, Robins Browne R, Lior et al. Characterization of enteroadherent-aggregative *Escherichia coli*, a putative agent of diarrheal disease. J Infect Dis 1988;158:70–79

34. Cover TL, Aber RC. *Yersinia enterocolitica*. N Engl J Med 1989;321:16–24

35. Development of vaccines against cholera and diarrhoea due to enterotoxigenic *Escherichia coli*: memorandum from a WHO meeting. Bull WHO 1990;68:303–312

36. Tauxe RV, Blake PA. Epidemic cholera in Latin America. JAMA 1992;267:1388–1390

37. San Joaquin VH. *Aeromonas, Yersinia* and miscellaneous bacterial enteropathogens. Pediatr Ann 1994;23:544–548

38. Young LS. *Mycobacterium avium* complex infections. J infect Dis 1988;157:863–867

39. Pickering LK, Matson DO. Therapy for diarrheal illness in children. In: Blaser MJ, Smith PD, Greenberg HB, Guerrant RL, Eds. Infections of the Gastrointestinal Tract. New York: Raven Press, 1995;1404–1406

19

CELIAC DISEASE

DAVID A. FERENCI

Celiac disease, celiac sprue, or gluten-sensitive enteropathy is defined as a permanent intolerance to wheat gliadin associated with mucosal disease of the proximal small bowel. It is one of the most common causes of malabsorption in childhood. It is characterized by intestinal malabsorption, histologic abnormalities of the small bowel mucosa, clinical and histologic improvement on a gluten-free diet, and relapse on a gluten-containing diet.

The world prevalence of celiac disease varies by location and can be as high as 1 in 300 in western Ireland.[1] A recent study in Olmsted County, MN, shows a U.S. prevalence of about 1 in 5,000.[2] Both environmental and genetic factors play a role in the disease. The incidence is high with increased exposure to gluten and significantly higher among white persons living in a similar environment. It is rare among native Africans, Japanese, and Chinese[3] populations. There is yearly variability in the incidence of celiac disease, suggesting nondietary environmental factors.[4] Concordance among twins is 70%.[5] There is an approximately 10% first-degree family incidence.[6] Family studies suggest an inherited susceptibility associated with human leukocyte antigens (HLA). Class II antigens HLA-DQw2[7] and HLA-DW3[8] have been implicated, yet these may be markers for other genes conferring susceptibility.

PATHOGENESIS

Grain proteins in wheat, rye, barley, and usually oats are toxic to people with celiac disease. Oats have typically been considered toxic, but a recent well-controlled adult study brought this into question.[9] Corn and rice are clearly nontoxic. Alpha-gliadin is considered the puta-

tive protein in wheat; prolamin, in other cereals. A sequence homology has been described between alpha-gliadin and an early protein of adenovirus-12, suggesting that a virus may trigger the disease in susceptible people.[10]

Both biochemical and immunologic theories exist as to the mechanism of the toxicity of gliadin. A peptidase deficiency is now thought to be a secondary phenomenon, and gliadin is considered a true lectin.[11] Current evidence suggests that celiac disease is an immunologic disorder associated with both cell- and humoral-related immunity.[3] Circulating antibodies are well described but may not be specific for celiac disease. It appears that celiac disease patients develop IgG antibodies, cell-mediated immunity (sensitized lymphocytes), and a secretory IgA response that targets the enterocyte for a cell-mediated cytotoxic reaction[12] and activates complement.[13] The activated T cell may be the mediator of the mucosal damage.[14]

Susceptible persons exposed to gluten develop proximal small bowel damage (Fig. 19-1). Increased shedding of enterocytes leads to a flattened mucosa (villous atrophy) with marked reduction in absorptive surface area. Histologically, small bowel cellular infiltration of the lamina propria with plasma cells and lymphocytes occurs, as well as elongation of crypts (crypt hyperplasia) and increased mitotic activity in crypt epithelial cells, resulting in a villus height-to-crypt length ratio of 1:1 or less.[15]

CLINICAL PRESENTATION

The classic patient with celiac disease presents at 1 to 3 years of age. The most common symptoms are diarrhea, anorexia, poor growth, abdominal distention,

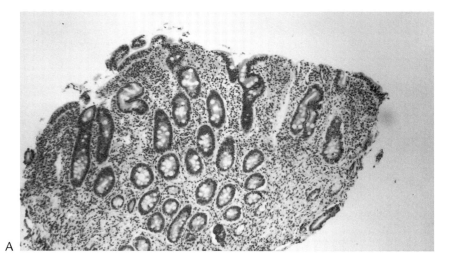

A

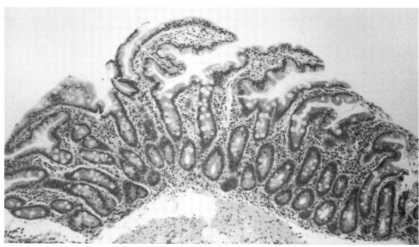

B

FIGURE 19-1. (*A*) Endoscopic small bowel biopsy demonstrating villous atrophy, crypt hyperplasia, and lamina propria inflammation. (*B*) Endoscopic small bowel biopsy after 6 months on a gluten-free diet. (Courtesy of Blair Chrenka, M.D., Department of Pathology, Children's Healthcare, Minneapolis, MN.)

abdominal pain, muscle wasting, and irritability (Fig. 19-2). The clinical symptoms and signs can vary widely and are especially dependent on the age of presentation and length of bowel affected (Table 19-1). The age of presentation is associated with the introduction of solid feedings in infants. There is generally a lag between the onset of symptoms and the introduction of gluten into the diet. The mode of presentation varies, with diarrhea occurring most commonly and failure to thrive another common occurrence. Infants and toddlers usually present with acute symptoms. Typically, they produce foul-smelling, bulky, greasy stools within weeks or months after the introduction of gluten. In rare cases, the patient will present in celiac crisis (see below) with severe diarrhea, dehydration, and potentially shock.

Other symptoms include vomiting, constipation, short stature, iron deficiency anemia, and behavioral problems in older children. Siblings or first-degree relatives of a child diagnosed with celiac disease may have asymptomatic villous atrophy.

Physical Examination

Physical findings include abdominal distention, malaise, weight loss, abdominal pain, edema, muscle wasting, weakness, dental erosion, and rectal prolapse (Table 19-1, Fig. 19-2). Short stature and failure to thrive have been well described in celiac disease. It is extremely important for the physician to plot a child's weight and height on an appropriate growth curve, as deviation from the growth curve may initially be the only clue to the diagnosis of celiac disease.[16]

Differential Diagnosis

Celiac disease occurs with an increased incidence in juvenile diabetes,[17] IgA deficiency,[18] and Down's syndrome.[19] Another associated disease (Table 19-2)[20] is dermatitis herpetiformis, a papulovesicular symmetric pruritic rash usually involving the knees, elbows, shoulders, buttocks, and scalp. Subepidermal blisters are seen on biopsy with IgA deposits in the dermal papillae. Ce-

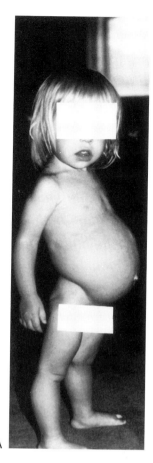 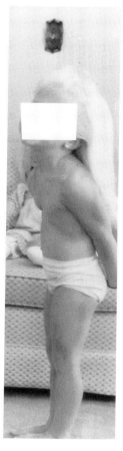

FIGURE 19-2. Child diagnosed with celiac disease. (*A*) Age 19 months at presentation. Note the distended abdomen and muscle wasting of the extremities. (*B*) Age 5 years on gluten-free diet. (Courtesy of Children's Healthcare, Minneapolis, MN.)

liac disease also comingles with various autoimmune diseases such as IgA nephropathy and thyroiditis. Rarer associations include cryptogenic hepatitis, arthritis, and epilepsy with occipital calcification.[21]

Malignancy is increased in patients with celiac disease.[22] T-cell lymphoma of the small bowel is the most common condition seen usually after long-standing disease in adults. It has been suggested that the risk of malignancy is reduced in patients who adhere to a gluten-free diet.[23]

DIAGNOSIS

Classically, the diagnosis of celiac disease is made by the demonstration of abnormal small bowel mucosa (villous atrophy, crypt hyperplasia, and plasma cell infiltrate) on initial presentation and clinical remission and histologic improvement after dietary gluten withdrawal, followed by another gluten challenge, again demonstrating small bowel pathology (Fig. 19-1).

More recently, the necessity of documenting histologic improvement and relapse with gluten challenge has been questioned. The most recent criteria reported by European Society of Pediatric Gastroenterology and Nutrition (ESPGAN) were updated in 1990[24] (Table 19-3) to include the use of serum antibody screening. This report stated that in cases demonstrating a typical history, a characteristic small bowel biopsy, and prompt response to diet, further biopsies or challenge are no longer mandatory. Most pediatric gastroenterologists in the United States continue to stress the importance of at least two biopsies (initial and on gluten withdrawal).

Elevated antibody titers, including antigliadin antibody (AGA), antiendomysial antibody (EMA), and antireticulin antibody (ARA) (see below), may be adequate for the diagnosis. Certain conditions may suggest a gluten challenge with repeat biopsy, including an uncharacteristic initial biopsy, an equivocal response to diet or in patients found by screening without gastrointestinal (GI) symptoms. Since conditions that mimic celiac disease (Table 19-4), such as milk/soy protein sensitivity and infectious and postinfectious enteritis, are common in infancy, it is generally advised that all patients diagnosed under the age of 2 years be challenged with gluten later in childhood.

A gluten challenge should be medically supervised. It should not be done before the age of 3 years because of associated dental defects and is usually not attempted during the first year of presentation. Typically, 10 g gluten flour is added (daily) to the gluten-free diet. This

TABLE 19-1. Signs and Symptoms Associated With Celiac Disease

Diarrhea
Distended abdomen
Muscle wasting
Decreased weight
Vomiting
Anorexia
Short stature
Irritability
Abdominal pain
Rectal prolapse
Constipation
Edema
Malaise
Delayed puberty
Osteopenia
Rickets
Aphthous ulcers
Dental enamel hypoplasia

TABLE 19-2. Associated Disorders in Celiac Disease

Firm Association, Numerous Reports	Probable Association, Some Reports	Possible Association, Mainly Case Reports
Dermatitis herpetiformis[a]	Autoimmune thyroid diseases	Addison's disease
Insulin-dependent diabetes mellitus	Asthma and atopic diseases	Dementia
Selective IgA deficiency	Epilepsy with cerebral calcifications	Inflammatory bowel disease
Lymphoma	Sjögren's syndrome	Sarcoidosis
Small intestinal cancer	Pharyngeal and esophageal cancer	Primary biliary cirrhosis and other chronic liver diseases
		Pancreatic insufficiency
		Rheumatoid arthritis and other connective tissue diseases

[a] Can be regarded as same disease.
(From Collin and Maki,[20] with permission.)

approach will not disrupt the imposed dietary restrictions to which the child has become accustomed. A repeat biopsy is performed within 3 to 6 months of the gluten challenge, and earlier if significant GI symptoms occur. Laboratory testing and serum antibodies may guide the timing of repeat biopsy. After the gluten challenge, if the biopsy shows only minimal changes, the diet is liberalized, and a repeat biopsy is performed 2 years later or sooner, if laboratory findings or symptoms become abnormal.[25] Although celiac disease is considered a permanent intolerance to gluten, certain persons may not relapse on an unrestricted diet. This has been generally estimated below 5%.[27] This finding suggests that clinical expression may vary with environment and age of pre-

sentation. If the diet is discontinued, repeat biopsies are suggested every 2 years into adulthood, since relapses can be extended.[26]

LABORATORY TESTS

Antibody Testing

Antibody testing has become a significant adjuvant in the screening and diagnosis of celiac disease. In the past, antigliadin IgG antibodies were reportedly very sensitive, with most studies conferring greater than 90% sensitivity.[28] Their specificity is more problematic; the antibody can be positive in other associated mucosal diseases (e.g., Crohn's disease, allergic gastroenteritis) and even in normal persons. Antigliadin IgA antibodies appear to be more specific but less sensitive.

More recently, other antibody tests appear to be more sensitive and specific than the AGA screen. ARA are highly specific for diagnosis of celiac disease.[29] EMA, a connective tissue antibody, is also highly specific for ce-

TABLE 19-3. Practical Clinical Diagnosis of Celiac Disease

Gluten challenge is not mandatory when
    There is characteristic small intestinal mucosal abnormality on histologic examination of a biopsy specimen
    There is clear-cut clinical remission on a strict gluten-free diet within weeks
    There are circulating IgA gliadin, reticulin, and endomysial antibodies present at diagnosis and disappearing in parallel to clinical response to a gluten-free diet

Control (follow-up) biopsy is indicated
    In asymptomatic patients (i.e., family members) to prove mucosal recovery
    When the clinical response to GFD is equivocal

Gluten challenge is indicated
    There is any doubt of original diagnosis
    No initial diagnostic biopsy
    Uncharacteristic biopsy
    Diagnosis made under age 2 years
    In those intending to abandon the GFD

(Adapted from ESPGAN Revised criteria for diagnosis of celiac disease,[26] with permission.)

TABLE 19-4. Conditions That Mimic Celiac Disease

Cow/soy milk sensitivity
Viral enteritis
Bacterial overgrowth
Eosinophilic enteritis
Giardiasis
Lymphoma
Autoimmune enteropathy
Tropical sprue
Severe malnutrition

TABLE 19-5. Laboratory Abnormalities Associated With Celiac Disease

More specific
    Antigliaden antibodies IgG/IgA (AGA)
    Antiendomysial antibodies (EMA)
    Antireticulin antibodies (ARA)
    Villous atrophy
    Decreased *d*-xylose absorption
    Abnormal sugar permeability test

Less specific
    Iron deficiency anemia
    Hypoalbuminemia
    Increased fecal fat
    Decreased cholesterol
    Decreased carotene
    Elevated alkaline phosphatase
    Increased protime
    Elevated fecal alpha-1-antitrypsin
    Folate deficiency
    Decreased calcium
    Decreased magnesium
    Delayed bone age
    Flocculation on barium study

liac disease. The data are now supportive of EMA as the best reflection of long-term dietary exposure to gluten and intestinal histopathology.[31] All IgA-based antibodies (AGA, EMA, ARA) may be negative as a secondary IgA deficiency can occur in celiac disease patients.[32]

The levels of all three antibodies decrease and normalize with gluten elimination and rise with reintroduction. These antibody tests can aid in the evaluation of children with GI symptoms, of those with short stature, and of family members of celiac disease patients,[33,34] as well as screening large population groups. They are especially useful in monitoring compliance with the gluten-free diet, although small amounts of gluten may not induce a rise in antibody levels, and timing the follow-up biopsy in those undergoing gluten challenge.[35] While some have advocated that following antibody titers after challenge may obviate the need for rebiopsy,[36] most pediatric gastroenterologists believe that repeat biopsies need to be performed to make the definitive diagnosis.[37]

Malabsorption Tests

As malabsorption is common in symptomatic celiac disease, multiple tests can be used in its evaluation. A complete blood count (CBC) with indices can indicate iron, folate, and B_{12} deficiencies. Decreased calcium, phosphorus, magnesium, iron, albumin, and increased alkaline phosphatase are clues for malabsorption. An elevated prothrombin time (PT) suggests fat-soluble vitamin deficiency and should be corrected before biopsy.

Once malabsorption is suspected, more formal assessments can be done. The most common is the *D*-xylose test (for further details, see Ch. 79).[38] While fat malabsoption is not as pronounced in celiac disease as it is in cystic fibrosis, fecal fat testing may indicate disease. Fat malabsorption is most easily tested by a 72-hour fecal fat quantitative collection (for further discussion, see Ch. 79).[38] A random fecal level of alpha-1-antitrypsin may be elevated and may signify a protein-losing enteropathy. Sweat chloride tests for cystic fibrosis should be done, as symptoms may overlap and, in rare cases, a patient may have both conditions. Permeability tests based on the differential absorption of mannitol compared to lactulose[39] can determine abnormalities of small bowel mucosa but are not specific to celiac disease.

Radiography

Signs of generalized mucosal disease can be demonstrated by barium small bowel series. These include demonstration of mucosal thickening, flocculation, segmentation, and dilation. Radiography can also reveal rickets secondary to malabsorption.

Small Bowel Biopsy

Once the diagnosis of celiac disease is clinically or biochemical suspected, the small bowel biopsy is the only way to confirm or exclude the diagnosis. At our institution, we use endoscopy, which permits the evaluation of other diagnoses. Per oral capsule biopsy (Crosby capsule) can also be done under fluoroscopic guidance. Most recent studies have supported the use of endoscopy[40] (for further discussion, see Ch. 71).

TREATMENT

With the discovery in 1953 that gluten is the etiologic or putative agent in the pathogenesis of celiac disease,[41] a strict gluten-free diet has been the mainstay of treatment of celiac disease. This includes a diet without wheat, rye, barley, and usually oats. Corn and rice products are allowed. The issue of oat restriction was recently questioned by a well-controlled study in adults,[20] in which serial biopsies showed that 50 g oats in the daily diet does not delay healing (up to 12 months) or induce relapse in celiac patients (up to 6 months). Nonetheless, oats are currently excluded in a gluten-free diet for children. Some reportedly gluten-free foods were found to have an unacceptable gluten content, probably representing secondary contamination. Clearly dietary counseling is very important.[42]

Once the diet is initiated, a rapid clinical response is seen (Fig. 19-2). Diarrhea, mood, and appetite may improve within days to weeks. Weight gain may be rapid, with height gain proceeding more slowly. Catch-up growth is typically rapid in the first year after diagnosis and complete after 2 to 3 years.[43] Intestinal villous abnormalities on biopsy normally improve after 6 months (Fig. 19-1); however, as improvement can occur rapidly, the gluten-free diet should not be initiated before the initial biopsy.

A secondary disaccharide intolerance often develops in conjunction with small bowel inflammation. In patients who demonstrate symptoms after consuming a lactose-containing meal, a lactose-reduced diet or lactase supplementation should be recommended. Fruit juices may need to be discontinued, as they can also exacerbate diarrhea. Some infants may demonstrate a sensitivity to cow's milk protein.

The effects of chronic malabsorption and malnutrition will not be immediately reversed by the gluten-free diet, so attention should be paid to these issues. Vitamin therapy may be necessary (especially fat-soluble vitamins). Vitamins may be given, with D, E, A, K in a single preparation. Multivitamins including trace elements are generally prescribed until the intestine heals. Care should be given when prescribing medications as many pharmaceutical compounds contain gluten fillers. Iron deficiency should also be corrected. Bone disease, such as rickets, osteopenia, and osteomalacia, may be evident and should be addressed.

Celiac disease is a lifelong disease, for which the gluten-free diet is mandated as permanent therapy. This approach is supported by data indicating that the mucosa eventually becomes abnormal upon re-exposure to gluten and that the clinical symptoms during a relapse may not become as apparent as at initial presentation. Minimal symptoms (e.g., malaise and lassitude), as well as decreased growth velocity and biochemical changes (e.g., anemia or bone disease) may not be appreciated by the patient or parent. The risk of malignancy of the small bowel seems to be reduced by adherence to the gluten-free diet, but this has not been clearly established.[23]

Compliance to the GFD is fairly difficult secondary to the universal presence of gluten in the Western diet. Young children tend to be more compliant, but adolescents are known to be significantly noncompliant.[44] Follow-up management is suggested, as there is little correlation in individual subjects between the presence of symptoms, severity of histologic findings, biochemical and immunologic abnormalities, and the amount of dietary gluten ingested.[45]

Antibody testing with the gluten sensitivity profile (AGA, EMA, and ARA) are helpful in monitoring dietary compliance. Testing may aid patients and families understand the chronicity of the disease if antibodies rise secondary to noncompliance with diet.

Other Family Members

Family members who are symptomatic should be evaluated aggressively for celiac disease; however, even those who are asymptomatic may benefit from antibody screening. Latent celiac disease has been used to describe persons with positive antibody and normal or minimal changes in intestinal biopsies who may later present with villous atrophy.

Celiac Crisis

Celiac crisis is not a common feature of celiac disease; however, some people may develop severe electrolyte disturbance with volume depletion and potential shock. In those who do not respond promptly to a gluten-free diet after rehydration, a short course of prednisone, 1 to 2 mg/kg/day for 1 to 2 weeks, and of parenteral nutritional support may be required.

REFERRAL PATTERN

Once the diagnosis of celiac disease is seriously entertained, the child should be referred to a pediatric gastroenterologist, who can evaluate the disease thoroughly and confirm the diagnosis with a small bowel biopsy. If the diagnosis is confirmed, the patient can be counseled and followed closely for symptomatic improvement. With restitution of weight and height, the GI follow-up can be set up on a once- to twice-yearly basis. Questions often arise as to the necessity of the gluten-free diet in the reportedly asymptomatic older child and adolescent. The gastroenterologist can assess biochemical and histologic indications of disease and help the family to maintain compliance. Access to good dietary advice and support groups is essential.

ROLE OF THE NUTRITIONIST

The dietitian plays a vital role in the treatment of the child with celiac disease. Gluten is a prevalent feature of many commercially prepared foods. It may not be apparent on labels as "vegetable protein" or it may be introduced into the diet inadvertently through fried foods or in medications. A dietitian well versed in the gluten-free diet is extremely helpful to most families in planning diets, balancing nutrition, and providing current information on gluten-free diets and products. A dietitian can also address vitamin and mineral deficiencies and supplementation, as well as growth and nutritional assessment. Prototype antibody (monoclonal antibody) kits have been described to aid patients with compliance with the gluten-free diet.

ROLE OF SUPPORT GROUPS

Since the dietary restrictions can be burdensome for the family of a patient with celiac disease support groups are especially helpful. The Celiac Sprue Association, USA (P.O. Box 31700, Omaha, NE 68131-0700) and the Gluten Intolerance Group of North America (P.O. Box 23053, Seattle, WA 98102-0353), are national support groups that provide information about research, food products, recipes, and companies selling gluten-free foods and referral services with thousands of members. Our local Midwest Gluten Intolerance Group, with 375 members, meets regularly and publishes newsletters offering medical information and dietary advice. Additionally, commercial companies cater to people with celiac disease, while certain supermarkets have dedicated gluten-free sections.

REFERENCES

1. Mylotte M, Egan-Mitchell B, McCarthy CF, McNicholl B. Incidence of coeliac disease in the West of Ireland. BMJ 1: 703–705

2. Talley NJ, Valdovinos MV, Petterson TM et al. Epidemiology of celiac sprue: a community-based study. Am J Gastroenterol 1994;89:843–846

3. Trier JS. Medical progress: celiac sprue, review article. N Engl J Med 1991;325:1709–1719

4. Ascher H, Krantz I, Kristiansson B. Increasing incidence of coeliac disease in Sweden. Arch Dis Child 1991;66:608–611

5. Polanco I, Biemond I, van Leeuwen A et al. Gluten sensitive enteropathy in Spain: genetic and environmental factors. In: McConnell RB, Ed. Genetics of Coeliac Disease. (Proceedings of International Symposium, 1979.) Lancaster: MTP Press, 1981:211–231

6. Mylotte M, Egan-Mitchell B, Fottrell PF et al. Family studies in celiac disease. Q J Med 1974;43:359–369

7. Tosi R, Visamara D, Tanigaki N et al. Evidence that coeliac disease is associated with a DC locus allelic specificity. Clin Immunol Immunopathol 1983;28:359–404

8. Keuning JJ. Pena AS, van Leeuwen A et al. HLA-DW3 associated with coeliac disease. Lancet 1976;1:506–508

9. Janatuinen EK, Pikkarainen PH, Kemppainen TA et al. Comparison of diets with and without oats in adults with celiac disease. N Engl J Med 1995;333:1033–1037

10. Kagnoff MF, Austin RK, Hubert JJ, Kasarda DD. Possible role for a human adenovirus in the pathogenesis of celiac disease. J Exp Med 1984;160:1544–1557

11. Colyer J, Farthing MJG, Kumar PJ et al. Reappraisal of the "lectin hypothesis" in the aetiopathogenesis of coeliac disease. Clin Sci 1986;71:105–110

12. Levenson SD, Austin RK, Dietler MD et al. Specificity of antigliadin antibody in celiac disease. Gastroenterology 1985;89:1–5

13. Brandtzaeg P, Farstad IN, Halstensen TS et al. Immune function in the normal and diseased human gut. In: Tsuchiya M, Nagura H, Hibi T, Moro I, Eds. Frontiers of Mucosal Immunology. Amsterdam: Excerpta Medica, 1991:29–36

14. MacDonald TT, Spencer J. Evidence that activated mucosal T-cells play a role in the pathogenesis of enteropathy in human small intestine. J Exp Med 1988;167:1321–1349

15. Stocker T, Dehner LP, Eds. Pediatric Pathology. Philadelphia: JB Lippincott 1992;678–679

16. Bonamico M, Scire G, Mariani P et al. Short stature as the primary manifestation of monosymptomatic celiac disease. J Pediatr Gastroenterol Nutr 1992;14:12–16

17. Maki M, Hallstrom O. Huupponen T et al. Increased prevalence of coeliac disease in diabetes. Arch Dis Child 1984; 59:739–742

18. Savilahti E, Pelkonen P, Visakorpi JK: IgA deficiency in children. A clinical study with special reference to intestinal finding. Arch Dis Child 1971; 46:665–670

19. Amil Dias J, Walker-Smith J. Down's syndrome and celiac disease. J Pediatr Gastroenterol Nutr 1990;10:41–43

20. Collin P, Maki M. Associated disorders in coeliac disease: Clinical aspects, review Scand J Gastroenterol 1994;29: 769–775

21. Ainne L, Maki M, Collin P, Keyrilainen O. Dental enamel defects in celiac disease. J Oral Pathol Med 1990;19:241–245

22. Logan RFA, Rifkind EA, Turner ID, Ferguson A. Mortality in celiac disease. Gastroenterology 1989;97:265–271

23. Holmes GKT, Prior P, Lane MR et al. Malignancy in coeliac disease—effect of a gluten free diet. Gut 1989;30:333–338

24. Walker-Smith JA, Guandalini S, Schmitz J et al. Revised criteria for diagnosis of coeliac disease. Arch Dis Child 1990; 65:909–911

25. Mayer M, Greco L, Troncone R et al. Early prediction of relapse during gluten challenge in childhood celiac disease. J Pediatr Gastroenterol Nutr 1989;8:474–479

26. Walker-Smith JA. Celiac disease. In: Walker WA, Durie PR, Hamilton JR, Walker-Smith JA, Watkins JB, Eds. Pediatric Gastrointestinal Disease. Philadelphia: BC Decker, 1991: 700–718

27. Shmerling DH. Questionnaire of the European Society for Paediatric Gastroenterology and Nutrition on Coeliac Disease. In: McNicholl B, McCarthy CF, Fottrell PF, Eds. Perspectives in Coeliac Disease. Lancaster: MTP Press, 1978: 245

28. Troncone R, Ferguson A. Antigliadin antibodies. J Pediatr Gastroenterol Nutr 1991;12;150–158

29. Maki M, Hallstrom O, Vesikari T, Visakorki JK. Evaluation of serum IgA-class reticulin antibody test for the detection of childhood celiac disease. J Pediatr 1984;105: 901–905

30. Chorzelski TP, Beutner EH, Suley J et al. IgA antiendomysium antibody. A new immunological marker of dermatitis herpetiformis and celiac disease. Br J Dermatol 1984;111: 395–402

31. Lerner A, Kumar V, Iancu TC. Immunological diagnosis of childhood coeliac disease: comparison between antigliadin, antireticulin and antiendomysial antibodies. Clin Exp Immunol 1994;95:78–82

32. Collin P, Maki M, Keyrilainen O et al. Selective IgA deficiency and coeliac disease. Scand J Gastroenterol 1992;27: 367–371

33. Corazza G, Valentini RA, Frisoni M et al. Gliadin immune reactivity is associated with overt and latent enteropathy in relatives of celiac patients. Gastroenterology 1992;103: 1517–1522

34. Vitoria JC, Arrieta A, Astigarraga I et al. Use of serological markers as a screening test in family members of patients with celiac disease. J Pediatr Gastroenterol Nutr 1994;19: 304–309

35. Grodzinsky E, Jansson G, Skogh T et al. Anti-endomysium and anti-gliadin antibodies as serological markers for coeliac disease in childhood: a clinical study to develop a practical routine. Acta Paediatr 1995;84:294–298

36. Wauters EAK, Jansen J, Houwen RH et al. IgG and IgA anti-gliadin antibodies as markers of mucosal damage in children with suspected celiac disease upon gluten challenge. J Pediatr Gastroenterol Nutr 1991;13:192–196

37. Not T, Ventura A, Peticarari S et al. A new, rapid, noninvasive screening test for celiac disease. J Pediatr 1993;123: 425–427

38. Leavelle DE, Ed. 1996 Test Catalog: Rochester, MN: Mayo Medical Laboratories, 1996

39. Juby LD, Rothwell J, Axon ATR. Lactulose/mannitol test:

an ideal screen for celiac disease. Gastroenterology 1989;96: 79–85

40. Oderda G, Ansaldi N. Comparison of suction capsule and endoscopic biopsy of small bowel mucosa. Gastrointest Endosc 1987;33:265–266

41. Dicke WK, Weijers HA, van de Kamer JH. Coeliac disease. The presence in wheat of a factor having a deleterious effect in cases of coeliac disease. Acta Paediatr 1953;42:34–42

42. Skerritt JH, Hill AS. Self-management of dietary compliance in coeliac disease by means of ELISA "home test" to detect gluten. Lancet 1991;337:379–382

43. Damen GM, Boersma B, Wit JM, Heymans HSA. Catch-up growth in 60 children with celiac disease. J Pediatr Gastroenterol Nutr 1994;19:394–400

44. Mayer M, Greco L, Troncone R et al. Compliance of adolescents with coeliac disease with a gluten free diet. Gut 1991; 32:881–885

45. Bardella MT, Molteni N, Prampolini L et al. Need for follow up in coeliac disease. Arch Dis Child 1994;70:211–213

20

CLOSTRIDIUM DIFFICILE

WENDY JESHION
CHRIS A. LIACOURAS

Clostridium difficile is an anaerobic spore-forming bacterium that causes a number of diseases, ranging from antibiotic-associated colitis to pseudomembranous colitis (PMC). PMC was first recognized in 1893, when J. M. Finney described a patient whose gastrointestinal (GI) surgery was complicated by the development of severe diarrhea, with eventual death on the 15th postoperative day. At autopsy, the patient was found to have a "diphtheritic membrane" in the stomach and small bowel.[1] Prior to the antibiotic era, this syndrome was reported and thought to be associated with a number of risk factors, including abdominal surgery, vascular insufficiency, uremia, neoplasia, and heavy metal toxicity.[2] Cases of PMC were diagnosed by their characteristic pathologic features, including the presence of plaque-like pseudomembranes in the intestinal mucosa.

During the 1950s, as the incidence of PMC increased, antibiotic agents were implicated as the cause of PMC. *Staphylococcus aureus* was the initial suspected pathogen, as it was often recovered in the stools of patient's with PMC. During the 1970s, Tedesco et al.[3] prospectively studied 200 patients treated with clindamycin and reported that 21% developed diarrhea; 10% had evidence of PMC on colonoscopy. This caused major concern in the medical community, as antibiotics were used quite frequently, and clindamycin was often used following abdominal surgery; however, *S. aureus* was not frequently recovered in the stools, and it became obvious that another organism might be responsible for the disease.

C. difficile was originally identified in 1935 by Hall and O'Toole and was found to be a normal member of the colonic flora in healthy infants. While it was later isolated from pediatric and adult patients who had no specific GI symptoms, *C. difficile* continued to be associated with a severe colitis, especially after prolonged antibiotic use.[4] In 1977, Larson et al.[5] isolated a cytopathic toxin in the stool specimens of patients with PMC; in 1978 *C. difficile* was identified as the source of the toxin.[2]

PATHOGENESIS

The requirements for *C. difficile*–associated colitis include a disturbance in the balance of normal colonic flora, the presence of *C. difficile* in the colon, and the production of toxin by the organism. Many investigators speculate that the environmental homeostasis of the colon is maintained by fatty acids and other products of anaerobic bacteria. Antibiotics presumably alter the colonic flora, allowing *C. difficile* spores, which are heat and acid resistant, to form vegetative forms that flourish and produce toxins.[4] The antibiotics most frequently implicated are ampicillin, clindamycin, and cephalosporins; however, PMC has been linked to almost any antibiotic (oral or parenteral) as well as to chemotherapeutic agents which have antimicrobial activity.

The colitis is caused by toxins produced and released by the *C. difficile* organism. There are at least two recognized toxins, toxin A and toxin B, which are antigenically different. Both toxins appear to play an important role in the disease, although their pathogenesis has not

151

been fully determined. Toxin A is a lethal enterotoxin that produces mucosal changes in the gastrointestinal tract.[4] It has been shown to cause fluid secretion, mucosal damage, hemorrhage, and inflammation in the intestines of rodents. Toxin B is noted for its cytotoxic effects in tissue culture cells. While both toxins have cytotoxic activity, toxin B is 100 to 1,000 times more potent a cytotoxin.[6]

EPIDEMIOLOGY

Approximately 30% to 70% of asymptomatic healthy neonates and infants harbor the organism and its toxins, in contrast to 1% to 3% of normal adult carriers. The cause of the relative resistance of infants to *C. difficile* toxin is unknown. It is speculated that either (1) the infants develop immunity secondary to placental maternal antibodies; (2) they are protected by maternal colostrum, which neutralizes the toxin; or (3) the toxins are unable to attach to neonatal mucosa.[6] The inability of the toxin to adhere to neonatal mucosa has been suggested to occur secondary to a deficiency of cell membrane toxin receptors on neonatal cells.[6,7]

Although most infants harbor the organism without developing the disease, infants who have undergone abdominal surgery or whose immune system has been compromised by other diseases may develop *C. difficile*.[6] In addition, a small percentage of infants and toddlers have chronic diarrhea secondary to *C. difficile*. Gryboski et al.[8] evaluated these infants and found that a significant number of patients had low levels of immunoglobulin, as compared to patients with chronic diarrhea unrelated to *C. difficile* and to patients who were asymptomatic carriers of *C. difficile*. It is hypothesized that these children are unable to produce an adequate local antibody response to the organism, thereby enabling it to act as a pathogen.[8] Warny et al.[9] demonstrated that some patients with relapsing *C. difficile*–associated diarrhea have a defective antibody response to toxin A.

Most cases of *C. difficile* infections in adults result from nosocomial infection. Only 1% to 3% of healthy adults are chronic carriers, as compared to 13% to 25% of adult hospital inpatients.[10] In inpatients, the organisms are released into the hospital environment and have been isolated from clothing and toilets. Studies have also documented the transmission of the organism from patient to patient through hospital personnel and by roommates. *C. difficile* spores can contaminate patient's rooms and survive for months. All efforts should be made to minimize the possibility of cross-contamination through strict adherence to enteric precautions and environmental decontamination.[10]

CLINICAL PRESENTATION

The spectrum of disease ranges from minor self-limited diarrhea to a severe intestinal illness that simulates toxic megacolon. Patients with antibiotic associated diarrhea can present with diarrhea occurring at a frequency of 3 to 20 times per day. The symptoms usually occur 3 to 10 days after the initiation of antibiotics, although several reports suggest that symptoms begin as late as 2 to 10 weeks after discontinuation of antibiotics.[7] *C. difficile*–associated diarrhea has also been reported to occur after a single dose of intravenous antibiotics.[7]

C. difficile can cause a severe colitis, manifested by profuse green, watery, foul-smelling diarrhea. Blood and mucus-streaked stools may be present. While diarrhea may be the only symptom, many patients will develop crampy abdominal pain, fever, and leukocytosis. Approximately 10% of patients with *C. difficile* develop severe PMC. These patients present with high fever, abdominal tenderness, leukocytosis, hypoalbuminemia, hypovolemia, and severe dehydration. Cases without diarrhea will often delay the diagnosis. Fecal leukocytosis is present in most patients with PMC. Complications include toxic megacolon and perforation.[11] Histology indicates isolated colonic involvement without evidence of small bowel disease.[4]

DIAGNOSIS

A number of diagnostic techniques are available to detect toxigenic *C. difficile*. One of the earliest methods of diagnosis is by obtaining an anaerobic culture of the organism from the stools. The disadvantage of this method is that it will also isolate nontoxigenic strains, which presumably are not the cause of the diarrheal illness. It is therefore necessary to confirm the diagnosis with an assay specific for *C. difficile* toxin. The gold standard is the tissue culture assay, which confirms the neutralization of the cytotoxic activity of toxin B by specific antisera. Although this method is expensive and time-consuming, it has excellent sensitivity and specificity.[7]

Enzyme-linked immunosorbent assay (ELISA) can detect toxins A or B, or both, depending on the specific antibody. These assays are excellent diagnostic alternatives to the cytotoxic assays, as they have good sensitivity and specificity and are less expensive and more rapidly performed. There is also a latex agglutination assay, which detects a protein other than A or B, but this technique has a high rate of false-positive and false-negative results.[7] The most definitive diagnosis of PMC is established by endoscopy (see below). For an in-depth discussion of diagnostic techniques, see Ch. 78.

PATHOLOGIC FEATURES

A wide spectrum of gross pathologic features are seen on endoscopic examination. Pseudomembrane are the most distinctive and appear as adherent focal, white or yellow plaques, surrounded by raised hyperemic mucosa. Histopathologically, the characteristic pseudomembrane has the appearance of a volcano erupting from the superficial colonic epithelium. This eruption of material consists of mucus, fibrin, and inflammatory cells. A milder form of the disease may exhibit colonic mucosa that is edematous, friable, and granular. On gross examination, it may be difficult to distinguish the mild form of *C. difficile* colitis from early inflammatory bowel disease; therefore, testing for the toxin should always be performed.[2] Additionally, individuals with inflammatory bowel disease are often superinfected with *C. difficile*.

TREATMENT

Primary Treatment

Primary treatment of *C. difficile* diarrheal illness consists of discontinuing the offending antibiotics and treating any associated illnesses. Approximately 25% to 50% of patients will respond to this form of therapy.[11] If symptoms persist or if the patient develops dehydration or a severe colitis, treatment should begin with antimicrobial therapy against *C. difficile*.

Oral vancomycin is considered the ideal therapy, as it is not absorbed and has the highest minimum inhibitory concentration (MIC) in the colon, giving excellent response rates. Approximately 95% of patients have complete resolution within 10 to 14 days. In addition, vancomycin typically has minimal side effects (i.e., bitter taste and the expense of treatment). The major disadvantage is its expense. Recently, the use of vancomycin has decreased secondary to the fear of inducing resistant strains of *Enterococcus*.

Metronidazole is an excellent alternative treatment and has the advantage of being less expensive than vancomycin. Theoretically, it appears to be an inferior therapy, as it is almost completely absorbed in the upper GI tract, resulting in poor colonic levels. However, a comparison of metronidazole to vancomycin showed similar response rates in patients.[12] The disadvantages of metronidazole include nausea and paresthesias. Bacitracin, cholestyramine, and rifampin can also be used in the treatment of *C. difficile* (Table 20-1). Antiperistaltic agents should be avoided in patients with PMC, as these medications could cause toxic megacolon.

There is no consensus on how to manage patients who are unable to take oral medication; however, there are two commonly recommended therapies. The first in-

TABLE 20-1. Treatment of *Clostridium difficile*–Associated Illness

Medication	Dose	Duration
Vancomycin	10 mg/kg/dose qid for children	10–14 days
	Maximum 250 mg qid 125–250 mg qid for adults	10–14 days
Metronidazole	5–7 mg/kg/dose qid for children	10–14 days
	Maximum 250 mg qid 250 mg qid for adults	10–14 days
Bacitracin	20,000 IU qid for adults	10–14 days
Rifampin	600 mg qd for adults	10–14 days
Cholestyramine	80 mg/kg/dose tid for children	2–4 wk
	4 g tid for adults	

cludes the administration of intravenous vancomycin and metronidazole. The second approach is often used in conjunction with parenteral therapy and consists of the administration of vancomycin by a nasogastric, intestinal, or colonic tube. Emergency ileostomy and cecostomies have also been performed for instillation of vancomycin when the patient is not responding to routine therapies.[11]

Relapse

Symptomatic relapse of *C. difficile* colitis occurs in approximately 10% to 20% of patients, with the onset of symptoms occurring at 1 to 4 weeks after the discontinuation of therapy.[11] While most patients respond to a second course of antibiotics, some will have multiple relapses. The frequency of relapse does not appear to be related to the specific antibiotic, the dose or to the length of treatment. Relapse is thought to be due to the germination of *C. difficile* spores that have persisted despite treatment; reinfection with *C. difficile*, the presence of an underlying disease, or the chronic use of antibiotics. Patients with relapsing *C. difficile* infections should be referred to a gastroenterologist for colonoscopy.

Other Therapies

Numerous therapies have been advocated for relapsing *C. difficile* infections. Some therapies are based on modifications of vancomycin therapy and include prolonged use of vancomycin (1 to 3 months), gradually tapering over 1 to 2 months[13]; with pulse-dose vancomycin every other day[14]; and vancomycin in combination with other drugs (bacitracin, rifampin, cholestyramine).[15] Alternative therapies based on repopulating the normal colonic bacterial flora include the rectal instillation of stool from donor patients[16] or broth cultures of stool flora.[17]

Some therapies involve the administration of substances that inhibit the growth of C. difficile. For example, oral administration of Lactobacillus has been used for therapy secondary to the ability of Lactobacillus to produce an antimicrobial substance that inhibits the growth of C. difficile.[18] Saccharomyces boulardii, a yeast found on lychee fruit, has also been used to treat chronic C. difficile. The efficacy of this organism is believed to be due to its production of a protease that destroys the receptor site for the C. difficile toxin A.[19] Relapsing C. difficile has also been treated with oral nontoxigenic isolates of C. difficile.[20]

Chronic intractable C. difficile has also been treated with whole-bowel irrigation with a polyethylene glycol solution (Golytely) in combination with oral Lactobacillus treatment or vancomycin, or both.[22] Another form of therapy is the administration of intravenous gamma-globulin.[23] This therapy is based on studies showing that some patients with chronic C. difficile have low antitoxin A antibody levels, suggesting a defective antibody response[9,23] or hypogammaglobulinemia.[8]

CONCLUSION

C. difficile infections often result from disturbances of the normal gut flora by antibiotics. The organism can produce a broad spectrum of disease activity, ranging from asymptomatic carnage to PMC and toxic megacolon.

REFERENCES

1. Finney JMT. Gastroenterostomy for cicatrizing ulcer of the pylorus. Bull Johns Hopkins Hosp 1893;4:S3–55

2. Freeman HJ. Antibiotic-induced pseudomembranous colitis: new approaches. Hosp Ther 1985;86–92

3. Tedesco FJ, Barton RW, Alpers DH. Clindamycin-associated colitis. A prospective study. Ann Intern Med 1974;81: 429–33

4. Bartlett J. Clostridium difficile: history of its role as an enteric pathogen and the current state of knowledge about the organism. Clin Infect Dis 1994;18:S265–S272

5. Larson HE, Parry JV, Price AB et al. Undescribed toxin in pseudomembranous colitis. BMJ 1977;1:1246–1248

6. Lyerly D, Krivan HC, Wilkins TD. Clostridium difficile: its disease and toxins. Clin Microbiol Rev 1988;1:1–18

7. Knoop F. Clostridium difficile: clinical disease and diagnosis. Clin Microbiol Rev 1993;6:251–265

8. Gryboski J, Pellerzno R, Young N, Edberg S. Positive role of Clostridium difficile infection and diarrhea in infants and children. Am J Gastroenterol 1991;86:685–68?

9. Warny M, Vaerman JP, Avesani V, Delmee M. Human antibody response to Clostridium difficile toxin A in relation to clinical course of infection. Infect Immun 1994;62:384–389

10. McFarland L. The epidemiology of Clostridium difficile infections. Viewpoints Dig Dis 1990;22(5):19–24

11. Fekety R, Shah AB. Diagnosis and treatment of Clostridium difficile colitis. JAMA, 1993;269:71–75

12. Teasley D, Gerding DN, Olson MM et al. Prospective randomized trial of metronidazole versus vancomycin for Clostridium difficile-associated diarrhea and colitis. Lancet 1983; 2:1043–1046

13. Tedesco FJ. Treatment of recurrent antibiotic-associated pseudomembranous colitis. Am J Gastroenterol 1982;77: 2201–2221

14. Tedesco FJ, Gordon D, Fortson WC. Approach to patients with multiple relapses of antibiotic-associated pseudomembranous colitis. Am J Gastroenterol 1985;80:867–868

15. Biggy BP. Therapy of relapsing Clostridium difficile associated diarrhea and colitis with the combination of vancomycin and rifampin. J Clin Gastroenterol 1987;9:155

16. Schwan A. Relapsing Clostridium difficile enterocolitis cured by rectal infusion of normal faeces. Scand J Infect Dis 1984; 16:211–215

17. Trede M. Bacteriotherapy for chronic relapsing Clostridium difficile diarrhea in six patients. Lancet 1989;6:1156–1160

18. Gorbach SL, Chang TW, Goldin B. Successful treatment of relapsing Clostridium difficile colitis with Lactobacillus, letter. Lancet 1987;2:1519

19. McFarland L. A randomized placebo-controlled trial of Saccharomyces boulardii in combination with standard antibiotics for Clostridium difficile disease. JAMA 1994;271:1913–1918

20. Seal D, Borriello SP, Barclay F et al. Treatment of relapsing Clostridium difficile diarrhea by administration of a non-toxigenic strain. Eur J Clin Microbiol 1987;6:51–53

21. Kreutzer E, Milligan FD. Treatment of antibiotic-associated pseudomembranous colitis with cholestyramine resin. Johns Hopkins Med J 1978;143:67–72

22. Liacouras C, Piccoli DA. Whole-bowel irrigation as an adjunct to the treatment of chronic relapsing Clostridium difficile colitis. J Clin Gastroenterol 1996;22:186–189

23. Leung D, Kelly CP, Boguniewicz M et al. Treatment with intravenously administered gamma globulin of chronic relapsing colitis induced by Clostridium difficile toxin. J Pediatr 1991;118:633–637

CONGENITAL ANOMALIES OF THE INTESTINE

CELESTE M. HOLLANDS

MARK A. HOFFMAN

ESOPHAGEAL ATRESIA

Pathophysiology

The precise etiology of esophageal atresia has not been resolved. The incidence is approximately 1 in 3,000 live births. Esophageal atresia occurs with or without a tracheoesophageal communication. A distal tracheoesophageal fistula with a proximal esophageal pouch is the most common configuration, occurring in 85% of cases. Associated anomalies are frequent and have been described and classified as VATER and VACTERL representing vertebral, alimentary, cardiac, renal, anal, and limb anomalies. The "TE" represents tracheoesophageal fistula.

Clinical Presentation

Characteristic features of esophageal atresia occurring during the immediate newborn period include excessive salivation, as well as coughing, choking, and cyanosis secondary to aspiration. Acute gastric dilation and pulmonary complications, including atelectasis and pneumonitis[1] also occur. On physical examination, a scaphoid abdomen (absent gastric air) may be noted if no distal tracheoesophageal fistula is present.

Diagnosis

A firm, radiopaque catheter should be passed through the nose and advanced into the esophagus until resistance is met. An anteroposterior and lateral chest and abdominal radiograph is then obtained. The catheter will be seen to end in the proximal esophageal pouch (Fig. 21-1). The presence of distal bowel gas on the abdominal radiograph confirms the presence of a distal tracheoesophageal fistula. Chest radiography or echocardiography is useful in indicating the position of the aortic arch, so that the side for thoracotomy can be determined, but these should not be ordered if they will delay the referral.

Treatment

A Replogle catheter (firm, single-lumen, nasoenteric catheter) should be left in the proximal pouch on continuous suction. The head of the infant's bed should be elevated 30 degrees. If the infant weighs less than 2,000 g or has significant associated anomalies, sepsis, or pneumonia, a gastrostomy is performed. Division of the fistula is occasionally necessary as well, with repair delayed until the patient's condition improves. If the infant is able to undergo a definitive operation, a thoracotomy with division of the fistula and primary repair is undertaken. In pure esophageal atresia, the distance between the proximal and distal pouches precludes early repair. There are several options[2]: (1) leave a Replogle tube in the proximal pouch, place a gastrostomy, perform bougienage, "stretching," of the pouches, and eventual re-exploration with anastomosis or (2) perform an esophagostomy and gastrostomy with eventual colon or gastric tube interposition.

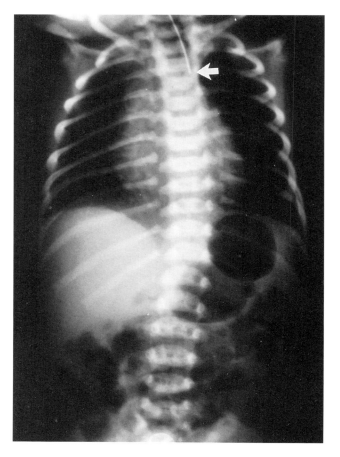

FIGURE 21-1. Catheter in proximal esophageal pouch (arrow).

Referral Pattern

The risk of aspiration mandates emergent surgical referral. As there are different management styles in treating this condition, contrast studies should be performed in consultation with a surgeon and a radiologist.

ENTERIC DUPLICATIONS

Pathophysiology

Duplications of the gastrointestinal (GI) tract are rare. The exact etiology is unknown, but several hypotheses have been proposed.[3] They can be located from the mouth to the anus and may be cystic or tubular. Tubular duplications usually communicate with the GI tract. Enteric duplications may contain gastric mucosa or pancreatic tissue.

Clinical Presentation

Most patients will present within the first few weeks of life. The clinical presentation is varied and depends on the site of the duplication. Esophageal duplications may

present with respiratory symptoms or as an asymptomatic mediastinal mass found incidentally on chest radiography. Intra-abdominal duplications may present as an asymptomatic mass or as an incidental finding on barium study, abdominal radiography, or ultrasound. Conversely, a variety of abdominal symptoms may predominate, including abdominal pain, GI bleeding, intestinal obstruction, or intussusception.

Diagnosis

In patients with an esophageal duplication, a chest radiograph may indicate a mediastinal mass. Barium swallow may show external compression of the esophagus (Fig. 21-2), and computed tomography (CT) may define a cystic mass and its relationship to surrounding structures. Intra-abdominal duplications are more difficult to evaluate and are usually diagnosed at laparoscopy or laparotomy performed for abdominal mass, abdominal pain, GI bleeding, or intussusception. There are no specific radiographic studies. Abdominal radiography or ultrasound may suggest a mass. Barium studies may demonstrate the duplication if there is communication with the GI tract. Patients with GI bleeding may have a positive technetium pertechnetate radionuclide scan if gastric mucosa is present.

Evaluation for vertebral anomalies (spinal radiographs), associated GI anomalies (ultrasound, barium study), and genitourinary anomalies (intravenous pyelogram, ultrasound) should be performed for all patients.

Treatment

The management of enteric duplications is surgical. Esophageal duplications are "shelled out" without mucosal entry. Abdominal enteric duplications are usually excised and a primary anastomosis performed. However, when an extensive tubular duplication exists sharing a common muscular wall and blood supply, drainage into the contiguous bowel and mucosal stripping should be performed.

Referral Pattern

Most patients are referred to a surgeon early during the diagnostic workup because of an abnormal radiographic study or because of signs and symptoms of abdominal pain, abdominal mass, intussusception, obstruction, or GI bleeding. For those patients with esophageal duplications, once the diagnosis is suspected, referral should be made for surgical evaluation and treatment.

HYPERTROPHIC PYLORIC STENOSIS

Pathophysiology

Pyloric stenosis occurs in approximately 3 of every 1,000 live births and is five times more common in males. It is more likely in infants with affected siblings or mothers.

A multifactorial mode of inheritance with some gender influence is generally postulated. Although the exact etiology is unknown, several hypotheses have been proposed.[4] The end result is hypertrophy of both the longitudinal and circular muscle layers of the pylorus, leading to elongation and thickening of the pylorus into the shape of an olive and gastric outlet obstruction.

Clinical Presentation

The hallmark of pyloric stenosis is nonbilious, projectile emesis that typically begins at 3 weeks of age, increasing in frequency. The infant remains hungry. About 2% of patients have an associated indirect hyperbilirubinemia that resolves with release of the pyloric obstruction. Constipation is not infrequent. Electrolyte abnormalities include a hypochloremic, hypokalemic alkalosis.

Classically, a visible peristaltic wave moving from left to right across the upper abdomen is described. More reliably, 70% to 90% of infants will have a palpable mass in the right epigastrium about the size and consistency of an olive. It is best palpated when the stomach is empty and the child is resting quietly. The left hand is placed under the child's back and the right hand is used to palpate the epigastrium in a bimanual fashion. Another technique for palpation is to place the child in the prone position and bimanually palpate the epigastrium.

Diagnosis

The diagnosis can be made with confidence if the history is reliable and an olive is palpated. If there is uncertainty, ultrasound examination is the test of choice. Ultrasound criteria with 100% positive predictive value for pyloric stenosis include muscle thickness greater than 5 mm, muscle diameter greater than 15 mm, or a combination of a 14-mm diameter and a 4-mm wall thickness.[5] However, in some cases ultrasound criteria will be borderline. In these cases, an upper GI contrast study or upper endoscopy may aid in the diagnosis. Typical upper GI findings include a string sign (Fig. 21-3), delayed gastric emptying, a shoulder sign, and an upturned pyloric curve.

Treatment

Operation for pyloric stenosis is not emergent. Fluid and electrolyte deficits must be corrected prior to surgical intervention. Most infants present with mild or moderate

FIGURE 21-2. Barium swallow with external compression due to esophageal duplication (arrow).

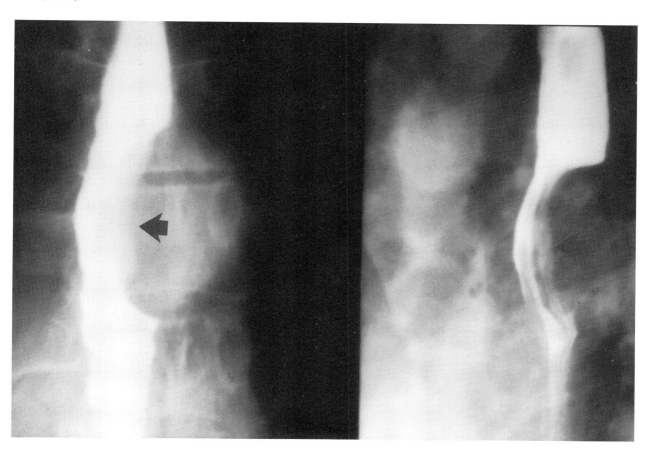

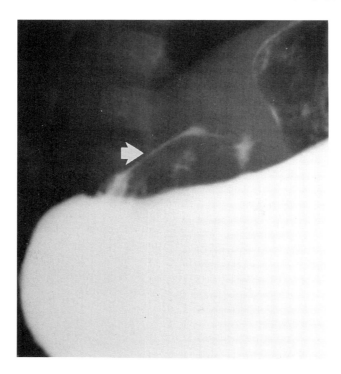

FIGURE 21-3. Upper GI contrast study of pyloric stenosis showing string sign (arrow).

dehydration and can be prepared for operation within 24 hours.

Referral Pattern

The infant should be referred to a surgeon once the diagnosis is suspected. Many surgeons will proceed to operation based on a suggestive history and a clearly palpable olive. Therefore, referral prior to radiologic intervention may be the most cost-effective management.

DUODENAL OBSTRUCTION

Pathophysiology

Duodenal obstruction may be complete (due to atresia) or partial (due to a web, annular pancreas, or preduodenal portal vein). Malrotation may also be a cause of both partial and complete duodenal obstruction. Failure of recanalization of the duodenum during embryogenesis produces atresia and webs. Annular pancreas is due to abnormal rotation of the pancreatic anlage. Obstruction with a preduodenal portal vein is thought to be due to either vein compression or associated malrotation with obstructing Ladd's bands. There is a significant association of other anomalies in infants with duodenal atresia.[6] Approximately 30% have Down's syndrome (trisomy 21) with associated cardiac and neurologic defects.

Clinical Presentation

Infants usually present with bilious emesis during the first 24 hours of life. Findings on examination are usually related to associated anomalies.

Diagnosis

Prenatal ultrasound may demonstrate maternal polyhydramnios, or proximal intestinal obstruction in the fetus. Plain abdominal radiographs show a characteristic "double bubble" sign (Fig. 21-4) with or without distal bowel gas, signifying partial or complete duodenal obstruction. Barium enema or upper GI series, or both, should be performed in consultation with a surgeon and a radiologist.

Treatment

A nasogastric tube should be placed for gastric decompression. Fluid and electrolyte abnormalities should be corrected expeditiously. Surgical exploration is mandatory, and correction is by duodenoduodenostomy or duodenojejunostomy for duodenal atresia, annular pancreas, preduodenal portal vein, and a web extensively involving the ampulla. Duodenotomy with resection of the web may be performed if the ampulla is not involved. Evaluation for additional intestinal abnormalities should be performed at surgery.

FIGURE 21-4. Double bubble of duodenal obstruction.

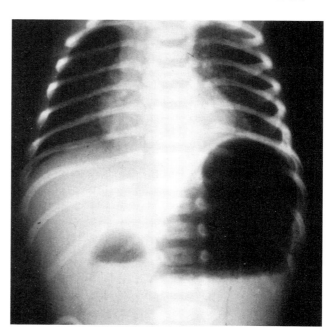

Referral Pattern

Duodenal obstruction requires immediate surgical evaluation and a briskly paced diagnostic workup. If the prenatal ultrasound point to duodenal obstruction, referral and counseling should be considered prior to delivery.

INTESTINAL ATRESIA

Pathophysiology

Intestinal atresia may occur at the jejunal, ileal, or colonic level, leading to complete bowel obstruction. The etiology is believed to be an in utero vascular accident.[7]

Clinical Presentation

Most patients present within the first few days of life with signs and symptoms of high-grade intestinal obstruction. The degree of abdominal distention relates to the level of obstruction. Atresia associated with gastroschisis may be difficult to diagnose if the bowel is thickened and heavily matted.

Diagnosis

Intestinal atresia should be suspected in newborns with bilious emesis and abdominal distention. Plain abdominal radiographs show dilated intestinal loops with air-fluid levels and no distal bowel gas. In general, the obstruction is distal if many loops are visible. Peritoneal calcifications may be visible on radiography and are indicative of intrauterine intestinal perforation. Barium enema results vary with the level of the atresia. In jejunoileal atresia, the barium enema indicates a microcolon. In colonic atresia, the barium enema shows a windsock deformity if the atresia is incomplete, and an abrupt "cutoff" if the atresia is complete.

Treatment

A nasogastric tube should be placed for gastric decompression. Fluid and electrolyte disturbances should be corrected. Repair includes resection of the affected segment and primary anastomosis for jejunoileal atresias and some colonic atresias.[8] A temporary colostomy may be necessary for some colonic atresias.[9,10]

Referral Pattern

Emergent surgical referral is necessary in instances of intestinal obstruction.

MECKEL'S DIVERTICULUM

Pathophysiology

A Meckel's diverticulum is the result of a persistent vitelline (omphalomesenteric) duct (Fig. 21-5). The incidence is about 2%. It is a true diverticulum that contains

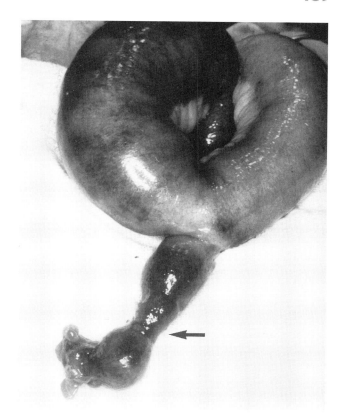

FIGURE 21-5. Meckel's diverticulum (arrow).

all three intestinal layers. The diverticulum occurs along the antimesenteric border of the ileum usually within 2 ft of the ileocecal valve. Gastric mucosa (44%) or pancreatic tissue (5%) may be present. The gastric mucosa may lead to ulceration and hemorrhage. Attachment to the umbilicus may persist and predispose to obstruction secondary to internal herniation around the offending band. The diverticulum may serve as a lead point for intussusception or may become inflamed with the possibility of perforation.

Clinical Presentation

The clinical presentation is varied but 95% are asymptomatic. For those that are symptomatic, painless lower GI bleeding (melena) is the most common presentation.[11] Other clinical presentations include intestinal obstruction, diverticulitis (indistinguishable from acute appendicitis), umbilical cysts and/or sinuses, or a palpable abdominal mass.

Diagnosis

The approach to diagnosis will depend on the presentation. For lower GI bleeding, a technetium pertechnetate radionuclide scan (Meckel's scan) will detect gastric mucosa, while a tagged red cell scan may demonstrate active blood loss. To counter the significant false-negative rate associated with this technique, accuracy may be improved by preparation with cimetidine or gastrin analogue. A barium enema is useful if intussusception is suspected. A small bowel contrast study occasionally demonstrates the diverticulum. Laparotomy and laparoscopy may demonstrate an inflamed Meckel's diverticulum as a cause of right lower quadrant pain, or they may show an incidental finding of a Meckel's diverticulum when either is performed for other pathology.

Treatment

Symptomatic patients require surgical referral. Patients with lower GI hemorrhage should be resuscitated. Most bleeding episodes will cease spontaneously. The diverticulum may then be resected semielectively, generally during the same hospital stay. If bleeding persists, the diverticulum is resected on an emergent basis. Those with inflammation will present as appendicitis, and at operation the diverticulum will be discovered and resected along with the appendix. Intussusception secondary to Meckel's diverticulum usually will not respond to attempted hydrostatic reduction. If it can be reduced at operation, resection is limited to the diverticulum. If it cannot be reduced, resection with primary anastomosis is required. Patients with obstruction will require relief of the obstruction and resection of the Meckel's diverticulum. When a Meckel's diverticulum is found incidentally at laparotomy or at laparoscopy, it should be resected if (1) abdominal pain is the reason for the surgery, (2) heterotopic mucosa or a mass is palpable within the diverticulum, or (3) its presence predisposes to obstruction by umbilical attachment.

Referral Pattern

Patients should generally be referred for surgical evaluation early in the course of symptoms. Radiologic workup can then be pursued in an expeditious manner in consultation with a radiologist.

MALROTATION

Pathophysiology

Intestinal malrotation is an anomaly of rotation and fixation of the intestine.[2,12,13] Normally, the mesentery possesses a broad base extending from the ligament of Treitz to the left of the spine down to the cecum in the right lower quadrant. With malrotation, the mesentery originates from a narrow pedicle, with the superior mesenteric artery coursing radially through it to the bowel wall from its aortic origin. This narrow pedicle is subject to volvulus, placing the entire mid-gut at risk of infarction. Peritoneal bands (Ladd's bands)[14] are also present and may obstruct the duodenum.

Clinical Presentation

The clinical presentation varies with age.[15] Most newborns characteristically present with bilious emesis. Older children have a more diverse clinical presentation. Acute duodenal obstruction, chronic abdominal pain, intermittent vomiting, chronic diarrhea, malabsorption, and failure to thrive may all be caused by malrotation with intermittent volvulus.[16,17] Patients may present at any age with an incidental finding of a malrotation on radiographic contrast studies. Physical findings range from an unremarkable examination, to abdominal distention, or peritonitis in an infant or child in severe shock. Intestinal ischemia classically presents with pain out of proportion to the physical examination.

Diagnosis

Once the diagnosis of malrotation is suspected, it must be rapidly evaluated. It is surgical dogma that bilious vomiting in the newborn is an emergency until proved otherwise. Abdominal radiographs may show duodenal obstruction ("double bubble," paucity of bowel gas distally). Upper GI and barium enema examinations have characteristic findings, including a right-sided jejunum, duodenal obstruction with characteristic beak shape, or patent corkscrew duodenum and a midline cecum. The diagnosis is based on the location of the ligament of Treitz[12] (for further discussion, see Ch. 64).

Treatment

Bilious emesis in the newborn mandates an emergency upper GI or barium enema, or both. A diagnosis of malrotation dictates surgical correction by Ladd's procedure.[14]

Referral Pattern

A symptomatic patient with malrotation should be referred emergently for surgical treatment. For a truly asymptomatic patient who is found incidentally to have a malrotation on a GI contrast study, counseling should be sought for medical attention, should worrisome abdominal symptoms develop.

ANORECTAL ANOMALIES

Pathophysiology

Anorectal anomalies occur due to abnormal formation of the urorectal septum. Classification of these anomalies is complex.[2] In general, the classification is based on the

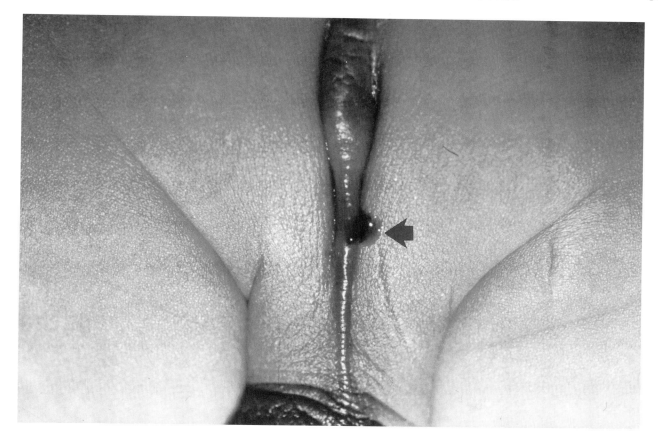

FIGURE 21-6. Male infant with imperforate anus and meconium staining at site of perineal fistula (arrow).

relationship of the anorectal anomaly to the puborectalis sling of the levator ani (low, intermediate, or high). The relationship to the puborectalis sling has significant anatomic, physiologic, and surgical implications. Anomalies that occur at or above the puborectalis sling are high or intermediate anomalies and generally have fistulas to the bladder or urethra (male), and vagina or cloaca (female). Anomalies that traverse the puborectalis sling are considered low and fistulize to the perineum or urethra (male) and to the vulva or vestibule (female).

Clinical Presentation

Patients with imperforate anus generally present with signs and symptoms of intestinal obstruction in the first few days of life. Patients with fistulas will discharge meconium from the perineum, scrotum, vaginal vestibule, or urethra (Fig. 21-6). An abnormal anus is usually obvious and is discovered shortly after delivery. Further examination may be consistent with intestinal obstruction. A fistulous connection along the perineum may not be immediately obvious but should become evident by 24 hours of life. Careful evaluation for associated anomalies, specifically the VATER and VACTERL associations, should be performed.

Diagnosis

Diagnostic workup includes a prone cross-table lateral radiograph and an "invertogram" (Rice and Wangensteen view) in an attempt to characterize the level of obstruction.[18] These studies should be delayed 12 to 18 hours to allow bowel gas to reach the distal rectum. Computed tomography (CT) and magnetic resonance imaging (MRI) may help determine the relationship of the atresia to the levator ani. Water-soluble contrast studies through the bladder, vagina, urethra, and perineal fistulas will be very useful in delineating the anatomy of the anomaly.

Treatment

The initial management goal is to relieve intestinal obstruction and define the anorectal and urogenital anatomy. A nasogastric tube should be placed. Evaluation for associated anomalies should be undertaken. Patients with a fistula amenable to dilation should not require colostomy unless refractory constipation develops. Those patients without a satisfactory external fistula will require a colostomy with eventual anorectoplasty.[18,19]

Long-term management of constipation and soiling is the major challenge with these patients.[19-21]

Referral Pattern

Patients with intestinal obstruction require emergent surgical referral. Those without obstruction will require surgical referral less urgently, but certainly within the first few days of life.

MESENTERIC/OMENTAL CYSTS

Pathophysiology

An uncommon entity, mesenteric and omental cysts are of lymphatic origin. These benign unilocular or multilocular cysts are lined with endothelium. They contain either chyle or serous fluid (Fig. 21-7).

Clinical Presentation

The presentation is varied,[2] and many patients have no discernible symptoms—only a coincidentally discovered mass. Others present with peritonitis or intestinal obstruction. However, the most common complaint is abdominal pain. Examination may demonstrate a palpable, freely movable mass.

Diagnosis

The precise diagnosis is generally made at laparotomy. Plain abdominal films may show a mass effect, and the walls of the homogeneous mass may be calcified. Ultrasound or CT scan may show a cystic structure.

Treatment

Laparotomy with complete resection of the cyst is the treatment of choice. In some cases, partial bowel resection may be necessary if the cyst is intimately adherent to the bowel wall.

Referral Pattern

Referral to a surgeon should be made once the diagnosis is suspected. For many of the presenting signs and symptoms, referral will be made before the precise diagnosis is suspected. The definitive diagnosis will most likely be made at laparotomy for those presenting with peritonitis and obstruction.

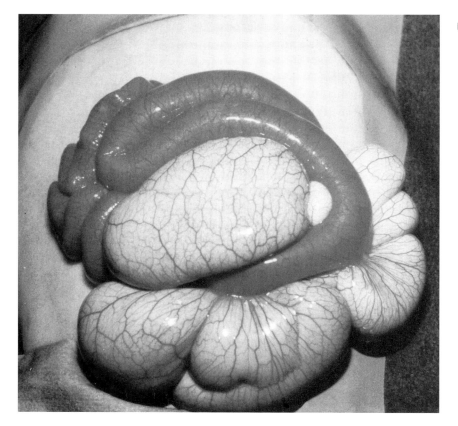

FIGURE 21-7. Large omental cyst.

REFERENCES

1. Grosfeld JL. Alimentary tract obstruction in the newborn. Curr Probl Pediatr 1975;5:3–47

2. Welch KJ, Randolph JG, Ravitch MM et al. Pediatric Surgery. Chicago: Year Book, 1986;682–1037

3. Holcomb GW III, Ghessari A, O'Neill JA Jr et al. Surgical management of alimentary tract duplications. Ann Surg 1989;209:167–174

4. Garcia VF, Randolph JG. Pyloric stenosis: diagnosis and management. Pediatr Rev 1990;11:292–296

5. Bowen AD. The vomiting infant's recent advances and unsettled issues in imaging. Radiol Clin North Am 1988;26: 377

6. Bailey PV, Tracy TF Jr, Connors RH et al. Congenital duodenal obstruction: a 32-year review. J Pediatr Surg 1993;28: 92–95

7. Louw JH, Barnard CN. Congenital intestinal atresia: observation of its origin. Lancet 1955;2:1065–1066

8. Rescorla FJ, Grosfeld JL. Intestinal atresia and stenosis: analysis of survival in 120 cases. Surgery 1985;98:668–676

9. Powell RW, Raffensperger JG. Congenital colonic atresia. J Pediatr Surg 1982;17:166–170

10. Pohlson EC, Hatch EI Jr, Glick PL, Tapper D. Individualized management of colonic atresia. Am J Surg 1988;155: 690–692

11. Brian JE Jr, Stair JM. Noncolonic diverticular disease. Surg Gynecol Obstet 1985;161:189–195

12. Ford EG, Senac MO, Srikanth MS, Weitzman JJ. Malrotation of the intestine in children. Ann Surg 1992;215: 172–178

13. Bill AH Jr, Grauman D. Rationale and technic for stabilization of the mesentery in cases of nonrotation of the midgut. J Pediatr Surg 1966;1:127–136

14. Ladd WE. Congenital duodenal obstruction. Surgery 1:1937; 878–885

15. Rescorla FJ, Shedd FJ, Grosfeld JL et al. Anomalies of intestinal rotation in childhood: analysis of 447 cases. Surgery 1990;108:710–716

16. Brandt ML, Pokorny WJ, McGill CW, Harberg FJ. Late presentations of midgut malrotation in children. Am J Surg 150: 1985;767–771

17. Pelucio M, Haywood Y. Midgut volvulus: an unusual case of adolescent abdominal pain. Am J Emerg Med 1994;12: 167–171

18. Pena A. Current management of anorectal anomalies. Surg Clin North Am 1992;72:1393–1415

19. Pena A. Anorectal malformations. Semin Pediatr Surg 1995; 4:35–47

20. Bender TM, Ledesma-Medina J, Sang K. Radiographic manifestations of anomalies of the gastrointestinal tract. Radiol Clin North Am 1991;29:335–349

21. Rintala R, Lindahl H, Marttinen E, Sariola H. Constipation is a major functional complication after internal sphincter-saving posterior sagittal anorectoplasty for high and intermediate anorectal malformations. J Pediatr Surg 1993;28: 1054–1058

22

CONSTIPATION AND ENCOPRESIS

WILLIAM J. WENNER

Up to 10% of all children will present to their physician with a chief complaint of constipation; 10% to 25% of referrals to pediatric gastroenterologists are for constipation.[1] Constipation is, however, a symptom, not a disease. The causes of constipation in the pediatric population can be categorized as due to either an anatomic or a physiologic impediment to defecation. Anatomic causes include Hirschsprung's disease, imperforate or malpositioned anus, ileal atresia, meconium ileus/plug, or a colonic stricture. Physiologic causes include hypothyroidism, spinal cord defects, prune-belly syndrome, ascariasis, infant botulism, diabetes, lead poisoning, medications, and the most common cause of constipation—functional constipation syndrome.

Functional constipation is a self-perpetuating condition that arises from voluntary withholding or decreased colonic motility. This condition occurs when the rectal vault continues to distend with stool without formal defecation. Eventually, the normal physiologic "urge" to defecate is lost. Most children with functional constipation voluntarily withhold secondary to pain on defecation as a result of anal fissure or the passage of large, hard stools. Often in the older child, the environment plays a crucial role, as many children develop constipation because they will not use "public" restrooms.

Encopresis has been found to occur in 1% to 2% of children.[2] It is characterized as soiling (involuntary defecation into clothing) of at least 1 month's duration. Three to four times more common in boys, this condition is an aberration of the complex blend of behavioral and physiologic factors that allow for bowel control. A definitive etiology has not been determined, but poor coordi-

nation of the bowel movement has been demonstrated, as has decreased sensation to rectal distention.

NORMAL STOOL PATTERN

A precise definition of constipation is not possible, as the normal stooling pattern differs greatly among individuals. Constipation is usually defined in terms of frequency, although it can include aberrations in size, consistency, and ease of passage. While norms have not been clearly quantified, some studies show that infants average about 1.5 bowel movements on the first day of life and by 1 week have four per day.[3] Normal breast-fed infants may have as many as seven per day or as few as one every 7 days. By 16 weeks of age, the average has decreased to two per day.[4] At 1 year of age, infants reportedly average 1.6 bowel movements per day, and at 4 years of age this has dropped to one per day. The range of normal in toilet trained children has less than 4% have less than one bowel movement every other day.[5] Adult norms fall between three per day to three per week.[6]

CLINICAL PRESENTATION

The typical presentation of constipation in children begins when parents notice that the child complains about painful defecation. Other common signs are "withholding" behaviors such as squeezing the legs together or "dancing" around the room when children feel the urge to defecate. Constipation is easily diagnosed when hard, large, and more infrequent stools occur; however, because of the wide range of normal and the uniqueness of constipation in each child, it is possible that these symptoms may not be the chief complaint for constipation. Often, children may present with diarrhea (encopresis) or abdominal pain as the initial complaint. In functional constipation, the parents may report daily bowel movements, but evaluation may demonstrate retained stool due to incomplete evacuation.

A diagnosis of constipation can be readily made by history, and attention should be paid to certain historic details. Age of onset, relationship to "toilet training," frequency of bowel movements, soiling, blood in stool, failure to thrive, fever, perception of the urge to defecate, and previous therapeutic maneuvers are important clues for the diagnosis. While the cause of constipation is most commonly functional, anatomic and physiologic etiologies such as Hirschsprung's disease, hypothyroidism, and sacral neurologic dysfunction should always be considered.

Blood in stool, failure to thrive, emesis, and persistent abdominal distention suggest anatomic etiology. Soiling, withholding behavior, and loss of the urge to defecate suggest a physiologic etiology. Soiling has been reported in less than 3% of patient's with Hirschsprung's disease, and only in those with limited rectal involvement. Symptoms of Hirschsprung's disease are demonstrated in 83% of patients within the first month of life, and in 96% by 1 year of age.[7] Failure to pass meconium on the first day of life has been reported in 94% of a series of 501 children with Hirschsprung's disease.[8] By 48 hours of life, only 57% of infants with Hirschsprung's disease failed to pass meconium. In normal infants, 94% will pass meconium in the first 24 hours of life. This finding gives a reassuring 99.7% predictive value that the child does not have Hirschsprung's disease if stool is passed within the first 24 hours. Failure to pass stool in the first 24 hours is only 0.1% predictive of Hirschsprung's disease. However, any child who has delay in the passage of meconium should be considered for evaluation for anatomic cause. Physical examination and the child's development are important in the assessment of Hirschsprung's disease, hypothyroidism, and spinal cord lesions.

PHYSICAL EXAMINATION

The physical examination is an important and valuable tool to determine the correct diagnosis. Emphasis should be placed on abdominal findings, anal tone and location, and contents of the rectum. A rectal examination should be performed in all patients with the complaint of constipation or diarrhea. In typical functional constipation, the rectal examination indicates a distended rectum filled with a large mass of stool. An empty, nondistended

rectum or a rapid expulsion of gas and stool following digital rectal examination may suggest Hirschsprung's disease. Abdominal distention that does not resolve may suggest an anatomic etiology; however, a palpable mobile mass may occur in all types of constipation. An anal wink should be elicited. Its absence may suggest a spinal or neurologic etiology. A wink in an area separate from the anal opening suggests a misplaced anus. A patulous anus suggests neurologic etiology, while a tight, almost glove-like sphincter suggests anatomic etiology.

DIAGNOSIS

Because of possible risk of enterocolitis and perforation, whenever the suspicion of an anatomic etiology is considered, a full evaluation should be performed. Hirschsprung's disease should be considered in all infants with constipation or bloody diarrhea (enterocolitis). In one series, 33% of the patients who presented with enterocolitis died.[9] The findings of fever, emesis, or blood in the stools are cause of concern and should be evaluated with urgency. Absence of gas in any section of the bowel on a flat plate of the abdomen suggests anatomic etiology, as does the finding of air-fluid levels. A flat plate is often useful to demonstrate to the parents the presence of stool retention when the history is not of infrequent stools. Evidence of diabetes or other pathologic entity should be investigated. Most states require neonatal thyroid screening, and the results of this testing should be viewed and evaluated. No screen is perfect, and strong suspicion should lead to re-evaluation.

A single-contrast unprepped barium enema is usually sufficient to make the diagnosis of Hirschsprung's disease in more than 80% of patients; however, the pathognomonic finding of a transition zone may not be fully developed during the first few months of life or may be missed if enemas or suppositories were given prior to performance of the test. Thus, lack of findings on barium enema should be interpreted with caution during the first months of life or in patients who have a strong clinical history despite a normal contrast study. Contrast studies are important in demonstrating other anatomic causes, such as stricture, malrotation, stenosis, and meconium obstruction.

Anal manometry has proved helpful in the diagnosis of Hirschsprung's disease, with a reported sensitivity of about 95%.[10] This study demonstrates the failure of the internal sphincter to relax in Hirschsprung's disease. Other studies have reported higher false-positive and false-negative results.[11] Manometric studies can confirm the suspicion of functional constipation, as large volumes are often required for the perception of rectal fullness or even the reflexive relaxation of the internal sphincter. It should be noted that anal manometry requires patient compliance—a crying, thrashing infant or child would make interpretation difficult. Consequently, manometry is not commonly used for diagnosis.

TABLE 22-1. Medications Used for Pediatric Constipation

Medication	Dosage
Oils (emollients)	
Mineral oil[a]	1–6 tbs/day
Kondremul[a]	1–6 tbs/day
Agarol[a]	1–6 tbs/day
Hyperosmolar	
Maltsupex[a]	1 tsp–3 tbs/day
Lactulose[a]	1–8 tbs/day (10 g/tbs)
Sorbitol[b]	25–50 ml of a 25% solution
Polyethylene glycol (GoLYTELY, Colyte)	1–4 L over 4 hr
Stimulants	
Castor oil[a]	1–6 tbs/day
Haley's MO[a]	1–6 tbs/day
Milk of Magnesia[a]	1–6 tbs/day
Diphenylmethanes	
Bisacodyl	5-mg dose
Phenophthalein	Use with great caution in children
Anthraquinones	
Cascara sagrada	Use with great caution in children
Senna[b]	Dose in children not well defined
Aloe[b]	Dose in children not well defined

[a] Dose should be adjusted, depending on the age of the child.

[b] Use in children is not well defined.

The gold standard for diagnosis of Hirschsprung's disease is the demonstration of absence of ganglion cells in the myenteric (Auerbach's) and submucous (Meissner's) plexus by rectal suction biopsy. As the normal hypoganglionic segment occurs from 3 mm (premature infants) to 8 mm (young children) from the pectinate line,[12] the biopsy should be taken 2 to 4 cm from the pectinate line. Acetylcholinesterase staining improves the reliability of the biopsy.[13] The biopsy is easily performed by a rectal thermometer–size instrument. No sedation and minimal preparation is necessary for the procedure. Magnetic resonance imaging (MRI) is the appropriate test for suspected spinal cord anomalies.

TREATMENT

Anatomic etiologies generally require surgical correction of the defect. Short-segment aganglionosis may be successfully treated with medical therapy. Medical disorders that cause physiologic constipation should be identified, and any pathologic entity should be treated.

A number of therapeutic agents are available for the treatment of functional constipation (Table 22-1). How-
ever, all are not appropriate for the child with constipation. Agents that irritate the bowel or that provoke an unnatural stimulus for defecation can have a counterproductive effect if used for more than the briefest period of time in children with mild constipation. Such agents often interfere with the re-establishment of a normal pattern and can result in dependency. Enemas are most useful for distal rectosigmoid cleanout but will not in themselves establish a normal self-generated pattern of defecation. Lubricants such as mineral oil should be avoided in infants or in any child at risk of aspiration. Long-term (more than 1 to 2 years) use of lubricants can result in fat-soluble vitamin deficiency. A multivitamin supplement may be indicated with long-term lubricant use.

Functional constipation and encopresis can be successfully treated in most cases. This condition requires a significant investment of the physician's time. The crucial element of success is to keep the bowel clean for a period of time sufficient to allow for resolution of the distention and return of normal sensation. This may be accomplished by the five-step process outlined in Table 22-2. Therapeutic success should be monitored by close

TABLE 22-2. Five-Step Approach to Functional Constipation and Encopresis

1. **Educate**
   Families often have incorrect or an unclear understanding of the process. Frustration with the condition is common. Guidance as to the etiology, therapy, and prognosis increases the likelihood of success.

2. **Clean out bowel**
   This is crucial to success. The distal rectosigmoid bowel must be emptied. Enemas are first-line therapy. Children under 2 years of age should be given pediatric-size enemas, while children older than 2 years require adult-size enemas. Consecutive enemas should be used; proper cleanout may require up to 5 consecutive days of enema administration. Frequent follow-up is needed to evaluate success of cleanout and progress of therapy.

3. **Maintenance**
   Oral medication is the mainstay of treatment. Oils, hyperosmolar agents, or stimulants should be given daily to promote one to two soft, painless stools per day with no associated withholding behavior.

4. **Restrain**
   Children should sit on toilet for 5 minutes, in morning and after evening meal.

5. **Record-keeping/reward system**
   Patient and family will record daily results of therapy. This provides visual feedback to the patient and allows the physician to monitor progress. Young children should not be forcibly "toilet trained" until the physiologic problem is corrected. Behaviors such as difficulty in using public restrooms should be addressed.

follow-up. During the initial period of therapy, weekly evaluations may be required. These routine visits are necessary to evaluate the adequacy of oral medication and to be sure that the initial colonic cleanout was successful. The dosage of lubrication should be adjusted as needed, but all leakage of oil may not be due to a high dose. Rather, the oil may be leaking around retained stool in the rectum. Often repeated evaluations are needed to determine the precise reason. Progress should be steady, but it is often accompanied by relapses that must be aggressively treated. Occasionally, outpatient treatment failure may require the use of polyethelene glycol lavage (GoLYTELY, Colyte) to obtain complete cleaning.

REFERRAL PATTERN

The initial evaluation, diagnosis, and treatment of constipation can be performed by the primary physician. Radiologic evaluation of suspected anatomic abnormalities should be done by a radiologist who has experience performing and interpreting these tests, as subtle nuances may be missed by less experienced practitioners. Similarly, manometric testing and biopsy require referral to a specialist. Functional constipation and encopresis that is unresponsive to therapy should be referred for further evaluation.

REFERENCES

1. Fleischer PR. Diagnosis and treatment of disorders of defecation in children. Pediatr Ann 1976;5:71–101

2. Nolan T, Oberklaid F. New concepts in the management of encopresis. Pediatr Rev 1993;14:447–451

3. Nyhan WL. Stool frequency of normal infants in the first week of life. Pediatrics 1952;10:414–425

4. Weaver LT, Ewing G, Taylor LC. The bowel habit of milk-fed infants J Pediatr Gastroenterol Nutr 1988;7:568–571

5. Weaver LT, Steiner J. The bowel habit of young children. Arch Dis Child 1984;59:649–652

6. Martelli H, DeVroede G, Arhan P et al. Some parameters of large bowel function in normal man. Gastroenterology 1978;75:612–618

7. Tobon F, Schuster MM. Megacolon: special diagnostic and therapeutic features. Johns Hopkins Med J 1978;135:91–105

8. Swenson O, Sherman JO, Fisher JH. Diagnosis of congenital megacolon: an analysis of 501 patients. J Pediatr Surg 1973; 8:587–594

9. Bill AH, Chapman ND. The enterocolitis of Hirschsprung's disease—its natural history and treatment. Am J Surg 1962; 103:70–74

10. Tobon F, Reid NCR, Talbert JL, Schuster MM. Nonsurgical tests for the diagnosis of Hirschsprung's disease. N Engl J Med 1968;278:188–194

11. Frenckner B. Anorectal manometry in the diagnosis of Hirschsprung's disease in infants. Acta Paediatr 1978;67:187

12. Aldridge RT, Campbell PE. Ganglion cell distribution in the normal rectum and anal canal. A basis for the diagnosis of Hirschsprung's diseases by anorectal biopsy. J Pediatr Surg 1968;3:475–489

13. Morikawa Y, Donahoe PK, Hendren WH. Manometry and histochemistry in the diagnosis of Hirschsprung's disease. Pediatrics 1979;63:865–871

23

CYSTIC FIBROSIS–RELATED GASTROINTESTINAL AND LIVER DISEASE

HELEN A. JOHN
ANDREW E. MULBERG

Cystic fibrosis (CF) affects approximately 1 in 2,500 white Americans and is associated with multisystem disease of the pancreas, liver, and intestinal and respiratory tracts. It remains the most common life-shortening autosomal recessive disease of white people in the United States.[1] Gastrointestinal (GI) manifestations of CF are among the most common presentations of this disease and greatly impact the treatment, diagnosis, and prognosis in children and adults.

PATHOPHYSIOLOGY

In 1989, Francis Collins, Lap-Chee Tsui, and Jack Riordan cloned the gene and identified the defect in CF.[2] These investigators established that the gene on chromosome 7 encodes a protein, termed the cystic fibrosis transmembrane conductance regulator (CFTR)[2] (Fig. 23-1). The CFTR gene contains 27 exons and spans more than 230 kilobases. The primary sequence of CFTR encodes a multimeric protein with 12 transmembrane-spanning domains, referred to as TM1-TM12, and two adenosine triphosphate (ATP)-binding domains, referred to as NBF1 and NBF2, which reversibly bind ATP and adenosine diphosphate (ADP). The predicted protein structure also has a highly polarized segment, the R domain, which

is believed to have a regulatory role. The primary evidence that CFTR is the gene product associated with CF has been derived from mutation analysis.

Mutations

Approximately 70% of CF chromosomes harbor a 3-base-pair deletion in CFTR of the phenylalanine residue at amino acid position 508 of the predicted CFTR polypeptide, and this has been named DF508. According to the most recent data from the Cystic Fibrosis Genetic Analysis Consortium, more than 400 presumptive mutations have been identified in the CFTR gene.[3] Most of the mutations have been identified among patients of caucasian ancestry, but some are unique to populations of non-caucasian origin. Different types of mutations affect the CFTR molecule, including the ATP-binding sites, the R domain, as well as the membrane-spanning portions[3] (Fig. 23-2).

The association of abnormal genotype, notably the presence of the DF508 haplotype, with clinical disease has been established for respiratory disease and pancreatic insufficiency.[4,5] By contrast, the genetics of CF-related hepatobiliary disease are not established. A study by Mowat and collaborators[6] at Kings College Hospital, London, demonstrated poor correlation between liver

FIGURE 23-1. Schematic model of the cystic fibrosis gene product based on sequence analysis. The segments have been labelled as TM1, TM2 (transmembrane, helical), NBF1, NBF2 (nucleotide-binding domains) and R (unique domain containing the phosphorylation sites). The Phe 508 deletion, the mutation found in 68% of patients, and most of the other mutations observed so far, occur in NBF1. The transmembrane helix mutations occur in TM1.

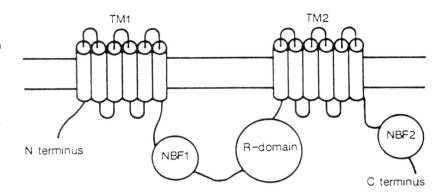

disease and specific genotypes. This review of 111 patients with CF defined three cohorts of patients: 29 children with liver disease with portal hypertension, 19 children with clinical and biochemical evidence of liver disease, and 63 with no liver disease. Screening was performed for at least three different mutations, including the DF508 mutation, and no increased prevalence of liver disease could be correlated with the CF genotype. In contrast to these data, Colombo et al.[7] of the University of Milan suggested that the DF508 haplotype may be slightly increased in patients with CF-related liver disease. Colombo's group established an association between liver function test and hepatobiliary scintigraphy abnormalities and meconium ileus at birth, but they were unable to confirm an association between these and the CF haplotype (DF508, G551D, or R553X mutations).

The pathophysiology of CFTR function in epithelial tissues has been closely correlated with its role as a cyclic adenosine (cAMP)-responsive chloride channel (Fig. 23-3). CFTR is an apical chloride channel; its abnormal function leads to decreased paracellular water movement, a concomitant increase in cellular sodium absorption, and the development of inspissation of mucus within the ductular lumina of pancreas, intestine, and liver.[1] Other factors relating to the pathogenesis of GI disease are discussed below.

CLINICAL PRESENTATION

Table 23-1 outlines a variety of clinical presentations of CF in children.

FIGURE 23-2. Types of mutations affecting the CFTR molecule.

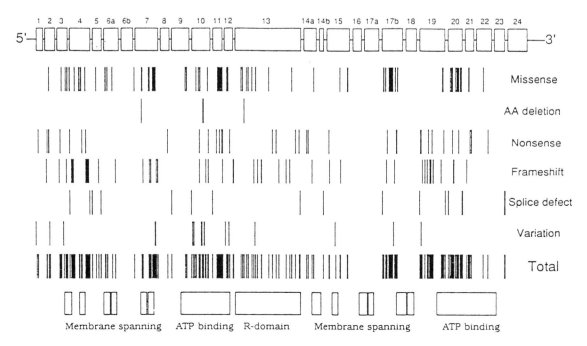

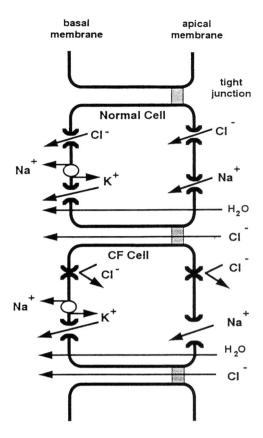

FIGURE 23-3. CFTR role as a cyclic adenosine–responsive chloride channel.

Intestinal Disorders

MECONIUM ILEUS

Meconium ileus is the presenting sign in 10% to 15% of patients with CF.[8] Intestinal obstruction within the first 48 hours of life is classic. There is no passage of meconium, and progressive abdominal distention eventually leads to bile-stained emesis. Physical examination demonstrates the presence of visible, firm loops of bowel that may be best palpated in the right lower quadrant. In these patients, a sweat test should be performed. Radiologic findings include distended loops of bowel with absent or minimal air-fluid levels. Barium enema demonstrates a microcolon and may outline the obstructing mass of meconium in the distal ileum. Abdominal calcification may represent meconium peritonitis. In uncomplicated meconium ileus, Gastrografin enemas are employed to relieve the inspissation. Surgery is recommended in complicated and sicker infants, since colonic perforation has been reported in meconium ileus.

DISTAL INTESTINAL OBSTRUCTION SYNDROME

Meconium ileus equivalent is now recognized as distal intestinal obstruction syndrome (DIOS). Since there is no meconium in the older child, this new term has been proposed by Richard J. Grand.[9] DIOS occurs in 10% to 15% of patients with CF. Signs and symptoms include recurrent colicky abdominal pain associated with a palpable fecal mass that may also represent appendicitis or intestinal obstruction. The pain is due to constipation or fecal impaction. Radiographically, dilated small bowel loops and a bubbly ileocecal soft tissue mass are seen. Management plans can include modification of pancreatic enzyme doses, stool softeners, and an oral poly-

TABLE 23-1. Clinical Manifestations of Cystic Fibrosis in the Gastrointestinal Tract

Esophagogastric

Gastroesophageal reflux

Peptic ulcer disease

Altered intraduodenal pH

Small intestine and colonic

Meconium ileus

Volvulus

Peritonitis

Ileal atresia

Distal intestinal obstruction syndrome
  Fecal masses
  Intussusception
  Obstruction

Rectal prolapse

Fibrosing colonopathy

Pancreas

Insufficiency causing steatorrhea and azotorrhea

Diabetes, glucose intolerance

Maldigestion and malabsorption

Vitamin deficiencies

Hepatobiliary

Mucous hypersecretion

Gallstones

Atrophic gallbladder

Focal biliary cirrhosis

Multilobular cirrhosis

Portal hypertension
  Esophageal varices
  Hypersplenism

Gastrointestinal malignancy

Esophagus

Intestine

Colon

Rectum

Biliary

Pancreas

ethylene glycol solution. Complications may include perforation and intussusception.

In some cases, the terminal ileum or the right colon, or both, may be completely obstructed by fecal material. The fecal bolus can be identified on barium enema. Treatment in uncomplicated DIOS includes the use of regular oral doses of pancreatic enzymes and stool softeners, oral or rectal administration of 10% N-acetylcysteine, and Gastrografin enemas. Maintenance treatment with oral doses of N-acetylcysteine, pancreatic enzymes, and stool softeners is used to prevent recurrence.

INTUSSUSCEPTION

Intussusception is usually ileocolic in location and is a complication of DIOS. Presumably, a tenacious fecal bolus adherent to the intestinal mucosa acts as the lead point for the intussusception. Clinical symptoms include intermittent, severe, cramping abdominal pain. The treatment includes hydrostatic or pneumatic reduction using Gastrografin; occasionally, a patient will require surgery.[10]

RECTAL PROLAPSE

Rectal prolapse may be the presenting complaint in 20% of patients with CF, frequently under the age of 3 years. Contributing factors include bulky stools, diminished muscle tone, and increased intra-abdominal pressure from coughing and pulmonary hyperinflation. Other factors responsible for the increased frequency of rectal prolapse include frequent bowel movements, malnutrition, and increased intra-abdominal pressure. Replacement with pancreatic enzymes often results in rapid improvement, but surgical correction may be necessary.

FIBROSING COLONOPATHY

Colonic stricture is now a recognized cause of DIOS. Between January 1990 and December 1994, 35 histologically confirmed cases of colonic stricture were reported to the Cystic Fibrosis Foundation.[11] The precise etiology of this increased incidence of strictures may be related to higher dosing forms of pancreatic enzymes and increased protease activity. Another recent hypothesis regarding pathogenesis of colonopathy relates to the Eudragit copolymer coating that causes submucosal fibrosis in a pig model system.[12]

GASTROINTESTINAL MALIGNANCY

A retrospective cohort study (1985–1992) of the occurrence of cancer in 28, 511 patients with CF in the United States and Canada identified the same risk as compared to the general population. There is, however, an increased risk of digestive tract tumors, including esophagus, rectum, pancreas, biliary tract, and bowel.[13] The etiology may relate to antioxidant injury, mislocalization, and function of the CFTR or to some other pathogenic process.

Pancreatic Disorders

Approximately 80% to 90% of patients with CF show evidence of exocrine pancreatic insufficiency. Pancreatic involvement is progressive. Pancreatic insufficiency shows a distinct relationship to genotype; 99% of patients who are homozygotes for DF508 mutation and 72% of heterozygotes with other mutations have pancreatic insufficiency. In affected individuals, the pancreas may appear shrunken, cystic, fibrotic, and fatty. The pancreatic lesions are usually caused by obstruction of small ducts with thickened secretions and cellular debris. Calcifications may also be present and be seen on plain radiographs.

Clinically, protein and fat maldigestion and their fecal losses are the main features seen in pancreatic insufficiency. Most of these patients present with inadequate weight gain and failure to thrive. Recurrent acute pancreatitis is an added complication. Very often abdominal pain with elevated lipase and amylase levels may be the only presenting feature. However, not all patients with pancreatitis are pancreatic insufficient. In some of these patients, pancreatic insufficiency develops later. Plain film of the abdomen may show pancreatic calcifications. Ultrasonography may indicate pancreatic enlargement or pancreatic pseudocysts.

ENDOCRINE DYSFUNCTION

Glucose intolerance has been reported in 30% to 40% of patients with CF. Carbohydrate intolerance in these patients is accompanied by insulinopenia.

PANCREATIC ENZYME REPLACEMENT

Pancreatic enzyme replacement is standard thereapy for pancreatic insufficiency. The goal is to deliver these enzymes into the duodenum. Fat malabsorption may not completely revert to normal despite therapy. Initial therapy should consist of pancreatic extract with 3,000 to 15,000 units lipase activity, given before a meal and with snacks. The exact dose depends on the patient's age, the degree of pancreatic insufficiency, the amount of fat ingested, and the commercial preparation. In infants and small children, the capsules are opened and the spheres are mixed with applesauce (jelly, Jell-O, ketchup, pureed fruits) to provide an acid medium. Care should be taken not to crush or chew the beads. In patients who receive large doses of enzymes, the total dose may be split before and during the meal, but before the end of the meal. Perioral and perianal irritation is not uncommon in infants and occur because of the effects of the protease effect on mucous membranes. Because of the link between large doses of pancreatic enzyme supplementation and the development of fibrosing colonopathy, newer

TABLE 23-2. Factors Involved in the Pathogenesis of Hepatobiliary Disease in Cystic Fibrosis

Biliary obstruction

Abnormal viscous secretions
  Mucous plugs
  Sludge

Lithogenic bile

Stones (extrahepatic, intrahepatic)

Stenosis of the common bile duct

Meconium ileus

Nonhepatic disease

Hypoperfusion/hypoxemia

Cor pulmonale

Pancreatic fibrosis

Nutritional

Taurine deficiency

Fatty acid deficiency

Vitamin E deficiency

Hepatotoxicity

Bile acids (hydrophobic-hydrophilic imbalance)

Drugs
  Antibiotics (e.g., carbenicillin, erythromycin)
  N-Acetylcysteine

Immune mechanisms—sensitization

---

enzyme products are being produced that promote a delayed release, thereby enhancing the efficacy of encapsulated lipase, which reduces the overall amount of administered enzyme replacement.

Hepatobiliary Disease and Manifestations

Hepatobiliary disease, which has been increasing in prevalence, will affect more children and adults as the longevity of CF patients increases to adult age, with many patients living into the third, fourth, or fifth decade.[17] Liver disease often begins in childhood and can have a protracted course. The pathognomonic hepatic lesion is focal biliary cirrhosis and is seen in 25% to 30% of CF patients. Focal biliary cirrhosis, one of the more common manifestations of liver disease, affects more than 70% of adults older than 24 years of age. Multilobular cirrhosis, often leading to portal hypertension and the need for organ transplantation, afflicts a smaller number of patients. Cholestasis in the newborn period and gallbladder disease are also common, affecting 5% to 20% of children. The prevalence of symptomatic liver disorder is 2% to 18% and can be the presenting or predominant feature of this disorder.[7] It appears that the risk of acquiring liver disease is increased almost fourfold in patients with a

history of meconium ileus or its equivalent. In a recent study of histocompatibility antigens, a significant increase in the frequency of HLA-A2, -B7, -DR2, and -DQw6 was found in CF patients with liver disease. Other factors considered important in the pathogenesis of hepatobiliary disease are listed in Table 23-2.

PATHOGENESIS

The site of CFTR mRNA and protein expression in humans is the intrahepatic bile duct epithelium.[18] This supports the fact that the pattern of hepatic injury in CF is predominantly of bile duct origin. Other factors that could contribute to the pathogenesis of liver disease in CF are biliary sludge, an increase in the ratio of hydrophobic to hydrophilic bile acids, oxidative injury to the liver, stasis, and infection of cytotoxic bile acids (Table 23-2).

HISTOPATHOLOGY

The typical findings on liver biopsy are bile duct proliferation, inspissated material within the portal tracts, chronic inflammatory infiltrate, and variable fibrosis.

CLINICAL PRESENTATION OF HEPATOBILIARY DISORDERS

Hepatic Disease

Hepatobiliary disease in children and adolescents can be asymptomatic for many years.[19] Liver enzymes may be elevated without any other symptoms. In the newborn, CF may present as neonatal cholestasis. Clinical signs and symptoms can mimic extrahepatic biliary atresia; meconium ileus can also occur. The cholestatic liver disease often improves spontaneously. CF can present with hepatomegaly and abdominal pain. Fat-soluble vitamin deficiency may be present. The end-stage liver disease is biliary cirrhosis. Patients with biliary cirrhosis can present with features of hypersplenism, recurrent variceal bleeding, ascites, jaundice, and ultimately liver failure.

Biliary Disease

Complications include microgallbladder, containing inspissated mucus or gelatinous material; gallbladder atony, subepithelial cysts, and cholelithiasis occurs commonly in CF. Gallstones can occur in 12% to 24% of patients with an increased prevalence in older age groups: 60% in the 15 to 20-year-old group. However, the stones are radiolucent and consist of calcium bilirubinate and other proteins. Gallstones occur primarily in patients with pancreatic insufficiency. Acute or recurrent episodes of abdominal pain that is diffuse or localized to the right upper quadrant may relate to bile duct obstruction from gallstones, sludge, stricture, or infection and can result in cholecystitis and cholangitis. Biliary obstruction may be associated with pancreatitis and severe fat malabsorption.

DIAGNOSIS OF HEPATOBILIARY DISORDERS

Physical examination is crucial to assess the size of the liver and spleen. Cutaneous markers of liver disease such as palmar erythema and spider nevi may be present. Sweat testing is very often used as a screening test. The diagnosis of esophageal and gastric varices is best confirmed by upper endoscopy. Pancreatic calcifications and radioopaque gallstones can be detected on a plain film of the abdomen. Ultrasonography is useful in detecting fatty infiltration of the liver, ascites, and severe cirrhosis of the liver associated with nodularity and irregular margins. Furthermore, portal hypertension can be diagnosed by the presence of a dilated portal vein, splenomegaly, esophageal varices, and the presence of hepatofugal flow in severe cirrhosis. Ultrasonography is very useful in evaluating the biliary tract and can be used to screen for cholecystitis.

Endoscopic retrograde cholangiopancreatography (ERCP) can detect intrabile duct obstruction due to gallstones, stenosis, or strictures. Hepatobiliary scintigraphy is employed to image bile flow and to determine hepatocyte function, liver size, and gallbladder filling. Histopathologic evaluation of the liver is usually performed in patients with liver disease in whom the diagnosis of CF cannot be readily made and may be important for prognostic implications. All patients with known or possible CF should have genotype analysis.

LABORATORY FINDINGS

Liver aminotransferases may be elevated and can fluctuate over the course of the illness. Injury to bile duct cells may be reflected by elevated serum alkaline phosphatase and gamma-glutamyltransferase (GGT) levels. Hypoalbuminemia, prolonged prothrombin time, and direct hyperbilirubinemia may also be present. Serum bile acids may prove to be a better screening test.[20,21]

TREATMENT OF HEPATIC DISEASE

For CF-related liver disease the drug, ursodeoxycholic acid (UDCA) has shown promising results. The dose used is between 10 to 30 mg/kg/day. UDCA has shown to decrease levels of serum aminotransferases, GGT, and alkaline phosphatase levels.[22] The long-term impact of this drug in CF-related liver disease is unknown. Newer products that are being developed include buffered microencapsulated form of UDCA, URSOCARB (Digestive Care, Bethlehem, PA) which has been shown in laboratory animals to produce greater bioavailability. Clinical studies identifying dose response and efficacy in children with CF are currently under way and being

designed at the Children's Hospital of Philadelphia and other medical centers.

In patients with bleeding from esophageal varices, sclerotherapy or endoscopic esophageal variceal ligation has been employed. Prophylactic sclerotherapy is performed in an effort to prevent and minimize recurrent variceal bleeds. There are no data to support the successful use of beta-blockade in children. In patients who continue to bleed, a portosystemic shunt should be considered. More recently, the transjugular intrahepatic portacaval shunt (TIPS) has been used in those patients for short-term portal decompression. At the Children's Hospital of Philadelphia, three children with CF and recurrent variceal hemorrhage unresponsive to sclerotherapy and conservative management underwent TIPS as a bridge toward orthotopic liver transplantation. Splenectomy is generally not indicated, as both operative morbidity and mortality with the associated risk of infection are very high in these patients.

Liver transplant has been performed in selected patients with CF.[23,24] Most patients with symptomatic cholelithiasis will require laparoscopic or surgical removal of the gallbladder. Overall improving the nutritional status of these patients plays a very important role in their survival as manifested for other patients with cholestatic and chronic liver diseases, including biliary atresia. These patients should have high-calorie diets with pancreatic enzyme replacement along with fat-soluble vitamins. Growth in addition to biochemical parameters and fat-soluble vitamin levels should be periodically assessed.

CONCLUSIONS AND PROSPECTS FOR THE FUTURE

In light of the increasing longevity and decreased morbidity of lung disease in CF patients, GI disease will cause more morbidity and mortality for these children and young adults. Gene therapy designed to treat lung manifestations is currently under way but still are not mainstays of clinical management. Initial attempts at treating the hepatobiliary complications with gene therapy have been undertaken in biliary epithelium in tissue culture.[25] Our awareness of GI manifestations in CF patients must assume a greater proportion of our clinical acumen and responsibility.

ACKNOWLEDGMENTS

A.E.M. is grateful for the support and encouragement of his wife, F. Elyse Kopp, D.O.

REFERENCES

1. Boat T, Welsh M, Beaudet A. Cystic fibrosis. In: Scriver C, Beaudet A, Sly W, Valle D, Eds. The Metabolic Basis of Inherited Disease. New York: McGraw-Hill 1989:2649–2860

2. Rommens JM, Iannuzzi MC, Kerem B et al. Identification of the cystic fibrosis gene: chromosome walking and jumping. Science 1989;245:1059–1065

3. Tsui L-C. The spectrum of cystic fibrosis mutations. Trends Genet 1992;8:392–398

4. Kristidis P, Bozon D, Corey M et al. Genetic determination of exocrine pancreatic function in cystic fibrosis. Am J Hum Genet 1992;50:1178–1184

5. Couper RTL, Corey M, Moore DJ et al. Decline of exocrine pancreatic function in cystic fibrosis patients with pancreatic sufficiency. Pediatr Res 1992;32:179–182

6. Duthie A, Doherty DG, Williams C et al. Genotype analysis for D508, G551D and R553X mutations in children and young adults with cystic fibrosis with and without chronic liver disease. Hepatology 1992;15:660–664

7. Colombo C, Apostolo MG, Ferrari M et al. Analysis of risk factors for the development of liver disease associated with cystic fibrosis. J Pediatr 1994;124:393–399

8. Holsclaw D, Eckstein H, Nixon HH. Meconium ileus: a 20 year review of 109 cases. Am J Dis Child 1965;109:101–113

9. Park RW, Grand RJ. Gastrointestinal manifestations of cystic fibrosis. Gastroenterology 1981;81:1143–1161

10. Agrons GA, Corse WR, Markowitz RI et al. Gastrointestinal manifestations of cystic fibrosis: radiologic-pathologic correlation. Radiographics 1996;16:871–893

11. Borowitz DS, Grand RJ, Durie PR, Committee C. Use of pancreatic enzyme supplements for patients with cystic fibrosis in the context of fibrosing colonopathy. J Pediatr 1995; 127:681–684

12. Van Velzen DV, Dezfulian AR, Southgate A et al. Fibrosing colonopathy-like submucosa fibrosis in adolescent pigs exposed to Eudragit L30 D55. Pediatr Pulm Supplement 1996; 13:315

13. Neglia J, Fitzsimmons SC, Maisonneuve P et al. The risk of cancer among patients with cystic fibrosis. N Engl J Med 1995;332:494–499

14. Cleghorn G, Benjamin L, Corey M et al. Age-related alterations in immunoreactive pancreatic lipase and cationic trypsinogen in young children with cystic fibrosis. J Pediatr 1985; 107:377–381

15. Morre DJ, Forstner GG, Largman C et al. Serum immunoreactive cationic trypsinogen: a useful indicator of severe exocrine dysfunction in the paediatric patient without cystic fibrosis. Gut 1986;27:1362–1368

16. Cleghorn G, Benjamin L, Corey M et al. Serum immunoreactive pancreatic lipase and cationic trypsinogen for the assessment of exocrine pancreatic function in older patients with cystic fibrosis. Pediatrics 1986;77:301–306

17. Grand RJ. Recommendations for management of liver and biliary tract disease in cystic fibrosis: summary of a consensus conference. In: Grand RJ, Ed. Cystic Fibrosis Consensus Conference. Chicago, 1989

18. Cohn JA, McGill J, Basavappa S et al. Bile duct epithelial cells are the predominant site of CFTR in liver. Cystic fibrosis. Washington, DC: Wiley-Liss, 1992:249

19. Williams SGJ, Westaby D, Tanner MS, Mowat AP. Liver and biliary problems in cystic fibrosis. Br Med Bull 1992;48: 877–892

20. Setchell KDR, Smethurst P, Giunta AM, Colombo C. Serum bile acid composition in patients with cystic fibrosis. Clin Chim Acta 1985;151:101–110

21. Colombo C, Zuliani G, Rochi M et al. Biliary bile acid composition of the human fetus in early gestation. Pediatr Res 1987;21:197–200

22. Colombo C, Crosignani A, Assaisso M et al. Urosdeoxycholic acid therapy in cystic fibrosis-associated liver disease: a dose-response study. Hepatology 1992;16:924–930

23. Sharp HL. Cystic fibrosis liver disease and transplantation. J Pediatr 1995;127:944–946

24. Mack DR, Traystman M, Colombo JL et al. Clinical denouement and mutation analysis of patients with cystic fibrosis undergoing liver transplantation for biliary cirrhosis. J Pediatr 1995;127:881–887

25. Grubman SA, Fang SL, Mulberg AE et al. Correction of the cystic fibrosis defect by gene complementation in human intrahepatic biliary epithelial cell lines. Gastroenterology 1995;108:584–592

24

EOSINOPHILIC ENTERITIS

KURT A. BROWN

Eosinophilic enteritis is a chronic idiopathic disorder characterized by gastrointestinal (GI) symptoms and eosinophilic infiltration of the intestine. Intestinal eosinophilia may be mucosal, muscular, or serosal and may affect the esophagus, stomach, small intestine, or colon, individually or in combination. Symptoms are related to the layer and location of the intestinal infiltrate. No evidence of parasitic or extraintestinal diseases may be present simultaneously. Eosinophilic enteritis most likely represents a heterogeneous group of immunologic abnormalities that remain ill-defined but have the final common pathway of histologic intestinal eosinophilia.

PATHOPHYSIOLOGY

The etiology of eosinophilic enteritis remains unclear. Considerable controversy surrounds the overlap between intestinal allergies and eosinophilic enteritis; 50% of patients with eosinophilic enteritis have a personal or family history of atopy, asthma, or elevated serum IgE, which may support an allergic etiology. Food allergies have been defined in a small number of eosinophilic enteritis patients who have demonstrated clinical and histologic resolution of disease on elimination diets.[1] Another small fraction of eosinophilic enteritis patients exhibits neither a clinical nor a histologic response to restriction diets; however, they may demonstrate clinical improvement with antihistamine therapy. Antihistamine response suggests histamine, and possibly mast cells, as mediators of this intestinal abnormality. Most eosinophilic enteritis patients do not respond to elimination or restricted diets or to antihistamines. These different responses to thera-

peutic interventions underscore the concept that eosinophilic enteritis most likely represents a heterogeneous group of disorders with histologic eosinophilic infiltration of the intestine.

The failure of physicians to comprehend eosinophilic enteritis fully may arise from limited data surrounding eosinophils and their function. Although primarily a tissue-dwelling cell, eosinophils are derived from the bone marrow and travel via the circulation. Most research has involved blood-derived eosinophils in the peripheral circulation. Data generated from studies of peripheral eosinophils may not be applicable to the form and function of tissue-dwelling eosinophils.

Eosinophils are named secondary to their characteristic cytoplasmic granules, which stain with the acid dye eosin. The major constituent functional proteins of eosinophils are major basic protein, eosinophil-derived neurotoxin, eosinophilic cationic protein, and eosinophilic peroxidase. The exact function of these proteins is not totally understood. In addition, cell mediators such as leukotrienes, cytokines, and platelet-activating factor have been shown, under certain circumstances, to be elaborated by eosinophils. Although the eosinophilic proteins have been isolated, their role, and the role of the eosinophil in host defense, intestinal allergy, and protection against parasitic infections, has not been clearly elucidated.[2]

CLINICAL PRESENTATION

Kaijer[3] initially described intestinal eosinophilia in 1937. Subsequently, Klein characterized eosinophilic enteritis patients into three distinct forms; mucosal, muscular, or serosal.[4] Although Klein's classification method may be helpful for conceptually thinking of eosinophilic enteritis, in reality, tissue eosinophilia is probably not discrete and most likely affects multiple bowel layers.

The most common presenting symptoms in eosinophilic enteritis patients are nonspecific (Table 24-1). In the largest review of pediatric patients to date, Whitington and Whitington[5] demonstrated that regardless of affected tissue layer or site, most patients presented with emesis and/or abdominal pain (Table 24-2). Patients with mucosal eosinophilia commonly have growth failure, weight loss, or diarrhea, all presumably related to malabsorption; however, D-xylose and fat malabsorptive studies have failed to demonstrate consistent small bowel abnormalities.[6] Chronic gastrointestinal occult blood loss, with or without anemia, has been rarely reported. Frank bloody stools and colitis have also been reported but are uncommon.[6] Peripheral edema secondary to hypoproteinemia or hypoalbuminemia associated with protein-losing enteropathy may be a presenting feature.[1]

The muscular form of eosinophilic enteritis may present with symptoms of either intestinal obstruction or GI dysmotility. Intestinal muscular hypertrophy or edema from eosinophilic infiltration most commonly affects the gastric antrum or pylorus. Gastric emptying is impaired in this form of eosinophilic enteritis that commonly results in emesis or abdominal pain. Obstructive symptoms of the terminal ileum have been described, but in general obstructive lesions of the small intestine and colon are less common.[6]

The least common form of eosinophilic enteritis involves the intestinal serosal surface. Pediatric serosal eosinophilic enteritis appears in the literature chiefly as case reports. Patients present with complaints of abdominal distention secondary to ascitic fluid collection or may

TABLE 24-2. Clinical Findings

Finding	Percentage
Emesis	53
Abdominal pain	35
Growth failure/weight loss	35
Edema/anasarca	23
Hematochezia (occult and frank)	12
Diarrhea	12
Colic	12
Anemia	12
Gastroesophageal reflux/esophagitis	6
Bowel obstruction	6
Ascites (isolated)	6

(Adapted from Whitington and Whitington,[5] with permission.)

have associated intestinal abnormalities. Intestinal perforation has also been reported in pediatric patients with serosal eosinophilic enteritis.[7] Eosinophilic infiltration can occur in extraintestinal organs such as the urinary bladder, liver, spleen, gallbladder, and visceral and parietal peritoneum.

Because eosinophilic enteritis is rare, it is difficult to characterize the typical patient. There appears to be equal sex distribution. While the most common age of presentation occurs in the second or third decade of life, infant and preschool-aged children can develop eosinophilic enteritis.[1] However, because so few patients are represented by the literature and because of eosinophilic enteritis's ability to mimic almost any intestinal disorder, the disease is most likely underreported.

TABLE 24-1. Clinical Manifestations of Eosinophilic Gastroenteritis

Intestinal Layer Involved	Manifestation
Mucosal	Abdominal pain
	Emesis
	Failure to thrive
	Diarrhea
	Hematochezia—mostly occult, possible associated anemia
	Hypoalbuminemia
Muscular	Abdominal pain
	Emesis
Serosal	Abdominal pain
	Emesis
	Failure to thrive
	Ascites
	Abdominal distention

(Adapted from Klein[4], with permission.)

LABORATORY EVALUATION

While no single test is diagnostic for eosinophilic enteritis, several laboratory studies have been used to support or shape the diagnosis of eosinophilic enteritis. Histologic eosinophilic intestinal infiltration is the single essential element required for diagnosis. In the mucosal form of the disease, eosinophilia has been demonstrated to occur in the esophagus, gastric antrum, and proximal portion of the small intestine, which are areas easily accessible via upper endoscopy. However, interpreting tissue eosinophilia can be confounding as eosinophils may be seen in the colon and small intestine in Crohn's disease and in the distal esophagus in gastroesophageal reflux disease.[8] Recent work suggests the greater the number of eosinophils per high powered field, the more likely the diagnosis of eosinophilic enteritis.[9] Multiple endoscopic biopsies should be obtained as eosinophilic enteritis may affect the bowel in a "patchy" distribution.[10]

Elevated peripheral blood eosinophilia reportedly ranges from 20% to 90% of eosinophilic enteritis patients in the adult literature. In a large review of pediatric eosinophilic enteritis patients, peripheral eosinophilia was found in 70% of patients.[5] Elevated serum IgE has been noted in some eosinophilic enteritis patients, but it is not a consistent finding, and the implication is not well understood.

Radiographic findings in eosinophilic gastroenteritis demonstrate extreme heterogeneity; eosinophilic gastroenteritis must be considered in the differential diagnosis of any intestinal lesion that produces thickened folds, intestinal edema, or even polypoid lesions. Gastric outlet obstruction or narrowing is the most common region of muscular eosinophilic enteropathy.[6] Ascitic fluid containing large numbers of eosinophils may be present in the serosal form of the disease.[7]

DIAGNOSIS

Eosinophilic enteritis should be considered in the differential diagnosis of severe, unexplained gastrointestinal symptoms, even in the absence of peripheral eosinophilia. The varied clinical presentations of eosinophilic enteritis often pose a diagnostic dilemma. The disease can affect any area of the GI tract from the mouth to the anus. Because of both the nonspecific and varied presentations of eosinophilic enteritis, eosinophilic enteritis must be included in the differential diagnosis of virtually all intestinal abnormalities. The diagnosis is based on clinical history, possible blood eosinophilia, and eosinophilic infiltration of intestinal biopsy specimens.

TREATMENT

Because eosinophilic enteritis most likely represents a heterogeneous group of disorders, varied therapies have been initiated with varied clinical responses. When specific foods appear to exacerbate the symptoms of eosinophilic enteritis, dietary restrictions should be imposed. The most common dietary constituents that may exacerbate eosinophilic enteritis include milk protein, peanuts, or fish.[11] However, random elimination diets have generally failed in most patients. Strict elimination diets (i.e., diets exclusively using elemental formulas as the sole form of nutrition) have demonstrated some promise in treating probable eosinophilic enteritis; however, these diets are usually poorly tolerated when used over the long term, especially in children.[11]

Antihistamine therapy has uniformly failed patients with eosinophilic enteritis. Oral cromolyn sodium therapy has met with mixed success. The rationale to treat eosinophilic enteritis with mast cell degranulation inhibitors is based on the histologic finding of variable numbers of mucosal mast cells in patients with eosinophilic enteritis.[12] Initial reports provided evidence that enteral cromolyn could be employed as an alternative to corticosteroid therapy.[13] Since those initial reports, not all eosinophilic enteritis patients have met with uniform response to enteral cromolyn sodium. Enteral cromolyn sodium is usually administered at 100 mg PO tid, regardless of the size of the pediatric patient. This medication is generally felt to be benign and without reported side effects.

Corticosteroids remain the mainstay of therapy for eosinophilic enteritis. There is usually a rapid and complete response to oral prednisone administered at 1 to 2 mg/kg/day. Corticosteroids are tapered with clinical response. Endoscopic reevaluation may be needed to verify the status of tissue eosinophilia if there is not a rapid clinical response to the initiation of corticosteroids. Low-dose or alternate-day corticosteroids may be used as a maintenance medication in resistant cases of eosinophilic enteritis. Eosinophilic enteritis exacerbations may be treated with brief pulses of steroids. Eosinophilic enteritis related ascites has also been successfully treated with steroids.

Spontaneous remission in eosinophilic enteritis is common, even in the absence of treatment. Waxing and waning of symptoms underscore eosinophilic enteritis not as a static process, but one that waxes and wanes without regard to diet, season, or other external stimuli. In addition, patients commonly experience exacerbations and remissions of disease, regardless of therapy. There is no reported risk of GI cancers, nor are there reports of malignant transformations in eosinophilic enteritis patients.

REFERRAL PATTERN

Eosinophilic enteritis is a chronic disorder that requires close clinical monitoring, especially in children where growth and development are critical. Therefore, eosinophilic enteritis should be monitored by a gastroenterologist, as the need for repeat biopsies to evaluate the disease and modulate therapy may be required.

REFERENCES

1. Katz AJ, Twarog FJ, Zeiger RS et al. Milk-sensitive and eosinophilic gastroenteropathy: similar clinical features with contrasting mechanisms and clinical course. J Allergy Clin Immunol 1984;74:72

2. Gleich GJ. The eosinophil leukocyte: structure and function. Adv Immunol 1986;39:177

3. Kaijer R. Zur Kerintnis der allergischen affectionen des Ver-

dauungs-Kanals von Standpunkt des Chirurgen aus. Arch Klin Chirurg 1937;188:36

4. Klein NC, Hargrove MD, Sleisenger MH et al. Eosinophilic gastroenteritis. Medicine (Baltimore) 1970;49:299

5. Whitington PF, Whitington GL. Eosinophilic gastroenteritis in childhood. J Pediatr Gastroenterol Nutr 1988;7:379

6. Caldwell JH, Mikhjian PE, Beman FM et al. Eosinophilic gastroenteritis with obstruction. Immunological studies of seven patients. Gastroenterology 1978;74:825

7. Hyams JS, Treem WR, Schwartz AN. Recurrent abdominal pain and ascites in an adolescent. J Pediatr 1988;113:569

8. Winter HS, Madara JL, Stafford RJ. Intraepithelial eosinophils: a new diagnostic criterion for reflux esophagitis. Gastroenterology 1982;83:818

9. Ruchelli E, Voytek T, Wenner W et al. Severity of esophageal eosinophilia predicts response to conventional reflux therapy. Mod Pathol 1996;9:6P

10. Johnstone JM, Morson BC. Eosinophilic gastroenteritis. Histopathology 1978;2:335–348

11. Kelly KJ, Lazenby AJ, Rowe PC et al. Eosinophilic esophagitis attributed to gastroesophageal reflux: improvement with an amino acid-based formula. Gastroenterology 1995;109:1503

12. Heatley RV. The gastrointestinal mast cell. Scand J Gastroenterol 1983;18:449

13. Di Giocchino M, Pizzicannella G, Fini N et al. Sodium cromoglycate in the treatment of eosinophilic gastroenteritis. Allergy 1990;45:161

25

GASTROESOPHAGEAL REFLUX

STEPHEN E. SHAFFER

Gastroesophageal reflux (GER) is a term that describes the intermittent regurgitation of stomach material into the esophagus and has been applied to a variety of clinical disorders frequently encountered in the care of pediatric patients. Since its first characterization in children in the 1950s by Carre,[1] our understanding of its pathophysiology, natural history, and management has dramatically progressed. GER not only denotes the typical "spitting up" observed in infancy, but an entire spectrum of associated signs, symptoms, and disease, partly the result of our improved technologic and diagnostic capabilities.

PATHOPHYSIOLOGY

The esophagus is essentially a conduit composed of involuntary smooth muscle in its distal half that functions to propel food from the mouth to the stomach by peristaltic contractions. A specialized, tonically contracted region of the distal esophagus, the lower esophageal sphincter (LES), works as a functioning gateway at the gastroesophageal junction. Under primarily neural control, the LES relaxes in response to swallowing, as well as with esophageal distention or contractions in the absence of deglutition. Spontaneous transient relaxations of the LES (TLESRs) not associated with a corresponding esophageal event may also occur and relate to the physiologic function of venting swallowed air through belching. GER occurs when there is loss of an esophagogastric pressure gradient maintained by the LES. Until recently, a low basal LES pressure was thought to be the

primary factor responsible for increased reflux in pediatric patients. However, more recent studies support the role of TLESRs and, to a lesser degree, transient increases in gastric pressure in mediating most reflux events. Further characterization of TLESRs and the contribution of other mechanisms are needed if we are to understand what makes clinically evident reflux truly "pathologic," differentiating it from physiologic reflux.

CLINICAL PRESENTATION

Much of the confusion surrounding pediatric GER in the literature and that has filtered into the practice of pediatrics has evolved from a lack of a proper system with which to categorize patients diagnostically. As GER is only a descriptive term, a strategy for its classification must account for a wide variety of related clinical signs and symptoms and also impart information about normal physiology and pathogenic mechanisms. Boyle[2] has suggested such a scheme, which is useful in the diagnosis and management of the spectrum of pediatric GER presentations (Table 25-1).

A certain degree of GER is normal or physiologic in infants and children. Such episodes of reflux typically occur during the immediate postprandial period, are of short duration, and are usually clinically insignificant, although episodic regurgitation may be apparent. As its name implies, infants and children with functional GER are otherwise healthy, without conditions that predispose to reflux, and exhibit frequent emesis or regurgitation with no sequelae. When GER results in disease, it

TABLE 25-1. Classification of Gastroesophageal Reflux in Infants and Children

Physiologic GER

Functional GER
    Symptomatic
    Occult

Pathogenic GER
    Esophagitis
    Chronic pulmonary disease
    Apnea
    Failure to thrive
    Neurobehavioral manifestations

Secondary GER
    Neurologic impairment
    Hiatal hernia
    Esophageal atresia

(Adapted from Boyle,[2] with permission.)

becomes pathogenic GER. Patients with pathogenic GER manifest signs and symptoms that reflect compromise in respiratory function, esophageal barrier function, or nutrition, or that can be characterized as neurobehavioral. The term secondary GER has been applied to patients with specific conditions, such as severe neurologic impairment or hiatal hernia, in whom reflux is common and often follows a course very different from that in children with functional GER.

Functional GER

Functional GER is the form of reflux most commonly encountered in the general care of infants and young children. This condition differs from that seen in older children and adults in its natural history and expression of symptoms. Reports in the literature suggest that it is a common finding, with daily emesis occurring in some 45% to 50% of well infants by 2 months of age. Unlike reflux in adults, which tends to persist, complete resolution is by far the most likely outcome in infants, although the time course to this end may vary considerably from patient to patient. In considering infants with functional GER in a general care setting, most have sufficiently resolved their regurgitation by 6 months.[3] Other sources in the literature suggest that the majority (60%) no longer experience symptoms by the age of 9 to 18 months, coincident with upright posturing and the transition to a solid diet.[1,4]

Early in life, reflux is manifested primarily by effortless, painless regurgitation, as opposed to the condition in older children and adults, who rarely exhibit this overt emesis. At times the regurgitation may be more forceful or projectile in nature and at other times silent, as in oral regurgitation. Episodes of regurgitation tend to occur most frequently during the hour or so following feedings, but some infants seem to manifest reflux almost constantly throughout the day. Experience suggests that regurgitation during quiet sleep is rare; when it does occur, it is during periods of wakefulness or active sleep.[5] The volume of emesis may also be quite variable and appears to be inversely related to the frequency of episodes.[4] Infants and young children with functional GER also exhibit quite typical patterns of regurgitation over the time course of the disorder.

Pathogenic GER

Complications and actual disease may result from reflux when there is delayed clearance of or increased noxiousness of the refluxate, when respiratory function is compromised, if regurgitation results in significant caloric loss, or when specific neurobehavioral symptoms are evident. Pathogenic GER may evolve in patients with frequent overt emesis or in situations where reflux is occult or physiologic, emphasizing that the increased frequency or volume of reflux may not correlate with its development. Several complications can occur.

ESOPHAGITIS

Numerous studies have confirmed that esophagitis, typically diagnosed histologically, is apparent in the vast majority of infants and children who manifest clinical findings of pathogenic GER. The intraepithelial eosinophil is now recognized as the essential feature in esophageal biopsies from such patients. Gross findings of esophageal erosions or ulcerations are rare in the younger pediatric patient experiencing symptomatic reflux.

Symptoms that may suggest underlying pain from reflux esophagitis in infants are crying, generalized irritability or fussiness, "colicky" behaviors, or sleep disturbance. Feeding difficulties or behavior, such as outright refusal or pulling away from the bottle, may also indicate esophageal pain with swallowing. Older children often complain of heartburn, epigastric abdominal or substernal chest pain, or swallowing difficulties similar to those of adults with reflux disease. Odynophagia, or pain with swallowing, suggests irritation of the esophagus, sometimes attributed to reflux esophagitis. The symptom of dysphagia, or difficulty in swallowing, is less specific for esophagitis, but it may also represent a complication of long-standing reflux esophagitis, peptic stricture. Gastrointestinal (GI) bleeding, evidenced by hematemesis, guaiac-positive stools, iron deficiency anemia, or melena, may further suggest esophagitis. Lastly, it is important to recognize that on occasion, patients with significant reflux esophagitis may not experience any pain or symptom referable to esophageal inflammation. Long-standing severe reflux esophagitis may rarely culminate in metaplastic change to a columnar epithelium, known as Barrett's esophagus, which poses a subsequent risk of esophageal adenocarcinoma.

RESPIRATORY DISEASE

One of the most important as well as controversial sequelae of GER is chronic pulmonary disease. The association between GER and recurrent aspiration pneumonia is obvious. Yet, not until the advent of esophageal pHmetry has reflux been linked to a variety of other chronic respiratory disorders, including cough, bronchospasm, bronchitis, laryngospasm, and hoarseness. Esophageal pHmetry has afforded the opportunity to demonstrate and quantify subclinical episodes of acid reflux in patients with pulmonary symptoms, yet is limited in its ability to establish a cause-and-effect relationship between the two.

Mechanisms that might account for a causal role of GER in chronic pulmonary disease include microaspiration and neurally mediated reflex bronchospasm. Microaspiration involves contamination of the upper airway by amounts of refluxate insufficient to produce pneumonia. Pulmonary sequelae result from the effects of direct irritation, triggering of local neural pathways that control airway tone, and stimulation of an inflammatory cascade. Reflex responses (e.g., bronchospasm or laryngospasm) involving acid stimulation of esophageal afferents are also known to occur, but on an order of magnitude much lower than that caused by microaspiration.

Although GER should not be viewed as a primary etiology for the vast majority of cases involving asthma or chronic cough, it is important to consider in certain clinical situations. Patients whose asthma symptoms occur primarily at night will often have problematic reflux. Likewise, GER should be suspected when chronic cough or wheezing is apparent during infancy or in the absence of a family history of asthma or atopy. The presence of subclinical GER should also be actively sought in any patient with wheezing that is difficult to control medically. Reflux is likely the cause of chronic hoarseness or laryngitis in selected cases, when other etiologies have been excluded. Most importantly, a careful history aimed at eliciting signs or symptoms of GER should always be taken in any child with chronic respiratory symptoms.

APNEA

Another issue that stimulates much discussion is the association of GER with apnea. Although infant apnea, generally of the obstructive type, has been documented following acid reflux into the esophagus, the premise that GER is etiologic in sudden infant death syndrome remains controversial. Mechanisms that might account for the association of acid reflux with obstructive apnea include laryngospasm induced by laryngeal or nasopharyngeal microaspiration or reflex laryngospasm mediated by stimulation of acid-sensitive esophageal receptors. Equally important in understanding this association is the suggestion that the apneic response represents a variation in normal vagal activity or airway-protective mechanisms.[2,6] Reflex central apnea or bradycardia provoked by GER has not been clearly demonstrated in humans, although some studies in immature animals support this theory. *Awake apnea* may be preceded by overt regurgitation and is manifested by a startled, rigid infant who subsequently becomes plethoric, pale, cyanotic, and limp.[7]

FAILURE TO THRIVE

Caloric deprivation occurs in two settings associated with GER in pediatrics. The first, and most obvious, is attributed to the frequent and voluminous emesis occasionally observed in infants and toddlers with functional GER. Food refusal or inadequate intake may also develop in complicated GER as an expression of pain from esophagitis or as a conditioned behavior.

NEUROBEHAVIORAL MANIFESTATIONS

Although infrequently encountered in the general care of children, neurobehavioral symptoms are an intriguing manifestation of pediatric GER disease. Sandifer's syndrome, the most well known of these behaviors, is a complex of maneuvers involving head tilting, neck cocking, and opisthotonic posturing, which is a specific response of the child to reflux. Infants may exhibit similar arching behavior or less specifically, generalized irritability even in the absence of reflux esophagitis or with concomitant acid-suppression therapy. Such behaviors in response to GER have been attributed to "visceral hyperalgesia" or to the perception of pain resulting from stimuli not expected to cause pain.[8] This theory may also partially account for the spectrum of aversive feeding behaviors associated with GER.[8] Rumination is a more complicated feeding disorder seen in infants and children with reflux, manifested by oral regurgitation and reswallowing of gastric contents, vomiting, gagging, and self-stimulatory behaviors. Psychosocial issues are pervasive in this disorder, ultimately making it difficult to determine whether the reflux is in fact a primary or secondary factor.

Secondary GER

A variety of underlying conditions have a well-known association with GER and comprise an important subcategory of pediatric reflux problems. A large proportion of children with significant neurologic impairment may be found to have GER. Reflux in these patients involves different mechanisms than in those with functional GER, which include frequent supine positioning, muscle spasticity, kyphoscoliosis, altered feeding patterns (e.g., through nasogastric or gastrostomy tubes), and altered central and enteric neural controls of GI motility. Similarly, the natural history of GER in neurologically impaired children is often protracted, resulting in pathogenic GER, which is usually difficult to control with medical means alone. Other conditions predisposing to secondary GER that are infrequently encountered include esophageal atresia and large hiatal hernias.

DIAGNOSIS

For most otherwise healthy infants in whom a history of effortless regurgitation beginning before 6 months of age can be elicited, no further diagnostic testing should be required to establish the diagnosis of functional GER. Further support for the diagnosis can be gained by screening for other known causes of vomiting, such as nutrient intolerance (complete blood count [CBC] for eosinophilia), metabolic disorders (electrolytes), or renal/urologic disorders (e.g., blood-urea nitrogen [BUN], creatinine, urinalysis, urine culture). However, concern for the development of pathogenic GER, an atypical history (e.g., onset beyond 6 months, projectile emesis), or failure of conservative management or to reassure the patient's parents generally dictates that further testing be performed.

Upper GI Series

The barium upper GI series should always be the first test ordered in the evaluation of complicated GER. The primary role of this series is not to diagnose reflux, but to exclude obstructive conditions in the differential diagnosis, such as pyloric stenosis, malrotation, antral web, intestinal atresia, peptic ulcer, and eosinophilic gastroenteropathy. Complications of GER, including peptic stricture, esophagitis, and, rarely, reflux with soiling of the airway, may also be detected by an upper GI series. For children with feeding difficulties or recurrent respiratory problems in whom pulmonary aspiration is a concern, we have found the videofluoroscopic barium swallow examination helpful in ruling out complicating oropharyngeal dysphagia as a cause of symptoms. For additional information refer to Chapter 64.

Scintigraphy

Gastroesophageal scintigraphy, also referred to as a "milk scan," is a radionuclide imaging technique that offers several advantages over contrast radiography in evaluating GER. The study is conducted using a radiolabeled liquid meal, providing a more functional or physiologic assessment for reflux. Imaging is usually performed for an hour, compared to a few minutes or so during an upper GI series, noting the frequency of reflux episodes in addi-

tion to quantifying the gastric emptying process. Scintigraphy continues to be the technique of choice when attempting to document pulmonary aspiration attributed to GER, although its overall sensitivity remains low (for an in-depth discussion, see Ch. 67).

Upper Endoscopy

Flexible upper endoscopy is the most sensitive modality for detecting mucosal disease in patients with clinical GER. Indications vary considerably among gastroenterologists but tend to include (1) overt evidence suggesting esophagitis, such as hematemesis or guiaic-positive stools; (2) feeding difficulties/failure to thrive; (3) failure or relapse after empirical acid suppression trial; or (4) the older child with symptoms such as heartburn, odynophagia, or dysphagia. In the hands of those experienced in dealing with children, pediatric endoscopy is quite safe and can be performed on an outpatient basis. Alternatively, "blind" suction esophageal biopsies can be obtained, but this method does not offer the ability to provide visual or biopsy surveillance of the entire upper GI tract (for an in-depth discussion, see Ch. 71).

pH Probe

Esophageal pHmetry is most useful in situations in which occult pathogenic reflux is suspected or as a means of establishing a temporal relationship between acid GER and a particular symptom. It provides little additional information in uncomplicated functional GER or in patients with documented reflux esophagitis (for a more comprehensive discussion, see Ch. 73).

Other Tests

Other modalities that address specific diagnostic questions in the evaluation of children with GER include intraluminal esophageal acid perfusion, known as the Bernstein test, and esophageal manometry. Esophageal acid perfusion studies are performed in an attempt to relate the presence of acid in the esophagus with chest pain or irritability, as in the classic Bernstein test, or other respiratory manifestations, such as wheezing, cough, or laryngospasm, referred to as a modified Bernstein test. Esophageal manometry has limited practical application in the diagnosis and management of reflux but is an important adjunct in characterizing peristaltic abnormalities in patients with dysphagic complaints and in those with esophageal atresia in whom surgical antireflux measures are contemplated.

TREATMENT

In most cases of functional GER in infants, overt emesis will resolve by a year or so. This consideration forms the cornerstone for management of such patients. Establish-

TABLE 25-2. Therapeutic Approach to Gastroesophageal Reflux

Type of Therapy	Strategy
Positional	Prone, upright with head elevated 20–30°
Dietary	Frequent, smaller volume feedings Thicken with 0.5–1.0 tbs/oz (cereal)
Antacid	0.5 ml/kg/dose (max: 1 tbs) 1 hr after meals qhs
Prokinetic	Bethanechol, 0.1–0.2 mg/kg/day tid or qid Metoclopramide, 0.15 mg/kg/dose qid Cisapride, 0.1–0.3 mg/kg/dose tid or qid
Acid blockade	Cimetidine, 10 mg/kg/dose qid Ranitidine, 2 mg/kg/dose bid Famotidine, 0.5–1.0 mg/kg/dose qd or bid Omeprazole, 0.7 mg/kg/dose qd or bid
Surgery and other alternatives	Fundoplication (open or laparoscopic) Gastrojejunal/surgical jejunal feeding devices

(Adapted from Boyle,[2] with permission.)

ing the diagnosis of GER, which can usually be accomplished in the office setting on clinical grounds alone, is the key initial aspect of treatment. Parents should be educated about the natural history and pathophysiology of GER and should also understand the signs and symptoms that suggest the development of pathogenic reflux. Once reassured by a positive diagnosis and the knowledge of what to expect for their child, most parents will readily accept a conservative treatment strategy appropriate for the infant with functional GER.

Management of GER in infants and younger children is best approached in a staged fashion that allows the physician to tailor therapy commensurate with the severity of the patient's symptoms and the presence of complications (Table 25-2). Stage 1, commonly referred to as conservative management of reflux, includes both positional and dietary therapy. The topic of infant sleeping position has become an area of intense debate since the American Academy of Pediatrics issued its recommendation that *healthy* infants be placed supine or on their sides for sleeping. Prone sleep positioning has been clearly shown to decrease the frequency of GER and should continue to be recommended for infants with GER. Upright positioning is also frequently advocated, although it is only practical in infants less than 3 to 4 months of age. Placing the infant in a car seat or in any upright sitting position after feedings may actually exacerbate GER by creating increased pressure on the abdomen. Thickening of formula feedings is a time-tested method that has been shown to significantly reduce overt regurgitation.[9,10] Individual cases may demonstrate increased emesis on thickened feeds, however; indeed, one recent study found increased cough and pul-

monary symptoms[11] associated with thickened feeds in refluxing infants.

Stage 2 therapy consists of pharmacologic options, which are generally indicated for infants and children with pathogenic GER or when conservative measures have failed to control emesis sufficiently in those with functional GER. Prokinetic agents are often initiated first, as they attempt to address, in theory, the pathophysiologic mechanisms that contribute to GER. Although they do not decrease the frequency of TLESR, prokinetics offer advantages in cases of clinical or subclinical reflux by augmenting tonic LES pressure, as well as enhancing both esophageal and gastric emptying. Bethanechol, a cholinergic agonist, was the first agent used for this purpose, although its availability for pediatric administration is limited and it is contraindicated in patients with a history of bronchospasm. Cisapride has recently become widely available and, for the most part, has replaced metoclopramide as the first-line choice in prokinetic drugs. Its primary advantage includes a more favorable therapeutic index than metoclopramide, as it acts at the local level to enhance the release of acetylcholine. Overall, the clinical response to any of these agents will vary greatly from patient to patient. Furthermore, it must be emphasized that prokinetic therapy has not been shown to alter the natural history of infant reflux or to diminish the likelihood of developing complications.

Medications that reduce gastric acid are often an important adjunct to prokinetic therapy in managing pathogenic GER, since esophagitis is present in most of these cases. Acid suppression is achieved through the use of either neutralizing agents (e.g., aluminum or magnesium hydroxide) or the antisecretory class of drugs, which includes histamine-2 (H_2)-receptor antagonists or the newer proton pump inhibitors. Although most pediatric gastroenterologists once reserved H_2-blockers, such as ranitidine, for cases of endoscopically proven esophagitis, experience has led to a less stringent set of indications for their use. The favorable safety and efficacy profiles of ranitidine, as well as its ease in dosing, justify its use as an alternative to simple antacids as empirical therapy in infants with symptoms suggesting reflux esophagitis. H_2-blockers are still considered first-line therapy for documented mild to moderate reflux esophagitis; however, a 6- to 8-week course of treatment is indicated for mild esophagitis or 3 to 4 months for moderate to severe cases. H_2-Antagonists are also indicated in the initial management of patients in whom reflux is probably contributing to pulmonary disease. Proton pump inhibitors, such as omeprazole, are potent antisecretory agents, as they exert their action directly at the acid-secreting parietal cell. Experience with their use in pediatrics is limited, but studies suggest that omeprazole is indicated for severe esophagitis that is refractory to ranitidine therapy or associated with Barrett's esophagus.[12,13]

TABLE 25-3. Indications for Antireflux Surgery in Infants and Children

Independent of medical therapy
  Esophageal stricture
  Barrett's esophagus
  Life-threatening apnea or aspiration
  Large hiatal hernia

After failure of maximal medical therapy
  Severe esophagitis
  Recurrent pneumonia, bronchospasm, or bronchopulmonary
    dysplasia exacerbated by GER
  Apnea
  Failure to thrive
  Intractable reflux symptoms in older child

(Adapted from Boyle,[2] with permission.)

Stage 3 management, or antireflux surgery, is warranted for severe complications of GER or failure of medical therapy. The indications for fundoplication are themselves straightforward (Table 25-3). Yet, as a consensus on the definition of medical refractoriness is lacking, the timing of antireflux surgery is often subjective.[2] Most gastroenterologists now include potent proton pump inhibitors as a necessary component of treatment for severe esophagitis and respiratory complications before they are willing to declare medical failure. The fundoplication procedure itself is very effective in controlling emesis. It involves augmenting the antireflux barrier by wrapping the gastric fundus partially (Thal fundoplication) or completely (Nissen fundoplication) around the lower esophagus. Success rates for correcting GER are generally good, although experience suggests that children with significant neurologic impairment are more susceptible to operative failure as well as suffer frequent complications. Short-term complications consist of dysphagia, gas-bloat syndrome, early satiety, or retching. Most of these complications resolve within several months, although they can become persistent. Long-term complications, such as dumping syndrome, gastric stasis, hiatal herniation of the wrap, and intestinal adhesions and obstruction, can be quite problematic, often requiring additional surgical intervention.

Occasionally, alternatives to antireflux surgery may be deemed more appropriate in situations in which a major operative procedure poses significant risk, when the patient is terminal, or when a previous fundoplication has failed. Alternative procedures typically involve placement of a supplemental feeding device in the jejunum, which bypasses the stomach and thereby diminishes the reflux potential.

REFERRAL PATTERN

For those with a clinical history compatible with physiologic or functional GER, parental education, conservative measures, medical therapy, and, most importantly, time are sufficient in most cases. Infants with symptoms suggesting reflux esophagitis should undergo an upper GI study. If the findings are normal, they may be started on an empirically based short course of H_2-blockers or antacids, but for those who do not respond or relapse upon discontinuing therapy, referral to a pediatric gastroenterologist for upper endoscopy is indicated.

REFERENCES

1. Carre IJ. The natural history of the partial thoracic stomach (hiatus hernia) in children. Arch Dis Child 1959;34:344–353
2. Boyle JT. Gastroesophageal reflux in the pediatric patient. Gastroenterol Clin North Am 1989;18:315–337
3. Kibel MA. Gastroesophageal reflux and failure to thrive in infancy. In: Gellis SS, Ed. Gastroesophageal Reflux. (Seventy-sixth Ross Conference of Pediatric Research.) Columbus, OH: Ross Laboratories, 1979;39–42
4. Herbst JJ. Gastroesophageal reflux. J Pediatr 1981;98:859–870
5. Jeffery HE, Heacock HJ. Impact of sleep and movement on gastro-oesophageal reflux in healthy, newborn infants. Arch Dis Child 1991;66:1136–1139
6. de Bethmann O, Couchard M, de Ajuriaguerra M et al. Role of gastro-oesophageal reflux and vagal overactivity in apparent life-threatening events: 160 cases. Acta Paediatr 1993;82(suppl 389):102–104
7. Spitzer AR, Boyle JT, Tuchman DN et al. Awake apnea associated with gastroesophageal reflux: a specific clinical syndrome. J Pediatr 1984;104:200–205
8. Hyman PE. Gastroesophageal reflux: one reason why baby won't eat. J Pediatr 1994;125:S103–S109
9. Orenstein S, Magill H, Brooks P. Thickening of infant feedings for therapy of gastroesophageal reflux. J Pediatr 1987;110:181–186
10. Vandenplas Y, Sacre L. Milk-thickening agents as a treatment for gastroesophageal reflux. Clin Pediatr 1987;26:66–68
11. Orenstein SR. Controversies in pediatric gastroesophageal reflux. J Pediatr Gastroenterol Nutr 1992;14:338–348
12. Karjoo M, Kane R. Omeprazole treatment of children with peptic esophagitis refractory to ranitidine therapy. Arch Pediatr Adolesc Med 1995;149:267–271
13. Gunasekaran TS, Hassall EG. Efficacy and safety of omeprazole for severe gastroesophageal reflux in children. J Pediatr 1994;123:332–334

26

HELICOBACTER PYLORI IN PEDIATRICS

KAREN LIQUORNIK
CHRIS A. LIACOURAS

Helicobacter pylori is a gram-negative microorganism that affects the gastric mucosa of susceptible individuals, causing an underlying chronic gastritis. The organism was first discovered in 1983 by Marshall and Warren[1] in Australia. Its discovery has radically altered the approach to management of patients with peptic ulcer disease. *Helicobacter* has been strongly associated with idiopathic duodenal and gastric ulcers.[2] It has also been implicated in the etiology of gastric cancer.[3] The association of gastritis and the presence of *H. pylori* in pediatrics has been documented.[4] Both animal and human studies have shown that these organisms are capable of inducing inflammation in otherwise healthy mucosa, helping to establish the cause-and-effect postulate, rather than the idea of *H. pylori* as a coincidental finding in inflamed mucosa.

The prevalence of *H. pylori* in select pediatric populations of developed countries is approximately 5% to 15% (North American studies); however, a greater incidence has been found (25% to 70%) in European countries such as Belgium.[5] These numbers are based on a select group of patients who were undergoing endoscopy because of gastrointestinal (GI) symptoms. Epidemiologic studies have shown that the bacteria affects men and women equally, with an increasing prevalence of *H. pylori* with increasing age. However, one study in 1994 from Peru followed the status of more than 100 infants, and found that the overall prevalence of the infection dropped from 72% to 48% from 6 to 18 months.[6] Individual children who had infection were seen to clear their infection and male infants acquired the infection more rapidly but cleared it less often. It was noteworthy that

this infection thought to persist lifelong without treatment did not do so in that study.

The reservoir for *H. pylori* is unknown. Evidence of intrafamilial clustering has been documented, suggesting either a common source or person-to-person transmission. Transmission is believed to be either fecal-oral or oral-oral. Overcrowded conditions, poor socioeconomic status, and endemic country origin are all associated risk factors for the development of *H. pylori* disease.

PATHOPHYSIOLOGY

It is clear that chronic inflammation is a critical component in initiating the progression from superficial gastritis to chronic atrophic gastritis and eventually to invasive adenocarcinoma of the stomach. It is also clear from numerous studies that *H. pylori* is a critical element in causing inflammation.[7] *H. pylori* has been found to withstand acid pH, as opposed to most other organisms, allowing it to live in the stomach. It can cause parietal cell dysfunction, leading to hypochlorhydria. The copious amounts of urease it produces are thought necessary to help the bacteria survive.[8] In addition, the bacteria possess one to five flagellae to help with motility, which has proved essential for gastric colonization and ensuing inflammation.[9] The bacteria tend to adhere solely to gastric mucosa and have been isolated in the duodenum but only when associated with metaplastic gastric tissue. Several adhesins have been postulated to allow for this adherence.

Although *H. pylori* infection induces an antibody response directed at many of its antigens, these antibodies do not result in eradication of the bacteria. It is therefore believed that the bacteria are protected in the gastric mucosa. *H. pylori* infection of the stomach is always found with an inflammatory infiltrate that resolves upon eradication of the bacteria. The bacteria do not appear to invade the gastric mucosa. Thus, postulates of inflammation include substances from the bacteria that may induce damage. An example is the urease produced, which has been found in the lamina propria, and can stimulate chemotaxis.[8] *H. pylori* also causes gastric inflammation by the stimulation of cytokine release after mucosal contact. There is evidence for increased interleukin-8 (IL-8), a peptide that has chemotactant and neutrophil stimulatory properties, in the gastric epithelium in *H. pylori* infection.[10]

The question as to why one person becomes symptoatic to *H. pylori* while another remains asymptomatic is an interesting issue. It is now believed that there are different strains of *H. pylori* [11] These may differ from one another in the expression of various proteins. Two of the more well known of these proteins with variable expression are products of the *vac*A and *cag*A genes. Strains of bacteria that do not possess the *cag*A gene, and thus do not produce its protein product, are less virulent, and tend to produce less damage. The specific mechanism whereby *H. pylori cag*A strains more often produce severe inflammation/ulceration is unknown.

H. pylori is well known to be associated with duodenal ulcer disease. The methods whereby *H. pylori* is thought to affect the duodenum include increased basal and peak acid output, lack of inhibition of gastrin release, and increased response to gastrin release. Additionally, somatostatin, which inhibits the release of gastrin, is decreased by *H. pylori*.[12] This organism can transform histamine into N-methyl histamine, a strong gastric secretogogue and inhibitor of somatostatin production.[13] Furthermore, duodenal bicarbonate secretion is diminished in patients with *H. pylori*, adding yet another method that this bacteria possesses to cause damage in the underlying mucosa.

CLINICAL PRESENTATION

H. pylori typically presents with abdominal pain (epigastric) and vomiting. The pain often occurs after meals, but it can also occur early in the morning. Younger children may present with severe irritability and decreased appetite, as it is difficult for them to pinpoint the exact location of their pain. Less frequent presenting symptoms include chest pain, heartburn, nausea, anorexia, or gastrointestinal bleeding (duodenal ulcer or gastric ulcer).[14] *H. pylori* is a known cause of duodenal ulceration and gastric ulceration, fulfilling all of Koch's postulates for causality.[15] *H. pylori* is found in more than 90% of adult

patients with duodenal ulcers, and in 60% to 90% of those with gastric ulcers. Chronic iron deficiency has been documented in children with gastritis or ulceration.

Many people with *H. pylori* are asymptomatic. Adults with GI symptoms and documented *H. pylori* infection but without mucosal ulceration are not commonly treated. Several serologic studies have shown that the bulk of pediatric patients with the infection are asymptomatic.[16] Various studies examining abdominal pain in children have not yet found a correlation with *H. pylori* when compared to controls. Other studies that look at clinical symptoms such as abdominal pain have shown no difference in improvement of the pain upon treatment for the *H. pylori* or placebo. One study done in Chile showed an 86% infection rate in children endoscoped for functional abdominal pain; it did not conclude that *H. pylori* was necessarily causing the abdominal pain in the bulk of these children with infection but no ulceration. However, other studies, although mostly case reports, have shown the occurrence of protein-losing enteropathy, hypoalbuminemia, and other symptoms that were associated with *H. pylori* that improved with treatment. Although these studies were uncontrolled, they do raise the possibility of *H. pylori* causing symptomatology even without peptic ulcer disease.

The role of *H. pylori* in the development of gastric carcinoma and even lymphoma is being investigated. The bacteria have been classified by the World Heath Organization (WHO) as a class 1 carcinogen, but clearly more studies in this area are warranted.

DIAGNOSIS

Current methods for the detection of *H. pylori* involve endoscopic and noninvasive techniques. The organism can be detected in biopsy material by culture, histology (with various special stains), or rapid urease assay methods. The histopathology method is currently considered the gold standard for detection. Most endoscopic protocols favor two specimens of the gastric antrum analyzed by an expert pathologist. All the above methods are considered highly sensitive and specific for *Helicobacter* organisms.[17]

Noninvasive methods include antibody detection and breath testing. Serum antibody tests can be utilized to detect past or current infection; however, it cannot distinguish between the two unless multiple blood tests are obtained before and after therapy, thus demonstrating a decrease in antibody titers.[18] Breath testing strategies have been well described, using ingested labeled urea. If *H. pylori* is present in the patient's stomach, the ingested urea is digested by bacterial urease, permitting CO_2 absorption in the blood and exhalation in the breath.[19]

The ^{13}C-urea breath test has recently been approved for use in adults.[20,21] Both the sensitivity and specificity of the ^{13}C-urea breath test have been found to be greater than 90% in adults. The use of the breath test as a tool for pediatrics has been studied in Belgium[22] and Japan[23]; however, no studies have been performed in North America.

TREATMENT

Who should be treated? Although various physicians believe that a patient's symptoms may be secondary to *H. pylori*, even without mucosal ulceration, the official recommendation for treatment of children affected with *H. pylori* is to treat only those with endoscopically proven peptic ulcer disease. Another controversy on leaving patients untreated is that untreated infection leads to an increased incidence of gastric carcinoma[24] as *H. pylori* has not only been associated with, but is now deemed a primary carcinogen. In contrast, other investigators fear that treatment of a colonized asymptomatic stomach may lead to more resistant and potentially carcinogenic bacteria emergence.

How successful is treatment? A study in adult patients showed that treatment of *H. pylori* infection with duodenal ulcer reduced the recurrence rate of ulceration from 80% to 20% at 1-year follow-up. A marked reduction was also seen in pediatric patients treated for the infection.[25] Treatment options include a variety of polytherapy regimens. Many monotherapy regimens have proven useless, with only suppression of the bacteria during treatment, and re-emergence of the bacteria and clinical symptoms upon cessation of treatment. Common combinations in the past have included a bismuth compound, amoxicillin, and metronidazole.[26] An alternative is an antihistamine, metronidazole, and amoxicillin. These have proven to be about 90% successful in eradication of metronidazole-sensitive strains. More recent therapies include amoxicillin and omeprazole, which has now been found to eradicate the organism in only about 60% of patients treated.[27] The advantages are compliance with only two medications to take and avoiding bismuth compounds that many children refuse. The most popular, and probably most successful, treatment is triple therapy with omeprazole and any two of clarithromycin, metronidazole, and amoxicillin.[28,29] Most studies suggest taking the antibiotics from 10 days to 2 weeks, and the proton-pump inhibitor from 3 to 6 weeks.

CONCLUSION

It has become increasingly evident that *H. pylori* involvement of the stomach is one of the underlying etiologies for chronic inflammation, peptic ulcer disease, and even carcinomas later in life. This concept is completely changing the notions previously held on the pathogenesis of peptic ulcer disease. Much more research on *H. pylori* in children is needed to help define the reservoir, transmission, and therapeutic options. In addition, the controversy surrounding the ability of *H. pylori* to cause clinical symptoms in the absence of ulceration needs to be resolved.

REFERENCES

1. Marshall BJ, Warren JR. Unidentified curved bacilli in the stomach of patients with gastritis and peptic ulceration. Lancet 1984;1:1311–1315

2. Rauws EAJ, Langenberg W, Houthoff HJ et al. *Campylobacter pyloridis* associated chronic antral gastritis. Gastroenterology 1988;94:33–44

3. Forman D, Newell DG, Fullerton F et al. Association between infection with *Helicobacter pylori* and risk of gastric cancer: evidence from a prospective investigation. BMJ 1991;302:1302–1305

4. Drumm B, Sherman P, Cutz E, Karmali M. Association of *Campylobacter pylori* on the gastric mucosa with antral gastritis in children. N Engl J Med 1987;316:1557–1561

5. Megraud F, Brassens RM, Denis F et al. Seroepidemiology of *Campylobacter pylori* infection in various populations. J Clin Microbiol 1989;27:1870–1873

6. Klein PD, Gilman RH, Leon-Barua R et al. The epidemiology of *Helicobacter pylori* in Peruvian children between 6 and 30 months of age. Am J Gastroenterol 1994;89:2196–2200

7. Peterson WL. *Helicobacter pylori* and peptic ulcer disease. NEJM 1991;324:1043–1048.

8. Eaton KA et al. Essential role of urease in pathogenesis of gastritis induced by *Helicobacter pylori* in gnotobiotic piglets. Infect Immun 1991;59:2470–2475

9. Eaton K, Morgan D, Krakowska S. *Campylobacter pylori* virulence factors in gnotobiotic piglets. Infect Immun 1989;57: 1119–1125

10. Crabtree J, Peichl P, Wyatt J et al. Gastric interleukin-8 and IgA IL-8 autoantibodies in *Helicobacter pylori* infection. Scand J Immunol 1993;37:65–70

11. Covacci A, Censini S, Bugnoli M et al. Molecular characterization of the 128 KOA immunodominant antigen of *Helicobacter pylori* associated with cytotoxicity and duodenal ulcer. Proc Natl Acad Sci USA 1993;90:5791–5795

12. Quelroz D, Mendex E, Rocha G et al. Effect of *Helicobacter pylori* eradication on antral gastrin- and somatostatin-immunoreactive cell density and gastrin and somatostatin concentrations. Scand J Gastro 1993;28:858–864

13. Courillon-Maller A, Lauray J, Roucayrol A et al. *Helicobacter pylori* infection: physiopathologic implication of N-a-methyl histamine. Gastroenterology 1995;108:959–966

14. Fiedorek SC, Casteel HB, Pumphrey CL et al. The role of *Helicobacter pylori* in recurrent, functional abdominal pain in children. Am J Gastroenterol 1992;87:347–349

15. Marshall B, Armstrong A, McGechie D et al. Attempt to

fulfill Koch's postulates for pyloric *Campylobacter*. Med J Aust 1985;142:436–444

16. Fiedorek SC et al. Factors influencing the epidemiology of *Helicobacter pylori* infection in children. Pediatrics 1991;88: 578–582

17. Marshall BJ, Warren JR, Francis GJ et al. Rapid urease test in the management of *Campylobacter pyloridis*-associated gastritis. Am J Gastroenterol 1987;82:200–210

18. Faigel D, Childs M, Furth E et al. New non-invasive tests for *H. pylori* gastritis (comparison with tissue-based gold standard). Dig Dis Sci 1996;41:740–748

19. Graham DY, Klein PD, Evans DJ et al. *Campylobacter pyloridis* detected non-invasively by 13C-urea breath test. Lancet 1987;1:1174–1177

20. Graham DY, Klein PD. What you should know about the methods, problems, interpretations, and use of urea breath tests. Am J Gastroenterol 1991;86:1118–1122

21. Klein PD, Graham DY. Minimum analysis requirements for the detection of *Helicobacter pylori* infection by the C13-urea breath test. Am J Gastroenterol 1993;88:1865–1869

22. Vandenplas Y, Blecker U et al. Contribution of the ^{13}C-urea breath test to the detection of *Helicobacter pylori* gastritis in children. Pediatrics 1992;90:608–611

23. Yamashiro Y, Oguchi S, Otsuka Y et al. *Helicobacter pylori* colonization in children with peptic ulcer disease. Diagnostic value of the ^{13}C-urea breath test to detect *H. pylori* colonization. Acta Paediatr Jpn 1995;37:12–16

24. Nomura A, Stemmermann G, Chyar P et al. *Helicobacter pylori* infection and gastric carcinoma in a population of Japanese-Americans in Hawaii. NEJM 1991;325:1132–1136

25. Israel DM, Hasall E. Treatment and long-term follow-up of *Helicobacter pylori*-associated duodenal ulcer disease in children. J Pediatr 1993;123:53

26. Mahony MJ et al. Management and response to treatment of *Helicobacter pylori* gastritis. Arch Dis Child 1992;67:940–943

27. Unge P, Ekstrom P. Effects of combination therapy with omeprazole and an antibiotic on *Helicobacter pylori* and duodenal ulcer disease. Scand J Gastroenterol 1993;228(suppl): 17–18

28. Tursi A et al. Evaluation of the efficacy and tolerability of four different therapeutic regimens for the *Helicobacter pylori* eradication. Panminerva Med 1996;38:145–149

29. Yousfi MM et al. One week triple therapy with omeprazole, amoxycillin and clarithromycin for treatment of *Helicobacter pylori* infection. Alimentary Pharmacol Ther 1996;10: 617–621

27

HEMOLYTIC UREMIC SYNDROME

KATHERINE MACRAE DELL
KEVIN E. C. MEYERS
BERNARD S. KAPLAN

Hemolytic uremic syndrome (HUS) is characterized by acute hemolytic anemia with fragmented erythrocytes, thrombocytopenia, and acute renal injury. Two broad clinical phenotypes are recognized: diarrhea-associated HUS (D+ HUS or typical HUS), in which there is a diarrheal prodrome, often with hemorrhagic colitis, and nondiarrheal (D− HUS, or atypical HUS), which occurs sporadically without a prodromal diarrheal illness.[1] D+ HUS is the most frequent cause of acute renal failure in children.[2] It is caused by intestinal infection with enterohemorrhagic *Escherichia coli* (EHEC) and, less commonly with *Shigella* species. D+ HUS occurs sporadically and in epidemics. The clinical course and prognosis of D+ and D− HUS differ considerably (Table 27-1). D+ HUS is the main focus of this review because it is more likely to be encountered by a primary care physician or gastroenterologist.

PATHOPHYSIOLOGY

D+ HUS is caused by toxin-producing bacteria, especially enterohemorrhagic *E. coli* (EHEC), which are also known as verocytotoxin-producing *E. coli* (VTEC). D+ HUS can also be caused by *Shigella dysenteriae*, *Salmonella typhi*, and *Aeromonas*.[3] As a result of improved isolation techniques, case identification, and reporting, *E. coli* O157 : H7, named for its somatic (O) and flagellar (H)

antigens, has emerged as the predominant pathogen in North America.[4] D+ HUS can be caused by other serotypes, especially in Europe, where the O111 serotype is more common.[5] EHEC produce one or more Shiga-like toxins (SLT), also known as verocytotoxins because of their ability to lyse cultured rabbit Vero cells. Shiga-like toxin I (SLT-I) has 100% homology with *Shigella* toxin. However, Shiga-like toxin II (SLT-II), which has 60% homology with *Shigella* toxin, is more likely to cause HUS.[5,6] The O157 : H7 serotype produces both SLTs, although it is somewhat more likely to produce SLT-II.[7] A new classification of the Shiga toxins has been proposed and is shown in Table 27-2.[8]

Most cases of D+ HUS that occur during epidemics are due to the ingestion of contaminated beef, in particular, undercooked ground beef. Approximately 1% of beef cattle in the United States harbor *E. coli* in the intestine.[9] In the processing of ground beef, organisms on the outside of carcasses may become incorporated within the meat. In addition, ground beef often contains meat from several different animals; therefore, one infected animal can contaminate a large quantity of ground beef.[4] Transmission of *E. coli* O157 : H7 has also been reported after swimming in contaminated lakes or after consumption of raw milk or fruits and vegetables soiled by manure.[5] Person-to-person transmission is important, especially in day care centers and nursing homes.[10,11]

The gastrointestinal (GI) tract, kidney, and central nervous system (CNS) are most severely affected. Al-

191

TABLE 27-1. Clinical Subgroups of HUS

Group	Typical D+ HUS	Atypical D− HUS
Escherichia coli infection	Common	Nil
Genetic factors	Rare	Common
Age	Mainly children	Older children/adults
Season	Summer	Year-round
Prodrome	Bloody diarrhea	Nil/nonspecific
Onset	Sudden	Insidious
Neurologic	Occasional	Common
Hypertension	Mild to moderate	Severe
Renal pathology	Glomerular	Arteriolar
Renal sequelae	Uncommon	Common
Relapses	Rare	Common
Death	<5%	Common

(Adapted from Frishberg et al.,[1] with permission.)

though GI symptoms were once considered nothing more than a prodrome to the syndrome, they are now considered an important manifestation of the underlying pathogenic process.[12] In the colon, the pattern is most consistent with ischemic or infectious injury, similar to that seen with other toxin-mediated diseases. Intestinal mucosa may show edema, hemorrhage, or ulceration with thickened bowel walls.[12–14] In more severe cases, frank infarction may be present.[15–17] Pseudomembranes can be difficult to distinguish from those caused by infection with *Clostridium difficile*.[4] Furthermore, secondary *C. difficile* infection has been reported as a complication of HUS.[18] Histologic examination may show thrombi and fibrin deposition in the submucosal and intramural vessels, and there may be focal ischemic necrosis or frank infarction.

TABLE 27-2. Uniform Nomenclature for the Shiga Toxin Family of Toxins

Current Name	Proposed Gene (Protein) Nomenclature
Shiga toxin (Stx)	stx (Stx)
Shiga-like toxin I (SLT-I) or verotoxin I (VT1)	stx1 (Stx1)
Shiga-like toxin II (SLT-II) or verotoxin II (VT-2)	stx2 (Stx2)
Shiga-like toxin IIc (SLT-IIc) or verotoxin IIc (VT2c)	stx2c (Stx2c)
Shiga-like toxin IIe (SLT-IIe) or verotoxin IIe (VT2e)	stx2e (Stx2e)

(Adapted from Calderwood et al.,[8] with permission.)

CLINICAL PRESENTATION OF D+ HUS

The highest incidence of D+ HUS is during the summer months, perhaps because of patterns of ground beef consumption and preparation. Children less than 5 years of age are most at risk.[7] Females are affected slightly more often than males.[2] D+ HUS is uncommon in blacks, both in Africa and in the United States. Typical D+ HUS begins with a diarrhea prodrome. The diarrhea is initially watery, then frequently becomes frankly bloody as the result of hemorrhagic colitis. Of those patients with *E. coli* O157 : H7 infection, 5% to 15% develop HUS.[4] Possible risk factors for the development of HUS are extremes of age, fever, leukocytosis, and treatment with antibiotics or antimotility agents.[4]

GASTROINTESTINAL MANIFESTATIONS

The diarrhea prodrome typically precedes the development of HUS by about 3 to 4 days, although HUS can occur up to 2 weeks later.[19] The hemorrhagic colitis can be striking with significant stool blood loss. Associated symptoms are abdominal pain, often crampy and severe, nausea, vomiting, jaundice, and low-grade fever.[2,5]

The abdomen is usually markedly tender and distended, and there may be overt peritoneal signs, hepatomegaly, and rectal bleeding. Less common findings include abdominal mass caused by hematoma, bowel infarction, or intussusception[19,20]; perianal erythema; anal sphincter dysfunction with alternating contraction and relaxation and a dilated orifice; and rectal prolapse.[12,21] Anal findings have been misdiagnosed as indicative of sexual abuse.[22] This constellation of findings can be confused with inflammatory bowel disease (regional enteritis or ulcerative colitis), acute appendicitis, intussusception, peritonitis, or cecal polyp.[12,14,19,23] Patients with severe GI manifestations may undergo barium enema and exploratory laparotomy before the diagnosis of HUS is apparent or even considered.

Colonic infarction is an important life-threatening complication.[15] Four of 37 children with HUS associated with an outbreak of *E. coli* O157 : H7 developed colonic necrosis that required partial or complete colectomy. Two of those patients died of multisystem organ failure and shock.[16] In another series of 134 patients, two developed colonic perforation and one had hemoperitoneum from pancolitis.[17] In some cases, infarction progresses to overt colonic gangrene, another important cause of mortality and morbidity. Intussusception occurs in fewer than 1% of cases, and rectal prolapse occurs in about 8% to 13% of patients.[19,24]

Pancreatitis, with variable elevations in pancreatic enzymes, occurs in 20% to 60% of patients. Diabetes

TABLE 27-3. Gastrointestinal Manifestations of D + HUS

Oropharynx/esophagus
    Parotitis
    Oral ulcers
    Esophageal stricture
Stomach
    Gastric hemorrhage
Pancreas
    Pancreatitis
    Diabetes mellitus with or without overt pancreatic necrosis
Liver
    Hepatomegaly with mild elevations in transaminases
    Cholestatic jaundice
    Gallstones
Colon
    Hemorrhagic colitis
    Intussusception
    Toxic megacolon
    Colonic ischemia/infarction with stricture
    Colonic gangrene
Rectum/anus
    Rectal prolapse
    Perianal excoriation
    Anal sphincter dysfunction

mellitus may occur in 2% to 5% of patients and may be transient or permanent. The hyperglycemia may first become apparent with the initiation of peritoneal dialysis, due to the dextrose content of the dialysate solution. There may be overt pancreatic necrosis.[25,26] At autopsy, fibrin deposition and hemorrhage are seen in the pancreas. Hepatomegaly is a common finding and is often associated with elevated transaminases, but overt hepatic failure has not been described. Cholestatic jaundice is rare,[19,27] as are gallstones. One case of esophageal stricture and one case of parotitis have been reported. Mucosal ulcerations occur rarely. GI manifestations are summarized in Table 27-3.

The onset of HUS often begins as the diarrhea is resolving, when the patient manifests signs and symptoms of hemolysis and renal insufficiency (Table 27-4).

TABLE 27-4. Signs of HUS in a Patient With Bloody Diarrhea

Increasing pallor

Petechiae, jaundice

Central nervous system changes

Decreasing urine volume during or after rehydration

Abnormal urinalysis

Increasing BUN and serum creatinine concentration during or after rehydration

There is pallor, and occasionally petechiae and purpura. Renal injury results in oliguria, edema, and cardiovascular signs of fluid overload, such as a gallop rhythm, hypertension, and pulmonary edema. Fluid overload usually occurs as the result of ongoing fluid replacement coupled with the failure to recognize the onset of oliguria.[28] The oliguria may not be appreciated early on in infants because of watery diarrhea.

Neurologic symptoms are frequent, and CNS catastrophes are now the main cause of morbidity and mortality. Most affected patients are irritable and lethargic. Seizures may occur in about 20% of patients as a result of metabolic derangements (hypocalcemia, hyponatremia), direct toxic injury, or thrombi.[23] Catastrophic CNS features, which include coma, delirium, ataxia, and stroke, are important acute and long-term problems.[19]

Cardiac dysfunction caused by myocarditis or cardiomyopathy can occur, as can lung involvement, with pulmonary hemorrhage, hypoxemia, and pulmonary edema. Petechiae and purpura are very uncommon. Autopsy findings have demonstrated abnormalities of the adrenal, thyroid, and ovary. These abnormalities generally do not correlate with clinical findings; however, one case of adrenal insufficiency has been reported.[29]

DIAGNOSIS

The diagnosis of diarrhea-associated HUS is based on history, physical examination, and laboratory findings. No definitive symptom or sign is diagnostic of HUS. The diagnosis is made when the patient exhibits acute hemolytic anemia with fragmented erythrocytes, thrombocytopenia, and acute renal injury. The differential diagnosis of D + HUS includes ulcerative colitis and intussusception. However, renal insufficiency and hemolysis do not occur in these disorders. Sepsis with multisystem organ failure, including renal failure, GI dysfunction, and hemolysis mimics HUS, although there is a disseminated, rather than localized, coagulopathy.

Radiographic findings on plain films may include bowel dilation, thickened bowel walls, and free air, if the bowel has perforated.[30] Invasive diagnostic procedures such as barium enema and colonoscopy are not recommended because of the risk of perforation. Nevertheless, patients sometimes undergo these procedures before the classic signs and symptoms of HUS are present. Barium enema studies may show a characteristic "thumbprinting" appearance, indicative of submucosal hemorrhage and ischemic bowel disease. Transverse ridging may be due to bowel spasm. Ulcerations, thickened mucosal folds, and colonic narrowing or dilation are also seen. At colonoscopy or sigmoidoscopy, colonic mucosa is edematous, friable, and ulcerated with yellow green exudate or "dirty-gray" pseudomembranes.[13] The latter may be indistinguishable from ulcerative colitis.[16,18] Ultrasound and computed tomography (CT) are occasionally performed and may show ascites and thickened bowel walls.[19]

LABORATORY TESTS

Laboratory tests can be grouped into three categories: those that evaluate acute renal injury, those that indicate hematologic abnormalities, and those that establish the infectious etiology. Laboratory findings in acute renal failure are a rising blood-urea nitrogen (BUN) and serum creatinine, hyponatremia (from overtreatment with hypotonic solutions in the face of oliguria), hyperphosphatemia, hyperkalemia, and metabolic acidosis. Serum uric acid concentrations may be elevated.[31] Urinalysis shows proteinuria, hematuria, and dysmorphic red blood cells; cellular and granular casts are occasionally seen, but red blood cell casts are infrequent. Hematologic abnormalities are Coombs-negative hemolytic anemia, a reticulocytosis and schistocytes on peripheral smear, thrombocytopenia, and leukocytosis. Prothrombin time (PT) and partial thromboplastin time (PTT) are usually normal, but serum fibrin degradation products may be elevated. There may be increases in serum transaminases, bilirubin, amylase, and lipase. Hypoalbuminemia occurs in most cases and is mainly the result of a protein-losing enteropathy.

The definitive diagnosis of *E. coli* O157 : H7 infection is made by a number of different methods. Commercially available tests as well as experimental techniques are summarized in Table 27-5.[32] The practitioner should be aware that many reference laboratories do not yet screen for the O157 : H7 serotype. Furthermore, the yield from a stool culture diminishes after 6 days of symptoms; therefore, the organism may not be recovered by the time the diagnosis of HUS is suspected.[5]

TABLE 27-5. Laboratory Diagnosis of *E. coli* O157:H7 Infection

Commercially available
   Stool culture—screening for sorbitol fermentation confirmed by serotyping
Experimental
   ELISA to detect SLT
   DNA probes for SLT-producing *E. coli*
   Colony blot assay with SLT monoclonal antibodies
   PCR to detect SLT genes
   Serology testing for antibodies against LPS (IgM)

Abbreviations: ELISA, enzyme-linked immunosorbent assay; LPS, lipopolysaccharide; PCR, polymerase chain reaction; SLT, Shiga-like toxin.

TREATMENT

There is no specific treatment for D+ HUS, and careful supportive care remains the mainstay of therapy. The improvement in survival over the past 40 years has resulted from earlier diagnosis of the disease, careful management of acute renal failure, and general advances in intensive care management. Meticulous attention to fluid and electrolyte balance is essential. Patients should be provided with replacement of insensible losses and any ongoing losses of urine or stool. We do not use furosemide and saline infusions because of the potential for inducing pulmonary edema in oliguric patients. Anuric patients rarely, if ever, respond to this challenge.

Dialysis is indicated in patients who develop anuria or electrolyte abnormalities that cannot be managed conservatively. About 50% of patients with D+ HUS require dialysis. Nutrition is also an important aspect of therapy. Total parenteral nutrition should be considered early. Patients sometimes develop intolerance to intralipids, so cholesterol and triglycerides should be monitored. Slow transfusions of small quantities of packed red blood cells are given when the hemoglobin decreases to less than 6 to 7 g/dl. We do not infuse platelets unless there is overt bleeding. There is no specific therapy for the diarrhea, and antibiotics and antimotility agents are contraindicated. We do not use fresh frozen plasma infu-

TABLE 27-6. Demographic Data for Patients With D+ HUS at the Children's Hospital of Philadelphia, 1987–1995

Age (yr)	5.5 ± 4.0
Sex (no)	Male, N = 23; female, N = 37
Ethnicity	Caucasian, 57
	African American, 1
	Hispanic, 1
	Other, 1
Duration of diarrhea prior to admission (days)	6.6 ± 4.3 (range 0–30)
Diarrhea source	Unknown, 54
	Fast foods, 3
	Barbecue, 1
	Affected sibling, 1
	Other, 1
Sibling with gastroenteritis	Yes, 6
	No, 53
Antibiotic for diarrhea	Yes, 29
	No, 30
Stool culture results	Positive—O157:H7, 11/59; other, 6/59
	Negative—41/59

TABLE 27-7. Gastrointestinal Findings in Patients With D+ HUS at the Children's Hospital of Philadelphia, 1987–1995

Finding	N	(%)
Bloody diarrhea	60	100
Vomiting	28	47
Jaundice	5	8.5
Diabetes	5	8.5
Edema	19	32
Acute abdomen/exploratory laparotomy	4	6.6
Intestinal gangrene	4	6.6
Stricture	1	1.6

TABLE 27-8. Causes and Associations of HUS

Infections
  Escherichia coli O157:H7
  Shigella dysenteriae
  Streptococcus pneumoniae
  Aeromonas hydrophila[a]
  Human immunodeficiency virus (HIV)[a]
Inherited
  Autosomal recessive
  Autosomal dominant
  Cobalamin C defect[a]
Drugs
  Cyclosporin A
  FK 506
  OKT3[a]
  Mitomycin-C
  Oral contraceptives[a]
  Quinine[a]
  Crack cocaine[a]
Additional causes and associations
  Pregnancy-associated HUS[a]
  Transplant-associated HUS[a]
  Cancer-associated HUS[a]
  Glomerulopathy-associated HUS[a]
  Systemic lupus–associated thrombotic microangiopathy (TMA)
  Systemic sclerosis–associated TMA
  Pancreatitis-associated TMA[a]

[a] Circumstantial evidence.
(Adapted from Kaplan,[3] with permission.)

sions, plasmapheresis, aspirin, dipyridamole, heparin, or intravenous gammaglobulin.

Newer therapies are currently in the investigational stage. A novel preventive therapy, an orally administered toxin binder called Synsorb-Pk is being evaluated in trials in Canada, and preliminary studies are encouraging. The decision to intervene surgically and perform an exploratory laparotomy is difficult. Indications are intestinal perforation, as suggested by free air on abdominal plain film, and gram-negative rod sepsis, which may indicate bowel necrosis. Peritoneal signs, however, may be an unreliable indicator of underlying bowel pathology. In one study, 5% of patients had physical examinations consistent with an acute abdomen, but only one-third of those had bowel gangrene on laparotomy.

The results of 60 cases seen at the Children's Hospital of Philadelphia (CHOP) from 1987 to 1995 are shown in Tables 27-6 and 27-7. Three of four who had exploratory laparotomies before referral to CHOP were found to have gangrene of the colon. All survived. One child, who died within 12 hours of admission, had multiorgan injury, including intestinal gangrene. One patient has had minor surgical sequelae from the intestinal injury.

ATYPICAL D– HUS

The causes of HUS are shown in Table 27-8. Although there are many causes of atypical D– HUS, these constitute less than 15% of all cases of HUS.

REFERRAL PATTERN

Patients with HUS complicated by anuric renal failure, intestinal gangrene, CNS catastrophes, or cardiac disease are best referred to a tertiary care center where modern forms of dialytic treatment, including continuous arteriovenous filtration, and intensive care facilities are available.

REFERENCES

1. Frishberg Y, Obrig TG, Kaplan BS. Hemolytic uremic syndrome. In: Holliday MA, Barratt TM, Avner ED, Eds. Pediatric Nephrology, 3rd Ed. Baltimore: Williams & Wilkins, 1994:871–889

2. Robson WLM, Leung AKC, Kaplan BS. Hemolytic-uremic syndrome. Curr Probl Pediatr 1993;23:16–33

3. Kaplan BS. Hemolytic-uremic syndrome in children. Curr Opin Pediatr 1992;4:254–258

4. Boyce TG, Swerdlow DL, Griffin PM. *Escherichia coli* O157:H7 and the hemolytic-uremic syndrome. N Engl J Med 1995; 333:364–368

5. Su C, Brandt LJ. *Escherichia coli* 0157 : H7 infection in humans. Ann Intern Med 1995;123:698–714

6. Taylor CM. Verocytotoxin-producing *Escherichia coli* and the haemolytic uraemic syndrome, editorial. J Infect Dis 1995; 30:189–192

7. Martin DL, MacDonald KL, White KE et al. The epidemiol-

ogy and clinical aspects of the hemolytic uremic syndrome in Minnesota. N Engl J Med 1990;323:1161–1167

8. Calderwood SB, Acheson DWK, Keusch GT et al. Proposed new nomenclature for SLT (VT) family. Am Soc Microbiol News 1996;62:118–119

9. Griffen PM, Tauxe RV. The epidemiology of infections caused by *Escherichia coli* 0157 : H7, other enterohemorrhagic *E. coli*, and the associated hemolytic uremic syndrome. Epidemiol Rev 1991;13:60–98

10. Belongia EA, Osterholm MT, Soler JT et al. Transmission of *Escherichia coli* 0157 : H7 infection in Minnesota child day-care facilities. JAMA 1993;269:883–888

11. Ryan CA, Tauxe RV, Hosek GW et al. *Escherichia coli* 0157 : H7 diarrhea in a nursing home: clinical, epidemiological, and pathological findings. J Infect Dis 1986;154:631–638

12. Chesney RW, Whitington PF. Gastrointestinal features of the hemolytic uremic syndrome. In: Kaplan BS, Trompeter R, Moake J, Eds. Hemolytic Uremic Syndrome and Thrombotic Thrombocytopenic Purpura. New York: Marcel Dekker, 1992:97–111

13. Tachen ML, Campbell JR. Colitis in children with the hemolytic-uremic syndrome. J Pediatr Surg 1977;12:213–219

14. Berman W. The hemolytic-uremic syndrome: initial clinical presentation mimicking ulcerative colitis. J Pediatr 1972;81:275–278

15. Van Stiegmann G, Lilly JR. Surgical lesions of the colon in the hemolytic uremic syndrome. Surgery 1979;85:357–359

16. Tapper D, Tarr P, Avner E et al. Lessons learned in the management of hemolytic uremic syndrome in children. J Pediatr Surg 1995;30:158–163

17. Brandt ML, O'Regan S, Rousseau E, Yazbeck S. Surgical complications of the hemolytic-uremic syndrome. J Pediatr Surg 1990;25:1109–1112

18. Burgner DP, Rfidah H, Beattie TJ, Seal DV. *Clostridium difficile* after haemolytic uraemic syndrome. Arch Dis Child 1993;69:239–240

19. Siegler RL. Spectrum of extrarenal involvement in postdiarrheal hemolytic-uremic syndrome. J Pediatr 1994;125:511–518

20. Gallo GE, Gianantonio CA. Extrarenal involvement in diarrhoea-associated haemolytic-uraemic syndrome. Pediatr Nephol 1995;9:117–119

21. Vickers D, Morris K, Coulthard MG, Eastham EJ. Anal signs in haemolytic uraemic syndrome, letter. Lancet 1988;998

22. Smith CD, Schuster SR, Gruppe WE, Vawter GF. Hemolytic-uremic syndrome: a diagnostic and therapeutic dilemma for the surgeon. J Pediatr Surg 1978;13:597–604

23. Bar-Ziv J, Ayoub JIG, Fletcher BD. Hemolytic uremic syndrome: a case presenting with acute colitis. Pediatr Radiol 1974;2:203–206

24. Grodinsky S, Telmesani A, Robson WLM et al. Gastrointestinal manifestations of hemolytic uremic syndrome: recognition of pancreatitis. J Pediatr Gastroenterol Nutr 1990;11:518–524

25. Andreoli SP, Bergstein JM. Development of insulin-dependent diabetes mellitus during the hemolytic-uremic syndrome. J Pediatr 1982;100:541–545

26. Burns JC, Berman ER, Fagre JL, Shikes RH, Lum GM. Pancreatic islet cell necrosis: association with hemolytic-uremic syndrome. J Pediatr 1982;100:582–584

27. Jeffrey A, Kibbler CC, Baillod R et al. Cholestatic jaundice in the haemolytic-uraemic syndrome: a case report. Gut 1985;26:315–319

28. Armstrong GD, Rowe PC, Goodyer P et al. A phase I study of chemically synthesized verotoxin (Shiga-like toxin) Pk-trisaccharide receptors attached to chromosorb for preventing hemolytic-uremic syndrome. J Infect Dis 1995;171:1042–1045

29. Wells RG, Sty JR, Brummond RA. Adrenal hyperechogenicity in hemolytic uremic syndrome. Wisc Med J 1994;93:467–468

30. Peterson RB, Meseroll WP, Shrago GG, Gooding CA. Radiographic features of colitis associated with the hemolytic-uremic syndrome. Pediatr Radiol 1976;118:667–671

31. Kaplan BS, Thomson PD. Hyperuricemia in the hemolytic-uremic syndrome. Am J Dis Child 1976;130:854–856

32. Kaplan BS, McGowan KL. Hemolytic uremic syndrome. Curr Opin Infect Dis 1994;7:351–357

28

HENOCH-SCHÖNLEIN PURPURA

GREGORY F. KEENAN

Henoch-Schönlein purpura (HSP), also referred to as anaphylactoid purpura, was originally described in the nineteenth century. Schönlein noted the association between the purpuric rash and arthritis in 1837. In 1874, Henoch described the triad of arthritis, rash, and colicky abdominal pain with gastrointestinal (GI) hemorrhage.[1] While the epidemiology of childhood vasculitides is not yet fully delineated, HSP appears to be the most common form of childhood vasculitis in the United States.[2,3] The syndrome typically occurs in children aged 2 to 12 years, with a peak incidence in children aged 4 to 7 years.[1,4,5] The annual incidence in children is estimated at 3 to 17 per 100,000.[5,6] However, there are seasonal variations, with peak incidence occurring in the spring.[1,4] It is rare in infants, adults, and black children.[1,5] Males are affected up to twice as commonly as females.[1,4] HSP is usually preceded by a viral or bacterial illness; however, no specific etiologic agent has been identified.

The classic triad consists of a nonthrombocytopenic purpuric rash, arthritis, and the presence of urinary sediment.[2] The full clinical complex includes dependent palpable purpura, edema, joint symptoms, gastroenterologic symptoms, fever, and renal involvement. The skin is the most commonly affected organ (Fig. 28-1). Management is directed toward symptoms, and no specific therapy has been shown to alter the ultimate outcome. The illness usually follows a benign course; however, gastroenterologic symptoms frequently mimic an acute surgical abdomen and, in a small minority of children, intussusception and/or perforation can occur. Renal complications are the feared chronic problem affecting outcome. However, only a few patients with persistent proteinuria will go on to develop renal insufficiency or failure.[6,7]

PATHOPHYSIOLOGY

HSP is thought to be an immune complex–mediated disease, with circulating IgA and activated complement immune complexes depositing in specific end organs and causing a specific clinical syndrome.[8] Biopsies of the skin demonstrate the presence of leukocytoclastic vasculitic lesions. The affected vessels are primarily capillaries and pre- and postcapillary vessels. Perivascular infiltrates of polymorphonuclear leukocytes (as well as occasional eosinophils and histiocytes) in various stages of lysis are present in biopsy specimens of affected skin, kidneys, and the GI tract. There may be vessel thrombosis, as well as perivascular hemorrhage. Epidermal edema may be present. Immune complexes composed of complement C3, IgA, and IgG can be detected within the lesions.[8]

CLINICAL PRESENTATION

Typically, the child with HSP will have had a brief antecedent illness. Subsequently, the manifestations of the syndrome (Fig. 28-1) will evolve over the span of a few days. Initially, the child will complain of vague abdominal pain, usually followed by loose stools. The typical lower extremity, gravity dependent, purpuric rash may develop just before the onset of abdominal symptoms or within 1 to 3 days of onset of abdominal pain. Rarely, abdominal complaints may precede the rash by up to 1 month.[9] Joint manifestations occur concomitantly. Approximately one third of affected children will have nephritis with proteinuria. A smaller minority will develop

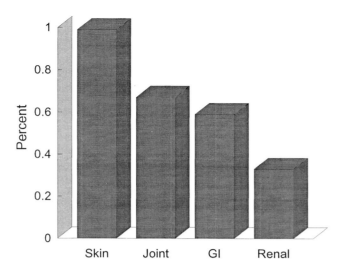

FIGURE 28-1. Prevalence of clinical findings.

hypertension. In most cases, the child will have a poor appetite for several days. Over the course of 1 to 3 weeks, the rash, GI symptoms, and joint complaints will resolve. Proteinuria will usually resolve over a period of 2 to 4 weeks. HSP manifestations recur in almost 50% of cases, usually within 4 to 6 weeks.

Cutaneous Manifestations

The rash associated with HSP is purpuric in nature and is usually seen in dependent areas, from the buttocks down the lower extremities. The skin of the arms and hands may be affected. The trunk is typically spared. Early in the evolution of the rash, there may be an ery-thematous, petechial, or urticarial appearance. Subsequently, discrete lesions may grow in size and may coalesce. As the lesions mature, they become brown and ecchymotic. Soft tissue edema of the lower extremities and face is common as well[1] (Fig. 28-2).

Joint Manifestations

The characteristic joint findings are periarticular, rather than articular, in nature. The most remarkable observation is that joint pain is markedly out of proportion to the physical findings. Affected joints are only slightly warm and have minimal effusions. Typically, the ankles are affected, but knee, elbow, wrist, and digit involvement has been described.[1,10] The vast majority of patients with joint complaints will have five or fewer joints affected.[11]

Gastroenterologic Manifestations

The gastroenterologic system is affected in most children with HSP. The most common feature is abdominal pain. It usually occurs within 1 week of the development of the rash and is usually diffuse and colicky in nature. On occasion, GI symptoms may precede the development of rash.[12,13] The pain usually persists for less than 1 week, with a range of 1 day to more than 30 days.[4,11,14]

A variety of GI phenomena may occur (Fig. 28-3). These are likely related to intestinal small vessel vasculitis and the resultant sequelae. Most of these features are relatively benign, but a few children will suffer from potentially lethal events. A survey of pediatric patients with HSP yielded 731 children in whom the presence

FIGURE 28-2. A 7-year-old with palpable purpura of the lower extremities. (From Glasier et al,[14] with permission.)

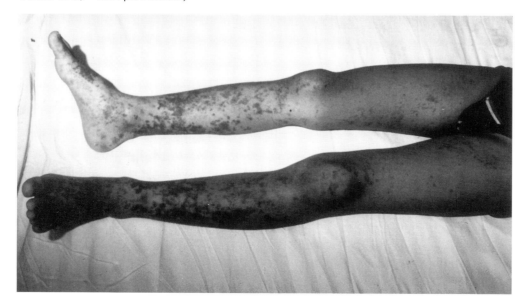

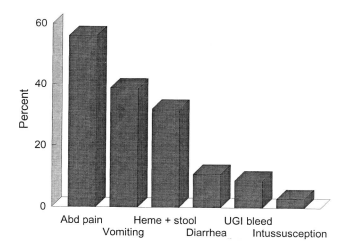

FIGURE 28-3. Gastrointestinal manifestations in HSP. Abd, abdominal; UGI, upper gastrointestinal.

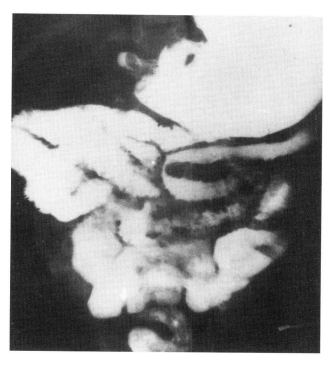

FIGURE 28-4. Thickened small bowel loops with jejunal thumbprinting consistent with submucosal edema. (From Glasier et al,[14] with permission.)

of GI manifestations had been documented. The survey determined that 2.3% of children developed hematochezia requiring transfusion; 4.8% required laparoscopy for evaluation of the intestine, surgical reduction of intussuscepted bowel, or bowel resection; and 2.9% developed intussusception, most of which were ileocolic (Table 28-1). Bowel necrosis occurred in 1.2% of cases.

Intra-abdominal catastrophes appear to occur later in the acute course. Bowel perforation was not reported in any of the series reviewed. However, isolated cases have been reported in the English literature.[12] Okano et al[15] collected 21 cases from the Japanese literature that were reported over a 30-year span. The 14 children in the series included 10 subjects aged 6 years or younger. The only child to die was a 1-year-old girl. Perforations occurred at any location from the stomach to the colon. The most common site of perforation was the ileum. Approximately

50% of affected children developed one or more lesions at this site.[15] In fewer than 5% of children, these events occurred before the development of the typical rash.[12] Death due to a GI event is extremely rare, with only one child of the 731 dying of irreducible intussusception.[1]

A barium swallow in children with abdominal pain may demonstrate bowel wall thickening as well as thumbprinting anywhere along the small bowel. These findings may be diffuse or isolated[14] (Fig. 28-4). Small

TABLE 28-1. Serious Gastrointestinal Manifestations of HSP[a]

	No. of Observations	No. Present	% with Finding
No. of HSP	731	731	100.0
Surgery	731	35	4.8
Intussusception	731	21	2.9
Ileocolic	667	12	1.8
Ileoileal	667	6	0.9
Jejunojejunal	667	1	0.1
Hematochezia, need transfusion	307	7	2.3
Bowel necrosis	731	9	1.2
Perforation	731	0	0.0
GI death	731	1	0.1

[a] Referral bias is minimized.

(References selected are series collected over several years from Gairdner,[10] Derham,[43] Allen et al,[1] Ansell,[27] Katz,[44] Glasier et al,[14] Hu,[45] Lopez et al,[21] Ilan and Naparstek,[4] Martinez-Frontanilla et al,[12] and Rosenblum.[46])

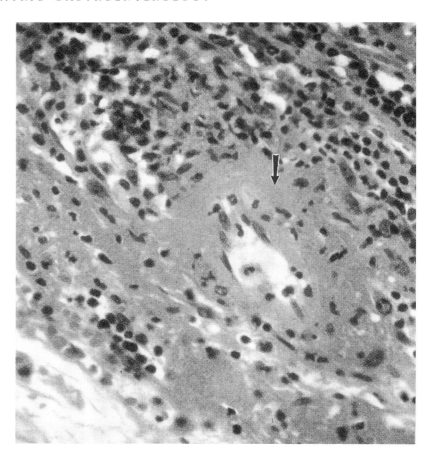

FIGURE 28-5. Biopsy specimen from jejunum demonstrates fibrinoid necrosis of a small submucosal artery (arrow).

bowel wall edema can also be demonstrated by ultrasound. Duodenal luminal enlargement and gall bladder hydrops may also be seen.[16,17] Upper endoscopy may reveal erythematous petechial lesions, erosions, and edema within the stomach and duodenum. Antral ulceration has also been seen. Esophageal lesions have not been described.[18,19] Colonic barium studies may demonstrate either bowel edema or intussuscepted bowel, or both.[14] Colonoscopy in isolated cases has detected focal petechial lesions with adjacent normal bowel.[20]

Histologic findings from endoscopic biopsies and from autopsy have exhibited evidence of leukocytic vasculitic changes in the mucosal vessels of the small intestine[21] (Fig. 28-5). Biopsy specimens of small intestine mural vessels and capillaries may contain areas of nonspecific inflammation in which IgA deposits may be exhibited by immunofluorescence studies. This may help confirm an atypical case.[19]

Rare complications reported in isolated cases include peritonitis,[21] pancreatitis,[22] ileal stricture,[23] and appendicitis.[24] Transient protein-losing enteropathy has been demonstrated in children with HSP.[25]

Renal Manifestations

Glomerular nephritis occurs in almost one-third of all children with HSP. Renal involvement occurs within 12 weeks of onset of HSP.[26] This is usually manifested as microscopic hematuria or proteinuria, or both. Hypertension will develop in 22% to 33% of children who have renal involvement.[1,6,27] However, the prevalence of the specific findings is dependent on the population studied. Consensus is lacking on whether the severity or duration of extrarenal manifestations correlates with severity of renal involvement.[26] Histopathologic findings by renal biopsy range from normal to severe crescentic glomerular nephritis. Electron microscopic examination may display mesangial, subendothelial, or subepithelial deposits. Immunofluorescence studies may demonstrate deposits of IgA, IgM, and IgG, as well as complement components.[26,28]

The occurrence of renal failure due to HSP is debated. However, in two recent reports of unselected children with HSP-associated nephropathy, the prevalence of ongoing active urinary sediment was 6% to 23%. Renal insufficiency occurred in 0% to 5% of cases. A total of two renal deaths occurred in the 94 patients (2%) reported in these two studies.[6,7]

Genitourinary Manifestations

Cases of scrotal symptoms and evidence of testicular vasculitis have been reported. In their series, Allen et al[1] noted the development of scrotal swelling and hemorrhage in 5 of 131 children. Other workers have reported boys presenting with symptoms mimicking testicular torsion.[9,29] One case of testicular torsion in a child with HSP and scrotal hematoma has been reported.[30] This uncommon manifestation may cause referred abdominal pain. Because torsion is unlikely but essential to recognize, radionuclide imaging should be obtained in suspicious situations. This diagnostic modality has shown an excellent ability to distinguish between torsion and edema/hemorrhage.[31]

Unusual Manifestations

The central nervous system (CNS) is rarely affected in HSP syndrome. Seizures, subarachnoid hemorrhage, cerebrovascular thrombosis, paresis, headache, and neuropathy have been described in conjunction with the syndrome.[32,33] Pulmonary alveolar hemorrhage, hemoptysis, and respiratory failure have been documented in case reports.[34]

DIAGNOSIS

The diagnosis of HSP is made on clinical grounds. Any combination of skin, joint, bowel, and renal manifestations may occur. A number of rheumatic and nonrheumatic diseases may mimic HSP (Table 28-2). The clinician should give consideration to these when generating a differential diagnosis. The American College of Rheumatology has developed a set of diagnostic criteria that are somewhat helpful in confirming the diagnosis[35] (Table 28-3).

Typically, the diagnosis will not be difficult with a young child presenting with a buttock and lower-extremity palpable hemorrhagic rash, fever, joint pain, and nausea and/or vomiting with heme positive stools. However, it is also common for a single manifestation to present one to several days before the full syndrome blossoms. Subtle manifestations such as a faint petechial rash or abdominal pain present in a child with periarthritis of the ankle should make the clinician suspicious of the diagnosis. Appropriate use of diagnostic modalities (Table 28-4) and laboratory studies is important.

The severity of the child's symptomatology should guide the extent of diagnostic evaluation and the level of monitoring. Many children will do well at home, with daily re-examinations during the acute phase of the illness. However, in the child exhibiting GI or renal manifestations, observation in the hospital setting is reasonable until the diagnosis has been established, and the severity of the acute illness has been determined and managed.

TABLE 28-2. Differential Diagnoses in the Evaluation of a Child With Possible HSP: Manifestations That May Mimic HSP

Disorders	Manifestations
Rheumatic	
Serum sickness	F, C, A
Kawasaki disease	F, C, A
Sarcoidosis	F, C, A, R
Löfgren's syndrome	
Infantile sarcoid	
Systemic lupus erythematosus	F, C, A, R, G, P
Juvenile rheumatoid arthritis	F, C, A, G
Dermatomyositis	F, C, A, G, P
Polyarteritis nodosa	F, C, A, R, G, T
Wegener's granulomatosus	F, C, A, R, P
Goodpasture's disease	F, R, P
Rheumatic fever	F, C, A
Cryoglobulinemia	F, C, A, R
Infectious	
Subcutaneous bacterial endocarditis	F, C, A, R
Disseminated gonococcal disease	F, C, A
Meningococcemia/meningococcal meningitis	F, C, A
Osteomyelitis	F, A
Gastroenterologic	
Inflammatory bowel disease	F, C, A, G
Intussusception (spontaneous)	F, G
Malignancy	
Acute lymphocytic leukemia	F, C, A
Neuroblastoma	F, C, A
Miscellaneous	
Left atrial myxoma	F, C, A

Abbreviations: F, fever; C, cutaneous; A, arthritis; R, renal; G, gastroenterologic; P, pulmonary; T, testicular.

LABORATORY STUDIES

Laboratory studies are nondiagnostic. Studies are done in order to exclude other entities in the differential diagnosis. The white blood cell (WBC) count is typically normal to slightly elevated. Hemoglobin level and platelet count are normal. The erythrocyte sedimentation rate is elevated. Electrolyte values reflect whether the affected child has been vomiting. Some children will have a hypokalemic metabolic alkalosis as a result. In the acute situation, serum creatinine will usually be normal. Urinalysis may indicate proteinuria or hematuria. Hemoccult testing may be positive.

Immunology studies including antinuclear antibodies

TABLE 28-3.   1990 American College of Rheumatology Criteria for Classification of HSP[a]

Criterion	Definition
Palpable purpura	Slightly raised hemorrhagic skin lesions unrelated to thrombocytopenia
Age <21 yr	Patient is ≤20 yr at onset of first symptoms
Bowel angina	Diffuse abdominal pain, worse after meals, or diagnosis of bowel ischemia, usually including bloody diarrhea
Vessel wall granulocytes	Histologic changes showing granulocytes in the walls of arterioles or venules

[a] The presence of two of four criteria indicates an 87.1% sensitivity of the classification schema; specificity is 87.7%.
(From Mills et al,[35] with permission.)

(ANA) and rheumatoid factor (RF) are negative. Complement C3, C4 studies are normal. On occasion, CH50 and properdin levels will be reduced, suggesting activation of the alternate complement pathway.[36,37] Anti-glomerular basement antibodies are not detectable. Antineutrophil cytoplasmic antibodies (ANCA) of the IgA type have been detected; however, none is anticytoplasmic (c type), and only rarely are they antimyeloperoxidase (p) type.[38,39]

TREATMENT

Therapeutic management is oriented toward two goals: symptom relief and outcome modulation. The child with joint pain can be managed with analgesics. Traditionally, acetaminophen or a nonsteroidal anti-inflammatory drug (NSAID) such as ibuprofen, or both, have been used to manage pain. Both are effective. Because abdominal complaints are common in these patients, NSAIDs are difficult to use in therapeutic levels over the course of joint pain. In addition, because of the risk of renal involvement, NSAIDs may be relatively contraindicated in certain patients. Systemic steroids work extremely well on articular complaints. Usually, a dose of prednisone within the range of 0.5 mg/kg/day will be sufficient. This can be tapered off over 7 to 14 days. Steroids do not appear to modify the evolution or severity of the cutaneous manifestations.[1]

Abdominal pain and nausea symptoms are also improved with corticosteroids. In a retrospective chart review performed by Rosenblum and Winter,[11] abdominal

TABLE 28-4.   Value of Diagnostic Study for HSP

Test	When Useful	Possible Finding in HSP
Skin biopsy	Atypical rash	Leukocytoclastic vasculitis IgA deposition by immunofluorescence
Arthrocentesis	Detect joint inflammation	Mild to moderate inflammatory synovitis
Abdominal flat plate	Quick/general assessment of obstruction	Ileus Perforation Air fluid levels
Ultrasound	Assessment of GI tract involvement	Bowel edema GB thickening Intussusception
UGI examination	Assessment of intra-abdominal involvement	Ulceration Spiculation of mucosal folds Intussusception
Barium enema	Assess for intussusception	Mucosal edema Intussusception Stricture
Esophagogastroduodenoscopy (EGD)	Findings potentially characteristic of HSP	Gastric hemorrhage Ulceration Intestinal petechiae
Colonoscopy	Rule out other causes of hematochezia	Bowel edema Colonic petechiae and hemorrhage
Testicular radionuclide scan	Rule out torsion	Increased flow

pain resolved 24 hours earlier when steroids were used, as compared to cases in which steroids were not used. There are theoretical reasons to support the use of steroids in an attempt to alter the likelihood of the development of intestinal vasculitis and hence intussusception, or perforation. However, no data have documented this effect.[1] Alternatively, systemic steroids could conceivably obscure the evolution of a surgical abdomen. Consequently, patients treated with steroids should be monitored closely.

Maintenance of hydration is the major management issue in a number of cases. For example, some children will be unable to tolerate enteral hydration; in these cases, parenteral hydration may be required. Under such circumstances, the use of systemic steroids can lessen the duration of required parenteral hydration in specific cases. However, this approach remains to be proved within study populations.[11]

Whether the outcome of HSP-associated nephropathy can be altered by steroids is debatable. Since the incidence of renal insufficiency is low in unselected populations,[6,7] it has been difficult to determine whether early steroid use alters or attenuates the incidence of renal insufficiency and failure. In a recent study by Mollica et al,[40] more than 12% of untreated children developed nephropathy. None of the patients treated with a 2-week course of 1 mg/kg/day developed nephropathy,[40] an observation that has been supported by other studies.[41] However, other studies have not detected a difference between steroid-treated and -untreated populations.[1,42] Reasonable use of steroids in HSP nephropathy should be based on evidence of severity of the renal lesion. This includes evidence of poor prognostic features such as nephrotic range proteinuria (greater than 3.5 g/24 hr/1.73 M^2), evidence of crescentic glomerular nephritis (more than 50% crescents), and/or elevations in serum creatinine and blood-urea nitrogen (BUN).[26] Cytotoxic therapy should probably be considered only in those patients who have deteriorating renal disease as well as pulmonary hemorrhage and CNS vasculitis.

REFERRAL PATTERN

Most patients with HSP are appropriately managed by the primary physician. Referrals should be obtained in cases of diagnostic uncertainty or of prolonged end-organ involvement. Atypical presentations of HSP are not uncommon; if the diagnosis is not fully apparent, referral to a rheumatologist, nephrologist, dermatologist, or gastroenterologist should be considered. Surgical consultation is warranted in the event of HSP presenting with an acute abdomen, for optimal assessment management of the possibility of intussusception or perforation, or both. After the acute illness has subsided, the child's

condition should be carefully monitored. If the proteinuria/hematuria does not resolve, a nephrologist should be consulted to consider the possibility of renal biopsy as well as additional medical therapy for hypertension.

REFERENCES

1. Allen DM, Diamond LK, Howell DA. Anaphylactoid purpura in children (Schönlein-Henoch syndrome): review with a follow-up of the renal complications. Am J Dis Child 1960;99:833–855

2. Cassidy JT, Petty RE. Textbook of Pediatric Rheumatology. 3rd Ed. Philadelphia: WB Saunders, 1995

3. Athreya BH. Vasculitis in children. Pediatr Clin North Am 1995;42:1239–1261

4. Ilan Y, Naparstek Y. Schönlein-Henoch syndrome in adults and children. Semin Arthritis Rheum 1991;21:103–109

5. Farley TA, Gillespie S, Rasoulpour M et al. Epidemiology of a cluster of Henoch-Schönlein purpura. Am J Dis Child 1989;143:798–803

6. Stewart M, Savage JM, Bell B, McCord B. Long term renal prognosis of Henoch-Schönlein purpura in an unselected childhood population. Eur J Pediatr 1988;147:113–115

7. Koskimies O, Mir S, Rapola J, Vilska J. Henoch-Schönlein nephritis: long-term prognosis of unselected patients. Arch Dis Child 1981;56:482–484

8. White RHR. Henoch-Schönlein purpura. In: Churg A, Churg J, Eds. Systemic Vasculitides. New York: Igaku-Shoin, 1991

9. Sahn DJ, Schwartz AD. Schönlein-Henoch syndrome: observations on some atypical clinical presentations. Pediatrics 1972;49:614–616

10. Gairdner D. The Schönlein-Henoch syndrome (anaphylactoid purpura). Q J Med 1948;17:95–122

11. Rosenblum ND, Winter HS. Steroid effects on the course of abdominal pain in children with Henoch-Schönlein purpura. Pediatrics 1987;79:1018–1021

12. Martinez-Frontanilla LA, Haase GM, Ernster JA, Bailey WC. Surgical complications in Henoch-Schönlein purpura. J Pediatr Surg 1984;19:434–436

13. Feldt R, Stickler G. The gastrointestinal manifestations of anaphylactoid purpura in children. Proc Mayo Clin 1962;137:465–483

14. Glasier CM, Siegel MJ, McAlister WH, Shackelford GD. Henoch-Schönlein syndrome in children: gastrointestinal manifestations. AJR 1981;136:1081–1085

15. Okano M, Suzuki T, Takayasu H et al. Anaphylactoid purpura with intestinal perforation: report of a case and review of the Japanese literature. Pathol Int 1994;44:303–308

16. Kagimoto S. Duodenal findings on ultrasound in children with Schönlein-Henoch purpura and gastrointestinal symptoms. J Pediatr Gastroenterol Nutr 1993;16:178–182

17. Amemoto K, Nagita A, Aoki S et al. Ultrasonographic gallbladder wall thickening in children with Henoch-Schönlein purpura. J Pediatr Gastroenterol Nutr 1994;19:126–128

18. Goldman LP, Lindenberg RL. Henoch-Schoenlein purpura:

gastrointestinal manifestations with endoscopic correlation. Am J Gastroenterol 1981;75:357–360

19. Kato S, Shibuya H, Naganuma H, Nakagawa H. Gastrointestinal endoscopy in Henoch-Schönlein purpura. Eur J Pediatr 1992;151:482–484

20. DiFebo G, Gizzi G, Biasco G, Miglioli M. Colonic involvement in adult patients with Henoch-Schoenlein purpura. Endoscopy. 1984;16:36–39

21. Lopez LR, Schocket RE et al. Gastrointestinal involvement in leukocytoclastic vasculitis and polyarteritis nodosa. J Rheumatol 1980;7:677–684

22. Garner JAM. Acute pancreatitis as a complication of anaphylactoid (Henoch-Schönlein) purpura. Arch Dis Child 1977;52:971–972

23. Lombard KA, Shah PC, Thrasher TV, Grill BB. Ileal stricture as a late complication of Henoch-Schönlein purpura. Pediatrics 1986;77:396–398

24. Mohammed R. Acute appendicitis: a complication of Henoch-Schönlein purpura. J Coll Surg Edinb 1982;27:367

25. Davin J, Mahieu P. Sequential measurements of intestinal permeability to [^{51}Cr] EDTA in children with Henoch-Schönlein purpura nephritis. Nephron 1992;60:498–499

26. Austin HA, Balow JE. Henoch-Schönlein nephritis: prognostic features and the challenge of therapy. Am J Kidney Dis 1983;11:512–519

27. Ansell BM. Henoch-Schönlein purpura with particular reference to the prognosis of the renal lesion. Br J Dermatol 1979;82:211–215

28. Lie JT, et al. Illustrated histopathologic classification criteria for selected vasculitis syndromes. Arthritis Rheum 1990;33:1074–1087

29. O'Regan S, Robitaille P. Orchitis mimicking testicular torsion in Henoch-Schönlein's purpura. J Urol 1981;126:834–835

30. Loh HS, Jalan OM. Testicular torsion in Henoch-Schönlein syndrome. BMJ 1974;2:96–97

31. Melloul MM, Garty BZ. Radionuclide scrotal imaging in anaphylactoid purpura. Clin Nucl Med 1993;18:298–301

32. Lewis IC, Philpott MG. Neurological complications in the Schönlein-Henoch syndrome. Arch Dis Child 1956;31:369–371

33. Belman AL, Leicher CR, Moshe SL, Mezey AP. Neurologic manifestations of Schönlein-Henoch purpura: report of three cases and review of the literature. Pediatrics 1985;75:687–692

34. Olson J, Kelly K, Pan C, Wortmann DW. Pulmonary disease with hemorrhage in Henoch-Schoenlein purpura. Pediatrics 1992;89:1177–1181

35. Mills J, Michel B, Bloch D et al. The American College of Rheumatology 1990 Criteria for the Classification of Henoch-Schönlein purpura. Arthritis Rheum 1990;33:1114–1121

36. Garcia-Fuentes M, Martin A, Chantler C, Williams DG. Serum complement components in Henoch-Schönlein purpura. Arch Dis Child 1978;53:417–419

37. Petersen S, Taaning E, Soderstrom T et al. Immunoglobulin and complement studies in children with Schönlein-Henoch syndrome and other vasculitic diseases. Acta Paediatr Scand 1991;80:1037–1043

38. Saulsbury FT, Kirkpatrick PR, Boulton WK. IgA antineutrophil cytoplasmic antibody in Henoch-Schönlein purpura. Am J Nephrol 1991;11:295–300

39. Ronda N, Esnault VLM, Layward L et al. Antineutrophil cytoplasm antibodies (ANCA) of IgA isotype in adult Henoch-Schönlein purpura. Clin Exp Immunol 1994;95:49–55

40. Mollica F, LiVolti S, Garozszo R, Russo G. Effectiveness of early prednisone treatment in preventing the development of nephropathy in anaphylactoid purpura. Eur J Pediatr 1992;151:140–144

41. Temmel AFP, Emminger W, Schroth B et al. Early prednisone treatment and nephropathy in anaphylactoid purpura. Eur J Pediatr 1993;152:782–783

42. Saulsbury F. Corticosteroid therapy does not prevent nephritis in Henoch-Schönlein purpura. Pediatr Nephrol 1993;7:69–71

29

HIRSCHSPRUNG'S DISEASE

CARLO DI LORENZO

Hirschsprung's disease is the most common cause of lower intestinal obstruction in neonates and is a rare cause of intractable constipation in toddlers and school-age children.[1] It is characterized by the total absence of ganglion cells in the myenteric and submucosal plexuses, with overgrowth of nerve trunks in the submucosa, muscularis mucosa, and lamina propria. The aganglionic segment begins at the internal anal sphincter and extends proximally for a variable distance. In 75% of cases, the disease is limited to the rectosigmoid area. It rarely extends beyond the colon. The smooth muscle of the aganglionic segment has a normal tone and a normal response to neurotransmitters, supporting the neurogenic nature of the disease.

PATHOPHYSIOLOGY

Hirschsprung's disease is characterized by a failure of the craniocaudal migration along the gastrointestinal (GI) tract of ganglion cell precursors deriving from neural crest cells. The normal migration of the neural elements begins in the proximal gut at about 5 weeks gestation and is completed by 12 weeks gestation. Recent studies have identified factors that control the migration, proliferation, maturation, and colonization of the neural crest cells in the fetal intestine. In some familial and sporadic cases of Hirschsprung's disease, mutations on the receptor tyrosine kinase RET proto-oncogene found on chromosome 10q 11.1 have been detected.[2] Receptor tyrosine kinase are cell surface molecules that control cell growth and differentiation. However, there are cases with no

abnormalities of this gene, suggesting that other factors must play a pathogenetic role. An animal model of Hirschsprung's disease has demonstrated an abnormal extracellular matrix of the GI tract, preventing normal neural cell migration into a segment of distal bowel.[3] This new "abnormal microenvironment" hypothesis explains both the congenital absence of ganglion cells in the colon and the range of other enteric neuronal abnormalities that may be found in children, including neuronal intestinal dysplasia, hypoganglionosis, and segmental aganglionosis.[4]

The loss of intrinsic innervation of the distal colon leads to overexpression of the extrinsic parasympathetic and sympathetic nerves, which stimulate unopposed contraction. As a result, the internal anal sphincter does not relax and the aganglionic segment is in a state of constant contraction. The bowel proximal to the aganglionic zone becomes dilated due to the functional distal obstruction.

CLINICAL PRESENTATION

The incidence of Hirschsprung's disease is approximately 1 in 5,000 live births, with approximately 700 new cases diagnosed every year in the United States. The incidence is equal for white and black infants. The overall male-to-female ratio is 3.8 : 1. When the aganglionosis extends beyond the sigmoid colon, the ratio is 2.8 : 1 and in total aganglionosis 2.2 : 1.[5] A family history of Hirschsprung's disease is reported in 7% of cases, increasing to 21% in cases of total colonic aganglionosis with or without small bowel involvement.[5] The incidence in siblings is approximately 3.5% overall, with a higher incidence in brothers of affected girls (18%) than in sisters of affected boys (0.6%). Hirschsprung's disease is not associated with prematurity, and the birth weight is usually appropriate for gestational age. Children with Hirschsprung's disease have a greater than expected incidence of Down's syndrome (2.9%) and cardiac anomalies (2.5%). Disorders associated with Hirschsprung's disease include Waardenberg syndrome, Laurence-Moon-Biedl syndrome, Smith-Lemli-Opitz syndrome, and congenital central hypoventilation (Ondine's curse). Chromosomal anomalies found with increased frequency in Hirschsprung's disease include trisomy 21 and deletion of chromosome 13q.[6]

More than 90% of normal neonates, as compared with less than 10% of children with Hirschsprung's disease, pass meconium during the first 24 hours of life.[7] Thus, a delayed passage of meconium by a full-term infant should raise the suspicion of Hirschsprung's disease. Other newborns with Hirschsprung's disease present with bilious vomiting, abdominal distention, and refusal to feed, suggesting intestinal obstruction. Perforation of the small intestine, appendix, or colon may follow. Rectal examination and radiologic studies are needed to rule out causes of mechanical obstruction, such as imperforate anus, meconium ileus, intestinal atresia, or tumors such as a teratoma.

Enterocolitis is a dreaded complication of Hirschsprung's disease. It occurs most often during the second and third month of life and is associated with 20% mortality. It is more common in children with long segment Hirschsprung's disease and is characterized by the sudden onset of fever; explosive, liquid and at times bloody stools; and abdominal distention. Enterocolitis may also occur after surgical treatment of Hirschsprung's disease. No specific organism has been isolated, and the pathogenesis of enterocolitis remains unclear. Treatment involves broad-spectrum antibiotics (including coverage for anaerobes), intravenous fluid resuscitation, nasogastric decompression, and saline enemas for colonic decompression. Serial radiographs of the abdomen are needed to monitor bowel distention and possible perforation. Enterocolitis and bowel perforation remain the major causes of mortality in Hirschsprung's disease.

Some infants with Hirschsprung's disease who pass meconium within the first day of life subsequently present with infrequent bowel movements and with recurrent obstructive crises or impaction. This is particularly common in exclusively breast-fed infants, who may remain asymptomatic until weaning. Subjects with a short segment Hirschsprung's disease may go undiagnosed until childhood. They have ribbon-like stools and an enlarged abdomen with prominent veins; many fail to thrive. In only 5% of patients, constipation is the only symptom. Encopresis is even more rare and occurs only when the aganglionic segment is extremely short (less than 5 cm).

DIAGNOSIS

The diagnosis of Hirschsprung's disease is made in 40% of infants during the first 3 months of life, and in 60% of infants by 12 months.[7] However, 8% to 20% remain unrecognized after the age of 3 years.[7,8] Physical examination reveals a distended abdomen and a contracted anal sphincter and rectum in most of the children. The rectum is devoid of stools, except in cases of short segment aganglionosis. As the finger is withdrawn, there is an explosive discharge of foul-smelling liquid stools, with decompression of the proximal normal bowel.

Radiographic Testing

During the neonatal period, a plain radiograph of the abdomen displays gaseous distention of the bowel, often with evidence of obstruction and absence of gas in the pelvis. In the older child, it may only show large amounts of gas and stools. Often, a single contrast barium enema demonstrates Hirschsprung's disease by exhibiting a "transition zone," a funnel-shaped area between the narrowed aganglionic distal segment and the dilated ganglionic proximal bowel (Fig. 29-1). The enema should be performed in an unprepared patient by introducing a small amount of radiopaque material in the colon, with the tip of the catheter placed just within the anal canal. A 24-hour film showing large amounts of retained barium increases suspicion of Hirschsprung's disease. The barium enema is less diagnos-

FIGURE 29-1. Anteroposterior view of a barium enema examination, showing a narrowed rectosigmoid, a transition zone, and a dilated left colon in a child with Hirschsprung's disease. (Courtesy of T. Bender, M.D.)

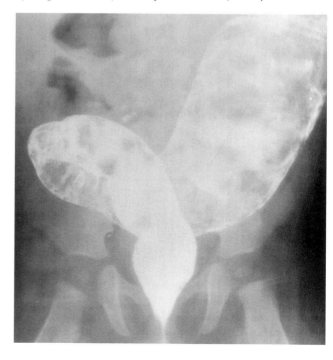

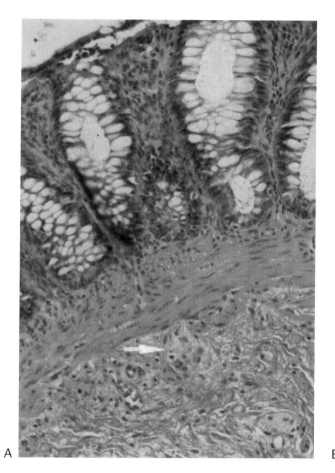 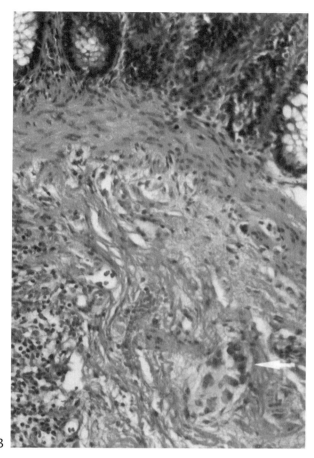

FIGURE 29-2. Rectal suction biopsies. (*A*) Hematoxylin-eosin staining (×100) in a child without Hirschsprung's disease. Ganglion cells in the submucosa are generally found in clusters (arrow). (*B*) Seen at higher magnification (×200) the ganglion cells have large nuclei and abundant cytoplasm (arrow) containing peripheral hematoxyphilic Nissl substance.

tic during the first 2 to 3 weeks of life, before severe dilation of the proximal bowel has occurred. It may also be difficult to interpret cases of total colonic or short segment Hirschsprung's disease in children whose transition zone is less evident.

Rectal Suction Biopsy

Rectal suction biopsies obtained 2 to 3 cm above the anal verge are diagnostic of Hirschsprung's disease. These biopsies demonstrate the absence of neuron cell bodies (ganglion cells) in the submucosal plexus. The biopsy should be deep enough to include adequate submucosa. Confirmation is obtained if the acetylcholinesterase staining is positive (Fig. 29-2). Interpretation of biopsies in short segment Hirschsprung's disease is difficult because there is normally a hypoganglionic area 2 to 3 cm proximal to the dentate line. Absence of neurons plus a negative acetylcholinesterase may indicate total colonic

aganglionosis. Bleeding and perforation are rare complications when a suction apparatus is used to obtain rectal biopsies. Occasionally, a suction biopsy is not diagnostic, and a full-thickness surgical biopsy is required.

Anorectal Manometry

In a cooperative child, anorectal manometry is a very sensitive and specific test for diagnosing Hirschsprung's disease. It is especially useful when the aganglionic segment is short. Manometry investigates the response of the anal sphincters to balloon distention of the rectum. Lack of relaxation of the internal anal sphincter upon rectal distention (rectoanal inhibitory reflex) is diagnostic of Hirschsprung's disease. In the presence of normal sphincter relaxation, further studies to diagnose Hirschsprung's disease are unnecessary. It should be emphasized that manometry is not readily available at most centers, and special expertise is needed to differentiate physiologic phenomena from artifacts.

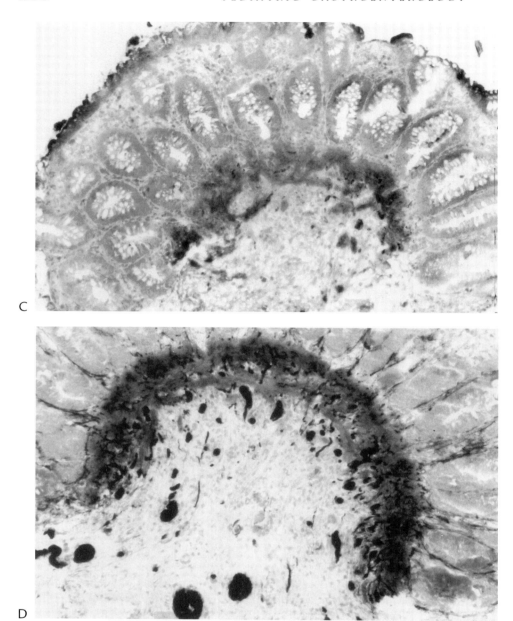

FIGURE 29-2. *(Continued) (C)* Acetylcholinesterase staining of a normal colon
(×75). There is no excess of thick submucosal nerve trunks, no increase in dark-stain-
ing neural fibers in the muscularis mucosa, and no excess of staining fibers in the
lamina propria. Profiles of neural units are not well seen at this magnification. *(D)*
Acetylcholinesterase staining of the aganglionic region of a child with Hirschsprung's
disease (×75), showing hypertrophic nerve trunks in the submucosa, thick neural fibers in the muscularis mucosae, and an excess of fine fibers in the lamina propria.
(Courtesy of R. Jaffe, M.D.)

Other Disorders

Rectal biopsies may also be used to diagnose more rare
colon neuropathies presenting with symptoms overlapping those of Hirschsprung's disease.[10] Both hypo- and
hyperganglionosis have been associated with constipa-

tion, although a pathologic diagnosis is often difficult due
to the lack of age and location of control specimens.[11,12]
Neuronal intestinal dysplasia is characterized by hyperplasia of the submucosal plexus and by increased numbers
of acetylcholinesterase-positive nerve fibers in the ad-
ventitia of submucosal blood vessels. It has been sug-

gested[13] that the incidence of neuronal intestinal dysplasia is similar to Hirschsprung's disease and that it can be associated with Hirschsprung's disease (proximal to the aganglionic segment).

In the older child presenting only with constipation, a careful history should be obtained with regard to the timing of the abnormal stool pattern, withholding behaviors, anal fissures (bleeding), and encopresis. A thorough physical examination is usually sufficient to differentiate functional constipation from Hirschsprung's disease (Table 29-1). In functional constipation, stool fills the colon, beginning with the distal segment. Rectal examination demonstrates the presence of a large amount of fecal material occupying a dilated rectal vault.

At times one may appreciate pigmented, vascular, or hairy patches over the lumbosacral spine, suggestive of occult spinal dysraphism, another cause of constipation not responsive to conventional medical management.[9] In children with low sacral lesions, constipation and urinary incontinence or retention may be the only symptoms. When the child is old enough to cooperate, light touch sensibility in the sacral dermatomeres can be tested using a wisp of cotton at the end of an applicator. Reflex contraction of the external anal sphincter in response to stroking of the perianal skin, the "anal wink," is evidence of the integrity of the sensorimotor apparatus of fecal continence.

LABORATORY STUDIES

Laboratory and radiologic studies are used to rule out other conditions that must be differentiated from Hirschsprung's disease. When enterocolitis is present, sepsis, necrotizing enterocolitis, cow's milk-induced colitis, and infectious colitis must be excluded. In infants in whom constipation is the main symptom, appropriate laboratory tests may be used to rule out hypothyroidism, hypokalemia, hypercalcemia, infant botulism, adrenal insufficiency, and tumors (e.g., neuroblastoma, lymphoma, rhabdomyosarcoma). In the older child with constipation, the differential diagnosis also includes diabetes mellitus, dermatomyositis, scleroderma, lead poisoning, and the use of constipating drugs, such as anticholinergics, opioids, iron, and aluminum-containing antacids.

TREATMENT

Surgery is the only safe and effective treatment of Hirschsprung's disease. The role of medical treatment is to stabilize the child during the preoperative period by correcting fluid and electrolyte imbalances, especially if enterocolitis is present. Before surgery, it is also important to decompress the bowel with warm saline irrigations through a carefully inserted rectal cannula. Bowel irrigations are carried out until the effluent is clear. This

TABLE 29-1. Distinguishing Features Between Childhood Functional Constipation and Hirschsprung's Disease

Feature	Functional Constipation	Hirschsprung's Disease
Onset	2–3 yr	At birth
Delayed passage of meconium	Rare	Common
Obstructive symptoms	Rare	Common
Withholding behavior	Common	Rare
Fear of defecation	Common	Rare
Fecal incontinence	Common	Rare
Stool size	Very large	Small, ribbon-like
Poor growth	Rare	Common
Enterocolitis	Never	Possible
Rectal ampulla	Enlarged	Narrowed
Stool in ampulla	Common	Rare
Barium enema	Massive amount of stools, no transitional zone	Transitional zone, delayed emptying
Anorectal manometry	Normal	Absent rectosphincteric reflex
Rectal biopsy	Normal	No ganglion cells, increased acetylcholinesterasic activity

procedure will almost immediately improve symptoms of abdominal distention and toxicity in infants with enterocolitis. Curative surgery consists of resection of the aganglionic bowel and reanastomosis of the proximal normal bowel to the anal canal. Traditionally, in infants a stoma is placed proximal to the aganglionic segment, above the transition zone. Intraoperative frozen sections are obtained to ensure that the ostomy is placed in the ganglionic bowel. Definitive surgery is then performed when the child is 6 to 12 months of age and weighs at least 15 pounds.

Other surgeons prefer a single-stage operative repair.[14] Laparoscopic pull-through for treatment of Hirschsprung's disease in children has also been reported.[15] In the older child presenting with an extremely dilated colon, placement of an ostomy allows the colon to return to a more normal size before it is pulled through the narrow pelvis. The three operations most often performed are those described by Swenson, Soave, and Duhamel (Fig. 29-3). In all these procedures, the goal is to leave the distal 1 cm of anorectum intact, preserving the sensitive anoderm and allowing for future continence and control of defecation. Most ostomies are removed at definitive surgery. Selection of the type of operation is based on the bias and experience of the surgeon. A detailed description of these techniques is beyond the scope of this discussion. Very short aganglionic segments can be treated successfully by anorectal myectomy and internal sphincterotomy.[16]

The most common immediate postoperative complications include anastomotic leaks and strictures. There may be a transient urinary incontinence secondary to pelvic dissection. In children with long segment disease involving the whole colon and much of the small intestine, problems of fluid loss, malabsorption, and electrolyte imbalance are common. These children should be managed as if they have short bowel syndrome. In a sizable minority of children, constipation persists after surgery.[17] This may be because of residual disease or an association with neuronal intestinal dysplasia.[13] Anorectal testing shows that most children with Hirschsprung's disease continue to have an abnormal internal anal sphincter pressure and relaxation.[18] Fecal incontinence has also been reported[19] in up to 80% of children regardless of the type of surgery received and the extent of the aganglionic segment. The prevalence of incontinence did not diminish with increasing age. A second surgery may succeed when the first surgery has failed,[20] but very careful assessment of intestinal and colonic motility is necessary before further surgery is planned.[21]

FIGURE 29-3. Surgical procedures most commonly used in the management of Hirschsprung's disease. Shaded areas identify normal colon. (*A*) Swenson procedure. The normal colon is anastomosed to the distal 1 to 2 cm of aganglionic rectum. An internal sphincterotomy is often performed. (*B*) Soave procedure. The mucosa of the aganglionic segment is stripped off, and the normal colon is pulled through the preserved muscular cuff and anastomosed about 1 cm above the dentate line. The internal sphincter remains intact and pelvic nerves are exposed to no damage. (*C*) Duhamel procedure. The normal colon is brought down through the retrorectal space and anastomosed obliquely to the posterior wall of the aganglionic rectum with a stapler.

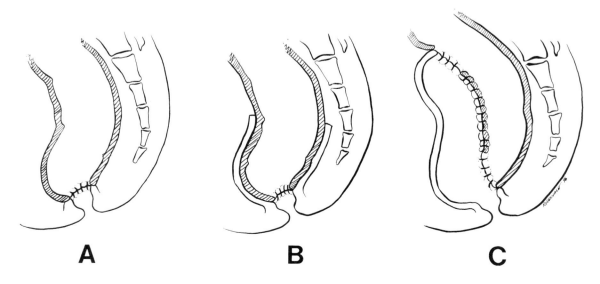

A   **B**   **C**

REFERRAL PATTERN

The most important factor in reducing the morbidity and mortality associated with Hirschsprung's disease is recognition of the condition before enterocolitis occurs. Any full-term infant who has not passed meconium during the first 24 hours of life, and who does not have a mechanical obstruction should not leave the hospital without being referred to a pediatric gastroenterologist or surgeon to rule out Hirschsprung's disease. Referral to a pediatric gastroenterologist is also indicated in older children with severe constipation[22] not responsive to conventional medical management.

REFERENCES

1. Hyman PE, Fleisher D: Functional fecal retention. Pract Gastroenterol 1992;16:29–37

2. Edery P, Lyonnet S, Mulligan LM et al. Mutation of the RET proto-oncogene in Hirschsprung's disease. Nature 1994; 367:378–380

3. Jacobs-Cohen RJ, Payette RF, Gershon MD, Rothman TP. Inability of neural crest to colonize the presumptive aganglionic bowel of Is/Is mutant mice: requirement for a permissive microenvironment. J Comp Neurol 1987;255:425–438

4. Sullivan PB. Hirschsprung's disease. Arch Dis Child 1996; 74:5–7

5. Klinhaus S, Boley SJ, Sheran M, Sieber WK. Hirschsprung's disease: a survey of the members of the surgical section of the American Academy of Pediatrics. J Pediatr Surg 1979; 14:588–600

6. Rudolph C, Benaroch L. Hirschsprung's disease. Pediatr Rev 1995;16:5–11

7. Swenson O, Sherman JO, Fisher JH. Diagnosis of congenital megacolon: an analysis of 501 patients. J Pediatr Surg 1973; 8:587–594

8. Landman GB. A five-year chart review of children biopsied to rule out Hirschsprung's disease. Clin Pediatr 1987;26: 288–291

9. Anderson, F. Occult spinal dysraphism: a series of 73 cases. Pediatrics 1975;55:826–835

10. Krishnamurthy S, Heng Y, Shuffler MD. Chronic intestinal pseudo-obstruction in infants and children caused by diverse abnormalities of the myenteric plexus. Gastroenterology 1993;104:1398–1408

11. Milla PJ, Smith VV. Aganglionosis, hypoganglionosis and hyperganglionosis: clinical presentation and histopathology. In: Kamm M, Lennard-Jones JE, Eds: Constipation. Petersfield, UK: Wrightson Biomedical, 1994:183–192

12. Schofield DE, Yunis EJ. Intestinal neuronal dysplasia. J Pediatr Gastroenterol Nutr 1991;12:182–189

13. Fadda B, Pistor G, Meier-Ruge W et al. Symptoms, diagnosis, and therapy of neuronal intestinal dysplasia masked by Hirschsprung's disease. Pediatr Surg Int 1987;2:76–80

14. Carassonne M, Morisson-Lacombe G, LeTourneau JN. Primary corrective operation without decompression in infants less than three months of age with Hirschsprung's disease. J Pediatr Surg 1982;17:241–243

15. Georgeson KE, Fuenfer MM, Hardin WD. Primary laparoscopic pull-through for Hirschsprung's disease in infants and children. J Pediatr Surg 1995;30:1017–1022

16. Lynn HB, van Heerdan JA. Rectal myectomy in Hirschsprung's disease. Arch Surg 1975;110:991–994

17. Helij HA, de Vries X, Bremer I et al. Long-term anorectal function after Duhamel operation for Hirschsprung's disease. J Pediatr Surg 1995;30:430–432

18. Mishalany HG, Wooley MM. Postoperative functional and manometric evaluation of patients with Hirschsprung's disease. J Pediatr Surg 1987;22:443–446

19. Catto-Smith AG, Coffey CMM, Nolan TM, Hutson JM. Fecal incontinence after the surgical treatment of Hirschsprung's disease. J Pediatr 1995;127:954–957

20. Velcek FT, Klotz DH, Friedman A, Kottmeier PK. Operative failure and secondary repair in Hirschsprung's disease. J Pediatr Surg 1982;17:779–785

21. Redmond JM, Smith GW, Barofsky I et al. Physiological tests to predict long term outcome of total abdominal colectomy for intractable constipation. Am J Gastroenterol 1995; 90:748–753

22. Powell RW. Hirschsprung's disease in adolescents. Am Surg 1989;55:212–218

30

INFLAMMATORY BOWEL DISEASE

JEFFREY S. HYAMS

Ulcerative colitis and Crohn's disease are idiopathic chronic conditions affecting the gastrointestinal (GI) system that are generically grouped under the term *inflammatory bowel disease* (IBD). Approximately 30% of all newly diagnosed cases of inflammatory bowel disease occur in people aged 20 years or younger; thus, clinicians dealing with children and adolescents need to be able to recognize the multifaceted presentations of these disorders.

ETIOLOGY

Despite decades of intensive research, the cause or causes of inflammatory bowel disease remain unknown. It is still not clear if ulcerative colitis and Crohn's disease represent entirely different diseases with similar clinical manifestations, or whether they are two forms of a single pathophysiologic disorder. A detailed discussion of the epidemiology and pathophysiologic mechanisms of IBD is beyond the scope of this book, and only a summary will be presented. Additional readings are suggested.[1–3]

EPIDEMIOLOGY

The incidence of IBD is highest in Scandinavian, western European, and North American countries and lowest in Asia, Africa, and South America. It is more common in Jews than non-Jews and in urban compared to rural areas. Smoking appears to be protective for ulcerative colitis and permissive for Crohn's disease.

GENETICS

Although ulcerative colitis and Crohn's disease are not inherited in a readily demonstrable recessive or dominant fashion, many studies have shown a strong genetic predisposition to these disorders.[4,5] At the diagnosis of either disorder, the likelihood of finding IBD in a first-degree relative is 10% to 25%. Approximately 7% of siblings of children in whom IBD develops will themselves also be affected during their lifetime. When more than one family member is affected with Crohn's disease, the distribution of affected bowel is often strikingly similar.

INFECTIOUS AGENTS

It has been suggested that IBD represents either a persistent infection with a fastidious organism or an abnormal and prolonged response to a common pathogen. Because of the granulomatous nature of the inflammatory process in Crohn's disease, aggressive attempts to identify mycobacterial agents have been made. To date, no definitive evidence has been demonstrated that a mycobacterium or any other infectious agent is of primary importance in the pathogenesis of IBD.

IMMUNOLOGIC FACTORS

Histologic examination of the normal large and small intestine demonstrates a modest degree of infiltration with monocytes, macrophages, lymphocytes, plasma cells, and eosinophils. These cells, as well as those found in lymphoid aggregates (Peyer's patches), represent what is termed *gut-associated lymphoid tissue* (GALT). This system constitutes an important component of the defensive barrier to the enormous antigenic load associated with normal diet, as well as to the micro-organisms that inhabit the intestinal lumen. The customary amount of inflammatory cells found here is said to be consistent with "physiologic" inflammation. This physiologic inflammation is controlled by the counterbalancing forces of a variety of glycosylated peptides referred to as cytokines. These peptides exert both a proinflammatory and an immunoregulatory role. It is currently believed that IBD may represent an aberration in this normal balance with exaggeration of "physiologic" inflammation into pathologic inflammation and tissue destruction. The defect may be at many levels, including increased antigen uptake through a leaky gut epithelium, defective antigen processing, abnormal vascular endothelial cell function, and abnormalities in the production of interleukins and eicosanoids.[6]

PATHOPHYSIOLOGY

Active inflammation in the small and large intestine leads to a number of physiologic abnormalities that result in diarrhea, protein-losing enteropathy, bleeding, abdominal pain, and stricture formation. Proinflammatory cytokines and eicosanoids increase vascular permeability and vasodilation, cause electrolyte secretion, and augment smooth muscle contraction. Inflamed epithelium leaks intravascular proteins. Many cytokines promote the recruitment and activity of collagen forming cells leading to fibrous tissue proliferation resulting in bowel wall thickening and stricture formation.

PATHOLOGY AND DISEASE DISTRIBUTION

While many similarities exist in the pathologic expression of ulcerative colitis and Crohn's disease, certain characteristics will always establish a firm diagnosis of Crohn's disease.

Crohn's Disease

Involvement of the small intestine establishes the diagnosis of Crohn's disease. The widespread use of endoscopy and advanced techniques of contrast radiography have now firmly demonstrated that the alimentary tract beyond the colon is involved in 90% of all affected individuals. Classically, the terminal ileum is the most common site, but other areas of the small intestine, as well

as esophagus and stomach, may be involved as well. The small bowel or colon is thickened and nodular, often with frank ulceration. Fistulas are thought to arise when transmural bowel inflammation extends through the serosa into adjacent structures such as bowel, bladder, vagina, or perineum. Colonic involvement may occur in isolation (Crohn's colitis, granulomatous colitis) in about 10% to 15% of patients and may involve the whole colon or isolated segments. Sixty per cent of all affected children have colonic and ileal disease (ileocolitis). Perirectal disease is seen in about 20% of cases and is usually accompanied by rectosigmoid inflammation. Noncaseating granuloma, the hallmark of Crohn's disease, is found in about 30% of all cases.

Ulcerative Colitis

In contradistinction to Crohn's disease where inflammation may become transmural, the process is generally limited to the mucosa in ulcerative colitis. Almost always starting in the rectum, the inflammatory process is homogeneous in appearance and extends proximally a variable distance. Approximately 5% of affected children have proctitis only, 10% to 15% proctosigmoiditis, 30% to 40% disease to the splenic flexure, and 50% pancolitis.[7] The findings of crypt abscesses, architectural distortion, and goblet cell depletion are typical of ulcerative colitis but nonspecific.

CLINICAL PRESENTATION

Gastrointestinal Manifestations

ULCERATIVE COLITIS

Bloody mucoid diarrhea is the most common initial symptom associated with ulcerative colitis. Occasionally, affected individuals will initially note more frequent and looser stools before they become bloody. Lower abdominal pain is usually mild at first and invariably associated with defecation. Nausea and vomiting at defecation may be reported, especially with more severe disease. Fulminant disease occurs in about 10% to 15% of patients and is defined by the presence of 6 or more bloody stools per day, abdominal tenderness, fever, tachycardia, anemia (hematocrit <30%), and hypoalbuminemia. Anorexia and weight loss may be seen but are less common than in Crohn's disease. In patients with proctitis, the stools are frequently formed and constipation may be reported.

Colonic carcinoma is a complication of longstanding ulcerative colitis with estimates putting the risk at 1% by 10 years of disease and then increasing in a cumulative fashion by 1% to 2% per year thereafter.

CROHN'S DISEASE

Abdominal pain and systemic symptoms are generally more severe in Crohn's disease than in ulcerative colitis, and the sites of GI involvement often dictate the particular mode of presentation. Abdominal pain is the most common symptom and tends to be severe enough to affect activity and may awaken the patient from sleep. With terminal ileal and right colon involvement, it is most prominent in the right lower quadrant; examination may indicate a tender fullness or mass. Gastroduodenal involvement produces a dyspeptic-type pain localized to the epigastrium and periumbilical region, and is often associated with vomiting. Diarrhea or rectal bleeding, or both, may or may not be present. With colonic involvement, diarrhea and rectal bleeding may be severe and may resemble ulcerative colitis. Recurrent aphthous lesions in the mouth are common. Perirectal disease including fissures, fistulas, and skin tags is present in 10% to 15% of subjects at the diagnosis.

Intestinal obstruction is common and results from the continued inflammation and scarring of involved bowel. Transmural bowel inflammation with fistulization and perforation may lead to the formation of abscesses that may be located in several areas, including interloop, intramesenteric, retroperitoneal-ileopsoas, or subdiaphragmatic. Recent observations suggest that carcinoma may develop in long-standing Crohn's colitis with similar frequency to that observed in ulcerative colitis.

Extraintestinal Manifestations

Extraintestinal manifestations may precede gastrointestinal ones, be present concomitantly, or may occur months to years after the diagnosis of IBD has been made. A partial listing of the more important ones is shown in Table 30-1.

SYSTEMIC

Fever may be a prominent finding in Crohn's disease, even in the absence of severe GI symptoms. In ulcerative colitis, the presence of fever is a sign of fulminant disease. Malaise is common in both disorders. Anorexia and weight loss may be present in 30% to 40% of subjects with Crohn's disease and in 10% of those with ulcerative colitis. Growth delay and delayed sexual development may be the presenting picture of Crohn's disease with GI symptoms mild or absent. Growth abnormalities are usually associated with chronic undernutrition. High-dose daily corticosteroid therapy may significantly impair linear growth.

LOCALIZED

More than 100 localized extraintestinal manifestations of IBD have been described.[8] The more common ones will be briefly discussed.

TABLE 30-1. Extraintestinal Manifestations of Inflammatory Bowel Disease

Skin	Liver/biliary tract
Erythema nodosum	Sclerosing cholangitis
Pyoderma gangrenosum	Chronic hepatitis
Perianal disease	Gallstones
Joints	Cirrhosis
Arthralgia	Bone
Arthritis	Osteopenia
Ankylosing spondylitis	Osteonecrosis
Sacroiliitis	Renal/urologic
Hypertrophic osteoarthropathy (clubbing)	Stones
Eyes	Hydronephrosis
Uveitis	Enterovesical fistula
Episcleritis	Vascular
Keratitis	Thrombophlebitis
Retinal vasculitis	Vasculitis
Cataract	Extraintestinal cancer
Hematologic	Lymphoma
Iron deficiency	Acute myelocytic leukemia
Anemia of chronic disease	
Folate deficiency	
Vitamin B_{12} deficiency	
Thrombocytosis	
Neutropenia	

Skin

The two most common dermatologic manifestations are erythema nodosum and pyoderma gangrenosum. The former is more common in Crohn's disease (3% to 5% of patients) and usually reflects increasing bowel activity. Pyoderma gangrenosum is more common in ulcerative colitis (1% of patients) and does not necessarily reflect disease activity. Rarely, patients with significant malabsorption and malnutrition may develop trace mineral and vitamin deficiencies resulting in rash.

Joints

The presence of either arthralgia or arthritis is the most common localized extraintestinal manifestation and is seen in 30% to 40% of subjects (10% to 15% with frank arthritis). Two forms of more significant joint involvement are seen. A peripheral arthritis may involve any joint but, in decreasing order of frequency, involves knees, ankles, hips, wrists, and elbows.[9] Peripheral arthritis is more common in the presence of colonic inflammation compared to that of the small bowel. Almost 50% of patients with peripheral arthritis also develop ocular inflammation or erythema nodosum. Axial arthropathy (ankylosing spondylitis, sacroiliitis) occurs in 1% to 2% of ulcerative colitis patients and in less than 1% of those with Crohn's disease. In more than 80% of cases, it is associated with HLA-B27. Progression is variable and does not appear to relate to severity of bowel disease.

Eyes

Inflammatory conditions such as uveitis, episcleritis, keratitis, and retinal vasculitis may occur. Patients may be asymptomatic or complain of eye pain, burning, headache, or blurred vision. Increased intraocular pressure and cataract formation may occur in the setting of chronic high-dose systemic corticosteroid therapy.

Liver/Biliary Tract

The two most worrisome hepatobiliary complications of IBD are sclerosing cholangitis and chronic active hepatitis. Sclerosing cholangitis occurs in about 3% of children with ulcerative colitis and in 1% of those with Crohn's disease.[10] Most patients are asymptomatic and diagnosis is based on initial findings of abnormal serum aminotransferases and gamma-glutamyltransferase, with subsequent confirmation of diagnosis by endoscopic retrograde cholangiopancreatography (ERCP). When symptoms develop, they may include jaundice, pruritus, abdominal pain, and evidence of portal hypertension. Chronic active hepatitis may be associated with either Crohn's disease or ulcerative colitis.

Bone

Bone demineralization can occur in the setting of chronic corticosteroid therapy, bed rest, vitamin D deficiency, inadequate calcium intake, protein-calorie malnutrition, and bowel inflammation with the production of cytokines that circulate systemically and interfere with bone metabolism.

Kidneys

Calcium oxalate, calcium phosphate, and uric acid stones may occur. Extensive terminal ileal disease or resection predisposes to oxalate stone formation. The right ureter may become entrapped in a phlegmonous inflammation of the ileum/cecum and result in hydronephrosis.

Vascular

Abnormalities in coagulation including thrombocytosis and activation of the clotting cascade with hyperfibrinogenemia may predispose to thrombophlebitis, rarely involving the CNS.

Hematologic

Anemia is common in both ulcerative colitis and Crohn's disease and may result from iron deficiency, folic acid deficiency, vitamin B_{12} deficiency, hemolysis, bone marrow suppression from medications (e.g., azathioprine), and the anemia of chronic disease. Proinflammatory cytokines have a potent suppressive effect on erythropoiesis by impairing iron metabolism and inhibiting erythropoietin production. An association between IBD

TABLE 30-2. Clinical and Laboratory Findings Used to Establish the Diagnosis of Crohn's Disease

History	Laboratory tests
Abdominal pain	Anemia
Diarrhea	Elevated erythrocyte
Rectal bleeding	sedimentation rate
Fever	(ESR)
Arthritis	Hypoalbuminemia
Rash	Thrombocytosis
Family history of inflammatory	Positive guaiac
bowel disease	Radiology
Physical examination	Nodularity
Abdominal tenderness	Skip areas
Mass	String sign
Perirectal disease	Fistula
Clubbing	Ulceration
Stomatitis	Endoscopy
Erythema nodosum	Ulcers
Pyoderma gangrenosum	Cobblestoning
Growth data	Rectal sparing
Height and weight velocity	
decreases for age	

(Adapted from Hyams,[22] with permission.)

and an increased likelihood of developing extraintestinal malignancy (e.g., lymphoma, acute myelocytic leukemia) has been suggested.

Diagnosis

The diagnosis of inflammatory bowel disease is suggested by a combination of clinical observations and confirmed by laboratory, radiologic, endoscopic, and histologic findings (Table 30-2). Most of the time the data strongly suggest a specific diagnosis of ulcerative colitis or Crohn's disease, but the data are inconclusive in about 10% of cases and the patient is temporarily labeled as having "indeterminate colitis."

HISTORY AND PHYSICAL EXAMINATION

Relevant historic observations are reviewed above. It is imperative that any child or adolescent being evaluated for chronic abdominal pain or diarrhea have careful inspection of the perianal region. Sexual maturity should be assessed and growth data plotted to detect any variance from expected values.

LABORATORY EVALUATION

In the presence of bloody or persistent diarrhea, a careful search for enteric bacterial and protozoal pathogens should be made. A complete blood count should be performed to look for evidence of anemia. A low hemoglobin is found in 40% to 70% of cases and often the mean corpuscular volume is low suggesting iron deficiency. The white blood cell (WBC) count is usually normal or minimally elevated but an increased number of immature band forms is common. Thrombocytosis is seen in 60% of cases and serves as an excellent acute-phase reactant. An elevated erythrocyte sedimentation rate (ESR) is found in 70% of cases of Crohn's disease and 40% of those with ulcerative colitis. A normal ESR never excludes a diagnosis of inflammatory bowel disease.[11]

Stool guaiac should be performed in all cases. Serum albumin is quite helpful in assessing nutritional status as well as monitoring protein-losing enteropathy. Breath hydrogen testing for lactose malabsorption may be helpful in defining the need for dietary restriction.

ENDOSCOPIC EVALUATION

Endoscopic evaluation of the colon should precede barium radiography in the presence of bloody diarrhea. Flexible sigmoidoscopy can be performed in minimally prepared patients and can immediately suggest a diagnosis of ulcerative colitis. The mucosa looks erythematous, granular, friable, and there is a loss of the normal vascular pattern (Fig. 30-1). Colonoscopy may be required to make a diagnosis of Crohn's colitis where rectal sparing

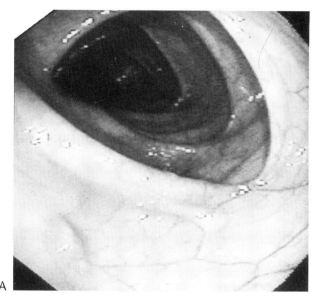

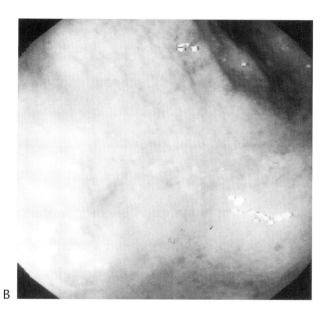

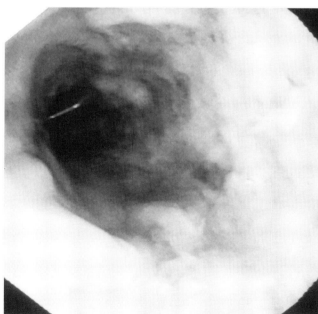

FIGURE 30-1. (*A*) Appearance of normal colonic mucosa with glistening mucosa and normal vascular pattern. (*B*) Colonic mucosa in ulcerative colitis with granularity, friability, and loss of vascular pattern. (*C*) Colonic mucosa in Crohn's colitis with irregular mucosal pattern, linear ulcers, and narrowed bowel lumen.

is common, and inflammation may be patchy in distribution. Normal-appearing colonic mucosa should always be biopsied, since microscopic inflammation and/or granuloma might be present with Crohn's disease. The presence of aphthous lesions, pseudo-polyps (heaped up mucosa), and interspersed normal-appearing mucosa is strongly suggestive of Crohn's disease in the proper clinical setting. If possible, intubation of the terminal ileum should be performed during colonoscopy to assess the ileal mucosa.

RADIOLOGIC EVALUATION

Barium enema is now used less frequently in the diagnosis of inflammatory bowel disease. Flexible sigmoidoscopy and colonoscopy are more sensitive and specific tests and allow for tissue sampling, which may facilitate the diagnosis of other disorders which may mimic inflammatory bowel disease (see below). Because small bowel involvement occurs in 90% of cases of Crohn's disease, a high-quality upper gastrointestinal series with small bowel followthrough is essential. Young children may be unwilling or unable to ingest sufficient barium; in these situations,

barium may need to be given by nasogastric tube. Careful fluoroscopy and abdominal palpation are used to identify irregular, nodular, and thickened bowel loops as well as stenotic areas, ulcers, and fistulas (Fig. 30-2). Abdominal ultrasound and computed tomography are used to evaluate complications of Crohn's disease such as intestinal phlegmon and abscess.

Differential Diagnosis

The multiple modes of presentation of inflammatory bowel disease create a lengthy differential diagnosis of symptoms (Table 30-3). In general, a careful history, physical examination, perusal of growth data, and basic laboratory studies will be able to quickly point the clinician in the correct diagnostic direction.

Therapy

No medical therapy is curative for either ulcerative colitis or Crohn's disease. Colectomy may cure ulcerative colitis, but surgery does not cure Crohn's disease. It is important to remember that treatment regimens should be directed toward relief of symptoms and quality of life,

FIGURE 30-2. (*A*) Terminal ileal nodularity and bowel wall thickening, and cecal deformity characteristic of Crohn's ileocolitis. (*B*) Extensive jejunal Crohn's disease.

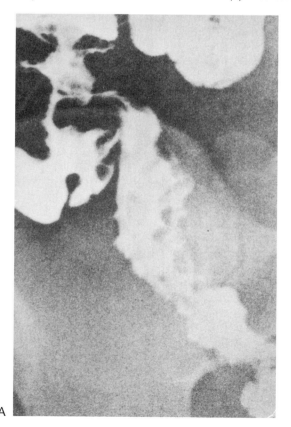

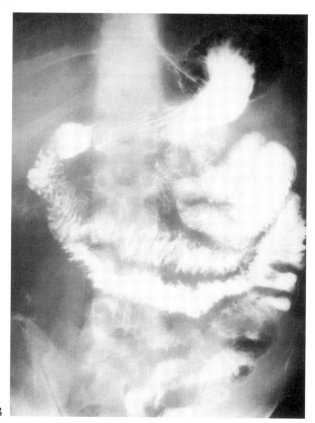

A   B

TABLE 30-3. Differential Diagnosis of Signs and Symptoms Suggesting Inflammatory Bowel Disease

Primary Presenting Symptom	Diagnostic Considerations
Right lower quadrant abdominal pain, with or without mass	Appendicitis, infection (e.g., *Campylobacter*, *Yersinia*), lymphoma, intussusception, mesenteric adenitis, Meckel's diverticulum, ovarian cyst
Chronic periumbilical or epigastric abdominal pain	Irritable bowel, constipation, lactose intolerance, peptic disease
Rectal bleeding, no diarrhea	Fissure, polyp, Meckel's diverticulum, rectal ulcer syndrome
Bloody diarrhea	Infection, hemolytic-uremic syndrome, Henoch-Schönlein purpura, ischemic bowel, radiation colitis
Watery diarrhea	Irritable bowel, lactose intolerance, giardiasis, cryptosporidium, sorbitol, laxatives
Perirectal disease	Fissure, hemorrhoid (rare), streptococcal infection, condyloma (rare)
Growth delay	Endocrinopathy
Anorexia, weight loss	Anorexia nervosa

(Adapted from Hyams,[22] with permission.)

and not necessarily normalization of all laboratory studies. Compliance must be carefully monitored, as failure to take medications correctly is often a cause of treatment failure, particularly in adolescents. A brief review of pharmacologic, nutritional, surgical, and psychosocial treatments will be given.

PHARMACOLOGIC

Currently, five main classes of medications are being used to treat inflammatory bowel disease.

5-Aminosalicylates

Sulfasalazine has been used to treat IBD for almost 50 years, but its use is limited in up to 30% of recipients by the development of GI problems (e.g., nausea, vomiting, abdominal pain, worsening bloody diarrhea) or extraintestinal complications (e.g., rash, Stevens-Johnson reaction, bone marrow toxicity).[12] It is appropriate therapy for mild to moderate ulcerative colitis and Crohn's colitis (dose 50 mg/kg/day). In order to avoid the toxicity associated with the sulfapyridine moiety of sulfasalazine, newer agents which contain only 5-ASA have been developed. Mesalamine may be broken down into its 5-ASA components either in the small bowel or large bowel depending upon the particular formulation. It is used for both ulcerative colitis and Crohn's disease (dose 40 to 60 mg/kg/day). Toxicities include watery or bloody diarrhea, pancreatitis, and nephritis.[13] Mesalamine may also be administered via enema for proctosigmoiditis. Both sulfasalazine and mesalamine are used to induce remission from active colonic disease and then in a prophylactic manner to prevent recurrence.

Corticosteroids

Prednisone remains the drug of choice for moderate to severe ulcerative colitis or Crohn's disease. It is usually initially given in a dose of 1 to 2 mg/kg/day, with a maximum of 40 to 60 mg. Once a patient is in a clinical remission attempts are made to wean the medication to an alternate-day regimen and then discontinue it completely. Side effects of high-dose daily administration may be severe and include cosmetic changes (moon facies, hirsutism, acne), hypertension, bone demineralization, cataracts, depression, insomnia, and growth retardation. Newer corticosteroids such as budesonide are being developed that undergo rapid metabolism in the liver, have lower systemic bioavailability, and fewer side effects.[14]

Antibiotics

Antibiotics are used both as primary therapy for IBD as well as to treat its complications. Metronidazole is primarily used to treat the perirectal fistulas associated with Crohn's disease but may also be effective in Crohn's colitis (dose 10 to 20 mg/kg/day). It may cause a peripheral neuropathy when used in higher doses for extended periods.[15] Ciprofloxacin is also used to treat perirectal disease in adolescents (250 to 500 mg bid). Both medications are used to treat pouchitis, an inflammatory condition occurring in surgically created small bowel reservoirs in the surgical management of ulcerative colitis.

Immunomodulators

The immunomodulators constitute a class of medication that is often used in patients who are refractory to, or dependent on, corticosteroids. 6-Mercaptopurine and azathioprine are the usual agents and given in doses of 1 to 2 mg/kg/day (maximum 100 mg). The duration between start of therapy and onset of action may range from 3 to 9 months.[16] Toxicities include bone marrow depression, pancreatitis, and drug fever.[17] Cyclosporine is now widely being used to treat fulminant ulcerative colitis as well as in limited situations of Crohn's disease.

While short-term efficacy has generally been seen, it does not appear to change the natural history of either disorder.[18]

Antidiarrheal Agents

Loperamide is the drug of choice for decreasing the frequency of diarrhea in patients with IBD. Its use should be considered adjunctive, and it is not used to control severe symptoms. Its use is contraindicated in the setting of severe colitis, as it may precipitate toxic megacolon.

SURGICAL

The indications for surgery in IBD include intractability, uncontrolled hemorrhage, perforation, obstruction, severe fistula formation, growth retardation, and carcinoma. Ten percent to 25% of children and adolescents with ulcerative colitis will require colectomy within 5 years of diagnosis.[19] The most commonly performed procedure is colectomy, mucosal proctectomy, and formation of an ileoanal pouch reservoir. While most patients do quite well, about 30% develop an inflammatory condition of the pouch known as pouchitis.[20]

Approximately 50% to 75% of children and adults with Crohn's disease require surgery within 10 to 15 years of diagnosis. Because resectional therapy is not curative, patients and their parents must be fully aware of the risks of recurrent disease. Areas of bowel which are narrowed but which do not contain active inflammation are often treated with strictureplasty rather than resection. A longitudinal incision is made through the stenotic bowel, and the opening is then closed transversely.

NUTRITIONAL THERAPY

Some evidence exists that elemental diet alone may induce remission in Crohn's disease. Since this diet is unpalatable for most children, it needs to be given via nasogastric tube. Children with growth delay because of chronic undernutrition may benefit greatly and establish catch-up growth following caloric supplementation.[21]

PSYCHOLOGICAL THERAPY

Ulcerative colitis and Crohn's disease are chronic conditions that may have a profound influence on the lives of affected children and their family members. Adolescents may have a particularly difficult time. Every effort should be made to facilitate normal age-appropriate activities and early intervention by psychologists or psychiatrists should be sought if problems develop.

REFERRAL PATTERN

Children and adolescents with inflammatory bowel disease should be treated with a team approach involving the pediatric gastroenterologist, nurse clinician, dieti-tian, and primary care provider. Initial diagnosis should be made with the minimum number of tests necessary and is probably best directed by the specialist. Since intercurrent viral and bacterial illnesses commonly exacerbate IBD, it is essential that there be frequent communication between the care providers.

REFERENCES

1. Jayanthi V, Probert CSJ, Sher KS, Mayberry JF: Current concepts of the etiopathogenesis of inflammatory bowel disease. Am J Gastroenterol 1991;86:1566–1572

2. Podolsky DK. Inflammatory bowel disease. N Engl J Med 1991;325:928–937

3. Brynskov J, Nielsen OH, Ahnfelt-Ronne I, Bendtzen K. Cytokines in inflammatory bowel disease. Scand J Gastroenterol 1992;27:897–906

4. Sofaer J. Crohn's disease: the genetic contribution. Gut 1993;34:869–871

5. Orholm M, Munkholm P, Langholz E et al. Familial occurrence of inflammatory bowel disease. N Engl J Med 1991; 324:84–88

6. Sartor RB. Cytokines in intestinal inflammation: pathophysiological and clinical considerations. Gastroenterology 1994; 106:533–539

7. Griffiths AM. Inflammatory bowel disease. In: Hyams JS, Ed. Gastrointestinal Disorders. Adolescent Medicine: State of the Art Reviews. Philadelphia: Hanley & Belfus, 1995: 351–368

8. Hyams JS. Extraintestinal manifestations of inflammatory bowel disease in children. J Pediatr Gastroenterol Nutr 1994; 19:7–21

9. Passo MH, Fitzgerald JF, Brandt KD. Arthritis associated with inflammatory bowel disease in children. Relationship of joint disease to activity and severity of bowel lesion. Dig Dis Sci 1986;31:492–497

10. Hyams J, Markowitz J, Treem W et al. Characterization of hepatic abnormalities in children with inflammatory bowel disease. Inflam Bowel Dis 1995;1:27–33

11. Thomas DW, Sinatra FR. Screening laboratory tests for Crohn's disease. West J Med 1989;150:163–164

12. Taffet SL, Das KM. Sulfasalazine. Adverse effects and desensitization. Dig Dis Sci 1983;28:833–842

13. Jarnerot G. New salicylates as maintenance treatment in ulcerative colitis. Gut 1994;35:1155–1158

14. Rutgeerts P, Lofberg R, Malchow H et al. A comparison of budesonide with prednisolone for active Crohn's disease. N Engl J Med 1994;331:842–845

15. Duffy LF, Daum F, Fisher SE et al. Peripheral neuropathy in Crohn's disease patients treated with metronidazole. Gastroenterology 1985;88:681–684

16. Markowitz J, Rosa J, Grancher K et al. Long-term 6-mercaptopurine in treatment of adolescents with Crohn's disease. Gastroenterology 1990;99:1347–1351

17. Present D, Meltzer SJ, Krumholz MP et al. 6-Mercaptopurine in the management of inflammatory bowel disease: short- and long-term toxicity. Ann Intern Med 1989;111:641–649

18. Sandborn WJ. A critical review of cyclosporine therapy in inflammatory bowel disease. Inflam Bowel Dis 1995;1:48–63

19. Hyams JS, Davis P, Grancher K et al. Clinical outcome of ulcerative colitis in children. J Pediatr 1996;129(1):81–88

20. Sandborn WJ. Pouchitis following ileal pouch-anal anasto-mosis: definition, pathogenesis, and treatment. Gastroenter-ology 1994;107:1856–1860

21. Kirschner BS, Klich JR, Kalman SS et al. Reversal of growth retardation in Crohn's disease with therapy emphasizing oral nutritional restitution. Gastroenterology 1981;80:10–15

22. Hyams JS. Crohn's disease. In: Wyllie R, Hyams J, Eds. Pediatric Gastrointestinal Disease: Pathophysiology, Diagnosis, Management. Philadelphia: WB Saunders, 1993:751

31

IRRITABLE BOWEL SYNDROME

EDISIO SEMEAO

STEVEN M. ALTSCHULER

Irritable bowel syndrome (IBS) describes a well-recognized disorder caused by a complex interaction between the gastrointestinal (GI) tract and central nervous system (CNS). It is generally referred to as a functional disorder because no anatomic or physiologic cause has been discovered. The diagnosis depends on the presence of subjective clinical symptoms in the patient. There is a consensus that the diagnosis not be made until symptoms, continuous or intermittent, are present for at least 3 months.[1] Most patients present with abdominal discomfort and altered bowel habits. More specifically, the intestinal symptoms include pain relief with bowel movements, abdominal distention usually associated with pain, and looser and more frequent stools with the onset of pain.[2] Manning et al.[3] noted six clinical symptoms seen more frequently with IBS than with organic causes of abdominal pain. These included pain relief with bowel movement, more frequent stools with pain, looser stools with pain, passage of mucus, feeling of incomplete evacuation, and abdominal distention.

Talley et al.[4] postulated that the more of these six symptoms the patient had the more likely it was that the diagnosis was IBS. In an attempt to differentiate other, organic causes of abdominal symptoms, Thompson et al.[5] defined symptomatic criteria (Table 31-1), reporting that if these criteria are strictly observed, 90% of those with at least two criteria will have IBS, and only 30% with two criteria will have some other, organic cause.

In defining IBS, it is also important to realize that symptoms may include other areas of the intestinal tract, as well as some extraintestinal manifestations.[3,6] Patients suffering from IBS are more likely to have gastroesophageal reflux, dysphagia, and biliary dyskinesia.[2] Extraintestinal symptoms involving organs with smooth muscle may also be affected.[6]

GI symptoms are very common and result in a high percentage of physician visits each year.[7,8] Using the above criteria, 10% to 20% of adults in the general population have reported symptoms compatible with IBS.[1] More than 50% of those diagnosed with IBS state their symptoms began before age 35, and as many as 33% trace these symptoms back to childhood. In fact, it has been theorized that nonspecific infantile diarrhea and infantile colic may be early manifestations of IBS.[2] Studies have also looked at the possible relationship between chronic abdominal pain in children and IBS. Appley and Naish[9] surveyed 1,000 school-age children for chronic abdominal pain. This was defined as at least three episodes of pain over at least a 3-month period severe enough to interfere with the child's activity. These investigators found that 10.8% of these children met the criteria. Girls were more likely than boys and many were noted to have "nervous" disorders.

PATHOPHYSIOLOGY

IBS is generally thought of as a complex clinical syndrome caused by altered GI motility and visceral sensation coupled with psychological stressors. Evidence of altered motility has been found to occur in both the upper and lower GI tract.[10] Initial evaluation of motility

TABLE 31-1. Clinical Criteria for the Diagnosis of IBS[a]

Abdominal pain
  Relieved with bowel movement
  Onset associated with a change in stool consistency
  Onset associated with a change in stool frequency
Altered bowel pattern
  Constipation
  Diarrhea
  Passage of mucus
  Straining or incomplete evacuation
Abdominal distention and/or bloated sensation

[a] Symptoms must be present for at least 3 months.

abnormalities focused on the colon because the pain frequently occurred in regions referable to the colon and many of the remaining symptoms could be attributed to colonic dysfunction. Snape et al.[11] showed an increase in slow wave activity of three cycles per minute (cpm) in the distal colon of patients with IBS, but not in controls. This activity is associated with nonpropulsive segment contraction of the colon, which can lead to constipation and pain.

Other investigators have demonstrated abnormal small bowel motility in patients with IBS. Pineiro-Carrero et al.[12] reported the following differences between patients with IBS and controls: (1) shorter duration of the migratory motor complex with poor antral contraction, (2) high pressure, nonpropagating duodenal contractions, and (3) disruption of the migratory motor complex.

More recently, investigation has focused on altered visceral sensation in patients with IBS. Studies using intraluminal balloon distention at a variety of sites have shown that patients with diarrhea-predominant IBS report abdominal pain at much lower levels of gas volume than do controls. Conversely, those with constipation-predominant IBS require a higher level of distention in order to report symptoms.[6]

On the basis of these and other findings, investigators have developed hypotheses that attempt to explain IBS as an abnormal or altered interaction between peripheral functioning of visceral afferent and the central processing of afferent information.[13] If true, this theory may allow therapy to be directed at the process or stimuli that alters the interaction between the visceral end organ and the CNS.

Other factors that may play a role in the development of IBS include luminal stimuli which irritate the small intestine or colon and lead to altered function. These factors can include exogenous dietary compounds such as lactose, sorbitol, and fructose and other foods that have been noted to trigger symptoms in a patient.[6] Abnormal levels of endogenous chemicals needed for the digestive process, such as bile acids and short-chain fatty acids, may also alter intestinal function and motility and result in symptoms of IBS.[14,15]

A final mechanism implicated in the pathophysiology of IBS is the presence of psychosocial stressors. Many patients with IBS do report exacerbation of symptoms at times of stress or psychological problems. Despite reports of stress and depression causing alterations in GI motor function,[16,17] it remains unclear whether these factors cause or only exacerbate the symptoms of IBS because of poorer coping capabilities and greater illness behavior demonstrated by patients with psychological disturbances.

CLINICAL PRESENTATION

Patients with IBS usually present with a constellation of symptoms, but the most common symptom is abdominal pain. The pain can be sharp, dull, crampy, or burning. It is commonly periumbilical or lower abdominal in nature, but not always. The pain usually is noted after meals and rarely wakes the patient from sleep. In a study of 50 children by Faull and Nicol,[18] the complaint of abdominal pain was commonly associated with other symptoms that included pallor, nausea, anorexia, and tiredness, which are not routinely seen in adult patients.

The next most common complaint of patients with IBS is a change in bowel habits. These changes appear to begin in early adolescence and tend to be progressive. Patients report alternating bouts of diarrhea and constipation with one symptom predominant during an episode. Each patient will usually have one of these symptoms more regularly.

Patients with constipation as the main symptom can go from several days up to a week with no stool passage. Abdominal pain may increase with delay in defecation but usually improves significantly after passage of stool. Some patients may be left with a feeling of incomplete evacuation that can lead to prolonged episodes of straining.[19]

In some instances, mucus can be a component of the stool in patients with IBS but the cause is unknown. However, blood is a rare finding, generally associated with local anal irritation or fissures secondary to constipation.

Abdominal distention and increased belching and flatulence are another set of symptoms that patients can present with.[6] This triad appears to be less common in children than in adults and has been reported only anecdotally.

Several less common symptoms have occasionally been reported in adults with IBS but appear to occur much less frequently in children. These complaints can include dyspepsia, nausea, vomiting, heartburn, urinary frequency, dysmenorrhea, and headache.[20]

The clinical expression of IBS is also affected by psychological factors in a large number of patients. Several investigations have found an increased prevalence of psychiatric disorders including personality disorders, anxiety, depression, hysteria, and somatization in patients with IBS.[1,21,22] Although, investigators agree that these psychological factors do not cause the symptoms of IBS, these factors appear to influence the way in which the illness is viewed and acted on by the patient. Patients with IBS and psychological symptoms have a higher frequency of seeking medical attention than patients with IBS and no associated psychological symptoms.[1]

A further clinical feature that is common in patients with IBS is the frequent report of some inciting event that exacerbates the symptoms. The most common inciting events include stressful situations, food intolerance, alcohol ingestion, and cigarette smoking. In a study of children, three major reasons were noted as initiating an episode of abdominal pain: (1) a stressful situation, especially related to school, (2) overeating or food intolerance, and (3) to attempt to "get out of something."[2]

DIAGNOSIS

The diagnosis of IBS is based on the presence of a number of subjective clinical symptoms and thus remains in large part a diagnosis of exclusion. As part of the evaluation of IBS, the physician should consider and exclude either by history, physical examination, or by use of certain studies a number of organic causes of recurrent abdominal pain associated with altered bowel habits (Table 31-2). The initial approach to a patient being evaluated for IBS should consist of a thorough review of the history. The features that should be focused on include the duration of symptoms and an assessment to determine the presence of the Manning criteria (previously listed in Table 31-1). Symptoms suggestive of organic disease also need to be excluded and these include pain awakening from sleep or interfering with the normal sleep pattern, fever, weight loss, and visible or occult blood in the stools. A dietary history should be obtained and features of lactose intolerance or excessive use of nonabsorbable sugars such as sorbitol or fructose should be examined. The use of medications should also be evaluated for possible GI side effects. Evaluation of psychosocial factors as possible inciting events should also be explored in all patients.

The physical examination in most patients with IBS will be unremarkable. Abdominal tenderness may be appreciated but is typically not pronounced. During the physical examination, findings such as a mass lesion, lymphadenopathy, hepatosplenomegaly, jaundice, ascites, and positive fecal blood are not consistent with the diagnosis of IBS, and further evaluation should be considered.

TABLE 31-2. Causes of Abdominal Pain and Altered Bowel Pattern

Inflammatory bowel disease

Chronic constipation
    Medications
    Pseudo-obstruction
    Functional
    Megacolon
    Encopresis
    Volvulus

Diarrhea
    Medications
    Infectious
        Bacterial overgrowth
        Enteric bacterial infections
        Parasitic infections

Malabsorption
    Lactose intolerance
    Excess sorbitol and fructose intake
    Celiac disease

Tumors
    Lymphoma
    Carcinoma

Other
    Psychiatric disorders
        Depression
        Anxiety
        Panic disorders
        Somatization
    Endometriosis
    Hyperthyroidism
    Urinary tract infections

LABORATORY TESTS

No laboratory tests are diagnostic for IBS, but several routine laboratory studies are used as a general screen to aid in the exclusion of specific disease processes. The initial evaluation should consist of a complete blood count (CBC), erythrocyte sedimentation rate (ESR), a chemistry panel with an albumin, and urinalysis. For patients in whom diarrhea is a predominant symptom, stool examination should include culture for enteric pathogens, *Clostridium difficile*, ova, parasites, and fecal leukocytes. In complicated cases a 24-hour stool collection may be helpful to differentiate between IBS and other disease processes. In IBS, stool weights of greater than 300 g/day are rare, as is excessive fecal fat content.[10]

In patients in whom lactose intolerance is suspected clinically, an empirical trial of lactose restriction may be initiated with close follow-up of symptoms. A lactose breath test may also be obtained in order to further evaluate lactose malabsorption.

In cases in which initial screening laboratory tests

are abnormal or in which there is suspicion of a potential disease process by history or physical examination, an endoscopy or colonoscopy may be indicated. Also, in patients in whom Crohn's disease is a concern, an upper GI study with small bowel follow through is indicated.

TREATMENT

Just as the diagnosis of IBS is somewhat subjective and complicated by the presence of a variety of symptoms, the treatment for IBS is also complicated by the large number of different approaches used by caregivers. The most important factor in treating a patient with IBS is to reassure both the parents and the child that although their symptoms may be significant, they are not dangerous and will leave no long-term sequelae.

In most cases of IBS, the initial therapeutic intervention is often a dietary change. Increasing fiber by dietary means or by supplementation or eliminating foods that appear to trigger episodes of IBS is in most cases sufficient to improve symptoms. Fiber in the diet may help prolong stool transit time to allow for more absorption of water, making it easier for the passage of stools in patients in which constipation is the predominant complaint. Fiber has also been demonstrated to decrease rectosigmoid pressures in both fasting and postprandial states, which may decrease the pain sensation experienced by patients.[2] While a trial of increasing dietary fiber is warranted in cases of IBS, clinical trials have reported mixed results.[2] More recently, investigators are discovering that the type of fiber used may be the important component in that it appears that soluble fiber preparations may be more therapeutic than insoluble fiber products.[23]

In cases in which dietary manipulation has not improved the symptoms, a variety of medications can be used to attempt to relieve symptoms. However, there is no one effective drug that is available for the treatment of IBS.

The most commonly used group of drugs in IBS are the antispasmodics/anticholinergics (dicyclomine, hyoscyamine) used to treat the abdominal pain reported by patients. The main mechanism of action is to cause smooth muscle relaxation. However, many of the drugs are associated with a number of unfavorable side effects, including headaches, epigastric fullness, and mild hypotension, which limit their use. A newer group of drugs that act more specifically on smooth muscle in the GI tract are calcium channel antagonist and an antimuscarinic agent.[19] In a recent metanalysis of the use of antispasmodics to treat IBS, the following five drugs were found to be more effective than placebo: cimetropium bromide, pinaverium bromide, trimebutine, octilium bromide, and mebeverine.[24]

Another class of drugs that in early trials appears to be helpful in decreasing pain and diarrhea is ondensetron.[25] This drug blocks the action of 5-hydroxytryptamine, which is a neurotransmitter in the gut. In adults with chronic pain symptoms that are refractory to other interventions, tricyclic antidepressants such as amitriptyline and desipramine may also be used.

When diarrhea is the predominant symptom an opioid agent, loperamide, which decreases intestinal transit, increases water absorption, and strengthens rectal sphincter tone, is frequently used. This drug does not cross the blood-brain barrier, so there are no central opioid effects. Cholestyramine may be helpful in rare cases especially if the diarrhea is related to idiopathic bile acid malabsorption.[21]

When the predominant symptom is constipation, the long-term intervention should be an increase in fiber intake. Pharmacologic agents should only be used in short-term exacerbations. Prokinetic agents such as cisapride have been used in limited fashion with some success in patients with IBS.[19] The use of stimulant laxatives in IBS is discouraged because of side effects and because they may exaggerate swings from constipation to diarrhea. In cases of severe constipation, an osmotic laxative to relieve the episode may be beneficial.

Alternative therapies such as psychotherapy, hypnotherapy, and biofeedback alone or in combination with other modalities have been shown to be effective in treating IBS.[10] These regimens appear to be especially helpful in cases in which psychosocial stressors are identified.

While there are many different approaches to treating IBS and in many cases pharmacological modalities are helpful, much of this experience comes from treating adults with IBS. There is still little information about the use of these drugs in children to treat IBS. As a result, a reasonable and usually effective approach to treating children is to combine dietary changes (the addition of fiber and restriction of foods that exacerbate the symptoms) with an identification and correction of psychosocial triggers.

REFERRAL PATTERNS

The role of the family physician, pediatrician, or general clinician in evaluating, treating, and following a patient with IBS is crucial. Such caregivers have the most important role because of the relationship that they have developed over time with the family and with the child. Thus, they are able to reassure the family that this process is not dangerous and provide them with a comfortable and continual source of information and support.

The initial screening laboratory evaluation consists of routine studies that are easily obtained through general clinical practice. No definitive set of criteria require a referral to a subspecialist for evaluation of IBS; however, several factors, if present in the history, physical examination, or screening laboratory studies, should serve as a red flag to general practitioners that further investigation and referral to a subspecialist is warranted.

Factors derived from the history that may be of concern are the presence of profuse diarrhea, involuntary weight loss or deceleration in linear growth, pain that regularly awakens a patient from sleep, fevers, regular episodes of joint pain, and significant alterations in daily activity. Also, while there are no strict criteria for age in the diagnosis of IBS, most investigators believe that initial onset may be in adolescence. Thus, preadolescent patients who have symptoms of IBS may require a more thorough evaluation at the outset, and consultation with a subspecialist may be helpful.

Findings on physical examination that would need further evaluation would include the presence of any abnormality, especially any findings of abdominal masses, guaiac-positive stools, perianal disease, or recurrent aphthous ulcers.

Abnormal results from screening laboratory studies also warrant further investigation. Specific findings of iron deficiency anemia, low albumin level, or elevated ESR would warrant further exploration.

REFERENCES

1. Lynn RB, Friedman LS. Irritable bowel syndrome: managing the patient with abdominal pain and altered bowel habits. Med Clin North Am 1995;79:373–390

2. Mezoff AG. Irritable bowel syndrome. In: Wyllie R, Hyams JS, Eds: Pediatric Gastrointestinal Disease: Pathophysiology, Diagnosis and Management. Philadelphia: WB Saunders, 1993:724–731

3. Manning AP, Thompson WG, Heaton KW, Morris AF. Towards positive diagnosis of the irritable bowel. BMJ 1978;2:653–654

4. Talley WJ, Phillips SF, Melton LJ et al. Diagnostic value of the Manning criteria in irritable bowel syndrome. Gut 1990;31:77–81

5. Thompson WG, Dotevall G, Drossman DA et al. Irritable bowel syndrome: guidelines for the diagnosis. Gastroenterol Int 1989;2:92–95

6. Camilleri M, Prather CM. The irritable bowel syndrome: mechanism and a practical approach to management. Ann Intern Med 1992;116:1001–1008

7. Everhart JE, Renault PF. Irritable bowel syndrome in office-based practice in the United States. Gastroenterology 1991;100:998–1015

8. Harvey RF, Salih SY, Read AE. Organic and functional disorders in 2,000 gastroenterology outpatients. Lancet 1983;1:632–634

9. Appley J, Naish N. Recurrent abdominal pain: a field survey of 1,000 school children. Arch Dis Child 1958;33:165–170

10. Lynn RB, Friedman LS. Irritable bowel syndrome. N Engl J Med 1993;329:1940–1945

11. Snape WJ, Carlson GM, Cohen S. Colonic myoelectric activity in the irritable bowel syndrome. Gastroenterology 1976;70:326–330

12. Pineiro-Carrero VM, Andres JM, Davis RH, Mathias JR. Abnormal gastroduodenal motility in children and adolescents with recurrent functional abdominal pain. J Pediatr 1988;113:820–825

13. McKee DP, Quigley EM. Intestinal motility in irritable bowel syndrome: IBS a motility disorder? Part 2. Motility of the small bowel, esophagus, stomach and gall-bladder. Dig Dis Sci 1993;38:1773–1782

14. Spiller RC, Brown ML, Phillips SF. Decreased fluid tolerance, accelerated transit and abnormal motility of the human colon induced by oleic acid. Gastroenterology 1986;91:100–107

15. Kamath PS, Hoepfner MT, Phillips SF. Short chain fatty acids stimulate motility of the canine ileum. Am J Physiol 1987;253:6427–6433

16. Almy TP, Tulin M. Alterations in man under stress. Experimental production of changes stimulating the "irritable colon." Gastroenterology 1947;8:616–626

17. Talley NJ, Camilleri M, Orkin BA, Kramlinger KG. Effect of cyclical unipolar depression on upper gastrointestinal motility and sleep. Gastroenterology 1989;97:775–777

18. Faull C, Nicol AR. Abdominal pain in six-year-olds: an epidemiological study in a new town. J Child Psychiat 1986;27:251–260

19. Boyle JT. Abdominal Pain. In: Walker WA, Durie PR, Hamilton JR, Walker-Smith JA, Watkins JD, Eds: Pediatric Gastrointestinal Disease: Pathophysiology, Diagnosis and Management. 2nd Ed. St. Louis: CV Mosby, 1996:205–226

20. Cann PA, Read NW, Brown C et al. Irritable bowel syndrome: relationship of disorders in the transit of a single solid meal to symptom patterns. Gut 1983;24:405–411

21. Drossman DA, Thompson WG. The irritable bowel syndrome: review and a graduated multicomponent treatment approach. Ann Intern Med 1992;116:1009–1016

22. Whitehead WE, Bosmajian L, Zonderman AB et al. Symptoms of psychologic distress associated with irritable bowel syndrome: comparison of community and medical clinic samples. Gastroenterology 1988;95:709–714

23. Snook J, Shephard HA. Bran supplementation in the treatment of irritable bowel syndrome. Aliment Pharmacol Ther 1994;8:511–514

24. Poynard T, Naveaus S, Mory B, Chaput JC. Meta-analysis of smooth muscle relaxants in the treatment of irritable bowel syndrome. Aliment Pharmacol Ther 1994;8:499–510

25. Steadman CJ, Talley NJ, Phillips SF, Mulvihill C. Trial of a selective serotonin type 3 (5-HT$_3$) receptor antagonist ondansetron (GR38032F) in diarrhea predominant irritable bowel syndrome. Gastroenterology 1990;98:A394

32

LACTOSE INTOLERANCE

JAY BARTH
MENNO VERHAVE

Lactose is a disaccharide, consisting of one molecule each of glucose and galactose. It is synthesized exclusively in the mammary gland of mammals during late pregnancy and lactation and is present as a free molecule only in milk. The digestion of lactose depends on the enzyme lactase phlorizin-hydrolase, or lactase, located on the microvillus membrane of the small intestine. When lactase is low, undigested lactose cannot be absorbed. It acts as an osmotic force in the small intestine, passing into the colon, where it is fermented by the intestinal flora, producing the symptoms of the condition known as lactose intolerance. Lactase deficiency occurs in a variety of situations, either as a primary or a secondary process.

TYPES OF LACTOSE INTOLERANCE

Congenital Lactase Deficiency

Primary congenital lactase deficiency is extremely rare. It is most likely an autosomal recessive condition in which lactase activity is absent or very low.[1] This condition was potentially lethal before the advent of lactose-free formulas.

Primary Lactase Deficiency

Primary lactase deficiency may occur in premature infants born prior to 35 weeks gestation. The specific activity of this enzyme increases during the last trimester of gestation, reaching maximal activity in the newborn period.[2] However, infants with lactase deficiency are usually not symptomatic because of colonic "salvage" of undigested lactose. The unabsorbed lactose can be converted by the colonic microflora to short-chain fatty acids, which are absorbable by the colonic mucosa.[3]

The most common cause of primary lactase deficiency is genetic late-onset lactase deficiency. This refers to the genetically determined decline in lactase levels, to approximately 10% of values at birth, occurring after 5 years of age and persisting throughout life.[4] The term lactase deficiency in this context is actually a misnomer, since worldwide most people have reduced lactase activity in adulthood (Tables 32-1 and 32-2); a more correct term would be lactase-non-persistence. Only a small percentage of the population, primarily those of northern European descent, have persistence of high enzyme levels throughout adulthood. Lactase persistence beyond childhood is thought to be an autosomal dominant trait.[4]

Secondary Lactase Deficiency

Since late-onset lactase deficiency only occurs after age 5 years, any child younger than this age with confirmed lactose intolerance must be investigated for a secondary cause of this condition.[5]

There are numerous secondary causes of lactase deficiency. Any process that causes mucosal injury may be implicated, including gastroenteritis (rotavirus most commonly), severe parasitic infection (giardiasis), celiac disease (gluten-sensitive enteropathy), radiation enteritis, drug-induced enteritis (e.g., colchicine), Crohn's dis-

TABLE 32-1. Distribution of Lactase Phenotype in Selected Populations in the United States

Population	Low Lactase (%)
Northern European	7
Whites	22
Blacks	65
American Indians	95
Vietnamese	100

(Data from Montgomery et al.[27])

ease involving the small intestine, and small bowel bacterial overgrowth.[6] The enzyme is found predominantly at the villus tip, which makes it especially sensitive to mucosal injury.[7] Lactase deficiency due to gastroenteritis generally resolves within 4 weeks.[8]

PATHOPHYSIOLOGY

The basis of symptoms in lactose intolerance is the same, regardless of the underlying cause of lactase deficiency. The presence of nonhydrolyzed lactose in the small intestine creates an osmotic force, moving water into the bowel. This stimulates peristalsis, leading to increased intestinal transit, further impairing absorption. The increased volume in the intestine causes borborygmi, bloating, pain, and cramps. Lactose passes into the colon, where it is fermented by the intestinal flora to hydrogen gas, carbon dioxide, and methane, and to short-chain fatty acids (butyrate, propionate, acetate). These events produce intestinal gas, causing flatulence and cramps. Diarrhea is the result of the osmotic effect of undigested

TABLE 32-2. Distribution of Lactase Phenotype in Selected Populations in Europe

Country	Population	Low Lactase (%)
Netherlands	Dutch	0
Sweden	Swedes	1
Austria	Austrian	20
France	French	32
	Southern French	44
Italy	Northern Italian	50
	Southern Italian	72
	Sicilian	71

(Data from Montgomery et al.[27])

lactose in the bowel and of peristalsis stimulated by the low pH level due to lactose fermentation.[5]

The nature and severity of symptoms can be quite variable between individuals because lactase activity and lactase intake are not the only determining factors in the clinical presentation of lactose intolerance. Other contributing factors include alterations in gastric emptying and intestinal transit, which in turn are influenced by luminal content and an individual's intestinal motility. Slower transit allows for increased absorption of lactose, while rapid transit leads to worsening symptoms.[9] Additionally, the composition of colonic microflora (which differs from person to person and can vary within an individual over time) may influence clinical manifestations because the predominant by-products of fermentation may be symptom-producing gas or absorbable molecules. Finally, patients have different subjective sensitivities to abdominal distention.

CLINICAL PRESENTATION

The variable clinical manifestations often make diagnosis difficult. Some patients experience symptoms shortly after the ingestion of lactose, making the association of symptoms with intake more obvious. Symptoms experienced within 30 minutes of ingestion include nausea and a sensation of abdominal fullness. Symptoms that occur 2 to 6 hours after ingestion include abdominal pain (which may be periumbilical or hypogastric), borborygmi, cramps, flatulence, and diarrhea. The typical diarrhea is characterized by watery, bulky, and frothy stools. In adolescents vomiting may predominate.

The correlation of lactose intake and symptoms can be difficult to establish on the basis of history, as many patients do not relate their symptoms to lactose ingestion. This is especially true in young children, who may be unable to express their complaints clearly and whose diet consists of a large quantity of lactose, ingested at various times of day. The physician should suspect lactose intolerance in children who present with recurrent abdominal pain, as studies have shown that lactose intolerance is a common underlying cause of this condition.[10] Older children and adolescents with the clinical pattern of irritable bowel syndrome should likewise be investigated for lactose intolerance.[3] Clinicians must maintain a high index of suspicion of lactose intolerance in children with gastrointestinal complaints.

DIAGNOSIS AND LABORATORY TESTS

The diagnosis of lactose intolerance is established by the presence of symptoms after lactose ingestion, combined with a confirmatory laboratory test. Physical examination is generally not helpful in establishing the diagnosis. Rarely, patients may show weight loss or, in severe cases (mostly in infants), signs of dehydration. The abdominal examination may indicate borborygmi. Because the association of symptoms to diet is often difficult to establish in children, laboratory testing assumes even greater importance. The use of testing to confirm the diagnosis avoids needlessly restricting the diet of a child who is, in fact, not lactose intolerant.

Currently, the preferred diagnostic test is the breath hydrogen test. It is simple to administer, noninvasive, and the most accurate method to diagnose lactose intolerance.[11] The test involves collecting the subject's breath samples and measuring the breath hydrogen content at 30-minute intervals for 2 to 3 hours after ingestion of a lactose load. In the lactose-deficient individual, fermentation of undigested lactase by colonic bacteria results in hydrogen gas production. A rise in breath hydrogen content of more than 20 ppm indicates lactose malabsorption. A rise of 10 to 20 ppm is considered positive if accompanied by symptoms; less than 10 ppm is considered negative.[3]

The breath hydrogen test does have several limitations. The test depends on the presence of colonic hydrogen-producing flora. Reports have demonstrated that 2% to 20% of patients are colonized with non-hydrogen-producing bacteria.[12] Recent use of antibiotics, smoking, or crying can influence the results.[13] In patients less than 5 years of age, an abnormal breath hydrogen test signifies the possibility of an underlying mucosal abnormality; in these cases, further testing, such as stool examination for parasites, radiologic studies, and small intestinal biopsy, must be considered.[9]

Low fecal pH and presence of reducing substances suggest lactose malabsorption, but fecal analysis is neither sensitive nor specific for lactase deficiency and has a number of limitations. It is valid only if lactose has been recently ingested, if intestinal transit time is rapid, and if stools are collected fresh and assayed immediately.[14]

The lactose absorption or lactose tolerance test consists of measuring blood glucose levels before and after lactose ingestion; a slight rise in the glucose level is consistent with malabsorption. The test actually measures lactose absorption, and not malabsorption. Results may be affected by the subject's insulin state or low renal threshold for glucose.[15] As the lactose tolerance test is invasive and time-consuming, it has been almost universally replaced by the breath hydrogen test.

Lactase activity can also be measured by small intestinal biopsy.[16] One indication for this assay is confirmation of the diagnosis of congenital lactase deficiency. It may also be helpful in evaluating the patient whose symptoms warrant small intestinal biopsy after noninvasive tests for carbohydrate malabsorption have proved inconclusive. In those situations, when direct measurement of lactase activity is indicated, jejunal biopsy is preferred, as lactase activity is normally low in the duodenum.[17] In the case of secondary lactase deficiency, the expression of duodenal lactase may be patchy; thus, a biopsy may not reflect the patient's true lactase status.[9]

TREATMENT

Therapy for primary lactose intolerance includes restriction of dietary lactose, substitution with alternative nutrient sources, provision of adequate calcium intake, and use of lactase enzyme substitutes.

The need for lactose restriction is based on individual tolerance. In adults, lactose comprises a small part of the diet. A recent blinded study showed that adult patients with self-reported "severe" lactose intolerance can tolerate 8 ounces of milk per day with negligible symptoms.[18] In infants and young children who consume an average milk intake, lactose constitutes 30% of daily calories,[3] so restriction has a major impact on their diet. The rare infant with congenital lactase deficiency must be treated with a lactose-free formula. Patients with late-onset lactase deficiency are often placed on a lactose-free diet at the time of diagnosis until symptoms subside. Lactose is then gradually reintroduced into the diet, to determine the quantity tolerated without causing symptoms. Enzyme supplements may be helpful in those who remain symptomatic even at low levels of intake.

Dairy products differ in lactose composition (Table 32-3). Milk has the highest lactose content. Commer-

TABLE 32-3. Lactose Content of Selected Foods

Food Source	Amount	Lactose (g)
Milk (whole, nonfat)	1 cup	11–12
Nonfat dry milk, instant	1½ cup	46
Evaporated milk	2 tbsp	3
Buttermilk	1 cup	10–12
Whipped cream	1 tbsp	0.4
Cottage cheese	1 cup	5–6
Cheese		
American (processed)	1 oz	0.8
Cheddar	1 oz	0.4–0.6
Cream	1 oz	0.8
Parmesan	1 oz	0.8
Swiss	1 oz	0.4–0.6
Cream (sour or sweet)	2 tbsp	1
Ice cream	1 cup	9
Yogurt	1 cup	12–14[a]

(Data from Grand et al.[3])

[a] Natural live yogurt will lose 50% to 100% of lactose in small intestine.

cially available low-lactose Lactaid milk (LactAid, Inc.), which is 70% lactose reduced, is generally acceptable to patients. Adding 5 drops of Lactaid enzyme to 1 quart of regular milk (24 hours before its ingestion) also lowers the lactose content by 70%, whereas adding 10 drops essentially digests all lactose.[19] Unfermented acidophilus milk, which contains *Lactobacillus acidophilus* cultures, is not effective in lactose intolerance.[20]

Certain dairy foods may be well tolerated by patients. Aged cheeses such as cheddar, Muenster, provolone, and Swiss, contain small amounts of lactose. Fermented milk products are also well tolerated. Live-culture yogurt contains endogenous beta-galactosidase, which is activated in the intestine, thus "autodigesting" the lactose it contains.[21] Yogurts that contain milk products added back after fermentation may produce symptoms.[3]

Patients must be instructed to read food labels for hidden sources of lactose, which may cause continued symptoms when the obvious milk products have been eliminated from the diet. Products containing whey, curds, caseinate, or lactoglobulin may also contain significant lactose. Lactose is used in many prepared foods, for bulk, texture, and taste; the most common of these are bread, baked goods, cereals, margarine, soups, luncheon meats, salad dressing, and candies.[22]

Provision of adequate calcium is essential for lactose-intolerant patients. A recent study demonstrated lower bone mineral content in lactose-intolerant children on a low-lactose, low-calcium diet as compared to controls.[23] Various foods other than dairy products are good sources of calcium, including vegetables (broccoli, collard greens), fish (oysters, salmon, sardines, shrimp), nuts, and tofu. Calcium supplementation, usually with calcium carbonate tablets (e.g., Tums [Norcliff Thayer] or Os-Cal [SmithKline Beecham]) should be given if the dietary intake does not meet the Recommended Dietary Allowance (RDA) of calcium (800 mg elemental calcium daily for children less than 10 years of age and 1,200 mg/day for those older than 10 years of age). For children who are unable to tolerate tablets, liquid calcium glubionate (Neo-calglucon Sandoz) is an alternative. Dietary counseling should be provided to ensure that the lactose-restricted diet contains adequate nutrients.

Enzyme substitution is often helpful in allowing patients to tolerate lactose-containing foods. Commercially available lactase substitutes are bacterial or yeast beta-galactosidases; some of these are listed in Table 32-4. These substitutes have been shown to reduce symptoms and breath hydrogen excretion when added to, or taken with, lactose[24]; however, they do not completely hydrolyze lactose, and each patient's response is variable. Lactase substitutes should be taken immediately before ingesting lactose. The effective dose is 1/2 tablet to 3 tablets per meal, depending on the patient and the amount of lactose ingested.[19]

TABLE 32-4. Commercial Lactase Enzyme Substitutes

Name	Dose Form	Supplier
Lactaid	Liquid/tablets	LactAid, Inc.
Lactase	Capsules	Kremers-Urban
LactAce	Capsules	Nature's Way Products, Inc.
DairyEase	Tablets	Glenbrook Laboratories
Lactrol	Caplets	Advanced Nutritional Technology

(From Grand et al,[3] with permission.)

The treatment of secondary lactose intolerance depends on its etiology. Infants who were previously healthy and well nourished and who develop acute mild gastroenteritis do not require any change from milk-based formula.[25] By contrast, infants with prolonged severe gastroenteritis have been shown to benefit from lactose-free formula for several weeks after the illness.[26] Hydrolysate formulas, though effective, are expensive; they are unnecessary, unless the infant has a concurrent protein sensitivity. In cases of lactose intolerance secondary to chronic mucosal disease, treatment is the same as proposed for those with genetic lactose intolerance until the underlying lesion has been treated or has resolved.

REFERRAL PATTERN

The key role of the primary care clinician is to rule out the diagnosis of genetic lactose intolerance, as it can cause a variety of gastrointestinal symptoms in children. If the child is less than 5 years old an underlying mucosal abnormality must be investigated, which may involve consulting a specialist. When lactose intolerance is suspected, the clinician should arrange for confirmatory testing with a breath hydrogen test. Although response to a trial of a lactose-free diet may be helpful, it does not establish the diagnosis. Appropriate testing will prevent unnecessary restriction of lactose-containing foods and the hidden cost of treating lactose intolerance, which may include the use of expensive enzyme substitutes, commercially prepared lactose-reduced milk, and calcium supplements. If long-term dietary restriction is expected, nutritional counseling must be provided to ensure that the diet is adequate in calcium content and nutrients. Referral to a specialist should also be considered if the diagnosis is uncertain, or if underlying intestinal disease is suspected.

REFERENCES

1. Savilathi E, Launiala K, Kuitunen P. Congenital lactase deficiency: a clinical study on 16 patients. Arch Dis Child 1983; 58:246–252

2. Mobassaleh M, Montgomery RK, Biller JA, Grand RJ. Development of carbohydrate absorption in the fetus and neonate. Pediatrics 1985;75:160–166

3. Grand RJ, Montgomery RK, Buller HA. Carbohydrate malabsorption. In: Bayless T, Ed. Current Therapy in Gastroenterology and Liver Disease. 4th Ed. St. Louis: Mosby-Yearbook, 1994:303–308

4. Flatz G. Genetics of lactose digestion in humans. In: Harris H, Hirschhorn K, Eds. Advances in Human Genetics. New York: Plenum Press, 1987:1–77

5. Buller HA, Rings EHHM, Montgomery RK, Grand RJ. Clinical aspects of lactose intolerance in children and adults. Scand J Gastroenterol 1991;26(suppl 188):73–80

6. Montgomery RK, Jonas MM, Grand RJ. Intestinal disaccharidases: structure, function, and deficiency. In: Lifshitz, Ed. Carbohydrate Intolerance in Infancy. New York: Marcel Dekker, 1982:75–94

7. Boyle JT, Celano P, Koldovsky O. Demonstration of a difference in expression of maximal lactase and sucrase activity in the adult rat jejunum. Gastroenterology 1980;79:503–507

8. Davidson GP, Goodwin D, Robb TA. Incidence and duration of lactose malabsorption in children hospitalized with acute enteritis: a study in a well-nourished urban population. J Pediatr 1984;105:587–590

9. Hyams JS, Stafford RJ, Grand RJ, Watkins JB. Correlation of lactose breath hydrogen test, intestinal morphology, and lactase activity in young children. J Pediatr 1980;97:609–612

10. Webster RB, DiPalma JA, Gremse DA. Lactose maldigestion and recurrent abdominal pain in children. Dig Dis Sci 1995;40:1506–1510

11. Maffei HVL, Metz G, Bampoe V et al. Lactose intolerance detected by the hydrogen breath test, in infants and children with chronic diarrhea. Arch Dis Child 1977;52:766–771

12. Arola H, Koivula T, Jokela H et al. Comparison of indirect diagnostic methods for hypolactasia. Scand J Gastroenterol 1988;23:351–357

13. Ostrander CR, Cohen RS, Hopper AO et al. Breath hydrogen analysis: a review of the methodologies and clinical applications. J Pediatr Gastroenterol Nutr 1983;1:525–533

14. Newcomer AD. Screening tests for carbohydrate malabsorption. J Pediatr Gastroenterol Nutr 1984;3:6–8

15. Newcomer AD, McGill DB, Thomas PJ et al. Prospective comparison of indirect methods for detecting lactase deficiency. N Engl J Med 1975;293:1232–1236

16. Dahlqvist A. Method for assay of intestinal disaccharidases. Anal Biochem 1968;22:99–107

17. Newcomer AD, McGill DB. Distribution of disaccharidase activity in the small bowel of normal and lactase-deficient subjects. Gastroenterology 1966;51:481–488

18. Suarez FL, Saviano DA, Levitt MD. A comparison of milk or lactose-hydrolyzed milk by people with self-reported severe lactose intolerance. N Engl J Med 1995;333:1–5

19. Sinden AA, Sutphen JL. Dietary treatment of lactose intolerance in infants and children. J Am Diet Assoc 1991;91:1567–1571

20. Newcomer AD, Parks HS, O'Brien PC, McGill DB. Response of patients with irritable bowel syndrome and lactase deficiency using unfermented acidophilus milk. Am J Clin Nutr 1983;38:257–263

21. Kolars JC, Levitt MD, Aouji M, Saviano DA. Yoghurt, an autodigesting source of lactose. N Engl J Med 1984;310:1–3

22. Scrimshaw NS, Murray EB. Milk and gastrointestinal symptoms. Am J Clin Nutr 1988;48(suppl):1099–1104

23. Stallings VA, Oddleifson NW, Negrini BY et al. Bone mineral content and dietary calcium intake in children prescribed a low-lactose diet. J Pediatr Gastroenterol Nutr 1984;18:440–445

24. Biller JA, King S, Rosenthal A, Grand RJ. Efficacy of lactase-treated milk for lactose-intolerant pediatric patients. J Pediatr 1987;11:91–94

25. Groothius JR, Berman S, Chapman J. Effect of carbohydrate ingested on outcome in infants with mild gastroenteritis. J Pediatr 1986;108:903–906

26. Rajah R, Pettifor JM, Noormohamed M et al. The effect of feeding four different formulae on stool weights in prolonged dehydrating infantile gastroenteritis. J Pediatr Gastroenterol Nutr 1988;7:203–207

27. Montgomery R, Buller HA, Rings EHHM et al. Lactose intolerance and regulation of small intestine lactase activity. In: Berdanier CD, Hargrove JL, Eds. Nutrition and Gene Expression. Boca Raton, FL: CRC Press, 1992:23–53

33

NECROTIZING ENTEROCOLITIS

KAREN D. FAIRCHILD
RICHARD A. POLIN

Necrotizing enterocolitis (NEC) is a leading cause of morbidity and mortality in the newborn intensive care unit. It is primarily a disease of the immature or injured intestine. Up to 90% of cases occur in preterm infants, and the remainder occur primarily in newborns at high risk of intestinal ischemia. Despite advances in our understanding of the pathophysiology and treatment of NEC, approximately 10,000 newborns are diagnosed with this disease each year in the United States, and 10% to 30% of affected infants die as a direct result of the disease.[1]

PATHOPHYSIOLOGY

As the name implies, NEC is characterized by ischemic and hemorrhagic necrosis, which, in severe cases, traverses the entire thickness of the intestinal wall, leading to perforation. The pathologic findings in NEC include mucosal edema and hemorrhage, bacterial overgrowth, inflammatory infiltration, and coagulation necrosis. The process may involve the entire bowel, or it may be focal. The most common region affected is the distal ileum and ascending colon, which constitutes a vascular "watershed zone" farthest from the major splanchnic blood supply.

The etiology of NEC is multifactorial. Early descriptions of the disease invoked intestinal ischemia as the primary pathogenic event. Asphyxia-induced autonomic vasoconstriction in the splanchnic circulation is rapidly reversed; this "autoregulatory escape" protects the intes-

tinal mucosa from severe ischemic damage.[2] Furthermore, several case control studies have not shown an association between asphyxia, hypoxia, or hypotension and the development of NEC.[3,4] This suggests that additional factors must be present in order for the compromised mucosa to become inflamed and necrotic.[5]

The presence of pneumatosis intestinalis implicates bacteria and feeding in the pathogenesis of NEC. Bacteria may invade the immature or damaged mucosa and ferment carbohydrates, producing hydrogen gas visible radiographically as bubbles of air within the bowel wall. Preterm infants commonly receive multiple courses of antibiotics, which can suppress the nonpathogenic bowel flora and permit the growth of more virulent bacteria. Further complicating the situation is gastrointestinal (GI) hypomotility, which prolongs exposure of the vulnerable GI mucosa to pathogens and hyperosmolar solutions.[6]

Epidemics of NEC have been described within intensive care nurseries and have been associated with common enteric pathogens such as enterotoxigenic *Escherichia coli*, *Salmonella*, *Clostridium difficile*, and rotavirus. Surprisingly, numerous studies have shown no consistent association of nonepidemic NEC with a particular infectious agent. It is likely that ischemic damage permits translocation of enteric bacteria into the bowel wall, leading to release of toxic, vasoconstrictive, and inflammatory mediators which, in combination with immature host defense, predispose some newborns to intestinal necrosis[7,8] (Fig. 33-1). Other possible contributors to the intestinal injury include toxic oxygen radicals, comple-

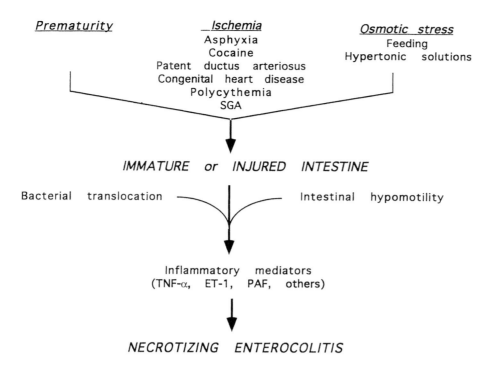

FIGURE 33-1. Pathogenesis of necrotizing enterocolitis. SGA, small for gestational age, TNFα, tumor necrosis factor–alpha; ET-1, endothelin-1; PAF, platelet activating factor.

ment, leukotrienes, and endothelin-1, a potent vasoconstrictor. Recent research has focused on platelet activating factor (PAF) as a possible mediator of NEC. PAF is rapidly degraded by acetylhydrolase, an enzyme present in human milk, but not in cow's milk or formula. This may in part explain the decreased incidence of NEC in preterm newborns fed with breast milk.[9,10]

Enteral feedings have been implicated in the pathogenesis of NEC for a variety of reasons: (1) about 90% of newborns who develop NEC have been fed, (2) the timing of NEC onset often corresponds with the beginning of enteral feeds, (3) the presence of pneumatosis requires a source of carbohydrate to produce hydrogen gas, and (4) enteral feedings (especially transpyloric feedings) promote the development of bacterial colonization. Mucosal injury may be precipitated or exacerbated by exposure to hyperosmolar solutions; this exposure is prolonged by intestinal hypomotility, a common occurrence in preterm infants. Enteral administration of hyperosmolar medications or electrolyte solutions can also cause mucosal damage and should be avoided in high-risk patients. Early institution and rapid advancement of enteral feeds increases the risk of NEC in extremely low-birth-weight infants. Delaying or eradicating gut colonization by administering antibiotics can also have adverse effects, including inhibition of enterocyte proliferation, decreased absorption and increased secretion of colonic fluids (osmotic diarrhea), and increased translocation of newly colonized bacteria. Institution of trophic

feeding or "gut priming" with small volumes of dilute formula or breast milk has been shown to have numerous physiologic benefits and does not increase the risk of NEC.[11]

CLINICAL ASSOCIATIONS

Clinical conditions predisposing to NEC include those in which GI perfusion or mucosal integrity is compromised. Premature newborns are particularly susceptible to mucosal injury because of impaired autoregulation of blood flow, increased permeability of the GI mucosa, and deficient local and systemic immune responses. The presence of a patent ductus arteriosus further increases the risk of NEC because of impaired systemic blood flow with left-to-right shunting during diastole. Polycythemia may be another predisposing risk factor for NEC. Increased oxygen-carrying capacity afforded by the increased red cell mass does not make up for the decreased blood flow from hyperviscosity, and studies have shown a 50% reduction in oxygen delivery to the tissues, with polycythemia.[5] Infants who are small for gestational age (SGA) are at increased risk of NEC, presumably from chronic asphyxia of the fetus due to placental insufficiency and from the associated polycythemia. A number of studies have linked in utero cocaine exposure to postnatal development of NEC in the full-term infant.[12,13] This may be due to ischemic damage from cocaine-induced vasoconstriction or to early disruption of vascular development in the GI tract.

CLINICAL PRESENTATION

The timing of onset of NEC is inversely proportional to gestational age: near-term infants commonly present during the first several days of life, while extremely preterm infants often develop the disease at several weeks of age. The clinical presentation of NEC ranges from a mild, indolent GI disturbance to a fulminant sepsis-like syndrome, which can be rapidly fatal. In the mild form of the disease, the infant often develops GI symptoms such as abdominal distention, increased gastric residuals, and guaiac-positive stools. Vomiting and loose stools are less common. Systemic signs may also be present, including lethargy, increased episodes of apnea and bradycardia, temperature instability, and poor color and perfusion. Taken individually, many of these findings are common in the preterm infant and may suggest other diagnoses, but a combination of these symptoms in a previously well child should alert the clinician to the possibility of NEC.

The newborn infant with fulminant NEC presents with the same signs and symptoms in a more severe and rapidly progressive form. The abdominal wall may become discolored with focal or diffuse erythema (sometimes referred to as the "red dot" sign), reflecting underlying peritonitis, or with a gray-green color from meconium, blood, or dead bowel in the peritoneal cavity. There is often evidence of shock with delayed capillary refill, tachycardia, and hypotension, which may be due to capillary leak or to abdominal distention causing compression of the inferior vena cava and decreased venous return to the heart.[14]

Another entity that is much less common is benign pneumatosis coli. This term describes the condition of a healthy, usually term or near-term infant in whom pneumatosis intestinalis is noted on an abdominal radiograph. The infant may be asymptomatic or have bloody stools. Laboratory studies are normal, and the pneumatosis usually resolves over several days. It is unclear whether the pathophysiology of benign pneumatosis coli is the same as that of NEC, with the disease severity limited by such factors as enhanced integrity of the gastrointestinal mucosa, more mature host defense mechanisms, or limited bacterial-virulence. Treatment of a newborn with benign pneumatosis coli is the same as for stage I NEC (Table 33-1), as continued enteral feedings can exacerbate the condition.[15]

DIAGNOSIS

A high index of suspicion and low threshold for instituting evaluation and treatment of NEC are necessary to detect the disease in its early stages and minimize mor-

bidity and mortality. Diagnosis is based on a combination of clinical, laboratory, and radiographic findings, as noted in Table 33-1.

Because of the wide range of severity of NEC, a staging system was devised by Bell et al.[16] in 1978 and later modified by Walsh and Kliegman.[17] The Modified Bell Staging Criteria for NEC (Table 33-1) distinguishes among suspected, proven, and advanced disease. Stage I NEC, sometimes referred to as suspected NEC or a NEC scare, describes the condition of an infant who has mild clinical signs but a normal abdominal radiograph and laboratory studies. In stage II NEC, pneumatosis intestinalis is seen on radiography and the infant may be mildly or moderately ill. Stage III NEC refers to advanced disease with peritonitis and shock. This classification facilitates communication among pediatricians, neonatologists, and surgeons caring for patients with NEC and simplifies interpretation of the literature on the disease.

Pneumatosis Intestinalis

The radiographic finding most commonly associated with NEC is pneumatosis intestinalis, or gas in the bowel wall. In an on-end view of an intestinal loop, this will appear as "train-tracking" or bubbles of air dissecting within the intestinal wall. When the bowel is seen in transverse section, pneumatosis may appear as a diffuse bubbly pattern that is indistinguishable from stool (Fig 33-2). Distention of the intestinal loops associated with an ileus is common and may be diffuse or localized. The presence of a single dilated loop whose position is unchanged on serial abdominal radiographs rays (the so-called "sentinel loop") is highly suggestive of NEC. In more advanced stages, air may dissect from the bowel wall into veins and may be seen as linear lucencies of air in the portal venous system within the liver. If intestinal perforation occurs, free air can be seen on radiography, the location of which depends on the position of the infant for the study. If the child is lying supine, an oval-shaped lucency may be seen overlying the abdomen. The free air may outline the falciform ligament in the liver, creating the "football sign" (oval lucency with a vertical stripe). The best positions to evaluate an infant for intestinal perforation are the left lateral decubitus position (left side down), with the free air visible above the liver, or the cross-table lateral view.[18]

Many of the signs and symptoms of NEC, taken individually, are associated with other disease processes in the newborn. Preterm infants often have GI hypomotility, and abdominal distention and gastric residuals are common findings. These signs, along with others, such as apnea or lethargy, can be observed in children with sepsis, many of whom will be found to have an ileus. Bloody stools should alert the clinician to the possibility of NEC, although anal fissures, milk protein allergy, or gastroenteritis may also be responsible. In the preterm

TABLE 33-1.   Clinical Features and Management of Necrotizing Enterocolitis Based on Bell's Staging

Bell's Stage	I (Suspect)	II (Mild–Moderate)	III (Severe)
Signs	Apnea, bradycardia Feeding intolerance Temperature instability Guaiac-positive stools (IA) Frank blood in stools (IB)	Same as stage I, plus: Abdominal tenderness Absent bowel sounds Abdominal wall discoloration (IIB) Right lower quadrant mass (IIB)	Same as stages I–II, plus: Severe peritonitis symptoms Hypotension, shock
Laboratory findings	Normal	Mild metabolic acidosis (IIB) Mild thrombocytopenia (IIB)	Severe metabolic acidosis DIC, neutropenia Hyponatremia
Radiographic findings	Normal or distended loops	Intestinal dilatation Pneumatosis intestinalis (IIA) Portal vein gas (IIB)	Same as stage II, plus: Ascites (IIIA) Pneumoperitoneum (IIIB)
Medical treatment	NPO; antibiotics ×3–4 days if symptoms resolve and cultures are negative; laboratory studies[a] and abdominal radiographs q24h	NPO; antibiotics ×10–14 days; laboratory studies[a] and abdominal radiographs q12h until stable	NPO; antibiotics ×14 days[b]; laboratory studies[a] and abdominal radiographs q6–8 h until stable; treat metabolic acidosis; fluid resuscitation; pressors; blood products as needed
Surgical treatment	None	None	Laparotomy, resection of necrotic bowel for perforation; peritoneal drain for extremely sick, extremely premature patient, as a temporizing measure

Abbreviations: DIC, disseminated intravascular coagulation; NPO, nothing per os.

[a] Laboratory studies: complete blood count with differential, serum electrolytes, blood gas (initial laboratory evaluation includes blood culture).

[b] Bowel rest may continue longer than 14 days, depending on clinical condition.

or high-risk full-term newborn with signs suggestive of NEC, feedings should be withheld until the diagnosis is ruled out by radiographs, laboratory studies, and physical examination.

LABORATORY FINDINGS

In the milder presentation or early stages of NEC, laboratory values are often normal. With more severe disease, laboratory abnormalities reflect the cytotoxic effects of ischemia, infection, and inflammation. Intestinal necrosis commonly results in a metabolic acidosis, which in some infants may stimulate a compensatory respiratory alkalosis. Cell death also results in the release of potassium, and hyperkalemia can be a life-threatening problem for the small preterm infant with renal insufficiency. Hyponatremia is a common finding in advanced NEC and is due to third-space fluid losses in the abdomen. The complete blood count (CBC) often indicates throm-

bocytopenia, which may or may not be associated with disseminated intravascular coagulation (DIC). Leukocytosis or leukopenia with a left-shifted differential count is commonly observed. Other indicators of infection or inflammation, such as the erythrocyte sedimentation rate (ESR) and C-reactive protein, are often elevated in NEC but are not specific for the disease.

Although 10% to 30% of infants with NEC have positive blood cultures, it is uncertain whether bacteremia is a cause or a consequence of NEC. Stool cultures should be obtained during NEC epidemics, both from patients and from staff who have symptoms referrable to the GI tract.

TREATMENT

Once the diagnosis of NEC is suspected, the two mainstays of therapy are bowel rest and parenteral antibiotics. Feedings should be discontinued and intravenous fluids

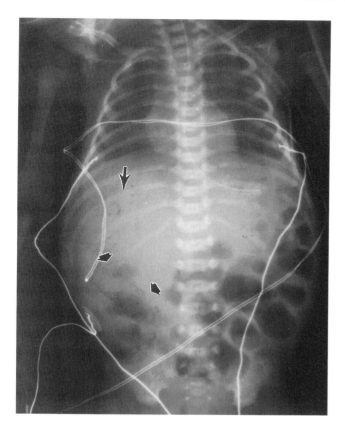

FIGURE 33-2. Radiographic appearance of pneumatosis intestinalis (small arrows) and portal venous air (large arrow).

started immediately. Any oral medications the child was receiving should be changed to intravenous dosing or discontinued. Choice of antibiotics depends to some extent on the condition of the infant and on the microbial flora of the unit during the illness, but generally ampicillin and gentamicin are effective. If the infant is at risk of staphylococcal infection, vancomycin should be considered in place of ampicillin until infection with a beta-lactamase-producing staphylococcus is ruled out. In severe cases of NEC, or in the face of intestinal perforation, clindamycin may be added to treat sepsis caused by anaerobic organisms.

An infant with stage III NEC may require more intensive therapy to treat shock or DIC. Fluid resuscitation should be accomplished with colloid solutions (5% albumin) or blood products, as required, to maintain adequate perfusion and blood pressure. Dopamine or other pressors should be used to support blood pressure and improve renal perfusion when capillary leak and abdominal distention are severe. Oliguria is often a sign of decreased intravascular volume and should be treated with vigorous fluid resuscitation to prevent prerenal failure. Treatment of metabolic acidosis, anemia, and thrombocytopenia is essential and may be difficult in the presence of extensive intestinal necrosis.[14]

Monitoring of the child with severe NEC includes frequent abdominal radiographs and laboratory studies, including a blood-gas determination, CBC, and serum electrolytes. This should be done every 6 to 8 hours during the acute stage of the illness. Children with mild disease require less frequent monitoring.

Indications for surgery in NEC vary somewhat from one institution and from one surgeon to the next. In general, the absolute indication for surgery is intestinal perforation diagnosed by radiography or paracentesis. Relative indications include persistent and severe metabolic acidosis or thrombocytopenia, refractory shock or oliguria, and abdominal mass. Surgical management of NEC commonly involves the resection of dead bowel and either primary anastomosis (when the process is localized and the remaining bowel appears healthy) or, more commonly, creation of an ostomy. Re-exploration is often necessary to ensure the removal of all necrotic bowel.[19] It is generally thought that survival is possible with as little as 25 cm of small bowel without an ileocecal valve or 11 cm of small bowel with an intact ileocecal valve.[20]

When an infant with perforated NEC is so sick or so small that general anesthesia and surgery carry a high risk of mortality, paracentesis and placement of a Penrose drain in the abdomen should be considered. This may decompress the abdomen and improve perfusion to the intestines and kidneys, giving the child a chance to stabilize enough to tolerate laparotomy at a later time.[21]

In cases not requiring surgery, also known as "medical NEC," duration of treatment depends on the degree of illness. Children with mild symptoms and minimal or no laboratory or radiographic abnormalities (stage I NEC) should be maintained on bowel rest for 2 to 4 days and treated with intravenous antibiotics, pending culture results and clinical improvement. For stage II NEC, treatment should continue for 14 days, or longer if radiographic abnormalities persist more than 3 or 4 days. Stage III NEC may require a longer duration of bowel rest to allow intestinal tissue to heal.[14]

Any infant kept on bowel rest for more than a few days should receive parenteral hyperalimentation to provide adequate nutrition. Often central venous access is necessary in order to provide enough glucose and calories for growth. The infant should be monitored for evidence of hyperalimentation-related complications, such as bacteremia, fungemia, cholestasis, and hepatitis. When the period of bowel rest is complete, enteral feedings should be reinstituted gradually, with close observation for signs of feeding intolerance. Protein hydrolysate formula or dilute formula may be better tolerated in some patients with decreased absorptive capacity.

Short-term complications of NEC include intestinal perforation, multiple-organ failure, extensive intestinal necrosis, and death. The most frequent long-term complication in both medically and surgically treated NEC is intestinal stricture or adhesions, which occur in 10% to 30% of cases. Any child with a history of NEC who develops abdominal distention or vomiting upon refeeding should undergo a contrast study to evaluate for possible obstruction. Another less frequent, but more serious, complication of NEC is short bowel syndrome, causing malabsorption and malnutrition.[22]

PREVENTION

On the basis of what is known and theorized about the pathophysiology of NEC, strategies for prevention have been proposed.[23,24] Since the vast majority of affected infants are premature, prevention of preterm delivery is an obvious priority. When delivery before 32 weeks gestation is anticipated, the mother should be treated with corticosteroids. Antenatal betamethasone therapy not only induces lung maturation but has also been shown to decrease the incidence of NEC by as much as threefold.[27] Once a baby is born prematurely, maintenance of adequate blood pressure, oxygen delivery, and acid-base balance and avoidance of polycythemia will help maximize GI blood flow and mucosal integrity. Careful consideration should be given to timing and method of feeding. Several studies have examined the use of minimal enteral feeding (trophic feeding) in preterm newborns and have found no correlation with the occurrence of NEC. In fact, trophic feeding, as the name implies, induces growth and maturation of the intestinal mucosa and may have a protective effect against NEC. Once the preterm infant is clinically stable and a decision is made to begin a feeding advance, the dictum "start low and go slow" is appropriate. The volume of feeds in this vulnerable group should not be increased by more than 20 ml/kg/day.[11] Signs of feeding intolerance or systemic illness should prompt discontinuation of feedings until a thorough evaluation is complete. Many neonatologists will elect to delay feedings for several days in a newborn with significant perinatal asphyxia and in those exposed to cocaine in utero.

Breast-milk feeding has long been known to have immunologic benefits. Recent studies have suggested a protective effect of breast milk in NEC. Many factors in human milk have the potential for playing a role in defense against bacterial infection, including secretory IgA, leukocytes, bifidus factor, which may promote the growth of non-pathogenic bacteria, and antibacterial molecules, such as lactoferrin, lactoperoxidase, and lysozyme.[25,26] Although it is unknown which of these factors is instrumental in decreasing the risk of NEC, much evidence points to a major role for immunoglobulins. Attempts have been made to prevent NEC with enteral administration of serum IgG and IgA in preterm infants; some clinical trials have shown a protective effect. Others have used prophylactic oral antibiotics to eliminate pathogenic bacteria, but this practice cannot be recommended because of the risk of selecting for resistant bacterial strains. Administration of bifidus or other nonpathogenic bacteria, especially to infants receiving prolonged courses of antibiotics, may overcome the problem of overgrowth of virulent bacterial strains. Acidification of the stomach with hydrochloric acid has also been investigated as a way to modulate the intestinal flora, and in one large study this was found to decrease the incidence of NEC.[28] Although none of these prophylactic strategies can be recommended routinely at this time, further clinical trials may prove their usefulness in preventing NEC in high-risk patients.

REFERRAL PATTERN

Newborns with NEC should be managed in an intensive care setting by neonatologists and pediatric surgeons.

REFERENCES

1. Stoll BJ. Epidemiology of necrotizing enterocolitis. Clin Perinatol 1994;21:205–218
2. Shepherd A, Granger J. Autoregulatory escape in the gut: a systems analysis. Gastroenterology 1973;65:77–81
3. Stoll B, Kanto W, Glass R et al. Epidemiology of necrotizing enterocolitis: a case control study. J Pediatr 1980;96:447–451
4. Kliegman R, Fanaroff A. Necrotizing enterocolitis. N Engl J Med 1984;310:1093–1103
5. Nowicki PT, Nankervis CA. The role of the circulation in the pathogenesis of necrotizing enterocolitis. Clin Perinatol 1994;21:219–234
6. Berseth CL. Gut motility and the pathogenesis of necrotizing enterocolitis. Clin Perinatol 1994;21:263–270
7. Willoughby RE, Pickering LK. Necrotizing enterocolitis and infection. Clin Perinatol 1994;21:307–315
8. Scheifele DW. Role of bacterial toxins in neonatal necrotizing enterocolitis. J Pediatr 1990;117:S44–46
9. Caplan MS, MacKendrick W. Inflammatory mediators and intestinal injury. Clin Perinatol 1994;21:235–246
10. Caplan MS, Sun XM, Hsueh W et al. Role of platelet activating factor and tumor necrosis factor-alpha in neonatal necrotizing enterocolitis. J Pediatr 1990;116:960–964
11. La Gamma EF, Browne LE. Feeding practices for infants weighing less than 1500 g at birth and the pathogenesis of necrotizing enterocolitis. Clin Perinatol 1994;21:271–306
12. Telsey A, Merrit T, Dixon S. Cocaine exposure in a term neonate. Clin Pediatr 1988;27:547–550
13. Czyrko C, DelPin C, O'Neil J. Maternal cocaine abuse and necrotizing enterocolitis. Pediatr Surg 1991;26:414–418
14. Kanto WP, Hunter JE, Stoll BJ. Recognition and medical

management of necrotizing enterocolitis. Clin Perinatol 1994;21:335–346

15. Leonidas JC, Hall RT. Neonatal pneumatosis coli: a mild form of neonatal necrotizing enterocolitis. J Pediatr 1976; 89:456–459

16. Bell MJ, Ternberg JL, Feigin RD et al. Neonatal necrotizing enterocolitis. Therapeutic decisions based upon clinical staging. Ann Surg 1978;187:1–7

17. Walsh MC, Kliegman RM. Necrotizing enterocolitis: treatment based on staging criteria. Pediatr Clin North Am 1986; 33:179–201

18. Morrison SC, Jacobson JM. The radiology of necrotizing enterocolitis. Clin Perinatol 1994;21:347–363

19. Ricketts RR. Surgical treatment of necrotizing enterocolitis and the short bowel syndrome. Clin Perinatol 1994;21: 365–387

20. Dorney SFA, Ament ME, Berquist WE et al. Improved survival in very short small bowel of infancy with use of long-term parenteral nutrition. J Pediatr 1985;107:521–525

21. Morgan LJ, Shochat SJ, Hartman GE. Peritoneal drainage as primary management of perforated necrotizing enterocolitis in the very low birth weight infant. J Pediatr Surg 1994; 29:30–34

22. Simon NP. Follow-up for infants with necrotizing enterocolitis. Clin Perinatol 1994;21:411–424

23. Vasan U, Gotoff SP. Prevention of neonatal necrotizing enterocolitis. Clin Perinatol 1994;21:425–435

24. Kliegman RM, Walker WA, Yolken RH. Necrotizing enterocolitis: research agenda for a disease of unknown etiology and pathogenesis. Clin Perinatol 1994;21:437–455

25. Lucas A, Cole TJ. Breast milk and neonatal necrotizing enterocolitis. Lancet 1990;336:1519–1523

26. Buescher ES. Host defense mechanisms of human milk and their relations to enteric infections and necrotizing enterocolitis. Clin Perinatol 1994;21:247–262

27. Crowley P, Chalmers I, Keirse MJNC et al. The effects of corticosteroid administration before delivery: overview of the evidence from controlled trials. Br J Obstet Gynaecol 1990;97:11–25

28. Carrion V, Egan EA. Prevention of necrotizing enterocolitis. J Pediatr Gastroenterol Nutr 1990;11:317–323

34

CANCER OF THE GASTROINTESTINAL TRACT

MICHAEL N. NEEDLE

The gastrointestinal (GI) tract is a common site of child-hood cancer. Nationwide, approximately 5% of cancer in children will be GI tumors, the overwhelming major-ity of which is non-Hodgkin's lymphoma (NHL). Pri-mary cancer (carcinoma) of the GI tract is a rare event in children and adolescents, compared to adults, in whom it is a major cause of morbidity and mortality, accounting for one-fourth of all cancer deaths. In the 25-year period ending in 1950, 1.05% (8 of 761) of the malignant tu-mors in patients less than 20 years of age encountered at Vanderbilt University Hospital were primary carci-noma of the GI tract.[1] Most of these arise in the colon and rectum. Carcinoma of the colon and rectum ac-counts for 1.5% of malignant solid tumors seen at the St. Jude Children's Research Hospital over a 15-year period beginning in 1962.[2] The Third National Cancer Survey reported an incidence of 1.3 cases of colorectal cancer per one million children.[3] These events are highly re-gional, and outside of the agricultural southeastern United States, colorectal carcinoma is an extraordinary event.

NON-HODGKIN'S LYMPHOMA

The most common malignant neoplasm of the GI tract in patients less than 20 years of age is lymphoma, often of the Burkitt's type, arising in Peyer's patches or the omentum. Like carcinoma of the alimentary tract, the presenting symptoms are rather nonspecific. Most pa-tients will complain of abdominal pain or distention. Some will have a palpable mass on physical examination. Others are taken to the operating room with the diagno-sis of intussusception. The onset is usually short and pa-tients can progress dramatically over a few days as these tumors can have a doubling time as short as 24 hours.

Pathophysiology

The most common histologic subtype is the diffuse small noncleaved cell type—Burkitt's lymphoma. This mature B-lymphocytic lymphoma expresses surface immuno-globulin. The defining cytogenetic abnormality is the t(8;14), which juxtaposes the c-myc oncogene and one of the immunoglobulin heavy chain loci.[4] Epstein-Barr virus (EBV) DNA has been associated with about 15% to 20% of sporadic Burkitt's lymphoma in the United States, as opposed to nearly all cases of endemic Burkitt's lymphoma in equatorial Africa.

Diagnosis

Most children with abdominal NHL will present with an abdominal mass or abdominal distention. For those taken to the operating room with intussusception, the only diagnostic pitfall is the failure to suspect lymphoma as the cause of the lesion, and not sending fresh tissue to the laboratory for cytogenetics and immunophenotyp-ing. Most patients will not present with an acute abdo-men. For those patients, laparotomy should be avoided as recovery from extensive surgery can delay the initiation of therapy in a patient with rapidly progressing disease. There is no need to attempt a radical resection, as extensive resection has no prognostic benefit in NHL. Bone marrow aspirate and biopsy is essential before taking a patient to the operating room, as patients with greater than 25% lymphoblasts in the marrow will be treated along the lines of a high-risk acute lymphoblastic leukemia (ALL). The yield is particularly high in patients who are anemic or thrombocytopenic, a sign of bone marrow replacement. Many patients will have ascites, and ascitic fluid can be obtained by paracentesis and used for cytology, immunophenotyping, and cytogenetics. If all these measures fail to confirm the diagnosis, a laparotomy should be performed.

Once the diagnosis is established, all patients will need a staging evaluation consisting of computed tomography (CT) of the chest and abdomen, bone scan, and bone marrow aspiration and biopsy. A lumbar puncture is required to evaluate possible central nervous system (CNS) involvement.

Therapy

An important consideration in the care of patients with Burkitt's lymphoma is tumor lysis syndrome, the metabolic consequence of high cell turnover and the release of uric acid, potassium, and phosphorus into the bloodstream. Careful monitoring of electrolytes, calcium, phosphorus, and uric acid is critical, once the diagnosis is established. Particular vigilance is required at the onset of chemotherapy, as treatment often exacerbates the level of metabolic disturbance. All patients should be started on high-dose intravenous fluids without supplemental potassium, usually at twice maintenance levels (125 ml/m^2/h). Bicarbonate should be added to the fluid to alkalinize the urine. A reasonable starting point is 5% dextrose with 35 mEq of sodium chloride and 35 mEq sodium bicarbonate per liter. Therapy with allopurinol should be instituted immediately and maintained until the level of uric acid stabilizes and returns to normal. The risk of tumor lysis and the need for these precautions are dependent on tumor bulk and may not be necessary in patients with localized small tumors.

Therapy is determined in large part by stage. Patients with disease limited to the abdomen can be treated with a brief, 6-month, course of four drugs; cyclophosphamide, vincristine, methotrexate, and prednisone.[5] Alternative regimens include the addition of doxorubicin, oral methotrexate, and 6-mercaptopurine.[6] All patients need prophylactic intrathecal chemotherapy to prevent CNS spread. Patients with disseminated disease require a longer course of more aggressive therapy, with the addition of cytosine arabinoside, doxorubicin, L-asparaginase, and high-dose methotrexate.[7] Most patients with Burkitt's lymphoma who are going to relapse will often do so within 6 months of initiation of therapy. Late relapses are particularly uncommon. Overall, prognosis is quite good, with greater than 70% survival for advanced-stage patients and greater than 90% survival for patients with localized disease.

COLORECTAL CARCINOMA

Of the primary malignant neoplasms of the GI tract, colorectal carcinoma is the most common; however, most children's hospitals will encounter this tumor rarely, if ever. There are no such cases in the tumor registry at the Children's Hospital of Philadelphia.

Pathophysiology

When evaluating a tumor as rare as colorectal carcinoma, there is little opportunity for epidemiologic investigations into possible etiology. It is noteworthy that the two largest series, which do not cover overlapping time periods, are both reported from Tennessee.[1,2] During a 2-year period, 13 patients with colorectal carcinoma were admitted to St. Jude Children's Research Hospital.[2] Eleven of the 13 children were from Tennessee, Mississippi, and Arkansas. Nine were from rural areas. Nine of 12 for whom data were available were exposed to either agricultural sprays, herbicides, or insecticides, suggesting exposure to these chemicals as a possible etiology. However, the tested pesticide levels in the blood of these patients were not generally higher than those in the blood of controls.[8]

Two conditions that predispose to colon cancer in adults are familial polyposis coli and inflammatory bowel disease (IBD). Although some investigators would recommend colectomy in patients with childhood onset of these diseases, none of the patients in the larger pediatric series had either of these conditions. This finding could reflect the long interval between onset of the predisposing condition and the diagnosis of cancer beyond adolescence.

Diagnosis

The major diagnostic pitfall in the evaluation of a patient with colorectal carcinoma is omitting colon cancer from the differential diagnosis. Most patients present in the second decade of life. Their presenting symptoms are nonspecific, with most children complaining of vague abdominal pain.[1,9] The next most common presenting symptom is alteration of bowel habits, both constipation and diarrhea, followed by anorexia and weight loss.[1,9,10] Rectal bleeding is an uncommon complaint. Median time from onset of symptoms to diagnosis is 2 to 6 months. Patients have been taken to the operating room with the presumptive diagnosis of acute appendicitis. In earlier series, the most common sign was an abdominal mass, followed by intermittent distention. In more recent series, these finding are less common. The common thread in reports from all investigators is that chronic, persistent, or recurrent abdominal pain requires a thorough investigation; malignancy should be considered along with the more common GI etiologies.

Initial workup begins with flexible endoscopy or barium enema. Lesions are often confirmed with CT or magnetic resonance imaging (MRI). Because of the common delay between onset of symptoms and definitive diagnosis, CT or MRI would be appropriate in any patient whose symptoms persist without an adequate diagnosis. Tumors are distributed throughout the ascending colon, the transverse colon, the descending colon, and the rectum. The rare patient with rectal bleeding will often have a tumor localized to the descending colon or rectum. Once the diagnosis is confirmed, staging evaluation should include a CT of the chest and bone scan.

Therapy

The mainstay of therapy is surgery. Laparotomy is essential to obtain adequate tissue for histologic examination in a disease for which the pediatric pathologist will demand certainty prior to making so rare a diagnosis. Careful staging, with sampling of regional lymph nodes and careful attention to seeding of the peritoneum and viscera, has tremendous prognostic value. Every attempt should be made to accomplish a complete surgical resection and primary reanastomosis if possible. Unfortunately, the majority of patients will have dissemination at the time of surgery (Dukes stages C and D) (Table 34-1).

The most common histology is a poorly differentiated mucin-producing type, in distinction to adults where this histology represents less than 15% of cases.[11] All series report that most patients will have evidence of distant spread at the time of operation. This is of crucial importance, as the few long-term survivors of colorectal carcinoma in adolescence are patients who were Dukes stage B at operation. Preoperative radiotherapy has been used to convert an unresectable tumor to one which was resectable.[10]

TABLE 34-1. Modified Dukes Classification of Colorectal Carcinoma

Stage	Description
A	Lesion confined to bowel wall
B	Direct extension to serosal fat without lymph node involvement
C	Lymph node involvement
D	Distant metastases

Experience with adjuvant chemotherapy has produced modest success. The choice of adjuvant chemotherapy is often guided by adult experience. Minor responses (less than 50% tumor shrinkage) have been observed following administration of the combination of 5-fluorouracil (5-FU), methyl-CCNU, and vincristine.[2] The combination of 5-FU and leucovorin produced one complete response and two partial responses in seven patients.[12] Although these responses are encouraging, most long-term survivors undergo complete surgical excision, which emphasizes that early diagnosis and radical surgery offer the best chance for cure.

GASTRIC CARCINOMA

Malignant tumors of the stomach are rare in childhood and adolescence. Most will be lymphomas and to a lesser extent sarcomas. Fewer than 20 cases of gastric carcinoma in children have been reported in the literature. There are two cases in the tumor registry at the Children's Hospital of Philadelphia. Presenting complaints include vomiting, abdominal pain, hematemesis, anorexia, and weight loss.[13–15] Most patients are more than 10 years of age. The most common diagnosis prior to discovery of malignancy is benign ulcer disease. As with colorectal cancer, a delay in definitive diagnosis is the norm, with a mean delay of 2.7 months from onset of symptoms to diagnosis.[14] The diagnosis is often made by endoscopy. CT scans of the chest and abdomen are useful for presurgical planning, and an attempt should be made at complete excision. Experience with adjuvant chemotherapy is limited and all effort should be made at complete resection. In circumstances militating against complete excision, radiation therapy and chemotherapy with 5-FU and leucovorin, modeled after colorectal carcinoma, is a reasonable alternative.

IMMUNE DEFICIENCY–RELATED CANCER

The increase in the incidence of immunodeficiency, both acquired and iatrogenic, has opened the potential for an increase in the incidence of cancer of the alimentary tract in children and adolescents. Acquired immunodeficiency syndrome (AIDS), human immunodeficiency virus (HIV), and immune suppression in the setting of solid organ or bone marrow transplantation predispose patients to GI neoplasms. Epstein-Barr virus–associated lymphoproliferative disease (EBV-LPD) is a life-treatening complication of immune suppression.[16] This condition is also referred to as post-transplant lymphoproliferative disease. Risk increases with the level of immune suppression and with the load of EBV in peripheral blood lymphocytes.[17] Patients infected follow-ing solid organ transplant are at greater risk than are those who have reactivation of latent EBV. The presen-tation is indistinguishable from de novo neoplasia. The primary diagnostic dilemma is establishing the grade of the tumor. Low-grade neoplasms, which are polymorphic and polyclonal, appear to be exuberant proliferative re-sponses to EBV infection. Most patients in this state can be treated with reduction or, if possible, with elimina-tion, of the offending agent, usually azathioprine, cyclosporin A, or FK-506. The result, when successful, is rapid spontaneous regression. In those cases in which the tumor is frankly malignant, in effect a B-cell (Bur-kitt's) lymphoma, reduction in immune suppression is usually inadequate. These tumors are histologically mo-nomorphic and consist exclusively of immunoblasts. They are usually monoclonal, as evidenced by immuno-globulin gene rearrangements, and must be treated as NHL. Efficacy of anti-B-cell monoclonal antibodies (mAb) has been reported as an alternative modality.[18] As the distinction between EBV-LPD and frank lym-phoma can be difficult, and carries tremendous prognos-tic and therapeutic implications, consultation with a pa-thologist familiar with these entities is essential. Patients with localized disease have been salvaged; patients with disseminated disease, particularly to the CNS, tend to fare poorly.

Leiomyoma of the GI tract is a rare soft tissue tumor. This entity has been reported in a number of children with AIDS.[19,20] Onset is insidious, with weight loss and abdominal tenderness reported as presenting signs. Tu-mors have been discovered at autopsy. Therapy is surgical excision when possible. Aggressive adjuvant therapy in patients with underlying immunodeficiency can be fraught with difficulty due to infectious complications. No long-term survivors have been reported to date.

SUMMARY

Cancer of the alimentary tract is an uncommon event, particularly primary carcinoma. As all these neoplasms are more likely to be treated successfully when localized, it is prudent for the diagnostician to include cancer in the differential diagnosis of patients with common GI complaints that are not readily explained by more com-mon diagnoses. Rapid consultation of the pediatric sur-geon, oncologist, and radiation oncologist will facilitate a rapid diagnostic evaluation and initiation of therapy.

REFERENCES

1. Sessions RT, Riddell DH, Kaplan HJ, Foster JH. Carcinoma of the colon in the first two decades of life. Ann Surg 1965; 162:279–284

2. Pratt, CB, Rivera G, Shanks E et al. Colorectal carcinoma in adolescents, implications regarding etiology. Cancer 1977; 40:2464–2472

3. Third National Cancer Survey: Incidence Data. In: Cutler SJ, Young JL, Ed. Monograph No. 41. Bethesda, MD: Na-tional Cancer Institute, 1975:102

4. Berger R, Bernheim A, DeLa Chapelle A. Chromosome rear-rangements in acquired malignant disease. Human gene mapping 6: sixth international workshop on human gene mapping. Cytogenet Cell Genet 1982;32:205

5. Meadows AT, Sposto R, Jenkin RDT et al. Similar efficacy of 6 and 18 months of therapy with four drugs (COMP) for localized non-Hodgkin's lymphoma of children: A report from the Children's Cancer Study Group. J Clin Oncol 1989; 7:92–99

6. Link MP, Donaldson SS, Berard CW et al. Results of treat-ment of childhood localized non-Hodgkin's lymphoma with combination chemotherapy with or without radiotherapy. N Engl J Med 1990;322:1169–1174

7. Finlay JL, Anderson JR, Cecalupo AJ et al. Disseminated nonlymphoblastic lymphoma of childhood: a Children's Cancer Group study, CCG-552. Med Pediatr Oncol 1994; 23:453–463

8. Caldwell GC, Cannon SB, Pratt CB, Arthur RD. Serum pesticide levels in patients with childhood colorectal carci-noma. Cancer 1981;48:774–778

9. Middlekamp JN, Haffner H. Carcinoma of the colon in chil-dren. Pediatrics 1963;32:558–571

10. Rao BN, Pratt CB, Fleming ID et al. Colon carcinoma in children and adolescents. Cancer 1985;55:1322–1326

11. Odone V, Change L, Caces J et al. The natural history of colorectal carcinoma in adolescents. Cancer 1982;49: 1716–1720

12. Pratt CB, Meyer WH, Howlett N et al. Phase II study of 5-fluorouracil/leucovorin of pediatric patients with malignant solid tumors. Cancer 1994;74:2593–2598

13. Murphy S, Shaw K, Blanchard H. Report of three gastric tumors in children. J Pediatr Surg 1994;29:1202–1204

14. McGill TW, Downey EC, Westbrook J et al. Gastric carci-noma in children. J Pediatr Surg 1993;28:1620–1621

15. Munck A, Bellaiche M, Ferkadji L et al. Carcinoma of the stomach in a child. J Pediatr Gastroenterol Nutr 1993;16: 334–336

16. Nalesnik MA. Lymphoproliferative disease in organ trans-plant recipients. Springer Semin Immunopathol 1991;13: 199–216

17. Savoie A, Perpete C, Carpentier L et al. Direct correlation between the load of Epstein-Barr virus-infected lymphocytes in the peripheral blood of pediatric transplant patients and risk of lymphoproliferative disease. Blood 1994;83: 2715–2722

18. Leblond V, Sutton L, Dorent R. Lymphoproliferative disor-ders after organ transplantation: a report of 24 cases observed in a single center. J Clin Oncol 1995;13:961–968

19. Chadwick EG, Connor EJ, Hanson ICG et al. Tumors of smooth-muscle origin in HIV-infected children. JAMA 1990;263:3182–3184

20. Mueller BU, Butler KM, Higham MC et al. Smooth muscle tumors in children with human immunodeficiency virus in-fection. Pediatrics 1992;90:460–463

35

PARASITES

MARK BAGARAZZI
LOUIS BELL

This chapter summarizes the pathophysiology, etiology, clinical manifestations, diagnosis, laboratory evaluation, and treatment of parasitic gastrointestinal (GI) infections in general. This discussion is followed by a description of the same features of the more common infections, both separately and in greater detail.

PATHOPHYSIOLOGY AND ETIOLOGY

Intestinal parasites are spread almost exclusively by the oral-fecal route, with the protozoa usually colonizing an unsuspecting host. The mechanisms that lead to the transition from asymptomatic carriage of protozoa to either a malabsorptive secretory diarrhea or the more invasive dysentery are poorly understood. Dysentery involves deeper mucosal invasion and is characterized by fever, more severe abdominal pain with tenesmus, and stool mixed with blood or mucus, or both.

Parasites have become an increasingly important consideration in children with GI disease as a result of several recent trends (Table 35-1). Increasing numbers of children are accompanying their families during international travel and are even more likely to develop parasitic infections because of their propensity for playing in soil (potentially fecally contaminated) and propensity for relatively poor hygiene. Immature immune responses and small physical size also contribute to increased symptomatology (e.g., dehydration). The same propensities and attributes also make children more susceptible to intestinal parasites at home, especially in child-care set-

tings. Immunosuppression not only increases the severity of any parasitic enteritis but also broadens the number of parasitic infections one needs to consider.

Parasitic causes of GI disease in the pediatric population range from the all-too-familiar pinworm, giardiasis, and amebiasis to exotic-sounding, yet rarely encountered, organisms such as *Diphyllobothrium latum* and *Angiostrongylus costaricensis*. The latter organism is actually a classic example of a very common parasite of South America that would be readily recognized by someone practicing there, but that is almost unheard of in the United States, except among travelers to that endemic area. This chapter describes the most common protozoa and helminths (worms) affecting children. Table 35-2 presents a brief outline of symptoms, diagnostic approaches, first-line therapy, and other features of slightly less common childhood parasitoses.

CLINICAL PRESENTATION

Parasitic infection is one of the leading considerations in the evaluation of any patient with GI symptoms (e.g., diarrhea) who has a history of recent immigration or travel from endemic areas with poor sanitation.[1] However, in the absence of historical clues, parasitic disease is not usually a primary consideration in the child who appears to be suffering from self-limited, presumably viral, enteritis. Persistence of the diarrhea is usually the first indication that leads to consideration of a parasitic cause. Although several parasitic diseases can be ac-

TABLE 35-1. Recent Trends Leading to Increased Parasitic Disease in Children

---

Acquired immunodeficiency syndrome (AIDS) and iatrogenic immunosuppression

Immigration from areas endemic for parasitic diseases, including adopted children

Day-care center attendance

International travel to areas endemic for parasitic diseases

---

quired in the United States,[2] a thorough travel history may provide the only clue to a parasitic diagnosis. As most parasites are found in a particular geographic distribution, questioning should include whether travel was limited to urban areas or included rural locales. Other important historical items are the length of visit and whether shoes were worn routinely. A dietary history can contribute in cases of *Trichinella* and the cestodes (tapeworms). GI symptoms are seen with fascioliasis, hookworm, and ascariasis. Urticaria is usually limited to tissue-invasive helminths but may point to infection with *Onchocerca volvulus*, hookworm, *Strongyloides stercoralis*, or trichinosis. Wheezing is seen rarely, as a result of pulmonary migration by helminths such as hookworm and *Ascaris*. The clinical manifestations of the most common childhood enteric parasites are described below.

DIAGNOSIS

Examination of the stool for ova and parasites should be done on at least three separate occasions to ensure adequate sensitivity due to the intermittent pattern of ova release by intestinal parasites (specifically the helminths). Fresh (less than 1-hour-old) stool specimens are preferred for observing live amebae and larvae but preservative containers with formalin and polyvinyl alcohol are available. Aspiration from the duodenum during endoscopy or the use of swallowed string tests (e.g., Entero-Test) may be useful in detecting *Giardia*, hookworm, *Strongyloides*, *Cryptosporidia*, or the liver flukes (*Clonorchis sinensis* and *Fasciola hepatica*) when stool ex-

TABLE 35-2. Less Common Gastrointestinal Parasitoses in Children[a]

Organism	Symptoms	Diagnosis	Complications	Therapy	Comments
Necator americanus, Ancylostoma duodenale (hookworm)	Absent to hoarseness, vomiting, colicky abdominal pain, diarrhea	Oocytes in stool or with concentration techniques, eosinophilia	Anemia, edema, malnutrition	Mebendazole, pyrantel pamoate, albendazole	Tropical and rural travel, bare feet
Trichuris trichiura (whipworm)	Abdominal pain, tenesmus, mucoid bloody diarrhea	Oocytes in stool or with concentration techniques	Rectal prolapse	Mebendazole, albendazole	Rural southeast U.S., prevalence 800 million worldwide
Ascaris lumbricoides (roundworm)	Mild or absent abdominal pain	Adult worm in feces or vomitus, eosinophilia	Intestinal or biliary obstruction, peritonitis, pneumonitis	Mebendazole, pyrantel pamoate, albendazole	Rural southern U.S., prevalence 1 billion worldwide
Clonorchis spp. (liver flukes)	Anorexia, epigastric pain, diarrhea	Oocytes in stool or biliary aspirate, eosinophilia	Cholangitis, cholelithiasis, pancreatitis	Praziquantel, albendazole	Southeast Asian immigrants, raw or pickled fish
Strongyloides stercoralis	Abdominal pain, distention, vomiting, mucoid voluminous diarrhea	Larvae in stool or duodenal aspirate, (Entero-test) serology, eosinophilia	Pruritic skin lesions in perianal and thigh areas, pneumonitis, gram-negative bacillary septicemia	Thiabendazole, ivermectin	Tropical and subtropical including southern and southwestern United States
Hymenolepis nana (dwarf tapeworm)	Usually asymptomatic, anorexia, abdominal pain and diarrhea with severe infection	Oocytes in stool		Praziquantel, niclosamide	Temperate and tropical worldwide, pet rodents

[a] Listed in order, from more to less common.

aminations are repeatedly negative but symptoms and suspicion persist.

LABORATORY EVALUATION

Eosinophilia (more than 500 eosinophils/μl) is far more common in helminthic than in protozoal infections, with the degree of tissue invasion correlating with the level of eosinophilia.[2] The positive predictive value of eosinophilia for parasitic infection has been measured to vary from 14% in expatriate Americans to 55% among Southeast Asian refugees.[3,4] The finding of less than 500 eosinophils/μl was shown to be more useful, with a negative predictive value of 96% and 73%, respectively, in the same populations. Consequently, the absence of eosinophilia is useful in ruling out parasitic diseases but its presence is less than diagnostic, even in an endemic population.

Protozoa

There may be considerable variability in the level of skill among microbiology technicians in detecting ova and parasites microscopically. Amebiasis, *Giardia*, and *Cryptosporidium* are now detectable using sensitive and specific enzyme-linked immunosorbent assay (ELISA) on stool specimens. Since the cost of an ELISA is one-third that of the ova and parasite examination, and the latter two organisms account for most parasitic infections in the United States, these assays have become a more cost-effective screen in specific clinical scenarios.[5] These situations would include persistent diarrhea in a child in a day-care setting or living on a farm (coming in contact with livestock), in association with a water-borne outbreak, after a camping trip, or in an immunosuppressed child. The examination of stool for ova and parasites is still the most cost-effective test in the patient returning from areas endemic for a variety of intestinal parasites. Clinicians using smaller laboratories should consult with their clinical microbiologists in determining if the newer tests would be better suited for their needs. These tests may also be useful as an adjunct to the traditional examination for ova and parasites in scenarios other than those listed above, since they are specific for only a handful of diseases.

Helminths

Serology is available for strongyloidiasis and trichinosis (latex agglutination). Other investigational diagnostic tests are available, free of charge, from the Division of Parasitic Diseases (DPD) Reference Immunodiagnostic Laboratory at the Centers for Disease Control and Prevention (CDC), once specimens have been processed

through one's state health department. They may be reached at (770) 488–4431 and (770) 488-4108 (FAX) for serology and at (770) 488–4474 for microscopic diagnostics. For a more detailed description of the laboratory techniques used to detect stool pathogen, see Chapter 79.

TREATMENT

Protozoa

Treatment is recommended for *G. lamblia* or *Isospora belli* infections, if symptomatic, and for all *Entamoeba histolytica* infections.[6] In 1% to 20% of stool ova and parasite examinations, *Blastocystis hominis* will be detected, although the significance of this finding is controversial, as an asymptomatic carrier state has been well described.[7] Treatment aimed at this organism should be considered only if other causes have been eliminated and symptoms persist. Metronidazole and iodoquinol have been used for this infection, although the evidence supporting their use is anecdotal. Table 35-3 lists other organisms that do not require specific therapy when encountered in a stool examination for ova and parasites. The latest recommendations from *The Medical Letter on Drugs and Therapeutics* include a complete listing of drugs and dosages for various parasitic GI infections.[8]

Helminths

Mebendazole and pyrantel pamoate are both effective against pinworms, hookworms, and ascarids, although only the former is effective for trichuriasis. *Hymenolepsis nana* and other intestinal cestodes (tapeworms) can be treated with niclosamide or praziquantel. Albendazole and thiabendazole are broad-spectrum antiparasitics related to mebendazole. The former became available in the summer of 1996, and the latter is limited by common side effects, including nausea, vomiting, and headache.

TABLE 35-3. Non-Pathogenic Stool Co-inhabitants Not Requiring Therapy

Endolimax nana

Entamoeba coli

Entamoeba hartmanni

Entamoeba polecki

Entamoeba gingivalis

Iodamoeba buetschlii

Chilomastix mesnili

Trichomonas hominis

GIARDIASIS

Pathophysiology and Etiology

The intestinal protozoa *Giardia lamblia*, arguably the most common parasitic cause of diarrhea in the United States and in other developed countries, was found in 7% of stool specimens in the United States in 1987.[9] It may be seen at any age but is especially prevalent in children attending nurseries or day-care facilities. Intestinal villi may become blunted with focal inflammation seen in the crypts during symptomatic infection.

Clinical Presentation

In a hypothetical sample of 100 people ingesting *G. lamblia* cysts, only 25% to 50% will become symptomatic, 5% to 15% will be asymptomatic carriers (reported up to 6 months), and the remainder will never demonstrate evidence of infection. The presence of persistent, and often intermittent, diarrhea is the most common clinical scenario associated with giardiasis. Steatorrhea and its associated foul smell is also common, as is flatulence, bloating, nausea, and anorexia. Impaired absorption of fat-soluble vitamins and weight loss may occur in cases in which the diagnosis is delayed. Lactase deficiency may occur, persisting several weeks after the infection has been cleared. The presence of mucus or blood should lead one to consider the presence of multiple organisms, as these are not features of isolated giardiasis.

Diagnosis

The diagnosis is usually established by the demonstration of the familiar owl's face of the trophozoite (usually only found in fresh liquid stool specimens) or cysts in more formed stool. Duodenal aspiration and the swallowed string test (e.g., Entero-Test) are performed less often but increase the diagnostic yield beyond that afforded by stool examination alone. Careful examination of a single stool is 50% to 70% sensitive, with some reports claiming up to 90% sensitivity on the basis of examination of three stools. At times, *G. lamblia* has been recovered only after seven or eight stool examinations, in cases of chronic diarrhea.

Laboratory Evaluation

Giardia antigens are now detectable in stool specimens, using monoclonal fluorescent and capture ELISA, which are both sensitive and specific. An ELISA detecting a glycoprotein of *G. lamblia* is reported to be 85% to 98% sensitive and 90% to 100% specific at a cost comparable to the traditional ova and parasites examination (see the section *Laboratory Evaluation*, above, in the introductory discussion).

Treatment

Treatment is only recommended for symptomatic *G. lamblia* infections. Metronidazole (15 mg/kg/day divided tid for 7 days) is effective in treating giardiasis but has become less popular than furazolidone (6 mg/kg/day divided qid) because of the more convenient liquid form of the latter agent. Patients also often complain of a metallic taste with metronidazole. Many older references list quinacrine for the treatment of giardiasis but, as those who have attempted to prescribe it may have learned, it is no longer available in the U.S. Children excreting *Giardia* without diarrhea should not be restricted from attending day care.[10]

AMEBIASIS

Pathophysiology and Etiology

As the third leading cause of parasitic mortality worldwide, *Entamoeba histolytica* is the only protozoan ameba of the seven that consistently causes disease, although differentiation from other amebae may be difficult. *Dientamoeba fragilis* is the only other ameba that occasionally produces symptomatic diarrhea, but silent infection is much more common. Table 35-3 lists the other commensal amebae. The cell wall of *E. histolytica* cysts typically dissolves in the small intestine, and the organism divides and is subsequently found in the colon. The characteristic flask-shaped ulcers form when cytolytic enzymes break down the mucosa, especially in areas of fecal stasis. Symptomatology is usually absent, but invasion of the bowel wall may herald the onset of significant disease.

Clinical Presentation

Symptoms range from dysentery to a fulminant picture in certain persons (e.g., pregnant women, corticosteroid recipients) infected with *E. histolytica*, while most remain clinically silent. The dysentery is characterized by cramping abdominal pain, flatulence, and intermittent (usually watery) foul-smelling diarrhea containing blood and mucus. More fulminant cases may be accompanied by fever, more severe abdominal pain, and profuse bloody diarrhea. Complications may include the classic hepatic abscess, secondary bacterial infection, postdysenteric colitis, and intestinal adhesions with or without fistula formation. The findings of fever and tender hepatic enlargement are classic for a solitary liver abscess located in the upper outer quadrant of the right lobe. The presentation of hepatic abscess may be either acute or insidious in roughly 5% of symptomatic patients. Hepatic abscess may extend locally into the pericardium, lung, or the unaffected hepatic lobe.

Diagnosis

Once again, trophozoites are more likely to be found in fresh liquid stool, while cysts may be present in more formed stools. Either form may be found by examination of wet mounts of fluid or stained tissue obtained endoscopically. Hepatic abscess should be apparent by abdominal ultrasound, which may be used in aspirating the characteristic reddish brown, odorless, acellular fluid.

Laboratory Evaluation

A test to differentiate pathogenic from co-inhabitant strains of E. histolytica is currently being developed. Serology may be positive in cases involving tissue invasion, especially in hepatic abscess, in which markedly elevated titers may be diagnostic.

Treatment

Metronidazole (35 to 50 mg/kg/day divided tid for 5 to 10 days) is the drug of choice for treating E. histolytica infections. Iodoquinol (30 mg/kg/day divided tid for 20 days) and paromomycin are both poorly absorbed but are currently recommended for use as immediate follow-up management of metronidazole therapy in amebic colitis, to reduce the incidence of relapse. Chloroquine at a dose of 10 mg/kg/day is recommended in addition to iodoquinol in extraintestinal amebiasis.[11] Family members of a patient with symptomatic amebiasis should undergo stool screening for asymptomatic carriage and receive iodoquinol to prevent spread to uninfected contacts, if cysts are found. Tinidazole has been shown to be superior to metronidazole in the treatment of amebiasis and giardiasis because it permits shorter courses and has fewer side effects but is not yet available in the U.S.[12]

PINWORM

Pathophysiology and Etiology

In contrast to most parasitic infections, the nematode Enterobius vermicularis is actually more common in temperate than in tropic climates, with more than 40 million Americans infected, mostly preschool and school age children. Eleven percent of tape tests performed by state laboratories in 1987 were positive for pinworm eggs,[9] making it the most common helminthic infection in the United States. Pinworm infection originates through hand-to-mouth ingestion of immature eggs, with larvae hatching and maturing to the adult form entirely within the intestines. Gravid females contribute to the cycle of auto-infection by migrating to the perianal region and releasing up to several thousand eggs. The oral hygiene habits of children play a role at this point, as a scratching hand picks up eggs, often catching them under fingernails, and eventually returns them to the mouth. Person-to-person spread is extremely efficient, with family members (especially mothers) and other co-inhabitants (i.e., institutionalized children) frequently becoming secondarily infected.

Clinical Presentation

Most pinworm infections are asymptomatic, with pruritus ani the sine qua non of a symptomatic infection.[13] The gravid female worm migrates to the perianal region more commonly at night, leading to the common complaint of nocturnal pruritus. Severe and/or prolonged pruritus may lead to perianal excoriation and subsequent bacterial superinfection. Even heavy infections rarely go on to cause abdominal pain or weight loss. Vulvovaginitis is a rare complication among girls.

Diagnosis

Pinworm cannot be diagnosed by standard ova and parasite stool examinations as the eggs are only rarely released into the bowel. Diagnosis is made by tape test, in which transparent tape is applied to the perianal region, preferably in the morning before bathing. The tape is then applied to a glass microscope slide, where the characteristic $55 \times 25\mu$ eggs may be seen under low magnification.

Laboratory Evaluation

The laboratory evaluation was described above.

Treatment

Treatment consists of an initial dose of pyrantel pamoate (11 mg/kg) or mebendazole (100 mg), followed 10 to 14 days later by a second dose. Experience is limited with either drug in children under the age of 2 years; the risks and benefits of treatment should be weighed in relation to the usually mild symptomatology. Treatment of the entire family should lessen the otherwise frequent occurrence of reinfection. Control of infections in day-care or institutional settings may be difficult, even with mass treatments of attendees and personnel. Subsequent reinfections probably do not reflect drug failure and may be treated with the initial regimen. No special hygienic measures are necessary. Excessive zeal in this area should be discouraged, to avoid inappropriate emphasis and the assignment of guilt.

CRYPTOSPORIDIOSIS

Pathophysiology and Etiology

Cryptosporidium parvum is a small (4 to 6 μ diameter) coccidian intestinal protozoan parasite that attaches to, and superficially invades, the microvilli of GI epithelial cells following fecal-oral transmission. The first human cases were reported in 1976 in two individuals who, in retrospect, were probably suffering from advanced AIDS. Infection has been demonstrated with as few as 10 oocysts and transmission is efficient with attack rates of 30% to 40% measured in day-care center outbreaks.[14] Children seem to be more easily infected, and outbreaks occur slightly more commonly in warmer humid months. The parasite is a common infection in cattle and may contaminate water reservoirs, such as occurred in Milwaukee, Wisconsin, in 1993, as it is unaffected by chlorination and most filters.

Clinical Presentation

Presentation depends largely on the immune status of the host. Symptoms in immunocompetent children vary from none to fever, vomiting, abdominal pain, and diarrhea (four to five watery foul-smelling stools per day) lasting from 1 day to more than a month (average ten days). In adults with more than 180 CD_4^+ lymphocytes per milliliter, cryptosporidia cleared spontaneously in 7 to 28 days, while 87% of patients with fewer than 180 CD_4^+ lymphocytes per milliliter developed persistent infection. Cellular immunity appears to be more important for protection, as several animal models have shown that antibody responses are not protective. In immunosuppressed children, especially those with AIDS, a chronic, cholera-like diarrhea often develops with subsequent severe dehydration and malnutrition, and often eventual death. The malabsorptive diarrhea is frequent (5 to 10 episodes per day), nonbloody, and watery (often referred to as frothy), often becoming chronic. The presence of blood or leukocytes in the stool of a patient known to be infected with C. parvum is unusual and may suggest the presence of more than one pathogen. Low-grade fever is the most common associated symptom, with crampy epigastric pain, nausea, vomiting, anorexia, and weight loss occurring as well. The infection is usually limited to the GI tract, including the bile duct system, but pulmonary and disseminated infection has been reported in rare cases in immunosuppressed patients.

Diagnosis

Standard ova and parasite examinations do not show the presence of the tiny oocysts. The diagnosis is usually made by the microscopic identification of red-stained (modified Kinyoun acid-fast) oocysts in concentrated stool, or occasionally in an intestinal biopsy specimen of a symptomatic patient. Oocyst shedding may be intermittent, so at least two separate specimens should be examined.

Laboratory Evaluation

Cryptosporidium is now detectable by monoclonal fluorescent and capture ELISA tests, both of which are sensitive and specific.

Treatment

The infection is usually self-limited in normal children, but it can be life-threatening in severely immunosuppressed patients, including adults living in the home of an infected child.[15] Many drugs have been tested in the treatment of cryptosporidiosis, but success has been elusive, especially in immunocompromised patients. Paromomycin (500 to 750 mg tid or qid in adults) is an essentially nonabsorbed aminoglycoside similar to neomycin that has shown limited effectiveness in patients with AIDS. Azithromycin at an adult dose of 1,250 mg/day for 2 weeks, followed by 500 mg/day, has shown some effectiveness as well. Antidiarrheal agents may provide some benefit to individual patients, but the mainstay of therapy is adequate hydration and nutrition by parenteral means if necessary. Patients with advanced AIDS should strongly consider using bottled drinking water, as the removal of cryptosporidia from the water supply cannot be guaranteed. Children excreting Cryptosporidium without diarrhea may attend day care.[14]

REFERRAL PATTERN

The CDC Disease Information System, (404) 639–1610, is periodically updated to provide information for international travelers and more detailed background information by FAX at (404) 332-4565. The CDC also provides information via its internet web page address of http://www.cdc.gov. The 1997 Red Book (Report of the American Academy of Pediatrics Committee on Infectious Diseases) may have additional details not covered in this brief synopsis. More difficult issues may be addressed by the pediatric faculty specializing in infectious diseases in the medical community or by U.S. government agencies such as the CDC, National Institutes of Health (NIH), or Armed Forces medical personnel. The National Center for Infectious Diseases DPD of the CDC is available for telephone consultation at (770) 488-7760 or 488-7761 (FAX). The CDC Drug Service, (404) 639-3670, also stocks several antiparasitics that are otherwise unavailable in the U.S.; these agents require an Investigational New Drug (IND) protocol.

REFERENCES

1. Baltazar J, Tiglao T, Tempongko S. Hygiene behavior and hospitalized severe childhood diarrhea: a case-control study. Bull WHO 1993;71:323–328

2. Wilson M. Eosinophilia. In: Wilson M, Ed. A World Guide to Infections: Diseases, Distribution, Diagnosis. New York: Oxford University Press, 1991:164–175

3. Nutman T, Ottesen E, Gam A et al. Eosinophilia in Southeast Asian refugees: evaluation at a referral center. J Infect Dis 1987;155:309–313

4. Markell E. Eosinophilia. In: Markell E, Voge M, Eds. Medical Parasitology. Philadelphia: WB Saunders, 1981:300–301

5. Rosenblatt JE. Laboratory diagnosis of parasitic infections. Mayo Clin Proc 1994;69:779–780

6. Richards FO. An overview of parasitic disease in children in the United States: What's old? What's new? Where's help? Pediatr Ann 1994;23:392–397

7. Rizack MA. Drugs for parasitic infections. Med Lett Drugs Ther 1995;37:99–108

8. Kappus K, Juranek D, Robert J. Results of testing for intestinal parasites by state diagnostic laboratories, United States, 1987. MMWR CDC, 1991;40(suppl):25–46

9. Addiss D, Juranek D, Spencer H. Treatment of children with asymptomatic and non-diarrheal *Giardia* infection. Pediatr Infect Dis J 1991;10:843–846

10. Pickering LK. Therapy for acute infectious diarrhea in children. J Pediatr 1991;118(suppl):S118–S128

11. White N. Antiparasitic drugs in children. Clin Pharmacokinet 1989;17(suppl):138–155

12. Russell L. The pinworm, *Enterobius vermicularis*. Prim Care 1991;18:13–24

13. Diekema D, Marcuse E. Information for parents and patients: cryptosporidiosis. Pediatr Infect Dis J 1992;11:689–690

14. Cordell R, Addiss D. Cryptosporidiosis in child care settings: a review of the literature and recommendations for prevention and control. Pediatr Infect Dis J 1994;13:310–317

15. Markell E, Udrow M. *Blastocystis hominis*: pathogen or fellow traveler? Am J Trop Med Hyg 1986;35:1023–1026

36

PEPTIC ULCER DISEASE

RANDOLPH M. MCCONNIE

The incidence and prevalence of acid peptic disease in children are not accurately known. Approximately 1 in 2,500 pediatric hospital admissions has been calculated to be due to peptic ulcer disease.[1,2] In adults, it is estimated to occur in 5% to 10% of the population. In children it is thought to be most commonly seen in those who have been under physical stress, such as a serious illness. Nonetheless, children who have not been under those severe conditions can also suffer from peptic problems.[3] Ulcers can be classified by their location (gastric versus duodenal), as well as by their presumed cause: primary ulcers have no known underlying predisposing etiology and secondary ulcers have a presumed underlying etiology. Secondary causes of peptic ulcers include nonsteroidal anti-inflammatory drug (NSAID) use, steroids, theophylline, tolazoline, sepsis, trauma, head injury, burns, acidosis, hypoglycemia, sickle cell anemia, cystic fibrosis, diabetes mellitus, systemic lupus erythematosus,[4] and *Helicobacter pylori*. The underlying mechanism responsible for ulcer formation is thought to be a breakdown in the gastric and duodenal mucosal antacid defense mechanism that makes the mucosa more susceptible to acid injury. Treatment of acid peptic disease aims to either decrease the production of acid in the stomach or to improve the mucosal antacid defense mechanisms. (For in-depth discussion of gastroesophageal reflux–induced esophageal peptic disease and *Helicobacter pylori*–induced gastritis and ulcer disease, see Chs. 25 and 26.)

PHYSIOLOGY AND PATHOPHYSIOLOGY[5–13]

The stomach can be divided into two regions for acid production purposes: the body, where acid is produced; and the antrum, where acid initiates a feedback mechanism that ultimately results in decreasing the formation of acid in the gastric body and fundus. Gastric secretions are regulated by local as well as central nervous system (CNS)–mediated stimuli. Ulcers form when the stomach's cytoprotective mechanism breaks down.

The CNS modulates gastric secretion with visual, olfactory, taste, or cortical (thought of food) stimuli, ultimately funneling through the vagus nerve and through the enteric nervous system within the stomach wall delivering a neurotransmitter (acetylcholine) to the acid-producing cells (parietal cells), as well as to acid-modulating cells (gastrin cells, D cells). This process is commonly known as the cephalic phase of digestion and is usually originated by the thought and taste of food. It is thought that vagal stimulation causes enterochromaffin cells to release histamines, which in turn stimulate the production of acid by stimulating the parietal cells via the histamine-2 (H_2)-receptors. The gastrin cells are also stimulated by gastrin-releasing peptides to produce gastrin (a hormone secreted by the gastrin cells in the pyloric gland of the antrum), which in turn stimulates the parietal cells to produce acid.

Functioning alone, acetylcholine, gastrin, or histamine only slightly stimulates acid production. It is postulated that all three receptors—acetylcholine, gastrin, and histamine receptors—on the parietal cell must be activated simultaneously in order for optimal gastric acid secretion stimulation to occur. It is understandable why H_2-receptor antagonists reduce gastric acid secretion.

Intragastric levels of pepsin and blood levels of gastrin are unchanged in patients with duodenal ulcers and gastric ulcers at 12 to 73 years of age. Furthermore, acid output appears to be unchanged with age at 12 to 73 years. Maximal and peak acid output appear to be higher in males than in females, and higher in duodenal ulcer patients than in gastric ulcer patients.[14]

In normal persons, when gastric acidity increases to a pH of 3.0, gastrin is blocked. This protects the stomach from excessive acidity and ulceration. It also helps maintain an optimal pH for peptic enzymatic activity to occur. Finally, pancreatic bicarbonate protects the duodenal mucosa from acid injury. Mucosal protection of the stomach is thought to be mediated by prostaglandins. The precise mechanism by which prostaglandins work is not entirely known. Prostaglandins are thought to stimulate the production of mucus and the secretion of bicarbonate. They are also thought to suppress acid secretion. The surface epithelium of the gastric and duodenal mucosa secretes bicarbonate. Its secretion is enhanced when the luminal duodenal pH is less than 3.

Gastroduodenal ulcers occur when the normal acid-pepsin balance and the mucosal defense mechanisms falter. Thus, ulcers may occur even in the presence of normal acid secretion. Nonetheless, the dictum "no acid, no ulcer" still holds. One situation in which this balance may be disrupted is in the NSAID-induced ulcers, where prostaglandin synthesis is suppressed. Patients with duodenal ulcer disease appear to have a blunted response to prostaglandin-stimulated bicarbonate secretion. *Helicobacter pylori* has also been implicated in the formation of ulcers (for further discussion, see Ch. 26).

Hydrochloric acid is found in normal premature and term infants, although its secretion is found to be much lower in premature than in term infants.[15] The acid output of newborns following histamine stimulation is very low and appears to increase through the third week of life,[12] continuing to rise thereafter.

EPIDEMIOLOGY[1,4,16–32]

The incidence and prevalence of peptic ulcer disease in children are unknown. The lifetime prevalence is 5% to 10%. The prevalence of gastric ulcers is the same in adult men and women. More boys have duodenal ulcers than occur in girls. In children, duodenal ulcers are thought to be more common than gastric ulcers, although this finding is dependent on the method used to detect the presence of the ulcers (i.e., endoscopic versus radiographic). The incidence of peptic ulcer disease increases with age. During the neonatal period, most of the ulcers (chiefly gastric) are of a secondary nature, usually associated with an underlying illness. Between the ages of 1 month and 6 years gastric ulcers continue to be more common than duodenal. By 10 years of age, the pattern is more similar to adult presentations, in which duodenal ulcers are more common in men than in women.

Abdominal pain is one of the hallmarks of peptic ulcer disease. The pain is typically periumbilical, relieved by food or antacids. Children who are old enough to provide a history describe the pain as having a burning character. Unfortunately, this is not the only way peptic ulcer disease presents in children. The pain may awaken the individual from sleep and be confused with night terrors or nightmares. A temporal relationship between pain and eating may not exist. It is not unusual for children, when asked, to fail to describe the character of the pain. Children are many times unable to localize the pain to any particular abdominal quadrant and will usually point to the periumbilical area as the location of the pain. Children who are able to localize the pain to a particular location other than the periumbilical region should be assumed to have abdominal pathology until proved otherwise. Even though vomiting, food intolerance, and gastrointestinal (GI) bleeding can be the presenting symptoms of peptic ulcer disease, not all ulcer patients vomit or bleed. Bowel perforation (gastric or duodenal) with GI bleeding can be the only presenting symptom some patients have. The pain of ulcer disease can come and go. Most untreated ulcers in adults resolve without treatment if followed long enough, and if lifestyle changes occur (e.g., stopping NSAIDs, alcohol, tobacco). Similar data are not available in children. *Helicobacter pylori* is thought to play a major role in the pathogenesis of ulcer disease in humans.

During the neonatal period, gastric or duodenal perforations can be the first signs of peptic ulcer disease, especially in children with a history of perinatal asphyxia or hypoxia. Other disorders, such as sepsis, respiratory distress syndrome, hypoglycemia, the use of nasogastric tubes, and CNS problems, can also predispose the neonate to ulcer disease. Formula intolerance, irritability, and vomiting are other manifestations of peptic ulcer disease.

In early childhood, secondary ulcers are seen with equal frequency in the duodenum and in the stomach. Underlying conditions, such as sepsis, meningitis, brain tumors, encephalitis, burns, and head injuries, can be predisposing factors. Other symptoms that can present at this age, especially with primary ulcers, include poor eating, anorexia, failure to thrive, abdominal distention, vomiting, irritability with crying spells in the postprandial period, and GI bleeding (melena, heme-positive stools, hematemesis). In older children, vomiting can also become a presenting symptom.

In children older than 6 years of age, abdominal pain is the most prominent symptom, usually in the periumbilical area. At times this pain can awaken the patient from sleep in the middle of the night or in the early morning. Schoolchildren and adolescents have more specific symptoms of epigastric burning and abdominal pain relieved by ingestion of food or antacids. The pain can be periodic and variable in character and severity. It is not unusual in adolescents for up to a year to elapse between the onset of the symptoms and the establishment of the diagnosis of peptic ulcer disease.

Nonulcer dyspepsia or functional dyspepsia is diagnosed in patients with symptoms of heartburn, biliary colic, and/or ulcer pain relieved by use of antacids and in those who have no detectable organic disease (i.e., no ulcers, gallbladder disease, or gastroesophageal reflux). The pain or discomfort these patients experience may be precipitated by stress, certain foods, alcohol ingestion, and NSAIDs that have caused no evidence of ulcer disease. In patients with occasional symptoms of dyspepsia, a short course of H_2-receptor antagonists is in order. If the symptoms become frequent or persistent, further investigation (radiographic or endoscopic) is warranted.

PHYSICAL EXAMINATION

Findings on physical examination can range from completely benign to an acute abdomen with peritoneal signs and hemodynamic instability. Patients with peptic ulcer disease may have tenderness to palpation of the epigastric area. Right upper quadrant pain, especially with a positive Murphy's sign, is more suggestive of gallbladder disease. The absence of bowel sounds should be taken as an ominous sign, which, in the case of GI bleeding, should raise suspicion of a perforated viscus. A rectal examination with guaiac of stool should be included in the evaluation of any individual with abdominal pain, unless there is strong contraindication. Rectal examination may help to understand presenting findings: GI bleeding with melena, constipation with a fecal impaction, and inflammatory bowel disease with perianal disease.

Examination of the vital signs, including checking the pulse and blood pressure in the supine and standing positions to assess for signs of orthostasis, can help determine the patient's intravascular volume status, especially in the case of an acute GI bleed. Even though patients with peptic ulcer disease can present with anemia, not all do. Moreover, patients with acute onset of severe GI bleeding and hemodynamic instability can present with a completely normal hemoglobin and hematocrit reading. Examination of the pharynx for signs of streptococcal pharyngitis, as well as examination of the chest for signs of

TABLE 36-1. Complications of Peptic Ulcer Disease

Gastrointestinal bleeding

Hemodynamic instability

Perforation

Pancreatitis

Fistulas into the gallbladder

Gastric outlet obstruction

Intra-abdominal abscess

pneumonia, should be included in the physical examination, as both can present with abdominal pain and vomiting.

COMPLICATIONS

Bleeding is by far one of the most common complications (Table 36-1) of peptic ulcer disease, and potentially one of the most life-threatening. In adults, 20% of patients with ulcer disease will bleed at some point in their lives. Similar data are not available in children. In adults, factors associated with poor outcome in bleeding ulcers include hemodynamic instability after a bleeding episode, age, presence of other disease, as well as continuation of bleeding during the same hospitalization. Presenting symptoms of bleeding include melena (dark/black tarry malodorous stools), dark red stools, coffee-ground emesis, and reddish emesis. Not all that is red or black is necessarily blood, and thus heme testing of the effluvia is an important diagnostic study to perform.

Perforation is a less common complication of ulcer disease, but it is by no means a benign problem. Patients with a perforated ulcer usually present with an acute abdomen, unless the ulcer has perforated in the pancreas, in which case the patient may present with abdominal pain radiating to the back, no free peritoneal air, and an elevated amylase. In adults, stress and NSAID use appear to be more commonly associated with perforation.

Gastric outlet obstruction is an uncommon complication of peptic ulcer disease and results from repeated episodes of ulceration and scar formation. Edema surrounding an ulcer may also cause gastric outlet obstruction, but the edema and the gastric outlet obstruction will usually resolve as the ulcer heals. Delayed gastric emptying, early satiety, nausea, and vomiting are symptoms that suggest outlet problems. Pharmacologic treatment of ulcer disease is believed to have decreased the prevalence of this now unusual complication.

DIFFERENTIAL DIAGNOSIS

Lesions that mimic peptic ulcer disease (Table 36-2) include malignancies such as gastric carcinomas and lymphomas, which are very rare in children, and Crohn's

TABLE 36-2. Differential Diagnosis of Gastric or Duodenal Ulcers

Infectious
Helicobacter pylori
Syphilis
Escherichia coli
Clostridium perfringens
Tuberculosis
Herpes simplex virus
Cytomegalovirus
Fungal infections

Stress related
Sepsis
Systemic illness with shock
Central nervous system injury
Burns (Curling's ulcers)
Neonatal stress
Cushing's ulcers
    Central nervous system lesions
    Surgery
    Trauma

Exogenous agents
Corrosives
NSAIDs
Ethanol
Antibiotics
    Penicillin
    Ampicillin
    Chloramphenicol
    Tetracycline
    Cephalosporin
Radiation
Mechanical trauma
    Nasogastric tubes
    Bezoars
    Foreign bodies
Potassium chloride
Clinitest tablets
Calcium salts
Iron sulfate
Acetylcysteine

Other conditions
Antral G-cell hyperfunction
Zollinger-Ellison syndrome
Mastocytosis
Cystic fibrosis
Alpha-1-antitrypsin deficiency
Sickle cell anemia
Chronic renal failure
Multiple endocrine neoplasia
Hyperparathyroidism
Crohn's disease
Chronic granulomatous disease
Cirrhosis
Malignancy
    Gastric adenocarcinoma
    Lymphoma

TABLE 36-3. Differential Diagnosis of Ulcer Symptoms

Gastric or duodenal ulcers

Gastroesophageal reflux and esophagitis

Parasitic infections

Streptococcal pharyngitis

Pneumonia

Urinary tract infection

Pancreatitis

Henoch-Schönlein purpura

Spinal lesion

Recurrent abdominal pain/irritable bowel syndrome

Biliary tract disease (cholelithiasis/biliary colic)

Constipation

Sarcoidosis

Protein sensitivity

Eosinophilic gastroenteritis

Diabetes

Ménétrier's disease

Atrophic gastritis (autoimmune)

Graft-versus-host disease

Lymphocytic gastritis

disease of the stomach and duodenum. Infections such as viral gastritis, tuberculosis, and syphilitic gastritis can also mimic peptic ulcer disease. Parasitic infections such as giardiasis and bacterial infections such as streptococcal pharyngitis and pneumonia can give pain symptoms similar to those of peptic ulcer disease. Eosinophilic gastroenteritis can present with abdominal pain and vomiting and thus can also be confused with the symptomatology of peptic ulcer disease. Other conditions can also present with symptoms similar to those of peptic ulcer disease (Table 36-3) and should also be considered in the differential diagnosis: pancreatitis, urinary tract infections, gallbladder disease, Henoch-Schönlein purpura, and spinal cord lesions. Constipation may present with symptoms of postprandial pain as the result of the gastrocolic reflex, which can lead to abdominal cramping after eating, especially in the child with functional constipation and stool withholding.

DIAGNOSIS

Some investigators have suggested that the sensitivity of double-contrast barium studies of the upper GI tract comes close to that of endoscopy in showing mucosal disease. Unfortunately, this observation is very operator dependent and is based on adult data. In children, the sensitivity of imaging studies of the upper GI tract is low for detecting mucosal disease. Nonetheless, barium studies are invaluable in defining anatomy and in ruling out conditions such as malrotation, fistulas, small bowel inflammatory disease, and obstruction.

Ultrasonography is not commonly used for defining or diagnosing peptic ulcer disease. It is nonetheless quite helpful in defining biliary tract disease, renal anomalies, as well as pyloric muscle hypertrophy seen in nonpeptic pyloric stenosis. Ultrasound may aid in ruling out conditions that can present with symptoms similar to those seen with peptic ulcer disease (pyloric stenosis, gallbladder disease).

Abdominal computed tomography (CT) with intestinal and intravenous contrast may be useful in identifying complications of peptic ulcer disease, such as a perforation into the head of the pancreas or an intra-abdominal abscess. CT imaging is also helpful in defining mass lesions such as bowel wall thickening seen in inflammatory bowel disease, intra-abdominal masses, and malignancies. It is not helpful in ruling in or ruling out mucosal anomalies of the stomach and duodenum.

Endoscopy is by far the most sensitive method available to identify mucosal disease of the upper GI tract. This technique not only affords an opportunity to inspect the appearance of the mucosa directly, but also allows the examiner to obtain biopsies of the tissue, obtain cultures, and assist in controlling GI bleeding.

TREATMENT[33-54]

Many ulcers in adults will heal on their own without treatment. Approximately 40% of adult duodenal ulcers heal without therapy by 8 weeks, and 50% to 60% of gastric ulcers heal without therapy by 8 weeks. This compares to approximately 80% of adult duodenal and gastric ulcers healing with H_2-blockers by 8 weeks. Comparable data are not available for children.

Dietary management of the nonobstructive ulcer has changed significantly since the days when the mainstay of ulcer treatment was the Sippy method with the Sippy diets. Most would agree that since the advent of H_2-receptor antagonists, the mainstay of therapy besides the H_2-receptor antagonists has been avoidance of alcohol and NSAIDs, and cessation of smoking. Thus, no specific food group is forbidden from the diet of peptic ulcer disease patients, unless one particular food item causes the individual patient to have GI problems.

The aims of therapy are to reduce acid secretion, increase the mucosal defenses against acid/pepsin, and neutralize acid. Ulcer healing is dependent on the amount of time that the gastric pH is above 3. H_2-Blockers can be used for the treatment of NSAID-induced ulcers, even while using the NSAID, although healing of the ulcer with concomitant use of NSAIDs is slower.

TABLE 36-4. Medications Used for Ulcer Therapy

Proton pump blockers*
  Omeprazole
    0.7 mg to 3.3 mg/kg/day to adult dose of 20 mg/day
  Lansoprazole
    No dosaging data for children

H_2-Receptor antagonists*
  Cimetidine
    Infants and neonates: 10 to 20 mg/kg/day IV/PO divided qid
    Children: 20 to 40 mg/kg/day IV/PO divided bid or qid to adult dose of 300 mg PO qid; 400 mg PO bid; or 800 mg PO qhs
  Ranitidine
    2 to 4 mg/kg/day PO divided bid or tid to adult dose of 150 mg PO bid or 300 mg PO qhs
    2 to 4 mg/kg/day IV divided q 8 h to maximum of 50 mg IV q 8
  Famotidine
    1 to 1.5 mg/kg/day PO divided bid to adult dose of 20 mg PO bid or 40 mg PO qhs
    0.6 to 0.8 mg/kg/day divided q 8 to 12 h to maximum of 40 mg/day
  Nizatidine
    No dosaging data for children

Cytoprotectors*
  Sucralfate
    40 to 80 mg/kg/day PO qid 30 to 60 min ac and hs for infants, to adult dose of 1 g PO 30 min ac and hs
  Antacids
    1–2 ml/kg at 1 and 3 h pc and at hs, to adult dose of 30 ml at 1 and 3 h pc and hs

* Doses may vary for renal insufficiency and renal failure.

Omeprazole has also been used to treat NSAID-induced ulcer disease with good results. If possible, it is best to stop using the NSAID. Acid reduction can be achieved by one of several routes (Table 36-4).

Proton Pump Blocker

Omeprazole and lansoprazole are commercially available in the United States. Of the two agents, omeprazole has the largest body of literature supporting its use in the pediatric age group. Omeprazole acts by irreversibly blocking the proton pump and thus disabling the mechanism for acid production in the stomach. It is a very potent drug. Some studies suggest that peptic ulcers heal somewhat faster with omeprazole than with H_2-receptor antagonists. The manufacturer and the Food and Drug Administration (FDA) suggest limiting the use of omeprazole to a few weeks, given the report of gastric carcinoid tumors in rats attributed to the prolonged achlorhydria produced by the drug. Such tumors have thus far not been associated with use of omeprazole in humans. There are reports supporting omeprazole long-term use in peptic esophagitis where H_2-blockers have failed to resolve the problem. There is a growing body of literature supporting the use of omeprazole in children. Very little has been published on the use of lansoprazole in the pediatric population.

H$_2$-Receptor Antagonists

The H$_2$-receptor antagonists block the histamine receptors on the surface of the parietal cell. Cimetidine was the first H$_2$-receptor antagonist to be commercially available in the United States. It is effective in decreasing acid production in the stomach, and its introduction into the GI pharmacopeia revolutionized the way ulcers were treated. Like any other drug, it has potential side effects and drug-drug interactions. It can inhibit cytochrome P-450, resulting in slowing the metabolism and elimination of drugs such as theophylline, phenytoin, warfarin, and any other drug metabolized by this cytochrome. It has been reported to cause drowsiness in older people, although some reports have suggested that this side effect is no different from that seen with other H$_2$-blockers. In younger men, it has been associated with reversible impotence. All H$_2$-blockers are thought to be equally effective in healing peptic ulcers. The choice of H$_2$-blocking agent is driven more by cost, palatability (and thus compliance), and side effects. Side effects with ranitidine include headaches, dizziness, bradycardia, drowsiness, and hyporeflexia; side effects with cimetidine include mental confusion, hallucinations, hepatotoxicity and hypotension. In adults, cimetidine has been associated with abnormal androgen and estrogen metabolism, leading to gynecomastia and oligospermia. In children, elevated prolactin levels have been reported with the use of cimetidine. Endocrine problems have thus far not been described with the use of famotidine or ranitidine. Continuous intravenous infusion of cimetidine and ranitidine is thought to be more effective in increasing gastric pH. Cimetidine, ranitidine, and famotidine may be added to hyperalimentation solutions.

Antacids

Aluminum and magnesium hydroxides used to be the mainstays of therapy before the advent of H$_2$-receptor antagonists. Acid neutralization required the use of high doses. Magnesium-based antacids usually precipitated an osmotic diarrhea in the patient. Aluminum-based antacids could cause constipation. Since both aluminum and magnesium are eliminated by the kidneys, their use is relatively contraindicated in renal failure. Today, antacids provide assistance in relieving acid-related symptoms not fully relieved by H$_2$-receptor antagonists.

Prostaglandins

In theory, synthetic prostaglandins should be helpful in providing mucosal protection, but in reality their use in adults has been disappointing. The only commercially available form for treatment of peptic ulcer disease is misoprostol, which is effective in treating mucosal disease caused by NSAIDs. It is not recommended for use in children or pregnant women.

Sucralfate

Aluminum sucrose sulfate is thought to be as effective in treating duodenal ulcers as H$_2$-receptor antagonists. It is not, however, as good for treatment of gastric ulcers or esophagitis. Sucralfate is an inhibitor of pepsin, but its mechanism of action is not completely understood. Some investigators postulate that it stimulates local production of bicarbonate, providing mucosal protection; others propose that it acts by stimulating the production of mucosal prostaglandins. The drug is not absorbed, and it can bind other medicines when given at the same time, making them not bioavailable. There is a relative contraindication for its use in renal insufficiency, given that it contains aluminum that may be absorbed leading to aluminum osteodystrophy, osteomalacia, and encephalopathy.

RECURRENCE

Ulcers should heal within 6 to 8 weeks of therapy. Failure to heal should raise the possibility of malignancy in gastric ulcers, Crohn's disease, and Zollinger-Ellison syndrome. Failure to heal with H$_2$-receptor antagonists should lead to treatment with a proton pump blocker and investigation of other causes of ulcers. Smoking and NSAID use may interfere with the healing of ulcers and should thus be avoided. For patients with duodenal ulcers whose symptoms have failed to improve and in whom the ulcer persists, a switch to a proton pump blocker should be considered.

Gastric and duodenal ulcers may recur. In adults, more than 50 % of patients whose ulcers heal have another ulcer within 12 months. These reports date from the pre-*H. pylori* era, and thus the numbers may differ in individuals who have had *H. pylori* diagnosed and treated. Recurrent ulcers should be treated with another course of 6 to 8 weeks of H$_2$-receptor antagonists. For patients who have frequent recurrent ulcers, long-term management has been suggested.

Prophylaxis for prevention of NSAID-induced ulcers in the duodenum is accomplished in adults by using standard ulcer healing doses of H$_2$-blockers. The same prophylaxis is not effective in preventing the formation of gastric ulcers. Misoprostol, a synthetic prostaglandin, has been used for treatment and prophylaxis of NSAIDs in adults. It is not recommended for use in children, young adults, or pregnant women.

ZOLLINGER-ELLISON SYNDROME[55–60]

The hallmark of Zollinger-Ellison syndrome is gastric acid hypersecretion. Patients suffering from this syndrome usually present with a history of severe peptic ulcer disease in a setting of gastric acid hypersecretion. These patients have a high concentration of circulating gastrin originating from a gastrinoma. Presenting symptoms associated with Zollinger-Ellison syndrome include peptic ulcers, gastroesophageal reflux, and diarrhea. Gastrinomas may be part of a multiple endocrine neoplasia (MEN) syndrome, including tumors of the pancreas, pituitary, and parathyroid. It is estimated that 1% of patients with duodenal ulcers have Zollinger-Ellision syndrome.

The diagnosis is established by documenting a high serum gastrin concentration in the presence of high gastric acid production. It is important to document both, since conditions such as achlorhydria and hypochlorhydria (e.g., chronic atrophic gastritis, pernicious anemia, gastric ulcers, gastric carcinoma, vitiligo, postvagotomy, drug-induced achlorhydria and hypochlorhydria) and other conditions with normal acid secretion or hyperchlorhydria (e.g., antral G-cell hyperplasia, gastric outlet obstruction, chronic renal failure, small intestinal resection, excluded gastric antrum, and, in rare instances, rheumatoid arthritis, diabetes mellitus, pheochromocytoma, hyperparathyroidism, and thyrotoxicosis) may also present with elevated gastrin levels. Gastric acid production is most accurately documented by gastric acid analysis that establishes a basal acid output (BAO) as well as a pentagastrin-stimulated peak acid output (PAO). Most untreated adult patients with Zollinger-Ellison Syndrome have BAO greater than 15 mmol hydrochloric acid per hour with a BAO-to-PAO ratio of greater than 50%. Most patients have gastrin levels greater than 1,000 pg/ml. In patients with elevated levels of gastrin of less than 1,000 pg/ml, a positive secretin (rise in serum gastrin concentration of at least 200 pg/ml above basal level after the injection of secretin) test is diagnostic.

In the pre-cimetidine era (before 1977 in the United States), surgical therapy offered the only alternative for controlling the disease. Early reports noted that tumor excision for cure was only possible in 2% to 5% of patients. Other surgical interventions included total gastrectomy. One pediatric series reporting on a 25-year follow-up of five patients with Zollinger-Ellison syndrome treated with total gastrectomies showed that one patient was dead from the tumor 14 years after gastrectomy, and the remaining four were alive at 30, 29, 28, and 27 years after total gastrectomy. Medical treatment became possible with the advent of H_2-receptor blocking agents, and later with proton pump blockers. More recent studies have reported an improved ability to find the gastrinoma by imaging with ultrasound, CT, magnetic resonance imaging (MRI), and/or selective angiographic imaging and blood sampling in an attempt to locate retroperitoneal, hepatic, duodenal, and pancreatic masses. These techniques have improved the yield of localizing the tumor and thus being able to remove it surgically to 30% to 53% in some series. In adults, tumors are found in 40% to 70% of patients at surgery, and in 20% to 30% of cases, a cure is achieved after resection of the gastrinoma.

Metastatic disease is a contraindication for surgery, as is multiple endocrine neoplasia I (MEN I) with no gastrinoma found before surgery. In patients with hyperparathyroidism, parathyroidectomy should be considered, as a reduction in serum calcium may reduce serum gastrin concentrations. Titration of gastric acid production post-treatment should be undertaken to ensure good gastric acid secretion control, which can be done by repeating a gastric acid analysis.

REFERENCES

1. Drumm B, Rhoads JM, Stringer DA et al. Peptic ulcer disease in children: etiology, clinical findings and clinical course. Pediatrics 1988;82:410–414

2. Shabib S, Sherman P. Peptic ulcer disease in children: a common disease in an uncommon setting. Can J Diagn 1992; 9:31

3. Goyal A, Treem W, Hyams JS. Severe upper gastrointestinal bleeding in healthy full-term neonates. Am J Gastroenterol 1994;89:613–616

4. George DE, Glassman M. Peptic ulcer disease in children. Gastrointest Endosc Clin North Am 1994;4:23–37

5. Behar J. Normal anatomy, histology, and physiology of the upper gastrointestinal tract. In: Molinoff PB, Ed. Peptic Ulcer Disease: Mechanisms and Management, Rutherford, NJ: The Healthpress Publishing Group, 1990:1–36

6. Flemstrom G. Gastric and duodenal mucosal bicarbonate secretion. In: Johnson LR, Ed. Physiology of the Gastrointestinal Tract. 2nd Ed. New York: Raven Press, 1987: 1055–1069

7. Guyton AC. Human Physiology and Mechanisms of Disease. Philadelphia: WB Saunders, 1992:490–493

8. Neutra MR, Forstner JF. Gastrointestinal mucus: synthesis, secretion, and function. In: Johnson LR, Ed. Physiology of the Gastrointestinal Tract. 2nd Ed. New York: Raven Press, 1987:975–1009

9. Peterson WL. Stomach and duodenum. In MKSAP in the Subspecialty of Gastroenterology and Hepatology. Philadelphia: American College of Physicians, 1993;48–73

10. Silen W. Gastric mucosal defense and repair. In: Johnson LR, Ed. Physiology of the Gastrointestinal Tract. 2nd Ed. New York: Raven Press, 1987:1055–1069

11. Wolfe MM, Soll AH. The physiology of gastric acid secretion. N Engl J Med 1988;319:1707–1715

12. Agunod M, Yamaguchi N, Lopez R et al. Correlative study of hydrochloric acid, pepsin, and intrinsic factor secretion in newborns and infants. Am J Dig Dis 1969;4:400

13. Reynolds JC. Pathophysiology and clinical aspects of peptic ulcer disease. In: Molinoff PB, Ed. Peptic Ulcer Disease: Mechanisms and Management. Rutherford, NJ: The Healthpress Publishing Group, 1990:37–82

14. Pilotto A, Vianello F, Di Mario F et al. Effects of age on gastric acid, pepsin, pepsinogen group A, and gastrin secretion in peptic ulcer patients. Gerontology 1994;40:253–259

15. Mignone F, Castello D. Ricerche sulla secrezione gastrica di acido cloridrico nell'immaturo. Min Pediatr 1961;13:1098 (Cited in Koldovsky O. Digestion and absorption. In: Stave U, Ed. Perinatal Physiology. New York: Plenum, 1978)

16. Bujanover Y, Konikeff F, Baratz M. Nodular gastritis and *Helicobacter pylori*. J Pediatr Gastroenterol Nutr 1990;11:41–44

17. Wen HH, Chen MH, Ho MM, Hwang KC. Fetal gastric ulcers presenting with bloody amniotic fluid. J Pediatr Gastroenterol Nutr 1992;15:455–457

18. Ament ME, Christie DL, Upper gastrointestinal fiberoptic endoscopy in pediatric patients. Gastroenterology 1977;72:1244–1248

19. Deckelbaum RJ, Roy CC, Lussier-Lazaroff J et al. Peptic ulcer disease: a clinical study in 73 children. Can Med Assoc J 1974;111:225–228

20. Tsang TM, Saing H, Yeung CK. Peptic ulcers in children. J Pediatr Surg 1990;25:744–748

21. Nord KS, Rossi TM, Lebenthal E. Peptic ulcer disease in children: the predominance of gastric ulcers. Am J Gastroenterol 1981;75:153–157

22. Eastham EJ. Peptic ulcer. In: Walker A, Drurie P et al, Eds. Pediatric Gastrointestinal Disease. Philadelphia: BC Decker, 1991:438–451

23. Acra S, Nakagawa N, Ghishan FZ. Peptic ulcer disease in children. Compr Ther 1991;17:22–26

24. Collen MJ, Santoro MJ, Chen YK. Giant duodenal ulcer: evaluation of basal acid output, nonsteroidal antiinflammatory drug use, and ulcer complications. Dig Dis Sci 1994;39:1113–1116

25. Rasquin-Weber A. Disorders of the stomach and duodenum. In: Roy CC, Silverman A, Alagille D, Eds. Pediatric Clinical Gastroenterology. St. Louis: CV Mosby, 1995:174–215

26. Gabriel S, Jaakkimainen L, Bombardier C. Risk of serious gastrointestinal complications related to use of nonsteroidal anti-inflammatory drugs: a meta-analysis. Ann Intern Med 1991;115:787–796

27. Kimura M, Uemura N, Inbe A et al. Characteristics of teenage patients with juvenile duodenal ulcer: relationship between inherited hyperpepsinogenemia I and duodenal ulcers. Scand J Gastroenterol 1993;28:25–30

28. Vuoristo M, Pikkarainen IM, Sipponem M et al. Functional characteristics of duodenal ulcer patients with their first degree relatives. Scand J Gastroenterol 1991;26(suppl 186):52–61

29. Petersen H, Kristensen P, Johannessen T et al. The natural course of peptic ulcer disease and its predictors. Scan J Gastroenterol 1995;30:17–24

30. Wolfe YG, Ryan T, Schropp KP, Harmel RP. Steroid therapy and duodenal ulcer in infants. JPGN 1991;12:269–271

31. McCarthy DM. NSAID-induced gastrointestinal damage: a critical review of prophylaxis and therapy. J Clin Gastroenterol 12(suppl 2):S13–S20

32. Rasquin-Weber A. Disorders of the stomach and duodenum. In: Roy C, Silverman A, Alagille D, Eds. Pediatric Clinical Gastroenterology. St. Louis: CV Mosby, 1995:174–215

33. Reynolds JC. The clinical importance of drug interactions with antiulcer therapy. J Clin Gastroenterol 1990;12(suppl 2):S54–S63

34. Karjoo M, Kane R. Omeprazole treatment of children with peptic esophagitis refractory to ranitidine therapy. Arch Pediatr Adolesc Med 1995;149:267–271

35. Kato S, Shibuya H, Hayashi Y et al. Effectiveness and pharmacokenetics of omeprazole in children with refractory duodenal ulcers. J Pediatr Gastroenterol Nutr 1992;15:184–188

36. Parente F, Bianchi Porro G et al. Double-blind randomized, multicenter study comparing aluminum phosphate gel with ranitidine in the short-term treatment of duodenal ulcer. Hepatogastroenterology 1995;42:95–99

37. Nauert C, Caspery WF. Duodenal ulcer therapy with low-dose antacids: a multicenter trial. J Clin Gastroenterol 1991;13(suppl 1):S149–S154

38. Feldman M, Burton ME. Histamine 2 receptor antagonists: standard therapy for acid-peptic disease. N Engl J Med 1990;323:1672–1680;323:1749–1755

39. Kelly DA. Do H2 receptor antagonists have a therapeutic role in childhood? J Pediatr Gastroenterol Nutr 1994;19:270–276

40. Kato S, Watanabe N, Harada Y. Pharmacokinetic study of cimetidine in pediatric duodenal ulcer. Clin Ther 1991;13:118–125

41. Peterson W. Pathogenesis and therapy of peptic ulcer disease. J Clin Gastroenterol 1990;12(suppl 2):S1–S6

42. McCarthy DM. Sucralfate. N Engl J Med 1991;325:1017–1025

43. Gunasekaran TS, Hassall EG. Efficacy and safety of omeprazole for severe gastroesophageal reflux in children. J Pediatr 1993;123:148–154

44. Alliet P, Raes M, Gillis P, Zimmermann A. Optimal dose of omeprazole in infants and children, letter to the editor. J Pediatr 1994;124:332–333

45. Atkinson AJ, Craig RM. Therapy of peptic ulcer disease. In: Molinoff PB, Ed. Peptic Ulcer Disease: Mechanisms and Management. Rutherford, NJ: The Healthpress Publishing Group, 1990:83–112

46. Dalzell AM, Searle JW, Patrick MJ. Treatment of refractory ulcerative oesophagitis with omeprazole. Arch Dis Child 1992;67:641–642

47. Festen HPM. Prevention of duodenal ulcer relapse by long term treatment with omeprazole. Scand J Gastroenterol 1994;29(suppl 201):S39–S41

48. Isenberg JI. Should safety concerns with available ulcer treatment influence drug selection? J Clin Gastroenterol 1990;12(suppl 2):S48–S53

49. Lysy J, Karmeli F, Wengrower D, Rachmelewits D. Effects of duodenal ulcer healing induced by omeprazole and ranitidine on the generation of gastroduodenal eicosanoids, platelet-activating factor, pepsinogen A, and gastrin in duodenal ulcer patients. Scand J Gastroenterol 1992;27:13–19

50. Maton PN. Omeprazole. N Engl J Med 1991;324:965–975

51. Von der Bruegge WF, Peura DA. Stress-related mucosal damage: review of drug therapy. J Clin Gastroenterol 1990; 12(suppl 2):S35–S40

52. Wilde MI, McTavish D. Omeprazole: an update of its pharmacology and therapeutic use in acid related disorders. Drugs 1994;48:91–132

53. Foulke G, Siepler J. Antiulcer therapy: an exercise in formulary management. J Clin Gastroenterol 1990;12(suppl 2): S64–S68

54. Wilhelmsen I, Tangen Haug T, Ursin H, Bersted A. Effect of short-term cognitive psychotherapy on recurrence of duodenal ulcer: a prospective randomized trial. Psychosomat Med 1994;56:440–448

55. Laine L. Upper gastrointestinal tract hemorrhage. West J Med 1991;155:274–279

56. Wolfe MM, Jensen RT. Zollinger-Ellison syndrome: current concepts in diagnosis and management. N Engl J Med 1987; 317:1200–1209

57. Berg CL, Wolfe MM. Zollinger-Ellison syndrome. Med Clin North Am 1991;75:903–921

58. Wilson S. Zollinger-Ellison syndrome in children: a 25-year follow-up. Surgery 1991;110:696–703

59. Webber HC, Venzon DJ, Lin JT et al. Determinants of metastatic rate and survival in patients with Zollinger-Ellison syndrome: a prospective long-term study. Gastroenterology 1995;108:1637–1649

60. Farley DR, Van Heerden JA, Grant CS et al. The Zollinger-Ellison syndrome: a collective surgical experience. Ann Surg 1992;215:561–570

37

PERITONITIS

DONNA ZEITER

Peritonitis is defined as inflammation of the peritoneal membranes lining the abdominal cavity. This inflammation may be categorized as either primary spontaneous bacterial peritonitis or secondary bacterial peritonitis. Spontaneous bacterial peritonitis (SBP) is defined as the presence of pathogenic bacteria, cultured from peritoneal fluid, without an identified intra-abdominal source of infection. Secondary bacterial peritonitis is an inflammation of the peritoneal cavity produced by an intra-abdominal source of infection, such as occurs with perforation of a hollow abdominal viscus or rupture of an abdominal abscess.

SPONTANEOUS BACTERIAL PERITONITIS

In children, SBP occurs more commonly in patients with chronic renal failure, with or without ascites. The incidence in patients with nephrotic syndrome is within the range of 2% to 17.3%.[1] Occasionally, SBP will occur in otherwise healthy children. Both gram-positive and gram-negative organisms lead to SBP in children. The most common organisms include *Streptococcus pneumoniae*, group A streptococci, and gram-negative enteric bacilli.[1]

In children and adults with advanced liver disease, SBP is recognized as a complication involving patients who have developed ascites as a result of poor hepatic synthetic function and cirrhosis. The cirrhosis may be of any cause. There have been isolated reports of patients developing spontaneous bacterial peritonitis with non-cirrhotic ascitic diseases, such as Budd-Chiari syndrome, congestive heart failure, systemic lupus erythematosus, and rheumatoid arthritis.[2]

In patients with cirrhotic ascites and SBP, most infections are monomicrobial. Aerobic gram-negative organisms accounts for most infections, with *Escherichia coli* causing approximately 50% and *Klebsiella* approximately 13%. Aerobic gram-positive organisms are the second most common, with *Streptococcus* occurring in approximately 19% of patients and *Enterococcus* in 5%. Anaerobes rarely cause SBP, and polymicrobial infections occur in relatively few patients (approximately 8%).[2]

Many potential mechanisms may account for the pathogenesis of SBP. The predominance of enteric organisms as the cause of the peritonitis suggests that translocation of organisms from the gut may be an important step in the development of the disease. The presence of portal hypertension has been shown to lead to increased translocation of organisms from the gastrointestinal (GI) tract into the portal veins or lymphatics.[3]

The patient's own host defenses may be ineffective in containing infections at other sites, leading to secondary seeding of the ascitic fluid from generalized bacteremia. Because of the diminished phagocytic activity of the hepatic reticuloendothelial system, patients with cirrhosis and ascites have impaired clearance of bacteria from the bloodstream. Additionally, complement, necessary for the opsonization of bacteria, is decreased in the ascitic fluid of patients with cirrhosis. In approximately 44% of patients, urine cultures have been found to be positive for the same organism as isolated from the ascites.[2] Pneumonias and soft tissue infections are other suggested sources.[4]

SECONDARY BACTERIAL PERITONITIS

Secondary bacterial peritonitis results from any process that leads to perforation of the GI tract (necrotizing enterocolitis, volvulus with ischemia, intussusception with ischemia, trauma, perforation from duodenal/gastric ulcers). In secondary bacterial peritonitis, the underlying bacterial infection tends to be a complex polymicrobial infection with an average of 2.9 to 3.9 different isolates. The most commonly isolated organisms are *E. coli* and *Bacteroides fragilis*. The most common gram-positive organisms are nonenterococcal streptococci and enterococci.[2]

Clinical Presentation

The prevalence of SBP ranges from 15% to 19% in patients with cirrhosis and ascites.[2] The diagnosis may be very difficult and must be carefully considered in the patient with ascites whose condition suddenly deteriorates clinically, even if peritoneal signs are absent. Approximately 10% of cases of SBP are completely asymptomatic.[2] When symptoms are present, the most common clinical features include fever and generalized abdominal pain. Other findings may include rebound tenderness, decreased bowel sounds, hypothermia, hypotension, diarrhea, increased ascites despite the use of diuretics, encephalopathy, and unexplained decrease in renal function.[2,4,5]

Diagnosis

The diagnosis of peritonitis must be confirmed with paracentesis. Abdominal ultrasonography may be used to pinpoint ascites, which are not detectable on physical examination. Once obtained, the fluid should be evaluated for polymorphonuclear leukocyte (PMN) count, total protein, lactate, glucose, and bacterial culture. Ascitic concentrations of glucose, protein, and lactate can be helpful in differentiating SBP from secondary bacterial peritonitis. In patients with SBP, the total protein of the ascitic fluid is usually less than 1 g/dl. The ascitic fluid from a patient with secondary bacterial peritonitis is usually higher in total protein (at least 1 g/dl), elevated in lactate (greater than 25 mg/dl), and lower in glucose (less than 50 mg/dl).[1,6]

An elevated ascitic PMN count is considered the most important laboratory indicator of SBP. Ascitic fluid cell counts of less than 250/mm³ are highly suggestive that SBP is not present. PMN counts of greater than 500/mm³ support the diagnosis in the appropriate clinical setting. PMN cell counts of 250 to 500/mm³ are compatible with the diagnosis in the appropriate setting; however, a follow-up paracentesis in 12 to 24 hours should be performed in the asymptomatic patient.[4–6]

When obtaining ascitic fluid for bacterial culture, 10 ml of fluid should be inoculated directly into blood culture bottles at the bedside. Bedside inoculation has been shown to increase the sensitivity of ascitic fluid cultures to 85%.[4,6] Gram stain of ascitic fluid appears to be helpful in the diagnosis of secondary bacterial peritonitis; however, it is insensitive in early SBP.[6]

Two variants of SBP have been described on the basis of ascitic fluid cell counts and culture results. Culture-negative neutrocytic ascites (CNNA) occurs when the PMN count is greater than 250 cells/mm³, ascitic fluid cultures are negative, no prior antibiotic treatment has been administered in one month, and no other explanation for the elevated PMN count can be identified. These findings may reflect an insensitivity of the fluid culture or a resolution of the SBP. Patients with culture-negative neutrocytic ascites should be treated as victims of SBP. Prognosis associated with culture-negative neutrocytic ascites is unknown.[4]

Monomicrobial nonneutrocytic bacterascites occurs when the fluid cultures are positive without an elevation in the PMN count. If bacterascites is truly asymptomatic, it rarely progresses to SBP and in most cases treatment is unnecessary. However, the patient must be monitored closely and a follow-up paracentesis performed if any suspicion of SBP develops.[4]

Management

Management of the patient with peritonitis involves controlling the underlying infection with antibiotics or surgery (in the case of secondary bacterial peritonitis) and supporting the patient's cardiovascular and respiratory systems (Fig. 37-1). An antibiotic regimen should be initiated as soon as the diagnosis is confirmed. In SBP, empirical antibiotic coverage should be directed primarily toward enteric gram-negative aerobes and gram-positive cocci. Ampicillin and an aminoglycoside have been found to be effective antibiotic coverage, although this regimen is associated with significant nephrotoxicity. Cefotaxime, a third-generation cephalosporin, has also been shown to be an effective therapy and is currently considered the antibiotic of choice in the acute setting.[4,5] Once the organism is identified, antibiotic coverage may be optimized according to the organism's sensitivity profile.

Many physicians advocate repeating a paracentesis approximately 48 hours after initiating antibiotic therapy. Most patients with SBP will demonstrate decreasing PMN counts and sterile fluid at this point. If PMN counts remain elevated or organisms continue to be isolated, antibiotic-resistant organisms or secondary bacterial peritonitis should be suspected.[4]

In secondary bacterial peritonitis no particular antibiotic regimen has been shown to be superior in controlled clinical trials. Both single agents and combination regimens have included cefoxitin, cefotetan, cefmetazole, and ticarcillin-clavulanic acid. Combination regimens

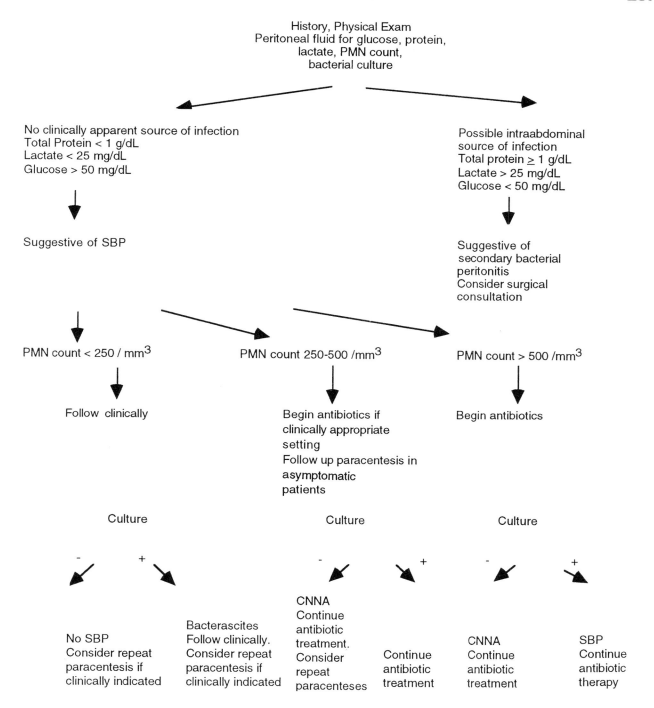

FIGURE 37-1. Suggested management of peritonitis.

that have been used include antianaerobe (Flagyl/clindamycin) plus aminoglycoside, antianaerobe plus third-generation cephalosporin, and clindamycin plus aztreonam. For severe infections, imipenem-cilastatin has also been used.[2,7] Hypovolemia results from extravascular extravasation and sequestration from the inflamed peritoneal membrane. The intravascular volume must be supported with crystalloids and blood products as needed.

Respiration may be mechanically impaired because of diaphragmatic spasm, abdominal rigidity, and increased permeability of the pulmonary vasculature in response to systemic inflammation. Despite detection and treatment of the underlying infection, SBP is associated with a high mortality of 30% to 40%. Prospective studies have documented that the probability of recurrence of SBP is 70% after 1 year.[5]

Predisposing factors to the development of SBP include advanced liver disease, decreased reticuloendothelial system activity, decreased serum complement levels, decreased ascitic protein and complement levels, and GI hemorrhage. In a recent prospective study by Andreu et al.,[8] low ascitic fluid total protein (1 g/dl or less) and elevated serum bilirubin (2.5 mg/d) were the most relevant predictive factors of patients at highest risk of a first episode of SBP. This study suggests a means of identifying the population most at risk of SBP, in order to most effectively intervene in preventing SBP. Recently, the effects of antibiotic prophylaxis on the risk of SBP have been studied in the adult population. These reports document a marked decrease in the incidence of SBP in patients given antibiotics such as norfloxacin to sterilize the gut. However, no decrease in the number of readmissions or mortality was demonstrated.[9,10] No studies have been performed in the pediatric population.

The role of surgery for secondary bacterial peritonitis is to gain control of the underlying source of the abdominal infection by repairing the affected bowel through laparotomy or laparoscopy. The degree of contamination may be decreased by intraoperative peritoneal lavage and by debridement of loculations and abscesses. Adding antibiotics to the lavage fluid has lost favor since the discovery that this procedure appears to impair neutrophil chemotaxis, to inhibit neutrophil bactericidal activity, and to increase the formation of adhesions. Catheters may be placed to drain a well-defined abscess cavity, to form a controlled fistula, or to provide access for continuous postoperative peritoneal lavage.[7]

REFERENCES

1. Baetz-Greenwalt B, Goske M. Intra-abdominal infection. In: Wyllie R, Hyams JA Eds. Pediatric Gastrointestinal Disease: Pathophysiology, Diagnosis, Management. Philadelphia: WB Saunders, 1993:220–240

2. Garcoa-Tsao G. Spontaneous bacterial peritonitis. Gastroenterol Clini North Am 1992;21:257–275

3. Sorell W, Quigley E, Jin G et al. Bacterial translocation in the portal-hypertensive rat: studies in basal conditions and on exposure to hemorrhagic shock. Gastroenterology 1993; 104:1722–1726

4. Bhuva M, Ganger D, Jensen D. Spontaeous bacterial peritonitis: an update on evaluation, management, and prevention. Am Med 1994;97:169–175

5. Gilbert J, Kamath P. Spontaneous bacterial peritonitis: an update. Mayo Clin Proc 1995;70:365–370

6. Runyon B. Care of patients with ascites. N Engl J Med 1994; 330:337–342

7. Nathans AB, Rotstein OD. Therapeutic options in peritonitis. Surg Clin North Am 1994;74:6577–6592

8. Andreu M, Sola R, Sitges-Serra A et al. Risk factors for spontaneous bacterial peritonitis in cirrhotic patients with ascites. Gastroenterology 1993;104:1133–1138

9. Salmeron J, Tito L, Rimola A et al. Selective intestinal decontamination in the prevention of bacterial infection in patients with acute liver failure. J Hepatol 1992;14:280–285

10. Soriano G, Guarner C, Teixido M et al. Selective intestinal decontamination prevents spontaneous bacterial peritonitis. Gastroenterology 1991;100:477–481

38

POLYPS

FRANCIS M. GIARDIELLO

A polyp is defined as any tissue protrusion above the normal, flat, gastrointestinal (GI) mucosal surface. Polyps are clinically important for two reasons. First, they can cause symptoms including bleeding and occasionally intussusception. Second, some polyps are premalignant lesions that can degenerate over time to adenocarcinoma, while others may already harbor adenocarcinoma.

It is essential to determine the histopathology of the polyp for proper patient management. Also, the number of polyps, as well as the patient and family history of polyps or colorectal cancer, should be ascertained. With these data, decisions concerning work-up, treatment, and follow-up can be made. Table 38-1 classifies polyps according to histopathology.

This chapter concentrates on the more common pediatric polyposis syndromes. Rare polyp syndromes not typically seen in the pediatric age group are described in Table 38-2.

HAMARTOMATOUS POLYPOSIS SYNDROMES

Hamartomatous polyps and polyposis syndromes occur more commonly in pediatrics, as compared to the adult population. Previously, these hamartomatous conditions were thought to harbor little if any malignant potential. However, recent evidence supports neoplastic sequelae in some of these syndromes.

Solitary Juvenile Polyps/Familial Juvenile Polyposis

CLINICAL ASPECTS

Juvenile polyps are hamartomatous lesions with a histopathology characterized by edematous mucosa and dilated mucus filled cysts. Most patients with solitary juve-

nile polyps present on average at 4 years of age with rectal bleeding or anal prolapse of a polyp. These solitary juvenile polyp patients (the vast majority of individuals affected by this lesion) have a nonfamilial condition and removal of polyp is sufficient treatment.

By contrast, patients with more than 2 rectosigmoid juvenile polyps or those with a family history of juvenile polyps should be suspected of having familial juvenile polyposis. These patients present on average at 9 years of age (but can be preschool age) with anemia, rectal bleeding, failure to thrive, and abdominal pain. In this syndrome, polyps, numbering from a dozen to hundreds, occur primarily in the colon, but also in the small intestine and stomach (Fig. 38-1). This condition may have autosomal dominant inheritance.

Of concern in familial juvenile polyposis patients is the high incidence of colorectal neoplasia (dysplasia and adenocarcinoma) found in up to 20% of patients at a relatively young age (average 37 years, but dysplasia has been found in the colectomy specimens of several patients younger than 5 years of age). Colorectal neoplasia can be found in the juvenile polyps as well as the flat mucosa. Gastric, duodenal, and pancreatic cancers have also been reported.

MANAGEMENT

Although rare, patients with solitary juvenile polyps have developed colorectal neoplasia. Therefore, these lesions should usually be removed, even if asymptomatic. In patients with a solitary juvenile polyp and no family history of juvenile polyps, this is sufficient treatment.

By contrast, we recommend that, when possible, patients with multiple juvenile polyps (three or more rectosigmoid polyps) or a family history of juvenile polyps should undergo complete upper and lower endoscopy and

TABLE 38-1. Histologic Classification and Inheritance of Polyps and Polyposis Syndromes

Adenomatous polyps (tubular, tubulovillous, villous)

Adenomatous polyposis syndromes
  Familial adenomatous polyposis coli[a] (familial polyposis/
    Gardner's syndrome)
  Turcot's syndrome[a]

Hamartomatous polyps
  Peutz-Jeghers syndrome[a]
  Solitary juvenile polyp/familial juvenile polyposis[a]
  Cronkhite-Canada syndrome
  Cowden's disease[a]
  Intestinal ganglioneuromatosis[a]

Hyperplastic polyps/hyperplastic polyposis

Nodular lymphoid hyperplasia

Lymphomatous/leukematous polyposis

Inflammatory polyps

Miscellaneous

[a] Inherited conditions.

small bowel radiography examinations to determine whether familial juvenile polyposis is present. In affected persons, periodic surveillance by colonoscopy with multiple random biopsies of both polyps and flat mucosa (as done in ulcerative colitis surveillance) every 1 to 3 years is recommended. The upper GI tract should probably also be surveyed. Removal of dysplastic juvenile polyps can be accomplished by endoscopic polypectomy in those with a small number of polyps. At times, colonoscopy surveillance may be difficult, especially in patients with numerous lesions. Colectomy is a consideration in these patients because neoplasia may not be sampled by biopsy and polypectomy. There do not appear to be sufficient data to justify prophylactic colectomy solely for the risk of colorectal carcinoma, as is done in familial adenomatous polyposis. However, in the presence of any other indications, such as persistent rectal bleeding or refractory protein loss, subtotal colectomy with ileorectal anastomosis is appropriate.

SCREENING

Initial screening of first-degree relatives at 12 years of age with colonoscopy is prudent because of the difficulty in recognizing asymptomatic affected persons. Some author-

TABLE 38-2. Rare Polyp Conditions

Condition	Inherited	Clinical Characteristics	Polyp Histology	Polyp Site
Cronkhite-Canada	—	Cutaneous hyperpigmentation, hair loss, nail dystrophy, diarrhea, malabsorption	Juvenile	Throughout
Cowden's disease	Autosomal dominant	Facial trichilemmomas, thyroid and breast cancer	Juvenile, lipoma inflammatory, lymphoid hyperplasia	Throughout
Intestinal ganglioneuromatosis	Autosomal dominant	von Recklinghausen neurofibromatosis	Neurofibromas	Throughout
Hyperplastic polyposis	—	Endoscopically confused with FAP	Hyperplastic	Colorectum
Nodular lymphoid	—	Associated with FAP, common variable immunodeficiency, lymphoma, healthy persons	Lymphoid hyperplasia	Terminal ileum
Inflammatory	—	Inflammatory bowel disease	Inflammatory	Colorectum
Pneumatosis cystoides intestinalis	—	Chronic obstructive pulmonary disease, scleroderma	Air-filled cysts	Intestine
Lipomas	—	Mimic cecal, colorectal polyps	Lipomas	Colorectum

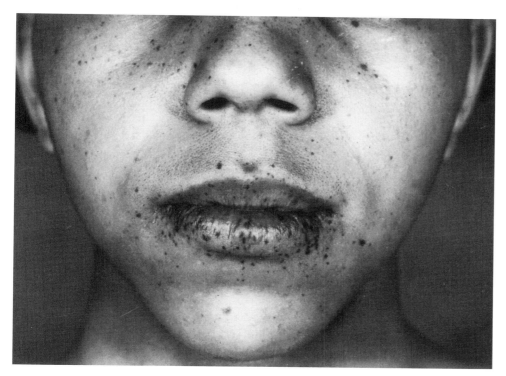

FIGURE 38-1. Patient with Peutz-Jeghers syndrome demonstrating characteristic melanin pigmentation of lips.

ities recommended subsequent screening with flexible sigmoidoscopy and hemoccult testing every 3 to 5 years.

Peutz-Jeghers Syndrome

CLINICAL ASPECTS

Peutz-Jeghers syndrome is an autosomal dominant condition in which Peutz-Jeghers polyps occur primarily in the small intestine, but they may also arise in the colon and stomach. The polyps usually number from 1 to 20 per intestinal segment and have a unique histopathology, with polyp epithelium supported by an arborizing framework of smooth muscle. The characteristic physical finding is macular melanin pigmentation on the lips and buccal mucosa, but also on the digits of the hands and feet and eyelids (Fig. 38-2). These findings can be present in infancy but tend to fade in adolescence.

The primary complication of this disorder in childhood is small intestine intussusception. Intestinal bleeding can also occur. Adults are at a strikingly increased risk at a relatively young age for both GI and non-GI cancers (e.g., breast, ovary, endometrium, pancreas). Subsets of patients have both intestinal adenomas and hamartomas. Unusual tumors found are Sertoli cell tumor of the ovary and adenoma malignum of the cervix in women and testicular cancer in prepubescent boys.

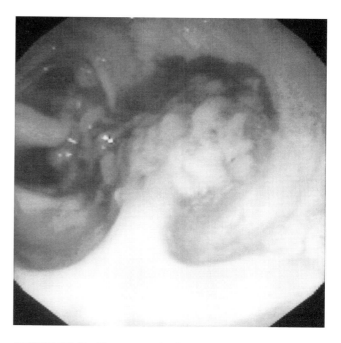

FIGURE 38-2. Air-contrast barium enema in patient with FAP demonstrating multiple filling defects consistent with diffuse colorectal polyposis.

MANAGEMENT

At-risk persons (first-degree relatives of affected individuals) should be screened at least once early in the second decade of life for Peutz-Jeghers syndrome with an upper GI series, with small bowel follow-through.

When diagnosed, affected patients should have at least an initial upper and lower GI endoscopy, biopsying all polyps to search for concomitant adenomas (the probable major source of GI neoplasm). All adenomas should be removed. Some investigators recommend repeating these endoscopic and small bowel radiographic studies every 2 years. These authorities suggest endoscopic polypectomy of any Peutz-Jeghers polyps that are hemorrhagic or greater than 1 cm. Surgery has been recommended for symptomatic small intestinal polyps or for those greater than 1.5 cm. At laparotomy, an attempt should be made to clear the small intestine of polyps by concomitant endoscopic polypectomy or, in the case of larger polyps, enterotomy.

Additional screening in affected patients should include annual history and physical examinations with routine laboratory testing. Mammography with a baseline examination at age 25 and then yearly at age 40, as well as yearly gynecologic examination with pelvic ultrasound starting in adolescence, are also recommended. Patient self-examination of the breast and testicles should be encouraged.

ADENOMATOUS POLYPS

Most authorities hold to the adenoma carcinoma sequence in which perhaps 10% to 30% of premalignant adenomas progress to carcinoma. In children, GI adenomas are almost always associated with hereditary polyposis syndromes, unlike in adults, in whom they can occur as solitary nonhereditary lesions. Since adenomas can progress to adenocarcinoma and may already harbor cancer, they should be removed. Whenever one colorectal polyp is discovered, total colonoscopy is mandatory to exclude synchronous lesions.

Adenomatous Polyposis Syndromes

FAMILIAL ADENOMATOUS POLYPOSIS (FAMILIAL POLYPOSIS/GARDNER'S SYNDROME)

Clinical Aspects

Familial adenomatous polyposis (FAP) is an autosomal dominant syndrome with high penetrance caused by mutation of the adenomatous polyposis coli (APC) gene on the long arm of chromosome 5. Patients develop hundreds to thousands of adenomas diffusely throughout the colorectum usually in teenage years (Fig. 38-3). Colorectal cancer is inevitable by the fifth decade of life if colectomy is not performed. Infrequently (7% of cases),

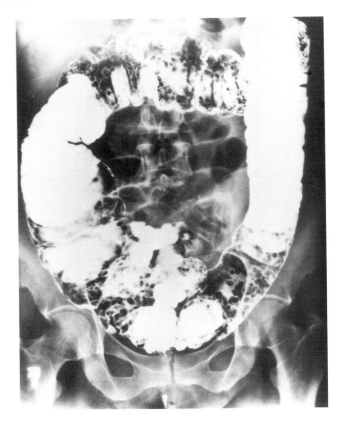

FIGURE 38-3. Endoscopic view of a juvenile polyp in patient with juvenile polyposis.

patients present with attenuated adenomatous polyposis coli (AAPC), in which oligopolyposis (fewer than 100 colorectal adenomas) occurs, rather than polyposis.

Extracolonic Lesions

FAP patients can develop both benign and malignant extracolonic lesions (previously, FAP without extracolonic manifestations was called familial polyposis and FAP with extracolonic manifestations was termed Gardner's syndrome) (Fig. 38-4). Benign lesions include osteomas of the jaw and long bones, skin lipomas, skin cysts, desmoid tumors of the abdomen and extremities, pigmented ocular fundus lesions, clinically occult osteosclerotic jaw lesions, gastric fundic gland retention polyps, gastric adenomas, and duodenal adenomas. FAP patients are at increased risk of malignancies of the duodenum, ampulla of Vater, thyroid, pancreas, and liver (exclusively, hepatoblastoma, a rapidly progressive hepatic tumor occurring before age 5). In fact, cancer of the duodenum is the 2nd most common cause of death in this population after colorectal cancer.

Diagnosis

In the setting of a family history of FAP, the diagnosis of FAP is confirmed by finding greater than 100 adenomatous polyps on endoscopic examination of the colon (sigmoidoscopy is usually sufficient, as FAP affects the

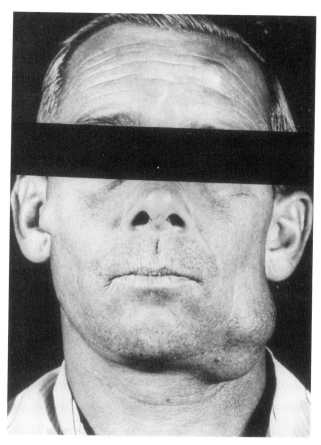

FIGURE 38-4. Familial adenomatous polyposis patient with left-sided mandibular osteoma and epidermoid cyst on forehead.

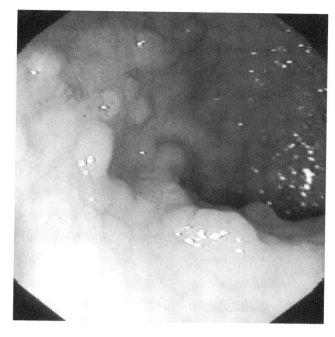

FIGURE 38-5. Endoscopic view of diffuse colorectal adenomatous polyposis in patient with FAP.

colon diffusely) (Fig. 38-3). Importantly, approximately one-third of newly diagnosed patients are new mutations with no family history of adenomatous polyposis. In an at-risk patient, the finding of more than 3 pigmented ocular fundus lesions on indirect ophthalmoscopic examination is associated with a 100% positive predictive value for the diagnosis of FAP. Recently, direct DNA genotypic analysis to diagnose presymptomatic cases has become available.

Screening

At-risk persons (first-degree relatives of affected patients) should undergo screening with yearly sigmoidoscopy starting at age 12. We reduce this frequency to every 2 years after age 25 and every 3 years after age 35. After age 50, patients are advised to follow the American Cancer Society guidelines for screening average-risk patients: flexible sigmoidoscopy at age 50 and, if negative at age 51, every 3 to 5 years; as well as three stool hemoccults every year starting age 50.

Direct genotypic testing in concert with formal genetic counseling should be done in all at-risk persons. If they do not have the mutated *APC* gene, screening by flexible

sigmoidoscopy can be reduced to two time points: age 18 and 30 years. Although DNA testing should have a virtually 100% positive and negative predictive value if the precise pedigree mutation is known, we still recommend several sigmoidoscopies as noted above to ensure that false-negative patients are diagnosed.

Hepatoblastoma occurs in about 1 in 300 at-risk persons under the age of 5 years. By defining which offspring actually have FAP by genetic testing, the risk is increased to about 1 in 150 persons. Because of the magnitude of hepatoblastoma risk and its potential curability by early surgery, screening with serum alpha-fetoprotein levels, and possibly abdominal ultrasound in genotypically positive infants and young children, may be prudent.

Treatment

Colectomy is the only effective therapy that eliminates the inevitable risk of colorectal cancer in FAP patients. Before surgery, upper endoscopy should be performed to assess the upper GI tract for adenomas (large adenomas of the duodenum may be removed during laparotomy for colectomy). In patients of older age (more than 25 to 30 years) with large polyps (greater that 1 cm) or with villous adenomas, colonoscopy is useful to evaluate for concomitant colorectal cancer, which might alter the choice of surgical procedure. Surgery should be done at the time of diagnosis of FAP to minimize any risk of colorectal cancer. However, if the patient is in the 2nd decade of life and the polyps are small (less than 5 mm) and infrequent, surgery could be delayed to accommodate work and school schedules. Surgical options include subtotal colectomy with ileorectal anastomosis, total colectomy with Brooke ileostomy (or continent ileostomy), and colectomy with mucosal proctectomy and ileoanal pull-through (with pouch formation).

Postoperative Follow-up

Patients with subtotal colectomy require routine endoscopic surveillance of the remaining rectum about every 6 months for recurrent adenomas or carcinoma, or both. Since the long-term risk of neoplastic transformation in the ileoanal pouch of patients with ileoanal pull-throughs is unknown, endoscopic biopsy surveillance at 3- to 5-year intervals should be considered.

Duodenal and periampullary carcinoma is estimated to occur over a lifetime in 1 of 21 FAP patients. Therefore, although the cost benefit has not been established, most authorities recommend upper endoscopic surveillance (with biopsy and brushing) of the stomach, duodenum, and periampullary region with front- and/or side-viewing endoscopes every 4 years. In patients with upper tract adenomas, surveillance is recommended at yearly intervals.

FAP patients are also at risk of neoplasms of the thyroid (usually in the 3rd decade of life) and pancreatic cancer (with a lifetime risk of about 1 in 47 and 1 in 59 persons, respectively). Screening for pancreatic cancer may not be worthwhile with currently available methods, but careful physical examination of the thyroid is warranted along with consideration for ultrasonography.

TURCOT'S SYNDROME

Clinical Aspects

Turcot's syndrome is clinically characterized by the concurrence of a primary brain tumor and multiple colorectal adenomas. Recently, the genetic basis of Turcot's syndrome has been defined. The association between brain tumors and colorectal adenomas can result from two distinct germline defects: mutation of the *APC* gene as in FAP or mutation of the DNA mismatch-repair genes or replication errors characteristic of hereditary nonpolyposis colorectal cancer (HNPCC).

Patients with mutation of the *APC* gene usually present with cerebellar medulloblastoma and colorectal polyposis (more than 100 colorectal adenomas). Patients with mutation of the mismatch-repair genes more often have cerebellar glioblastomas and oligopolyposis (fewer than 100 adenomas).

Management

Differentiation of Turcot's syndrome into FAP or HNPCC type by clinical characteristics and, if possible, genotyping should be accomplished. Management of patients and families with FAP-type Turcot's syndrome is identical to treatment of FAP with the addition of careful neurologic examinations as part of routine surveillance.

Affected and at-risk individuals with HNPCC type Turcot's syndrome are managed as for HNPCC, with additional regard for the development of central nervous system tumors. Right-sided colorectal cancer occurring at a young age is the hallmark of HNPCC. Therefore, first-degree relatives (at 50% risk of HNPCC) and those found to be affected by genotyping or in whom genotyping cannot be done should undergo colorectal surveillance by colonoscopy. Surveillance should start by at least 25 years of age or 5 to 10 years earlier than the earliest colorectal neoplasm noted in the pedigree. If colorectal cancer is found, patients should undergo at least colectomy with ileorectal anastomosis, to lessen the danger of unrecognized synchronous colorectal neoplasm and reduce the risk of future cancer or adenoma. With the advent of genetic testing, presymptomatic persons testing positive for HNPCC gene mutations could consider prophylactic colectomy. However, this cannot be given as a firm recommendation, since the penetrance of HNPCC is incomplete and the age of presentation can vary greatly.

Extracolorectal cancer is also a concern in HNPCC. Women at 50% or greater risk of HNPCC should undergo surveillance for endometrial carcinoma.

Rare Polyp Syndromes

Table 38-2 describes rare polyp syndromes not typically presenting in the pediatric age range.

SUGGESTED READINGS

Boland CR, Itzkowitz SH, Kim YS. Colonic polyps and the gastrointestinal polyposis syndromes. In: Sleisenger MH, Fordtran JS, Eds. Gastrointestinal Disease: Pathophysiology, Diagnosis, and Management. 4th Ed. Philadelphia: WB Saunders, 1989: 1500–1507

Burt RW. Polyposis syndromes. In: Yamada T, Ed. Textbook of Gastroenterology. Philadelphia: JB Lippincott, 1991: 1674–1695

Giardiello FM, Hamilton SR, Kern SE et al. Colorectal neoplasia in patients with juvenile polyposis or juvenile polyps. Arch Child Dis 1991;66:971–975

Giardiello FM, Welsh SB, Offerhaus GJA et al. Increased risk of cancer in Peutz-Jeghers syndrome. N Engl J Med 1987;316: 1511–1514

Luk GD. Colonic polyps: benign and premalignant neoplasm of the colon. In: Yamada T, Ed. Textbook of Gastroeterology. Philadelphia: JB Lippincott 1991;1645–1674

Offerhaus GJA, Giardiello FM, Krush AJ et al. The risk of upper gastrointestinal cancer in familial adenomatous polyposis. Gastroenterology 1992;102:1980–1982

39

PROTEIN-LOSING ENTEROPATHY

AZAM SOROUSH
ANDREW E. MULBERG

Protein-losing enteropathy (PLE) is a syndrome due to excessive loss of serum proteins into the gastrointestinal (GI) tract.[1–5] As a result, patients develop hypoalbuminemia, edema, diarrhea, and symptoms related to the loss of other serum proteins (please refer to clinical manifestation section for more details). PLE is associated with a variety of underlying pathophysiologic causes (Table 39-1).

PATHOPHYSIOLOGY

Albumin is a protein with a molecular weight of about 70,000 M_r. It maintains plasma oncotic pressure and binds drugs, hormones, bilirubin, toxic metabolites, and nutrients. Albumin is synthesized by the liver at a rate of 130 to 200 mg/kg/day; 31% to 42% of the total albumin is in plasma, and the rest remains in the extravascular space. The exchangeable pool is 4 g/kg in women and 4.5 to 5 g/kg in men; 7% to 11% of total albumin is degraded every day and corresponds to an albumin half-life ($t_{1/2}$) of 15 to 23 days. Up to 10% of normal turnover of plasma albumin and globulins can be attributed to GI protein loss; however, up to a 60% loss has been reported in patients who have pathologic conditions with excessive enteric protein loss.[6]

Whenever hepatic synthesis fails to compensate for the excessive protein loss, hypoproteinemia and hypoalbuminemia occur. The most dramatic change is observed in proteins with a long half-life, including albumin, hormone-binding proteins, and gamma-globulins (IgG, IgM,

IgA). Levels of alpha-2-macroglobulins, clotting factors, insulin, IgE, and other proteins remain close to normal because of their short half-life.[7]

In general, hypoproteinemia can result from pathologic processes as outlined in Table 39-2. These include very low intake of proteins, malabsorption of amino acid or proteins from the intestinal lumen, impaired protein synthesis, increased protein loss, increased catabolism of proteins and abnormal distribution of body fluid and proteins.[8,9]

Excessive Enteric Loss of Plasma Proteins

In contrast to nephrotic syndrome, protein loss in PLE is not selective. PLE has several different mechanisms: (1) increased enterocyte damage, resulting in increased permeability of the intestinal cell lining to plasma proteins or increased epithelial cell shedding without evidence of significant ulcer or erosion; (2) mucosal erosion and ulceration with leakage of inflammatory exudate into the intestinal lumen; and (3) lymphatic obstruction with leakage of lymph into the intestinal tract.[8] A wide variety of disorders can lead to PLE; these may be systemic, congenital, localized or generalized, transient or long-term, and benign or malignant (Table 39-1).

PRIMARY INTESTINAL LYMPHANGIECTASIA

Primary intestinal lymphangiectasia is a congenital disorder of the lymphatic system characterized by dilated intestinal lymphatics, PLE, hypoalbuminemia, edema, and

TABLE 39-1. Childhood Disorders Associated With Protein-Losing Enteropathy

Mucosal disease without ulceration
    Acute viral gastroenteritis
    Bacterial gastroenteritis
    Clostridium difficile colitis
    Helicobacter pylori gastritis
    Intestinal parasites: giardiasis, hookworm
    Intestinal tumors
    Drug-induced gastroenteritis
    Eosinophilic gastroenteritis
    Allergic gastroenteritis
    Reflux esophagitis
    Infectious esophagitis
    Giant hypertrophic gastropathy
    Hypertrophic gastropathy with hypersecretion
    Gastric bezoar
    Radiation enteropathy
    Enterocolitis: Hirschsprung's disease
    Bacterial overgrowth
    Post-measles diarrhea
    Varicella enteritis
    Celiac disease
    Cystic fibrosis
    Jejunal stenosis
    Hemangioma of the intestine
    Kwashiorkor
    Polyposis
    Systemic lupus erythematosus
    Henoch-Schönlein purpura
    Common variable immunodeficiency
    Nephrotic syndrome
    Burn
    Epidermolysis bullosa

Diseases with ulceration or diffuse erosion
    Esophageal, gastric, or duodenal ulcer
    Infectious esophagitis
    Erosive gastritis
    Infectious enteritis; shigellosis, HIV, salmonellosis, amebiasis, etc.
    Pseudomembranous colitis
    Crohn's disease
    Ulcerative colitis
    Malignancies of the GI tract
    Graft-versus-host disease (GYHD)

Lymphatic obstruction
    Congenital intestinal lymphangiectasia
    Cardiac disease: constrictive pericarditis
    Congestive heart disease, post-Fontan
    Tricuspid regurgitation, cardiomyopathy
    Thrombosis of the superior vena cava
    Retroperitoneal fibrosis
    Malrotation
    Lymphoenteric fistula
    Crohn's disease
    Intestinal tuberculosis
    Cirrhosis of the liver
    Necrotizing enterocolitis

TABLE 39-2. Hypoproteinemia

Low intake
    Malnutrition
    Chronic vomiting

Malabsorption
    GI disorders
    Trypsinogen deficiency
    Enterokinase deficiency

Impaired synthesis
    Liver disease
    Chronic illness
    Inborn errors of protein metabolism
    Analbuminemia
    Pleural effusion with or without chest tube
    Markedly increased plasma volume

Increased catabolism
    Chronic illness
    Severe infection
    Trauma
    Surgery
    Pregnancy
    Malignancy
    Hyperthyroidism
    Familial hypercatabolic hypoproteinemia

Altered distribution
    Third spacing of the body fluids
    Massive ascites
    Defective immunoglobulin synthesis
    Afibrinogenemia
    IV fluid
    SIADH
    Congestive heart failure

lymphopenia.[7,10] Most cases of intestinal lymphangiectasia are sporadic; however, involvement in several families has been reported, suggesting a genetic etiology. This disorder can present anytime from the newborn period to adulthood. It presents most commonly before 2 years of age, with a mean age of onset of 11 years and both sexes affected equally. The disease has been associated with other syndromes, including Turner's, Noonan-DiGeorge, peliosis hepatis, Charcot-Marie-Tooth, and Klippel-Trenaunay-Weber.[9] In rare cases, intestinal lymphangiectasia is associated with intestinal lymphangiomatosis, a malformation of the lymphatics arising from sequestration of lymphatic tissue, usually beyond the level of the lacteal lymphatics.[11,12] Intestinal lymphangiectasia does not normally communicate with the proximal part of the lymphatic system; it is able to proliferate and to accumulate a large amount of lymph, giving a cystic appearance to the lesion.

Occasionally, the lymphatic involvement in lymphangiectasia is generalized, resulting in peripheral edema (Milroy's syndrome), chylous ascites, or pleural or pericardial effusions. The lymphatic block may occur in the lamina propria, submucosa, or serosa.[10] In intestinal lymphangiectasia, lymphopenia is a characteristic finding not seen in PLE secondary to mucosal lesions.

SECONDARY INTESTINAL LYMPHANGIECTASIA

Intestinal lymphangiectasia may occur secondary to an elevated lymphatic pressure (i.e., obstruction). Cardiac lesions may lead to elevated central venous pressure, causing impaired drainage of the lymph at the level of the thoracic duct. Subsequently, the pressure in the lymphatics increases, and transmission of the raised pressure results in rupture of dilated lacteals, leading to the release of its lymphatic contents into the intestinal lumen, producing PLE. Constrictive pericarditis, tricuspid insufficiency, severe pulmonary stenosis, congestive heart failure (CHF), and cardiomyopathy all increase lymphatic pressure.[13] Palliative cardiac surgery for congenital heart disease (i.e., the Fontan, Glenn, or Mustard operation) often produces elevations in lymphatic pressure, causing protein loss into the GI tract.[14] Patients with cardiac disease often have cardiac cirrhosis and malnutrition, in addition to a high metabolic rate, further complicating the compensatory mechanisms for hypoalbuminemia.

Pathologic processes involving the chest or abdominal lymphatics can also cause obstruction of the lymphatic flow, resulting in a secondary intestinal lymphangiectasia. Crohn's disease or intestinal tuberculosis promotes protein loss due to mucosal erosions and inflammation of the lymphatics with secondary obstruction. Malrotation and volvulus may compromise venous and lymphatic drainage causing PLE.[15]

ACUTE TRANSIENT PLE

Children, usually those less than 3 years old, may present with sudden onset of hypoalbuminemia and edema. This is associated with acute nonspecific gastroenteritis, typically of viral origin, although it has been reported to occur in association with *H. pylori* gastritis.[16–18] The protein loss is usually transient, lasting a few weeks to a few months, until the intestinal mucosal insult is healed.

MENETRIER'S DISEASE

Menetrier's disease has an uncertain etiology, although an association has been noted between Menetrier's disease and cytomegalovirus (CMV) infection.[19] It is most commonly seen in men older than 50 years and is rare in children. Unlike in adult patients, the disease in the pediatric population usually has a short course with spontaneous recovery. It is associated with pronounced hypertrophic mucosal folds, visualized mainly in the fundus and body of the stomach. The histology is characteristic and demonstrates mucosal thickening, elongated gastric pits, and cystic dilation with a marked decrease in parietal and chief cells.

ALLERGIC GASTROENTERITIS

Waldmann et al.[20] described several infants with edema, iron deficiency anemia, eosinophilia, hypoalbuminemia, hypogammaglobulinemia, growth retardation, and other features suggestive of GI allergy. These patients had excessive fecal excretion of albumin, significantly improved after instituting a hypoallergenic formula; antigenic challenge produced a recurrence of intestinal protein loss. Patients with allergic gastroenteritis may have GI blood loss and an elevated IgE without evidence of lymphocytopenia or skin anergy.

CELIAC DISEASE

Approximately 20% to 50% of patients with celiac disease have hypoalbuminemia secondary to both malabsorption and leakage of plasma proteins into the intestinal lumen.[21] Patients may also present with hypocalcemia, hypoproteinemia, anemia, or vitamin deficiency. The duodenal and jejunal mucosa in these patients is atrophied; this is often demonstrated histologically by endoscopic biopsy. (For a detailed discussion of the features of celiac disease see Ch. 19.)

CLINICAL MANIFESTATIONS

Because of the large number of disorders causing PLE, the presenting signs and symptoms may vary. GI protein loss may be increased two- to fourfold without evidence of serum hypoalbuminemia and without other visible or GI signs and symptoms. As protein loss increases, a generalized, symmetric, fluctuating pitting edema will develop. By contrast, lymphedema in lymphangiectasia produces an asymmetric, constant nonpitting edema. Lymphedema can present at birth, but generalized edema usually presents after the newborn period.

Patients with PLE may have diarrhea, steatorrhea, nausea and vomiting, abdominal pain, growth failure, or anemia. These symptoms often present prior to generalized edema. In rare cases, chylous ascites and chylothorax are the presenting symptoms, causing respiratory compromise. Patients with chylous ascites are also at risk of the development of adhesions and intestinal obstruction. Hypocalcemia and tetany have been reported to occur in up to 12% of patients with PLE. Serum levels of magnesium, iron, folic acid, vitamin B_{12}, and fat-soluble vitamins may be decreased. Macular edema has been reported to cause blindness in patients with severe hypoalbuminemia.[22]

Patients with PLE may be at increased risk of infections secondary to alterations of the immune system and to accumulation of fluid in the serosal cavity. However, the risk is much lower in this group when compared to patients who have primary immunodeficiency.

DIAGNOSIS

Most proteins and polypeptides undergo complete proteolysis in the gut lumen. Exceptions to this rule include alpha-1-antitrypsin (α_1-AT), IgA, and intrinsic factor. The diagnosis of PLE should be made by measuring a macromolecule not absorbed, secreted, or degraded by the GI tract. Several radiolabeled proteins have been used to detect protein loss in the GI tract: (1) ^{131}I-labeled albumin, an inaccurate test secondary to salivary and gastric excretion and intestinal absorption; (2) ^{67}Cu-ceruloplasmin, which is difficult to use because of its short half-life and expense; and (3) ^{51}Cr-albumin, the most widely used test before the popularity of fecal alpha-1-antitrypsin measurements.

Fecal α_1-AT is a simple, safe method that does not require radioactive agents.[23,24] α_1-AT is a glycoprotein with broad-spectrum antiprotease activity that accounts for almost 80% of the serum alpha-1-fraction. It comprises approximately 4% of the total serum protein content. α_1-AT is increased during stress, infection, or chronic illness and is mainly synthesized in the liver; however, synthesis and secretion can occur in the intestinal mucosa, especially when inflamed. The molecular weight of α_1-AT is 50,000. It cannot be found in the diet because of its antiprotease activity. The fecal level of α_1-AT reflects proteins originating from the serum. Urinary contamination of the stool will not interfere with the results of the test, an important feature for pediatric population.

Because the level of α_1-AT is higher in meconium, fecal α_1-AT measurement is not an accurate test before the first week of life. Because α_1-AT is denaturated at a pH of less than 3, it is not an accurate test for assessment of PLE secondary to esophageal or gastric lesions. Some have recommended concurrent use of H_2-blockers when attempting to define a disease arising from the stomach.[25] Severe lower GI bleeding also alters the results of the fecal α_1-AT test. Approximately 40% of patients with infectious diarrhea, necrotizing enterocolitis, cow's milk protein allergy, and inflammatory bowel disease normally have an increased fecal α_1-AT level.[26–28]

When calculating α_1-AT clearance (C), the stools should be collected for one or more days, and the following formula should be used:

$$C = (F \times W)/P$$

where C = α_1-AT clearance (ml/day), F = fecal concentration of α_1-AT, W = weight of the stool (g/day), and P = plasma concentration of α_1-AT.

A random stool specimen can be measured and calculated as the concentration (mg) of α_1-AT per gram of dried stool or milliliter of loose stool. These values should be compared with control values because of the high chance of variability between different controls. When an underlying cause of PLE is apparent, a quantitative measurement may not be indicated. Testing may be done for follow-up evaluation of the disease process and response to therapy.

ENDOSCOPIC FINDINGS

In lymphangiectasia, scattered white spots may be apparent at the site of the tip of the villi representing markedly dilated lacteals or intraepithelial spaces filled with fat or chylomicron droplets. These endoscopic findings may be more evident after a fatty meal. In order to have a higher success rate in obtaining adequate tissue from these patchy lesions, large cup-shaped forceps should be used in order to obtain multiple deep specimens. Occasionally, laparotomy is indicated to confirm abnormal lymphatics in areas deeper than the mucosa.

PATHOLOGIC FINDINGS

Intestinal biopsy often demonstrates generalized edema of the interstitial area or submucosa. In patients with lymphangiectasia, a patchy involvement of the intestine (occasionally diffuse involvement) may be seen. Dilated lacteals within the villi, submucosa, or subserosa are characteristic lesions. While the small intestine is the usual site of involvement in primary intestinal lymphangiectasia, on rare occasions disease is limited to the colonic mucosa. Electron microscopy depicts gaps between basal epithelial cells that communicate directly with the edematous fluid in the lamina propria.

RADIOLOGIC FINDINGS

An upper GI series may demonstrate hypertrophic gastric rugae characteristic of Menetrier's disease, hypertrophic lymphocytic gastritis, or gastric lymphoid hyperplasia. In lymphangiectasia, the upper GI series may be completely normal or show a typical malabsorption pattern with thickened jejunal folds, fluid hypersecretion with barium dilution, punctate lucencies, or spiculation—all nonspecific findings. Bony abnormalities in the form of melorheostosis can be seen in generalized lymphangiectasia. A lymphangiogram, which is a difficult technique to perform in small children, should be performed only when the intestinal biopsy is inconclusive.

OTHER LABORATORY FINDINGS

The serum albumin may be normal or low, depending on the severity of PLE. Most patients with PLE suffer from steatorrhea demonstrated by measurement of fecal fat or fat-soluble vitamin deficiency. Carbohydrate absorption is usually unchanged. Serum iron, magnesium, calcium, copper, folic acid, and vitamin B_{12} may be decreased. Cholesterol may be normal or low. Levels of fibrinogen and alpha-2-macroglobulins are usually normal. Hormone-binding proteins may be decreased causing decrease in total hormone level with a normal free hormone level. Patients with severe edema may have hyperaldosteronism and sodium retention secondary to depleted intravascular volume. Serum levels of IgG, IgM, and IgA may be decreased and patients often have lymphopenia.[29] Patients may have an impaired cellular immunity with cutaneous anergy and impaired allograft rejection and impaired in vitro lymphocyte proliferative responses to mitogens.[30] Response to primary and booster immunizations may be abnormal. Hyposplenism, thymic hypoplasia, and impaired neutrophil function have also been described.[31] Analysis of the chylous drainage usually shows a milky fluid that has a high triglyceride and a high cholesterol level with up to 3% protein.

APPROACH TO THE PATIENT WITH HYPOPROTEINEMIA

When evaluating a patient with hypoproteinemia, common causes must be excluded (Table 39-1). A nutritional history as well as measurements of weight, height, and ideal body weight should be performed (skinfold measurements are inaccurate due to edema). A physical examination and urinalysis are needed to rule out renal protein loss. Serum liver function tests help evaluate the protein synthetic ability of the liver. If the patient has evidence of enteric protein loss, infectious causes must also be excluded.

Stool specimens should be sent for culture and for ova and parasitic analysis. Serum should be analyzed for evidence of lymphopenia and other nutrients (other proteins, fat, minerals, vitamins). An upper GI series with small bowel followthrough may indicate gastric, intestinal, or anatomic abnormalities or a malabsorption pattern. Whenever PLE is suspected, upper endoscopy should be performed. An echocardiogram, and possibly cardiac catheterization, should be performed whenever heart disease is suspected. Finally, abdominal or chest computed tomography (CT) may be useful when looking for a mass lesion, fibrosis, or enlarged lymph node.

TREATMENT

All patients with severe PLE and hypoalbuminemia benefit from temporary albumin infusions coupled with diuretics. However, the underlying cause must be diagnosed and treated whenever possible. Surgery should be performed to correct Hirschsprung's disease, jejunal stenosis, malrotation, hemangioma of the bowel, and localized lymphangiectasia. Few refractory cases of chylous ascites and chylothorax have achieved improvement with surgical shunts or pleurectomy.[32] Cardiac lesions with elevated right-sided heart pressure should be corrected by appropriate medical or surgical therapy.

Dietary therapy is the only successful therapy for lymphangiectasia.[33,34] The goal is to decrease lymphatic pressure and flow and subsequently decrease the amount of lymphatic leakage into the intestinal lumen. The diet should be supplemented with high-protein, high medium-chain triglyceride (MCT) components with vitamins and minerals whenever necessary.

MCT contains fatty acid chains with 8 to 12 carbon atoms. Long-chain triglyceride (LCT) has more than 16 carbons. It originates from coconut oil, butter, and kernel oil. It is more water soluble than LCT and can bypass the lymphatics and diffuse directly to portal system without the need for chylomicron formation. In the presence of high LCT, MCT can be incorporated in chylomicrons. Each gram of MCT provides 8.3 kcal, compared to 9.3 kcal/g LCT. In lymphangiectasia, the diet should be maintained indefinitely. In patients unresponsive to diet therapy, total parenteral nutrition (TPN) has been effective.

Antiplasmin has had a controversial effect in lymphangiectatic patients with elevated plasma fibrinolytic activity who were unresponsive to dietary therapy.[35,36] Steroids have been shown to control some of the primary disorders and are effective in controlling PLE following Fontan procedure.[37]

PROGNOSIS

Patients with lymphangiectasia who are compliant with their dietary and medical regimen, will improve both clinically and nutritionally. Patients with cardiac, anatomic, or other localized lesions may have complete resolution following resection of the affected organ system.

REFERENCES

1. Maimon SN, Bartlett JP, Humphreys EM et al. Giant hypertrophic gastritis. Gastroenterology 1947;8:397–428

2. Citrin Y, Sterling K, Halsed JA. Mechanism of hypoproteinemia associated with giant hypertrophy of gastric mucosa. N Engl J Med 1957;257:906–912

3. Gordon RS, Bartter FC, Waldmann TA. Idiopathic hypoalbuminemias. Ann Intern Med 1984;51:553–576

4. Waldmann TA, Peterson VP. Protein-losing enteropathy. Lancet 1961;1:417

5. Crossley JR, Elliot RB. Simple method for diagnosing protein-losing enteropathy. BMJ 1977;2:428–429

6. Anderson SB, Glenert J, Wallevik K. Gammaglobulin turnover and intestinal degradation of gammaglobulin in the dog. J Clin Invest 1963;42:1873–1881

7. Waldmann TA. Protein losing enteropathy. Gastroenterology 1966;50:422–443

8. Tunnessen WW Jr. Edema. In: Signs and Symptoms in Pediatrics. 2nd Ed. Philadelphia: JB Lippincott, 1987:56–64

9. Goldberg RI, Calleja GA. Protein losing enteropathy. In: Bockus Textbook of Gastroenterology. 5th ed. Vol 2. Philadelphia: WB Saunders, 1995:1072–1086

10. Vardy PA, Lebenthal E, Shwachman H. Intestinal lymphangiectasia: a reappraisal. Pediatrics 1975;55:842–851

11. Levine C. Primary disorders of the lymphatic vessels. J Pediatr Surg 1989;24:233–240

12. Walker-Smith JA, Reye RDK, Soutter GB et al. Small intestinal lymphangiectasia. Arch Dis Child 1969;44:527–532

13. Wilkinson P, Pinto B, Senior JR. Reversible protein losing enteropathy with intestinal lympangiectasia secondary to chronic constrictive pericarditis. N Engl J Med 1965;273:1178

14. Mulberg AE, Piccoli DA, Murphy JD. Severe enteric protein loss causes hypoproteinemia and hypogammaglobuinemia after the modified Fontan procedure. Circulation 1989;80(suppl):484

15. Burke V, Anderson CM. Chronic volvulus as a cause of hypoproteinemia, edema and tetany. Aust Paediatr J 1966;2:219

16. Maki M, Harmoines A, Vesikari T et al. Fecal excretion of α_1-antitrypsin in acute diarrhea. Arch Dis Child 1982;57:154–155

17. Hill ID, Sinclair-Smith C, Lastovica AJ et al. Transient protein-losing enteropathy associated with acute gastritis and *Campylobacter* infection. Arch Dis Child 1987;62:1215–1219

18. Cohen HA, Shapiro RP, Frydman M et al. Childhood protein-losing enteropathy associated with Helicobacter Pylori infection. J Pediatr Gastroenterol Nutr 1991;13:201–203

19. Leonidas JC, Beatty EC, Wenner HA. Menetrier's disease and cytomegalovirus infection in childhood. Am J Dis Child 1973;126:806–808

20. Waldmann TA, Wochner RD, Laster L. Allergic gastroenteropathy: a cause of excessive gastrointestinal protein loss. N Engl J Med 1967;276:761–769

21. Gaze H, Donath A, Rossi E. Albumin turnover studies in celiac disease with special reference to the loss of albumin to the GI tract. In: Proceedings of the Thirteenth International Congress on Pediatrics 243–248, 1971

22. Pomerantz M, Waldmann TA. Systemic lymphatic abnormalities associated with gastrointestinal protein loss secondary to intestinal lymphangiectasia. Gastroenterology 1963;45:703–711

23. Magazzu G, Jacono G, Di Pasquale G et al. Reliability and usefulness of random fecal α_1-antitrypsin concentration: further simplification of the method. J Pediatr Gastroenterol Nutr 1985;4:402–407

24. Hill RE, Comm B, Herez A et al. Fecal measurement of α_1-antitrypsin: a reliable measure of enteric protein loss in children. J Pediatr 1981;99:416–419

25. Florent CH, Vidon N, Flourie A et al. Gastric clearance of α_1-antitrypsin under cimetidine perfusion, a new test to detect protein-losing enteropathy. Dig Dis Sci 1986;31:12–15

26. Zuin G, Fontana M, Nicoli S et al. Persistence of protein loss in acute diarrhea. A follow up study by fecal α_1-antitrypsin measurement. Acta Paediatr 1991;80:961–963

27. Schulman RJ, Buffone G, Wise L. Enteric protein loss in necrotizing enterocolitis as measured by fecal α_1-antitrypsin excretion. J Pediatr 1985;107:287–289

28. Thomas DW, Sinatra FR, Russel JM. Fecal α_1-antitrypsin in young people with Crohn's disease. J Pediatr Gastroenterol Nutr 1983;2:491–496

29. Waldmann TA et al. The role of the gastrointestinal system in idiopathic hypoproteinemia. Gastroenterology 1961;41:197–207

30. Strober W, Wochner RD, Waldmann TA. Intestinal lymphangiectasia: a protein-losing enteropathy with hypogammaglobulinemia, lymphocytopenia and impaired homograft rejection. J Clin Invest 1967;46:1643–1645

31. Bolton RP, Cotter KL, Losowsky MS. Impaired neutrophil function in intestinal lymphocytes. J Clin Lab Immunol 1988;26:1–3

32. Lester LA, Rothberg R, Krantman HJ et al. Intestinal lymphangiectasia and bilateral pleural effusions: effect of dietary therapy and surgical intervention on immunologic and pulmonary parameters. J Allergy Clin Immunol 1986;78:891–897

33. Yssing M, Jensen H, Jarnum S. Dietary treatment of protein-losing enteropathy. Acta Paediatr 1966;56:306–308

34. Holt PR. Dietary treatment of protein loss in intestinal lymphangiectasia. Pediatrics 1964;34:629–635

35. Mine K, Matsubayashi S, Nakai Y et al. Intestinal lymphangiectasia markedly improved with antiplasmin therapy. Gastroenterology 1989;96:1996–1999

36. Cohen SA, Diuguid DL, Whitelock RT et al. Intestinal lymphangiectasia and antiplasmin therapy, correspondence. Gastroenterology 1993;102:2193

37. Rychik J, Piccoli DA, Barber G. Usefulness of corticosteroid therapy for protein-losing enteropathy after the Fontan procedure. J Cardiol 1991;68:819–821

40

PSEUDO-OBSTRUCTION

DELMA L. BROUSSARD

Intestinal pseudo-obstruction refers to a disorder of gastrointestinal (GI) motility characterized by signs and symptoms of intestinal obstruction without evidence of mechanical obstruction of the intestinal lumen.[1] Acute or transient intestinal pseudo-obstruction is a paralytic ileus described primarily in the elderly and chronically ill.[2,3] Chronic or recurrent intestinal pseudo-obstruction includes a heterogeneous group of motility disorders, which may be associated with other systemic diseases or drug ingestions.

PHYSIOLOGIC BACKGROUND

The smooth muscle cell is the final mediator of GI contractions. Individual smooth muscle cells are functionally coupled by low resistant junctions (gap junctions), which enable rapid spreading of electrical activity between the individual cells.[4] Smooth muscle cells have a fluctuating resting membrane potential that results in periodic smooth muscle depolarizations known as slow waves, electrical control activity (ECA), or basic electrical rhythm. These pacesetter potentials are below the threshold potential necessary to initiate a contraction. Contractions occur only when a slow wave, following chemical or electrical excitation, reaches the threshold voltage, resulting in electrical response activity (ERA) or a spike potential.[5] The slow wave is responsible for the timing, speed, and direction of gastrointestinal contractions, as a result of the ERA occurring intermittently against the slow wave background.[6]

Both neural and humoral stimuli contribute to the smooth muscle cell depolarization. The neural control of GI motor activity comes from both the central nervous system (CNS) and the intrinsic neural tissue to the intestinal wall, the enteric nervous system (ENS). The ENS is unique as compared to other nerve ganglia in the peripheral nervous system, because it is capable of mediating reflex activity independent of the CNS.[7] The ENS consists of two major plexuses, the myenteric (Auerbach's), located between the external circular and longitudinal muscle layers, and the submucosal (Meissner's). These neuronal groups regulate intestinal secretion, transport, mucosal blood flow, in addition to smooth muscle contractions. In pseudo-obstruction, there is hypomotility of the gut wall secondary to abnormal smooth muscle[8] or altered innervation of the intestine.[9]

HISTOPATHOLOGY

Chronic intestinal pseudo-obstruction in the adult and pediatric populations includes a group of heterogeneous disorders based on histopathology. In patients with primary intestinal pseudo-obstruction, the intestine may exhibit normal histology,[10–13] degeneration of the enteric neurons,[14–16] abnormal smooth muscle,[17–19] or both.[20] Careful histologic studies by Kirshnamurthy and Schuffler[8] have demonstrated changes in the morphology of enteric neurons in patients with chronic pseudo-obstruction.

Table 40-1 lists causes of both primary and secondary pseudoobstruction. Secondary pseudo-obstructive syndromes have been associated with a number of disease

TABLE 40-1. Causes of Intestinal Pseudo-Obstruction

Primary pseudo-obstruction
   Visceral myopathy
      Familial visceral myopathy
      Non-familial visceral myopathy
   Visceral neuropathy
      Familial visceral neuropathy
      Non-familial visceral neuropathy
Secondary intestinal pseudo-obstruction
   Diseases of gastrointestinal smooth muscle
      Collagen-vascular disease
      Muscular dystrophies
      Amyloidosis
      Hollow visceral myopathy
   Diseases of the nervous system
      Diabetic polyneuropathy
      Chagas disease
      Post-viral pseudo-obstruction
      Primary autonomic dysfunction
      Parkinson's disease
      Enteric nervous system diseases
   Endocrine diseases
      Hypoparathyroidism
      Hypothyroidism
      Pheochromocytoma
   Drug-related causes
      Antidepressants/Antianxiety drugs
      Antiparkinsonian drugs
      Cathartics
      Opiates
      Cytotoxic agents
      Anticholinergics
   Metabolic diseases
      Porphyria
      Uremia (or severe electrolyte imbalance)
   Miscellaneous
      Celiac sprue
      Jejunoileal bypass
      Paraneoplastic pseudo-obstruction
      Radiation enteritis
      Organ transplantation (Cytomegalovirus, Epstein-Barr virus, Herpes simplex virus)
      Intra-abdominal inflammation

states and drugs. Disease associated with primary pseudo-obstruction may be sporatic or familial. Secondary causes of pseudo-obstruction are more common in adults, so pediatric cases will most likely be a result of a primary motor disorder.[21]

DIAGNOSIS

Chronic intestinal pseudo-obstruction is a clinical diagnosis that includes signs and symptoms consistent with delayed transit or functional obstruction of the intestine.

Clinical complaints are secondary to motility disturbances in any region of the GI tract and include nonspecific symptoms, such as dysphagia, nausea, early satiety, vomiting, abdominal pain, altered bowel habits (constipation and diarrhea), and abdominal distention. Since pseudo-obstructive syndromes are associated with visceral neuromuscular dysfunction, other visceral systems may also be affected. Therefore these patients may have urologic symptoms in addition to intestinal symptoms. Secondary complications of pseudo-obstruction include diarrhea (steatorrhea) resulting from bacterial overgrowth in the small intestine and malnutrition secondary to malabsoption and/or decreased intake.

A history, physical examination, or laboratory study suggestive of chronic or recurrent episoides of intestinal obstruction should raise the suspicion of intestinal pseudo-obstruction. Clinical symptoms, however, may be mild. The initial workup should investigate conditions and diseases associated with secondary pseudo-obstruction, which may reduce the number of GI studies. However, in many cases, GI imaging will be necessary to exclude a mechanical obstruction, as the history and examination may not provide a complete explanation for the symptoms.

Plain radiographs are the study of choice to exclude mechanical obstruction. It is not uncommon to see dilation of the small and/or large intestine due to an increased amount of gas.[22] There may also be colonic distention with or without air fluid levels. Additionally, radiographs may not show gas in the rectum or colon, or there may be pneumatosis intestinalis or pneumoperitoneum. Although most cases will have abdominal radiographs demonstrating diffuse involvement of the GI tract, some patients will demonstrate segmental abnormalities. Contrast radiography can distinguish mechanical obstruction from pseudo-obstruction, as well as grossly evaluate GI contractility.[22]

Scintigraphic studies have been shown to be useful in the evaluation of GI transit.[23–25] In these studies, small amounts of gamma-emitting radioisotopes are used to label food in the GI tract. The total radioactivity within a lumen is determined serially throughout the study, in order to observe transit time of luminal contents from a given bowel segment (e.g., esophagus, stomach, small intestine, or colon). This technique is associated with less radiation than occurs with a barium radiograph and is quantitative and more physiologic. Therefore, scintigraphy is a useful test in the evaluation of patients with suspected intestinal pseudo-obstruction, once a mechanical obstruction is ruled out. Additionally, it is a safe and valuable tool in the evaluation of the efficacy of therapeutic agents. However, the experience with scintigraphic studies is more limited in the pediatric population than in the adult population.

Direct evaluation of intestinal motor function requires intubation for manometric evaluations. GI manometry documents contractile patterns and enables the differentiation between neuropathic and myopathic processes. Manometry shows normal amplitude contractions that are not coordinated in a neuropathic (extrinsic or intrinsic) disorder, and coordinated low-amplitude contractions in myopathic disorders.[26] Antroduodenal manometry can be helpful in confirming a clinical diagnosis of pseudo-obstruction. Additionally, small bowel manometry has been useful in further characterizing chronic intestinal pseudo-obstruction in children and in assessing the effectiveness of a prokinetic agent in this population.[27,28] Because of the invasiveness of antroduodenal manometry, this procedure is not done routinely in the evaluation of patients with possible motility disorders.

intestine bacterial overgrowth with antibiotics.[39] Surgical interventions include a venting enterostomy to relieve abdominal distention and bloating.[40] Additionally, patients with localized disease may be candidates for limited resections, if a more generalized motility disorder has been excluded. Diversionary stomas or myotomy may also be helpful in individual patients. However, surgery in most cases is only palliative.

Chronic idiopathic intestinal pseudo-obstruction is a rare diagnosis; however, it does occur in the pediatric age group.[11,31,41] A delay in diagnosis may have a significant impact on the growth of these patients, as well as their long-term outcome.[42] Physicians should therefore be aware of this disorder in order to prevent misdiagnosis.

TREATMENT

Identification of an underlying condition is important in the medical management of a patient with chronic intestinal pseudo-obstruction. Stabilization of the patient's hydration and metabolic status is necessary before nutritional intervention is begun. Gastrostomy feeds are commonly needed in patients with severe symptoms of food intolerance. However, jejunal feeds may be successful in select children with intestinal pseudo-obstruction when gastrostomy feeds fail.[29] Nutitional support within this heterogeneous population ranges from enteral nutrition with an elemental formula to total parenteral nutrition, depending on the severity of clinical symptoms. Parenteral nutrition has been very successful in both the adult[30] and pediatric[31] populations with intestinal pseudo-obstruction; however, it is not without significant morbidity.

Numerous pharmacologic agents have been tried to stimulate normal intestinal propulsion. Cholinergic agents have proved unsuccessful in the treatment of patients with pseudo-obstruction.[13,32] Metoclopramide, a cholinergic stimulant and a dopamine receptor antagonist, has been tried to treat a number of pseudo-obstruction disorders and has demonstrated limited efficacy.[3,10,33,34] Cisapride, a nondopaminergic prokinetic agent that stimulates acetylcholine release from myenteric neurons, has shown promise in the treatment of patients with intestinal pseudo-obstruction. It has been shown to stimulate small intestinal transit in children[27] and adults.[35] Cisapride can increase rates of gastric emptying.[36] Cisapride may be useful in the treatment of chronic constipation in a subgroup of patients with severe idiopathic constipation.[37] Other medical options include erythromycin, a motilin agonist, in combination with octreotide (a long-acting somatostatin analogue), which has been used successfully to relieve upper tract symptoms in patients with chronic pseudo-obstruction.[38]

An additional medical therapy is treatment of small

REFERENCES

1. Dudley HA, Sinclair ISR, McLaren IF et al. Intestinal pseudo-obstruction. JR Coll Surg Edinb 1958;3:206–217

2. Anuras S, Christensen J. Recurrent or chronic intestinal pseudo-obstruction. Clin Gastroenterol 1989;10:177–190

3. Faulk DL, Anuras S, Christensen J. Chronic intestinal pseudo-obstruction. Gastroenterology 1978;74:922–931

4. Gabella G. Gap junctions of the muscles of the small and large intestine. Cell Tissue Res 1981;219:469–488

5. Sarna SK. Gastrointestinal electrical activity: terminology. Gastroenterology 1975;68:1631–1635

6. Sarna SK. Cyclic motor activity; migrating motor complex: 1985. Gastroenterology 1985;89:894–913

7. Wood JD. Intrinsic neural control of intestinal motility. Annu Rev Physiol 1981;43:33–51

8. Kirshnamurthy S, Schuffler MD. Pathology of neuromuscular disorders of the small intestine and colon. Gastroenterology 1987;93:610–639

9. Camilleri M. Disorders of gastrointestinal motility in neurologic diseases. Mayo Clin Proc 1990;65:825–846

10. Lewis TD, Daniel EW, Sarna SK et al. Idiopathic intestinal pseudoobstruction. Report of a case, with intraluminal studies of mechanical and electrical activity, and response to drugs. Gastroenterology 1978;74:107–111

11. Byrne WJ, Cipel L, Euler AR et al. Chronic idiopathic intestinal pseudo-obstruction syndrome in children—clinical characteristics and prognosis. J Pediatr 1977;90:585–589

12. Sullivan MA, Snape WJ, Matarazzo SA et al. Gastrointestinal myoelectrical activity in idiopathic intestinal pseudo-obstruction. N Engl J Med 1977;297:233–238

13. Maldonado JE, Gregg JA, Green PA, Brown AL. Chronic idiopathic intestinal pseudo-obstruction. Am J Med 1970; 49:203–212

14. Dyer NH, Dawson AM, Smith BF, Todd IP. Obstruction of bowel due to lesion in the myenteric plexus. BMJ 1969;1: 686–689

15. Schuffler MD, Bird TD, Sumi SM. A familial neuronal disease presenting as intestinal pseudo-obstruction. Gastroenterology 1978;75:889–898

16. Schuffler MD, Jonak Z. Chronic idiopathic intestinal pseudo-obstruction caused by a degenerative disorder of the myenteric plexus: the use of Smith's method to define the neuropathology. Gastroenterology 1982;82:476–486

17. Faulk DL, Anuras S, Gardner GD et al. A familial visceral myopathy. Ann Intern Med 1978;89:600–606

18. Schuffler MD, Pope CE. Studies of idiopathic intestinal pseudo-obstruction. I. Hereditary hollow visceral myopathy: clinical and pathological studies. Gastroenterology 1977;73:327–338

19. Jacobs F, Ardichvili D, Perissiono A et al. A case of familial visceral myopathy with atrophy and fibrosis of the longitudinal muscle layer of the entire small bowel. Gastroenterology 1979;77:745–750

20. Smout AJPM, De Wilde L, Kooyman CD, Ten Thije OJ. Chronic idiopathic intestinal pseudo-obstruction: coexistence of smooth muscle and neuronal abnormalities. Dig Dis Sci 1985;30:282–287

21. Christensen J. The syndromes of intestinal pseudo-obstruction. J Pediatr Gastroenterol Nutr 1988;7:319–322

22. Rohrman CA, Ricci MT, Krishnamurthy S, Schuffler MD. Radiologic and histologic differentiation of neuromuscular disorders of the gastrointestinal tract. AJR 1981;143:933–941

23. Tolin RD, Malmud LS, Reilley J, Fisher RS. Esophageal scintigraphy to quanititate esophageal transit. Gastroenterology 1979;76:1402–1408

24. Mayer EA, Elashoff J, Hawkins R et al. Gastric emptying of mixed solid-liquid meal in patients with intestinal pseudo-obstruction. Dig Dis Sci 1988;33:10–18

25. Krevsky B, Malmud LS, D'Ercole F et al. Colonic transit scintigraphy—a physiologic approach to the quantitative measurement of colonic transit in humans. Gastroenterology 1986;91:127–132

26. Colemont LJ, Camilleri MD. Chronic intestinal pseudo-obstruction: diagnosis and treatment. Mayo Clin Proc 1989;64:60–70

27. Hyman PE, McDiarmid SV, Napolitano J. Antroduodenal motility in children with chronic intestinal pseudo-obstruction. J Pediatr 1988;65:899–905

28. Stanghellini V, Camilleri M, Malagelada J-R. Chronic idiopathic intestinal pseudo-obstruction: clinical and intestinal manometric findings. Gut 1987;28:5–12

29. Di Lorenzo C, Flores AF, Buie T, Hyman PE. Intestinal motility and jejunal feeding in children with chronic intestinal pseudo-obstruction. Gastroenterology 1995;108:1379–1385

30. Warner E, Jeejeebhoy KN. Successful management of chronic intestinal pseudo-obstruction with home parenteral nutrition. JPEN J Parent Ent Nutr 1985;9:173–178

31. Bagwell GE, Filler RM, Cutz E et al. Neonatal intestinal pseudo-obstruction. J Pediatr Surg 1986;19:732–739

32. Sullivan MA, Snape WJ, Matarazzo SA et al. Gastrointestinal myoelectric activity in idiopathic intestinal pseudo-obstruction. N Engl J Med 1977;297:233–238

33. Lipton AB, Knauer CM. Pseudo-obstruction of the bowel. Therapeutic trial of metoclopramide. Am J Dig Dis 1977;22:263–265

34. Schuffler MD. Chronic intestinal pseudo-obstruction syndromes. Med Clin North Am 1981;65:1331–1358

35. Camilleri M, Brown ML, Malagelda J-R. Impaired transit of chyme in chronic intestinal pseudo-obstruction: correct by cisapride. Gastroenterology 1986;91:619–626

36. Camilleri M, Malagelda J-R, Abell TL. Effect of six weeks of treatment with cisapride in gastroparesis and intestinal pseudo-obstruction. Gastroenterology 1989;96:704–712

37. Krevsky B, Maurer AH, Malmud LS, Fisher RS. Cisapride accelerates colonic transit in constipated patients with colonic inertia [see comments]. Am J Gastroenterol 1989;84(8):882–887

38. Verne GN, Eaker EY, Hardy E, Sninsky CA. Effect of octreotide and erythromycin on idiopathic and scleroderma-associated intestinal pseudo-obstruction. Dig Dis Sci 1995;40(9):1892–1901

39. Keshavarzian A, Isaacs P, McColl I, Sladen GE. Idiopathic intestinal pseudo-obstruction and contaminated small bowel syndrome: treatment with metronidazole, ileostomy, and indomethacin. Am J Gastroenterol 1983;78:562–565

40. Pitt HA, Mann LL, Berquist WE et al. Chronic intestinal pseudo-obstruction: management with total parenteral nutrition and venting enterostomy. Arch Surg 1985;120:614–618

41. Anuras S, Mitros FA, Soper RT et al. Chronic intestinal pseudo-obstruction in young children. Gastroenterology 1986;91:62–70

42. Glassman M, Spivak W, Mininberg D, Madara J. Chronic idiopathic intestinal pseudo-obstruction: a commonly misdiagnosed disease in infants and children. Pediatrics 1989;83:603–608

41

SHORT BOWEL SYNDROME

MICHAEL WILSCHANSKI
RAANAN SHAMIR

Short bowel syndrome (SBS) may be defined as the failure of the gastrointestinal (GI) tract to absorb nutrients in order to sustain normal growth and development. This may be due to an anatomic deficit of surface area due to massive small bowel resection, or it may be a functional abnormality, such as pathologic motility. The region of intestinal loss is as important as the length of bowel resected. Up to one-half of the small intestine may be resected without significant long-term nutritional problems, provided the duodenum, terminal ileum, and functional ileocecal valve (ICV) remain in situ. However, a distal resection, including the ICV, may result in nutritional deficits even though only 25% of the intestine has been lost.

ETIOLOGY

There has been a dramatic change in the etiology of SBS in children over the past 25 years. In earlier series, the major causes were intestinal atresia or midgut volvulus. However, the tremendous advances in neonatal intensive care have resulted in the most common etiology now being necrotizing enterocolitis (NEC). This is caused by a low blood flow state secondary to generalized hypovolemia or sepsis resulting in necrosis of the bowel. In a recent compilation of 238 patients,[1] NEC was responsible for 35% of cases (Table 41-1). Intestinal atresias were the second most common cause. Failure of the embryonic midgut to return to the abdominal cavity results in a foreshortened bowel, a condition known as gastroschisis.

If the gut fails to rotate and fixate to the posterior abdominal wall on return to the abdominal cavity, a midgut volvulus may develop. These two intrauterine catastrophes form two important causes of SBS. It should be noted that volvulus, with the resulting loss of intestine, may occur in older children and may follow the formation of adhesions after intra-abdominal surgery.

SBS may develop when the entire bowel is intact but is nonfunctional. Examples are long segment Hirschsprung's disease and idiopathic intestinal pseudo-obstruction. SBS may result from a combination of anatomic and functional etiologies (e.g., gastroschisis is often associated with dysfunctional peristalsis of the remaining small intestine). Rarer causes of SBS include complicated intussuseption, meconium ileus, vascular anomalies of the superior mesenteric artery, omphalocele, and congenital SBS. Congenital SBS may present as neonatal diarrhea as its only manifestation. The etiology of SBS in children is vastly different from that in adults, in whom mesenteric infarction, Crohn's disease, radiation enteritis, and trauma are the most common causes.

COMPLICATIONS

Diarrhea

The major loss of intestinal surface area and the disordered transit of intestinal contents compromise the major function of the small intestine—the digestion and

TABLE 41-1. Etiology of Pediatric SBS
(n = 238)

Disorder	Percent
Necrotizing enterocolitis	35
Atresias	28
Volvulus	18
Gastroschisis	14
Hirschsprung's disease	7
Other	3

(Adapted from Warner and Ziegler,[1] with permission.)

absorption of nutrients. Extensive jejunal resection causes an osmotic diarrhea, as dissacharidase activity is reduced. Loss of the ileum results in increased intestinal fluid volume and decreased transit time. Loss of the terminal ileum alone also results in diarrhea, as nonabsorbed bile acids irritate the colonic mucosa and produce watery diarrhea. This may result in bile salt depletion, as the liver is unable to compensate for this loss by increasing synthesis, producing steatorrhea. The presence of the ileocecal valve prolongs transit time and increases the duration of contact of the intestinal contents with the absorptive surface. It also serves as a barrier to prevent the reflux and overgrowth of colonic microorganisms in the ileum. Loss of the colon leads to loss of fluid absorption.

When both the ileum and colon are resected, the remaining bowel cannot concentrate the intestinal contents. This results in the jejunostomy syndrome: dehydration, hypokalemia, and hypomagnesemia. It must be noted that, at times, the presence of the colon aggravates the diarrhea. Bile acids reaching the colon not only irritate the mucosa but may stimulate electrolyte and water secretion, causing even more diarrhea. Deficiencies of divalent cations (e.g., Ca^{2+}, Mg^{2+}, Fe^{2+}, and Zn^{2+}) are not uncommon, as they are absorbed throughout the small intestine. Deficiencies of specific vitamins, both water-soluble and fat-soluble, occur (see Ch. 13).

Bacterial Overgrowth

Bacterial overgrowth frequently complicates SBS, especially when the ileocecal valve is absent and the dysmotility or stasis, or both, are present in the remaining bowel loops. This may cause structural and functional changes to the remaining mucosa and brush border. Etiologic organisms include facultative aerobes and anaerobes. This should be suspected when the patient experiences increased diarrhea, abdominal pain, and bloating, or when there is a period of poor weight gain. An interesting complication of bacterial overgrowth is the fermentation of carbohydrate to D-lactate. Patients may present with neurologic symptoms, metabolic acidosis with increased anion gap, and elevated plasma levels of D-lactate but normal levels of L-lactate.

Gastric Hypersecretion

Gastric hypersecretion is common in SBS and appears to be proportional to the length of small intestine resected. This condition may be due to the lack of an intestinal gastrin inhibitory factor. Together with this, the lowering of intraduodenal pH inactivates pancreatic digestive enzymes and stimulates peristalsis.

Gallstones

The incidence of cholelithiasis in SBS is increased due to the interruption of the enterohepatic circulation, resulting in lithogenic bile. Prolonged parenteral nutrition may also be an etiologic factor.

Renal Stones

Insoluble soaps are formed by calcium and malabsorbed fat. This results in the increased absorption of dietary oxalate, as calcium oxalate cannot be formed. Bile salts in the colon may also increase calcium oxalate absorption. Thus, the patient with a functional colon in situ is at increased risk of renal oxalate stones.

INTESTINAL ADAPTATION

Following massive intestinal resection, adaptive changes are detected in the remaining bowel after 48 hours. The compensatory changes include all layers of the bowel wall, leading to dilatation, lengthening, and thickening of the small bowel. Crypt and villous hyperplasia occur, and there is an increase in mucosal mass, as confirmed by greater protein, DNA and RNA content. If the distal bowel is exposed to a greater than normal nutrient load, the result is mucosal hyperplasia. Numerous studies have implicated the direct effects of casein,[2] long-chain tryglycerides (LCTs),[3] free-fatty acids,[4] and carbohydrates[5] on mucosal hyperplasia. Nutrients may act by direct stimulation of hyperplasia through contact with the mucosa, a stimulation of secretion of local gut hormones or through release of secretions that are trophic to the small intestine.

Numerous potential humoral mediators have been postulated. Pancreaticobiliary secretions,[6] enteroglucagon,[7] prostaglandin E_2 (PGE_2),[8] epidermal growth factor,[9] and insulin growth factor-1 (IGF-1)[10] have been shown to augment adaptation. There may be a role for other metabolic substrates for the enterocyte. Glutamine is a nonessential amino acid, the most abundant amino acid in the plasma. It is the major fuel for the small intestinal epithelium. It has been shown to have an effect on small intestinal growth in animal models; in a recent study in humans, its addition to parenteral nutrition prevented deterioration in gut permeability and preserved mucosal structure.[11] Glutamine provided enterally can enhance post-resection adaptation. Short-chain fatty acids, especially butyrate, have been shown to be the preferred substrates for colonocytes and are trophic to both the small intestine and the colon, possibly through the autonomic nervous system.[12] The noncellulose dietary fiber pectin has been shown to be fermented by colonic bacteria and leads to an increase in colonic short-chain fatty acid concentration. Pectin supplementation of an elemental diet in rats that underwent massive intestinal resection was associated with enhancement of colonic adaptation manifested by an increase in colonic water absorption and an increase in colonic crypt depth. This effect may be due to the physical stimulus, causing mucosal hyperplasia or due to the fermentation products of pectin, short-chain fatty acids, the metabolism of which leads to colonic mucosal proliferation.[13] There may also be a role in intestinal adaptation for polyamines.[14]

MEDICAL MANAGEMENT

The tremendous reduction in mortality of SBS in recent years is largely attributed to the development and refinement of nutritional support. Medical management of SBS focuses on three major goals: correction of acute and ongoing deficits and metabolic problems, utilization of maximum nutritional support, and promotion of intestinal adaptation. This management plan is outlined in Table 41-2.

Immediate postoperative management focuses on the replacement of fluid and electrolyte losses using isotonic solutions. Once stabilization is achieved, parenteral nutrition should be started through a central vein. Patients with a high-output proximal fistula require additional minerals in the parenteral nutrition. Intestinal losses should be monitored and carefully replaced. (For further discussion of parenteral nutrition and long-term problems, see Ch. 85.)

TABLE 41-2. Medical Management of SBS

Fluid/electrolytes postsurgery

Total parenteral nutrition by central venous line

Enteral nutrition

Decrease intestinal motility and output

Decrease bile acid–induced diarrhea

Treat gastric hypersecretion

Treat bacterial overgrowth

Enteral nutrition should commence as soon as possible, to aid in the adaptive response of the remaining intestine.[15] Intestinal adaptation will not occur without enteral feeding. The timing depends on the etiology of the SBS. Most patients can be started on some enteral nutrition a few days after surgery, but premature infants with NEC may require 2 to 3 weeks before the enteral route is used. The patient's ability to tolerate enteral feeding depends on the length of the remaining intestine, the presence of ICV, and whether the colon is in continuity with the remaining bowel. However, in every patient, enteral nutrition is mandatory for normal GI development and adaptation. Most centers routinely insert a gastrostomy tube with or without fundoplication at initial surgery for SBS.

Initially, an elemental or defined formula is infused. These formulas appear to be the most effective at stimulating adaptation, are more rapidly absorbed, and cause less diarrhea.[16] Increasing enteral infusion and decreasing parenteral nutrition depends on various clinical parameters, including stool volume, stool pH, and the presence of reducing substances in the stool. There is some debate based on animal experiments as to whether continuous or bolus feedings should be used.[17] With time, the parenteral nutrition is weaned to an intermittent schedule, eventually allowing delivery at night, providing the patient with freedom during the day. Enteral nutrition is increased until the patient's caloric requirements are achieved, or until diarrhea occurs.

The process of weaning off parenteral nutrition may take months, or even years, and the patient may return home still receiving parenteral nutrition. Many centers now have specialized home total parenteral nutrition nursing personnel to train families and follow up on the patient. Another important component in the management of SBS patients is feeding behavior. Young infants must be encouraged to continue to suck and swallow and, if possible, to take at least a small volume of feed by mouth. This can avoid feeding problems and frank food phobia later on. It is still debatable as to the type of formula to use in later management.[18,19] Recent research has lead to a re-evaluation of earlier practice that a high-carbohydrate, low-fat diet was ideal for SBS patients with no functioning colon. If the colon is present and functioning, a high-carbohydrate, high-calorie diet may be recommended. As more food is taken through the enteral route, the physician must follow vitamin and mineral blood levels; oral supplementation is frequently indicated.

Pharmacologic Therapy

Drug therapy for SBS is directed to the complications referred to above. H$_2$-receptor antagonists are used to decrease gastric acid secretion for up to 1 year postresection. In refractory cases, proton pump inhibitors may be used for limited periods. Pharmacologically retarding intestinal transit is another method to improve nutrient contact with the absorptive mucosa. Several antidiarrheal agents, including codeine, diphenoxylate, and loperamide, may be used as long-term therapy. Cholestyramine, an ion-exchange resin, is often used to reduce the effect of malabsorbed bile salts in the colon and to bind dietary oxalate. The disadvantages of cholestyramine include further depletion of the bile salt pool reducing its concentration to possibly a level below the minimal micellar concentration, worsening the diarrhea and steatorrhea. It also may worsen metabolic bone disease.

Octreotide, a somatostatin analogue, decreases gastric, biliary, and pancreatic secretion, as well as slowing gastrojejunal transit, and has been shown to reduce stool volume in secretory diarrhea.[20] However, it is beneficial only to patients who are in negative balance. Administration of octreotide to rats after only a 40% intestinal resection resulted in impaired adaptation of the remaining bowel. This drug should be given by injection; it is costly, but it has been used in adults and children with SBS.[21] However, the long-term effects of this drug are unknown, and there are concerns especially with regard to growth hormone level.

Bacterial overgrowth occurs when motility is slowed, the bowel is dilated, or the ICV is absent. Megaloblastic anemia due to vitamin B_{12} deficiency may occur, fat-soluble vitamins may be low, and hypoproteinemia is not uncommon. The gold standard for diagnosis is aspiration and culture of the small intestinal fluid. Fasting breath hydrogen tests are now used more often and are less invasive. An "early" peak in a lactulose breath test is highly suggestive of overgrowth. This problem can be treated with oral antibiotics. Often, cycling of agents (e.g., a course of metronidazole alternating with septrin, followed by gentamicin) may be useful. In many cases, patients may require continuous treatment. Novel therapies include the manipulation of dietary carbohydrate with restriction of monosaccharides and oligosaccharides.[22] The fungus in Brewer's yeast, Saccharomyces boulardii, has been reported to be useful particularly in patients with D-lactic acidosis.

SURGICAL MANAGEMENT

Additional surgical procedures are often indicated in SBS. These indications include the inability to advance enteral feeding, often in the face of complications associated with parental nutrition (e.g., hepatotoxicity, multiple central venous line infections and limited venous access, bacterial overgrowth unresponsive to therapy, bowel obstruction, and the inability of the remaining intestine to adapt further. Various surgical procedures have been used to address the special anatomic and

TABLE 41-3. Surgical Management of SBS

Procedures to Slow Intestinal Transit	Procedures to Increase Mucosal Surface Area
Intestinal valve construction	Tapering enteroplasty
Reversed intestinal segments	Intestinal lengthening
Colon interposition	Isolated bowel segments
Intestinal pacing	Small bowel transplantation

(Adapted from Warner and Ziegler,[1] with permission.)

pathophysiologic problems of SBS. Detailed descriptions of the various procedures are beyond the scope of this chapter (for excellent recent surgical reviews, see Warner and Ziegler,[1] Collins et al.,[23] and Bianchi[24]). There are two major categories of surgery as listed in Table 41-3. The first category includes ICV formation and the reversal of intestinal segments to slow transit time. More experimental methods in this category have been tried, including interposition of a segment of colon between two limbs of small intestine, and reversed electrical pacing of the distal valve. The second major category is to increase intestinal mucosal surface area. There has been some encouraging work on intestinal patching to stimulate the growth of new mucosa. Peristalsis may be improved by reducing the diameter of the dilated bowel—the "tapering enteroplasty" procedure. Intestinal lengthening pioneered by Bianchi involves transection of the bowel longitudinally, preserving the blood supply to both sides and creating a bowel segment twice the length, and one-half the diameter of the original.

Small Bowel Transplantation

Small bowel transplantation, if successful, eliminates the need for intravenous feeding within a relatively short time. It should be considered in all children with irreversible intestinal failure who are dependent on parenteral nutrition and who have severe liver disease. However, in practice, it is still experimental and is fraught with serious difficulties. There are problems in finding a suitably sized match donor, very heavy postoperative immunosuppression, and difficult and invasive monitoring postoperatively. In addition, infection and lymphoproliferative disease are still too common. The introduction of the new macrolide immunosuppressant drug, tacrolimus (FK 506) has been a major advance. It has produced a far greater graft survival than has been achieved with the conventional immunosuppressive agents (e.g., cyclosporine).[25] Early results are encouraging in some large centers. The largest published experience is from the University of Pittsburgh, which reported a 3-year review of intestinal transplantation. In pediatric patients, the 1-year survival was 75.6%, and graft survival was 68%.[26]

PROGNOSIS

With the advances discussed, the overall prognosis in SBS is now greater than 80%, reaching 94% in infants with up to 40 cm of bowel remaining.[27] The length of only 10 cm is the new low limit for achieving enteral nutrition,[28] and recently a 4-year-old girl left with only 12 cm of jejunum was managed without the use of total parenteral nutrition.[29]

FUTURE

Dietary formulations that improve adaptation and nutrient absorption are an exciting area of reseach. Drugs that delay gastric emptying or small intestinal transit time might improve absorption (e.g., peptide YY antagonists).[30] An oral somastotatin analogue might be helpful to both inhibit exocrine secretions and slow intestinal transit and new combinations of drugs and diet may be effective.[31] Newer imaginative surgical techniques in autologous GI reconstruction and fetal intestinal surgery offer great hope. However, small intestinal transplantation does provide the ultimate savior for the patient with persistent, resistant intestinal failure.

REFERENCES

1. Warner BW, Ziegler MM. Management of the short bowel syndrome in the pediatric population. Pediatr Clin North Am 1993;40:1335–1350

2. Vanderhoof JA, Grandjean CJ, Burkley KT, Antonson DL. Effect of casein versus casein hydrosylate on mucosal adaptation following massive bowel resection in infant rats. J Pediatr Gastroenterol Nutr 1984;3:262–267

3. Jenkins AP, Ghatei MA, Bloom SR, Thompson RPH. Effects of bolus doses of fat on small intestinal structure and on release of gastrin, cholecystokinin, peptide tyrosine-tyrosine, and enteroglucagon. Gut 1992;33:218–223

4. Grey VL, Garofolo C, Greenberg GR, Morin CL. The adaptation of the small intestine after resection in response to fatty acids. Am J Clin Nutr 1984;40:1235–1242

5. Weser E, Tawil T, Fletcher JT. Stimulation of small bowel mucosal growth by gastric infusion of different sugars in rats maintained on total parenteral nutrition. In: Robinson JWL, Dowling RH, Ricken EO, Eds: Mechanisms of Intestinal Adaptation. Falk Symposium No. 30. Lancaster, England: MTP Press, 1982:141–149

6. Weser E, Drummond A, Tawil T. Effect of diverting bile and pancreatic secretions into the ileum on small bowel mucosa in rats fed a liquid formula diet. JPEN 1982;6:39–42

7. Bloom SR. Gut hormones in adaptation. Gut 1987;28(suppl 1):31–35

8. Vanderhoof JA, Grandjean CJ, Baylor JM et al. Morphological and functional effects of 16,16-dimethyl prostaglandin E₂ on mucosal adaptation after massive distal small bowel resection. Gut 1988;29:802–808

9. Ulshen MH, Lynn-Cook LE, Raasch RH. Effects of intraluminal epidermal growth factor on mucosal proliferation in the small intestine of adult rats. Gastroenterology 1986;91:1134–1140

10. Lemmey AB, Ballard FJ, Martin AA et al. Treatment with IGF-1 peptides improves function of the remnant gut following small bowel resection in rats. Growth Factors 1994;10:243–252

11. Van der Hulst RRWJ, Van Kreel BK, Von Meyenfeldt MF et al. Glutamine and the preservation of gut integrity. Lancet 1993;334:1363–1365

12. Frankel WL, Zhang W, Singh A et al. Mediation of the trophic effects of short-chain fatty acids on the rat jejunum and colon. Gastroenterology 1994;106:375–380

13. Roth JA, Franfel WL, Zhang W et al. Pectin improves colonic function in rat short bowel syndrome. J Surg Res 1995;58:240–246

14. Wang JY, McCormack SA, Viar MJ, Johnson LR. Stimulation of proximal small intestinal mucosal growth by luminal polyamines. Am J Physiol 1991;261:G504–511

15. Bernard DKH, Shaw MJ. Principles of nutrition therapy for short bowel syndrome. Nutr Clin Pract 1993;8:153–162

16. Mukau L, Talamini MA, Sitzmann JV. Elemental diet may accelerate recovery from total parenteral nutrition induces gut atrophy. JPEN 1994;18:75–78

17. Shulman RJ, Redel CA, Stathos TH. Bolus versus continuous feedings stimulate small-intestinal growth and development in the newborn pig. J Pediatr Gastrointest Nutr 1994;18:350–354

18. Nordgaard I, Stenbaek Hansen B, Brobech Mortensen P. Colon as a digestive organ in patients with short bowel. Lancet 1994;343:373–376

19. Briet F, Flourie B, Achour L et al. Bacterial adaptation in patients with short bowel and colon in continuity. Gastroenterology 1995;109:1446–1453

20. Couper RTL, Berzen A, Berall G et al. Clinical response to the long acting somatostatin analogue SMS 201–995 in a child with congenital microvillus atrophy. Gut 1989;30:1020–1024

21. Ohlbaum PH, Galperine Ri, Demarquez Jl et al. Use of a long acting somatostatin analogue (SMS 201–995) in controlling a significant ileal output in a five year old child. J Pediatr Gastroenterol Nutr 1987;6:466–470

22. Mayne AJ, Handy DJ, Preece MA et al. Dietary management of D-lactic acidosis in short bowel syndrome. Arch Dis Child 1990;65:229–231

23. Collins JB, Georgeson KE, Vicente Y et al. Short bowel syndrome. Semin Pediatr Surg 1995;1:60–73

24. Bianchi A. Autologous gastrointestinal reconstruction. Semin Pediatr Surg 1995;1:54–59

25. Gruessner RWG, Fryer JP, Fasola C et al. A prospective study of FK506 versus CsA and pig ATG in a porcine model of small bowel transplantation. Transplantation 1995;59:164–171

26. Todo S, Tzakis A, Reyes J et al. Clinical intestinal transplan-

tation 3 year experience. Transplant Proc 1994;26:1407–1408

27. Goulet OJ, Revillon Y, Jan D et al. Neonatal short bowel syndrome. J Pediatr 1991;119:18–23

28. Kurkchubasche AG, Rowe MI, Smith SD. Adaptation in short bowel syndrome; reassessing old limits. J Pediatr Surg 1993;28:1069–1071

29. Surana R, Quinn FMT, Puri P. Short gut syndrome. Intestinal adaptation in a patient with 12 cms of jejunum. J Pediatr Gastroenterol Nutr 1994;19:246–249

30. Nightingale JMD, Kamm MA, van der Sijp JRM et al. Gastrointestinal hormones in short bowel syndrome. Peptide YY is the "colonic brake" to gastric emptying. Gastroenterology 1992;102:A230

31. Byrne TA, Persinger RL, Young LS et al. A new treatment for patients with short bowel syndrome growth hormone, glutamine and a modified diet. Ann Surg 1995;222:243–255

42

SUCRASE-ISOMALTASE DEFICIENCY

WILLIAM R. TREEM

Sucrase-isomaltase (SI) is one of four disaccharidases located on the brush border of the enterocytes that line the small intestine (Table 42-1). Three of the four disaccharidases, including SI, maltase-glucoamylase, and trehalase, are alpha-glucosidases involved in the digestion of sucrose and starch. After hydrolysis of starch by salivary and pancreatic alpha-amylases, the resulting products are glucose, alpha-1–4-linked maltose (two glucose molecules), maltotriose (three glucose molecules), malto-oligosaccharides (more than three glucose molecules), and alpha-limit dextrins (glucose polymers with at least one alpha-1-6-linked bond). In normal individuals, sucrase hydrolyzes the alpha-1–4-linked glucose bonds of maltose and maltotriose and the glucose-fructose linkage of sucrose. Isomaltase cleaves the alpha-1–6-glucose bonds of alpha-limit dextrins, the 1–6 linkage of isomaltose, as well as the 1–4 linkages of maltose. The SI complex also hydrolyzes glucose polymers with up to six glucose residues.[1]

The other brush-border alpha-glucosidase complex, maltase-glucoamylase, overlaps with SI activity by hydrolyzing the alpha-1–4-glucose linkages of maltose, maltotriose, starch, glycogen, and other oligosaccharides from their nonreducing ends with maximal affinity for medium-size polysaccharide chains with 5–10 glucose residues.[2] However, only 20% of maltase activity is accounted for by the maltase-glucoamylase complex and the remaining 80% by the SI enzyme complex. SI activity is distributed along the whole length of the small intestine. The highest activity occurs in the jejunum, with 20% to 30% less activity proximal to the ligament of Treitz and distally in the ileum.[3]

PATHOPHYSIOLOGY

In patients with congenital SI deficiency, malabsorption of dietary sucrose, glucose polymers, and starch in the proximal small intestine gives rise to an osmotic load that simulates peristalsis in the ileum and colon. The osmotic pressure generated inside the lumen of the small intestine by the malabsorbed carbohydrate solute induces the retention of a large volume of intraluminal isotonic fluid with a normal sodium concentration. When the retained carbohydrate, sodium, and fluid enter the colon, the capacity of the colonic bacteria to ferment carbohydrate to short-chain fatty acids and of the colonic enterocyte to absorb fluid, sodium, and the resulting short-chain fatty acids is overwhelmed and diarrhea ensues.

Congenital SI deficiency is not invariably associated with severe diarrhea. Whether sugar or starch malabsorption produces symptoms depends not only on the residual disaccharidase enzymatic activity, but on additional factors such as the quantity of ingested carbohydrate, the rate of gastric emptying, the effect on small bowel transit, the metabolic activity of colonic bacteria, and the absorptive capacity of the colon. For many of these parameters, the infant is at a disadvantage compared to the adult. This undoubtedly contributes to the increased severity of symptoms seen in many infants with congenital SI deficiency. In infants, the length of the small intestine is shorter and the reserve capacity of the colon to absorb excess luminal fluid is reduced compared to that of adults. Some infants may be consuming a high-carbohydrate diet in the form of juices, baby food fruits and vegetables, and cereals. In young infants with carbohydrate

TABLE 42-1. Role of Brush-Border Enzymes in Digestion of Disaccharides and Starch

Enzyme	Bond Cleaved	Substrate	Products
Lactase	β-(1-4) galactosidase (β-glucosidase)	Lactose	Glucose, galactose
Sucrase	α-(1-4)-glucosidase	Sucrose, maltose, maltotriose, α-limit dextrins with terminal α-1-4 links	Glucose, fructose malto-oligosaccharide with α-1–6 linkage
Glucomylase	α-(1-4) glucosidase	Maltose, maltotriosemalto-oligosaccharide (glucose polymers with maximal affinity for chains of 6–10 residues)	Glucose, malto-oligosaccharide with terminal α-1–6 linkage
Isomaltase	α-(1-6) glucosidase	Maltose, isomaltose, α-limit dextrins malto-oligosaccharide with terminal (1–6 links)	Glucose, malto-oligosaccharides
Trehalase	α- and β-glucosidase (tested on renal trehalase)	Trehalose (found principally in mushrooms)	Glucose

(From Treem,[5] with permission.)

malabsorption, small intestinal and colonic transit is likely to be more rapid, allowing less time for alternative paths of carbohydrate digestion, including the salvage of malabsorbed carbohydrate by colonic bacterial fermentation.

As is often the case with genetic-metabolic defects, both genetic heterogeneity and other host variables play a role in the phenotypic differences observed in patients with this disorder. The gene encoding human SI has been localized to the long arm of chromosome 3,[4] and the enzyme is synthesized on the rough endoplasmic reticulum as a long polypeptide chain carrying two similar, but not identical, active sites (pro-sucrase-isomaltase).[5] The polypeptide then undergoes complex glycosylation in the Golgi apparatus and is finally inserted into the enterocyte membrane, with the sucrase catalytic domain protruding farthest out into the lumen. Pro-SI is then rapidly processed by pancreatic trypsin, yielding the two subunits of isomaltase and sucrase associated by noncovalent strong ionic interactions. Although specific genetic mutations have not yet been identified, different molecular defects have been documented in patients with congenital SI deficiency that indicate abnormalities of intracellular processing (glycosylation and folding of the enzyme protein), intracellular transport, and homing and insertion of the enzyme into the brush-border membrane.[6,7]

In most patients with congenital SI deficiency, both sucrase and isomaltase activities are completely absent; however, in some cases, the mature enzyme is found inserted into the brush-border membrane and the mutation only affects the catalytic site of sucrase leaving sucrase activity absent and isomaltase activity reduced by 50% to 90%. In two recent series, 4 of 14 and 3 of 9 patients had residual isomaltase activity measured in small bowel biopsies.[8,9] Immunoelectrophoresis and immunoblotting experiments with biopsied tissue have revealed a single polypeptide with a molecular weight of 145,000 corresponding to residual isomaltase in some patients.

In addition to differences in residual isomaltase activity, another source of phenotypic heterogeneity in patients with congenital SI deficiency is a difference in the enzymatic activity of the other brush-border alpha-glucosidase complex responsible for the digestion of starch and oligosaccharides, maltase-glucoamylase.[10] Recent work has supported the concept that some patients with congenital SI deficiency have a primary deficiency in maltase-glucoamylase as well.[9,11] Polyacrylamide gel electrophoresis (PAGE) and immunoprecipitation experiments have shown that SI-deficient patients have greatly varying amounts of maltase-glycoamylase in their brush border.[9,11,12]

CLINICAL PRESENTATION

Congenital SI deficiency is considered a rare autosomal recessively inherited disease, but it is likely that the prevalence has been underestimated (Table 42-2). Previous studies have attempted to ascertain the number of heterozygote carriers in the general population based on measurements of sucrase enzymatic activity in small intestinal biopsies. Heterozygotes are defined as those with a level of sucrase activity below the lower limit for the normal population, with ratios of intestinal sucrase to lactase activity of less than 0.9, and with normal small bowel morphology. Based on these criteria, the best esti-

TABLE 42-2. Prevalence of Congenital SI Deficiency in Various Populations

Group	%
Greenland Eskimos	2–10
Native Alaskans	3.0
Canadian Native peoples	3.6–7.1
Danes	<0.1
North Americans	<0.2

(From Treem,[5] with permission.)

mate of the prevalence of heterozygotes in the North American and European white populations is approximately 1 in 50 persons.[13] The prevalence appears to be less in the African American population. Based on these data and studies in Europeans with abdominal pain and diarrhea, the incidence of homozygous congenital SI deficiency appears to be approximately 1 in 2,500.[5]

Presenting symptoms in patients with congenital SI deficiency are variable and can be grouped into three major categories (Table 42-3). The classic presentation is chronic watery diarrhea with a low pH in the infant, severe diaper dermatitis, and failure to thrive. Initiation of these symptoms depends in part on the introduction of sucrose into the diet. Breast-fed babies or infants consuming lactose-containing formulas will not manifest symptoms until they ingest juices, solid foods, or medications sweetened with sucrose. Baby cereals usually cause less severe symptoms because of the compensatory mechanisms for starch digestion. Other nonspecific findings in infants include abdominal distention, gassiness, colic, irritability, and at times, vomiting.[14]

Some severely affected patients require hospitalization for diarrhea and dehydration, malnutrition, muscle wasting, and weakness.[15] Often, the correct diagnosis is delayed, while other causes of severe chronic diarrhea are

TABLE 42-3. Presenting Symptoms in 23 Patients with Congenital SI Deficiency

Symptoms	Frequency	Mean Age at Diagnosis (yr)
Chronic diarrhea and failure to thrive	7/23	2.0 ± 1.1
Chronic diarrhea with normal growth	9/23	5.6 ± 3.5
Irritable bowel syndrome, abdominal pain	7/23	15.4 ± 7.3

(From Treem,[5] with permission.)

entertained. These infants may be presumed to have cow's milk or soy protein allergy and often are subject to multiple formula changes. In an effort to avoid cow's milk or soy protein, these infants are often given a protein-hydrolysate formula with carbohydrate in the form of glucose polymers. Many specialized formulas use glucose polymers in place of lactose because lactose intolerance is a relatively frequent problem, occurring as a secondary phenomenon in association with a variety of intestinal disorders. Although some infants with congenital SI deficiency will improve while taking these formulas, often the glucose polymers are poorly digested due to low levels of SI and reduced maltase-glucoamylase activity.[16] Carbohydrate nutritional supplements routinely given to infants (including prematures) in order to increase the caloric density of formulas are often composed of glucose polymers and can precipitate worsening diarrhea in affected patients. Mild steatorrhea due to rapid intestinal transit and chronic malnutrition with partial villous atrophy has been documented in some patients with congenital SI deficiency and may suggest cystic fibrosis or celiac disease. Transient hypoglycemia, acidosis, dehydration, and lethargy may lead to consideration of inborn errors of metabolism.

Children with less severe phenotypes of congenital SI deficiency may present later with chronic symptoms of intermittent diarrhea, bloating, and abdominal cramps. They attain normal growth and, as toddlers, may be considered to have chronic, nonspecific diarrhea of childhood.[5] The institution of a diet for this condition, including the avoidance of fruit juices, soft drinks, and fructose and sorbitol-containing beverages and fruits, may actually ameliorate symptoms by simultaneously reducing the sucrose load in the diet.[17] Dietary habits may mask symptoms and also delay the diagnosis of congenital SI deficiency. Of 20 Greenland Eskimos diagnosed in a study published in 1972, 7 were adults who denied having any gastrointestinal symptoms, presumably as a result of their habitually low-sucrose diet.[18]

Congenital SI deficiency has also been diagnosed in adult patients in industrialized countries.[19–21] These patients often give a history of feeding difficulties during infancy and intermittent symptoms since childhood. The symptoms that persist in adult life may be limited to some increase in bowel frequency and to abdominal distension and flatulence, especially at the end of the day. Episodic watery diarrhea is associated with a large sucrose intake. Many of these patients have been labeled with a diagnosis of irritable bowel syndrome.[22] Some investigators have noted a tendency for spontaneous improvement of symptoms with age. Possible explanations for this observation include self-regulation of the diet to limit sucrose ingestion and an adaptive increase in colonic salvage of carbohydrate through the stimulatory effects of chronic carbohydrate malabsorption on the fermentative activity of colonic flora.

DIAGNOSIS AND LABORATORY FINDINGS

An excess of reducing substances (>0.5%) may be demonstrated in liquid stool from a patient with congenital SI deficiency provided the fecal sucrose is hydrolyzed by boiling with 0.1 N hydrochloric acid. The pH of the stools in a patient with congenital SI deficiency classically should fall between 5.0 and 6.0. Both tests have a high degree of false-negative results.[23]

The sucrose breath hydrogen test has been extensively validated in children with sucrose malabsorption and normal controls,[24] and has become the main screening test for the diagnosis of congenital SI deficiency. This test is based on the principle that an oral sucrose load should be completely digested and absorbed in the small intestine in a normal person. In a patient with congenital SI deficiency, the ingested sucrose will not be hydrolyzed to glucose and fructose, and intact sucrose will arrive in the colon, where colonic bacteria will ferment the malabsorbed carbohydrate. The by-products of this fermentation process will be gases such as hydrogen and carbon dioxide and short-chain fatty acids, predominantly acetate, propionate, and butyrate. Excess colonic hydrogen will be absorbed, filtered in the lung and exhaled in the breath. Two previous studies of children with congenital SI deficiency have shown an elevation of greater than 20 parts per million (ppm) of breath hydrogen over baseline at 90 to 180 minutes after the ingestion of approximately 2 g/kg of oral sucrose.[24,25]

False-negative results have been reported with this test in patients who are nonhydrogen producers. The prevalence of an inability to produce colonic hydrogen in response to malabsorbed carbohydrate is probably less than 10% of the general population.[26] Another potential confounding variable is the acid milieu that may exist in the colon of patients with chronic sucrose and starch malabsorption due to the continued high level of bacterial fermentation and production of short-chain fatty acids and lactate. A chronically low intracolonic pH has been shown to inhibit colonic hydrogen production and the expected rise in breath hydrogen excretion after carbohydrate malabsorption.[27] These potential pitfalls suggest that care must be taken in the interpretation of sucrose breath hydrogen tests in patients with potential congenital SI deficiency. It is important to monitor the symptoms and stool pattern of these patients for 24 hours after the breath test. Patients who experience significant diarrhea and other symptoms in spite of seemingly negative sucrose breath hydrogen tests should be screened by other methods, including following their stool pH measurements.[28]

Measurement of intestinal disaccharidases from small bowel biopsy material has remained the gold standard for the diagnosis of congenital SI deficiency. A small bowel biopsy obtained either with a capsule placed in the proximal jejunum or with the endoscope in the second or third portion of the duodenum provides material not only for enzymatic activity determination but for histologic determinations as well. At least two biopsy specimens taken via a standard upper endoscope and three biopsy specimens taken with a pediatric upper endoscope should be obtained for disaccharidase determinations. The mucosa is usually normal histologically, but some patients with severe malnutrition may show mild partial villous atrophy.

SI deficiency is defined as the reduction of enzymatic activity to levels lower than at least two standard deviations (2 SD) below the mean for biopsy specimens from normal patients with normal small bowel histology. Most patients with congenital SI deficiency will have completely absent sucrase activity and isomaltase (palatinase) activity reduced to 10% of normal or less.[8] Maltase activity will also be markedly reduced to approximately 60% to 90% of normal. Lactase and bowel alkaline phosphatase activity should be normal.

Combining the actual measured values of sucrase, isomaltase, maltase, and lactase with a lactase to sucrase ratio can increase the diagnostic accuracy of this test for congenital SI deficiency. Provided the patient does not have primary lactase deficiency or secondary disaccharidase deficiency from partial or total villous atrophy, the normal sucrase to lactase ratio in adults is approximately 2.0 and 1.5 in children less than 3 years of age.[29,30] However, the ratio should never be less than 1.0 unless there is isolated decreased SI activity; it should actually increase in primary lactase deficiency or diffuse small bowel injury and secondary disaccharidase deficiency, where lactase levels are usually more severely depressed than SI activity.

TREATMENT

Adherence to a strict sucrose-free low-starch diet usually abolishes the symptoms of congenital SI deficiency; however, only a small percentage of patients adhere to this diet throughout their lives. The starch content of the diet must be reduced with special attention to foods having a high amylopectin content (alpha-1-6 bonds), such as wheat and potatoes. A recent report emphasizes that even formulas containing glucose polymers may cause symptoms because of the reliance on the SI complex for their digestion.[16] Dietary recommendations are illustrated in Table 42-4.

Compliance with this diet is difficult, and there appears to be a high incidence of chronic GI complaints, decreased weight for height, and decreased weight for age in patients with congenital SI deficiency followed after diagnosis.[14,15,31] Until recently, no reliable enzyme

TABLE 42-4. Sucrose-Free, Low-Starch Diet for Children With Congenital SI Deficiency

Food Group	Foods Allowed	Foods Excluded
Fruits (only 2 servings/day)	Blackberries, blueberries, cranberries, loganberries, currants, grapes, strawberries, raspberries, boysenberries, cherries, kadota figs, Damson plums, Bartlett pears	All others
Fruit juice (1/2 cup/day)	Juice from allowed fruits	All others
Vegetables	Asparagus, broccoli, Brussels sprouts, cauliflower, mushrooms, spinach, chard, collards, celery, radish, kale, kohlrabi pepper, okra, lettuce, water cress tomato, parsley, white potato	All others
Breads Cereals Grains	White rice, unsweetened puffed rice, cornflour, rice flour, and rice cakes	All others
Milk Milk products Cheese	Whole low-fat skim milk, plain yogurt, sugar-free yogurt, natural cheese, cottage cheese	Chocolate milk, milkshakes, sweetened milk, yogurt with fruit, ice cream, sherbet, ice milk, processed cheese
Meat Egg Protein	Beef, pork, veal, lamb, fish, chicken, turkey, shellfish, eggs	Breaded meats, cold cuts, cured meat, dried beans, dried peas, lentils, peanut butter
Fat	Butter, margarine, oil, sour cream, cream cheese, homemade salad dressing	Mayonnaise, commercial salad dressing, tarter sauce
Miscellaneous	Broth, bouillon, sugar-free Jell-O, sugar-free custard, homemade rice pudding, fructose, herbs and spices, soy sauce, vinegar, lemon, lime, salt, pepper	Canned soup, custard, pudding, cookies, cakes, pies, doughnuts, steak sauce, taco sauce, catsup, Tabasco sauce, barbecue sauce, sugar, brown sugar, molasses, jelly, jam, preserves, honey, pancake syrup, chewing gum, sugar breath mints, cough syrup

substitution therapy was available for children with congenital SI deficiency. It has long been known that invertase, a beta-fructofuranosidase with sucrose-splitting properties but no effect on malto-oligosaccharides, is an important exoenzyme in most cultivated and wild yeasts.[32] Recently, investigators capitalized on this by administering a small amount of lyophilized baker's yeast (*Saccharomyces cerevisiae*) to children with congenital SI deficiency and demonstrating a reduction in symptoms of diarrhea, cramps, or gas after an oral sucrose load.[33] However, baker's yeast is not palatable in this form and is poorly accepted, especially by young children.

This yeast-derived enzyme has recently been extensively studied both in the laboratory[34,35] and in clinical trials in patients with congenital SI deficiency.[8] As a by-product of the manufacture of belt-dried baker's yeast, a concentrated relatively odorless, tasteless, liquid preparation of invertase has been derived that has extremely potent sucrose-hydrolyzing activity and is stable with freezing, thawing, refrigeration, and even standing at room temperature. It is resistant to low pH but can be degraded by proteolytic enzymes such as pepsin in the intragastric environment.

Recently published and ongoing studies with this liquid yeast-derived enzyme preparation have shown that patients with congenital SI deficiency can tolerate a sucrose load without a marked rise in breath hydrogen or the occurrence of GI symptoms, if given in conjunction with the yeast invertase[8] (Fig. 42-1). Many of these patients can then go on to consume a more normal sucrose-containing diet with mealtime enzyme supplementation without engendering symptoms of abdominal pain, diarrhea, distention, or gas. Further studies are ongoing to determine the optimal dose and method of administration of this enzyme replacement therapy. Secondary SI deficiency caused by celiac disease, severe viral or parasitic GI infections, acquired immunodeficiency syndrome (AIDS), or the short bowel syndrome may also be amenable to treatment with liquid yeast invertase.

REFERRAL PATTERN

Infants with chronic diarrhea and failure to thrive present a challenging differential diagnosis. Historic information that links the onset of diarrhea with the introduc-

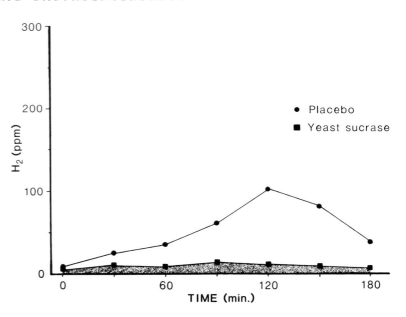

FIGURE 42-1 Two breath hydrogen (H₂) test results in a patient with congenital SI deficiency given a 2-g/kg sucrose load with yeast-derived concentrated liquid invertase (sucrase) (squares) versus a water placebo (circles). In the placebo test, there is a dramatic use in breath H₂ over the course of 180 minutes after the oral sucrose load, implying small bowel malabsorption of sucrose and colonic bacterial fermentation of malabsorbed sucrose to hydrogen, CO₂, and short-chain fatty acids. In the test accompanied by the ingestion of yeast invertase, there is no such rise in the breath H₂ excretion suggesting complete hydrolysis and absorption of sucrose.

tion of sucrose into the diet either in formulas, or in the form of juice or fruit, is a very important clue to the diagnosis. Specialized formulas containing glucose polymers (polycose, corn syrup solids) may also precipitate worsening diarrhea in these patients. The diagnosis of congenital SI deficiency should be considered in toddlers with chronic nonspecific diarrhea but normal growth, if they do not have evidence of a chronic enteric infection, are not lactose intolerant, have no blood in their stools, and have no other symptoms or laboratory findings that suggest protein-induced allergic gastroenteropathy. A trial of dietary therapy of chronic nonspecific diarrhea is warranted in those children with reduced total fluid intake; avoidance of sorbitol, fructose, and high-carbohydrate containing juices; an increased fat content in the diet; reduced carbohydrate-derived calories; and increased fiber intake.[17] However, if there is no response to this dietary intervention, the diagnosis of congenital SI deficiency should be entertained. Older children and adolescents with irritable bowel syndrome may also be candidates for screening for congenital SI deficiency under several conditions (1) their history dates back to an early age, (2) they have diarrhea-predominant irritable bowel syndrome, and (3) they are resistant to the usual dietary interventions for irritable bowel syndrome or the antispasmodic antimotility pharmacologic agents that are sometimes used.

These groups of patients should be referred to a pediatric gastroenterologist and screened with a sucrose breath hydrogen study. A positive test or even a "negative" study, followed by symptoms that suggest malabsorption of the sucrose load should prompt consideration of an upper GI endoscopy and small bowel biopsy with the examination of small bowel histology and the measurement of brush-border disaccharidases.

REFERENCES

1. Gray GM, Lally BC, Conklin KA. Action of intestinal sucrase-isomaltase and its free monomers on an alpha-limit dextrin. J Biol Chem 1979;254:6038–6043

2. Kelly JJ, Alpers DH. Properties of human intestinal glucoamylase. Biochim Biophys Acta 1973;315:113–120

3. Skovbjerg H. Immunoelectrophoretic studies on human small intestinal brush border proteins: the longitudinal distribution of peptidases and disaccharidases. Clin Chim Acta 1981;112:205–212

4. Green F, Edwards Y, Hauri HP, et al. Isolation of a cDNA probe for a human jejunal brush-border hydrolase, sucrase-isomaltase, and assignment of the gene locus to chromosome 3. Gene 1987;57:101–110

5. Treem WR. Congenital sucrase-isomaltose deficiency. J Pediatr Gastroenterol Nutr 1995;21:1–14

6. Sterchi EE, Lentze MJ, Naim HY. Molecular aspects of disaccharidase deficiencies. Bailleres Clin Gastroenterol 1990;4:79–96

7. Fransen JAM, Hauri HP, Ginsel LA, Naim HY. Naturally occurring mutations in intestinal sucrase-isomaltase provide evidence for existence of an intracellular sorting signal in the isomaltase subunit. J Cell Biol 1991;115:45–57

8. Treem WR, Ahsan N, Sullivan B et al. Evaluation of liquid yeast-derived sucrase enzyme replacement in patients with sucrase-isomaltase deficiency. Gastroenterology 1993;105:1061–1068

9. Skovbjerg H, Krasilnikoff PA. Maltase-glucoamylase and residual isomaltase in sucrose intolerant patients. J Pediatr Gastroenterol Nutr 1986;5:365–371

10. Treem WR. Clinical heterogeneity in congenital sucrase-isomaltase deficiency. J Pediatr 1996;128:727–729

11. Lebenthal E, Maung-U K, Zheng BY et al. Small intestinal glucoamylase deficiency and starch malabsorption: a newly recognized α-glucosidase deficiency in children. J Pediatr 1994;124:541–546

12. Hadorn B, Green JR, Sterchi EE et al. Biochemical mechanisms in congenital enzyme deficiencies of small intestine. Clin Gastroenterol 1981;10:671–690

13. Welsh JD, Poley JS, Bhatia M, Stevenson DE. Intestinal disaccharidase activities in relation to age, race and mucosal damage. Gastroenterology 1978;75:847–855

14. Antonowicz I, Lloyd-Still MB, Skaw KT, Shwachman H. Congenital sucrase-isomaltase deficiency. Pediatrics 1972; 49:847–853

15. Gudmand-Hoyer E. Sucrose malabsorption in children: a report of thirty-one Greenlanders. J Pediatr Gastroenterol Nutr 1985;4:873–877

16. Newton T, Murphy MS, Booth IW. Glucose polymer as a cause of protracted diarrhea in infants with unsuspected congenital sucrase-isomaltase deficiency. J Pediatr 1996;128: 753–756

17. Treem WR. Chronic non-specific diarrhea of childhood. Clin Pediatr 1992;31:413–420

18. McNair A, Gudmand-Hoyer E, Jarnum S, Orrild L. Sucrase malabsorption in Greenland. BMJ 1972;2:19–21

19. Ringrose R, Preiser H, Welsh JD. Sucrase-isomaltase (palatinase) deficiency diagnosed during adulthood. Dig Dis Sci 1980;25:384–387

20. Cooper BT, Scott J, Hopkins J, Peters TJ. Adult onset sucrase-isomaltase deficiency with secondary disaccharidase deficiency resulting from severe dietary carbohydrate restriction. Dig Dis Sci 1983;28:473–477

21. Sontag WB, Brill ML, Troyer WC et al. Sucrose-isomaltose malabsorption in an adult woman. Gastroenterology 1964; 47:18–25

22. Rosovsky A, Zheng B, Mehta D et al. Alpha-glucosidase deficiencies as a possible cause of irritable bowel syndrome (IBS), abstract. Gastroenterology 1994;104:A278

23. Soeparto P, Stobo EA, Walker-Smith JA. Role of chemical examination of the stool in diagnosis or sugar malabsorption in children. Arch Dis Child 1972;47:56–61

24. Perman JA, Barr RG, Watkins JB. Sucrose malabsorption in children: non-invasive diagnosis by interval breath hydrogen determination. J Pediatr 1978;93:17–22

25. Ford RPK, Barners GL. Breath hydrogen test and sucrase-isomaltase deficiency. Arch Dis Child 1983;58:595–597

26. Strocchi A, Corazza G, Ellis CJ et al. Detection of malabsorption of low doses of carbohydrate: accuracy of various breath H$_2$ criteria. Gastroenterology 1993;105:1404–1410

27. Perman JA, Modler S, Olsen AC. Role of pH in production of hydrogen from carbohydrates by colonic bacterial flora. J Clin Invest 1981;67:643–650

28. Moore D, Lichtman S, Durie P, Sherman P. Primary sucrase-isomaltase deficiency: importance of clinical judgment. Lancet 1985;2:164–165

29. Smith JA, Mayberry JF, Ansell ID, Long RG. Small bowel biopsy for disaccharidase levels: evidence that endoscopic forceps biopsy can replace the Crosby capsule. Clin Chim Acta 1989;183:317–322

30. Heitlinger LA, Rossi TM, Lee PC, Lebenthal E. Human intestinal disaccharidase concentrations: correlations with age, biopsy technique, and degree of villous atrophy. J Pediatr Gastroenterol Nutr 1991;12:204–208

31. Kilby A, Burgess EA, Wigglesworth S, Walker-Smith JA. Sucrase-isomaltase deficiency: a follow-up report. Arch Dis Child 1978;53:677–679

32. Rose AH, Harrison JS, Eds. The Yeasts. Vol 2: Physiology and Biochemistry of Yeast. San Diego: Academic Press, 1971

33. Harms H-K, Bertele-Harms R-M, Bruer-Kleis D. Enzyme-substitution therapy with the yeast Saccharomyces cerevisiae in congenital sucrase-isomaltase deficiency. N Engl J Med 1987;316:1306–1309

34. Trimble RB, Maley F. Subunit structure of external invertase from Saccharomyces cerevisiae. J Biol Chem 1977;252: 4409–4412

35. Chu FK, Takesek, Guarino D, Maley F. Diverse properties of external and internal forms of yeast invertase derived from the same gene. Biochemistry 1985;24:6126–6132

43

UNCOMMON INTESTINAL DISEASES

BACTERIAL OVERGROWTH OF THE INTESTINE

WILLIAM J. WENNER

Bacterial overgrowth of the small bowel is a condition in which the bacterial population of the upper intestine (duodenum, jejunum) contains large numbers of bacteria that typically reside only in the colon (coliforms, anaerobic bacteria). The presence of large numbers of bacteria in the small bowel is abnormal and usually results from an underlying intestinal disorder that has altered intestinal motility or anatomy, predisposing to bacterial overgrowth.

PATHOPHYSIOLOGY

While the human infant is born with a sterile gastrointestinal (GI) tract, the human bowel does not remain a sterile organ. Organisms from the birth canal, from the mother, and from other caretakers quickly colonize the infant's bowel. Within 48 hours of birth, fecal flora inhabit the colon in concentrations of 10^8 per ml.[1] For the remainder of life, only the stomach remains relatively sterile. The proximal small intestine contains less than 10^5 organisms per milliliter, while the distal small intestine has greater than 10^8 per milliliter and the colon greater than 10^{10} organisms per milliliter. Duodenal organisms are predominately aerobic and oral, while ileal organisms are mixed aerobic and anaerobic. Colonic organisms are anaerobic or facultative anaerobic.[2]

Certain anatomic and physiologic factors prevent the bacteria from interfering with GI function. These factors include peristalsis, an intact ileocecal valve, gastric acid, pancreatic enzymes, bile acids, immunoglobulin A (IgA), IgG, T cells, and macrophages. Disruptions of these protective factors allow the resident organisms to proliferate without restriction and create an environment that is pathologic to the child.

Bacterial overgrowth has specific effects on the mucosa and in the lumen that cause the disease process. Direct enterocyte damage results in protein loss, bleeding and loss of disaccharidases with resultant diarrhea. Direct binding of intrinsic factor can cause a B_{12} malabsorption. Certain bacteria such as *Escherichia coli* and *Bacteroides* produce B vitamins, vitamin K, and folic acid and may result in high serum levels.[3] Bile salt deconjugation and loss, small chain fatty acid fermentation and lipid malabsorption are specific causes of the symptoms of bacterial overgrowth.

ETIOLOGY

Anatomic predisposing factors include diverticula, duplication cysts, fistulas, intestinal stenosis, strictures, webs, or the absence of the ileocecal valve. A surgically constructed blind loop predisposes to overgrowth and provides a common name for this syndrome: blind loop syndrome. Physiologic disruptions include absence of the migratory motor complex (MMC), achlorhydria, autonomic neuropathy (especially diabetes induced), collagen vascular disorders, and pseudo-obstruction. Disruptions of the immune system such as acquired immunodeficiency syndrome (AIDS) or any immunodeficiency, malnutrition, and prematurity can predispose a child to bacterial overgrowth.

CLINICAL PRESENTATION

The classic symptoms of bacterial overgrowth are anemia, diarrhea, and steatorrhea. Classic symptoms have been observed in one of three adults diagnosed with bacterial overgrowth[4]; however, these symptoms probably occur less often in the pediatric population. Also associated are abdominal pain, arthritis, ataxia, edema, erythema nodosa, hepatitis, hepatic steatosis, nephritis, night blindness, Raynaud's phenomenon, elevated serum folic acid levels and weight loss. Any unexplained diarrhea with a predisposing history should be evaluated for bacterial overgrowth.

DIAGNOSIS

A complete history and physical examination may indicate the etiology of the symptoms. Particular attention should be directed to previous surgery, and signs or symptoms of diabetes. In the pediatric population, short bowel syndrome (SBS) is the most common historic element.

Screening tests such as fecal fat, Schilling's test with intrinsic factor, folic acid level, or upper gastrointestinal radiological examination with a small bowel follow through (UGI/SBFT) may suggest bacterial overgrowth. However, definitive tests are required for the diagnosis. The standard for diagnosis is a quantitative duodenal aspirate (fluid culture), usually obtained by upper endoscopy. A finding of greater than 10^6 organisms per milliliter is diagnostic. However, bacterial overgrowth may occur in segments of the intestine in which culture is not possible, such as a surgically created loop. Other diagnostic tests include breath tests (lactose, lactulose, D-glucose, [14]Cholylglycine or ^{14}C-d-xylose) and detection of bacterial metabolites in the urine (quantitation of deconjugated intraluminal bile salts and short-chain fatty acids). Interpretation of these tests can be influenced by many clinical factors and the tests should be conducted and interpreted by experienced personnel.

TREATMENT

Unless the underlying disorder can be corrected (revision of a blind surgical loop), oral antibiotics are the primary pharmacologic therapy for bacterial overgrowth. Some investigators believe that culture directed therapy is important for success.[5] Others believe that cultures are not helpful in directing therapy.[6] Improvement has been documented with metronidazole, kanamycin, neomycin, tetracycline, trimethoprim, and lincomycin. Evidence shows that in certain situations metronidazole may be superior to kanamycin.[7] Effectiveness against bacteroides is crucial to successful treatment.[8] Initial therapy should be for 2 to 4 weeks. If a relapse occurs, the second course should be for 4 to 8 weeks. Continued relapse may require continuous antibiotics. Resistance has been documented on kanamycin and neomycin.

Correction of the causative factors is helpful but is not always possible. Nutritional status should be optimized, using parenteral nutrition if necessary. Elemental formulas with medium-chain triglycerides (MCT), short-chain amino acids and monosaccharides are often helpful. Anemia and vitamin deficiencies should be addressed. Anemia, though rare in children, may not be noticeable prior to iron replacement. Pernicious anemia will not correct until the anaerobes are eradicated from the small bowel as they are such effective competitors for bound and unbound B_{12}. A case of pellagra was reported following treatment of bacterial overgrowth due to the elimination of nicotinamide-producing bacterial.[9] Fat-soluble vitamin supplementation may be required in patients with steatorrhea.

REFERRAL PATTERN

Diagnostic tests for bacterial overgrowth are generally available only at tertiary care centers staffed by gastroenterologists. Experience in the interpretation of breath tests is crucial in obtaining the correct diagnosis.

REFERENCES

1. Long SS, Swenson RM. Development of anaerobic fecal flora in healthy newborn infants. J Pediatr 1977;91:298–301

2. Drasar BS, Shiner M, McLeod GM. Studies on intestinal flora. I. The bacterial flora of the gastrointestinal tract in healthy and achlorhydric persons. Gastroenterology 1969;56:71–79

3. Hoffbrand AV, Tabaqchali S, Booth CC. Small intestinal bacterial flora and folate status in gastrointestinal disease. Gut 1971;12:27–33

4. King CD, Toskes PP. Small intestinal overgrowth. Gastroenterology 1979; 76:1035–1055

5. Goldstein F, Mandle RJ, Schaedler RW. The blind loop syndrome and its variants. Am J Gastroenterol 1973;60:255–264

6. Isaacs PET, Kim YS. Blind loop syndrome and small bowel bacterial contamination. Clin Gastroenterol 1983;12:395–414

7. Barry RE, Chow AW, Billesdon J. Role of intestinal microflora in colonic pseudo-obstruction complicating jejunoileal bypass. Gut 1977;18:356–359

8. Forstner G, Sherman P, Lichtman S. Bacterial overgrowth. In Walker WA, Durie PR, Hamilton JR, Walker-Smith JA, Watkins JB, Eds. Pediatric Gastrointestinal Disease. Philadelphia: BC Decker, 1991:697

9. Tabaqchali S, Pallis C. Reversible nicotinamide deficiency encephalopathy in a patient with jejunal diverticulosis. Gut 1970;11:1024–1028

BEZOARS

DONNA ZEITER

Bezoars are collections of swallowed foreign material that form in the GI tract. Most of these masses develop in the upper gastrointestinal tract, primarily the stomach. However, colonic bezoars have been reported in the literature.[1] Bezoars are classified by the material of which they are formed. The most frequently encountered include 1) lactobezoars (concretions of casein, fat, and calcium); (2) phytobezoars (formed from indigestible fruit and vegetable matter); and (3) trichobezoars (composed of the patient's own hair).

Medications may also cause bezoar formation. The most commonly implicated drugs include antacids, psyllium, sucralfate, cimetidine, nefedipine, and vitamins.[2] Other material reported to have formed bezoars includes foreign bodies, bubble gum, and Gummi Bears.[3]

CLINICAL PRESENTATION

The peak age of onset is 10 to 19 years, and approximately 90% of reported patients are women. The presentation of a bezoar is highly variable. Many bezoars are completely asymptomatic. Abdominal pain is the most common presenting symptom; however, other associated symptoms may include weight loss, anorexia, vomiting, constipation, diarrhea, melena, guaiac-positive stools, or perforation.[2,4] Physical examination may show the presence of abdominal distension, crepitus, or peritoneal signs. A palpable left upper quadrant abdominal mass is often detected with trichobezoars. An abdominal mass is palpable in less than one-half of patients with phytobezoars.[2,4]

Each type of bezoar has a unique presentation and usually occurs in a specific patient population. In patients with developmental delay who develop emesis and feeding intolerance, a trichobezoar or foreign body must be considered. Lactobezoars occur most commonly in premature, low-birth-weight infants. There are also reports of lactobezoar formation in full-term infants and in in-fants who are exclusively breast fed. Factors that have been found to contribute to lactobezoar formation include formulas with a high casein content, early and rapid feeding advancement in small infants, high-caloric density formulas, formulas with high calcium/phosphate content, continuous tube feedings, and altered gastric motility in low-birth-weight infants (Fig. 43–1).[2] Often, these infants develop difficulty with feeding intolerance with prolonged gastric residuals.

Phytobezoars occur most commonly in the adult population. Their formation tends to be associated with gastric dysmotility, poor gastric emptying (either primary or following gastric surgery), and hypochlorhydria. They are composed primarily of cellulose, hemicellulose, lignins, and tannins.[2,4] Trichobezoars are associated with trichotillomania and trichophagia (Fig. 43–2). These bezoars may become large and form a cast of the stomach. Occasionally, the bezoar may extend through the pylorus into the small bowel. This "tail" may obstruct the papilla of Vater, leading to jaundice and pancreatitis. Steatorrhea and protein-losing enteropathy have also been reported in these patients.[4]

DIAGNOSIS

Bezoars are often detected on plain abdominal radiography of the abdomen. Upper GI studies may also be helpful in outlining the mass. For the rare colonic bezoar, Hypaque enemas may help to define the obstruction more fully and to evaluate for the presence of perforation.[1] Endoscopy usually provides both the diagnosis of the specific type of bezoar and the method of treatment. Some bezoars may be manipulated into small fragments; these fragments can then be allowed to pass through the GI system or removed endoscopically.[4] Screening blood testing may document laboratory features of iron deficiency anemia and hypoproteinemia. Steatorrhea may also be documented on stool screening with Sudan stains and 72-hour fecal fat collections.

FIGURE 43-1. Upper gastrointestinal contrast study showing a lactobezoar (arrows).

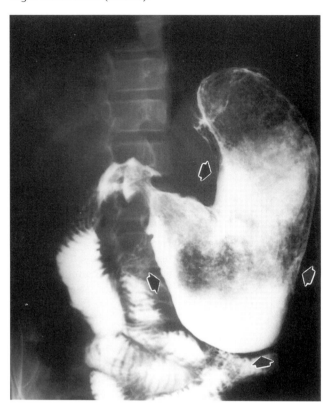

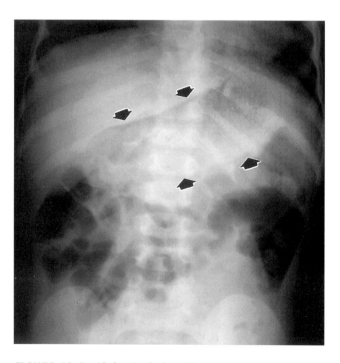

FIGURE 43-2. Abdominal plain film demonstrating an air-filled cast of the stomach (arrows) caused by a trichobezoar.

MANAGEMENT

Unless perforation has occurred, the treatment of a bezoar is linked to the type of material of which it is composed.

Lactobezoars

Lactobezoars almost always resolve spontaneously if feedings are withheld for approximately 2 days while the infant is maintained on intravenous fluids. Recurrence of a lactobezoar is rare.[2,4]

Phytobezoars

The treatment options for phytobezoars are more diverse and include institution of a low-fiber diet, the use of prokinetic agents to stimulate gastric motility, gastric lavage, enzyme therapy to help dissolve the material, endoscopic fragmentation or extraction, and surgical extraction. Case reports have documented some success at dissolving phytobezoars using acetylcysteine, papain, or meat tenderizers; however, complications of these therapies have included gastric ulceration and hypernatremia secondary to the high sodium content of the meat tenderizers. Cellulase was first used in 1968; the 19 reported cases in the literature document 100% efficacy. However, the enzyme formulation and trials were not controlled. This enzyme is currently very difficult to obtain in the United States.[5] We do not currently recommend the use of enzyme therapy. If diet alteration, prokinetic agents, and lavage fail to dissolve the mass, or if there is a question of malignancy, the patient should be promptly referred to a subspecialist for enzyme, endoscopic, or surgical therapy.

Trichobezoars

Trichobezoars are normally very large and pose a difficult management problem as hair is not dissolvable. Endoscopic fragmentation should not be performed, not only because endoscopic removal is nearly impossible but also because there is a risk of forming secondary small bowel lesions. Surgical removal is recommended.[4]

REFERRAL PATTERN

Except for a small lactobezoar, any child who is diagnosed with a bezoar should be referred to a pediatric gastroenterologist.

REFERENCES

1. Larson J, Vender R, Camuto P et al. Phytobezoar of pure vegetable matter causing colonic obstruction. J Clin Gastroenterol 1995;20:176–177

2. Byrne W. Foreign bodies and bezoars. In: Wyllie R, Hyams J, Eds. Pediatric gastrointestinal disease: Pathophysiology Diagnosis and Management Philadelphia: WB Saunders 1993: 174–175

3. Barron M, Steerman P. Gummi-bear bezoar: a case report. J Emerg Med 1989;7:143–144

4. Dodge J. Trauma and foreign substances. In: Walker W, Durie P, Hamilton J, Walker-Smith J, Watkins J, Eds. Pediatric Gastrointestinal Disease: Pathophysiology Diagnosis and Management. 2nd Ed. St. Louis, MO: Mosby-Yearbook, 1996: 529–531

5. Walker-Renard P. Update on medicinal management of phytobezoars. Am J Gastroenterol 1993;88:1663–1666

MALLORY WEISS TEAR

JANICE A. KELLY

Nearly 70 years have passed since the initial description of Mallory Weiss tear in four autopsy subjects.[1] A Mallory Weiss tear is a laceration of the mucosa at or near the gastroesophageal junction. Initially, an association was drawn between alcoholic binging and the findings of linear mucosal ulcerations (or Mallory Weiss tears) arranged circumferentially along the longitudinal axis of the esophagus.[2] We now know that many patients have no antecedent history of alcohol intake.

For many years, Mallory Weiss tears were thought to be an uncommon cause of GI bleeding in adults; however, the advent of endoscopy has shown that Mallory Weiss tears cause GI bleeding in 10% to 15% of adult patients.[3] It is the third most common cause of GI hemorrhage in adults.[4]

The natural history of Mallory Weiss tears is different in the pediatric population. The first Mallory Weiss tear in children was described during the late 1970s.[5,6] Mallory Weiss tears were not reported earlier because it was not a recognized cause for hematemesis before the use of pediatric fiberoptic endoscopy. The initial reported symptoms of Mallory Weiss tear in pediatric patients included a prodrome of fever, nonbloody emesis, or upper respiratory infection symptoms.[5,6]

Some investigators believed that Mallory Weiss tears did not occur in children secondary to a lack of "resistance to emesis,"[6] resulting in absence of the increased intragastric pressure needed to produce a mucosal tear. The majority of pediatric patients are also not exposed to the risk factors seen with Mallory Weiss syndrome in adults, such as alcohol abuse, blunt trauma to the abdomen, heavy lifting, Valsalva maneuver, seizures, upper endoscopy, childbirth, and closed-chest resuscitation. Recent studies have now shown that Mallory Weiss tears can occur anytime during or after vomiting from any cause.[3] One case involved a tear after postprandial hiccups in a 3-week-old infant.[7] Initially, the diagnosis may have been overlooked in some pediatric patients because in the 1970s, one out of every five patients with melena and hematemesis could not have a source of bleeding identified.[8] This is complicated by the rapid healing of Mallory Weiss tears that can occur in as little as 72 hours, thereby reducing endoscopic visualization of this lesion.[9]

PATHOPHYSIOLOGY

Mallory Weiss tears are believed to be caused by a transient, transmural pressure gradient between the intragastric pressure and the thoracic pressure at the gastroesophageal junction. When the gastroesophageal junction is vigorously raised above the diaphragm, the pressure gradient causes dilatation of the gastroesophageal junction and mucosal tearing. Mallory Weiss tear occurs more frequently in patients with an established hiatal hernia; these patients will tend to have a tear on the gastric side (specifically, the gastric cardia) of the gastroesophageal junction.[10] Some patients can have a retching episode that causes a transient mushrooming of the stomach into the esophagus,[2] akin to a reverse intussusception, witnessed on upper endoscopy.[11]

Alternatively, the pathogenesis of the Mallory Weiss lesion can be explained by thinking of the stomach as a cylinder. The rationale for the occurrence of a Mallory Weiss tear can be explained by the physical law that states that in a cylinder, the tension required to tear the mucosa in the longitudinal direction is one-half that required to produce a tear in the circumferential direction. A tear will occur at the site of the greatest intraluminal diameter subjected to a sufficiently great transmural pressure gradient. The location of greatest risk would be the gastric mucosa near the gastroesophageal junction. The risk is increased in those patients who have a hiatal hernia.[9]

In a hiatal hernia, the maximum mucosal tension would be at the point of widest diameter exposed to the transmural pressure gradient existing between the thorax and the abdomen, that is, the cardiac portion of the stomach when the stomach is located above the diaphragm.[9] In a series by Watts,[10] an observed difference in incidence of hiatus hernia between those cases where the tear was in the esophagus and where the tear was in the stomach was highly significant. Patients with hiatal hernia were more likely to have a gastric tear than an esophageal tear.[10] The GI tract in children, including the esophagus, has greater tensile circumferential strength than the adult GI tract, as has been documented by Powell et al.,[11] Burt,[12] and Kinsella et al.[13] Perhaps this contributes to the decreased reporting of this lesion in the pediatric population.

CLINICAL PRESENTATION

Classically, Mallory Weiss tears present as hematemesis after a bout of nonbloody vomiting, coughing, or retching. This presentation occurs in 30% to 80% of patients. Bloody vomitus can occur at the onset of the first emesis and has been reported in both adults (in 50% of cases in one series)[14] and children.

The syndrome is usually acute in presentation, with as many as 70% of patients admitted within 24 hours of initial symptoms. Delayed presentation of up to 48 hours has been reported in up to 20% of patients. Ten percent of patients in one series presented with melena.[15] One series of adult patients documented up to 40% of patients had antecedent complaints of dyspepsia and abdominal pain.[16] One out of five pediatric cases did not have antecedent vomiting.[17] A male to female predominance of 3 : 1 has also been reported.

Mallory Weiss syndrome has been documented in children as young as 3 weeks old,[7] although all age groups have been represented. The hemodynamic presentation in children is varied, with some only mildly anemic, while others are frankly hypotensive, anemic, and in shock.[16] Since no one clinical presentation is pathognomonic, endoscopy is required for diagnosis.

LABORATORY EVALUATION

Initial laboratory evaluation should include a complete blood count (CBC) (to assess for anemia), coagulation studies (to determine whether a bleeding disorder is present), reticulocyte count, chemistry panel with liver function enzymes (to rule out fulminant liver failure), and a type and screen (in case of need for a transfusion). Stool for hemoccult should be checked, and a Gastroccult should be checked from the nasogastric lavage as well.

A chest radiograph and upright abdominal radiograph should be obtained to rule out occult intestinal perforation.

DIAGNOSIS

Whenever a patient presents with a history of hematemesis, nasogastric suction is an important tool to define the severity of the bleeding episode. Bright red blood is returned by nasogastric tube in 90% of adult patients. If persistent bleeding is present, upper endoscopy is indicated.

Endoscopy shows a single tear in 80% to 100% of cases in adults (Fig. 43-3). More than one tear is seen in less than 10% of cases.[17] The most common site for the tear is at, or just distal to, the junction of the esophagus and stomach, on the posterior wall, in most pediatric cases (Fig. 43-4). The lesions could extend up to 2 cm inferiorly or superiorly. Lesions are less commonly seen on the gastric surface; this is more commonly noted in patients with hiatal hernia, as previously discussed. The diagnosis is rarely made by barium study, because barium studies are not as efficacious as endoscopy for mucosal lesions. Other mucosal lesions, related to alcohol or nonsteroidal anti-inflammatory drugs (NSAIDs),[15] are found in many adult cases. By contrast, the pediatric patient usually presents with a solitary mucosal tear.

TREATMENT

Therapy includes intravenous H_2-blockers, hydration, and transfusion, when indicated. Most patients can be managed conservatively. Rarely, when intractable hem-

FIGURE 43-3. Location of Mallory Weiss tears in order of decreasing frequency.

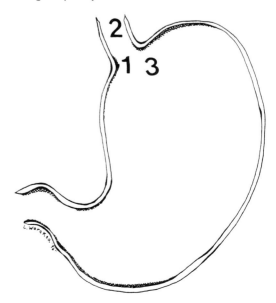

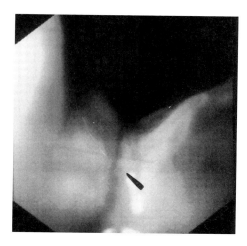

FIGURE 43-4. Mallory Weiss tear. (Photo courtesy of Dr. M. Zitin.)

orrhage occurs, a Pitressin infusion or electrocoagulation should be utilized prior to taking the patient to surgery.[11] Mallory Weiss tears almost never rebleed.[15]

REFERRAL PATTERN

Patients exhibiting signs and symptoms of significant GI bleeding should be admitted to a hospital setting that can provide an aggressive evaluation, supportive care, and appropriate diagnostic tests and therapy. The patient should be evaluated by a pediatric gastroenterologist for diagnosis and treatment.

REFERENCES

1. Mallory GK, Weiss S. Hemorrhages from laceration of the cardiac orifice of the stomach due to vomiting. Am J Med Sci 1929;178:506–515

2. Sugawa C, Benishek D, Walt AJ. Mallory Weiss Syndrome. A study of 224 patients. Am J Surg 1983;145:30–33

3. Schuman BM, Threadgill ST. The influence of liver disease and portal hypertension on bleeding in Mallory Weiss syndrome. J Clin Gastroenterol 1994;18:10–12

4. Yu PP, White D, Iannuccilli EA. The Mallory Weiss Syndrome in the pediatric population. BMJ 1982;65:73–74

5. Lamiell JM, Weyandt TB. Mallory Weiss syndrome in two children. J Pediatr 1978;92:583–584

6. Ross LA. Mallory Weiss syndrome in a 10 mos old infant. Am J Dis Child 1979;133:1069

7. Cannon RA, Lee G, Cox KL. Gastrointestinal hemorrhage due to Mallory Weiss syndrome in an infant. J Pediatr Gastroenterol Nutr 1985;4:323–324

8. Ament ME, Gans SL, Christie DK. Experience with esophagogastroduodenoscopy in diagnosis of 79 pediatric patients with hematemesis, melena, or chronic abdominal pain. Gastroenterology 1975;68:858

9. Graham DY, Schwartz JT. The spectrum of the Mallory-Weiss tear. Medicine Baltimore 1978;57:307–318

10. Watts HD. Lesions brought on by vomiting: the effect of hiatus hernia on the site of injury. Gastroenterology 1976; 71:683–688

11. Powell TW, Herbst CA, Ulshen M. Mallory Weiss syndrome in a 10 month old requiring surgery. J Pediatr Surg 1984;19: 596–597

12. Burt CAV. Pneumatic rupture of the intestinal canal. Arch Surg 1931;22:875–902

13. Kinsella TJ, Morse RW, Hertzog AJ. Spontaneous rupture of the esophagus. J Thoracic Surg 1948;17:613–631

14. Harris JM, DiPalma JA. Clinical significance of Mallory Weiss tears. Am J Gastroenterol 1993;88:2056–2058

15. Katz PO, Salas L. Less frequent causes of upper gastrointestinal bleeding. Gastroenterol Clin North Am 1993;22: 875–889

16. Kerlin P, Bassett D, Grant AK, Paull A. The Mallory Weiss lesion: a five year experience. Med J Aust 1978;1:471–473

17. Countryman D, Norwood S, Andrassy J. Mallory Weiss syndrome in children. South Med J 1982;75:1426–1427

RECTAL PROLAPSE

WILLIAM J. WENNER

Rectal prolapse can occur at any age. It is an uncommon illness, however, particularly in adequately nourished children. A major U.S. referral center identified only 54 cases of rectal prolapse over a 10-year period.[1] Observed most often before 3 years of age, the incidence occurs most frequently in children less than 1 year of age.

PATHOPHYSIOLOGY

Normal pediatric anatomy, including weak levator and anal support, a flat sacrum and coccyx, and the vertical course of the rectum, are all contributing factors.[2] In infancy, the predisposition to prolapse may be due to the loose attachment of the naturally redundant mucosa to the muscularis. Loss of rectal support due to an inadequate ischiorectal fat pad is believed to be the causative factor in malnourished children.[3]

ETIOLOGY

Rectal prolapse has been associated with cystic fibrosis, diarrheal diseases, celiac disease, ulcerative colitis, chronic constipation, malnutrition, Hirschsprung's disease, Ehlers-Danlos syndrome, meningomyelocele, rectal polyps, solitary rectal ulcer syndrome, and following anal rectal surgery. Infectious causes include *Clostridium difficile*, *Shigella*, hemolytic uremic syndrome (*Escherichia coli* O157:H7), pertussis, and a variety of parasites, including amebae, *Schistosoma*, *Trichiura*, and *Giardia*.

CLINICAL PRESENTATION

Rectal prolapse is quite easily recognized by parents. They often describe a deep red or purple, round mass of tissue passing through the canal and protruding out the anus. Occasionally a colonic polyp can be mistaken as rectal prolapse.

Two types of prolapse occur. Partial prolapse involves the mucosa alone and usually protrudes 1 to 2 cm beyond the anal verge.[4] Complete, or procidentia, is a full-thickness prolapse and may protrude 5 cm or more. They can be distinguished clinically as the presence of radial mucosal folds indicate partial prolapse, while the visualization of circular mucosal folds occurs with procidentia. Blood or mucus is commonly passed and occurs secondary to vascular engorgement. Ulceration and incarceration are rare.

DIAGNOSIS AND LABORATORY EVALUATION

While the majority (48%) of patients presenting with rectal prolapse have constipation or acute diarrheal diseases, cystic fibrosis (CF) must always be considered to be the etiology until proved otherwise. The incidence of rectal prolapse in CF has been reported to occur in as many as 18% to 23% of children with CF prior to diagnosis.[5,6] Anatomic causes were found in 24%. In some reports, up to 17% of patients have no definable etiology.[5,6]

Evaluation of rectal prolapse should include a sweat test, a barium enema, and, if the prolapse is associated with diarrhea, stool cultures for bacteria and ova/parasites ($\times$3) should be obtained.

TREATMENT

Manual replacement is the initial therapy. Placing the child in a knee-chest position may facilitate replacement as this decreases the anal and levator tone. Sedation may be required for replacement.

Further episodes may be prevented by stool softeners such as lactulose in a child under 1 year of age or with risk of aspiration, and mineral oil in older children. In patients who develop recurrent rectal prolapse, manual support to the perineum during defecation, placing the infant in a recumbent position, raising the potty, use of an adult size seat and strapping or taping the buttocks have been suggested; however, these maneuvers are often suggested without sufficient data reported in the literature. This medical therapy is almost always successful. In rare cases, a surgical consultation is needed. In these instances, injection of a sclerosing agent in the submucosal tissues surrounding the rectum may be required. Other surgical methods include linear cauterization of the anorectum and anal encirclement with catgut or Silastic.

REFERRAL PATTERN

Most patients with rectal prolapse should be evaluated and treated by the primary physician. Malnourished patients, patients diagnosed with CF or abnormal anatomy, or patients with recurrent prolapse should be evaluated by a gastroenterologist.

REFERENCES

1. Zempsky WT, Rosenstein BJ. The cause of rectal prolapse in children. Am J Dis Child 1988;142:338–339

2. Dudgeon DL, Colombani PM, Beaver BL. Colonic and anorectal lesions: surgical considerations. In: Rudolph AM, Hoffman JIE, Eds. Pediatrics. 18th Ed. Norwalk, CT: Appleton & Lange, 1987:949

3. Corman ML. Rectal prolapse in children. Dis Col Rectum 1989;28:535–538

4. Freeman NV. Rectal prolapse in children. J R Soc Med 1984; 77(suppl 3):9–12

5. Kulczyki LL, Shwachman H: Studies in cystic fibrosis of the pancreas: occurrence of rectal prolapse. N Engl J Med 1958; 259:409–412

6. Stern RC, Izant RJ Jr, Boat TF: Treatment and prognosis of rectal prolapse in cystic fibrosis. Gastroenterology 1982;82: 707–710

SHWACHMAN'S SYNDROME

TIMOTHY SENTONGO
CHRIS A. LIACOURAS

Shwachman's syndrome is a rare but important multiorgan disease of unknown etiology, occurring in 1 in 10,000 children. It is the second most common congenital disorder of the exocrine pancreas. The syndrome is characterized by short stature, skeletal abnormalities, and exocrine pancreas insufficiency despite a normal sweat chloride test.[1] Affected patients also often develop recurrent bacterial infections secondary to neutropenia and abnormal granulocyte function. Other less common associated features include renal tubular dysfunction, icthyosis, dental abnormalities, delayed puberty, liver disease, and diabetes mellitus. The syndrome appears to have an autosomal recessive inheritance pattern.[2]

CLINICAL PATHOLOGIC FEATURES

Growth Retardation

Short stature is the most common feature of Shwachman's syndrome.[2] Most affected children are of normal birth weight; however, during infancy, they develop failure to thrive secondary to fat malabsorption from pancreatic insufficiency. Other causes of poor growth include feeding difficulties, diarrhea, abdominal pain, and recurrent infections. By 2 years of age, almost all patients plot below the third percentile for height even though constant linear growth is usually maintained. Puberty is delayed in many adolescents.

Pancreatic Disease

Pancreatic hypoplasia secondary to fatty infiltration of the gland is one of the cardinal features of the syndrome.[1,3] Pancreatic ductular structures and islet cells characteristically remain intact. The degree of pancreatic secretory impairment is extremely variable. The most severe cases often present in the first 6 months when children present with diarrhea, steatorrhea, and associated fat-soluble vitamin deficiencies. In many patients, GI symptoms improve by the age of 3 to 6 years secondary to partial function of the pancreas. Exocrine pancreatic insufficiency in Shwachman's syndrome is characteristically associated with a normal sweat chloride. Pancreatic insufficiency may be determined by abnormal fecal fat collections and pancreatic stimulation testing. Fatty infiltration of the pancreas may be reliably detected by ultrasonography or computed tomography (CT) scan.[4] The differential diagnosis of pancreatic fatty infiltration includes all processes that lead to fibrosis of the pancreas (i.e., CF, chronic pancreatitis, prolonged treatment with steroids, Cushing's syndrome, or obesity).

Hematologic/Bone Marrow Disease

Bone marrow abnormalities can occur in one or all three blood cell lines and may present as neutropenia, thrombocytopenia, hypoplastic anemia, or pancytopenia.[5] These abnormalities may be transient or persistent. Recurrent bacterial infections are a common feature of Shwachman's syndrome. Otitis media, sinusitis, osteomyelitis, and recurrent skin infections may occur. Overwhelming sepsis is the leading cause of death, and mortality rates from infections have been reported as high as 25%. Immunoglobulin deficiency may also be present. The number of infectious episodes diminishes with age. Lymphoproliferative and myeloproliferative malignancies have also been reported.[6]

Skeletal Abnormalities

Early features of Shwachman's syndrome include thoracic dystrophy manifested by abnormally short ribs with flared anterior end "cup deformities." This may be so pronounced as to result in a narrow thoracic cage causing persistent respiratory difficulty during infancy.[7] Older children may have short long bones, hypoplasia of the iliac bones, and short wide femoral necks. Metaphyseal chondroplasia is characterized by irregular defects of epiphyseal cartilage mineralization and widening of the metaphysis, mainly localized at the anterior ends of the ribs and at the knees. Clinodactyly of the fifth finger is present in up to one-half of those affected in some series. The most frequent radiologic abnormality is delayed bone age. Typically, these abnormalities are mild and require no medical treatment.

DIAGNOSIS

Shwachman's syndrome should be considered in all patients with fat malabsorption with hematologic or bone abnormalities and a normal sweat test. The diagnosis is more difficult in older children as the exocrine pancreatic deficiency may not present clinically. Thus, any child with short stature, intermittent or persistent blood cell line abnormalities, repeated bacterial infections, or skeletal anomalies should be evaluated for Shwachman's syndrome. Quantitative pancreatic enzyme analysis is most useful for determining the diagnosis; however, this test is usually only offered at tertiary care centers, is cumbersome and unpleasant and is difficult to perform on infants and young children. Noninvasive studies such as quantitative fecal fat analysis, serum trypsinogen, and radiography may be helpful in these children.

TREATMENT

Treatment of Shwachman's syndrome is supportive. Whenever pancreatic insufficiency is present, pancreatic enzyme replacement should be used. The dose of enzymes required to achieve adequate absorption is one-third to one-half that required by patients with CF (see Ch. 23). Concurrent administration of fat-soluble vitamins is recommended. Patients with neutropenia generally require no treatment when asymptomatic; however, patients who develop fevers or a clinically toxic appearance should be treated similarly to an immunosuppressed patient consisting of routine cultures with provision of appropriate antibiotics until cultures are negative or the infection resolves.

REFERENCES

1. Shwachman H, Diamond LK, Oski FA et al. The syndrome of pancreatic insufficiency and bone marrow dysfunction. J Pediatr 1964;65:645–663

2. Aggett PJ, Cavanagh NPC, Matthew DJ et al. Shwachman's syndrome: a review of 21 cases. Arch Dis Child 1980;55:331–347

3. Bodian M, Sheldon W, Lightwood R. Congenital hypoplasia of the exocrine pancreas. Acta Paediatr 1964;53:282–293

4. Kurdziel JC, Dondelinger R. Fatty infiltration of the pancreas in Shwachman's syndrome: computed tomography demonstration. Eur J Radiol 1984;4:202–204

5. Burke V, Colebatch JH, Anderson CM et al. Association of pancreatic insufficiency and chronic neutropenia in childhood. Arch Dis Child 1967;42:147–157

6. Woods WG, Roloff JS, Lukens JN et al. The occurrence of leukemia in patients with Shwachman's syndrome. J Pediatr 1981;99:425–428

7. Michels VV, Donovan GK. Shwachman syndrome: unusual presentation as asphyxiating thoracic dystrophy. Birth Defects 1982;18:129–134

44

ALAGILLE SYNDROME

ELIZABETH B. RAND

GENETICS

Alagille syndrome is a clinically defined disorder characterized by cholestatic liver disease, peculiar facies, structural heart defects (predominantly pulmonic stenosis), vertebral anomalies, and ocular abnormalities.[1–4] Additional findings may include growth retardation, long bone abnormalities, and renal disease.[1–3] There is a wide range of clinical expression even among close family members, as well as in each independent organ system within a given person.[1–3,5] The incidence is approximately 1 in 70,000 live births, with equal numbers of males and females.[6] There is no known ethnic association.

The full syndrome was first described in the English literature by Alagille in 1975; however, it had been previously described incompletely by Watson and Miller[7] in 1973 and in the French literature by Alagille et al.[8] in 1969. The syndrome has been variously referred to as arteriohepatic dysplasia, Alagille syndrome, Watson-Alagille syndrome, intrahepatic atresia, and syndromic paucity of the interlobular bile ducts. Early pedigree analysis suggested that its inheritance is autosomal dominant with variable penetrance.[1,2] Many cases are thought to be new mutations, as parents of probands usually appear to be clinically unaffected.

The association between Alagille syndrome and chromosome 20p was first noted in a case report describing a patient with del(20)(p11.23-pter) and a phenotype consistent with Alagille syndrome.[9] This large deletion included almost the entire short arm of chromosome 20 and was therefore easily visible by cytogenetic analysis.

A total of eight Alagille probands with del(20p) have since been described since that report.[9–15] In one instance, an affected mother of a proband carried the same del(20p) as her child.[13] The size of the deletions seen in the reported cases has varied between families, and the overlap of the deletions allowed the definition of a smaller Alagille region at 20p12.[13,15] The identification of these overlapping deletions gave rise to the generally accepted hypothesis that Alagille is a contiguous gene syndrome.[13] Contiguous gene syndromes are postulated to be caused by the deletion of a finite but variable number of genes, with the extent of the deletion correlating with the range and severity of disease.[16] The contiguous gene deletion hypothesis is attractive because it can explain the highly variable clinical presentation and the diversity of organ involvement by invoking numerous genes. If a single gene abnormality underlies this disorder, it must have a basic role, not only in the growth and regulation of biliary epithelium, but also in formation of the heart, vertebrae, and eyes, in order to explain the major features alone.

Despite the identification of the Alagille region, molecular characterization of the (gene) causing the syndrome has not been achieved. Studies aimed at reaching this goal have thus far used two basic modalities to investigate the region of interest. First, high-resolution cytogenetic studies of several series of Alagille probands have been performed.[12,17] The results of these surveys have demonstrated a low percentage of cytogenetic deletions in Alagille syndrome (less than 5%), as compared to other contiguous gene syndromes. For example, cytogenetically visible deletions are present in 50% to 60% of patients with Prader-Willi syndrome[18] and in 20% of patients with velocardiofacial syndromes.[19] Second, molecular testing of several series of cytogenetically normal patients has been performed and has identified only a single submicroscopic deletion.[15,17,20] The absence of significant numbers of detectable deletions makes the designation of this disorder as a contiguous gene deletion syndrome less likely, but not impossible.[15] Small shared 20p12 deletions below the current level of detection may exist, or abnormalities not on chromosome 20 may cause an indistinguishable phenotype. Ongoing efforts within the 20p12 locus should ultimately result in the cloning of the gene(s) whose abnormalities cause the Alagille syndrome phenotype at this locus.

Identification of the Alagille gene has been reported simultaneously by several groups and has been submitted for publication in early 1997.[21] It appears that the gene (jagged-1) encodes a transmembrane protein that binds a receptor (notch) on neighboring cells and thereby allows for cell-to-cell communications during differentiation. Although the homologues of this gene and its product have been studied in various invertebrates, nothing is known regarding its function in human development of the organs involved in Alagille syndrome. Identification of the gene should allow the development of specific genetic testing in the near future as well as the opportunity to study new aspects of hepatic development.

CLINICAL PRESENTATION

Most Alagille patients present in infancy with a history and physical examination consistent with a diagnosis of biliary atresia. In addition, the distinctive hepatic histologic feature of Alagille syndrome, intrahepatic bile duct paucity, may be absent during the first 6 months of life.[4,22] Portal inflammation and intrahepatic cholestasis sometimes seen on liver biopsy of Alagille infants are also characteristic of extrahepatic biliary atresia and may contribute to this common misdiagnosis.[4,22] The difficulty in differentiating Alagille syndrome from biliary atresia is compounded by the often benign nature of the extrahepatic manifestations of Alagille syndrome in infancy. For example, pulmonary arterial stenosis, the most common cardiac finding in Alagille syndrome, often manifests as a simple murmur indistinguishable from the benign peripheral pulmonic stenosis frequently heard in normal infants, as well as in Alagille syndrome patients.[1,3,4] Unless the diagnosis of Alagille syndrome is specifically considered, posterior embryotoxon in the eye, as well as vertebral anomalies (if present), are unlikely to be discovered.[4,23] Finally, the Alagille facies, which are difficult to discern even in some older children and adults, are often not recognizable in infancy when facial features are still indistinct.[4]

Taken together, these factors can lead to early misdi-agnosis of biliary atresia, generally followed by a Kasai procedure. This standard surgical approach to atresia of the extrahepatic biliary tree links a loop of small bowel directly to the porta hepatis (portoenterostomy) to provide enteric bile drainage. The procedure is not indicated in Alagille syndrome, in which the extrahepatic biliary tree is generally patent, except for in those rare cases in which true extrahepatic biliary atresia is also present.[4] If extrahepatic biliary drainage is achieved in the course of an unindicated Kasai, the procedure will generally lead to recurrent episodes of ascending bacterial cholangitis, which accelerate the progression to biliary cirrhosis. If unsuccessful, the Kasai procedure results in complete extrahepatic biliary obstruction and rapid progression to biliary cirrhosis.

Although Alagille syndrome generally presents in infancy as described above, it may not come to medical attention until school age. Infants with the syndrome may undergo spontaneous resolution of jaundice without intervention (or evaluation) and may present later with xanthomata or pruritis with or without jaundice. Occasionally these patients present to a dermatologist with these complaints; xanthomata may even be biopsied before liver disease is suspected.

As Alagille syndrome is variably expressed, it is often difficult to determine whether parents and siblings of probands are unaffected or have subclinical disease.[5,6] For example, the liver function of a mother of an infant with Alagille syndrome was evaluated by serologic analysis of liver enzymes, prothrombin and partial thromboplastin times, physical examination, and arteriogram and found to be normal. This evaluation was conducted prior to living related liver transplantation, during which the mother's left lateral hepatic lobe would be donated to her infant. Despite the normal findings, histologic examination of a biopsy of the partial hepatectomy specimen demonstrated ductal paucity consistent with Alagille syndrome and the transplantation was aborted (Whitington PF: personal communication, 1992). Obviously, liver biopsy samples are not generally available from the healthy relatives of an affected patient, making the diagnosis extremely difficult. The issue is most important with respect to genetic counseling, as patients with Alagille syndrome have a 50% chance of transmission of the disorder with each conception, and the severity of disease in the next generation is unpredictable.

DIAGNOSIS

The frequency of the five major features of the syndrome described by Alagille have been compiled in two large series, summarized in Table 44-1[2,3] Less common findings associated with the syndrome are listed in Table 44-2. Alagille syndrome presents the clinician with numer-

TABLE 44-1. Alagille Syndrome: Major Clinical Features

Characteristic	Alagille et al.[2] (n = 80)		Deprettere et al.[3] (n = 27)	
	n	%	n	%
Chronic cholestasis (with intrahepatic bile duct paucity by biopsy)	73	91	25	93
Congenital heart disease (usually PPS or pulmonic stenosis)	68	85	26	95
Ophthalmic anomalies (usually posterior embryotoxon)	55/62	88	9/16	56
Vertebral anomalies (usually butterfly vertebrae)	70	87	6/18	33
Peculiar facies (frontal bossing, deep-set eyes, bulbous nose tip, pointed chin)	76	95	19	70

(Data from Alagille[2] and Deprettere.[3])

ous diagnostic and therapeutic challenges. Diagnostic errors lead to clinical mismanagement and inappropriate therapy, both of which could be avoided if specific testing were available.

In order to assign the diagnosis of Alagille syndrome the patient must have cholestatic liver disease with a characteristic biopsy, demonstrating intrahepatic bile duct paucity, and at least two additional major features, excluding facies. Bile duct paucity is determined by examining the liver biopsy for number of bile ducts per portal triad, with paucity defined by an average of up to 0.5 ducts/triad over 10 triads. Given the difficulty of providing genetic counseling to affected families, healthy nonjaundiced first-degree relatives have been considered by some to be affected if they express even a single feature of the disease.[6] Considering the nontrivial frequency of some features in the normal population (i.e., posterior embryotoxon 10% to 15%), this may be inaccurate. Prenatal diagnosis is not available.

MANAGEMENT

Clinical management of the child and young adult with Alagille syndrome is also problematic. Probably fewer than 10% of Alagille patients will develop liver disease that progresses to cirrhosis and liver failure, but these patients pose special therapeutic challenges.[4] Management of these patients is essentially indistinguishable from children with other cholestatic disorders leading to end-stage liver disease (see Chs. 48 and 58). An equal proportion of children with Alagille syndrome have

complex congenital heart disease requiring surgical intervention, but the vast majority have pulmonic stenosis, small septal defects, or other minor structural abnormalities not requiring surgery.[2,4] Cardiac and hepatic disease vary independently in each patient, so that only one or both may be severe in a given individual.

Patients with Alagille syndrome who do not have liver failure or profound cardiac disease present with a different constellation of therapeutic difficulties. The liver disease that presents in infancy generally worsens over the first few years of life and then gradually improves if fibrosis and cirrhosis did not intervene. Serum bile salts become increasingly elevated during the early cholestatic phase, accompanied by severe pruritis.[4] Before the devel-

TABLE 44-2. Alagille Syndrome: Reported Extrahepatic Findings

Heart
　Generally right-sided disease (pulmonic artery stenosis or PPS)
　Ventricular septal defect
　Atrial septal defect
　Tetralogy of Fallot

Bones/joints
　Butterfly vertebrae
　Scoliosis
　Incomplete spina bifida
　Lack of progressive widening of interpedicular distance of the lumbar spine
　Shortening of the ulna
　Shortening of the distal phalanges
　Seronegative polyarticular arthritis

Eyes
　Posterior embryotoxon
　Prominent Schwalbe's line
　Axenfeldt's anomaly
　Microcornea
　Anomalous optic discs
　Peripapillary retinal depigmentation

Kidneys
　Membranous nephropathy with lipid deposits
　Duplication renal pelvis
　Interstitial renal fibrosis
　Medullary cysts

Skin
　Xanthomata
　Lichenification
　Lichen amyloidosis
　Nevus comedonicus

Growth
　Decreased height for age
　Decreased weight for age

Pancreas
　Pancreatic insufficiency
　Nesidioblastosis

opment of newer choleretic agents, pruritis was generally treated unsuccessfully with antihistamines, barbiturates, benzodiazepines, baths, and nighttime restraints. If allowed to scratch, many patients produce excoriations and bleeding. More effective therapies include rifampin (by an unknown mechanism action) and ursodeoxycholate (which induces choleresis and downregulates the synthesis of toxigenic bile acids).[24] Ursodeoxycholate should be administered at a dose of 15 to 30 mg/kg/day, divided at least twice a day. The primary side effect of oral ursodeoxycholic acid therapy is diarrhea, caused by malabsorption of this bile acid. The diarrhea can be minimized by decreasing the dose while simultaneously increasing the frequency of administration. Ursodeoxycholate is currently available only as a 300-mg capsule, an inappropriate dose for small pediatric patients. The contents of the capsule dissolve readily in water, but the solution is unstable and cannot be stored for later use. In most cases, it is convenient for parents to open the capsule and sprinkle an estimated fraction of the contents on spoon feeding. Alternatively, the entire contents of the capsule can be dissolved in 10 ml water and an appropriate fraction of the solution administered orally with the remainder discarded. Rifampin is generally less effective then ursodeoxycholate for the pruritis associated with chronic cholestasis, and those patients who achieve an initial response may notice declining efficacy over time. If the starting dose of 5 mg/kg/day (administered qd or divided bid) is ineffective, or if symptoms worsen after an initial response, the dose can be progressively increased to 15 mg/kg/day. Given that rifampin can itself alter serum aminotransferase levels and cause discoloration of bodily fluids, at least monthly monitoring of liver enzymes and family anticipatory guidance must be provided.

External biliary drainage by a partial cutaneous biliary diversion is another therapeutic option for patients with profound cholestasis.[25] This procedure uses a jejunal loop with mesentery as a conduit for external drainage of bile. The proximal end of the intestinal loop is attached by a side-to-side anastomosis with the gallbladder, and the distal end of the jejunal loop is used to create a cutaneous stoma. This process diverts approximately 30% of bile flow and depletes the bile salt pool of tertiary toxigenic bile salts in favor of benign primary equivalents. Although this procedure has been shown to be effective in stimulating choleresis and in halting the progression of biliary fibrosis to cirrhosis in patients with persistent familial intrahepatic cholestasis (Byler's disease), it has had mixed results in patients with Alagille syndrome.[25]

Impaired growth in patients with Alagille syndrome generally exceeds that expected for the degree of liver disease, and even patients with very mild or subclinical disease are frequently small for age. Alagille patients studied have normal growth hormone levels, and, if treated with additional recombinant growth hormone do not respond with increased levels of insulin-like growth factor 1 as do growth hormone-deficient persons.[25] These findings suggest that the small stature of these patients is not solely the result of cholestasis or hepatic dysfunction but is an independent feature of Alagille syndrome. Growth failure will be exacerbated in patients with profound cholestasis, resulting in malabsorption of fat and fat-soluble vitamins. All patients with Alagille syndrome presenting in childhood should receive supplements of vitamins A, E, D, and K. Vitamin A, E, and D levels should be monitored every 4 to 6 months in patients with evolving cholestasis, and the prothrombin time should be monitored at least that frequently to determine whether vitamin K deficiency exists. Complications of fat-soluble vitamin deficiencies in patients with Alagille syndrome who have normal hepatic synthetic function can include visual problems (vitamin A), ataxia and/or developmental delay (vitamin E), osteopenia with frequent fractures (vitamin D), and coagulopathy (vitamin K), just to name a few. (For further discussion of fat-soluble vitamins, see Ch. 13.)

REFERRAL PATTERN

In general, the diagnosis of Alagille syndrome will be made by a specialist in pediatric gastroenterology. Although the diagnosis of the syndrome may be suspected in an infant with cholestasis and heart disease, heart defects are also found in a subset of biliary atresia patients; therefore, liver biopsy will generally be required to determine the presence of the characteristic bile duct paucity. Even an infant with cholestasis, heart disease, and additional findings of Alagille syndrome (e.g., butterfly vertebrae) should undergo liver biopsy because of the possibility of coexisting extrahepatic biliary atresia. In short, all jaundiced infants should be evaluated with total and direct serum bilirubin measurements, all of those with evidence of cholestasis warrant referral to a pediatric gastroenterologist. Any infant with a nonexcreting diisopropyl iminodiacetic acid (DISIDA) scan (or equivalent) requires liver biopsy to rule out biliary atresia, and a diagnosis of Alagille syndrome may well be made as part of this evaluation. Patients with mild cholestasis may not require frequent subspecialty follow-up evaluation; however, signs of worsening cholestasis (e.g., increasing jaundice, pruritis, xanthomata), progressive liver disease (e.g., splenomegaly, GI bleeding, hypoalbuminemia, coagulopathy, rickets), or fat-soluble vitamin deficiency (e.g., coagulopathy, rickets, visual disturbances, ataxia) should stimulate prompt referral.

REFERENCES

1. Alagille D, Odievre M, Gautier M, Dommergues JP. Hepatic ductular hypoplasia associated with characteristic facies, vertebral malformations, retarded physical, mental, and sexual development, and cardiac murmur. J Pediatr 1975;86:63–71

2. Alagille D, Estrada A, Hadchouel M et al. Syndromic paucity of interlobular bile ducts (Alagille syndrome or arteriohepatic dysplasia): review of 80 cases. J Pediatr 1987;110: 195–200

3. Deprettere A, Portmann B, Mowat AP. Syndromic paucity of the intrahepatic bile ducts: diagnostic difficulty; severe morbidity throughout early childhood. J Pediatr Gastroenterol Nutr 1987;6:865–871

4. Mueller RFM. The Alagille syndrome (arteriohepatic dysplasia). J Med Genet 1987;24:621–626

5. Shulman SA, Hyams JS, Gunta R et al. Arteriohepatic dysplasia (Alagille syndrome): extreme variability among affected family members. Am J Med Genet 1984;19:325–332

6. Dhorne-Pollet S, Deleuze J-F, Hadchouel M et al. Segregation analysis of Alagille syndrome. J Med Genet 1994;31: 453–457

7. Watson GH, Miller V. Arteriohepatic dysplasia: familial pulmonary arterial stenosis with neonatal liver disease. Arch Dis Child 1973;48:459–466

8. Alagille D, Borde J, Habib EC, Thomassin N. Tentatives chirurgicales au cours des atrésies des voies biliares intrahépatiques avec voie biliare extra-hépatique permeable. Arch Pediatr 1969;26:51–71

9. Byrne JLB, Harrod MJE, Friedman JM, Howard-Peebles PN. Del(20p) with manifestations of arteriohepatic dysplasia. Am J Med Genet 1986;24:673–678

10. Schnittger S, Hofers C, Heidemann P et al. Molecular and cytogenetic analysis of an interstitial 20p deletion associated with syndromic intrahepatic ductular hypoplasia (Alagille syndrome). Hum Genet 1989;83:239–244

11. Legius E, Fryns JP, Eyskens B et al. Alagille syndrome (arteriohepatic dysplasia) and del(20)(p11.2). Am J Med Genet 1990;35:532–535

12. Zhang F, Deleuze JF, Aurias A et al. Interstitial deletion of the short arm of chromosome 20 in arteriohepatic dysplasia (Alagille syndrome). J Pediatr 1990;116:73–77

13. Anad F, Burn J, Matthews D et al. Alagille syndrome and deletion of 20p. J Med Genet 1990;27:729–737

14. Teebi AS, Murthy DS, Ismail EA, Redha AA. Alagille syndrome with de novo del(20) (p11.2). Am J Med Genet 1992; 42:35–38

15. Rand EB, Spinner NB, Piccoli DA et al. Molecular analysis of 24 Alagille syndrome families identifies a single submicroscopic deletion and further localizes the Alagille region within 20p12. Am J Hum Genet 1995;57:1068–1073

16. Emanuel BS. Molecular cytogenetics: toward dissection of the contiguous gene syndromes. Am J Hum Genet 1988;43: 575–578

17. Desmaze C, Deleuze JF, Dutrillaux AM et al. Screening of microdeletions of chromosome 20 in patients with Alagille syndrome. J Med Genet 1992;29:233–235

18. Nicholls RD, Knoll JHM, Glatt et al. Restriction fragment length polymorphisms within proximal 15q and their use in molecular cytogenetics and the Prader-Willi syndrome. Am J Med Genet 1989;33:66–77

19. Driscoll D, Spinner NB, Budarf ML et al. Deletions and microdeletions of 22q11.2 in velo-cardio-facial syndrome. Am J Med Genet 1989;44:261–268

20. Deleuze J-F, Hazan J, Dhorne S et al. Mapping of microsatellite markers in the Alagille region and screening of microdeletions by genotyping 23 patients. Eur J Hum Genet 1994; 2:185–190

21. Li L, Krantz ID, Deng Y, et al. Alagille syndrome is caused by mutations in hJagged1, a ligand for notch. Nature Genetics 1997 (submitted)

22. Dahms BB, Petrelli M, Wyllie R et al. Arteriohepatic dysplasia in infancy and childhood: a longitudinal study of six patients. Hepatology 1982;2:350–358

23. Wells KK, Pulido JS, Judisch GF et al. Ophthalmic features of Alagille syndrome (arteriohepatic dysplasia). J Pediatr Ophthalmol Strabismus 1993;30:130–135

24. Caestecher JS, Jazrawi PP, Petroni ML, Northfield TC. Ursodeoxycholic acid in chronic liver disease. Gut 1991;32: 1061–1065

25. Whitington PF, Whitington GL. Partial external diversion of bile for treatment of intractable pruritis associated with intrahepatic cholestasis. Gastroenterology 1988;95:130–136

26. Bucuvalas JC, Horn JA, Carlsson L et al. Growth hormone insensitivity associated with elevated circulating growth hormone-binding protein in children with Alagille syndrome and short stature. J Clin Endocrinol Metab 1993;76: 1477–1482

45

ALPHA-1-ANTITRYPSIN DEFICIENCY

EMIL CHUANG

Homozygous PiZZ alpha-1-antitrypsin (α_1-AT) deficiency is the most common inherited cause of liver disease in infants and children[1] and is one of the most common metabolic disorders for which children undergo liver transplantation. It is thought to affect approximately 1 in 1,600 to 2,000 live births of white children in North America and Scandinavia but is rare in Asians and African Americans.[1,2] Population screening studies in Sweden have prospectively followed newborns with PiZZ phenotype α_1-AT deficiency for 18 years.[3–5] Only 10% to 15% have been found to develop symptomatic liver disease in infancy, and most improve over time. Sometimes, patients may not present until their teenage years. There is also an increased risk of liver cirrhosis and hepatocellular carcinoma in older adults.[6,7] Even though hepatic injury is almost always associated with the PiZZ phenotype, numerous phenotypic variants of α_1-AT deficiency may result in emphysema in adults.

PATHOPHYSIOLOGY

The α_1-AT protein belongs to the superfamily of *serine protease inhibitors* (serpins). Its principal physiologic action is to inhibit neutrophil elastase in the lung, through the formation of a covalent complex between α_1-AT and the protease.[1,8] α_1-AT is a 52-kDa glycosylated single polypeptide consisting of 394 amino acids. It is folded into a globular structure that consists of nine alpha-helices, three beta-pleated sheets, and three internal salt bridges.[8] The normal serum level is 150 to 350 mg/dl but, because it is an acute-phase reactant, the serum level

may increase fourfold in response to systemic inflammation or stress.[1,9]

The gene is located on the long arm of chromosome 14 at q31–32.2 and is expressed predominantly by hepatocytes, but some epithelial cells and mononuclear phagocytes also express the gene.[8] Inheritance of α_1-AT is co-dominant, with each parental gene contributing to its own protein activity. More than 100 variants of this monomeric glycoprotein have been identified, each differing in amino acid sequences and/or the three asparaginyl-linked carbohydrate side chains. The classification system of this protease inhibitor (Pi) is alphabetic according to its isoelectric point, as identified by agarose electrophoresis or isoelectric focusing.[10] Allelic variants with the highest mobility complexes are assigned letters near the beginning of the alphabet. For example, the most common variant M_1, migrates to an intermediate isoelectric point, whereas the most common allele associated with severe deficiency migrates to the highest isoelectric point, designated Z. Variants with similar or identical electrophoretic properties are subclassified by either a number or geographic location of the proband. Minor differences are distinguished by restriction fragment-length polymorphism (RFLP) or direct DNA sequence analysis, or both.

The α_1-AT protein may be grouped as normal, deficient, null/absent, or dysfunctional based on the serum level or activity (Table 45-1). The predominant alleles are M_1, M_2 and M_3, which together represent 90% to 95% of α_1-AT alleles.[11–13] Serum α_1-AT levels are normal with these variants and cause no disease. The next most common allele, PiS, is associated with a reduction in α_1-AT protein. The PiSZ phenotype may cause em-

315

TABLE 45-1. Classification of Common Variants of α_1-AT Deficiency and Their Clinical Significance

Variants	Common Alleles	Serum α_1-Antitrypsin (mg/dl)	Variants With Lung Disease	Variants With Liver Disease
Normal	M_1, M_2, M_3, F, P, R, N, B, C, D, E, G, X, V_{Munich}	150–350	—	—
Deficient	Z, S, $M_{Procida}$, $M_{Heerlen}$, M_{Duarte}, $M_{Maltone}$, P_{Duarte}	15–200	Z, $M_{Procida}$, $M_{Heerlen}$, D_{Duarte}, M_{Malton}, P_{Duarte}	Z, M_{Duarte} (?), M_{Malton} (?), P_{Duarte} (?)
Null/absent	$Null_{Bellingham}$, $Null_{Granite\ Falls}$	—	$Null_{Bellingham}$, $Null_{Granite\ Falls}$	—
Dysfunctional	Pittsburgh	150–350	—	—

physema and mild liver disease. The PiZ variant has a gene frequency of approximately 1% among whites. It codes for a dysfunctional protein that is profoundly deficient in the serum. Null variants are those in which no detectable α_1-AT protein is present in serum. Other variants are caused by insertions, deletions, or substitutions of amino acids in the molecular sequence of the gene; they sometimes produce unstable or abnormal proteins that may or may not lead to clinical disease. In clinical practice, almost all disease associated with α_1-AT deficiency will have PiZZ, PiZ(null), PiSZ, or Pi(null)(null) phenotypes.[11] Liver disease has been reported with each of these phenotypes, except for the Pi(null)(null) phenotype, which only causes emphysema.

The pathophysiology of hepatic disease is not fully understood, although it is widely accepted that the cellular damage is a result of abnormal accumulation of α_1-AT protein in the endoplasmic reticulum of hepatocytes. The PiZ allele results in a single base substitution of lysine for glutamic acid at amino acid 342 that prevents the formation of one of the structural salt bridges important in the formation of the tertiary structure of the protein. It is not folded into its usual configuration, and the abnormal protein is trapped in the cytoplasm; only a small fraction translocate from the endoplasmic reticulum to the Golgi apparatus for final processing and excretion. The remainder accumulates in the rough endoplasmic reticulum of hepatocytes and provokes an inflammatory response.[14] However, this does not explain why only 10% to 15% of children with the PiZZ phenotype develop liver disease.

Perlmutter and colleagues[15] made an interesting observation that may help explain this apparent incongruity. α-AT degradation was studied in cultured fibroblasts obtained from PiZZ patients with and without liver disease. The fibroblasts were transduced with recombinant retroviral particles containing a viral promoter and either wild-type or mutant a_1-AT complementary DNA (cDNA). It was observed that fibroblasts from patients with diseased liver have a lag in the degradation of α_1-AT protein, in comparison to protected hosts without liver disease who had normal degradation rates. This raises the possibility that other genetic traits, such as the rate of α_1-AT degradation in the common endoplasmic degradation pathway, may at least in part determine susceptibility to liver disease. Alternatively, it has been proposed that the serpin-enzyme complex receptors mediate neutrophil chemotaxis and that activation of these receptors may have a putative role in hepatotoxicity.[16]

In contrast to PiZZ, patients with the Pi(null)(null) phenotype do not synthesize α_1-AT. There is no accumulation of protein in hepatocytes and liver disease does not occur. Significant emphysema has been associated with phenotypic variants with a serum α_1-AT level less than 35% of normal.[17] Like elastase, proteases are capable of cleaving many connective tissue proteins of the extracellular matrix, including elastin, alveolar interstitium, proteoglycans, and major components of the cellular basement membrane.[8,18,19] α_1-AT provides a major defense in the lower respiratory tract against the proteolytic effects of this powerful serine protease. Smoke may have a direct oxidative effect on α_1-AT and at the same time increases the oxidation of substrates such as methionine residues; both reactions may interfere with the complex formation of α_1-AT with elastase.

CLINICAL PRESENTATION

The mode of presentation of α_1-AT deficiency is age dependent (Table 45-2). The most common hepatic manifestation of α_1-AT deficiency is an acute icteric hepatitis during the neonatal period. This occurs in approximately 10% to 15% of infants with the PiZZ form of the disease.[3] The usual age of onset is at 2 to 3 weeks of life, but jaundice may present anytime during the first 4 months of life. The diagnosis of α_1-AT deficiency must be considered in any infant with a conjugated hyperbilirubinemia. The jaundice typically peaks during the neonatal period with levels in the range of 4 to 21 mg/dl. Acholic stool is seen with severe cholestasis; this presentation may be indistinguishable from extrahepatic biliary atresia. Unlike the latter condition, improvement in the jaundice and in liver function tests is often seen over the next 3 months. About 25% of infants who present

TABLE 45-2. Clinical Presentation of α_1-AT Deficiency at Different Age Groups

Age Group	Clinical Manifestations
Neonates and early infancy	Prolonged cholestatic jaundice, elevated transaminases
Early childhood	Elevation of transaminases with hepatomegaly, severe liver dysfunction
Late childhood and adolescence	Hepatosplenomegaly with portal hypertension, severe liver dysfunction
Adulthood	Liver cirrhosis and portal hypertension, hepatoma; chronic bronchitis or chronic obstructive pulmonary disease

(Adapted from Perlmutter,[30] with permission.)

with neonatal cholestasis will progress to liver failure before 5 years of age, and 50% will develop liver cirrhosis by adolescence (Fig. 45-1). Jaundice will resolve completely in about one-half of the infants, but only 25% will have complete normalization of their transaminases.[3,20]

The outcome of infants whose jaundice resolves spontaneously in infancy is variable. Hepatomegaly is present in all symptomatic infants, and by 1 year of age, one-half will also have splenomegaly. Transaminases are rarely normal at 1 year, although 25% will continue to show clinical and biochemical improvement, and laboratory studies normalize at 3 to 10 years of age.[3–5,21–24] Liver biopsies in these patients are limited to minimal liver fibrosis and to widening of the portal tracts. Survival to the third decade without cirrhosis has been reported. Another 25% will have a period of well-being for months to years but will then develop cirrhosis, hepatic decompensation, and failure to thrive. These patients commonly develop glomerulonephritis manifesting as hematuria and proteinuria and will be at increased risk of hypertension after liver transplantation.[25] The remainder of children will have persistently elevated liver function tests throughout the first decade, and one-half will have cirrhosis on liver biopsy. Liver function tests may eventually return to normal in the absence of cirrhosis, but the remainder will probably require liver transplantation.

For reasons that are not fully understood, newborns with α_1-AT deficiency are often small for gestational age

FIGURE 45-1. Outcome of patients with α_1-AT deficiency at different age groups from birth to adulthood. Neonatal cholestasis develops in 10% to 15% of affected newborns, and abnormal transaminases are found in another 50% in infancy. By adulthood, 75% to 85% will have normal liver function test results and 10% will still have elevated transaminases. Dashed line represents an insidious progression to liver cirrhosis. (Data from Sveger[3–5] and from Mowat and colleagues.[20,26])

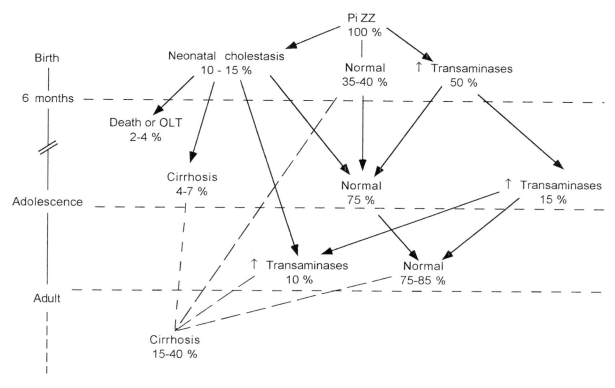

(SGA) and demonstrate poor growth in infancy.[21] An improvement in growth parameters usually coincides with a resolution of the hepatitis. In approximately 2% of affected newborns, the presenting feature is a severe bleeding episode at 2 to 6 weeks of age, as a result of vitamin K malabsorption.[26] It may be a mild exsanguinating bleed from the umbilicus or superficial bruising and, at worse, intracranial bleeding may occur. Invariably, all these infants have jaundice and elevated transaminases. The prothrombin time is greatly prolonged, but intravenous vitamin K will quickly reverse the clotting abnormality. Early diagnosis and treatment will prevent this occurrence.[21]

About one-half of newborns with PiZZ phenotype will develop mild asymptomatic elevations in transaminases in early infancy.[3] These and the remainder of infants with normal liver function tests generally have a good prognosis, and only 2% of these children will develop liver cirrhosis before adulthood.[26] The usual presentation in older children and adolescents is hepatosplenomegaly, elevated transaminases, and/or complications of portal hypertension. There may be no prior history of jaundice in infancy. The reported risk of liver cirrhosis in patients with the PiZZ phenotype is 15% to 47%[21,22]; 15% to 29% of adults are also at risk of developing hepatoma.[26] The tumor occurs more commonly in males and may develop in the absence of liver cirrhosis, but rarely before the sixth decade of life.[27]

PULMONARY DISEASE

Chronic obstructive pulmonary disease, specifically emphysema, is the most prevalent clinical disorder associated with α_1-AT deficiency. Clinical manifestations are generally not seen in the pediatric age population. The mean age of onset of emphysema is the third decade of life in smokers and the fifth decade in nonsmokers. Affected individuals, and in particular female patients who avoid smoking, are likely to have a normal life span.[28] Wide population studies suggest that 1% to 2% of all cases of emphysema are related to α_1-AT deficiency, but the proportion increases to 18% in adults who develop more severe emphysema or who present at a younger age.[22] Emphysema associated with α_1-AT deficiency usually involves the basal lobes, rather that the apices, where smokers are typically affected. Asthma and chronic bronchitis are also common manifestations of α_1-AT deficiency, but the onset of such symptoms in the pediatric age group is probably coincidental. Significantly, affected individuals with a history of childhood asthma are at increased risk of emphysema. The development of emphysema in heterozygotes with PiMZ is controversial.[22] In the absence of asthma, it is doubtful whether there is an increased risk, whereas PiSZ phenotypes are susceptible to emphysema, even in the absence of asthma or smoking.

DIAGNOSIS

α_1-AT deficiency is part of the differential diagnosis of neonatal cholestasis syndrome. Direct hyperbilirubinemia in neonates must be investigated aggressively, as certain metabolic disorders, such as galactosemia and tyrosinemia, are potentially life-threatening. Furthermore, the surgical success for extrahepatic biliary atresia is better in young infants less than 10 to 12 weeks of age. The clinical presentation, and sometimes the histologic appearance on liver biopsy of α_1-AT deficiency, are sometimes indistinguishable from that of biliary atresia and therefore must be excluded prior to any exploratory surgery.

Serum α_1-AT level and Pi typing should be obtained for any patient in whom the diagnosis of α_1-AT deficiency is being considered. The serum level is a useful screening tool but, because it is an acute-phase reactant, the level alone has no diagnostic value. Therefore, Pi typing is essential to confirm the diagnosis of PiZZ α_1-AT deficiency.

A percutaneous liver biopsy is an invaluable diagnostic tool for investigating neonatal cholestasis and cryptogenic cirrhosis. However, pediatric hepatologists disagree as to the value of a liver biopsy, once the diagnosis of α_1-AT deficiency has been made. Some consider monitoring serial liver transaminases alone adequate in most cases,[22] while others believe that liver biopsy has some value for prognostication. Significant scarring at diagnosis is associated with a poorer prognosis and with an increased likelihood of progressing to end-stage liver disease.[21]

LABORATORY FINDINGS

Homozygous individuals with PiZZ phenotype typically have serum α_1-AT levels about 10% to 15% of normal.[17] Although serum values at this level are suggestive of α_1-AT deficiency, Pi typing is essential to make the definitive diagnosis, since other variants may have low serum levels, yet cause no disease. Furthermore, a low normal or moderately depressed serum α_1-AT level does not exclude the diagnosis of α_1-AT deficiency. Pi typing is tested from plasma by agarose electrophoresis or isoelectric focusing in a polyacrylamide gel.[22] Unlike the serum α_1-AT level, which is available in many commercial laboratories, Pi typing requires testing in a specialized laboratory.

Liver biopsy of all patients with PiZZ and many PiSZ and PiMZ phenotypes will demonstrate distinctive dia-

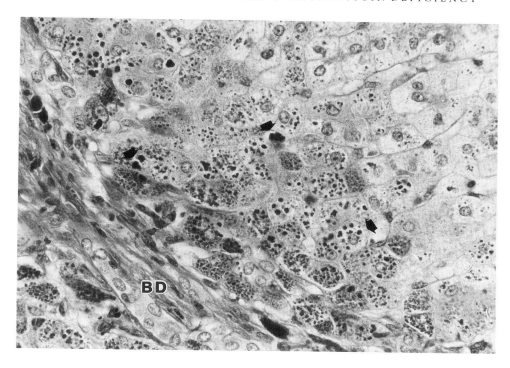

FIGURE 45-2. Photomicrograph of ex-plant liver from a 2-year-old patient with α_1-AT deficiency, who required liver transplantation for end-stage liver disease. PAS-positive diastase-resistant granules are prominent in the cytoplasm of periportal hepatocytes (arrows). Bile ducts (BD) are seen in the portal tract. (Courtesy of Dr. Eduardo Ruchelli.) ($\times$ 50.) (Original magnification)

stase-resistant, periodic acid Schiff (PAS) reagent-positive cytoplasmic inclusions in the periportal hepatocytes (Fig. 45-2). These inclusions appear on electron microscopy as membrane-bound moderately electron-dense amorphous deposits within the cisternae of the endoplasmic reticulum. These inclusions are uncommon in liver biopsies of infants less than 3 months of age. They are not specific and should be distinguished from bile droplets, giant lysosomes, megamitochondria, and Councilman bodies. Many hepatocellular tumors, embryonal liver sarcoma, and yolk sac tumors can be PAS positive as well. The presence of α_1-AT protein in cells is confirmed by immunofluorescence, immunoperoxidase, and/or monoclonal antibody techniques. The histologic findings in infants with α_1-AT deficiency on liver biopsy are nonspecific. The most common finding is an acute hepatitis with or without giant cell transformation. Cholestasis is a frequent finding associated with any significant insult to the liver in infants. There may also be bile duct paucity and, with progression of disease, ductular proliferation and portal fibrosis may be seen.

TREATMENT

No specific treatment is available for the hepatic disease associated with α_1-AT deficiency. Management is that of chronic cholestasis and of liver cirrhosis. Maintenance of good nutrition is essential in infants, as many who present in infancy are SGA and demonstrate failure to thrive. Cholestatic patients in particular are susceptible to fat-soluble vitamin and essential fatty acid deficiencies. There is no evidence that anti-inflammatory agents (e.g., prednisone and penicillamine), immune-modulating agents (e.g., cyclosporine), or antioxidants (e.g., vitamin E) will alter the course of the liver disease. Liver transplantation remains the only option for children with end-stage liver failure. The 5-year survival following transplantation is comparable to that noted with other causes of liver failure in childhood, although there is an increased incidence of systemic hypertension because of the association with glomerulonephritis.

The single most effective therapy for the lung destruction seen in α_1-AT deficiency is prevention. All susceptible people should avoid smoking and smoke exposure. Therefore, household members should be strongly advised against smoking in the same environment as affected patients. Since α_1-AT is inactivated by oxidation, antioxidant activity should be maximized in the lung. Antioxidants such as vitamin E may be important in protecting against lung destruction, and patients should maintain normal serum levels of vitamin E. The data are insufficient to suggest that supraphysiologic doses of vitamin E or other antioxidants provide additional benefit.

Gene therapy offers the best hope for cure in affected persons in the future. Direct Pi MM gene targeting to the hepatocyte ex vivo or in vivo is now possible in animal models.[29] Another theoretical possibility is the correction of the hepatic secretory problem by inserting a gene that modifies the α_1-AT polypeptide, to allow it to assume a normal tertiary configuration to facilitate secretion.

REFERRAL PATTERN

α_1-AT deficiency is in the differential diagnosis of any cholestatic syndrome in neonates or the older child who presents with hepatomegaly or liver cirrhosis. Although most biochemical tests are available through commercial laboratories, any neonate with documented cholestatic jaundice should be referred on an urgent basis to a tertiary center for evaluation. Rapid diagnosis and treatment may be life-saving in some metabolic disorders, and an experienced pediatric hepatobiliary surgeon should be available if extrabiliary atresia is suspected. The same level of urgency does not apply to the older child who presents with an enlarged liver but who is otherwise well and not in liver failure. It may be reasonable to perform screening biochemical tests, including serum α_1-AT levels and Pi typing, prior to referral. If the diagnosis of PiZZ α_1-AT deficiency is confirmed in a symptomatic patient, referral to a pediatric hepatologist at a liver transplant center is indicated, as there is a possibility that the patient will ultimately require transplantation.

Once diagnosed, subspecialty care is not essential for the routine management of the PiZZ variant of α_1-AT deficiency in children. Affected patients require periodic monitoring for deteriorations in liver function, as manifested by serum biochemistry tests or poor growth, or both. Cholestatic patients should be followed closely for clinical and biochemical evidence of fat-soluble vitamin deficiency. All patients with significant progression of liver disease, or of portal hypertension, or both, should be referred for evaluation at a liver transplantation center.

Referral to a pulmonologist is indicated for the child with α_1-AT deficiency who develops asthma or recurrent bronchitis. Poor control with ongoing bronchial and alveolar inflammation may hasten the onset of lung disease in this condition.

REFERENCES

1. Perlmutter DH. The cellular basis for liver injury in alpha$_1$-antitrypsin deficiency. Hepatology 1991;13:172–185
2. Silverman EK, Miletich JP, Pierce JA et al. Alpha$_1$-antitrypsin deficiency: Prevalence estimation from direct population screening. Am Rev Respir Dis 1989;140:961–966
3. Sveger T. Liver disease α_1-antitrypsin deficiency detected by screening of 200,000 infants. N Engl J Med 1976;294: 1216–1221
4. Sveger T. The natural history of liver disease in α_1-antitrypsin deficient children. Acta Paediatr Scand 1988;77: 847–851
5. Sveger T, Eriksson S. The liver in adolescents with alpha 1-antitrypsin deficiency. Hepatology 1995;22:514–517
6. Eriksson S, Carlson J, Velez R. Risk of cirrhosis of primary liver cancer in α_1-antitrypsin deficiency. N Engl J Med 1986; 314:736–739
7. Eriksson S. Alpha$_1$ antitrypsin deficiency and liver cirrhosis in adults. Acta Med Scand 1987;221:461–467
8. Brantly M, Nukiwa T, Crystal RG. Molecular basis of alpha-1-antitrypsin deficiency. Am J Med 1988;84:13–31
9. Sifers RN, Finegold MJ, Woo SL. Molecular biology and genetics of alpha 1-antitrypsin deficiency. Semin Liver Dis 1992;12:301–310
10. Sharp HL. The current status of alpha-1 antitrypsin deficiency, a protease inhibitor in gastrointestinal disease. Gastroenterology 1976;70:611–621
11. Morse JO. Alpha$_1$-antitrypsin deficiency. First of two parts. N Engl J Med 1978;299:1045–1048
12. Kueppers F, Black LF. Alpha$_1$-antitrypsin and its deficiency. Am Rev Respir Dis 1974;110:176–194
13. Silverman EK, Miletich JP, Pierce JA et al. Alpha-1-antitrypsin deficiency. High prevalence in the St. Louis area determined by direct population screening. Am Rev Respir Dis 1989;140:961–966
14. Brind AM, Bassendine MF. Molecular genetics of chronic liver diseases. Baillieres Clin Gastroenterol 1990;4:233–253
15. Wu Y, Whitman I, Molmenti E et al. A lag in intracellular degradation of mutant alpha 1-antitrypsin correlates with the liver disease phenotype in homozygous PiZZ alpha 1-antitrypsin deficiency. Proc Natl Acad Sci USA 1994;91: 9014–9018
16. Perlmutter DH. The SEC receptor: a possible link between neonatal hepatitis in alpha 1-antitrypsin deficiency and Alzheimer's disease. Pediatr Res 1994;36:271–277
17. Gadek JE, Crystal RG. Alpha$_1$-antitrypsin deficiency. In: Stanbury JB, Wyngarrden JB, Fredricksen DS, et al., Eds. The Metabolic Basis of Inherited Metabolic Diseases. New York: McGraw-Hill, 1982:1450–1467
18. Birrer P, McElvaney NG, Chang-Stroman LM, Crystal RG. Alpha 1-antitrypsin deficiency and liver disease. J Inher Metab Dis 1991;14:512–525
19. Crystal RG. Alpha 1-antitrypsin deficiency, emphysema, and liver disease. Genetic basis and strategies for therapy. J Clin Invest 1990;85:1343–1352
20. Mowat AP. Alpha 1-antitrypsin deficiency (PiZZ): features of liver involvement in childhood. Acta Paediatr 1994; (suppl)393:13–17
21. Mowat AP. Alpha-1-antitrypsin deficiency (PiZZ) and other glycoprotein storage diseases. In: Liver Disorders in Childhood. Oxford: Heinemann Butterworth, 1994:335–348
22. Cox DW, Beaudet AL, Sly AL, Valle D. α_1-Antitrypsin deficiency. In: Scriver CR et al, Eds. Metabolic and Molecular

Bases of Inherited Disease. New York: McGraw-Hill, 1995: 4125–4158

23. Filipponi F, Soubrane O, Labrousse F et al. Liver transplantation for end-stage liver disease associated with alpha-1-antitrypsin deficiency in children: pretransplant natural history, timing and results of transplantation. J Hepatol 1994;20: 72–78

24. Sveger T, Piitulainen E, Arborelius M Jr. Lung function in adolescents with alpha 1-antitrypsin deficiency. Acta Paediatr 1994;83:1170–1173

25. Stauber RE, Horina JH, Trauner M et al. Glomerulonephritis as late manifestation of severe alpha 1-antitrypsin deficiency. Clin Invest 1994;72:404–408

26. Hussain M, Mieli-Vergani G, Mowat AP. Alpha 1-antitrypsin deficiency and liver disease: clinical presentation, diagnosis and treatment. J Inher Metab Dis 1991;14:497–511

27. Cohen C, Derose PB. Liver cell dysplasia in alpha-1-antitrypsin deficiency. Mod Pathol 1994;7:31–36

28. Larsson C. Natural history and life expectancy in severe $alpha_1$-antitrypsin deficiency. Acta Med Scand 1978;204: 345–353

29. Alino SF, Crespo J, Bobadilla M et al. Expression of human alpha-1-antitrypsin in mouse after in-vivo gene transfer to hepatocytes by small liposomes. Biochem Biophys Res Commun 1994;204:1023–1030

30. Perlmutter DH. Liver diseases in α_1-AT deficiency. Prog Liver Dis 1993;11:139–165

46

ASCITES

DROR WASSERMAN

Ascites is defined as accumulation of fluid in the abdominal cavity. It is a common complication of cirrhosis. It is also associated with acute and chronic processes, such as liver dysfunction, as well as other systemic, metabolic, inflammatory or neoplastic processes. Ascites can be congenital or acquired[1–14] (Table 46-1). Acquired ascites is most commonly associated with cirrhosis; however, other etiologies should always be considered.

PATHOPHYSIOLOGY

The occurrence of ascites in cirrhosis is due to portal hypertension, which causes an increase in hydrostatic pressure at the sinusoidal level which alters splanchnic and systemic hemodynamics. Excessive peritoneal fluid formation is a consequence of abnormalities in the dynamic steady-state process between peritoneal fluid production and absorption. In the process of ascites formation, oncotic pressure, portal venous pressure, and direct lymphatic flow not only dictate the fluid balance between the intravascular and extravascular spaces but also the quality of the accumulated fluid.[14] In cirrhosis of the liver, structural distortion of sinusoidal vessels is the major factor responsible for the increase in portal venous pressure and the development of ascites. The mechanisms by which advanced liver cirrhosis leads to widespread changes in the circulation are unclear but may include vasodilation, increased cardiac output, expanded plasma volume and activation of the renin-angiotensin axis and its associated antidiuretic and natriuretic factors.

Three main hypotheses have been proposed to explain the pathophysiologic process, including the under filling hypothesis, the overflow hypothesis, and the peripheral arterial vasodilatation hypothesis.[15] Ascitic fluid can develop either acutely or insidiously. Whenever a sudden accumulation of fluid occurs, other nonhepatic etiologies should be considered. In addition, a similar presentation may occur when acute hepatic dysfunction develops in a patient with an already marginally compensated liver (secondary to infection, shock, malignancy, hepatic toxins, or hemorrhage).

Chyle is a fluid rich in triglycerides, characterized by the presence of chylomicrons. Chylous ascites occurs when abdominal lymphatics are obstructed or distorted (i.e., intestinal lymphangiectasis or postoperatively after abdominal surgery), as an unusual complication of malignant neoplasms, especially secondary to lymphoma,[16] or as a complication of mesenteric adenitis or intra-abdominal tuberculosis. Perforation of the common bile duct commonly leads to insidious onset of bilious ascites.[12]

CLINICAL PRESENTATION

In children, the development of ascites can be rapid or insidious. Newborns can also present with congenital ascites of unclear etiology. If isolated ascites develops, a full metabolic, hemolytic, and anatomic workup should be performed (Table 46-1). In some children, the accumulation of ascites may be slow and occur over a prolonged period of time. In these cases, early diagnostic indicators include poor nutrition and growth failure or

TABLE 46-1. Etiology of Ascites

Congenital Ascites[1]	Acquired Ascites
Lysosomal storage disease[2]	Cirrhosis[5]
Hydrops fetalis	Hypoalbuminemia
Congenital anomalies of lymphatics	Portal vein flow obstruction
Congenital heart disease	Inflammation of peritoneum
Congenital urinary anomalies	Lymph flow obstruction
Meconium peritonitis[3]	Rupture of intra-abdominal cyst
Perforation of common bile duct[4]	Mesenteric lymphadenitis
	Intra-abdominal TB[6]
	Neoplastic diseases[7]
	Severe pancreatitis
	Hepatic veno-occlusive disease[8]
	Nephrogenic ascites in end stage renal disease[9]
	Serosal eosinophilic enteropathy[10]
	Myxedema ascites[11]
	Post-abdominal aortic surgery[12]
	Eosinophilic ascites-parasites[13]

(Data from Machin,[1] with permission.)

inappropriate weight gain. Peripheral edema usually does not occur in children.

PHYSICAL EXAMINATION

Signs on physical examination include shifting dullness to percussion and increasing abdominal girth. In advanced stages, ascites can be detected by inspection with the patient showing abdominal distention, fullness of the flanks, the formation of hernias (femoral, inguinal, or incisional), and an inverted umbilicus. Scrotal edema may accompany congenital forms of ascites. The physical examination may demonstrate decreased total body muscle mass, as well as signs of the underlying disease process, including (1) liver disease with signs of portosystemic shunting (distended abdominal wall vessels, around gastrostomy tube and ileostomies) and striae; (2) heart disease with a murmur and pleural effusions; (3) and metabolic or hemolytic conditions. Edema is present in children with hypoalbuminemia.[17]

Clues that help in the assessment of the etiology of ascites include splenomegaly and prominent abdominal wall veins (portal hypertension), cor pulmonale (chronic heart failure), a pericardial friction rub (pericarditis and possible Budd-Chiari syndrome), diffuse abdominal pain (peritonitis), abdominal pain radiating to the back (pan-

creatitis), and lymphedema (lymphatic obstruction or trauma to the thoracic duct).

DIAGNOSIS

Imaging Methods

While plain abdominal radiographs may show signs of ascites, abdominal ultrasound remains the study of choice.[18] An ultrasound examination identifies free fluid versus a loculated fluid collection and may demonstrate the presence of intra-abdominal masses, vascular anomalies and malignancies. Computed tomography (CT) and magnetic resonance imaging (MRI) are not necessary for confirming the diagnosis of ascites but may be helpful in determining the etiology of the ascites (see Chs. 66 and 68).

ABDOMINAL PARACENTESIS

Paracentesis is a safe procedure and is the procedure of choice in the evaluation of ascites.[19] Possible complications of this procedure are perforation of the bowel, puncture of abdominal organs (bladder, uterus, ovary), and hemorrhage. The technique is performed under sterile conditions using a narrow bore angiocatheter. The puncture is done in the midline at the linea alba, 2 cm below the umbilicus, using a Z technique. (The skin entrance should be shifted in the figure of a Z from the entrance to the peritoneal cavity to minimize the risk of peritoneal leak.) Peritoneal fluid is collected for routine studies, including white blood cell (WBC) count, culture, lactate dehydrogenase (LDH), total protein, albumin, glucose, Gram stain, amylase, cholesterol, triglycerides, and cytology. These tests require approximately 10 to 20 ml of fluid. (For further details on the evaluation of peritoneal fluid, see Ch. 37.) Fluid can be evaluated for infection, chyle or blood. Cytology is the single best test when peritoneal carcinomatosis is suspected.[7]

THERAPY

While the management of ascites should always be directed toward its underlying etiology, acute decompensation in marginally compensated liver disease should be promptly investigated and immediately treated with supportive care. Supportive treatment involves bed rest, a low-sodium diet and the administration of aldosterone antagonists and loop diuretics. Furosemide, a loop diuretic, is often used in the acute management of severe ascites in a dose of 1 to 2 mg/kg/dose up to 6 mg/kg/day. Adverse effects of loop diuretics include headache, fever, lethargy, rash, gynecomastia, nausea, and diarrhea. Rarely, boluses of 25% albumin can be given in association with a loop diuretic in the presence of hypoalbuminemia. Spironolactone, in a usual dose of 1.5 to 3.5 mg/kg/day in divided doses, is often used as a maintenance diuretic and is administered once the acute effects of ascites have been controlled. The diuretic effect of spironolactone may be delayed for 2 to 3 days. Management with diuretics should be based on a step-by-step progressive addition of more potent drugs as this is the best way of controlling ascites while minimizing potentially dangerous biochemical side effects.[20] Once diuretics are begun, electrolytes, renal function, and blood pressure changes need to be closely monitored.

Patients who fail to respond to the above treatment are said to have refractory ascites and require therapeutic paracentesis, surgical portosystemic shunting or a transjugular intrahepatic portcaval shunt (TIPS) procedure.[21,22] TIPS was introduced in 1989. TIPS provides a side-to-side portosystemic shunt without a major abdominal operation, and has become an effective therapy for the treatment of intractable ascites. TIPS has poor long-term patency (months) and requires frequent ultrasound-doppler evaluation for assessment of patency. TIPS is especially useful in patients anticipating liver transplant. There is limited information on TIPS in children. The pediatric experience has been derived chiefly from cystic fibrosis patients with end-stage liver disease.

REFERRAL PATTERN

Any patient suspected of having ascites should be evaluated by a pediatric gastroenterologist. The goals of the evaluation should be both to treat the ascites and to determine the underlying etiology.

REFERENCES

1. Machin GA, Diseases causing fetal and neonatal ascites. Pediatr Pathol 1985;4:195–211
2. Gillan JE, Lowden JA, Gaskin K et al. Congenital ascites as a presenting sign of lysosomal storage disease. J Pediatr 1984; 104:225–231
3. Sukcharoen N. Prenatal sonographic diagnosis of meconium peritonitis: a case report. J Med Assoc Thai 1993;76(3): 171–176
4. Holland RM, Lilly JR. Surgical jaundice in infants: other than biliary atresia. Semin Pediatr Surg 1992;1(2):125–129
5. Bac DJ, Siersema PD, Wilson JH. Paracentesis. The importance of optimal ascitic fluid analysis. Neth J Med 1993;43: 147–155
6. Marshall JB. Tuberculosis of the gastrointestinal tract and peritoneum. Am J Gastroenterol 1993;88:989–999
7. Runyon BA. Malignancy-related ascites and ascitic fluid "humoral tests of malignancy." J Clin Gastroent 1994;18(2): 94–98
8. Shulman HM, Hinterberger W. Hepatic veno-occlusive disease-liver toxicity syndrome after bone marrow transplantation. Bone Marrow Transplant 1992;10(3):197–214
9. Hammond TC, Takiyyuddin, MA. Nephrogenic ascites: a poorly understood syndrome. J Am Soc Nephrol 1994;5: 1173–1177
10. Kuri K, Lee M. Eosinophylic gastroenteritis manifesting with ascites. South Med J 1994;87:956–957
11. de Castro F, Bonacini M, Walden JM, Schubert TT. Myxedema ascites. Report of two cases and review of literature. J Clin Gastroenterol 1991;13:411–414
12. Williams RA, Vetto J, Quinones-Baldrich W et al. Chylous ascites following abdominal aortic surgery. Ann Vasc Surg 1991;5:247–252
13. Lambroza A, Dannenberg AJ. Eiosinophylic ascites due to hyperinfection with Strongyloides stercoralis. Am J Gastroenterol 1991;86:89–91
14. Garcia-Tasco G. Cirrhotic ascites: pathogenesis and management. Gastroenterologist 1995;3:41–54
15. Gentilini P, La Villa G, Romanelli M, Laffi G. Pathogenesis and treatment of ascites in hepatic cirrhosis. Cardiology 1994;84(suppl 2):68–79
16. Oosterbosh L, Leloup A, Verstraeten P, Jordens P. Chylothorax and chylous ascites due to malignant lymphoma. Acta Clin Belg 1995;50:20–24
17. Fitzgerald JF. Ascites. In: Wyllie R, Hyams J, Eds. Pediatric Gastrointestinal Disease. Philadelphia: WB Saunders, 1993: 151–160
18. Wasserman D. Ascites. In: Schwartz W, Bell L, Bingham, Chung E, Friedman D, Mulberg A, Sinai L, Eds. Five Minutes in Pediatrics. Maryland: Williams & Wilkins, 1996:808–809
19. Runyon BA. Refractory ascites. Semin Liver Dis 1993;13: 343–351
20. Gerbes AL. Medical treatment of ascites in cirrhosis. J Hepatol 1993;17(suppl 2):S4–S9
21. Wong F, Blendis L. Transjugular intrahepatic portosystemic shunt for refractory ascites; tipping the sodium balance, editorial. Hepatology 1995;22:358–364
22. Skeens J, Semba C, Dake M. Transjugular intrahepatic portosystemic shunts. Annu Rev Med 1995;46:95–102

47

CHRONIC AUTOIMMUNE HEPATITIS

KARAN MCBRIDE
ERIC S. MALLER

Autoimmune chronic hepatitis or more commonly known now simply as autoimmune hepatitis (AIH) is an uncommon but important cause of progressive inflammatory liver disease. The major features of this idiopathic disorder are female predominance, presence of hyperglobulinemia, an association with a variety of autoantibodies and a response to corticosteroid or other immunosuppressive therapy.[1] Unless controlled by immunosuppressive therapy, AIH is often progressive and may result in cirrhosis and end-stage hepatic dysfunction.

ETIOLOGY AND PATHOGENESIS

The cause of AIH is unknown. The conceptual framework for the pathogenesis hypothesizes that several factors need to occur for the initiation of AIH, including an environmental agent (i.e., a virus or toxin) that triggers an autoimmune process directed at liver antigens and a genetic predisposition among those harboring a defect in immunoregulatory T-cell function (which may be mediated by certain HLA haplotypes and non-HLA genes).[2]

Investigators postulate that environmental agents may initiate a process that leads to immunologic changes, resulting in the activation of cytotoxic T cells as mediators of the hepatic injury. Although viruses were initially suspected to be possible initiators, limited evidence implicates any virus as a cause. For example, it has been of interest that titers of antibodies to measles virus in pa-

tients with AIH are significantly higher than those occurring after natural measles infections.[1] There is also considerable debate about the possible role of hepatitis C as an initiator of an autoimmune response. This debate is based on the finding that a certain percentage of patients with AIH test positive for hepatitis C virus (HCV). A study done by Lenzi in 1990[3] found an overall incidence of 78% positivity for HCV in type II AIH, characterized by the presence of anti–liver-kidney microsomal (LKM) antibodies. It is postulated that HCV infection may lead to an altered expression of the LKM antigen, which may result in loss of tolerance and induction of anti-LKM antibodies that lead to autoimmune liver disease.[2]

There is considerable evidence supporting the role of genetic factors in predisposing a patient to the development of AIH. As in other autoimmune diseases, there are primary associations with major histocompatibility complexes on chromosome 6 (i.e., A1, B8, DR3). There is also an increased incidence of autoantibodies and other autoimmune disorders in the family members of patients with AIH.[4]

There also appear to be a variety of immunologic abnormalities in patients with AIH. Almost all known autoantibodies have been reported to occur in patients diagnosed with AIH. Anti-actin (anti-smooth muscle) and anti-nuclear antibodies (ANA) are commonly present. Antimitochondrial antibodies are found in 10% to 30%[6] of affected patients but are usually present in low titers. New evidence suggests that most patients with AIH have a defect in suppressor T-cell activity, which is also found

TABLE 47-1. Autoantibodies in the Subtypes of AIH

Subtype of AIH	Autoantibodies	Characteristics
Type I	Antinuclear antibody (ANA), anti-actin antibody or anti-smooth muscle antigen antibody	Most common (classic AIH)
Type II	Anti-liver kidney microsomal (LKM) antibody (ANA, smooth muscle antigen)	Less common (usually pediatric patients)
Type III	Anti-soluble liver antigen/antibody	

in 50% of healthy first- and second-degree relatives of these patients.[2] The defect appears to be inherited in an autosomal dominant fashion, independent of HLA type.

SUBDIVISIONS OF AIH

Several distinct subdivisions of AIH are defined by the pattern of autoantibodies. All subgroups occur predominantly in females.[4]

Type I AIH

Type I AIH is the most prevalent form and is characterized by the presence of anti-actin (formerly designated anti-smooth muscle) antibodies and ANA.

Type II AIH

Type II is characterized by the presence of antibodies to microsomal antigens. The major markers are the presence of anti-LKM antibodies type 1 (anti-LKM 1) and the absence of ANA or anti-actin antibodies.[5] The antigenic target of the anti-LKM antibody is cytochrome p450 db1 as described by Manns in 1989.[6] Anti-LKM and anti-actin antibodies are mutually exclusive.

Type II AIH is less prevalent and the patients tend to be younger. Type II is also the form of AIH which may be related to HCV infection. When type II patients were tested for the presence of HCV by recombinant immunoblot assay, many of them were positive. This suggested that HCV may lead to the production of anti-LKM antibodies, which cause AIH.[7] There is also an additional antibody, called anti-GOR, which is found in type II AIH patients and is thought to be secondary to infection with HCV. This antibody was found in most type II patients who were HCV positive, but in none of the type I AIH or other autoimmune disorders (e.g., primary biliary cirrhosis). Anti-GOR may be induced by HCV infection but be independent of the formation of anti-LKM. These differences lead to further subdivisions: type IIA patients are negative for anti-HCV and anti-

GOR, whereas type IIB are positive for anti-HCV and anti-GOR.[5]

Other Types

The third subdivision of AIH is characterized by the presence of antibodies to a soluble liver antigen. This group is the least common, and the average age of the patients is older. Most patients are female with hyperglobulinemia and high aminotransferases, but with no ANA or anti-LKM antibody.[8]

CLINICAL PRESENTATION

The clinical features of autoimmune hepatitis are extremely heterogeneous. The spectrum of clinical disease extends from absence of symptoms (in which disease is discovered by high levels of aminotransferases on routine screening) to severe acute hepatitis and even liver failure. Patients often present with insidious onset of malaise, anorexia, and fatigue. Seventy-five percent of these patients are female, with onset at age 10 to 40 years.[1] Associated menstrual abnormalities are frequent. Jaundice is often not a predominant feature. Very often many of these patients have other autoimmune disorders (e.g., Sjögren's syndrome, ulcerative colitis, arthritis, or autoimmune hemolytic anemia).

Occasionally AIH is characterized by profound jaundice, an elevated prothrombin time (PT), and elevated aminotransferases. In such cases, the presentation is very similar to that of an acute viral hepatitis. It is important to distinguish the two by testing for hepatitis A, B, C, Epstein-Barr virus (EBV), and cytomegalovirus (CMV). In general, elevated aminotransferases are more striking than the elevated bilirubin and alkaline phosphatase (ALP). Rarely, AIH presents with a cholestatic picture. There are also patients who present with advanced AIH who already have ascites, portal hypertension, and hepatic encephalopathy, indicating that the progression of the disease can be insidious with little clinical evidence initially.[4]

DIAGNOSIS

The clinical picture of AIH may vary from a benign clinical presentation to fulminant hepatic failure. The diagnosis of AIH is initially one of exclusion. It is critical to first rule out the most common viral causes of hepatitis. If the investigation for infectious causes is negative, the patient should be evaluated for exposure to hepatotoxic drugs (i.e., nitrofurantoin or Isoniazid) and for evidence of the common metabolic disorders such as Wilson's disease or alpha-1-antitrypsin deficiency.

The characteristic liver biopsy features of AIH include periportal hepatitis and "piecemeal necrosis" of varying severity, appearing as a portal mononuclear cell infiltrate invading the hepatocyte boundary surrounding the portal triad and entering the surrounding lobule (usually with individual necrotic hepatocytes).[9] The histological picture of AIH may vary from minimal changes to severe disruption of the hepatic architecture with widespread necrosis. In all but the mildest cases, fibrosis is present.

Until recently, chronic hepatitis has been divided by pathologic classification into two major subdivisions: chronic active hepatitis (CAH) and chronic persistent hepatitis (CPH). In the past, AIH has most often been classified as CAH. This classification system was designed in order to provide guidelines for predicting the disease course in chronic hepatitis. CPH was considered a benign, nonprogressive injury characterized by inflammation confined to the portal triad without periportal inflammation. CAH was characterized by hepatocellular necrosis and fibrosis secondary to progressive injury leading to cirrhosis. More recently, this distinction has been abandoned in favor of a more descriptive classification categorized by severity of inflammation, degree of fibrosis, type (as outlined above), and lobular location of cellular infiltrate.[10] The older classification is mentioned because it appears widely in much of the existing literature regarding AIH.

Histologically, AIH is a more aggressive disorder than many other forms of hepatitis. The features of unresolving active hepatitis for more than 4 to 6 months on liver biopsy, coupled with the findings of hyperglobulinemia and autoantibodies is characteristic of the diagnosis of AIH.[9] The histopathology of the liver biopsy is crucial in determining the severity of the disease. The coexistence of another autoimmune disorder (e.g., autoimmune thyroiditis, ulcerative colitis, hemolytic anemia, celiac disease, myasthenia gravis, or mixed connective tissue disorders) in these patients is also a clue to the diagnosis.

LABORATORY EVALUATION

The essential laboratory evaluation begins with screening for hepatic synthetic dysfunction prothrombin time, partial thromboplastin time (PTT), serum albumin, and total protein. Liver transaminases, bilirubin, and gamma-glutamyltransferase phosphate (GGTP) may indicate hepatocyte damage or biliary dysfunction, respectively. If the findings do not indicate the need for supportive measures — which is the priority — the pursuit of the etiology of the hepatitis may begin. Initial serologic screening for hepatitis A, B, and C and for EBV and CMV as well as for metabolic diseases such as Wilson's disease and alpha-1-antitrypsin deficiency is the first priority. When these possibilities have been excluded, specific laboratory tests for AIH should be obtained, including quantitative globulins and autoantibodies. The autoantibody panel should include ANA, anti-actin (anti-smooth muscle) antibody, and anti-LKM 1 antibody. The presence of antimitochondrial antibodies is rare, but in isolation they usually signify the presence of primary biliary cirrhosis; depending on the commercial assay, it may also be confused with the actual presence of anti-LKM antibodies. Anti-LKM antibody suggests type II.

TREATMENT

Despite the spectrum of disease severity, AIH is generally responsive to corticosteroid therapy. Without treatment, most adults and adolescents with severe AIH die within 3 years.[11] In general, the prognosis is inversely correlated with the histologic severity of the disease.[12] Of the adult patients who had bridging necrosis on initial biopsy, 19% developed cirrhosis. The remission rate induced by initial corticosteroid therapy is reported to be approximately 80%. Reports show that approximately 50% of treated patients remain in remission or only have mild disease activity when medication is withdrawn (after initial treatment); however, most require long-term maintenance therapy. Treatment failures are estimated at 20% and occur more frequently in patients whose initial biopsies had established cirrhosis, in patients diagnosed at a young age, and in patients with HLA B8 or DR3 phenotypes.[1]

Treatment with prednisone (2 mg/kg/day to a maximum of 60 mg/day orally) should be instituted in patients with AIH in which the liver histology indicates severe hepatitis, with or without cirrhosis. In patients with mild hepatitis on biopsy, treatment may not be required immediately. The clinical and histologic disease must be carefully monitored. Rarely does a patient with AIH enter remission spontaneously. Although corticosteroids are the backbone of therapy for AIH, some cases require a limitation of the dose secondary to the long-term side effects of steroids (i.e., hypertension, cataracts, diabetes mellitus, severe growth failure or decreased bone density). A reduction in the steroid dose can be accomplished by concomitant administration of azathioprine (steroid-sparing therapy). In many patients, maintenance therapy with low-dose prednisone alone (5 to 15 mg) or in combination with azathioprine (50 to 150 mg) is successful. Some patients do well on long-term maintenance therapy with azathioprine alone at a dose of 2 mg/kg. Azathioprine carries with it the side effects of bone marrow suppression and immunosuppression and other rare side effects, such as pancreatitis, alopecia, and hypersensitivity skin rash.

PROGNOSIS

The prognosis and likelihood of response to medication appear to be similar for all subdivisions of AIH, with a slightly higher response rate in patients with type I who have anti-actin antibodies. A study from the Mayo Clinic explored the pattern of response to therapy in AIH and found that if remission does not occur within 4 years of beginning therapy the patient was highly unlikely to respond later. Patients who were nonresponders and received liver transplants had a 5-year survival rate of 92% without evidence of recurrence of AIH.[13]

There are no firm guidelines for withdrawal or reduction of immunosupressant medications, particularly because histologic changes may lag behind biochemical and clinical changes. However, one reliable index for adequate therapy is to follow the serum aminotransferase levels and to attempt to control them within two times the upper limit of normal. Decreased inflammation or mild histologic activity on biopsy is not predictive of long-term remission after treatment has been discontinued. When treatment fails, increasing inflammation results in worsening cirrhosis with eventual need for liver transplantation, or death.

REFERRAL PATTERN

Patients who are diagnosed with, or are suspected of having, AIH should be monitored closely for progressive disease, with medications needing to be titrated accordingly. These patients should be referred to a gastroenterologist.

REFERENCES

1. Maddrey WC. Chronic hepatitis. Disease-a-Month St Louis: Mosby-Year Book, Inc. 1993;57–125

2. Poley JR. Chronic hepatitis (HB surface-antigen negative). In: Gracey M, Bunke V, Eds. Pediatric Gastroenterology and Hepatology. Boston: Blackwell Scientific Publication 1993: 685–695

3. Lenzi M, Ballardini G, Fusconi M, et al. Type 2 autoimmune hepatitis and Hepatitis C infection. Lancet 1990;335: 258–259

4. Czaja AJ. Natural history, clinical features and treatment of autoimmune hepatitis. Semin Liver Dis 1984;4:1

5. Maddrey WC. Subdivisions of idiopathic autoimmune chronic active hepatitis. Hepatology 1987;7:1372

6. Manns M. Autoantibodies and antigens in liver disease—updated. J Hepatol 1989;9(2):272–280

7. Friedman LS, Patel KP, Munoz SJ. Hepatitis C virus and autoimmune chronic active hepatitis: closing the ring. Gastroenterology 1992;102:1436–1438

8. Mews C, Sinatra F. Chronic liver disease in children. Pediatr Rev 1993;14:998–1005

9. Krawitt EL, Wiesner R. Autoimmune Liver Disease. New York: Raven Press, 1991:21–42

10. Desmet VJ, Gerber M, Hoofnagle JH et al. Classification of chronic hepatitis: diagnosis, grading and staging, review. Hepatology 1994;19:1513–1520

11. Geall MD, Schoenfield JJ, Summerskill WHJ. Classification and treatment of chronic active liver disease. Gastroenterology 1968;55:724

12. Krawitt EL. Autoimmune hepatitis. N Engl Med 1996;334: 897–903

13. Sanchez-Urdazpal L, Czaja AJ, Van Hoek B. Prognostic features in the role of liver transplantation in severe corticosteroid-treated autoimmune chronic active hepatitis. Hepatology 1991;15:215

48

BILIARY ATRESIA

KAREN F. MURRAY
MAUREEN M. JONAS

Extrahepatic biliary atresia (EHBA) is a disorder that results in progressive destruction of the extrahepatic biliary system with variable involvement of intrahepatic bile ducts. It is the most common hepatic surgical disorder in infancy and is a major cause of childhood cirrhosis and liver failure.[1] The incidence is 1 in 10,000 to 20,000 live births, and it is 1.4 times more common in females than males.[2] Between 10% and 25% of cases are associated with congenital anomalies. Although medical management is important in the care of these patients, surgical intervention is required for long-term survival. The surgical outcome is in part dependent on early diagnosis and referral to a tertiary care facility skilled in the management of EHBA. Consequently, a high index of suspicion is required for pediatricians who encounter jaundiced infants in the first weeks of life. With prompt identification and referral, expert surgical care, and liver transplantation, long-term survival and quality of life in these patients have been markedly improved.

ETIOLOGY AND PATHOPHYSIOLOGY

In the embryo, the biliary system develops from two primary components of the hepatic diverticulum, a foregut-derived bud of cells arising at 4 weeks gestation. The intrahepatic and proximal extrahepatic portions of the biliary tree arise from the cranial portion of the hepatic diverticulum, and the caudal portion of the diverticulum gives rise to the gallbladder and the cystic and common bile ducts.[3] Despite the separate origins of the intrahe-

patic and extrahepatic ducts, there appears to be luminal continuity between them throughout organogenesis.[4] Approximately 20% to 25% of cases of EHBA have a primitive embryonic shape to their interlobular ducts, suggesting that the abnormality starts early in fetal life in these cases.[3,4]

The etiology of EHBA is unknown. There is no race predilection, and twin studies are inconclusive. The low incidence in dizygotic twins makes perinatal autoimmune processes or infection unlikely. The latter, however, continues to be actively investigated, and several viral agents have been studied. No association with hepatitis A or B, cytomegalovirus (CMV), or rubella has been found.[5] Serologic testing and immunohistochemical staining of hepatobiliary tissue for reovirus 3 have provided conflicting results,[6,7] but more recently the lack of detection of reoviral RNA, using polymerase chain reaction (PCR), in the tissue from many patients, has indicated that reovirus 3 is not likely a causative agent.[8] A vascular accident resulting in fibrosis, or malunion of the pancreatic and biliary ducts resulting in pancreatic reflux, has been suggested, but lack of related abnormalities and anatomic corroboration make these unlikely. There is some evidence that immunogenetic factors may be involved in susceptibility to EHBA. There is a significantly higher frequency of HLA-B12, and of haplotypes A9-B5 and A28-B35, as compared to controls, especially among patients without associated malformations (relative risk of 2.61 among all patients, and 3.23 among patients without associated extrahepatic anomalies).[9]

EHBA is a progressive disease that, if left untreated,

advances over months to years until bile duct obliteration results in biliary cirrhosis and liver failure. The disease process may affect both the intra-and extrahepatic ducts. In 10% to 15% of cases, only the distal biliary tree is affected, whereas in 85% to 90% there is fibrosis of the entire extrahepatic biliary tree.[2] Histologically, initially there is preservation of the basic hepatic architecture, but periductal mononuclear inflammation causes progressive epithelial damage. For approximately 6 months after birth, intrahepatic bile duct hyperplasia is seen, followed by bile duct degeneration.[2] Obstructed bile flow results in cholestasis within the hepatic parenchyma. Eventually, the bile ducts are replaced with fibrous tissue. At presentation, the degree of hepatic damage and biliary obstruction varies from patient to patient.

CLINICAL PRESENTATION

Typically, infants with EHBA are born full term after a normal pregnancy and are usually normal at birth. The conjugated bilirubinemia of EHBA generally develops at 2 to 6 weeks. Because this is after the peak incidence of physiologic jaundice, it is relatively easy to miss, unless there is a high index of suspicion. Consequently, any infant who has persistent hyperbilirubinemia after 2 weeks of age should have the conjugated component of the total bilirubin determined.

Despite their jaundice, patients with EHBA usually appear healthy. Initially, their weight gain and development are normal. Hepatomegaly, with a firm or hard liver, can be present early, and splenomegaly is sometimes present. Because of the high conjugated component of the bilirubin, the skin will frequently have a greenish hue. Dark urine and clay-colored, acholic stools are occasionally present at birth; however, these more commonly develop over the first 6 weeks.

Associated anomalies are found in 10% to 25% of patients with EHBA. Approximately 30% of these, or 4% to 12% of all EHBA patients, have some features of the polyasplenia sequence: polysplenia, cardiovascular malformations, abdominal heterotaxia, intestinal malrotation, and anomalies of the portal vein and hepatic artery.[1] Another 12% of all EHBA patients have anomalies that do not follow a recognizable pattern. The organ systems most commonly involved are the cardiovascular, GI, and urinary systems.[1]

DIAGNOSIS

In any infant with persistent hyperbilirubinemia beyond 2 weeks of age, determination of the conjugated bilirubin component is required. A direct bilirubin level greater than 2.0 mg/dl or greater than 15% of the total bilirubin

level warrants evaluation for infectious, metabolic, and anatomic abnormalities; close observation with appropriate consultation should be obtained.[10] Since the treatment outcome of many conditions causing cholestasis is reliant on early diagnosis, the evaluation should not be delayed.

There are no unique clinical signs of EHBA. Clay-colored stools, often associated with EHBA, are not pathognomonic of this condition but are also seen in patients with a variety of anatomic abnormalities, infections, and metabolic liver diseases.[11] Consequently, laboratory and radiographic studies are required to distinguish EHBA from other causes of infantile cholestasis (Fig. 48-1).

After consideration of infectious and relevant metabolic disorders, the first radiographic study for possible structural biliary abnormalities is ultrasonography. Although this study is important to rule out other obstructive abnormalities, such as a choledochal cyst, it is frequently nondiagnostic in EHBA. The gallbladder may or may not be visualized despite a 4-to 6-hour fast, and the common bile duct, although never dilated, may appear normal in caliber or may not be visualized. Suggestive associated abnormalities, such as polysplenia or heterotaxia, may be detected by ultrasonography.

The patency of the extrahepatic biliary system may be demonstrated by radionuclide scanning, a technique that has become standard in the radiographic diagnosis of EHBA. Technetium-99-labeled diisopropyl iminodiacetic acid (DISIDA) and other derivatives are taken up by hepatocytes and excreted by the bile. The excretion of DISIDA can be enhanced with phenobarbital, administered for 3 to 5 days prior to the study, at 5 mg/kg/day in two daily doses. Biliary obstruction is suggested by uptake of the radionuclide by the liver, but failure to excrete it into the duodenum (Fig. 48-2). Uptake of the radionuclide is generally reflective of hepatocellular function; decreased uptake, although usually seen in hepatitis, can also be seen in advanced EHBA, where hepatic dysfunction is already established. If no isotope is detected in the intestinal lumen, even after delayed scanning (4 to 24 hours), EHBA remains a possibility, and the workup must continue. However, false-positive DISIDA scans may occur with severe cholestasis of any etiology.

Although some have reported the use of endoscopic retrograde cholangiopancreatography in diagnosing EHBA,[12] experience with this technique in neonates is limited, and nonvisualization of the extrahepatic tree does not constitute specific evidence of the condition.[13]

When the DISIDA scan does not demonstrate patency of the extrahepatic biliary system, percutaneous liver biopsy is frequently performed for histologic diagnosis. Bile duct proliferation with cholestasis and fibrosis are the characteristic features of the disease (Fig. 48-3). These features may not be well established and diagnos-

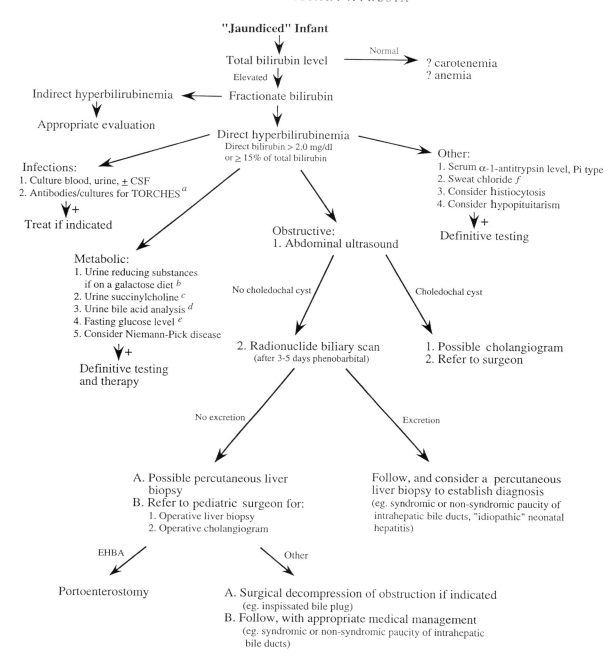

"Jaundiced" Infant

Total bilirubin level — Normal → ? carotenemia / ? anemia

Elevated ↓

Fractionate bilirubin

Indirect hyperbilirubinemia ←
↓
Appropriate evaluation

Direct hyperbilirubinemia
Direct bilirubin > 2.0 mg/dl
or ≥ 15% of total bilirubin

Other:
1. Serum α-1-antitrypsin level, Pi type
2. Sweat chloride *f*
3. Consider histiocytosis
4. Consider hypopituitarism
↓ +
Definitive testing

Infections:
1. Culture blood, urine, ± CSF
2. Antibodies/cultures for TORCHES *a*
↓ +
Treat if indicated

Metabolic:
1. Urine reducing substances
   if on a galactose diet *b*
2. Urine succinylcholine *c*
3. Urine bile acid analysis *d*
4. Fasting glucose level *e*
5. Consider Niemann-Pick disease
↓ +
Definitive testing
and therapy

Obstructive:
1. Abdominal ultrasound

No choledochal cyst / Choledochal cyst

2. Radionuclide biliary scan
(after 3-5 days phenobarbital)

1. Possible cholangiogram
2. Refer to surgeon

No excretion / Excretion

A. Possible percutaneous liver
   biopsy
B. Refer to pediatric surgeon for:
   1. Operative liver biopsy
   2. Operative cholangiogram

Follow, and consider a percutaneous
liver biopsy to establish diagnosis
(eg. syndromic or non-syndromic paucity of
intrahepatic bile ducts, "idiopathic" neonatal
hepatitis)

EHBA / Other

Portoenterostomy

A. Surgical decompression of obstruction if indicated
   (eg. inspissated bile plug)
B. Follow, with appropriate medical management
   (eg. syndromic or non-syndromic paucity of intrahepatic
   bile ducts)

FIGURE 48-1. Evaluation of the infant with hyperbilirubinemia. *a* Toxoplasmosis, rubella, cytomegalovirus, herpes, syphilis; *b* galactosemia; *c* tyrosinemia; *d* bile acid disorders; *e* glycogen storage disease III or IV; *f* cystic fibrosis.

tic during the first few weeks, occasionally making early diagnosis problematic. In this circumstance, if a specific diagnosis has not been made through other means, either repeat liver biopsy or surgical cholangiography is indicated.

When radiographic and histologic evidence is suggestive of EHBA surgical exploration is indicated for definitive diagnosis and therapeutic intervention. Direct visualization usually depicts a nodular, greenish brown liver with a small fibrous gallbladder. An intraoperative cholangiogram is performed by injecting contrast into the gallbladder, to elucidate the extent of the ductular patency. The findings of the intraoperative cholangiogram and biopsy dictate the subsequent therapeutic intervention. If patency of the extrahepatic biliary tree is not demonstrated, careful dissection to the porta hepatis is undertaken until bile flow is established. A portoenterostomy (described below) is then performed.

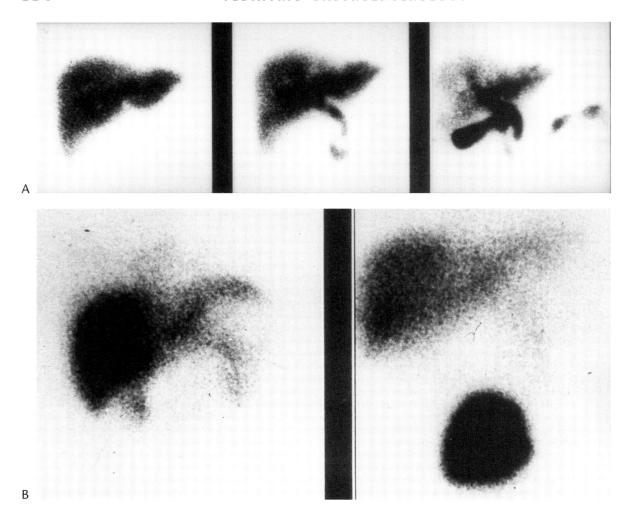

FIGURE 48-2. Characteristic radionuclide (DISIDA) scan findings in EHBA. (*A*) Normal DISIDA scan showing good hepatic uptake of the radioisotope, excretion into the gallbladder and extrahepatic bile ducts, and subsequent excretion into the intestine. (*B*) DISIDA scan in an infant with EHBA showing uptake of the radioisotope into the liver, but failure of excretion into the extrahepatic bile ducts or intestine. Radioisotope is seen in the kidneys and urinary bladder.

LABORATORY STUDIES

There are no diagnostic or specific laboratory tests for EHBA. The hallmark of the condition is cholestasis with resultant jaundice. Despite complete obstruction of biliary outflow, the total bilirubin level is usually initially 5 to 15 mg/dl and is 50% to 80% conjugated. As the disease progresses and hepatocellular injury ensues, however, the total bilirubin level can increase to 30 mg/dl. At diagnosis, the serum aminotransferases are usually moderately elevated, up to two to three times normal. As a result of the biliary obstruction, alkaline phosphatase and gamma-glutamyl transpeptidase (GGTP) are frequently markedly elevated early in the course of the disease. Initially, the prothrombin time (PT) and partial thrombo-plastin time (PTT) are normal, but as fat malabsorption causes vitamin K deficiency, elevation of both values, but predominantly the PT, occurs. As the synthetic capacity of the liver decreases, the PT is no longer responsive to vitamin K administration. Additionally, the serum albumin level decreases with progressive hepatic dysfunction. When hypersplenism complicates splenomegaly, thrombocytopenia and neutropenia result.

TREATMENT

The first suggestion that EHBA could be surgically corrected by anastomosis of the biliary tract to the bowel was in 1916.[14] However, this report by Holmes was based on postmortem observations, and it was not until 1928 that the first reported surgical correction was attempted.[15] The next 30 years saw little advancement in treatment until, in 1955, Kasai et al.[16] described a procedure that could be applied to all patients with EHBA, regardless of the extent of bile duct involvement. Although there have been several modifications of this procedure since its initial description, the basic portoenterostomy described by Kasai and colleagues remains the standard surgical therapy for EHBA.

Portoenterostomy

Surgery entails dissection of the biliary remnant proximal to the level of the porta hepatis, as necessary to achieve bile flow. The exposed hepatic tissue in the hilum of the liver is then anastomosed to a 20 to 45-cm Roux-en-Y loop of jejunum (Fig. 48-4). In this way, drainage of bile directly into the intestine is achieved.

When the rare patient who has atresia only of the distal biliary tree is encountered, a choledochojejunostomy may be performed, which allows anastomosis of the unaffected proximal bile duct or gallbladder to the Roux-en-Y jejunal loop.

Some modifications of the original Kasai procedure included exteriorization of biliary drainage, in attempts to avoid the complication of ascending cholangitis. However, this practice was complicated by stomal variceal bleeding, increased malabsorption, stomal prolapse, and increased morbidity with subsequent surgery. Consequently, this practice has been largely abandoned, and now, with the routine use of liver transplantation, exteriorization of biliary drainage should not be performed.[2] More recent modifications have involved the creation of an antireflux valve in the intestinal conduit, again in an attempt to decrease the incidence of ascending cholangitis after surgery. Some investigators have reported a decrease in the incidence of postoperative cholangitis,[2] but this remains controversial.

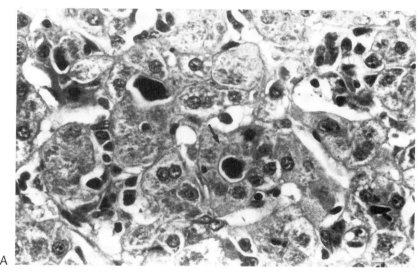

A

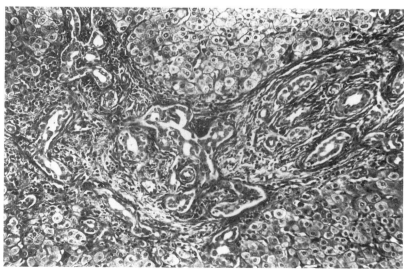

B

FIGURE 48-3. Histologic features of EHBA. (*A*) Pseudoacinar formation (arrow) with dilated bile-filled canaliculi (H&E, × 250). (*B*) Portal fibrosis and bile duct hyperplasia (Masson trichome, × 40).

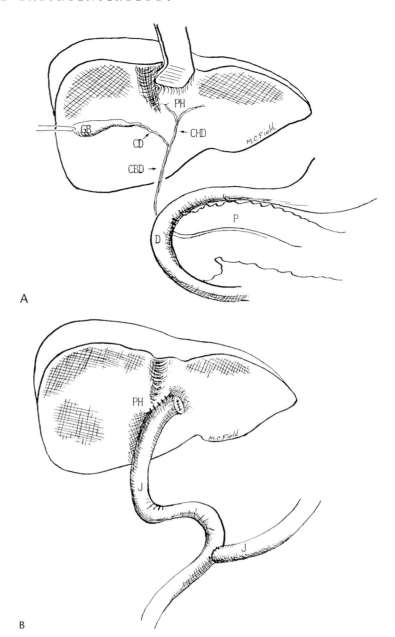

FIGURE 48-4. (*A*) Schematic diagram of the underside of the liver with the fibrotic biliary system in EHBA showing involvement of the entire extrahepatic biliary system. (*B*) Portoenterostomy, with the Roux-en-Y jejunal loop anastomosed to the porta hepatis. PH, porta hepatis; GB, gallbladder; CD, cystic duct; CHD, common hepatic duct; CBD, common bile duct; D, duodenum; J, jejunum; P, pancreas. (Illustrations by Marcia C. Field.)

The short-term prognosis after portoenterostomy, although somewhat dependent on a number of variables, is determined primarily by the age of the patient at surgery. In almost all studies correlating age at surgery with the rate of becoming jaundice-free postsurgery, there is a higher rate of success at younger patient age. Surgery performed before 60 days of age is successful in 70% to 80% of cases, whereas if surgery is delayed to 90 days the success rate drops to 20% to 30%.[2,17,18] Hence the importance of prompt diagnosis and referral of patients suspected of having EHBA. Successful outcome also correlates with less hepatic fibrosis and with a larger size of remaining ductules at the porta hepatis.[17] Although ductal size correlates with surgical success in achieving bile flow, there is controversy as to whether the degree of ductal patency correlates with survival. One study of 191 patients found that there was no linear correlation between the probability of survival and the ductal diameter at the porta hepatis, but total obliteration of the ducts and absence of inflammation were associated with poor prognosis. Interestingly, there was no correlation between the degree of portal inflammation and patient age.[19]

COMPLICATIONS

Cholangitis

The most common complication after portoenterostomy is ascending cholangitis, which occurs in 50% to 100% of cases.[2,10,18] It usually occurs within 2 years of surgery and is more common in those patients in whom bile drainage is achieved. Patients with cholangitis are usually febrile (greater than 38°C), but only 75% of patients will have a rise in bilirubin level. Most will develop an increase in serum alkaline phosphatase and aminotransferase levels, but this may occur late in the course of infection. Although blood cultures should be obtained, they will be positive in the minority of cases. Definitive diagnosis can be made only by histologic examination and culture of the liver tissue. With blood and hepatic tissue cultures, an organism may be identified in up to 75% of cases. Most organisms identified are gram-negative rods, including *Pseudomonas*, although gram-positive cocci, *Candida*, and *Haemophilus influenzae* have been reported. Cholangitis is believed to be a polymicrobial infection, and aggressive antibiotic therapy is indicated with broad spectrum coverage, to include treatment for anaerobes, for three to six weeks, intravenously. The use of prophylactic antibiotics, although advocated by some, has not been shown to reduce the incidence of cholangitis.

Portal Hypertension

Portal hypertension is frequently present at the diagnosis of EHBA. Not surprisingly then, approximately 70% of patients will develop esophageal varices after the portoenterostomy, with a 40% to 80% prevalence by 5 years of age.[2,10] Recurrent bleeding is a major problem in these patients. Obliterative sclerotherapy or band ligation of esophageal varices is currently the therapy of choice. The use of beta-adrenergic antagonist agents to decrease portal pressure has been used with some success.[20] In patients with recurrent bleeding despite these maneuvers, surgical or transjugular intrahepatic portosystemic shunting may be palliative until a liver transplant is available.[20]

Malnutrition

Chronic cholestasis results in fat malabsorption, and consequently caloric and fat-soluble vitamin deficiencies. Vitamin D deficiency can result in rickets. Supplementation with ergocalciferol, 5,000 to 8,000 IU/day, is usually required in these patients. Approximately three-fourths of patients will develop vitamin E deficiency,[2] which can result in progressive neurologic symptoms. Supplementation with D-alpha-tocopherol is rarely effective in repleting stores, and a special preparation such as D-alpha-tocopheryl-polyethylene glycol-1000 succinate (TPGS) is often required. Vitamin K deficiency contributes to the coagulopathy in these patients. Supplementation with 2.5 to 5 mg/day with mephyton or phytonadione can be provided; however, intramuscular injections are frequently required. Vitamin A deficiency can be prevented by supplementing with water-soluble vitamin A, 5,000 to 15,000 IU/day. Levels of vitamins A, D, and E should be monitored, and vitamin K moni-

tored with PT values. Additionally, patients with EHBA have altered metabolism of some micronutrients and increased energy requirements. Their growth and weight gain should be monitored regularly, since supplemental tube feedings are often needed. Maintaining an optimal nutritional status is important, especially in anticipation of possible hepatic transplantation.

Portoenterostomy has provided a therapeutic option for patients with EHBA However, even if surgery is performed within 60 days of birth, the overall 5-year survival is approximately 50%,[21] and the 10-year survival is 30% to 36%.[2,18,22] This decrease in survival over time reflects not only mortality from complications, but also progression of the hepatic disease despite surgery. Disease progression may be the result of repeated bouts of cholangitis, an underlying panhepatic inflammatory process, or a consequence of ongoing extrahepatic biliary obstruction despite the decompressing surgery.[23] Overall, no more than 20% to 30% of patients will reach adult life and be cured of their disease. Approximately 30% of patients will have their disease palliated by the portoenterostomy and live an extended life. However, they will become liver transplant candidates at 5 to 15 years of age. In the remaining 30% to 40% of patients the Kasai procedure will not be successful; without a liver transplant, these patients will die of liver failure before age two.[18]

With ongoing hepatocellular damage, fibrosis progresses to cirrhosis, leading to failure of the liver's ability to synthesize clotting factors, albumin, and other vital proteins. Signs of hepatic failure may appear as early as 3 months of age in patients in whom the diagnosis has been delayed, or in whom adequate biliary drainage has not been secured surgically. The resultant hypoalbuminemia causes edema and ascites; decreased synthesis of the clotting factors I (fibrinogen), II (prothrombin), V, VII, IX, and X, exacerbated by hypersplenism with thrombocytopenia, and fat malabsorption (vitamin K), causes a coagulopathy. Portal hypertension is present in approximately 70% of patients by 2 to 4 months of age, and commonly at diagnosis. Portal hypertension is initially manifest as splenomegaly, but can later contribute to GI bleeding.

Left untreated, the average life expectancy of the patient with EHBA, is approximately 11 months,[10] with death occurring most commonly from massive gastrointestinal bleeding, or overwhelming bacterial infection. Fewer than 10% of untreated patients survive beyond 3 years.

Transplantation

Approximately 80% of patients with biliary atresia will eventually require liver transplantation despite timely portoenterostomy. It is not surprising that EHBA is the most common indication for liver transplantation in the pediatric age group, and accounts for approximately 50% of transplants performed in major series.[18] Indications for transplantation after portoenterostomy include hepatic insufficiency, portal hypertension with recurrent bleeding and/or ascites, hepatopulmonary syndrome, irreversible failure to thrive, repeated cholangitis, intractable pruritis, and persistent cholestasis.

Because of the frequent need for transplantation among patients with EHBA, some investigators have advocated primary transplantation in this disorder. Portoenterostomy, however, will be curative in roughly 20% of patients. Furthermore, it provides a longer pretransplant interval for family education, development of optimal nutrition and growth in the patient, and, most significantly, a larger donor pool associated with increased recipient size.[24] Consequently, most investigators consider the two procedures complementary.

The long-term survival of patients after transplantation is 80% to 88%, when performed electively.[18,25] This decreases to approximately 65% when the procedure is required urgently.[18] With the newer techniques of using split livers and living-related donors for pediatric recipients, the donor pool for these patients has increased. This allows more patients to undergo transplantation electively, when in optimal condition, with a better chance for long-term survival.

REFERRAL PATTERN

The pediatrician's role is critical in the early identification and initial evaluation of these patients. Any infant suspected of having EHBA should be promptly referred to a facility experienced in the diagnosis and management of the disease. As most of these patients ultimately require a liver transplant, it is also important that the patient be evaluated by a center experienced in anticipating the timing of a transplant. Given the complicated nature of EHBA, the chronic care of these patients requires the combined efforts of the pediatrician, pediatric gastroenterologist, and pediatric surgeon.

ACKNOWLEDGMENTS

Dr. Murray was in part supported by the NIH Training Grant in Pediatric Gastroenterology and Nutrition, T32-DK07477.

REFERENCES

1. Carmi R, Magee CA, Neill CA, Karrer FM. Extrahepatic biliary atresia and associated anomalies: etiologic heterogeneity suggested by distinctive patterns of associations. Am J Med Genet 1993;45:683–693

2. Stein JE, Vacanti JP. Biliary atresia and other disorders of the extrahepatic biliary tree. In: Suchy FJ, Ed. Liver Disease in Children. St. Louis: CV Mosby, 1994:426–442

3. Desmet VJ. Congenital disease of intrahepatic bile ducts: variations on the theme "ductal plate malformation." Hepatology 1992;16:1069–1083

4. Tan CEL, Moscoso GJ. The developing human biliary system at the porta hepatis level between 11 and 25 weeks of gestation: a way to understanding biliary atresia, Part 2. Pathol Int 1994;44:600–610

5. Balistreri WF, Schubert WK. Liver disease in infancy and childhood. In: Schiff L, Schiff ER, Eds. Diseases of the Liver 7th Ed. Philadelphia: JB Lippincott, 1993:1099–1203

6. Brown WR, Sokol RJ, Levin MJ et al. Lack of correlation between infection with reovirus 3 and extrahepatic biliary atresia or neonatal hepatitis. J Pediatr 1988;113:670–676

7. Morecki R, Glaser J. Reovirus 3 and neonatal biliary disease: discussion of divergent results. Hepatology 1989; 10:515–517

8. Steele MI, Marshall CM, Lloyd RE, Randolph VE. Reovirus 3 not detected by reverse transcriptase-mediated polymerase chain reaction analysis of preserved tissue from infants with cholestatic liver disease. Hepatology 1995;21:697–702

9. Silveira TR, Salzano FM, Donaldson PT et al. Association between HLA and extrahepatic biliary atresia. J Pediatr Gastroenterol Nutr 1993;16:114–117

10. Piccoli DA, Witzleben CL. Disorders of the extrahepatic bile ducts. In: Walker WA, Durie PR, Hamilton JR et al., Eds. Pediatric Gastrointestinal Disease; Pathophysiology, Diagnosis, Management. Philadelphia: BC Decker, 1991: 1140–1151

11. Lai M-W, Chang M-H, Hsu S-C et al. Differential diagnosis of extrahepatic biliary atresia from neonatal hepatitis: a prospective study. J Pediatr Gastroenterol Nutr 1994;18: 121–127

12. Guelrud M, Jaen D, Torres P et al. Endoscopic cholangiopancreatography in the infant: evaluation of a new prototype pediatric duodenoscope. Gastrointest Endosc 1987; 33:4–8

13. Heyman MB, Shapiro HA, Thaler MM. Endoscopic retrograde cholangiography in the diagnosis of biliary malformations in infants. Gastrointest Endosc 1988;34:449–453

14. Holmes JB. Congenital obliteration of the bile ducts. Am J Dis Child 1916;11:405–430

15. Ladd WE. Congenital atresia and the stenosis of the bile ducts. JAMA 1928;91:1082

16. Kasai M, Kimura S, Asakura Y et al. Surgical treatment of biliary atresia. J Pediatr Surg 1968;3:665–675

17. Miyano T, Fujimoto T, Ohya T, Shimomura H. Current concept of the treatment of biliary atresia. World J Surg 1993;17:332–336

18. Otte J-B, de Goyet JdV, Reding R et al. Sequential treatment of biliary atresia with Kasai portoenterostomy and liver transplantation: a review. Hepatology 1994;20:41S–48S

19. Tan CEL, Davenport M, Driver M, Howard ER. Does the morphology of the extrahepatic biliary remnants in biliary atresia influence survival? A review of 205 cases. J Pediatr Surg 1994;29:1459–1464

20. Hassall E. Nonsurgical treatments for portal hypertension in children. Gastrointest Endosc Clin North Am 1994;4: 223–258

21. Emblem R, Stake G, Monclair T. Progress in the treatment of biliary atresia: a plea for surgical intervention within the first two months of life in infants with persistent cholestasis. Acta Paediatr 1993;82:971–974

22. Toyosaka A, Okamoto E, Okasora T et al. Outcome of 21 patients with biliary atresia living more than 10 years. J Pediatr Surg 1993;28:1498–1501

23. Nietgen GW, Vacanti JP, Perez-Atayde AR. Intrahepatic bile duct loss in biliary atresia despite portoenterostomy: a consequence of ongoing obstruction? Gastroenterology 1992;102:2126–2133

24. Ryckman F, Fisher R, Pedersen S et al. Improved survival in biliary atresia patients in the present era of liver transplantation. J Pediatr Surg 1993;28:382–386

25. Kalayoglu M, D'Alessandro AM, Knechtle SJ et al. Long-term results of liver transplantation for biliary atresia. Surgery 1993;114:711–717

49

CONGENITAL ANOMALIES OF THE PANCREAS AND BILIARY TRACT

JANICE B. HEIKENEN
STEVEN L. WERLIN

ANNULAR PANCREAS

The incidence of annular pancreas is unknown. An autopsy series in adults found only 3 cases in 20,000 autopsies. Annular pancreas may be associated with Down's syndrome, malrotation, intrinsic duodenal obstruction, cardiac disease, intestinal atresia, imperforate anus, and pancreatitis.

Pathophysiology

Annular pancreas results from incomplete rotation of the left (ventral) pancreatic anlage. The obstruction is caused by a flat band of tissue partially or completely surrounding the second portion of the duodenum.[1] Anatomically, there may be an associated pancreas divisum (see below) or other ductal abnormalities.[2]

Clinical Presentation

Annular pancreas may present at any age from infancy to adulthood. In a review of 281 cases, Kiernan reported that one-half of these patients presented in childhood and one-half in infancy.[3] In this study, 86% of pediatric cases presented in the newborn period. The age of presentation is dependent on the degree of obstruction and associated congenital anomalies. When presenting in infancy, patients with annular pancreas typically manifest symptoms of complete or partial bowel obstruction, such as bilious vomiting and abdominal distention. Many patients have a history of maternal polyhydramnios. After infancy, children may present with abdominal pain, feeding intolerance, chronic vomiting, pancreatitis, biliary colic, gastric outlet obstruction, and peptic ulcer disease.

Physical Examination

Physical examination in the child may be normal or may demonstrate abdominal distention, abdominal tenderness, and jaundice. Infants are typically distended.

Diagnosis

Plain abdominal radiographs show the classic "double bubble," characteristic of duodenal obstruction in the infant. An upper gastrointestinal (GI) examination done cautiously with a small amount of water-soluble contrast will confirm the presence of duodenal obstruction (Fig. 49-1). The differential diagnosis of duodenal obstruction in the newborn includes duodenal atresia and stenosis, duodenal web, and volvulus. Prenatal diagnosis has been made by ultrasonography. In the older child, an upper GI series is required to make the diagnosis. Typical findings include dilation and reverse peristalsis of the proximal duodenum and a filling defect in the second portion of the duodenum. Diagnosis of difficult cases has been aided by endoscopic retrograde cholangiopancreatography (ERCP).

Treatment

The treatment of choice is duodenojejunostomy. Division of the pancreatic ring is not attempted, since a duodenal diaphragm or duodenal stenosis frequently accompanies annular pancreas. Morbidity and mortality is related to associated congenital anomalies.

PANCREAS DIVISUM

Pancreas divisum, which occurs in 5% to 15% of the general population, is the most common developmental anomaly of the pancreas.

Pathophysiology

As a result of failure of the dorsal and ventral pancreatic anlagen to fuse, the tail, body, and part of the head of the pancreas drain through the smaller accessary duct of Santorini, rather than through the main duct of Wir-

sung.[1] It has been proposed that relative obstruction of the accessory duct of Santorini may lead to the development of pancreatitis.

Clinical Presentation

While the clinical importance of this anomaly remains controversial, most investigators believe that pancreas divisum may be associated with recurrent pancreatitis, possibly due to relative obstruction ventral pancreas outflow.[4] Thus, patients present with recurrent episodes of pancreatitis.

Physical Examination

The child with acute pancreatitis has steady epigastric abdominal pain, with or without persistent vomiting and fever. The child may assume an antalgic position with hips and knees flexed, sitting upright or lying on the side. The abdomen may be distended and quite tender, and a mass may be palpable. The pain increases in intensity for 24 to 48 hours, during which vomiting may increase; the patient may require hospitalization for dehydration and fluid and electrolyte therapy. Between attacks, the physical examination is normal.

FIGURE 49-1. Annular pancreas. Classic "double bubble" finding of dilated stomach (S) and proximal duodenum (D). (*A*) Plain film. (*B*) Contrast study. (Courtesy of John R. Sty, M.D.)

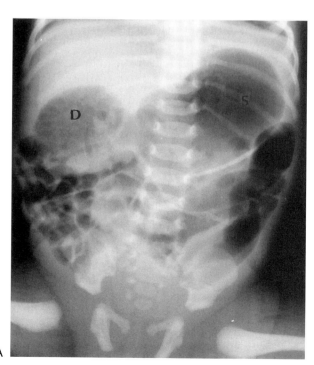

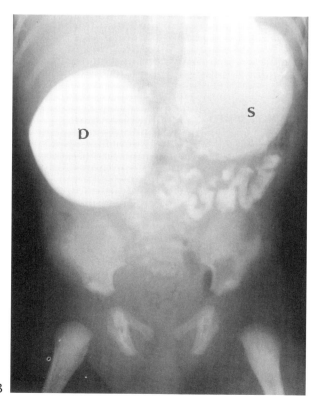

A

B

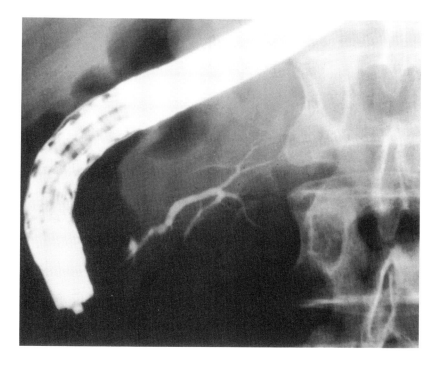

FIGURE 49-2. Pancreas divisum. Injection of the major papilla fills the rudimentary ventral duct of Wirsung, which only drains the head of the pancreas. (From Werlin[15] with permission.)

Diagnosis

The diagnosis of pancreas divisum can be made only by ERCP (Fig. 49-2).

Treatment

Management of patients with pancreas divisum and recurrent pancreatitis remains controversial.[4,5] While a variety of surgical and therapeutic endoscopic procedures have been attempted with only mixed success, recent data suggest that for adults, endoscopic sphincterotomy or surgical sphincteroplasty is beneficial in selected patients. Unfortunately, the long-term consequences of sphincterotomy in children are unknown. We recommend endoscopic insertion of a stent into the minor papilla in children with recurrent pancreatitis and pancreas divisum. If episodes of pancreatitis stop occurring or occur only when the stent becomes dislodged or occluded, we recommend surgical sphincteroplasty.

ECTOPIC PANCREAS

Ectopic pancreatic rests in the stomach or small intestine occur in about 3% of the population. Aberrant pancreatic tissue has also been found in a variety of intra-abdominal locations, including gallbladder, liver, and omentum. Most cases (70%) are found in the upper intestinal tract.[6,7] Recognized on barium contrast studies by their typical umbilicated appearance or at endoscopy, they are rarely of clinical importance. Endoscopic exami-

nation shows typically irregular yellow, submucosal nodules 2 to 4 mm in diameter. A pancreatic rest may, however, be the lead point of an intussusception or bleed or may cause bowel obstruction. Unless a complication develops, no treatment is necessary.

PANCREATIC DYSGENESIS

Varying degrees of pancreatic dysgenesis have been reported.[1] The most severe form, complete agenesis, is not only rare but is incompatible with life. Other forms, including partial agenesis, dysplasia, and hypoplasia, have been reported.

Pathophysiology

Complete and partial agenesis result from a primary defect early in pancreatic organogenesis. In partial agenesis, the pancreatic tissue present is normal, but the gland is defective in size and shape due to lack of development of one of the pancreatic anlagen. Dorsal agenesis is the most common form of partial agenesis. Partial agenesis is also referred to as congenital short pancreas.

By contrast, in pancreatic hypoplasia, the gland develops a normal size and shape, but cellular proliferation proceeds abnormally. The normal pancreatic structures are replaced by fatty tissue. Terminal ductal differentiation is abnormal, causing a reduction in the number of ducts and their terminal differentiation. In pancreatic dysplasia, the parenchyma is disorganized and the ducts are dilated. The underlying etiology of these conditions is unknown, although associated congenital anomalies are common.

Clinical Presentation

Pancreatic agenesis is associated with a fulminant neonatal course, including intrauterine growth retardation (IUGR), diabetes, acidosis, and death. Patients with pancreatic partial agenesis, hypoplasia, and dysplasia may present with signs of pancreatic insufficiency, such as malabsorption and growth failure, or may be completely asymptomatic, depending on the amount of tissue present.[8] Adults with partial agenesis have presented with recurrent pancreatitis. A number of syndromes, including Shwachman's syndrome, Pearson's syndrome, Johanson-Blizzard syndrome, Beckwith-Wiedemann syndrome, and hepatic renal pancreatic dysplasia syndrome, are associated with pancreatic hypoplasia.

Diagnosis

Definitive diagnosis of pancreatic agenesis can be made only at surgery or autopsy. The diagnosis of partial agenesis can made on the basis of computed tomography (CT), (MRI), or ERCP. The diagnosis in most cases was made by chance during evaluation of abdominal pain. The fatty pancreas seen in pancreatic hypoplasia can be detected by CT. Pancreatic function can be determined indirectly by stool collection for fecal fat analysis or directly by intubation of the duodenum and collection of pancreatic juice following stimulation by secretin.

Treatment

Patients with malabsorption due to pancreatic insufficiency are treated with pancreatic enzyme preparations. Associated endocrine insufficiency is treated with insulin.

CHOLEDOCHAL CYST

Choledochal cysts, segmental cystic dilations of the common bile duct, are uncommon congenital abnormalities. Choledochal cysts were initially classified into four anatomic types by Alonzo-Lej (Table 49-1) and have subsequently been modified.[9]

Pathophysiology

While the etiology of choledochal cysts is unknown, the most widely held belief is that an anomalous connection between the pancreatic and common bile ducts may lead to reflux of pancreatic juice into the common bile duct, with resultant ductal irritation and dilation. An alterna-

TABLE 49-1. Types of Choledochal Cyst

Type	Description
I	Fusiform dilation of the common bile duct
II	Diverticulum of the common bile duct
III (choledochocele)	Dilation of the terminal portion of the common bile duct
IV	Dilation of the extra and intrahepatic bile ducts

tive theory proposes dysgenesis of the pancreatobiliary duct results in ineffective biliary drainage with increased intraluminal pressure and dilatation.

Clinical Presentation

The classic triad of jaundice, abdominal pain, and a right upper quadrant mass occurs in only 6% to 9% of patients.[10] Two of these findings are present in 82% of patients with a choledochal cyst. Other less common presentations are cholangitis due to biliary obstruction, pancreatitis due to pancreatic duct obstruction, biliary cirrhosis leading to portal hypertension, and cystic rupture. More than 60% of patients present before 10 years of age. Some patients present in adulthood or are incidentally diagnosed; 70% to 84% of patients are female. The occurrence rate in the Western hemisphere is estimated to be 1 in 100,000 to 150,000 live births, with a higher incidence in Asia.

Diagnosis

With the advent of prenatal ultrasound, choledochal cysts are now often detected in the fetus. Choledochal cysts are usually diagnosed by abdominal ultrasound or CT scan (Fig. 49-3) as part of the evaluation of the patient with jaundice, an abdominal mass, or pancreatitis. Intrahepatic and extrahepatic dilation of the bile ducts may be seen by ultrasonography and by CT. Scintigraphy may provide physiologic information regarding uptake and accumulation in the dilated ducts. ERCP and cholangiography, which provide anatomic details of the biliary system, may be necessary prior to surgical repair. Small choledochal cysts may be missed on imaging studies and found only when ERCP is performed to evaluate a patient with recurrent pancreatitis.

Conjugated hyperbilirubinemia is present in 56% of patients. Mild elevations of the transaminases, alkaline phosphatase and gamma-glutamyltransferase (GGT) are found in 70% of cases. Pancreatitis due to ductal obstruction is accompanied by elevations in serum amylase and lipase. Impaired hepatic synthetic function, reflected in a

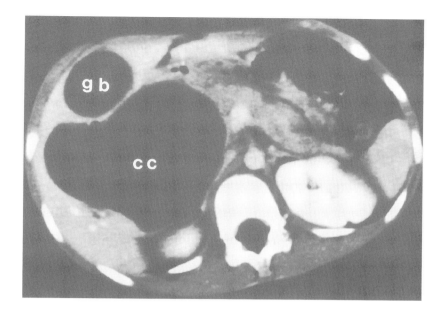

FIGURE 49-3. Choledochal cyst. CT scan of abdomen with intravenous contrast delineates normal gallbladder (gb) and massive choledochal cyst (cc). (Courtesy of John R. Sty, M.D.)

low serum albumin or prolonged prothrombin time (PT), may occur due to secondary biliary cirrhosis.

Treatment

The treatment of choice is complete surgical excision with drainage of the biliary tract into the jejunum. Carcinoma, particularly adenocarcinoma, is a well-recognized complication of incompletely resected choledochal cysts.

CAROLI DISEASE AND CAROLI SYNDROME

Both Caroli disease, a congenital segmental nonobstructive dilation of the intrahepatic bile ducts, and Caroli syndrome, the association of Caroli disease with periportal fibrosis, especially in more peripheral levels of the biliary tree, are due to malformation of the ductal plates.[11]

Pathophysiology

Ductal plates are embryonic cisterns that surround the portal structures and normally remodel into mature tubular forms. Lack of involution of these ductal plates results in abnormal dilated ducts, often with an associated increase in periportal tract fibrous tissue. Caroli disease, ectasia of the intrahepatic bile ducts, is less common than Caroli syndrome, with its associated periportal fibrosis. Both may be associated with renal cysts. Both conditions may be inherited in an autosomal recessive manner.

Clinical Presentation

Patients with Caroli disease most commonly present with fever, abdominal pain, and jaundice. Elevations in bilirubin and transaminase reflect cholestasis. Dilation of the bile ducts causes biliary stasis, lithiasis, obstruction, cholangitis, and liver abscess. In Caroli syndrome, fibrosis can lead to hepatomegaly, portal hypertension splenomegaly, and bleeding from the esophageal varices. Associated renal disease and, in adults, cholangiocarcinoma, can lead to unusual clinical presentations. Although most commonly diagnosed in young adults, manifestations can occur at any age, including the neonatal period. A proportion of affected people will remain asymptomatic.

Diagnosis

Caroli disease is usually diagnosed by radiologic imaging of the liver and biliary tract as part of an evaluation for jaundice, hepatomegaly, or abdominal pain. Ultrasound and CT delineate the severity, location, and extent of liver involvement. Transhepatic cholangiography or ERCP, or both, are useful in providing anatomic detail (Fig. 49-4).

Treatment

Management depends on the extent and type of liver involvement. In the asymptomatic unobstructed patient, ursodeoxycholic acid (Actigall), 10 to 15 mg/kg/day, is given to improve bile flow. Obstruction is treated by interventional radiologic procedures, such as percutaneous drainage or endoscopic stone removal. Surgical techniques, including enterostomy, and segmental or lobar hepatic resection may be required. Liver transplant is the

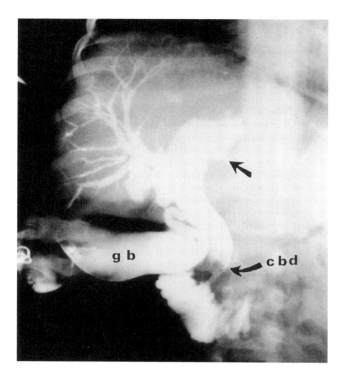

FIGURE 49-4. Caroli disease. Operative cholangiogram demonstrates distention of the gallbladder (gb) and dilation of the common bile duct (cbd) and the left hepatic duct. The cbd contains two calculi (curved arrow); note numerous calculi in the left hepatic duct (straight arrow). (From Hermansen et al.[16] with permission.)

treatment of choice for intractable obstruction leading to chronic or recurrent cholangitis and biliary sepsis.

CONGENITAL HEPATIC FIBROSIS

In congenital hepatic fibrosis, bands of noninflammatory fibrous tissue, containing multiple bile ductules, link the portal tracts. Most cases are associated with polycystic kidney disease; renal dysplasia and adult polycystic kidney disease occur less commonly. Associated malformations include Caroli disease and choledochal cyst. The mode of inheritance is autosomal recessive.

Pathophysiology

Although the etiology is uncertain, it is proposed that immature bile duct structures are subject to a variable progressive process of cholangitis, leading to involution and resultant periportal fibrosis.

Clinical Presentation

Clinical expression is variable due to the spectrum of hepatic and renal involvement.[12] Although congenital hepatic fibrosis can present at any age, it is primarily encountered in children and young adults. Renal manifestations are most common in the young child, while hepatosplenomegaly, portal hypertension, and variceal bleeding more frequently occur in the older child or adult. Although hepatomegaly is noted in 93% and splenomegaly in 89% at presentation, standard tests of liver function are usually normal. When splenomegaly is present, thrombocytopenia is a common finding. Renal findings include an abnormal intravenous pyelogram (IVP) (89%) and polycystic kidney disease (37%). The mean age at time of diagnosis is 10 years. There is a slight female preponderance.

Diagnosis

The diagnosis of congenital hepatic fibrosis is based on histologic evidence of fibrous bands containing dysmorphic bile ducts, with areas of normal lobar architecture on biopsy specimen. Renal abnormalities are best evaluated by ultrasonography.

Treatment

Treatment is directed at the prevention and treatment of variceal bleeding. Beta-blockers have been shown to prevent bleeding from esophageal varices. Treatment of bleeding varices is discussed elsewhere and may include injection sclerotherapy, banding and portosystemic shunting. Prognosis is largely based on associated biliary and/or renal involvement.

MALFORMATIONS OF THE GALLBLADDER

A variety of malformations of the gallbladder occur as a result of embryologic dysgenesis. Congenital absence of the gallbladder affects 1 in 2,500 to 6,000 live births and is possibly inherited as a non-sex-linked trait with variable penetration.[13]

Pathophysiology

Absence of the gallbladder is usually associated with other malformations, particularly extrahepatic biliary atresia. Congenital heart disease, gastrointestinal (GI), genitourinary, and anterior wall anomalies, and central nervous system (CNS) defects may also occur. Anatomic malposition, such as intrahepatic, retrohepatic, and retroperitoneal ectopic sites, has been reported. Dysgenesis, including hypoplasia, duplication, and single or multiple septation, is rare. Heterotopic tissue in the gallbladder from the gastric or hepatic mucosa and the adrenal, pancreatic, and thyroid glands has been reported.

Clinical Presentation

Although congenital anomalies of the gallbladder may be responsible for biliary symptoms in adults, they are usually asymptomatic in the pediatric population, unless accompanied by stone formation and/or cholecystitis.

Diagnosis

Gallbladder malformations are generally diagnosed when ultrasonography is performed during evaluation for unrelated problems.

Treatment

In the absence of symptoms or complications due to cholelithiasis, treatment is unnecessary.

MISCELLANEOUS DISORDERS OF THE BILE DUCTS

A multitude of uncommon hepatic excretory duct anomalies due to embryologic dysgenesis have been described, including accessory bile ducts draining individual segments of the liver, accessory bile ducts communicating between major biliary channels, hepatocholecystic ducts (sinuses of Luschka) arising from the liver and entering the gallbladder wall, anomalies of the cystic duct including agenesis, hepatic duct anomalies, and anomalous insertions of the bile duct into the duodenum.[14]

Clinical Presentation

Although the incidence of acute and chronic biliary tract disease is higher in persons with congenital anomalies of the biliary tract, these uncommon abnormalities are usually found incidentally.

Diagnosis

Biliary tract anomalies are often incidentally diagnosed when radiologic imaging (ultrasound, CT) or surgery is performed for unrelated problems.

Treatment

No treatment is required, although surgical procedures may require modification to preserve biliary tract patency.

REFERENCES

1. Kozu T, Suda K, Toki F. Pancreatic development and anatomical variation. Gastrointest Endosc Clin North Am 1995; 5:1–30
2. England RE, Newcomer MK, Leung JWC, Cotton PB. Case report: Annular pancreas divisum—a report of two cases and review of the literature. Br J Radiol 1995;68:324–328
3. Kiernan PD, ReMine SG, Kiernan PC, ReMine WH. Annular pancreas. Arch Surg 1980;115:46–50
4. Lehman GA, Sherman S. Pancreas divisum. Gastrointest Endosc Clin North Am 1995;5:145–170
5. Siegel JH, Ben-Zvi JS, Pullano W, Cooperman A. Effectiveness of endoscopic drainage for pancreas divisum: endoscopic and surgical results in 31 patients. Endoscopy 1990;22: 129–133
6. Thoeni RF, Gedgaudas RK. Ectopic pancreas: usual and unusual features. Gastrointest Radiol 1980;5:37–42
7. Armstrong CP, King PM, Dixon JM, Macleod IB. The clinical significance of heterotopic pancreas in the gastrointestinal tract. Br J Surg 1981;68:384–387
8. Winter WE, Maclaren NK, Riley WJ et al. Congenital pancreatic hypoplasia: a syndrome of exocrine and endocrine pancreatic insufficiency. J Pediatr 1986;109:465–468
9. Forbes A, Murray-Lyon IM. Cystic disease of the liver and biliary tract. Gut 1991;(suppl):S116–S122 Vol 32
10. Stringer MD, Dhawan A, Davenport M et al. Choledochal cysts: lessons from a 20 year experience. Arch Dis Child 1995;73:528–531
11. Desmet VJ. Congenital diseases of intrahepatic bile ducts: variations on the theme "Ductal plate malformation." Hepatology 1992;4:1069–1083
12. Alvarez F, Bernard O, Brunelle F et al. Congenital hepatic fibrosis in children. J Pediatr 1981;99:370–375
13. Bennion RS, Thompson JE, Tompkins RK. Agenesis of the gallbladder without extrahepatic biliary atresia. Arch Surg 1988;123:1257–1260
14. Goor DA, Ebert PA. Anomalies of the biliary tree. Arch Surg 1972;104:302–309
15. Werlin SL. ERCP in children. Pediatr Clin North Am 1994; 4:161
16. Hermansen M, Starshak R, Werlin S. Caroli disease: the diagnostic approach. J Pediatr. 1979;94:879

50

DRUG HEPATITIS

EVE A. ROBERTS

Although drug hepatitis is uncommon in children, perhaps due to differences between children and adults with respect to hepatic drug metabolism, it can lead to clinically important illness. Drug hepatitis implies drug-induced liver damage with inflammation and damage to hepatocytes. There may be some degree of cholestasis, mainly as a result of hepatocellular injury, but possibly due to damage to bile duct epithelial cells. It may be asymptomatic, evident only biochemically by elevated serum aminotransferases. More severe drug hepatitis is symptomatic with anorexia, nausea, vomiting, abdominal pain, and hepatomegaly. When damage is very severe and widespread, acute liver failure, with coagulopathy and hepatic coma, may occur. Alternatively, a chronic process may evolve with the histopathologic features of chronic active hepatitis (Table 50-1); cirrhosis can also develop.

Drug-induced liver disease includes other types of damage besides hepatitis (Table 50-2): isolated or bland cholestasis, steatosis, hepatic venous occlusion (Budd-Chiari syndrome, veno-occlusive disease), granulomatosis, and neoplasms are some other possible patterns of liver injury. In some cases, cells other than hepatocytes are the main target of injury; in others, a specific immune mechanism is prominent. Some drugs can cause more than one pattern of liver damage.

The view that all hepatotoxins either are intrinsically toxic or act exclusively on an unpredictable, "allergic" basis is gradually being abandoned. The mechanism of hepatotoxicity often involves abnormalities in hepatic drug biotransformation that lead to an imbalance between production of toxic metabolite(s) and intrinsic cytoprotective defenses (Fig. 50-1). Drug interactions, for example, by induction of drug-metabolizing enzymes,

may enhance production of toxic intermediates. Genetic defects in drug detoxification, apparent only when a specific drug or class of chemicals is administered, may provide inadequate defenses against ordinary concentrations of toxic metabolites. The target of the toxic metabolite determines many of the clinical features of drug hepatotoxicity. Damage to hepatocellular organelles may cause cytotoxicity directly. Damage to hepatocellular membranes may initiate an immune response leading to an immunoallergic reaction resembling hypersensitivity. Greater understanding of these mechanisms, including the pattern of immune response in specific patients, makes it possible to predict drug hepatotoxicity. However, for many drugs this knowledge is still very sketchy, especially for those which occasionally cause transient elevations in serum aminotransferases without further evolution of the hepatotoxic process.

A high level of clinical suspicion is often required to identify drug hepatitis. Direct questioning is required regarding prescription and nonprescription medications, as well as herbal drugs. Teenagers may be at equivalent risk of drug hepatotoxicity as adults.

SPECIFIC CAUSES OF DRUG HEPATITIS IN CHILDREN

Antipyretics

ACETAMINOPHEN

In large doses, acetaminophen is a potent hepatotoxin in children and adults. The clinical course of acute severe acetaminophen toxicity is quite characteristic. Immedi-

TABLE 50-1. Drugs Associated With Features of Chronic Active Hepatitis on Liver Biopsy

Methyldopa

Sulfonamides

Propylthiouracil

Nitrofurantoin

Isoniazid

Oxyphenisatin

ately after the drug is taken, nausea and vomiting occur. After these symptoms resolve, there is an asymptomatic interval of 1 to 2 days before hepatic damage becomes clinically apparent. Then jaundice with elevated serum aminotransferases and coagulopathy develops. Finally, coma and renal failure may develop. Serum aminotransferases may be extremely high but still do not predict outcome. Predictors of catastrophic outcome include extremely prolonged prothrombin time (PT), renal failure, hepatic coma, and acidosis.[1] Treatment with N-acetylcysteine should be initiated as soon as possible and may be continued beyond the conventional 17 doses without untoward effect.[2]

The classic acute type of hepatotoxicity typically occurs in toddlers who ingest pills from the medicine cabinet or in teenagers attempting suicide. Therapeutic misadventure is responsible for an important alternative pattern of acetaminophen hepatotoxicity in children. This occurs when comparatively large doses of acetaminophen (approximately 30 to 70 mg/kg) are administered at regular intervals (usually every 2 to 4 hours) for two to three days or longer, before hepatotoxicity becomes evident. This happens when adult tablets are substituted for children's elixir or when proper dosing practice is ignored. Acute liver failure develops, but without the usual systemic signs of toxicity. Moreover, the classic asymptomatic interval does not occur. The serum concentration of acetaminophen is often *not* in a toxic range. Diagnosis is difficult unless a very careful drug history is obtained. The nomogram for treatment with N-acetylcysteine does not easily apply in such situations. Estimating the elimination half-life of acetaminophen may be helpful. In general, it seems reasonable to treat with N-acetylcysteine as soon possible.

Young children appear to be quite resistant to acetaminophen hepatotoxicity and tend to recover when it does occur.[3,4] This may be due to differences in acetaminophen metabolism in children. Nevertheless, there are many reported cases of severe acetaminophen hepa-

TABLE 50-2. Patterns of Drug-Induced Liver Disease

Pattern of Injury	Associated Drugs
Acute hepatitis	Phenytoin, isoniazid, halothane, pemoline, diclofenac
Hepatitis-cholestasis	Erythromycin, chlorpromazine, azathioprine, nitrofurantoin, sulfonamides
Zonal liver necrosis	Acetaminophen, cocaine
Bland cholestasis	Estrogens, cyclosporine
Steatohepatitis	Perhexiline, amiodarone, methotrexate
Phospholipidosis	Amiodarone
Macrovesicular steatosis	Prednisone, dexamethasone
Microvesicular steatosis	Valproic acid, tetracycline
Glycogenosis	Prednisone
Granulomatosis	Sulfonamides, phenylbutazone, carbamazepine
Interlobular ductopenia (vanishing bile ducts)	Nafcillin, oxacillin, Augmentin, sulfonamides, clindamycin, carbamazepine
Biliary cirrhosis	Chlorpropamide
Sclerosing cholangitis	Floxuridine infused through the hepatic artery
Peliosis hepatis	Estrogens, androgens
Hepatic vein thrombosis (Budd-Chiari syndrome)	Estrogens (oral contraceptives)
Veno-occlusive disease	Thioguanine, busulfan, pyrrolizidine alkaloids
Nodular regenerative hyperplasia	Azathioprine
Liver cell adenoma	Estrogens (oral contraceptives), anabolic steroids
Hepatocellular carcinoma	Estrogens (oral contraceptives), anabolic steroids
Porphyria	2,3,7,8-Tetrachlorodibenzo-p-dioxin, chloroquine

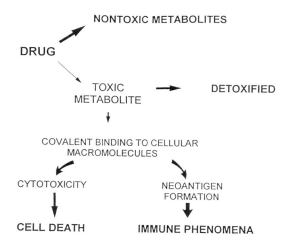

FIGURE 50-1 Possible outcomes of hepatic drug metabolism. Nontoxic metabolites are favored (broad arrow). Drug interactions leading to enzyme induction might increase importance of an otherwise minor route (thin arrow) forming toxic metabolites. Saturation of detoxification pathways or genetic inadequacy of these pathways increases extent of binding to cellular macromolecules and its consequences.

totoxicity in children. Some children require liver transplantation to survive.

Anti-inflammatory Drugs

ASPIRIN

Hepatotoxicity is dose dependent, mainly associated with high-dose treatment. Hepatotoxicity is not limited to patients with rheumatoid disease, although most cases are associated with juvenile rheumatoid arthritis. Clinical hepatitis and elevated serum aminotransferases are usually found.[5,6] Signs of severe liver damage such as jaundice and coagulopathy are rarely found. Serum aminotransferase levels may exceed 1000 IU/L.[7] In some cases, encephalopathy (unrelated to Reye's syndrome) has been reported.[8] Clinical and laboratory abnormalities resolve when aspirin is stopped.

METHOTREXATE

Chronic low-dose treatment with methotrexate frequently causes hepatic fibrosis with steatosis, resembling alcoholic hepatitis with fibrosis.[9] Cirrhosis can develop, and liver transplantation has been performed in some adult patients. Although this toxicity has been reported more often in adults than in children, it is still a risk among children.[10] Regular monitoring of liver function tests during treatment may be more reasonable then repeated liver biopsies.[11] However, serum aminotransferases may not reflect ongoing liver damage and may be

normal even when fibrosis or cirrhosis has developed.[12] For children, a biochemical surveillance strategy may suffice. Methotrexate should be stopped if persistent aminotransferase abnormalities develop. A pretreatment baseline biopsy may be informative, especially if the child is obese or there is reason to suspect ongoing liver disease. High-dose methotrexate treatment used in some antineoplastic treatment regimens may cause acute hepatitis as shown by a sudden rise in serum aminotransferases.[13]

Anti-neoplastic Agents

Many drugs used to treat childhood cancers can cause hepatotoxicity.[14] However, these drugs are rarely used separately, and patients receiving them are often susceptible to many types of liver damage. Hepatitis, often asymptomatic with elevation in serum aminotransferases and no other evidence of severe liver toxicity, is common. Antineoplastic drugs that frequently produce asymptomatic elevation of serum aminotransferases include nitrosoureas, 6-mercaptopurine, cytosine arabinoside, cisplatinum, and dacarbazine (DTIC). Cyclophosphamide may cause a dose-related drug hepatitis.[15] L-Asparaginase can cause severe damage characterized by severe steatosis, hepatocellular necrosis, and fibrosis. This is usually reversible after the L-asparaginase is stopped.[16] Thrombocytopenia and acute liver failure were reported in an 18-year-old patient receiving carboplatin.[17]

Adriamycin and vinca alkaloids are infrequently associated with hepatotoxicity. Although dactinomycin is infrequently associated with hepatotoxicity, it has caused severe hepatic dysfunction, with extremely elevated serum aminotransferases and coagulopathy, all of which resolved spontaneously off drug. Dactinomycin hepatotoxicity may be enhanced by irradiation. Adriamycin may enhance the hepatotoxic potential of 6-mercaptopurine.

Anti-epileptics

PHENYTOIN

Phenytoin hepatotoxicity is relatively common.[18] It presents as a hepatitis associated with a drug hypersensitivity syndrome. Serum aminotransferases are elevated, and the patient may be moderately jaundiced. In severe cases, clinical features of liver failure (e.g., coagulopathy, ascites, altered level of consciousness) are also present. The drug hypersensitivity syndrome includes fever, rash (morbilliform rash, Stevens-Johnson syndrome, or toxic epidermal necrolysis), lymphadenopathy, leukocytosis, eosinophilia, and atypical lymphocytosis. Liver biopsy in phenytoin hepatotoxicity usually shows scattered necrosis of hepatocytes but sometimes looks like mononucleosis or viral hepatitis. In severe cases, treatment with high-dose corticosteroids has appeared effective in some patients, although this has not been tested in a controlled trial and anecdotal reports do not consistently show a clear benefit.

CARBAMAZEPINE

Carbamazepine hepatotoxicity in children is usually a hepatitis, sometimes associated with a drug hypersensitivity syndrome similar to that of phenytoin. Clinically, this may resemble mononucleosis, with rash, lymphadenopathy, hepatosplenomegaly, and neutropenia.[19] Severe hepatotoxicity has also been reported.[20] Four children with fatal acute liver failure were taking carbamazepine, phenytoin, and primidone.[21]

Like phenytoin and phenobarbital, carbamazepine may be metabolized via arene oxides, reactive intermediates which are detoxified via epoxide hydrolase. A pharmacogenetic problem, lack of epoxide hydrolase, may account for susceptibility to this toxicity. This metabolic idiosyncrasy places these persons at risk of phenytoin and phenobarbital hepatotoxicity.

PHENOBARBITAL

In relationship to its widespread use, phenobarbital hepatitis is rare; however, more than one-half of reported cases were children. It is usually associated with a multisystemic drug hypersensitivity syndrome, but hepatitis may be the main finding.[22] In cases with hepatitis, jaundice began within 8 weeks of starting phenobarbital, with generalized rash and fever. Usually the liver disease was moderately severe but self-limited; however, one child died of acute liver failure. One child developed chronic liver disease.

The mechanism of phenobarbital-induced hepatotoxicity remains unclear. An inherited defect in epoxide hydrolase has been corroborated in in vitro rechallenge. People who develop phenobarbital hepatotoxicity may be sensitive to other barbiturates, for example, those used for sedation for diagnostic procedures. They may also develop hepatitis from phenytoin or carbamazepine.

VALPROIC ACID

Valproic acid causes hepatotoxicity more often in children than adults. A certain proportion of patients, estimated at 11%,[23] develop abnormal serum aminotransferases, usually within a short time of starting treatment. This dose-responsive biochemical abnormality resolves when the dose of valproic acid is decreased.

Some patients develop progressive liver failure, clinically resembling Reye's syndrome.[24] This severe hepatotoxicity usually does not improve when the drug is withdrawn, and it is frequently fatal.[25] Unfortunately, it cannot be predicted by regular monitoring of serum aminotransferases and other liver function tests.[26] The time from initiating treatment with valproic acid and onset of liver disease is usually, but not always, less than 4 months. Specific risk factors include age under 2 years, multiple anticonvulsant treatment along with valproic acid, and coexistent medical problems, such as severe developmental delay or congenital abnormalities.

The clinical presentation of the severe hepatotoxicity is hepatitis; seizure control may also deteriorate. Coagulopathy develops early. Clinical jaundice occurs later, with other features of progressive liver failure, such as ascites and hypoglycemia. Liver transplantation may be life-saving, although the course of the underlying neurologic disease is unpredictable.

The mechanism of valproic acid hepatotoxicity remains unclear, although it appears to involve generation of toxic metabolite(s) plus some type of metabolic idiosyncrasy, rendering the patient susceptible. Mitochondrial ω-oxidation is important in the metabolism of valproic acid, which can also undergo metabolism by cytochrome P-450. Decreased serum carnitine has been found in valproic acid hepatotoxicity.[27] Serum carnitine may be low in patients treated chronically, without any clinical evidence of hepatotoxicity, as conjugation to carnitine is a minor detoxification pathway for valproic acid. It remains uncertain whether carnitine repletion constitutes effective treatment for severe hepatotoxicity, but limited reported experience suggests that it is not.[28,29]

Antibiotics

SULFONAMIDES

Sulfanilamide, trimethoprim-sulfamethoxazole, and pyrimethamine-sulfadoxine have all been reported to cause significant hepatotoxicity.[30] Sulfasalazine has been associated with severe liver disease in adolescents and young adults.[31] In some cases, acute liver failure occurred, sometimes fatal. The spectrum of sulfa-associated liver toxicity also includes asymptomatic elevation of serum aminotransferases and granulomatous hepatitis. Sulfa hepatotoxicity is often associated with a systemic drug hypersensitivity reaction. Fever, significant rash, periorbital edema, atypical lymphocytosis, lymphadenopathy, and proteinuria all may occur.

Sulfonamide hepatotoxicity involves an electrophilic toxic metabolite in the liver. The toxic metabolite is a reactive species, possibly the nitroso, derived from the hydroxylamine metabolite of the particular sulfonamide.[32] Being a slow acetylator (in the rapid/slow polymorphism for N-acetyltransferase-2), as well as being unable to detoxify this reactive metabolite, may predispose to hepatotoxicity.[30]

ERYTHROMYCIN

All erythromycins are potentially hepatotoxic, usually causing a mixed hepatitic-cholestatic process.[33] Regardless of which erythromycin ester is involved, clinical features include clinical hepatitis and abdominal pain, predominantly in the right upper quadrant. The latter may be severe enough to suggest biliary tract obstruction. Hepatomegaly, sometimes accompanied by splenomegaly, appears to be common in children. Erythromycin ethylsuccinate hepatotoxicity reported in a child was a relatively mild self-limited disease.

NITROFURANTOIN

Fatal cholestatic hepatitis with severe pulmonary toxicity was reported in a teenage girl.[34] In adults, nitrofurantoin has been associated with chronic active hepatitis.[35]

ISONIAZID

Isoniazid is a well-known cause of drug hepatotoxicity in adults. Most patients have an asymptomatic elevation of serum aminotransferases.[36] Overt symptoms of hepatitis indicate severe disease; mortality is greater than 10% in patients with jaundice. Isoniazid hepatotoxicity is also common in children. There are numerous reports of isoniazid hepatotoxicity, including fatal hepatic necrosis, in children treated for tuberculosis or in those receiving prophylaxis.[37] As with adults, hepatotoxicity typically develops during the first 2 to 3 months of treatment. Children with more severe tuberculosis seem to be at greater risk of hepatotoxicity.[38]

Isoniazid hepatotoxicity appears to be due to a toxic metabolite, but the mechanism has not yet been determined. Several reports in children show no clear pattern of hepatotoxicity in relation to acetylator status.[39]

KETOCONAZOLE

Ketoconazole causes significant hepatotoxicity. An initial major report of ketoconazole hepatotoxicity included two children (a 17-year-old boy and a 5-year-old boy, both with chronic mucocutaneous candidiasis).[40] In most cases, clinical hepatitis occurred within 6 to 8 weeks of starting treatment (range: 5 days to 6 months).

Anesthetics

HALOTHANE

Halothane hepatotoxicity is nearly always hepatitis. Either asymptomatic hepatitis (elevated serum aminotransferases) occurs in the first or second week after the anesthetic exposure, or severe hepatitis with extensive hepatocyte necrosis and liver failure develops.[41] Although halothane hepatitis is uncommon in children, it definitely can occur, and acute liver failure may develop.[42]

Drugs Used in Treating Attention-Deficit Disorder

PEMOLINE

Pemoline appears to be quite hepatotoxic, causing at least asymptomatic elevation of serum aminotransferases. Recent reports describe acute hepatitis of variable severity, including one patient who died with fulminant hepatitis.[43,44] Two other deaths associated with hepatic dysfunction while the patients were receiving pemoline have been reported; one may have had previous chronic liver disease and the other may have taken an overdose of pemoline.[45] Another death occurred in a boy taking pemoline and methylphenidate concomitantly.[46] This hepatitis is reported more commonly in boys. The mechanism of this hepatotoxicity is not known. Serum aminotransferases should be monitored during treatment with pemoline. If they become elevated, pemoline should be discontinued.

Antithyroid Drugs

PROPYLTHIOURACIL

Propylthiouracil hepatotoxicity has been reported in children: it is more common in girls.[47] The clinical presentation is usually hepatitis with jaundice. Serum aminotransferases are moderately elevated. Symptoms typically begin within 2 to 3 months of starting treatment but may occur much later.[48] Asymptomatic elevation of serum aminotransferases may be the earliest sign of hepatotoxicity, and these levels should be checked regularly throughout the first 3 to 6 months of treatment.

A case of propylthiouracil hepatotoxicity associated with chronic active hepatitis was reported in a child who developed urticaria on methimazole and then nonicteric hepatomegaly with elevated serum aminotransferases after more than 1 year of treatment with propylthiouracil only.[48] Anti-smooth muscle antibodies and anti-liver-kidney microsomal (anti-LKM 1) antibodies were not detected.

METHIMAZOLE

Hepatotoxicity from methimazole is rare. When it occurs, the main feature is cholestasis,[49] unlike propylthiouracil, which produces a cholestatic-hepatitic picture. Nevertheless, drug hepatitis from methimazole may occur.

Non-medicinal Drugs

COCAINE

Cocaine hepatotoxicity has not been reported in children, but adolescents may be at risk. A clinically severe hepatitis was reported in young adults: the main histologic finding was extensive zonal necrosis of perivenular hepatocytes, and some steatosis.[50] Acute liver failure occurred in some patients. The histologic pattern of hepatic injury in humans is consistent with the generation of a toxic metabolite, probably by cytochrome P-450. Glutathione appears to protect against cocaine-induced hepatic injury.[51] Ethanol and phenobarbital-type inducers increase cocaine hepatotoxicity.

Herbal Medications

Comfrey, germander, chaparral leaf, and jin bu huan have all been associated with significant drug hepatitis in adults.

TREATMENT

The first step in treatment is to make the diagnosis of drug-induced hepatitis. Stopping the drug may be all the treatment necessary. Use of an antidote, usually to supplement cytoprotective mechanisms, may be effective. The classic example is N-acetylcysteine for acetaminophen hepatotoxicity. The effectiveness of administering corticosteroids remains unproved and is therefore controversial. Corticosteroids have appeared effective in hastening recovery from phenytoin and phenobarbital hepatotoxicity. In acute liver failure, liver transplantation may be the only effective option.

REFERRAL PATTERN

Patients who show no improvement after stopping the drug suspected to cause drug hepatitis, who show signs of chronic liver disease, or who have acute liver failure should be referred to a specialist. Any patient who requires a liver biopsy may need referral. Prospective assessment for risk of drug hepatitis may be indicated in some patients. In vitro susceptibility studies are still largely a research tool.

REFERENCES

1. Pereira LM, Langley PG, Hayllar KM et al. Coagulation factor V and VIII/V ratio as predictors of outcome in paracetamol induced fulminant hepatic failure: relation to other prognostic indicators. Gut 1992;33:98–102
2. Smilkstein MJ, Knapp GL, Kulig KW, Rumack BH. Efficacy of oral N-acetylcysteine in the treatment of acetaminophen overdose. N Engl J Med 1988;319:1557–1562
3. Rumack BH. Acetaminophen overdose in young children. Treatment and effects of alcohol and other additional ingestants in 417 cases. Am J Dis Child 1984;138:428–433
4. Peterson RG, Rumack BH. Age as a variable in acetaminophen overdose. Arch Intern Med 1981;141:390–393
5. Benson GD. Hepatotoxicity following the therapeutic use of antipyretic analgesics. Am J Med 1983;75:85–93
6. Hamdan JA, Manasra K, Ahmed M. Salicylate-induced hepatitis in rheumatic fever. Am J Dis Child 1985;139:453–455
7. Doughty R, Giesecke L, Athreya B. Salicylate therapy in juvenile rheumatoid arthritis. Am J Dis Child 1980;134:461–463
8. Ulshen MH, Grand RJ, Crain JD, Gelfand EW. Hepatotoxicity with encephalopathy associated with aspirin therapy in rheumatoid arthritis. J Pediatr 1978;93:1034–1037
9. Whiting-O'Keefe QE, Fye KH, Sack KD. Methotrexate and histologic hepatic abnormalities: a meta-analysis. Am J Med 1991;90:711–716
10. Keim D, Ragsdale C, Heidelberger K, Sullivan D. Hepatic fibrosis and the use of methotrexate for juvenile rheumatoid arthritis. J Rheumatol 1990;17:846–848
11. Kremer JM, Alarcón GS, Lightfoot RWJ et al. Methotrexate for rheumatoid arthritis. Suggested guidelines for monitoring liver toxicity. Arthritis Rheum 1994;37:316–328
12. Newman M, Auerbach R, Feiner H et al. The role of liver biopsies in psoriatic patients receiving long-term methotrexate treatment. Arch Dermatol 1989;125:1218–1224
13. Perez C, Sutow WW, Wang YM, Pearson HA. Evaluation of overall toxicity of high-dosage methotrexate regimens. Med Pediatr Oncol 1979;6:219–228
14. Menard DB, Gisselbrecht C, Marty H et al. Antineoplastic agents and the liver. Gastroenterology 1980;78:142–164
15. Honjo I, Suou T, Hirayama C. Hepatotoxicity of cyclophosphamide in man: pharmacokinetic analysis. Res Commun Chem Pathol Pharmacol 1988;61:149–165
16. Pratt CB, Johnson WW. Duration and severity of fatty metamorphosis of the liver following l-asparaginase therapy. Cancer 1971;28:361–364
17. Hruban RH, Sternberg SS, Meyers P et al. Fatal thrombocytopenia and liver failure associated with carboplatin therapy. Cancer Invest 1991;9:263–268
18. Shear NH, Spielberg SP. Anticonvulsant hypersensitivity syndrome. In vitro assessment of risk. J Clin Invest 1988;82:1826–1832
19. Brain C, MacArdle B, Levin S. Idiosyncratic reactions to carbamazepine mimicking viral infection in children. BMJ 1984;289:354
20. Hadzic N, Portmann B, Davies ET et al. Acute liver failure induced by carbamazepine. Arch Dis Child 1990;65:315–317
21. Smith DW, Cullity GJ, Silberstein EP. Fatal hepatic necrosis associated with multiple anticonvulsant therapy. Aust NZ J Med 1988;18:575–581
22. Roberts EA, Spielberg SP, Goldbach M, Phillips MJ. Phenobarbital hepatotoxicity in an 8-month-old infant. J Hepatol 1990;10:235–239
23. Powell-Jackson PR, Tredger JM, Williams R. Hepatotoxicity to sodium valproate: a review. Gut 1984;25:673–681
24. Suchy FJ, Balistreri WF, Buchino J et al. Acute hepatic failure associated with the use of sodium valproate. Report of two fatal cases. N Engl J Med 1979;300:962–966

25. Scheffner D, Konig ST, Rauterberg-Ruland I et al. Fatal liver failure in 16 children with valproate therapy. Epilepsia 1988; 29:530–542

26. Green SH. Sodium valproate and routine liver function tests. Arch Dis Child 1984;59:813–814

27. Böhles H, Richter K, Wagner-Thiessen E, Shaefer H. Decreased serum carnitine in valproate induced Reye syndrome. Eur J Pediatr 1982;139:185–186

28. Laub MC, Paetzke-Brunner I, Jaeger G. Serum carnitine during valproic acid therapy. Epilepsia 1986;27:559–562

29. Murphy JV, Groover RV, Hodge C. Hepatotoxic effects in a child receiving valproate and carnitine. J Pediatr 1993; 123:318–320

30. Shear NH, Spielberg SP, Grant DM et al. Differences in metabolism of sulfonamides predisposing to idiosyncratic toxicity. Ann Intern Med 1986;105:179–184

31. Gremse DA, Bancroft J, Moyer SA. Sulfasalazine hypersensitivity with hepatotoxicity, thrombocytopenia, and erythroid hypoplasia. J Pediatr Gastroenterol Nutrit 1989;9:261–263

32. Rieder MJ, Uetrecht J, Shear NH et al. Diagnosis of sulfonamide hypersensitivity reactions by in-vitro "rechallenge" with hydroxylamine metabolites. Ann Intern Med 1989;110: 286–289

33. Zafrani ES, Ishak KG, Rudzki C. Cholestatic and hepatocellular injury associated with erythromycin esters. Report of nine cases. Dig Dis Sci 1979;24:385–396

34. Mulberg AE, Bell LM. Fatal cholestatic hepatitis and multisystem failure associated with nitrofurantoin. J Pediatr Gastroenterol Nutr 1993;17:307–309

35. Sharp JR, Ishak KG, Zimmerman HJ. Chronic active hepatitis and severe hepatic necrosis associated with nitrofurantoin. Ann Intern Med 1980;92:14–19

36. Mitchell J, Zimmerman H, Ishak K et al. Isoniazid liver injury: clinical spectrum, pathology and probable pathogenesis. Ann Intern Med 1976;84:181–196

37. Tsagaropoulou-Stinga H, Mataki-Emmanouilidou T, Karadi-Kavalioti S, Manios S. Hepatotoxic reactions in children with severe tuberculosis treated with isoniazid-rifampin. Pediatr Infect Dis 1985;4:270–273

38. O'Brien RJ, Long MW, Cross FS et al. Hepatotoxicity from isoniazid and rifampin among children treated for tuberculosis. Pediatrics 1983;72:491–499

39. Seth V, Beotra A. Hepatic function in relation to acetylator phenotype in children treated with antitubercular drugs. Ind J Med Res 1989;89:306–309

40. Lewis JH, Zimmerman HJ, Benson GD, Ishak KG. Hepatic injury associated with ketoconazole therapy. Analysis of 33 cases. Gastroenterology 1984;86:503–513

41. Moult PJ, Sherlock S. Halothane-related hepatitis. A clinical study of twenty-six cases. QJ Med 1975;44:99–114

42. Kenna JG, Newberger J, Mieli-Vergani G et al. Halothane hepatitis in children. BMJ 1987;294:1209–1211

43. Pratt DS, Dubois RS. Hepatotoxicity due to pemoline (Cylert). A report of two cases. J Pediatr Gastroenterol Nutr 1990;10:239–241

44. Nehra A, Mullick F, Ishak KG, Zimmerman HJ. Pemoline-associated hepatic injury. Gastroenterology 1990;99: 1517–1519

45. Jaffe SL. Pemoline and liver function. J Am Acad Child Adolesc Psychiatry 1989;28:457–458

46. Berkovitch M, Pope E, Phillips J, Koren G. Pemoline-associated fulminant liver failure: testing the evidence for causation. Clin Pharmacol Ther 1995;57:696–698

47. Jonas NM, Edison MS. Propylthiouracil hepatotoxicity: two pediatric cases and review of the literature. J Pediatr Gastroenterol Nutr 1988;7:776–779

48. Maggiore G, Larizza D, Lorini R et al. PTU hepatotoxicity mimicking autoimmune chronic active hepatitis in a girl. J Pediatr Gastroenterol Nutr 1989;8:547–548

49. Arab DM, Malatjalian DA, Rittmaster RS. Severe cholestatic jaundice in uncomplicated hyperthyroidism treated with methimazole. J Clin Endocrinol Metab 1995;80: 1083–1085

50. Perino LE, Warren GH, Levine JS. Cocaine-induced hepatotoxicity in humans. Gastroenterology 1987;93:176–180

51. Boelsterli UA, Goldlin C. Biomechanisms of cocaine-induced hepatocyte injury mediated by the formation of reactive metabolites. Arch Toxicol 1991;65:351–360

51

PORTAL HYPERTENSION

WILLIAM J. COCHRAN
ROBERT N. BALDASSANO

Portal hypertension is the abnormal condition of sustained elevated pressure in the portal venous system. In the normal state, portal pressure is 5 to 10 mmHg. Unlike systemic blood pressure, portal pressure measurements rarely are made in clinical practice because they are difficult to obtain and are invasive. Several studies have documented that complications of portal hypertension do not occur until the portal pressure gradient (i.e., gradient between the portal vein and the hepatic veins or the inferior vena cava) exceeds 12 mmHg.[1] Because portal and hepatic veins do not have valves, increased portal pressure results in increased blood flow and simultaneously increased pressure in the splanchnic system. This prompts the formation of portosystemic collaterals through existing veins, which diverts portal blood away from the liver to the systemic circulation. In severe cases of cirrhosis, as much as 90% of the portal blood enters the systemic circulation through these collaterals and bypasses the liver.

Portal hypertension is more prevalent in adult patients than in pediatric patients. As a result of this and the fact that clinical studies are more difficult to perform in the pediatric population, most of the knowledge we have on the etiology and treatment of portal hypertension comes from animal experiments and adult studies.

ETIOLOGY AND PATHOPHYSIOLOGY

Several factors contribute to the development and maintenance of portal hypertension; the two major factors are increased portal blood flow and increased portal resistance. In most situations, the initiating factor in the development of portal hypertension is an increase in vascular resistance. There are three major sites of increased vascular resistance: prehepatic, intrahepatic, and posthepatic (Table 51-1).

The two most common causes of prehepatic portal hypertension are portal vein thrombosis and splenic vein thrombosis, with the former the most frequent cause in the pediatric population.[2] Portal vein thrombosis develops as a result of sepsis, dehydration, pancreatitis, umbilical vein catheterization, or omphalitis. As this condition evolves, many small tortuous collateral veins develop in order to transport portal blood to the liver. This condition is referred to as cavernous transformation of the portal vein. Patients with cavernous transformation of the portal vein can present at any time in life with splenomegaly or variceal bleeding, or both. Classically, the frequency of variceal bleeding is thought to decrease after adolescence, but it can occur at any age and can result in massive bleeding.[3] For more information, refer to the chapter on cavernous transformation.

Intrahepatic portal hypertension can be presinusoidal, sinusoidal, or postsinusoidal in origin. Hepatic schistosomiasis is the most common etiology of presinusoidal portal hypertension on a world-wide basis, although it is exceedingly rare in North America. Patients with hepatic schistosomiasis develop portal hypertension as the result of ova deposited in the portal venules and the subsequent periportal granulomatous reaction. Overall, hepatic schistosomiasis is second only to cirrhosis as the most common cause of portal hypertension. Neoplasms

TABLE 51-1. Causes of Portal Hypertension

Prehepatic origin

Portal vein thrombosis

Splenic vein thrombosis

Intrahepatic origin

Presinusoidal
    Schistosomiasis
    Neoplasms
    Hepatic cysts

Sinusoidal
    Cirrhosis

Postsinusoidal
    Veno-occlusive disease

Posthepatic origin

Hepatic vein thrombosis (Budd-Chiari syndrome)

Right ventricular heart failure

Constrictive pericarditis

---

and hepatic cysts, as seen in polycystic disease or Caroli's disease, may compress the portal venules, resulting in presinusoidal portal hypertension.

The primary cause of sinusoidal portal hypertension in pediatric and adult patients is cirrhosis, the most common etiology of portal hypertension. Numerous pediatric disorders can lead to cirrhosis. The major etiologic categories of pediatric cirrhosis include biliary tract disease, genetic and metabolic disorders, infection, immune disorders, nutritional, drug and toxin, cardiac, and miscellaneous (Table 51-2).

Veno-occlusive disease is an example of intrahepatic postsinusoidal portal hypertension. This is relatively uncommon in children but occurs most commonly following bone marrow transplantation or in patients with immune deficiency.[4,5] Histologically, veno-occlusive disease is characterized by sclerosis of the terminal hepatic veins, which results in increased resistance and the development of portal hypertension.

The classic cause of posthepatic portal hypertension is Budd-Chiari syndrome, a condition that occurs when a thrombus develops in the hepatic vein at the entry to the inferior vena cava.[6] Posthepatic portal hypertension also can develop as a result of severe right heart failure or constrictive pericarditis.

While increased vascular resistance in the portal system may be the initiating factor in the development of portal hypertension, other hemodynamic changes contribute to the maintenance of portal hypertension.[7] A hyperdynamic circulatory state exists in patients with portal hypertension characterized by increased cardiac output and heart rate and a decrease in systemic blood pressure. Arterial vasodilation, especially in the splanchnic system, occurs secondary to a rise in several circulat-

ing vasodilators, including glucagon, nitric oxide, prostacyclin, and vasoactive intestinal polypeptide (VIP). The increased levels of these vasodilators are thought to be secondary to reduced catabolism of these substances by the liver due to blood bypassing the liver by portosystemic collaterals or secondary to hepatic dysfunction. The vasodilation noted in these patients may also be the result of decreased responsiveness of vascular endothelium to various vasoconstrictors.

This vasodilation results in renal sodium retention

TABLE 51-2. Etiology of Cirrhosis in Pediatric Patients

Biliary tract disorders

Biliary atresia

Intrahepatic bile duct paucity/cholestatic syndromes
    Alagille's syndrome
    Byler's disease
    Nonsyndromatic

Choledochal cyst

Congenital hepatic fibrosis

Sclerosing cholangitis

Cystic fibrosis

Genetic and metabolic disorders

α_1-Antitrypsin deficiency

Wilson's disease

Hemochromatosis

Tyrosinemia

Glycogen storage disease

Galactosemia

Hereditary fructose intolerance

Wolman's disease

Niemann-Pick disease

Infection

Hepatitis B

Hepatitis C

Autoimmune hepatitis

Nutritional

Hepatic steatosis

TPN

Drug and toxin

Methotrexate

Alcohol

Cardiac

Miscellaneous

Peroxisomal disorders

Neonatal hepatitis

Indian childhood cirrhosis

Histiocytosis

increasing plasma volume. Cardiac output is then increased secondary to decreased vascular resistance and increased venous return. The splanchnic vasodilation, increased plasma volume, and increased cardiac output combine to increase portal blood flow and thus contribute to the maintenance of portal hypertension.

CLINICAL MANIFESTATIONS

Portal hypertension can present as gastrointestinal (GI) bleeding, splenomegaly, ascites, or prominent abdominal vascular markings. GI bleeding is the presenting manifestation of portal hypertension in 50 to 90% of cases and can occur as early as in infancy. The bleeding is most commonly from esophageal varices but can occur from gastric,[8] duodenal, or colonic varices. The presence of rectal hemorrhoids in an infant or young child should raise the possibility of the presence of portal hypertension. Portal gastropathy[9] and portal colopathy[10] are other sources of GI bleeding in patients with portal hypertension.

Splenomegaly is the next most common mode of presentation, occurring in 25% of cases. Most patients with portal hypertension will eventually develop splenomegaly. The presence of upper GI bleeding in a patient with splenomegaly should be considered secondary to portal hypertension until proved otherwise.

Ascites, a frequent problem in patients with sinusoidal and postsinusoidal portal hypertension, is uncommon in patients with presinusoidal hypertension. Ascites may be minimal and may only be detected incidentally on ultrasonic examination of the abdomen. Massive ascites can result in respiratory insufficiency (Fig. 51-1).

Uncommonly, portal hypertension presents with prominent abdominal vasculature (Fig. 51-2). The prominence of abdominal vasculature is the result of diversion of portal blood as in the case of varices. When these vessels radiate from the umbilicus, the condition is referred to as caput medusae.

DIAGNOSIS

Portal hypertension can be determined by several modalities (Table 51-3) but is diagnosed most frequently by physical examination. The most common physical manifestations of portal hypertension are splenomegaly (Fig. 51-3), ascites, prominent abdominal vasculature, hemorrhoids, or rectal varices. When portal hypertension is secondary to chronic liver disease, other physical manifestations may be present, such as icterus, a firm to hard liver, asterixis, spider hemangiomas, palmar erythema, encephalopathy, and malnutrition.

LABORATORY EVALUATION

Various laboratory studies are important to obtain in patients with portal hypertension in order to assess hepatic function and the patient's nutritional status and to pro-

FIGURE 51-1. Infant with severe neonatal hepatitis and massive ascites. Note the abdominal distention, ascitic fluid collection in areas of abdominal wall defects, and scrotal swelling.

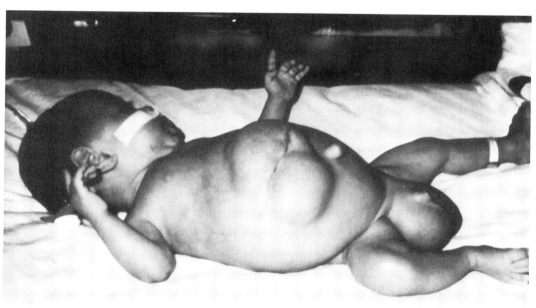

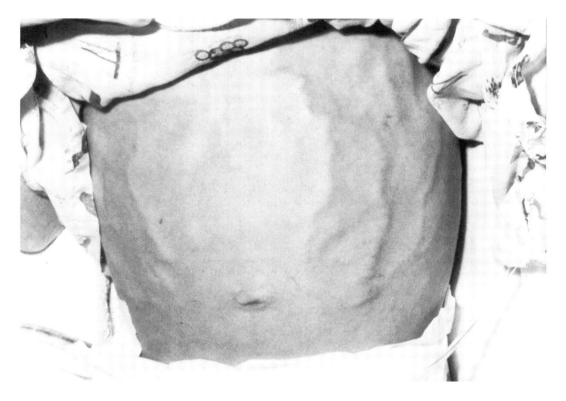

FIGURE 51-2. Patient with chronic granulomatous disease and portal vein obstruction. Note prominent abdominal vasculature.

vide evidence of hypersplenism. These studies should consist of a complete blood count, serum electrolytes, biochemistry profile, and coagulation profile.

Several invasive and noninvasive techniques can be used to document portal hypertension.[11] The two major noninvasive techniques are the barium swallow and ultrasonography. Invasive techniques to determine the presence of portal hypertension include endoscopy, direct measurement of portal pressure, measurement of hepatic venous pressure gradient, angiography, and splenoportography.

Barium Swallow

Before the advent of flexible endoscopy, the barium swallow was the test performed most commonly to detect portal hypertension and its major complication, esophageal varices. Because most patients with long-standing portal hypertension have esophageal varices, barium swallow may demonstrate varices by the displaying worm-like structures adjacent to the esophageal wall (Fig. 51-4). However, because therapy is often indicated, esophageal varices are usually diagnosed by upper endoscopy.[12]

Abdominal Ultrasound

Ultrasonography can also be useful in evaluating children with portal hypertension. In addition to predicting the presence of portal hypertension, ultrasonography is helpful in evaluating the cause of portal hypertension such as cirrhosis, hepatic cysts, or portal vein thrombosis. Ultrasonography can also assess spleen size, detect the presence of ascites, and determine whether there are any associated renal abnormalities (seen in congenital hepatic fibrosis). A classic ultrasonographic finding of por-

TABLE 51-3. Diagnosis of Portal Hypertension

Physical examination
  Splenomegaly
  Ascites
  Prominent abdominal vasculature
  Hemorrhoids
Noninvasive techniques
  Barium swallow
  Ultrasonography
Invasive techniques
  Endoscopy
  Direct measurement of portal pressure
  Measurement of hepatic venous pressure gradient
  Angiography
  Splenoportography

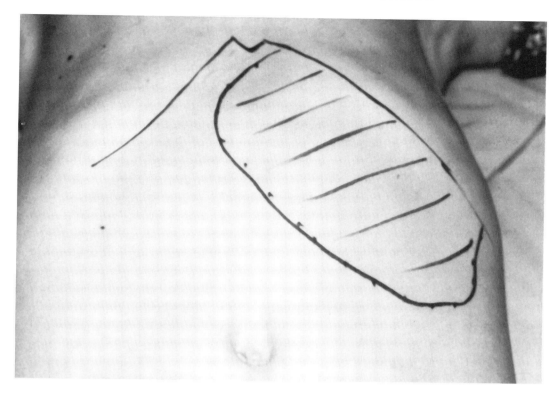

FIGURE 51-3. Patient with cavernomatous transformation of the portal vein with splenomegaly.

tal hypertension in adult patients is an enlarged portal vein diameter. The portal vein should also be assessed in relation to respiration. In normal patients, the portal vein increases in diameter with inspiration. This increase does not occur with inspiration in patients with portal hypertension, and its absence may be a more reliable indicator of portal hypertension than the actual diameter of the portal vein.

In pediatrics, a more reliable marker of portal hypertension is the ratio of portal vein diameter (in mm) to surface area (in m^2). If this ratio exceeds 12, esophageal varices are likely. Another useful parameter is the ratio of the lesser omentum thickness to aortic diameter. In patients with portal hypertension, there is increased blood flow through the lesser omentum, increasing its thickness and thus increasing this ratio. A ratio of greater than 1.9 is a good predictor of the presence of esophageal varices.[13]

Doppler ultrasound has the ability to assess blood flow within the portal vein. Blood flow decreases as portal hypertension increases due to increasing vascular resistance; in severe cases, the direction of the blood flow may be reversed. In cases of cavernomatous transformation of the portal vein, color Doppler can help in determining the presence of the small collaterals around the obstructed portal vein. Finally, a recent study using Doppler ultrasound in children suggests that portal vein

pulsativity is a sensitive and specific finding indicative of portal hypertension in children.[14]

Upper Endoscopy

Endoscopy can be performed safely in pediatric patients and is usually more sensitive in detecting esophageal varices than the barium swallow or ultrasonography. Endoscopy provides direct visual inspection of the varices and is required to determine their size and color and the risk of bleeding (Fig. 51-5). Endoscopy can also determine the presence of portal gastropathy, gastric and duodenal varices.

Vascular Studies

While direct measurement of portal pressure can be done by percutaneous puncture of an intrahepatic branch of the portal vein or during abdominal surgery by inserting a needle directly into the portal vein, it is difficult to perform in pediatric patients. It is generally considered an unacceptable procedure to render for the diagnosis of portal hypertension. These measurements are most commonly performed in a research setting.

Hepatic venous pressure gradient is measured by placing a catheter in the hepatic vein under fluoroscopic control. The hepatic venous pressure (free) is obtained;

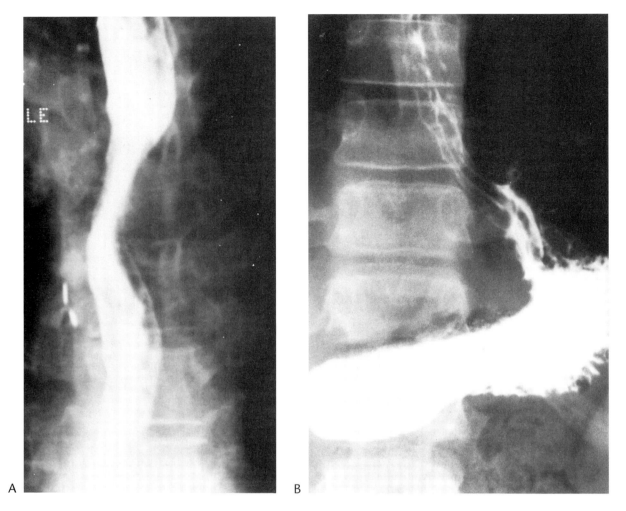

A   B

FIGURE 51-4. *(A)* Barium swallow in patient with esophageal varices, seen as "worm-like" filling defects. *(B)* Esophageal varices following partial emptying of the barium.

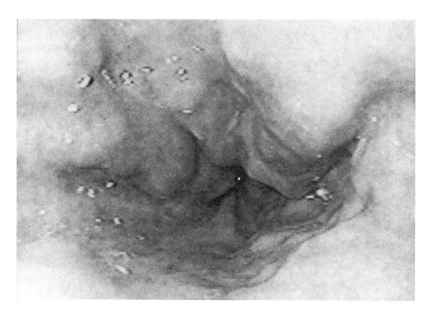

FIGURE 51-5. Endoscopic view of esophageal varices.

the catheter is then advanced until the catheter occludes a small hepatic vein. The pressure is obtained in this position and is referred to as the wedged hepatic venous pressure. The hepatic venous pressure gradient is the difference between the wedged hepatic venous pressure and the free hepatic venous pressure. This gradient is normally less than 5 mmHg; a value greater than 10 mmHg is indicative of portal hypertension. Complications of portal hypertension typically do not occur until the hepatic venous pressure gradient exceeds 12 mmHg. Patients with prehepatic portal hypertension such as portal vein thrombosis will have a normal hepatic venous pressure gradient. This procedure is invasive and complicated; it is most commonly used in adult studies assessing the efficacy of pharmacologic agents to reduce portal pressure.

The major role of angiography in patients with portal hypertension is to rule out vascular thrombosis (Budd-Chiari syndrome) and portal vein thrombosis or to define the vascular anatomy if surgery is contemplated. Splenoportography can be performed by the direct puncture of the spleen percutaneously with the subsequent administration of a contrast agent under direct pressure. Because of the high risk associated with this procedure, and because the portal system can be visualized with less invasive techniques, it is rarely performed. It should not be done unless surgery can be performed immediately, in the event that complications occur.

COMPLICATIONS AND TREATMENT

There are four major complications of portal hypertension: variceal bleeding, ascites, portosystemic encephalopathy (PSE), and splenomegaly.

Varices

Variceal bleeding is the most severe and potentially life-threatening complication of portal hypertension. Varices are present in 50 or 60% of patients with cirrhosis, and 30% will have an episode of variceal hemorrhage within 2 years of diagnosis. In adults with esophageal variceal bleeding, the mortality rate is 40 to 50%. The mortality rate in children is lower (12 to 21%) but still significant. After a patient has experienced an episode of variceal bleeding, 80 to 100% will have another bleed within 2 years. Most episodes of variceal bleeding are esophageal in origin but can also be from gastric, small intestinal, or colonic varices (for a discussion on the management of varices, see Ch. 51).

Ascites

Ascites, a frequent problem in patients with sinusoidal and postsinusoidal portal hypertension, is uncommon in patients with presinusoidal portal hypertension. The pathogenesis of ascites in patients with portal hypertension is multifactorial. The portal hypertension results in increased hydrostatic pressure; in those with associated liver disease with hypoalbuminemia, there is a decreased oncotic pressure. These alterations in Starling forces cause fluid to move from the intravascular space to the extravascular space. When the rate of extravascular fluid production exceeds the ability of the lymphatic system to reabsorb this fluid and transport it back to the vascular system, the fluid accumulates in the peritoneal cavity, causing ascites. Another factor contributing to the development of ascites in patients with cirrhosis is renal sodium retention and subsequent plasma volume expansion. This increase in intravascular volume increases the hydrostatic pressure in the hepatosplanchnic circulation resulting in fluid extravasation into the peritoneal space.

Portal hypertension is the most common cause of ascites in North America, but ascites can also result from hypoalbuminemia, infections, renal disease, and other GI causes.[15] Patients noted to have ascites are best evaluated with an abdominal ultrasound to confirm the presence of ascites and make sure it is not pseudoascites. If a paracentesis is performed, the fluid typically is clear or straw colored with a total protein of less than 2.5 to 3 g/dl or less than one-half the plasma total protein concentration. The leukocyte count is less than 250 to 500 cells/mm^3 with less than one third of the cells being neutrophils. The concentrations of electrolytes, urea, creatinine, triglyceride, and glucose approximate the plasma levels.

Ascites can be minimal, detected only incidentally on ultrasonic examination, or it can be massive, resulting in early satiety and malnutrition or respiratory distress. Medical therapy for ascites consists of normalization of the patient's nutritional status, salt restriction, and the use of diuretics such as spironolactone. If the patient is having acute symptoms (i.e., respiratory distress), a large volume therapeutic paracentesis can be done or intravenous albumin 1 g/kg administered over 1 to 2 hours, along with intravenous furosemide 1 mg/kg halfway through the infusion. For refractory ascites, patients can undergo placement of a peritoneovenous shunt, LeVeen or Denver shunt, or transjugular intrahepatic portosystemic shunt (TIPS).[16]

Another potential complication of ascites with portal hypertension is spontaneous bacterial peritonitis (SBP).[17] The organisms most commonly involved are *Escherichia coli, Klebsiella, Streptococcus,* and *Enterococcus.* Cefotaxime is considered the drug of choice for SBP and therapy should be continued for 10 to 14 days. SBP is associated with a mortality rate of 25 to 50%. There is also a high recurrence rate of SBP in those who survive, with a probability of recurrence of 70% in 1 year. Because of this high mortality rate and the rate of recurrence, patients with cirrhosis who recover from the initial episode of SBP should be considered for liver transplantation. Trimethoprim-sulfamethoxazole appears to be effective prophylaxis in patients with cirrhosis and ascites for the prevention of SBP.[18]

Portosystemic Encephalopathy

Portosystemic encephalopathy is a neuropsychiatric disorder characterized by alterations in consciousness, impaired intellectual abilities, and several neuromuscular signs such as asterixis.[19] Laboratory evaluation of affected patients reveals elevated ammonia levels, and an electroencephalogram (EEG) demonstrates diffuse slowing. This condition develops most often in patients with severe liver disease who have portosystemic shunts. These shunts can develop spontaneously or may be the result of transjugular intrahepatic portacaval shunt (TIPS) or surgically created portosystemic shunts. Although multiple theories have tried to explain its pathogenesis, the exact cause of portosystemic encephalopathy is unknown. Therapy is directed toward a reduction in serum ammonia levels by decreasing dietary protein, controlling any ongoing GI hemorrhaging, and removing blood from the GI tract. Neomycin can be administered to decrease enteric bacterial ammonia production, and lactulose is used to trap ammonia in the gut. Any precipitating cause of portosystemic encephalopathy, such as bacterial infection, should be treated.

Splenomegaly

Splenomegaly and associated hypersplenism is a frequent problem in patients with portal hypertension. The patients may have massive splenomegaly, predisposing them to splenic rupture after blunt abdominal trauma. The patient's symptoms vary from moderate left upper quadrant pain or left shoulder pain to overt shock. Patients with hypersplenism have a reduction in one or more hematologic components. Thrombocytopenia secondary to hypersplenism is typically within the range of 50,000 to 150,000/mm^3. If the condition is severe, treatment consists of splenectomy, liver transplantation, or the creation of a portosystemic shunt.

If splenectomy is required, it is better to wait, until the child is at least 5 years of age if possible, to try and avoid overwhelming sepsis. Pneumococcal vaccine and meningococcal vaccine in children greater than 2 years of age should be given before splenectomy and prophylactic penicillin administered after splenectomy.

PREVENTION

Preventive measures in patients with portal hypertension are directed at primary or secondary prevention of variceal bleeding.[20,21] The risk of variceal hemorrhage for patients with esophageal varices is 25 to 40%. Owing to the frequency of variceal hemorrhage, the high morbidity and mortality rates associated with variceal hemorrhage, and the high rate of rebleeding, the physician should attempt to prevent initially hemorrhage. Available therapeutic modalities include medical and surgical approaches.

Products that can precipitate or worsen variceal bleeding should be avoided in children with portal hypertension. Aspirin is a potentially aggravating factor in variceal bleeding. Because aspirin is part of several medications, patients and parents should be taught to read the label of medications to avoid inadvertent consumption of aspirin. Prophylaxis with acid suppressing agents, H$_2$-blockers, and proton pump inhibitors offers no benefit in the prevention of variceal bleeding and should be used only if the patient has acid peptic disease or gastroesophageal reflux. Theoretically, agents which increase lower esophageal sphincter pressure may be beneficial by decreasing blood flow in esophageal varices; however, no benefit of these agents has been documented.

Pharmacologic therapy for the prevention of variceal hemorrhage is directed at reducing portal pressure. This can be accomplished either by decreasing blood flow into the portal system or by decreasing vascular resistance in the vessels at the site of origin of the portal hypertension and its collaterals, or both. Propranolol, a nonselective beta blocker, is the agent most commonly employed in the prevention of primary and secondary variceal hemorrhage. Propranolol reduces splanchnic blood flow and portal pressure by blocking vasodilatory splanchnic beta-adrenergic receptors and by decreasing cardiac output. Propranolol has been shown to be more effective at reducing portal pressure than atenolol, a cardio-selective beta-1-blocker. A reduction in intravariceal pressure has been documented in patients on propranolol, as well as a 30% reduction in azygous blood flow.

It has been well documented that propranolol significantly reduces the incidence of initial variceal bleeding and the frequency of fatal hemorrhage compared to placebo. There may also be improved mortality rate in patients treated with propranolol. Because of this reduction in the incidence of bleeding and fatal bleeding, patients with portal hypertension should be screened for esophageal varices and, if present, therapy with propranolol should be instituted. Typically, the dose administered is that sufficient to cause a reduction in heart rate by 25%.

In addition to reducing the incidence of initial variceal bleeding, propranolol is effective at reducing the risk of rebleeding. However, there is no associated reduction in mortality rate. Propranolol helps prevent acute and chronic bleeding from portal hypertensive gastropathy.

Isosorbide mononitrate is a vasodilator that acts by increasing nitrous oxide formation in vascular smooth muscle cells. This vasodilation results in a decrease in venous return, and possibly in a reduction in arterial pressure, leading to splanchnic vasoconstriction and decreased portal blood flow. There is no role for isosorbide mononitrate as a single agent in the treatment of portal hypertension. When combined with propranolol, isosorbide mononitrate has been shown to cause a further reduction in portal pressure, as compared to propranolol by itself. Some patients who do not respond to propranolol alone will have a reduction in portal pressure with the combination of propranolol and isosorbide mononitrate. Clinical trials are under way to assess the efficacy of combination pharmacologic therapy, compared with propranolol alone at preventing variceal bleeding.

Spironolactone has been shown to reduce the hepatoportal venous gradient in cirrhotic patients with ascites. There are no studies evaluating the use of spironolactone in preventing variceal bleeding; however, its use should be considered in patients with ascites. Other potential benefits of spironolactone are decreased ascites and increased protein content in ascitic fluid, which may decrease the incidence of SBP. Low-sodium diets exert no beneficial effect on portal pressure but high sodium intake should be avoided.

Potential surgical modalities available to prevent variceal bleeding include endoscopic sclerosis of varices, TIPS, portosplenic shunt surgery, and liver transplantation. None of these therapeutic modalities is recommended for primary prevention of variceal hemorrhage. Prophylactic endoscopic sclerotherapy is probably the surgical procedure of choice in the prevention of recurrent variceal hemorrhage. Sclerotherapy and propranolol appear to be equally effective at preventing recurrent variceal bleeding. Because of the invasiveness of sclerotherapy, many feel that this should be considered second-line therapy, except in those who do not tolerate propranolol.

TIPS placement is a relatively new therapeutic modality available for the management of portal hypertension.[22] This procedure functions on the same principle as other surgically created portosystemic shunts to decrease portal pressure. This is accomplished by passing a catheter through the internal jugular into the hepatic vein under fluoroscopic control. The hepatic vein is punctured and the catheter advanced into a branch of the portal vein. A metallic mesh stent is then placed between the portal vein and the hepatic vein. This results in a decrease in absolute portal pressure and an increase in vena cava pressure. The combined effect is a reduction in the portal pressure gradient. TIPS is also associated with an increase in cardiac output, increased right atrial pressure, and a decrease in systemic vascular resistance (SVR). TIPS is contraindicated in patients with portal vein thrombosis. TIPS is effective at decreasing the risk of recurrent esophageal variceal bleeding. Because of the high stenosis and occlusion rate along with the risk of developing portosystemic encephalopathy, TIPS is rec-

ommended for those patients who are unresponsive to or do not tolerate propranolol or sclerotherapy.

Portosystemic shunt[23] surgery appears to be very effective at decreasing the risk of recurrent bleeding, but shunt surgery is invasive, is associated with a high incidence of PSE, and may make subsequent liver transplantation more difficult. The distal splenorenal shunt is as effective as nonselective shunts in reducing the incidence of rebleeding. It is associated with a lower frequency of encephalopathy, and it does not have as much impact on subsequent liver transplantation, making it the preferred shunting procedure. This may be the preferred therapeutic modality for patients who do not have ready access to centers with the ability to manage acute variceal bleeding in pediatric patients.

Liver transplantation is the therapeutic modality of choice for preventing recurrent bleeding in pediatric patients with end-stage liver disease.[24] The current survival rate for pediatric patients undergoing elective liver transplantation is upward of 85%.

REFERENCES

1. Boyer TD. Portal hypertensive hemorrhage: pathogenesis and risk factors. Semin Gastrointest Dis 1995;6:125–133

2. Alvarez F, Bernard O, Brunelle F et al. Portal obstruction in children: Clinical investigation and hemorrhage risk. J Pediatr 1983;103:696–702

3. Webb LJ, Sherlock S. The aetiology, presentation and natural history of extrahepatic portal venous obstruction. Q J Med 1979;48:627–639

4. Meresse V, Hartman O, Vassal G et al. Risk factors for hepatic veno-occlusive disease after high-dose busulfan-containing regimens followed by autologous bone marrow transplantation. Bone Marrow Transplant 1992;10:135–141

5. Etziomi A, Benderly A, Rosenthal E et al. Defective humoral and cellular functions associated with veno-occlusive disease of the liver. J Pediatr 1987;110:549–554

6. Gentil-Kocher S, Bernard O, Brunelle F et al. Budd-Chiari syndrome in children: report of 22 cases. J Pediatr 1988;113:30–38

7. Ready J, Rector WG Jr. Systemic hemodynamic changes in portal hypertension. Semin Gastrointest Dis 1995;6:134–139

8. Sarin SK, Lahoti D, Saxena SP et al. Prevalence, classification and natural history of gastric varices: A long-term follow-up study in 568 portal hypertension patients. Hepatology 1992;16:1343–1349

9. Hashizume M, Sugimachi K. Classification of gastric lesions associated with portal hypertension. J Gastroenterol Hepatol 1995;10:339–343

10. Kozarek RA, Botoman VA, Bredfeldt JE et al. Portal colopathy: prospective study of colonoscopy in patients with portal hypertension. Gastroenterology 1991;101:1192–1197

11. Lebrec D. Methods to evaluate portal hypertension. Gastroenterol Clin North Am 1992;21:41–59

12. Ginai AZ, Van Buuren HR, Hop WC, Schalm SW. Oesophageal varices: how reliable is a barium swallow? Br J Radiol 1993;66:322–326

13. DeGiacomo C, Tomasi G, Gatti C et al. Ultrasonographic prediction of the presence and severity of esophageal varices in children. J Pediatr Gastroenterol Nutr 1989;9:431–435

14. Westra SJ, Zaninovic AC, Vargas J et al. The value of portal vein pulsatility on duplex sonograms as a sign of portal hypertension in children with liver disease. AJR 1995;165:167–172

15. Cochran WJ. Ascites. In: Oski FA et al, Eds. Principles and Practice of Pediatrics. Philadelphia: JB Lippincott, 1994:1902–1907

16. Ochs A, Rossle M, Haag K et al. The transjugular intrahepatic portosystemic stent-shunt procedure for refractory ascites. N Engl J Med 1995;332:1192–1197

17. Bhuva M, Ganger D, Jensen D. Spontaneous bacterial peritonitis: an update on evaluation, management, and prevention. Am J Med 1994;97:169–175

18. Singh N, Gayowski T, Yu VL, Wagener MM. Trimethoprim-sulfamethoxazole for the prevention of spontaneous bacterial peritonitis in cirrhosis: a randomized trial. Ann Intern Med 1995;122:595–598

19. Conn HO. Hepatic encephalopathy. In: Schiff L, Schiff ER, Eds. Diseases of the Liver. 7th ed. Philadelphia: JB Lippincott, 1993:1036–1060

20. Grace ND. Prevention of initial variceal hemorrhage. Gastroenterol Clin North Am 1992;21:149–161

21. Burroughs AK, McCormick PA. Prevention of variceal rebleeding. Gastroenterol Clin North Am 1992;21:119–147

22. Crecelius SA, Soule MC. Transjugular intrahepatic portosystemic shunts for portal hypertension. Gastroenterol Clin North Am 1995;24:201–219

23. Orloff MJ, Orloff MS, Rambotti M. Treatment of bleeding esophagogastric varices due to extrahepatic portal hypertension: results of portal systemic shunts during 35 years. J Pediatr Surg 1994;29:142–154

24. Henderson JM. Liver transplantation for portal hypertension. Gastroenterol Clin North Am 1992;21:197–213

52

GAUCHER'S DISEASE AND NIEMANN-PICK DISEASE

JEFFREY E. MING
ALICE T. MAZUR
PAIGE KAPLAN

Lysosomes degrade macromolecules derived from normal turnover and from exogenous sources. Defects in lysosomal enzymatic reactions result in specific substrate accumulation, depending on the affected enzymatic reaction. Commonly, the reticuloendothelial organs of the gastrointestinal (GI) tract (liver, spleen) are involved, and patients often present first with organomegaly. However, patients also develop neurologic, visceral, skeletal, and/or ocular abnormalities. Extensive variation in the clinical presentation can occur even among persons affected by the same enzyme defect. Hepatomegaly and splenomegaly are generally most pronounced in two of these lysosomal disorders: Gaucher's disease and Niemann-Pick disease. This chapter discusses the pathophysiology, clinical presentation, diagnosis, and management of these two disorders.

GAUCHER'S DISEASE

Gaucher's disease is a lysosomal glycolipid storage disorder characterized by the accumulation of glucosylceramide (glucocerebroside) primarily in the spleen, liver, and bones, and also in lungs and brain.[1] This systemic disease affects children and adults and has an autosomal recessive inheritance pattern.[2]

There are three types of Gaucher's disease (Table 52-

1) All are characterized by hepatosplenomegaly and hypersplenism; however, type 1 (by far the most common type) does not have neuronopathic (brain) involvement.[3] There is a wide spectrum of phenotypes in all subtypes of the disease, even among members of the same family.[4,5]

Pathophysiology

Glucocerebrosidase (glucosidase) deficiency is the enzymatic defect in Gaucher's disease. The lack of sufficient glucocerebrosidase activity leads to the accumulation of glucosylceramide (glucocerebroside), a complex lipid, which is normally metabolized to its two components, glucose and ceramide. Glucocerebroside accumulates in the lysosomes of tissue macrophages (i.e., reticuloendothelial cells). Macrophages, engorged with glucocerebroside, are the storage cells of Gaucher's disease. They are referred to as Gaucher cells and present a distinctive "wrinkled tissue paper" appearance upon microscopic examination.[6] Although typical of Gaucher's disease, they may occur in other disorders, such as thalassemia[7] and multiple myeloma.[8]

Macrophages develop from bone marrow-derived monocytes that migrate into tissues and mature. These macrophages are present in the liver as Kupffer cells, in bone as osteoclasts, in the lungs as alveolar macrophages,

TABLE 52-1. Gaucher's Disease: Clinical Types

Clinical Features	Type 1	Type 2	Type 3
Age at onset	Childhood/adulthood	Infancy	Childhood
Splenomegaly	+ to + + +	+ +	+ to + + +
Hepatomegaly	+ to + + +	+ +	+ to + + +
Skeletal disease/bone crises	− to + + +	—	+ + to + + +
Primary central nervous system disease	Absent	+ + +	+ to + + + (1st to 5th decade)
Life span	6–80 + yr	~2 y	2–60 y
Ethnicity/demographic group	Pan-ethnic/Ashkenazi Jewish(AJ)	Pan-ethnic	Pan-ethnic/Norrbottnian
Frequency	~1/60,000–1/200,000 ~1/500–1/1,000 (AJ)	<1/100,000	<1/50,000

and as bone marrow and spleen tissue macrophages. This distribution of macrophages in tissue explains the organ involvement in patients with Gaucher's disease.

Clinical Presentation

Three different types of Gaucher's disease have been described. All have liver and spleen enlargement, but type 1 does not have brain involvement.

TYPE 1 (NON-NEURONOPATHIC)

Type 1 Gaucher's disease is the most common (95%) form of the disease. It is pan-ethnic, with the highest incidence in the Ashkenazi (Eastern European) Jewish population. In the general population, the incidence of type 1 is estimated at about 1 in 60,000, and in the Ashkenazi Jewish population, its incidence is approximately 1 in 500 to 1 in 1,000.[2]

The clinical manifestations of type 1 Gaucher's disease result from engorged macrophages causing enlargement and dysfunction of the liver and spleen, as well as displacement of normal bone marrow and damage to bone leading to infarctions and fractures. In about 50% of symptomatic children, poor growth and delayed puberty occur.[9]

The disorder is markedly variable in expression, even within the same family.[4,5] Some individuals present in early childhood with massive hepatosplenomegaly combined with severe abnormalities of spleen function, pancytopenia, and extensive skeletal abnormalities. At the other end of the spectrum, affected adults may not be symptomatic; their condition may be diagnosed only when family studies are done, and they may have only mild thrombocytopenia. Approximately one-half of affected people have little or no symptoms throughout most or all of their lives. Thirty percent may have moderate disease, and 20% are severely affected.

Painless splenic enlargement is present in almost all patients and is often the first sign in children.[10] Spleno-megaly may range from minimal to marked, with the spleen filling most of the abdominal cavity. Splenic bulk may interfere with normal food intake. Splenic infarctions may occur, causing an acute abdomen with fever, metabolic acidosis, and hyperuricemia.

Thrombocytopenia is the most common peripheral blood abnormality.[11] Early in the course of the disease, it is usually due to splenic sequestration of platelets. Bleeding secondary to the thrombocytopenia occurs frequently. Anemia can also occur and is usually mild but occasionally can be very severe. Leukopenia appears in some patients. These changes are caused by a combination of increased splenic sequestration and decreased production because of marrow replacement by Gaucher cells.[1]

Liver enlargement is found in all patients.[12] Liver function tests may be abnormal with increases in plasma transaminases and gamma glutamyltransferase activity. Severe liver function abnormalities are rare because hepatocytes are not affected. Frank hepatic failure and/or cirrhosis with portal hypertension and ascites are uncommon.

The skeletal disease, due to marrow infiltration with Gaucher cells, can be very painful and disabling. Nearly all patients, even children, have bony lesions on radiographic, scintigraphic, computed tomographic (CT), or magnetic resonance imaging (MRI) scans.[13] The classic "Erlenmeyer flask deformity" of the distal femur is a common radiographic finding but is not universally present nor is it pathognomonic. Many patients have generalized bone loss and may complain of dull aches in joints or shafts of long bones.

Bone crises occur in 20% to 40% of patients. They can occur at any age but are more frequent in children and adolescents. They are episodic and extremely painful, usually affecting the humeral heads, vertebral bodies, and ischium of the pelvis.[1] They can occur spontaneously or can follow a febrile syndrome, beginning with a deep, aching pain in the involved area, followed by severe pain. These crises have been misdiagnosed as osteomyelitis. Although radiographs may appear normal in the first few weeks, areas of ischemia are usually present on technetium-99m bone scans. Bed rest and analgesics are required to control the intense pain, which subsides to a dull ache within a few days. Recurrence is usually at a different location.

Children with acute hip lesions have been misdiagnosed as having Legg-Calvé-Perthes disease.[1] Most severe bone lesions appear during childhood and adolescence followed by a slowly progressive process in adulthood. Pathologic fractures of the femoral neck occur in the later decades of life in areas of pre-existing bone lesions.

Gaucher cells may infiltrate the lung, but clubbing is rare.[1] Pulmonary failure resulting from right to left intrapulmonary shunting secondary to severe liver disease occurs infrequently.

Patients with type 1 Gaucher's disease do not have primary central nervous system involvement. However, massive systemic fat emboli in the brain and lung have been reported rarely. Compression of the spinal cord secondary to vertebral collapse may also occur.

TYPE 2

Onset of symptoms is in infancy, with marked liver and spleen enlargement and a neurodegenerative course that results in death by 2 years of age. This disorder is pan-ethnic. The frequency is fewer than 1 in 100,000 live births.[2] Oculomotor abnormalities, such as bilateral fixed strabismus or oculomotor apraxia, are usually the first symptoms to manifest. Extensive hepatosplenomegaly is present. Hypertonia, primarily involving neck muscles with retroflexion of the head, bulbar signs, limb rigidity, seizures, and choreoathetoid movements occur. Rarely, the disease manifests at birth with ichthyosis or hydrops fetalis.

TYPE 3

The subacute neuronopathic form of Gaucher's disease usually manifests in early childhood with liver and spleen enlargement, similar to severe cases of type 1, and, in late childhood, with neurologic symptoms similar to those in type 2, but less severe.[1] This type is often referred to as the Norrbottnian form with ethnic predilection for those of northern Swedish ancestry. The frequency of this type of Gaucher's disease is estimated at 1 in 50,000 live births, but no accurate figures are available.[2]

The first symptoms are usually visceral involvement followed by neurologic degeneration during the first decade of life. Oculomotor abnormalities are the first symptoms that herald the onset of chronic neurologic degeneration. There is a wide spectrum of neurologic abnormalities, including ataxia; spastic paraparesis; myo-

clonic, grand mal, or psychomotor seizures; and dementia. Death usually occurs by the second to the fourth decade of life.

Diagnosis

Gaucher's disease should be suspected in any child presenting with abdominal organomegaly, particularly painless splenomegaly or any combination of hypersplenism or hepatomegaly and decreased platelets, anemia, fatigue, bleeding diathesis, recurrent bone pain, Legg-Calvé-Perthes disease, bone lesions on radiography or MRI, and growth retardation and/or delayed puberty. Patients presenting with splenomegaly and hematologic abnormalities are often mistakenly misdiagnosed as having lymphoma, leukemia, or a bleeding disorder.

Blood testing for enzymatic and molecular abnormalities are noninvasive and widely available and should be obtained initially in all patients suspected of having Gaucher's disease; liver or bone marrow biopsies usually are not required for the diagnosis.[14]

Laboratory Evaluation

ENZYMATIC DIAGNOSIS

Assay of β-glucosidase activity in peripheral blood leukocytes is a specific and reliable technique for the diagnosis of Gaucher's disease.[1] There is a wide range of variability in activity, even within a given morphologic type, so selection of a reliable laboratory is necessary to obtain optimal results. Diagnosis can also be made in cultured skin fibroblasts, amniotic fluid cells, and chorionic villus samples.

Heterozygotes (carriers) for Gaucher's disease average half-normal β-glucosidase activity in leukocytes and cultured skin fibroblasts. However, there may be considerable overlap between the low normal range and values in heterozygotes. Differentiation between neuronopathic disease (types 2 and 3) and nonneuronopathic disease cannot be done on the basis of enzymatic activity.

MOLECULAR DIAGNOSIS

The gene for glucocerebrosidase, on chromosome 1q21, contains approximately 7,000 base pairs in 11 exons and 10 introns.[15] Multiple point mutations and a frameshift mutation have been identified in the glucocerebrosidase gene, and several mutations are frequently observed. Four of the mutations, located at either nucleotide 1226 (amino acid N370S), 1448 (L444P), IVS-2, or 84GG, account for nearly 95% of the disease-producing alleles in Ashkenazi Jewish patients.[3] In non-Jewish patients, 75% of the disease-producing alleles have been identified as mutations at nucleotide 1448 (L44P) and 1226 (N370S). Several other uncommon mutations have been found.[3]

Mutation analysis has some predictive value with

respect to disease prognosis, although there are exceptions.[16] Many people have two different mutations, making them "compound heterozygotes." Patients homozygous for the L444P mutation all have severe visceral disease, and most have neurologic disease (types 2 and 3). The N370S mutations are associated with mild to moderate disease phenotypes, whereas mutation 84GG has a more severe phenotype.

Carriers can be diagnosed if the person has one of the four common mutations.

MORPHOLOGIC DIAGNOSIS

Histologic diagnosis of Gaucher's disease has been a means of diagnosis in patients in whom Gaucher's disease has not previously been suspected. This method relies upon the identification of the specific storage cell, the Gaucher cell, in organ tissue. Similar appearing cells, pseudo-Gaucher cells, have been described in a number of other disorders, but they do not contain the typical tubular structures of true Gaucher cells.

Treatment

ENZYME REPLACEMENT THERAPY

Macrophage-directed exogenous enzyme therapy, using alglucerase and imiglucerase, is available for treatment of patients with type 1 Gaucher's disease.[17] In order for exogenous enzyme to be effective, it must reach the lysosome in the macrophage. The discovery that macrophage receptors recognize and bind mannose when it is the terminal sugar residue on the glycoprotein's oligosaccharide chain provided the rationale for macrophage-targeted enzyme replacement therapy. The carbohydrate portion of glucocerebrosidase is modified to expose the mannose terminal, facilitating the recognition and uptake of glucocerebrosidase into macrophages. Alglucerase (Ceredase) is the enzyme extracted from placental tissue, which has been purified so that known viruses, such as human immunodeficiency virus (HIV), are destroyed. Recombinant enzyme, imiglucerase for injection (Cerezyme), is also available.

Intravenous treatment with Ceredase and Cerezyme is used only for moderately or severely affected type 1 Gaucher's disease patients and results in positive clinical response with increased hemoglobin concentration and platelet count, and reduction in spleen and liver size after several months. Bone lesions also improve, but more slowly. Ten percent to 15% of treated patients will develop antibodies against the enzyme protein, but these usually do not interfere with clinical response.

A few untoward reactions have been reported with enzyme therapy. Most are not serious, and symptoms include abdominal pain, tightness of the chest, and hives. These reactions usually have been due to too-rapid intra-venous infusion of the drug, especially during the initial phase of infusion. Slow infusion early in the course with incremental increases in rate have resulted in fewer side effects of the medication. There has been one report of severe anaphylaxis.

The optimal dose and frequency of treatment with enzyme replacement are under debate.[18] Generally, patients with severe disease respond favorably to doses of 60 U/kg of body weight given every 2 weeks.[17] Less severely affected individuals may require only 15 to 40 U/kg every 2 weeks for good response. As clinical, hematologic, and radiologic improvements occur, the dose of enzyme can be decreased while the patient is closely monitored. Some physicians are using doses of 2.3 U/kg given at a frequency of 3 times weekly and report favorable response in clinical, hematologic, and organ volume parameters. Importantly, however, skeletal improvement with use of smaller doses has not yet been documented.

The use of enzyme replacement therapy in patients with type 2 disease has not proven satisfactory. The neurologic manifestations do not respond to enzyme therapy, although there is reduction in spleen and liver size. In type 3, there is not sufficient experience to know if enzyme replacement is of long-term value.

SPLENECTOMY

Splenectomy should be considered only in patients with mechanical cardiopulmonary compromise in whom enzyme replacement therapy has not decreased the size of the organs sufficiently to facilitate medical management.[1] Until enzyme replacement therapy was available for widespread use, splenectomy was an effective treatment for thrombocytopenia and, to a lesser extent, anemia.[3] There is no evidence that splenectomy will result in accelerated deposition of glucosylceramide and progression of the disease in other organs, like the skeleton. However, in Norrbottnian patients, splenectomy resulted in increased accumulation in plasma and brain and a more rapid clinical deterioration.

Partial splenectomy was proposed as a means of obtaining the therapeutic benefits of splenectomy, while avoiding the side effects of total removal of the organ. With few controlled studies on the use of this therapeutic adjunct, there is little justification for its use.

BONE DISEASE

In many patients, especially in older patients, the most debilitating consequence of the disease is the bone involvement.[19] Orthopedic procedures can relieve pain and promote better use of affected joints. These procedures should be considered along with enzyme replacement therapy to achieve optimal outcome, especially in patients with cortical thinning.[20] Joint replacement therapy should not be considered in children because of its interference with limb growth. Aminohydroxypropylidine bisphosphonate administration has been used in a few patients with Gaucher's disease, with improved calcium balance and bone density and reversal of bone disease.[21] There are no controlled studies on its use; however, it may prove a valuable adjunct in the treatment of patients with severe bone disease or older patients.

Patients who manifest severe bone disease or who have grossly enlarged liver and spleen should avoid activities that could result in pathologic fractures of bone or rupture of organ. Bone crisis is a severe manifestation of the disease that usually requires hospitalization for intravenous hydration and administration of analgesics for pain control. Blood cultures and bone scans should be done to ensure that there is no osteomyelitis.

GROWTH

In symptomatic children with Gaucher's disease, linear growth is usually normal in the first 1–2 years of life and then decelerates. One-half of children with type 1 have growth retardation (at or below the 5th percentile), and another 25% are below mid-parental height before treatment. Normalization of growth occurs in 72% within a few years after starting enzyme therapy.[9] Menarche is delayed in untreated or undertreated adolescent females. In girls treated during the first decade with alglucerase, puberty can occur at a normal age.[9] Delayed puberty in untreated males has not been reported.

Genetic Counseling

Gaucher's disease is inherited as an autosomal recessive condition. In the Ashkenazi Jewish population, the carrier (heterozygote) rate is estimated to be 1 in 10 to 1 in 15 persons, and in the non-Ashekenazi Jewish population, 1 in 120.[2] Carriers do not manifest any signs or symptoms of the disease. When both parents are heterozygotes, each child they conceive together will have a 1 in 4 chance of inheriting both abnormal genes and being affected. In the Ashekenazi Jewish population, there may be apparent autosomal dominant inheritance if a parent and child are both affected. In this type of family, the other (unaffected) parent must be a carrier, so the affected child has inherited a mutant gene from each parent, in an autosomal recessive mode.

Prenatal diagnosis by enzyme assay or DNA mutation analysis is reliable. Molecular diagnosis is feasible if the mutations have been identified in both parents. It is controversial whether there should be prenatal diagnosis or heterozygote screening in communities at risk.

Referral Pattern

Children with either hematologic, visceral, or orthopedic abnormalities should be referred to the appropriate specialist for further confirmatory diagnosis and management. Evaluation should include a thorough history of familial diseases, bleeding (gums, nose), and easy bruisability. Complete physical examination of the patient should include liver and spleen size, bruises, and bone pain or tenderness. Initial laboratory evaluation should include a complete blood count (CBC), liver transaminases, total acid phosphatase, and enzymatic activity in leukocytes. If the glucocerebrosidase activity is low, confirming the diagnosis, the patient should be referred to a Gaucher's treatment center for further evaluation including DNA mutation analysis.

These centers, usually in hematology or biochemical genetics departments, have the experienced personnel to evaluate and monitor the patient's disease. Enzyme replacement therapy, costly from both a financial and time commitment perspective, is warranted if the disease is moderate or severe. Most affected children need treatment. Serial evaluations at the treatment center include continuous patient and family history, physical examination, and laboratory evaluation, including liver and spleen volumes (by MRI/CT) to accurately determine the degree of enlargement and bone MRI or CT to determine extent of bone involvement. Bone density studies (DXA) are useful in assessing bone loss and degree of replacement by infiltrates. The dose and frequency of enzyme is individualized.

The centers participate in the International Collaborative Gaucher Group Registry. Through this, the best monitoring techniques, optimal treatment schedules, and natural history of Gaucher's disease are reported and evaluated.

NIEMANN-PICK DISEASE

Niemann-Pick disease is a rare condition that is also characterized by an accumulation of lysosomal products in different organs. The age at presentation can vary from the neonatal period to adulthood. Several classifications of subtypes have been proposed, but there is overlap of features among the groups. The most commonly used classification divides this disease into three categories (Table 52-2). In types A and B, a mutation in acid sphingomyelinase is present. The biochemical defect in type C prevents cholesterol esterification; the specific enzyme has not yet been determined.

Pathophysiology

In Niemann-Pick disease types A and B, decreased activity of acid sphingomyelinase leads to lysosomal accumulation of sphingomyelin up to 70 times normal levels. Tissue cholesterol levels are increased by an unknown mechanism and probably reflect a secondary effect. Bis-(monoacylglycero)phosphate and other sphingolipids also accumulate. The enzymatic activity level in cultured

TABLE 52-2. Features of Types of Niemann-Pick Disease

	Type A	Type B	Type C
Enzyme defect	Sphingomyelinase	Sphingomyelinase	Cholesterol esterification
Age at diagnosis	Infancy	Infancy–adulthood	Variable
Life expectancy	<5 yr	Adulthood	Variable, usually <20 yr
Sphingomyelinase activity	0–5% of normal	2–10% of normal	Normal
CNS involvement	Present, severe	Absent	Present, variable severity
Hepatosplenomegaly	Neonatal period	Infancy/childhood	Neonatal/childhood

fibroblasts ranges from undetectable to 5% of normal in type A, and from 2% to 10% in type B. In general, patients with type B have higher levels of residual enzyme activity than individuals with type A Niemann-Pick disease.

The biochemical defect underlying Niemann-Pick disease type C has not been determined. Esterification of exogenously derived cholesterol is greatly decreased, leading to accumulation of unesterified cholesterol. Intracellular transport or trafficking of free cholesterol may be defective. The severity of the defect in cholesterol esterification correlates with the degree of clinical disease. Sphingomyelinase activity may be reduced, owing to an uncharacterized secondary effect of cholesterol accumulation.

Epidemiology and Genetics

All forms of Niemann-Pick disease are inherited in an autosomal recessive manner. The incidence of type A and type B Niemann-Pick disease is increased in the Ashkenazi Jewish population, but Niemann-Pick disease is pan-ethnic.[22] The sphingomyelinase gene is on chromosome 11p15.1–11p15.4.[23] Point mutations leading to amino acid substitutions, deletions leading to a premature stop codon, and a three-nucleotide deletion have been described. There seems to be a correlation between the specific type of mutation and the severity of disease in the Ashkenazi Jewish population. However, in non-Jewish individuals, each family tends to have a unique mutation, making genotype-phenotype correlations difficult.

Type C is also pan-ethnic, although an increased carrier frequency has been identified in populations in Nova Scotia (Acadian) and southern Colorado (Hispanic). There are two distinct complementation groups,[24] and the gene for the major group has been mapped to chromosome 18 by linkage analysis.[25] The location of the gene for the minor complementation group is unknown.

Clinical Presentation

Type A is the most severe form, with both neurologic and visceral abnormalities. Typically, patients with type A are normal at birth. Hepatosplenomegaly is noted only occasionally in the neonatal period, but is generally present by 6 months of age. The spleen may be enlarged ten-fold and the liver two-fold. Liver function is usually normal or mildly impaired, although prolonged neonatal jaundice has been reported.[26] Feeding difficulties, which may be secondary to hypotonia, and severe failure to thrive manifest in infancy. The children have a wasted appearance with protuberant abdomens. Early neurologic manifestations include hypotonia and muscular weakness. By 6 months, psychomotor retardation becomes apparent and is followed by loss of developmental milestones. Neurologic deterioration is relentless, and spasticity and loss of awareness of the environment occur. A macular cherry-red spot is seen in about 50% by the second year. Alternatively, a gray granular-appearing macula or corneal opacification may be present.[27] The electroretinogram may be abnormal, although vision loss is rare. Some features found in other lysosomal diseases, such as seizures, hyperacusis, and macrocephaly, are not typical in Niemann-Pick disease. Chest radiography may show diffuse granular infiltrates. Generalized osteoporosis is common, although deformities due to marrow expansion are unusual. Moderate microcytic anemia and thrombocytopenia can occur. Death generally occurs by 3 years.

Type B disease presents more variably, even within families, with little or no central nervous system manifestations. Splenomegaly followed by hepatomegaly is noted incidentally during infancy, childhood, or even adulthood. The liver is usually more enlarged than the spleen, in contrast to the case in Gaucher's disease. Cirrhosis and/or portal hypertension has been reported in an adolescent (personal observation) and two adult women.[28,29] Pancytopenia due to hypersplenism may occur. Progressive pulmonary disease due to alveolar infiltration can lead to dyspnea on exertion, pneumonia, and asthma. The rate of progression is quite variable. Short stature is another finding. Intellectually normal patients with cherry-red spots or gray pigmentation near the fovea have been reported.[30] Two unrelated patients were mentally retarded at the ages of 9 and 18 years, respectively,[31] and other individuals with cerebellar ataxia have been reported.[32] The survival of these patients into late childhood or adolescence is unusual. From biochemical evaluations performed on these patients, it is unclear whether their disease represents a longer-surviving variant of type A, an unusual form of type B with mental retardation, or type C Niemann-Pick disease.

Type C Niemann-Pick disease has an extremely variable presentation but generally involves the central nervous system. Most frequently, abnormalities manifest in mid-childhood. Hepatosplenomegaly is usually detected, but not always. Neurologic manfestations are progressive and include ataxia, hypotonia, dementia, dysarthria, dystonia, and seizures. Supranuclear vertical gaze paresis is very typical. Affected children usually die by 20 years of age. A self-limiting neonatal cholestatic jaundice occurs in one-half of patients[33]; severe neonatal hepatic dysfunction or fetal ascites occurs rarely.[34] In another form, onset is in adolescence or adulthood, with psychiatric symptoms and dementia predominating. Affected adults also have vertical supranuclear ophthalmoplegia.

Diagnosis

Type A should be considered in an infant with hepatosplenomegaly, feeding problems, and developmental delay or loss of milestones. A macular cherry-red spot will distinguish Niemann-Pick disease from type 2 Gaucher's disease. Splenomegaly is generally the first manifestation of type B. The finding of hepatosplenomegaly in a child with developmental delay, especially if there is a history of neonatal jaundice or supranuclear ophthalmoplegia, should raise suspicion for type C.

Laboratory Evaluation

ENZYMATIC DIAGNOSIS

Types A and B

Direct enzymatic testing in blood, the most appropriate, definitive, and least invasive test, should be done in preference to bone marrow biopsy or aspiration. Types A and B will have markedly decreased activity of acid sphingomyelinase in leukocytes, cultured fibroblasts, or lymphoblasts. Heterozygote detection is difficult by enzymatic means because heterozygotes may have activity that falls within the low normal range of normal.

Type C

The enzymatic defect in type C Niemann-Pick disease is unknown. Filipin-stained cultured fibroblasts will show intense perinuclear fluorescence, indicating intralysosomal accumulation of unesterified cholesterol. When taken in combination with a demonstration of abnormal intracellular cholesterol esterification, the diagnosis of type C disease can be made.[35] Similar tests can be per-

formed on chorionic villus or cultured amniotic cells. The combination accurately detected affected fetuses in which a family member had a severe defect.[36] However, the general applicability of this technique to less severely affected families is uncertain. Accurate heterozygote identification is not available because of the overlap between normal and heterozygote values.

A gene, *NPC1*, with insertion, deletion, and missense mutations has been identified recently in type C Niemann-Pick patients.[37] The gene has been shown to regulate intracellular cholesterol trafficking.[38]

HISTOLOGIC DIAGNOSIS

Liver biopsy may be nondiagnostic in some cases of Niemann-Pick disease type A, B, or C. The presence of foam cells and sea-blue histiocytes in the bone marrow supports the diagnosis, but they are not always present. In all forms of Niemann-Pick disease, there are histiocytes filled with sphingomyelin, termed "foam cells" or "Niemann-Pick cells." The distinct "sea-blue histiocytes" derive their color from the bluish intracellular material found in bone marrow cells. The cells stain for cholesterol, in contrast to Gaucher cells. These cells occur in all affected organs (bone marrow, spleen, tonsils, lymph nodes, liver, lung, and brain) and distort the organs. The microscopic architecture shows infiltration of laden macrophages, and parenchymal cells may become vacuolated. The sinuses are affected first, followed by the portal areas. Niemann-Pick and vacuolated epithelial cells occur in the stomach and colon wall. In type C with early onset, there may be cholestasis with variable liver parenchymal damage and lobular inflammation. In adults, only a few foamy cells are found in the sinusoids without significant storage in hepatocytes.

MOLECULAR DIAGNOSIS

Ashkenazi Jewish individuals may benefit from molecular analysis of DNA, as a few common mutations make up the vast majority of defects in this group. Prenatal diagnosis is done by measuring acid sphingomyelinase activity in cultured amniocytes or chorionic villi.

Treatment

There is no specific treatment for Niemann-Pick disease. Liver, bone marrow, and amniotic cell transplantation have been attempted in type A and type B Niemann-Pick disease, and none has shown significant long-lasting effects. Liver transplantation in a type C patient did not affect neurologic disease. Dimethylsulfoxide (DMSO), which improves partial sphingomyelinase deficiency and partially reverses the cholesterol trafficking abnormalities in Niemann-Pick type C fibroblasts, has not shown consistent success. Interventions are largely supportive, and symptomatic management of seizures and dystonia is important.

Referral Pattern

Patients who are suspected of having Niemann-Pick diease should be referred to an experienced biochemical geneticist so that proper enzymatic testing can be performed. Evaluations of organ systems that may be involved and supportive treatment can be coordinated between the subspecialist and the primary physician.

Genetic Counseling

Niemann-Pick disease is inherited as an autosomal recessive condition. Carriers do not show abnormal signs or symptoms. Each child of two heterozygote parents has a 1 in 4 chance of inheriting both abnormal genes and being affected. Genetic counseling regarding the recurrence risk for future pregnancies of the affected family and their relatives should also be provided.

CONCLUSION

Two diseases, Gaucher's disease and Niemann-Pick disease, caused by defects in lysosomal enzymatic activity, can manifest in childhood with liver or spleen enlargement, or both. In each condition, some subtypes may have central nervous system involvement. The presentation and severity of disease of the non-neuronopathic forms vary widely. The diagnosis in an individual with splenomegaly with or without hepatomegaly is best established by the less invasive measurement of enzyme levels in peripheral blood leukocytes. For type 1 Gaucher's disease, enzyme replacement therapy is effective in reversing organomegaly, growth retardation, and bone involvement. No effective treatment exists for any of the neuronopathic forms.

REFERENCES

1. Beutler E, Grabowski GA. Gaucher disease. In: Scriver CR, Beaudet AL, Sly WS, Valle D, Eds. The Metabolic and Molecular Bases of Inherited Disease. Vol. II. New York: McGraw-Hill, 1995:2641–2670

2. Grabowski GA. Gaucher disease, enzymology, genetics, and treatment. Adv Hum Genet 1993;21:377–441.

3. Beutler E. Gaucher's disease. Review article. N Engl J Med 1991;325:1354–1360

4. Shahinfar M, Wenger DA. Adult and infantile Gaucher disease in one family: mutational studies and clinical update. J Pediatr 1994;125:919–921

5. Sidransky E, Ginns EI. Clinical heterogeneity among patients with Gaucher's disease. JAMA 1993;269:1154–1157

6. Parkin JL, Brunning RD: Pathology of the Gaucher cell. Prog Clin Biol Res 1982;95:151–175

7. Zaino EC, Rossi MB, Pham TD, Azar HA. Gaucher's cells in thalassaemia. Blood 1971;38:457–462

8. Scullin DC Jr, Shelburne JD, Cohen HJ. Pseudo-Gaucher cells in multiple myeloma. Am J Med 1979;67:347–352

9. Kaplan P, Mazur A, Manor O et al. Acceleration of retarded growth in children with Gaucher disease after treatment with alglucerase. J Pediatr 1996; 129:149–153

10. Lee RE. The pathology of Gaucher disease. In: Desnick RJ, Gatt, S, Grabowski GA, Eds. Gaucher Disease: A Century of Delineation and Research. New York: Alan R. Liss, 1982: 177–217

11. Medoff AS, Bayrd ED. Gaucher's disease, in 29 cases: hematologic complications and effect of splenectomy. Ann Intern Med 1954;40:481–492

12. James, SP, Stromeyer FW, Stowens DW, Barranger JA. Gaucher disease: Hepatic abnormalities in 25 patients. In: Desnick RJ, Gatt S, Grabowski GA, Eds. Gaucher Disease: A Century of Delineation and Research. New York: Alan R. Liss, 1982:131–145

13. Stowens DW, Teitelbaum SL, Kahn AJ et al. Skeletal complications of Gaucher disease. Medicine (Baltimore) 1985; 64:310–322

14. Beutler E, Saven A. The misuse of marrow examination in the diagnosis of Gaucher disease. Blood 1990;76:646–648

15. Shafit-Zagardo B, Devine EA, Smith M et al. Assignment of the gene for acid beta-glucosidase to human chromosome 1. Am J Hum Genet 1981;33:564–575

16. Theophilus B, Latham T, Grabowski GA, Smith FA. Gaucher disease: molecular heterogeneity and phenotype-genotype correlations. Am J Hum Genet 1989; 45:212–225

17. Barton NW, Brady RO, Dambrosia JM et al. Replacement therapy for inherited enzyme deficiency—macrophage-targeted glucocerebrosidase for Gaucher's disease. N Engl J Med 1991;324:1464–1470

18. Figueroa ML, Rosenbloom EB, Kay AC et al. A less costly regimen of alglucerase to treat Gaucher's disease. N Engl J Med 1992;327:1632–1636

19. Mankin HJ et al. Metabolic bone disease in patients with Gaucher's disease. In: Avioli LV, Krane SM, Eds. Metabolic Bone Disease and Clinically Related Disorders. 2nd Ed. Philadelphia: WB Saunders, 1990:730–752

20. Mankin HJ. Indications for and complications of skeletal surgery in patients with Gaucher disease. In: Barranger JA, Barton NW, Grabowki GA Eds. Gaucher Clinical Perspectives. Molecular Medicine and Therapeutics. Vol. 4, No 1. Califon, NJ: SynerMed, 1996:7–11

21. Samuel R et al. Aminohydroxypropylidene bisphosphonate (APD) treatment improves the clinical skeletal manifestations of Gaucher's disease. Pediatrics 1994;94:385–389

22. Goodman RM. Genetic Disorders Among the Jewish People. Baltimore: Johns Hopkins University Press, 1979

23. Pereira LV, Desnick RJ, Adler DA et al. EH Regional assignment of the human acid sphingomyelinase gene by PCR anal-

ysis of somatic cell hybrids and in situ hybridization to 11p15.1–p15.4. Genomics 1991; 9:229–234

24. Steinberg SJ, Ward CP, Fensom AH. Complementation studies in Niemann-Pick disease type C indicate the existence of a second group. J Med Genet 1994;31:317–320

25. Carstea ED, Polymeropoulos MH, Parker CC et al. Linkage of Niemann-Pick disease type C to human chromosome 18. Proc Natl Acad Sci USA 1993;90:2002–2004

26. Wenger DA, Barth G, Githens JH. Nine cases of sphingomyelin lipidosis, a new variant in Spanish-American children. Am J Dis Child 1977;131:955–961

27. Walton DS, Robb RM, Crocker AC. Ocular manifestations of group A Niemann-Pick disease. Am J Ophthalmol 1978; 85:174–180

28. Putterman C, Zelingher J, Shouval D. Liver failure and the sea-blue histiocyte/adult Niemann-Pick disease. Case report and review of the literature. J Clin Gastroenterol 1992;15: 146–149

29. Tassoni JP Jr, Fawaz KA, Johnston DE. Cirrhosis and portal hypertension in a patient with adult Niemann-Pick disease. Gastroenterology 1991;100:567–569

30. Lipson MH, O'Donnell J, Callahan JW et al. Ocular involvement in Niemann-Pick disease type B. J Pediatr 1986;108: 582–584

31. Takada G, Satoh W, Komatsu K et al. Transitory type of sphingomyelinase deficiency in Niemann-Pick disease: clini-cal and morphological studies and follow-up of two sisters. Tohoku J Exp Med 1987;153:27

32. Elleder M, Cihula J. Niemann-Pick disease (variation in the sphingomyelinase deficient group): neurovisceral phenotype (A) with an abnormally protracted clinical course and variable expression of neurological symptomatology in three siblings. Eur J Pediatr 1981;140:323

33. Vanier MT, Wenger DA, Comly ME et al. Niemann-Pick disease group C: clinical variability and diagnosis based on defective cholesterol esterification. A collaborative study on 70 patients. Clin Genet 1988;33:331–348

34. Maconochie IK, Chong S, Mieli-Vergani G et al. Fetal ascites: an unusual presentation of Niemann-Pick disease type C. Arch Dis Child 1989; 64:1391–1393

35. Vanier MT, Rodriguez-Lafrasse C, Rousson R et al. Type C Niemann-Pick disease: biochemical aspects and phenotypic heterogeneity. Dev Neurosci 1991;13:307–314

36. Vanier MT, Rodriguez-Lafrasse C, Rousson R et al. Prenatal diagnosis of Niemann-Pick type C disease: current strategy from an experience of 37 pregnancies at risk. Am J Hum Genet 1992;51:111–122

37. Loftus SK, Morris JA, Carstea ED et al. Murine model of Niemann-Pick C disease: mutation in a cholesterol homeostasis gene. Science 1997;277:180–181

38. Carstea ED, Morris JA, Coleman KG et al. Neimann-Pick C1 disease gene: homology to mediators of cholesterol homeostasis. Science 1997;277:228–231

53

GLYCOGEN STORAGE DISEASES

STEVEN M. WILLI

The glycogen storage diseases (GSDs), or glycogenoses, represent a heterogeneous group of disorders of considerable import to clinical pediatric gastroenterologists. These disorders result from at least 10 different genetic defects governing glycogen metabolism. The common thread that ties these disorders together is simply a qualitative or quantitative abnormality in the accumulation of glycogen in various tissues. The liver's involvement in most of the glycogenoses provides the rationale for the inclusion of this chapter in a gastroenterology text.

The prevailing classification scheme for the glycogenoses (Table 53-1), initially proposed by Cori,[1] numbers the disorders consecutively in chronologic order of their initial clinical description.[2] The subsequent appreciation of subtypes of many of the glycogenoses[3,4] has led to considerable complexity, which this archaic strategy is ill-equipped to deal with. Although several of the glycogenoses affect glycogen metabolism in both liver and muscle, a useful distinction can be drawn between those that have primarily hepatic versus muscular effects.

PATHOPHYSIOLOGY

Glycogen is a glucose polymer that provides an efficient and accessible intracellular depot of energy, even under anaerobic conditions. While glycogen is particularly abundant in liver and muscle, it exists in smaller quantities in almost all animal cell types. The tree-like structure of glycogen (Fig. 53-1) is made possible by a combination of straight[1,4] and "branched"[1,6] disaccharide linkages. In this way, glycogen is more efficiently "packaged" in a soluble globular form. As only terminal glucose moieties are directly available for enzymatic activity, this structural organization maximizes glycogen's degradative (and synthetic) capacity by providing as much as 7% to 10% of the molecule in this form.

In the fed state, glucose is absorbed through the gastrointestinal (GI) tract. Through the action of insulin, glucose is metabolized directly or is stored in the liver as glycogen. Upon fasting, blood glucose levels fall, leading to an inhibition of insulin release. If this fall in serum glucose remains unchecked, counterregulatory hormone secretion ensues.[5] This combination of events (decreased insulin secretion and counterregulatory hormone production) causes a shift in metabolism toward the breakdown of available substrates, including glycogen.

Hepatic glycogen represents the most immediate source of carbohydrate for the maintenance of normal glucose homeostasis. In the liver, glucagon and epinephrine stimulate glycogenolysis through a cascade of phosphorylation reactions, eventually leading to glucose 6-phosphate (G6P) (Fig. 53-2). This substrate may enter glycolysis directly, but most of it is converted to glucose for utilization in distant sites. In muscle, insulin favors glycogen synthesis by facilitating intracellular transport of glucose and through activation of glycogen synthetase. As muscle cells lack glucagon receptors, catecholamines provide the primary signal for glycogen breakdown. The G6P thus produced cannot exit the myocyte and therefore enters glycolysis directly.

Almost all mammalian cell types possess a secondary system for glycogen metabolism in the lysosomes. The function of this alternative system is to hydrolyze glycogen, which has been engulfed by autophagic vacuoles in

TABLE 53-1. Classification and Major Features of the Glycogen Storage Diseases

Enzyme Defect	Type	Alternative Name	Tissues Affected	Clinical Characteristics
Glycogen synthase	0	Aglycogenosis	Liver[a]	Fasting hypoglycemia and accelerated ketosis, postprandial hyperglycemia, no hepatomegaly
Glucose 6-phosphatase	Ia	Von Gierke disease	Liver[a], kidney, intestine	Hepatomegaly, short stature, hyperlipidemia, hyperuricemia, fasting hypoglycemia, and lactic acidosis
Glucose 6-phosphate translocase	Ib		Above + neutrophils	Same as GSD Ia, with the addition of profound neutropenia, frequent infections and stromal ulcerations
Inorganic phosphate transporter	Ic		Liver[a]	Hepatomegaly, diabetes mellitus, with recurrent fasting hypoglycemia
Acid α-glucosidase (lysosomal)	IIa,b	Pompe disease	Generalized (WBC[a])	Glycogen deposition in all tissues leading to hepatomegaly, cardiomegaly, macroglossia, and hypotonia
Amylo-1,6-glucosidase, "debrancher enzyme"	III	Cori disease, limit dextrinosis	Liver,[a] WBC,[a] muscle, heart	Hepatomegaly, fasting hypoglycemia, hyperlipidemia, borderline glycemic response to glucagon, myopathy in adults, cardiomyopathy rare
Amylo-1,4→1,6-transglucosidase "branching enzyme"	IV	Andersen disease, Amylopectinosis	Generalized (liver[a] most severely affected)	Hepatosplenomegaly, failure to thrive, cirrhosis, portal hypertension, ascites, hypoglycemia (only in the presence of cirrhosis); muscular weakness and cardiomyopathy less prominent than hepatic manifestations
Phosphorylase (muscle)	V	McArdle disease	Skeletal muscle[a]	Exercise intolerance and muscle cramps (esp. in adulthood); rhabdomyolysis and myoglobinuria with stress
Phosphorylase (liver)	VI	Hers disease	Liver,[a] WBC	Hepatomegaly, mild hypoglycemia, no hyperglycemic response to glucagon or epinephrine
Phosphofructokinase	VII	Tauri disease	Skeletal muscle,[a] RBC[a]	Similar to GSD V (but more severe and earlier onset), also hemolysis, hyperbilirubinemia, and hyperuricemia
Unknown (phosphorylase present, but in inactive form)	VIII		Liver,[a] brain	Hepatomegaly, ataxia, nystagmus, and gradual neurologic deterioration to spasticity and decerebration
Phosphorylase kinase	IXa		Liver[a]	Hepatomegaly, short stature resolving in childhood
	b		Liver,[a] RBC,[a] WBC[a]	Hepatomegaly, mild fasting hypoglycemia, short stature (X-linked recessive inheritance)
	c		Liver,[a] muscle, RBC[a]	Hepatomegaly, failure to thrive, hypotonia, and mild weakness
	d		Cardiac muscle[a]	Infantile dilative or hypertrophic cardiomyopathy
cAMP-dependent kinase	X		Liver,[a] muscle[a]	Hepatomegaly, mild recurrent myalgia and weakness, poor glycemic response to glucagon
Unknown	XI		Liver, kidney	Hepatomegaly, severe growth retardation, vitamin D–resistant rickets, hyperlipidemia and renal Fanconi syndrome

[a] Represents the biopsy tissue type most suitable for procuring a definitive diagnosis.

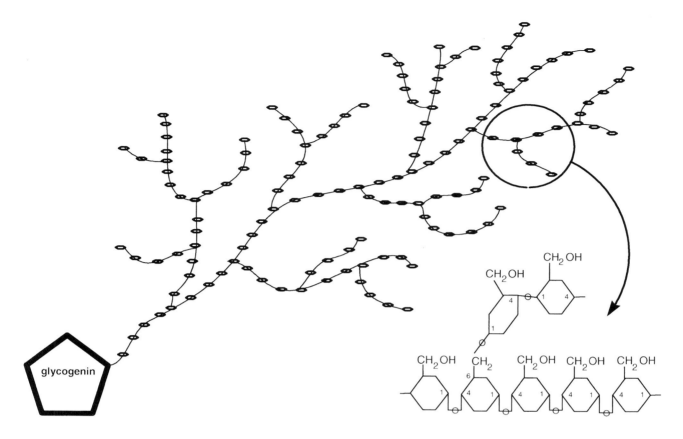

FIGURE 53-1. Schematic representation of a single glycogen molecule (actual size within the range of 20,000 to 30,000 glucose residues). This structure permits efficient mobilization of glucose, as nearly 60% of glucose moieties lie in straight chains immediately proximal to nonreducing ends (which are available for phosphorylation or chain lengthening).

the process of cell remodeling. A single lysosomal enzyme (alpha-glucosidase) is responsible for this process of acid hydrolysis.[6]

The GSDs result from a deficiency of one of the enzymes responsible for glycogen metabolism (Fig. 53-2). However, an additional level of complexity results from the fact that several of these enzymes exist in various isoforms (i.e., different enzymes with the same function, expressed in different tissue types). For example, phosphorylase activity may be deficient in muscle, leading to muscle cramping and fatigability, but no generalized metabolic derangements (GSD V). The same enzyme deficiency in liver leads to hepatomegaly, mild fasting hypoglycemia and an inability to mount a hyperglycemic response to glucagon, but muscular manifestations are absent (GSD VI). Furthermore, the deficiency of at least one of the glycolytic enzymes (phosphofructokinase), results in excess glycogen deposition in affected tissues.

CLINICAL PRESENTATION

As the glycogenoses are a heterogeneous group of disorders, their clinical presentation may differ considerably from one to the next. However, several clinical syndromes are shared by a number of the glycogenoses, though there may be considerable variation in the severity of disease. The single clinical feature most frequently exhibited by these disorders is hepatomegaly. This clinical sign is evident in all the hepatic glycogenoses, in part due to the presence of excess hepatic glycogen deposition. However, affected livers rarely contain more than 12% glycogen[7] (about two times normal). Most cases of liver enlargement result from fatty infiltration. Under certain circumstances, the local effects of the metabolic derangement result in hepatotoxicity and eventually cirrhosis.

Generalized metabolic disturbances are particularly common in the hepatic glycogenoses, especially GSD 0,

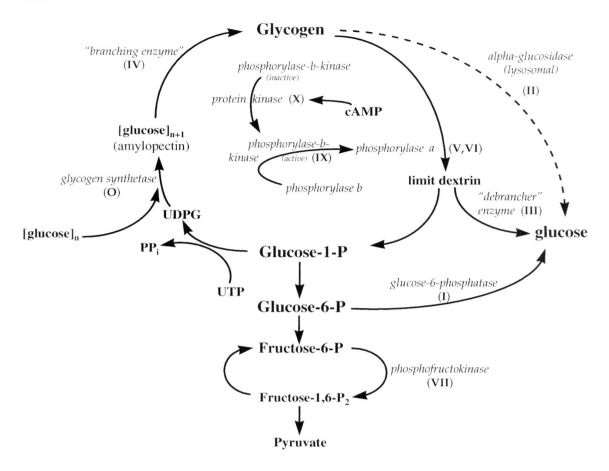

FIGURE 53-2. Metabolic pathways in carbohydrate metabolism affected by the various glycogen storage diseases. Enzyme names are given in italics, with related glycogenoses identified by Roman numerals.

I, III, and VI. In the early postabsorptive phase, the affected liver is unable to release sufficient glucose from hepatic glycogen to meet peripheral tissue demands. This state of accelerated fasting results in a number of generalized metabolic consequences that are common to many of the glycogenoses. The most immediate and potentially life-threatening of these manifestations is hypoglycemia, which frequently occurs within 4 to 6 hours of a meal. In response to this "accelerated fasting," profound elevations of counterregulatory hormones regularly invoke lipolysis and gluconeogenesis. In the untreated patient, this phenomenon may result in hyperlipidemia and hyperuricemia (from increased protein turnover).

The most common of the GSDs, GSD I, is not a defect in glycogen storage at all. The enzymatic deficiency responsible for GSD I (G6Pase) involves virtually all forms of hepatic glucose production. During fasting, excess quantities of G6P are produced. As the liver is incapable of releasing glucose into the periphery, the accumulated substrate enters glycolysis, producing a lactic acidosis.[8] As lactate can serve as an alternative fuel for brain metabolism,[9] patients with untreated GSD I may

not manifest clinical signs of hypoglycemia, even when blood glucose levels fall below 20 mg/dl. The negative effect of this chronic metabolic acidosis is growth failure. Furthermore, lactic acidosis, as well as other metabolic derangements specific to type I glycogenosis, has been implicated in the development of platelet dysfunction,[10] hepatic adenomata,[11] and renal disease[12] in these patients.

Skeletal muscle disease is present in many of the glycogenoses as well. This effect is most striking in GSD V and GSD VII, which present with muscle cramping, and even myoglobinuria, with exercise. However, muscle disease may also manifest as mild weakness (as in GSD I, III, and IXc) or hypotonia (as in GSD II).[13,14] The heart is frequently affected, albeit less severely, in the muscle glycogenoses. Normally, cardiac muscle stores only one-tenth the amount of glycogen, as compared to skeletal muscle. In the absence of ischemia, cardiac function is greatly dependent on the provision of exogenous substrates (especially fatty acids), rather than utilization of endogenous glycogen. As a result, the level of myocardial involvement appears to be more dependent on the accumulation of excess glycogen, rather than on impaired energy utilization from a defect in metabolism. Not surprisingly, GSD II represents the most severe of the glycogenoses affecting the heart.

DIAGNOSIS

The diagnostic approach to the glycogen storage diseases will depend upon the clinical manifestations of the disease. The most frequent manifestation is hepatomegaly, with or without hypoglycemia. While liver biopsy is frequently necessary for a definitive diagnosis, the astute clinician should narrow the field of investigation in an effort to avoid the need for multiple tissue samples. The presence of various metabolic abnormalities can suggest the presence of GSD I. As GSD I represents a defect in the conversion of G6P to glucose, hypoglycemia in this condition may be severe. Lactic acidosis, hyperlipidemia, hyperuricemia, and hypophosphatemia may all complicate this disorder when the patient is in poor metabolic control. The concomitant occurrence of neutropenia suggests the presence of the subtype of GSD I affecting white blood cells (WBCs) (GSD Ib).

In any of the hepatic glycogenoses, an assessment of fasting adaptation may be helpful. This evaluation can be achieved through frequent monitoring of blood glucose levels in the inpatient setting. Such a study should be attempted only in the presence of experienced medical personnel. The fast should be timed in a manner that ensures that the acute hypoglycemic episode occurs at a time when adequate medical attention is available (typically, between 09:00 and 16:00 hours). Glucose and lactate levels should be monitored at least every 2 hours, and with greater frequency as the blood sugar falls.

The fasting study can be terminated with a dose of intravenous glucagon (0.03 mg/kg), which prompts a glycemic increment of greater than 40 mg/dl in most normal children.[15] A rise in lactate above 2.4 mmol/L (especially in the absence of a significant rise in serum glucose) strongly suggests the diagnosis of GSD I (or some other disorder of gluconeogenesis).[16] By contrast, when a glucagon challenge fails to elicit a rise in glucose (30 mg/dl or greater) and lactate levels are normal, GSD 0, III, VI, and X are likely. The remaining hepatic glycogenoses (GSD IV, VIII, and IX) show moderately impaired glycemic response to the fasted glucagon challenge test, which may overlap with normal results.[16,17] The muscle specific glycogenoses (GSD V and VII) as well as GSD II demonstrate no metabolic abnormalities upon glucagon challenge.

While the fasted glucagon challenge test may "narrow the field" of possible diagnoses, liver biopsy and enzymatic assay of fresh tissue remains the definitive diagnostic procedure for the hepatic glycogenoses. Typically, less than 100 mg of tissue is required for each assay, so a single percutaneous biopsy may be sufficient for microscopic analysis, measurement of glycogen content, and one or two specific assays. A number of these enzymes are expressed in more accessible tissues (e.g., leukocytes, fibroblasts, erythrocytes), which can be assayed as well. Owing to the existence of isoenzymes, however, the presence of normal activity in these tissues cannot rule out the possibility of hepatic involvement. Recently, genetic testing has become available for GSD Ia, circumventing the need for liver biopsy.

LABORATORY ABNORMALITIES

GSD I is unique among the glycogenoses, in that it represents a combined defect in glycogenolysis and gluconeogenesis. As such, this disorder presents a myriad of laboratory abnormalities resulting from the liver's inability to produce glucose from various substrates. Hypoglycemia occurs after relatively short periods of fasting. In the immediate postabsorptive state, blood glucose levels frequently drop below 40 mg/dl. In the absence of exogenous glucose, high levels of counterregulatory hormones[18] result in remote effects on several metabolic pathways. The intrahepatic accumulation of G6P leads to trapping of inorganic phosphate, and often hypophosphatemia. Lactic acidosis, during fasting, results from glycolysis of this excess G6P.

Serum triglyceride and cholesterol levels are profoundly elevated in untreated patients with GSD I. Intensive nutritional therapy may improve the hyperlipidemia, but moderate hypertriglyceridemia typically persists.[19] Hyperuricemia and gout frequently occur with this condition as well. The etiology of this metabolic consequence remains unclear, but it is readily reversible with dietary therapy. Hematologic abnormalities, especially anemia, are not uncommon in GSD I as well. Neutropenia is pathognomonic of the b subtype, as this disorder affects the ability of WBCs to derive energy from glycolysis.

By contrast, the glycogenoses which directly impair hepatic glycogenolysis (i.e., GSD III, VI, IX, and X) and glycogen synthetase deficiency (GSD 0) are frequently accompanied by fasting hypoglycemia, but lactic acidosis only occurs after oral administration of glucose.[17] These defects in glycogenolysis typically cause elevations in lipid levels which are in proportion to the degree of fasting hypoglycemia observed. Uric acid abnormalities have not been reported, but hepatocellular damage may be evident from variable elevations in transaminases (AST, ALT).

The glycogenoses involving muscle (especially GSD III, V, and VII) can lead to elevated creatine kinase levels, but normal values do not rule out muscle disease.

Intense exercise causes excessive increases in serum ammonia and uric acid, in the absence of a normal rise in lactate.[20] Rarely, exercise-induced rhabdomyolysis and myoglobinuria may precipitate acute renal failure.

TREATMENT

A complete understanding of the pathophysiology of the glycogenoses has led to considerable development in the area of therapy. As GSD I represents a defect in hepatic glucose production, maintenance of the fed state would seem to avoid many of the metabolic consequences of this disease. This supposition has been validated with the use of overnight intragastric feedings in combination with frequent feedings during the daytime.[21] The goal of therapy should be to maintain the blood glucose level at 70 to 100 mg/dl. This goal is typically achieved through the use of a formula whose predominant calorie source is from glucose or glucose polymers. Initial infusion rates should simulate rates of hepatic glucose production, which are age dependent.[22] If high fat formulas are avoided, a 10-hour overnight infusion provides only 25% to 35% of total caloric requirements, permitting ample opportunity for daytime feedings. A continuous pump, equipped to alarm in the event of failure, is used in combination with a nasogastric tube to facilitate delivery. The infusion is begun within 3 hours of the last meal and, if possible, is continued until after the first meal of the day is consumed.

A frequent schedule of small high-starch feedings during the daytime has also proved effective in the management of GSD I. Starchy vegetables and grains are digested almost entirely to glucose and are more suitable than galactose- or fructose-containing carbohydrate sources. Restriction of fruits and dairy products may result in inadequate intake of certain nutrients (especially vitamin C and calcium), necessitating supplementation. Between meals, uncooked cornstarch (1.5 to 2.5 g/kg) can effectively support blood sugars above 70 mg/dl, as it is absorbed very slowly. Several investigators have advocated the use of cornstarch in place of overnight nasogastric infusion,[23] but this approach requires validation with glucose monitoring and may have limitations in young children. As young children with GSD III are also susceptible to hypoglycemia, nocturnal infusions and frequent feedings can be helpful. Increased dietary protein may be beneficial in GSD III as well, as these patients do not have a defect in gluconeogenesis.[24]

The remaining hepatic glycogenoses, with the exception of GSD IV, are relatively mild and no specific dietary therapy is generally required. GSD IV leads inexorably to hepatic failure, and is not responsive to dietary manipulations. The glycogenoses that affect muscle (GSD III, V, VII, and IX) can be responsive to a diet high in protein.[25] The dietary management of GSD II has been relatively unrewarding. No therapy for the severe infantile form of this disease has proved effective, but high protein diets have been palliative when used for milder forms of the disease.[26]

Several adjuvant medical therapies have been used to address the metabolic and hematologic complications of the glycogenoses, especially GSD I. Allopurinol can be used to prevent gout and uric acid nephropathy.[27] As in diabetes mellitus, the nephropathy associated with GSD I is preceded by hyperfiltration,[12] prompting the suggestion that angiotensin converting enzyme inhibitors may have a role in treatment. Mild persistent hyperlipidemia has been successfully treated with diet or gemfibrozil.[14] The course of infectious complications of GSD Ib can be ameliorated by granulocyte colony-stimulating factor.[28] Liver transplantation has been utilized for GSD I and GSD IV, with positive preliminary results.[29] The long-term outcome and effects of transplantation on complications are as yet undetermined.

REFERRAL PATTERN

Many of the glycogenoses are of sufficient rarity and severity in pediatric practice to warrant referral to a specialty center when a diagnosis appears likely. This is especially true in GSD I and III, which may have profound metabolic consequences if not treated aggressively. In the case of infantile GSD II, supportive care is only palliative. Referral to a geneticist may be of benefit for genetic counseling and subsequent prenatal testing of chorionic villi or amniocytes. As GSD IV leads inexorably to liver failure, prompt referral to a pediatric transplant center is advisable. The mild hepatic glycogenoses (GSD VI, IX and X) carry a favorable prognosis, and specialized treatments may not be necessary. As rhabdomyolysis may develop in several of the glycogenoses, referral to a neurologist is warranted whenever muscle disease is suspected.

REFERENCES

1. Cori GT. Glycogen structure and enzyme deficiencies in glycogen storage disease. Harvey Lect 1954;48:145–171

2. Fernandes J. The history of the glycogen storage diseases. Eur J Pediatr 1995;154:423–424

3. Beudet AL, Andersen DC, Michels VV et al. Neutropenia and impaired neutrophil migration in type Ib glycogen storage disease. J Pediatr 1980;97:906–913

4. Huijing F, Fernandes J. X chromosomal inheritance of liver glycogenosis with phosphorylase kinase deficiency. Am J Hum Genet 1969;21:275–284

5. Cryer PE, Tse TF, Clutter WE, Shah SD. Roles of glucagon

and epinephrine in hypoglycemic and nonhypoglycemic glucose counterregulation in humans. Am J Physiol 1984;10: E198–205

6. Beratis NG, Labadie GU, Hirschhorn K. Characterization of the molecular defect in the infantile and adult acid α-glucosidase deficiency fibroblasts. J Clin Invest 1978;62: 1264–1274

7. Hug G. The glycogen storage diseases. In: Behrman RE, Vaughan VC, Eds. Nelson Textbook of Pediatrics. Philadelphia: WB Saunders, 1983:455–468.

8. Sadeghi-Nejad A, Presente E, Binkiewiez A, Senior B. Studies in type I glycogenosis of the liver. The genesis and deposition of lactate. J Pediatr 1974;85:49–53

9. Fernandes J, Berger R, Smit GPA. Lactate as a cerebral metabolic fuel for glucose-6-phosphatase deficient children. Pediatr Res 1984;18:335–339

10. Ambruso DR, McCabe ERB, Anderson D, Beaudet MD. Infections and bleeding complications in patients with glycogenosis Ib. Am J Dis Child 1985;139:691–697

11. Parker P, Burr I, Slonim A et al. Regression of hepatic adenomas in type Ia glycogen storage disease with dietary therapy. Gastroenterology 1981;81:534–536

12. Baker L, Dahlem S, Goldfarb S et al. Hyper filtration and renal disease in glycogen storage disease, type I. Kidney Int 1989;5:1345–1350

13. DiMauro S, Hartwig GB, Hays A et al. Debrancher deficiency: neuromuscular disorder in 5 adults. Ann Neurol 1979;5:422–436

14. Talente GM, Coleman RA, Alter C et al. Glycogen storage disease in adults. Ann Intern Med 1994;120:218–226

15. Vasella F. Die Glukagonbelastungsprobe beim gesunden Kind. Helv Paediatr Acta 1957; 12:331–360

16. Dunger DB, Leonard JV. Value of the glucagon test in screening for hepatic glycogen storage disease. Arch Dis Child 1982;57:384–389

17. Fernandes J, Koster JF, Grose FA, Sorgedrager N. Hepatic phosphorylase deficiency: Its differentation from other hepatic glycogenoses. Arch Dis Child 1974;49:186–191

18. Slonim AE, Lacy WW, Terry AB et al. Nocturnal intragastric therapy in type I GSD: effect on hormonal and amino acid metabolism. Metabolism 1979; 28:707–715

19. Greene HL, Swift LL, Knapp HR. Hyperlipidemia and fatty acid composition in patients treated for type Ia GSD. J Pediatr 1991;119:398–403

20. Mineo I, Kono N, Takao S et al. Excess purine degradation in exercising muscles of patients with glycogen storage disease types V and VII. J Clin Invest 1985;76:556–560

21. Greene HL, Slonim AE, Burr IM, Moran JR. Type I GSD: five years of management with nocturnal intragastric feeding. J Pediatr 1980;96:590–595

22. Bier DM, Leake RD, Haymond MW et al. Measurement of "true" glucose production rates in infancy and childhood with 6,6-dideuteroglucose. Diabetes 1977;26:1016–1023

23. Wolfsdorf JI, Plotkin RA, Crigler JF. Continuous glucose for treatment of patients with type I GSD: comparison of the effects of dextrose and uncooked cornstarch on biochemical variables. Am J Clin Nutr 1990;52:1043–1050

24. Slonim AE, Coleman RA, Moses SW. Myopathy and growth failure in debrancher enzyme deficiency: improvement with high-protein nocturnal enteral therapy. J Pediatr 1984;105: 906–911

25. Slonim AE, Coleman RA, McElligot MA et al. Improvement of muscle function by high protein therapy. Neurology 1983;33:34–38

26. Umpleby AM, Trend P, Chubb D et al. The effect of high protein diet on leucine and alanine turnover in acid maltase deficiency. J Neurol Neurosurg Psychiatry 1989;52:954–961

27. Fernandes J, Leonard JV, Moses SW et al. Glycogen storage disease: recommendations for treatment. Eur J Pediatr 1988; 147:226–228

28. Schroten H, Roesler J, Breidenbach T et al. Granulocyte and granulocyte-macrophage colony-stimulating factors in the treatment of neutropenia in GSD type Ib. J Pediatr 1991; 119:748–754

29. Selby R, Starzl TE, Yunis E et al. Liver transplantation for type I and type IV glycogen storage disease. Eur J Pediatr 1993;152 (suppl 1):S71–76

54

IRON OVERLOAD CONDITIONS

PATRICIA A. DERUSSO

HEREDITARY HEMOCHROMATOSIS

The most common inherited liver disease is caused by a disorder of iron metabolism known as hereditary hemochromatosis.[1,2] Although the metabolic defect is present at birth, hemochromatosis rarely manifests before adulthood. Many years of excessive iron absorption are necessary before toxic accumulation occurs in the liver and other organs. The disorder occurs in individuals of northern European ancestry and is due to the autosomal recessive inheritance of an abnormal gene closely linked to the HLA-A locus on the short arm of chromosome 6. In the United States, approximately 12.5% of individuals are heterozygous and 4.5 per 1,000 are homozygous for the hemochromatosis gene.[3] Expression of the disease is influenced by dietary iron intake and by both physiologic and pathologic blood loss. Women are affected less frequently than men, probably because menstruation and childbearing decrease the iron burden. The precise biochemical abnormality responsible for excessive iron absorption and subsequent accumulation has not been defined. Significant iron loading can occur without clinical manifestations of the disorder.[4]

Because heterozygosity for the abnormal gene is common and early treatment can prevent complications, screening for the disorder in children of individuals with hemochromatosis is recommended.[5,6] The natural history of the disease from birth to clinical presentation is unknown, and the optimal age to begin screening is debatable. Studies in adults have established that early diagnosis and treatment is essential to prevent the complications of liver cirrhosis, organ failure, and primary hepatocellular carcinoma.[7]

Pathophysiology

In healthy individuals, total body iron is regulated by controlling the amount of iron absorbed. Absorption must be tightly regulated because significant amounts of iron are not excreted. There are small losses of iron from mucosal epithelial cells, sweat, urine, and exfoliation of skin. Substantial iron losses are seen in females who lose blood during menstruation. In addition, high iron requirements are associated with pregnancy and childbirth.[8]

The pathway involved in regulating iron absorption is unknown, but when total body iron is high there usually is a concomitant decrease in the amount absorbed. An increase in iron absorption occurs when iron stores are low. After absorption, iron is transported in the blood bound to the protein transferrin.[8]

Experimental evidence suggests that the abnormality in hemochromatosis ultimately leads to excessive absorption of iron in the intestinal mucosa. The primary defect may be in the intestinal mucosal cell or involve the liver or reticuloendothelial system.[2] Individuals with hemochromatosis continue to absorb inappropriately high amounts of iron despite elevated stores.[9] When excess iron is absorbed, circulating transferrin becomes saturated, and deposition of iron occurs in the parenchymal cells of various organs of the body, especially the liver.

Clinical Presentation

Children of individuals with hemochromatosis are brought to the physician because parents are concerned that their child will inherit the disease. The prevalence

TABLE 54-1. Organ System Involvement in Individuals With Hemochromatosis With Onset Before or After 30 Years of Age

Organ System	Onset <30 yr	Onset ≥30 yr
	% (n = 53)	% (n = 787)
Liver involvement	83	94
Skin pigmentation	85	86
Diabetes mellitus	34	82
Hypogonadism	64	30
Cardiomyopathy	58	35
Arthritis	10	N/A

(Adapted from Lamon et al,[15] with permission.)

of hemochromatosis in children of one affected parent is estimated as high as 1 in 20.[5] This estimate incorporates the likelihood that a homozygote will mate with a heterozygote. An affected offspring must inherit an abnormal gene from each parent. When both parents are homozygous for the disorder, all the offspring are at risk of the development of hemochromatosis, unless a rare recombination event occurs. When a sibling has the disorder, there is a 1 in 4 probability that another sibling is homozygous for hemochromatosis.

Family studies have permitted earlier detection of homozygous individuals. Screening family members of 93 individuals with hemochromatosis in one study led to the identification of 37 homozygotes.[10] Nearly 50% of these homozygotes were asymptomatic. Symptomatic adults will see a physician with complaints of abdominal pain, joint pain, and weakness. Hepatomegaly, abnormal serum transaminases, and arthritis are some of the clinical findings in individuals with the disorder. The classic triad of diabetes mellitus, liver cirrhosis, and hyperpigmentation is less prevalent, now that homozygous individuals are identified before significant iron loading has occurred. The clinical presentation of hemochromatosis in adults has been discussed in detail elsewhere.[7,10,11]

There are rare reports of symptomatic hemochromatosis in children and adolescents.[12–18] Males and females are equally affected. Cardiomyopathy and hypogonadism are seen more frequently in young individuals with hemochromatosis than older individuals (Table 54-1). It is unclear whether young individuals with iron overload have a more severe form of the adult HLA-linked disease or a different disease process.[2]

Diagnosis

All first-degree relatives of an affected individual should be evaluated for hemochromatosis. A history and physical examination should be performed. Laboratory studies should include a transferrin saturation and serum ferritin measurement. Serum aminotransferase levels should be included, although they may not be elevated. When the transferrin saturation is elevated, a repeat level should be obtained after an overnight fast. When transferrin saturation or serum ferritin is abnormal for no apparent reason, the patient should be referred to a specialist for diagnostic confirmation. A liver biopsy may be necessary to analyze tissue for evidence of iron storage in parenchymal cells, extent of liver disease, and presence of hepatomas.

When a sibling has the disorder, HLA typing can be helpful in predicting the risk of iron loading in other siblings. When two siblings share identical haplotypes and one is affected, the other sibling is considered homozygous for the disorder. This individual must be closely monitored for iron loading with biannual laboratory tests.

Other causes of iron overload must be excluded especially in children with organ system involvement. A history of numerous red blood cell transfusions would suggest parenteral iron overload with deposition in reticuloendothelial cells. Tissue distribution of iron is an important consideration because iron in the parenchymal cells causes organ damage. In the absence of transfusion therapy, disorders of ineffective erythropoiesis, such as thalassemia syndromes and sideroblastic anemia, can result in excessive absorption of iron from the gastrointestinal (GI) mucosa.[2,11] The physician must exclude these anemias as causes of parenchymal iron overload. Furthermore, there are data to suggest that individuals with hereditary spherocytosis and heterozygous thalassemia can develop iron overload from increased GI absorption if they are also heterozygous for hemochromatosis.[2] Hematologic studies such as a complete blood count (CBC), red cell indices, reticulocyte count, and analysis of the peripheral smear should be included in the investigation.

Laboratory Evaluation

Two laboratory tests are used for hereditary hemochromatosis: transferrin saturation and serum ferritin.[6] When elevated, these are phenotypic markers of affected individuals with hemochromatosis. Serum iron concentrations have not been reliable in detecting this disorder.[2] Serum iron aminotransferases may or may not be elevated.[7]

Transferrin saturation is elevated early in the course of iron accumulation and is the most useful screening test for hemochromatosis. Transferrin saturation is calculated from the serum iron divided by the total iron binding capacity. When excessive iron is absorbed, an abnormally high percentage of transferrin becomes saturated with iron. A value of greater than 60% in men and of 50% in women is considered abnormal for adults.[2,6] The transferrin saturations of affected children homozygous for hemochromatosis may be lower. When the transferrin saturation is above normal, a repeat value after an overnight fast should be done. A morning sample is necessary because there is a diurnal variation in serum iron concentrations. Also, recent ingestion of iron can elevate the value. In addition, transferrin saturations are unreliable during acute illness.

Serum ferritin concentration provides an indication of total body iron stores. The concentration varies depending on age and sex. Serum ferritin may not be elevated in individuals with hemochromatosis until there is significant stainable hepatic iron or clinical manifestations of disease.[4] The value must be interpreted with caution because serum ferritin is an acute-phase reactant and may be elevated for reasons other than iron overload. A combination of both transferrin saturation and serum ferritin provides more accurate information than either test alone.[19]

Family studies have shown that hemochromatosis in populations of northern European origin is HLA linked. Thus, hemochromatosis genes and HLA haplotypes are inherited together. HLA typing can be helpful when evaluating siblings of an individual with hemochromatosis. When a sibling has inherited the same HLA haplotypes, they are both presumed to be homozygous for the disorder. HLA testing is not indicated in the management of children of one affected parent because one abnormal gene must be inherited from each parent in order to be homozygous for the condition. HLA typing is expensive and provides no information regarding the iron status of an individual.

Treatment

When a patient has been diagnosed with hereditary hemochromatosis, treatment should begin immediately. Data from adult studies indicate that iron removal prior to development of liver cirrhosis results in improved survival.[7] Since hemochromatosis rarely occurs in children, no consensus regarding a phlebotomy regimen is available. Escobar et al[18] recommend the removal of 5 to 7 ml/kg of blood every 7 to 10 days for an affected child. In adults, removal of excess iron is achieved by weekly removal of 500 ml of blood once or twice a week.[6] Serum ferritin, transferrin saturation, and hemoglobin values are obtained while on a phlebotomy regimen to determine progress and future phlebotomy requirements. In adults, phlebotomy is performed until an early iron deficiency anemia develops and the serum ferritin concentration is very low. Lifelong maintenance phlebotomy is individualized to prevent the reaccumulation of iron. Liver transplantation is done when diagnosis and treatment are initiated after severe liver disease has occurred.

Referral Pattern

The primary care physician should perform laboratory studies for all first-degree relatives of individuals with hemochromatosis. Any child or adolescent with an ele-

vated transferrin saturation or serum ferritin should be referred to a pediatric gastroenterologist for confirmation of the disorder. A liver biopsy will most likely be necessary. A phlebotomy regimen would be started for anyone with hepatic iron overload. Individuals with hemochromatosis on a phlebotomy regimen have been monitored by their primary physician with annual visits to the specialist.

NEONATAL IRON STORAGE DISEASE

Neonatal iron storage disease (NISD) is a rare disorder characterized by severe hepatic insufficiency of intrauterine onset and marked iron deposition in multiple organs, including the liver. It has also been called perinatal and neonatal hemochromatosis. Although NISD and hereditary hemochromatosis are different diseases, the striking similarity is that iron deposition is found in parenchymal cells, rather than in reticuloendothelial cells, in both disorders. No HLA association exists in NISD, and the disorder has occurred both sporadically and in siblings. NISD is recognized by a phenotype in which no biochemical defect or etiology has been identified. Often the disease is unrecognized unless a sibling was similarly affected. Identifying this disorder is essential, as survival is rare unless the infant receives a liver transplant soon after presentation.[20,21] The use of an iron chelator with antioxidants has had some favorable results in a few individuals.[22] Evaluation of this treatment is under way.

Pathophysiology

The pathophysiology of NISD remains obscure. Several theories have been proposed to explain the phenotype of iron overload. There are a number of case reports in which iron overload is seen in neonates who have had an infectious or metabolic disorder.[23,24] This would suggest that injury to the fetal liver can result in dysregulation of iron metabolism.

Thus, iron overload is a consequence of fetal liver injury. It is also possible that a primary defect in iron metabolism involving fetoplacental iron handling leads to iron overload. It should be noted that biosynthesis of iron proteins, transferrin receptor, and ferritin is appropriately regulated by iron in fibroblasts from neonates with the disorder.[25] In addition, mothers of neonates with NISD have normal iron studies. The occurrence of NISD in multiple siblings suggests the disorder is inherited, but a specific inheritance pattern is not evident. The etiology of NISD remains elusive, probably because it is a rare disorder and there is inadequate evidence supporting any one theory.

Clinical Presentation

In 1981 Goldfischer et al[26] described two infants with neonatal iron storage disease and reviewed 10 additional cases. Since then more than 100 cases have been reported.[20–25,27–30] NISD is seen both sporadically and in multiple siblings. A history of early stillbirths and of in utero hydrops is common. Affected individuals are born just before term or at term. They are often small for gestational age (SGA). Males and females are affected equally. Affected individuals are usually ill within the first few days of life. Infants may initially present with lethargy, irritability, and feeding intolerance. The disease is often mistaken for viral sepsis or disseminated intravascular coagulopathy. Impaired liver function leads to coagulopathy and hyperbilirubinemia. Infants become edematous from hypoalbuminemia. Some infants also have respiratory and renal insufficiency secondary to decreased perfusion and poor oncotic pressure. The liver size is either normal or small as a result of hepatic necrosis. Splenomegaly may already be present from portal hypertension. The disorder is often fatal due to renal or hepatic failure.

Diagnosis

The diagnosis is based on clinical and pathologic findings and requires the exclusion of all other causes of neonatal liver failure. Large hepatic iron stores are also seen in tyrosinemia and in Zellweger's disease. In addition, cytomegalovirus (CMV) infection and Δ^4-3-oxosteroid-5β-reductase deficiency, a bile acid metabolism defect, has been associated with NISD.[23,24] These disorders, as well as other causes of neonatal liver failure, must be excluded.

In an infant suspected of having NISD on the basis of clinical findings or family history, the demonstration of iron deposition in multiple organs is essential for the diagnosis. Large iron stores are found in the liver of neonates without liver disease.[28] In individuals with NISD, excessive parenchymal iron has been seen in the liver, pancreas, heart, and other organs with sparing of the spleen, bone marrow, and other sites of the reticuloendothelial system. Several investigators have reported usefulness of a lip or gingival biopsy to assess iron deposition in minor salivary glands especially when coagulopathy precludes liver biopsy.[29]

Laboratory Evaluation

No laboratory test is available to confirm the diagnosis of NISD. Elevated serum ferritin levels have been found in neonates with the disorder. The transferrin saturation level is usually elevated until 2 months of age and is therefore less helpful. Laboratory studies mostly reflect marked hepatocellular dysfunction (see *Laboratory Studies*, in Ch. 9). Severe coagulopathy, conjugated hyperbilirubinemia, hypoalbuminemia, thrombocytopenia, and hypoglycemia are common. Serum transaminases are often normal or low, reflecting long-standing liver injury.

Treatment

Treatment of infants with NISD includes supportive care, iron chelation, antioxidant therapy, and liver transplantation. While providing supportive care, the infant suspected of having NISD should be evaluated for orthotopic liver transplant. Reports indicate transplantation has been successful.[20,21] However, the etiology of the disorder remains obscure, and long-term follow-up in such patients is not available.

Iron chelation therapy in the form of subcutaneous deferoxamine in one individual revealed no change in clinical, biochemical, or histologic findings, and the infant subsequently died at 3 months of age.[30] There have been more favorable results reported in three individuals treated with a combination of iron chelation and antioxidant therapy. N-Acetylcysteine, alpha-tocopherol polyethylene glycol succinate (TPGS), and selenium, in addition to prostaglandin E_1 (PGE$_1$) and deferoxamine, were given to infants aged 1 to 14 days, with subsequent recovery.[22] Evaluation of this treatment is in progress.

Referral Pattern

Infants with NISD are critically ill and are treated in a neonatal intensive care unit. A pediatric gastroenterologist should be consulted for diagnostic evaluation, management, and treatment. The neonate should be evaluated by a liver transplant team.

For parents considering subsequent pregnancies, early prenatal diagnosis is not yet available because no specific biochemical marker or gene defect has been identified. Fetal hydrops detected on ultrasound has identified some affected individuals, but this method is not specific. It may not be until the precise defect is known before we are able to offer more informative counseling and effective therapy.

REFERENCES

1. Powell LW. Hemochromatosis: the impact of early diagnosis and therapy. Gastroenterology 1996;110:1304–1307

2. Powell LW, Jazwinska E, Halliday JW. Primary iron overload. In: Brock JH, Halliday JW, Pippard MJ, Powell LW, Eds. Iron Metabolism in Health and Disease. London: WB Saunders, 1994:228–309

3. Edwards CQ, Griffen LM, Goldgar D et al. Prevalence of hemochromatosis among 11,065 presumably healthy blood donors. N Engl J Med 1988;318:1355–1362

4. Edwards CQ, Carroll M, Bray P, Cartwright GE. Hereditary hemochromatosis: diagnosis in siblings and children. N Engl J Med 1977;297:7–13

5. Adams PC, Kertesz AE, Valberg LS. Screening for hemochromatosis in children of homozygotes: prevalence and cost-effectiveness. Hepatology 1995;22:1720–1727

6. Edwards CQ, Kushner JP. Screening for hemochromatosis. N Engl J Med 1993;328:1616–1620

7. Niederau C, Fischer R, Purschel A et al. Long-term survival in patients with hereditary hemochromatosis. Gastroenterology 1996;110:1107–1119

8. Bothwell TH, Charlton RW, Motulsky AG. Hemochromatosis. In: Scriver CR, Beaudet AL, Sly WS, Valle D, Eds. The Metabolic and Molecular Bases of Inherited Disease. 7th Ed. New York: McGraw-Hill, 1995:2237–2269

9. Williams R, Manenti F, Williams HS, Pitcher CS. Iron absorption in idiopathic haemochromatosis before, during, and after venesection therapy. BMJ 1966;2:78–81

10. Adams PC, Kertesz AE, Valberg LS. Clinical presentation of hemochromatosis: a changing scene. Am J Med 1991;90: 445–449

11. Rouault TA. Hereditary hemochromatosis. JAMA 1993; 269:3152–3154

12. Kaikov Y, Wadsworth LD, Hassall E et al. Primary hemochromatosis in children: report of three newly diagnosed cases and review of the pediatric literature. Pediatrics 1992; 90:37–42

13. Haddy TB, Castro OL, Rana SR. Hereditary hemochromatosis in children, adolescents, and young adults. Am J Pediatr Hematol Oncol 1988;10:23–34

14. Perkins KW, McInnes IWS, Blackburn CRB, Beal RW. Idiopathic hemochromatosis in children. Am J Med 1965;39: 118–126

15. Lamon JM, Marynick SP, Rosenblatt R, Donnelly S. Idiopathic hemochromatosis in a young female: a case study and review of the syndrome in young people. Gastroenterology 1979;76;178–183

16. Cazzola M, Ascari E, Barosi G et al. Juvenile idiopathic hemochromatosis: a life-threatening disorder presenting as hypogonadotropic hypogonadism. Hum Genet 1983;65: 149–154

17. De Bont B, Walker AC, Carter RF et al. Idiopathic hemochromatosis presenting as acute hepatitis. J Pediatr 1987; 110:431–434

18. Escobar GJ, Heyman MB, Smith WB, Thaler MM. Primary hemochromatosis in childhood. Pediatrics 1987;80:549–554

19. Bassett ML, Halliday JW, Ferris RA, Powell LW. Diagnosis of hemochromatosis in young subjects: predictive accuracy of biochemical screening tests. Gastroenterology 1984;87: 628–633

20. Rand EB, McClenathan DT, Whitington PF. Neonatal hemochromatosis: report of successful orthotopic liver transplantation. J Pediatr Gastroenterol Nutr 1992;15:325–329

21. Lund DP, Lillehei CW, Kevy S et al. Liver transplantation in newborn liver failure: treatment for neonatal hemochromatosis. Transplant Proc 1993;25:1068–1071

22. Shamieh I, Kibart PK, Suchy FJ, Freese DK. Antioxidant therapy for neonatal iron storage disease (NISD). Pediatr Res 1993;33:109A

23. Kershisnik MM, Knisely AS, Sun C-C J et al. Cytomegalovirus infection, fetal liver disease, and neonatal hemochromatosis. Hum Pathol 1992;23:1075–1080

24. Shneider BL, Setchell KDR, Whitington PF et al. Δ^4-3-Oxosteroid 5β-reductase deficiency causing neonatal liver failure and hemochromatosis. J Pediatr 1994;124:234–238

25. Knisely AS, Harford JB, Klausner RD, Taylor SR. Neonatal hemochromatosis: the regulation of transferrin-receptor and ferritin synthesis by iron in cultured fibroblastic-line cells. Am J Pathol 1989;134:439–445

26. Goldfischer S, Grotsky HW, Chang CH et al. Idiopathic neonatal iron storage involving the liver, pancreas, heart and endocrine and exocrine glands. Hepatology 1981;1:58–64

27. Silver MM, Beverley DW, Valberg LS et al. Perinatal hemochromatosis: clinical, morphologic, and quantitative iron studies. Am J Pathol 1987;128:538–554

28. Witzleben CL, Uri A. Perinatal hemochromatosis: entity or end result? Hum Pathol 1989;20:335–340

29. Knisely AS, O'Shea PA, Stocks JF, Dimmick JE. Oropharyngeal and upper respiratory tract mucosal gland siderosis in neonatal hemochromatosis: an approach to biopsy diagnosis. J Pediatr 1988;113:871–874

30. Jonas MM, Kaweblum YA, Fojaco R. Neonatal hemochromatosis: failure of deferoxamine therapy. J Pediatr Gastroenterol Nutr 1987;6:984–988

55

HEPATIC FIBROSIS

DAVID A. PICCOLI

OVERVIEW OF FIBROSIS AND CIRRHOSIS

Fibrosis of the liver is due to the formation of new collagen fibers as a result of inflammation, metabolic disease, toxic insult, or collapse of the pre-existing connective tissue framework. It is found in a wide variety of disorders. Generally, the prognosis of the fibrosis is associated with the outcome of the causative process. Fibrosis may be diffuse, perisinusoidal, or bridging portal-to-portal tract. Fibrosis—even bridging fibrosis—should be distinguished from cirrhosis. Cirrhosis is a diffuse process in which the normal acini are replaced by nodules separated by fibrous tissue. These nodules are most commonly the result of the regenerative hyperplasia that follows certain hepatocellular insults. In these regenerative nodules, there is a severe disturbance of the vascular flow through the lobule, resulting in portal hypertension.

Many hepatocellular insults result in fibrosis, which may progress to cirrhosis, but this sequence is not inevitable, nor is the degree of fibrosis or cirrhosis directly related to the level of hepatocellular unrest or necrosis. Some processes will result in minimal inflammation, with severe fibrosis, while others may cause complete massive lobular necrosis, with eventual recovery without fibrosis. The factors that govern these processes are incompletely understood. The diagnosis of fibrosis or cirrhosis must be accompanied by the investigation for a cause. Most forms of hepatic fibrosis are the result of a primary process that causes a progressive deposition of collagen fibers. The time course is variable. Hepatitis C may be present for decades before progressing to signifi-

cant fibrosis and then cirrhosis. In biliary atresia, profound fibrosis and cirrhosis may be present by 4 months of age. Thus, in most clinical situations, the etiology of the fibrosis is more likely to dictate therapy and outcome than the status of the fibrosis. In its advanced stages, severe fibrosis and cirrhosis are accompanied by portal hypertension and chronic liver failure. Therapy for patients is directed toward those clinical manifestations of the disease.

Congenital hepatic fibrosis (CHF) is the result of a distinct pathophysiologic process. It has unique histologic, genetic, and clinical features, discussed in the remainder of the chapter.

CONGENITAL HEPATIC FIBROSIS

The term CHF was first used by Kerr et al.[1] to describe a disorder composed of a characteristic hepatopathology, cystic disease of the kidneys, portal hypertension, and increased risk of ascending cholangitis. In many pedigrees, the disease appears to be inherited in an autosomal recessive manner.[2,3] Common usage of the term CHF has now been extended by many gastroenterologists to include all patients with the hepatic histopathologic lesion of ductal plate malformation (DPM) (Fig. 55-1). Thus, the clinical constellation of CHF describes the hepatic manifestation of many unique disorders. The overwhelming majority of patients with ductal plate malformation of the liver have autosomal recessive polycystic kidney disease (ARPKD); some of these patients have the marked intrahepatic dilation of the bile duct consid-

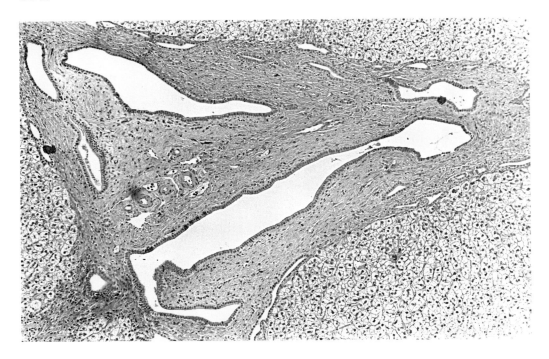

FIGURE 55-1. Ductal plate malformation in 4-year-old patient with CHF due to ARPKD. There are giant, bizarre, ectatic duct elements in the portal tract, with numerous smaller abnormal duct structures in the periphery of the tracts. These ducts communicate proximally and distally with the bile drainage system. The same (or very similar) portal tract lesions are also seen in a number of malformation syndromes (see text). Hematoxylin & eosin, ×20.

ered to be the communicating cystic spaces described by Caroli, now termed Caroli disease.

Because imprecise usage of each of these terms has led to significant confusion, it is important to characterize these processes either by the histopathologic picture (DPM) or by the genetically distinct etiologies (e.g., ARPKD). Thus, prognosis and complications of the disorders can be appropriately categorized.

THE DUCTAL PLATE AND THE DUCTAL PLATE MALFORMATION

The intrahepatic ducts develop primarily by differentiating from the hepatocytes at the margins of the developing portal tracts. This differentiation results in the formation of the ductal plate (Fig. 55-2), which is initially a layer of cytokeratin-staining cells. This cell layer thickens, and duct elements form from it at the margin of the portal tract. This process takes place in a centripetal fashion beginning from the hilus, through a process termed by Desmet as *remodeling*.[4] Duct elements form, and the majority of the ductal plate margin disappears. The duct elements become incorporated within the portal tract, and at the completion of this process in the

normal infant the ductal plate has disappeared, leaving only the centrally located highly differentiated interlobular duct. The ductal plates make their first appearance at 7 to 8 weeks gestation, and a few persisting elements of the plates may be present at or beyond term in the normal infant. Persistence of the ductal plate in the postnatal liver creates a lesion known as the DPM,[5] also termed biliary dysgenesis and congenital hepatic fibrosis (Fig. 55-2). DPM consists of plates or cisternae of duct elements characteristically found at the circumference of the portal tracts and is associated with increased portal tract fibrous tissue (Fig. 55-2). Jorgensen[5] recognized the similarity between these portal tracts and those seen in fetal life and coined the term ductal plate malformation to signify that the lesion represents an arrest in the development of normal portal tract and bile duct structures or a disruption of the normal remodeling of the embryonic bile duct and portal tract structures into their mature forms. This postnatal abnormal histology resembles the prenatal normal histopathology of the ductal plate; hence the term *malformation* may actually signify an abnormal lack of remodeling rather than a progressive and unique lesion. The extrahepatic ducts, which develop from a separate embryologic origin, are usually normal.

The lesion of DPM is found in combination with renal

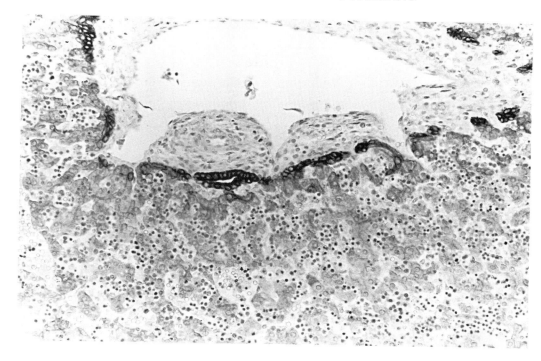

FIGURE 55-2. Fetal ductal plate. Cells at the ductal plate stained with cytokeratin stain, arranged in single and double layers at the periphery of the portal tract, which includes a large branch of the portal vein and loose connective tissue. Some areas of the ductal plate are interrupted. Hematoxylin & eosin, ×40.

abnormalities (usually cysts) in a number of heritable conditions. In addition to these heritable disorders, Desmet[4] suggested that persistence of the ductal plate can occasionally be associated with extrahepatic biliary atresia (EHBA), which is not heritable and not associated with renal disease. The factors that control ductal plate remodeling (and the commonly associated renal abnormalities) are unknown.

DPM is seen in a number of distinct clinical abnormalities (Table 55-1). The most common disease associated with DPM is autosomal recessive polycystic kidney disease. DPM is also rarely seen, however, in autosomal dominant polycystic kidney disease, which is genetically and clinically distinct from recessive polycystic kidney disease. The typical hepatic lesion in dominant polycystic kidney disease is a noncommunicating cyst rather than DPM, but the overlap causes diagnostic problems for the gastroenterologist. As the gene for recessive polycystic kidney disease (known to be on chromosome 6) is identified, this confusion will be resolved. The DPM lesion of ARPKD has clinical consequences that can be predicted on the basis of the histopathology. Patients with DPM have a "congenital" fibrosis, with preservation of the lobular architecture and normal hepatocytes in most cases. This severe fibrosis causes portal hypertension, usually accompanied by preserved synthetic function. The ductal plate remnants are large, bizarre duct elements which in three dimensional configuration may

TABLE 55-1. Diseases With Ductal Plate Malformation Histology and Congenital Hepatic Fibrosis Clinically

Autosomal recessive polycystic kidney disease

Autosomal dominant polycystic kidney disease, rarely

Juvenile nephronophthisis

Meckel-Gruber syndrome

Jeune syndrome

Ivemark syndrome

Laurence-Moon-Biedl syndrome

With vaginal atresia

With tuberous sclerosis

With choledochal cyst

"With" (as) Caroli disease (see text)

resemble large communicating cysts or cylinders seen at the periphery (plate margin) of the portal tract (Fig. 55-1). These can be detected by ultrasound, which generally cannot discriminate communicating from noncommunicating "cysts" in the liver. These large communicating cysts were described by the pathologist Caroli, who noted the association with renal disease (probably ARPKD).[6] More recently, the term Caroli disease has been redefined by radiologists and invasive cholangiographers to signify any type of communicating duct dilation, regardless of the association with extrahepatic disease. These large communicating spaces may have stasis and develop bacterial cholangitis. The abnormal development of the portal tract and portal vein and the portal fibrosis contribute to the severe portal hypertension seen in many of these patients.

ASSOCIATION WITH RENAL DISEASE AND SYSTEMIC DISEASE

The major heritable renal conditions characterized by intrahepatic bile duct cysts and hepatic fibrosis are ADPKD and ARPKD. The latter is intimately related to, if not identical with, CHF. There are also a number of heritable malformation syndromes characterized by hepatic and renal disease, and the ductal plate malformation is seen in all of these conditions (least commonly in ADPKD). For most purposes, the clinical hepatic process termed congenital hepatic fibrosis is equivalent to the hepatic manifestation of ARPKD. Since gastroenterologists tend to characterize all patients with DPM as CHF, some investigators have taken to separating the diseases with terms such as CHF-ARPKD, CHF-ADPKD, CHF-nephronophthisis, and CHF associated with syndromes such as Ivemark syndrome, Zellweger syndrome, Meckel syndrome, Jeune syndrome, Elejalde syndrome, and others (Table 55-1). Although it appears likely that ARPKD and CHF are manifestations of the same abnormal process, typically one or the other manifestation is predominant clinically. In patients who present in infancy, the polycystic kidney disease predominates, with renal failure, renal insufficiency, hypertension, and palpable kidneys as possible manifestations. If the renal disease is mild or inapparent, the patient may present later with hepatic disease (see below). These manifestations are not exclusive, however, and some patients will have severe disease in both kidneys and liver. Patients have been successfully transplanted for either organ or both.

HEPATIC DISEASE IN CONGENITAL HEPATIC FIBROSIS

Portal Hypertension

Among older patients with CHF, the most significant and common hepatic abnormality is portal hypertension. The precise pathogenesis is unknown but is thought to be associated with the hepatic fibrosis and/or portal vein abnormalities. Clinically, hematemesis or melena is the presenting sign of CHF in 30 to 70% of cases.[7] In children, the age for presentation of hematemesis may be as early as the first year of life,[8] but it usually ranges from 5 to 13 years. Firm or hard hepatomegaly is present in nearly all patients, often with a prominent left lobe, and this may be one of the presenting findings. Splenomegaly occurs in most cases, accompanied by hypersplenism with thrombocytopenia. Splenic pressure is elevated, and naturally occurring splenorenal or gastrorenal shunts are occasionally documented. Portal vein abnormalities, such as duplication of the intrahepatic branches are common.[9]

Biliary Lesions and Ascending Cholangitis

Dilation of the abnormal intrahepatic ducts is common in CHF,[10] leading to increased risk of cholangitis, presumably due to stasis in the ectatic ductular structures.[11–13] The cholangitis may be occult, acute, or chronic. Because of the abnormal drainage, the cholangitis can be refractory to therapy, and it can contribute significantly to both the morbidity and mortality of CHF.

Vascular Abnormalities

Abnormalities of the development of the intrahepatic portal veins have been identified in patients with CHF. There may be a nearly parallel duplication of portal vein branches, which may itself contribute to the substantial portal hypertension seen in many patients. The reason for this vascular abnormality is unknown but may have to do with the number of or remodeling of early ductal plate structures. In addition to the duplication of the intrahepatic portal venous system, other vascular abnormalities and congenital heart disease[14] are recognized associations. These include cerebral,[15] hepatic, splenic, and renal aneurysms, and cerebellar hemangioma. The reason for these associations is likewise unknown, but they may contribute to the mortality of the disease.

CLINICAL MANIFESTATIONS OF CHF

Patients with CHF typically are identified by physical examination or following unexplained gastrointestinal (GI) bleeding. Routine examination of the well child may reveal organomegaly. The liver is enlarged, commonly with a prominent left lobe extending well below the xyphoid and across the midline. The edge is typically hard and sharp. The spleen is usually enlarged and firm in texture. In some cases, the kidneys are palpable as well, although much less commonly than in infancy. The other presentation is unsuspected massive GI bleeding from esophageal varices. Commonly, the patient has been well and the hepatosplenomegaly unrecognized on previous examination. Just after a significant bleed, the spleen may decrease markedly in size, at times not palpable even on careful examination. In either presentation, the majority of patients have laboratory evidence of normal synthetic function, as measured by albumin and coagulation factors. The aminotransferases are likewise typically normal or mildly elevated, and the bilirubin is commonly normal. Occasionally, the albumin may be low and the bilirubin elevated following a significant esophageal bleed. CHF-ARPKD may be suggested by an elevated creatinine or a decreased creatinine clearance as evidence of intrinsic renal disease. An ultrasound will typically demonstrate hepatomegaly with intense echogenicity, and associated splenomegaly. The Doppler flow study may demonstrate reversed flow in the portal or splenic veins in advanced cases.

The kidneys may be abnormal in size or may demonstrate increased echogenicity. An intravenous pyelogram may identify polycystic disease. A percutaneous liver biopsy will demonstrate DPM in most patients, although in some mild and older cases the biliary dysgenesis will not be evident. This DPM is consistent with, but not exclusively diagnostic of, ARPKD. The final diagnosis associated with the clinical CHF will require formal assessment of the renal histology, renal pedigree, systemic features, or the genetic identity of the causative disease. The biopsy is also diagnostic for cholangitis, with polymorphonuclear leukocytes at the margin of, or in, the ducts. It is prudent to take a liver sample for bacterial culture in all patients with leukocytosis, fever, or hyperbilirubinemia.

THERAPY FOR CONGENITAL HEPATIC FIBROSIS AND ITS COMPLICATIONS

Most patients with mild CHF will require no hepatic therapy. Prophylactic antibiotics or sclerotherapy have not been shown to have any clinical value for these patients. If variceal bleeding occurs, standard therapy at the time of bleeding should be implemented. Although the coagulation times are commonly normal, these patients may still have life-threatening bleeds, and resuscitation may be hampered by diminished intrinsic renal function. Care should be taken with vasopressin therapy if renal function is compromised. Sclerotherapy may have a beneficial role in caring for patients who have bled. It appears that some patients may form spontaneous decompressing portosystemic shunts. For patients with aggressive or refractory bleeding, portosystemic shunting has been the treatment of choice. There appears to be a low incidence of postoperative encephalopathy or hyperammonemia.[2] Selective shunts, such as a mesocaval shunt, should be considered. Most patients with shunts will not require transplantation subsequently, but consideration should be given to early transplant if there is evidence of hepatic synthetic compromise.

Although rare, cholangitis can be severe and intractable. A transhepatic biliary aspirate and direct culture of a portion of the biopsy specimen may guide therapy by identifying a specific organism and its antibiotic sensitivities. Therapy may need to be administered for weeks or longer. The role of choleretic agents is unstudied, but such drugs may be beneficial in patients with stasis or infection. Surgical or transhepatic drainage may be indicated for refractory cases. ERCP, however, is probably contraindicated, as it may cause a cholangitis in the susceptible biliary system.[16]

REFERENCES

1. Kerr DNS, Harrison CV, Sherlock S et al. Congenital hepatic fibrosis. Q J Med 1961;30:91–117

2. Alvarez F, Bernard O, Brunelle F et al. Congenital hepatic fibrosis in children. J Pediatr 1981;99:370–375

3. Pereira Lima J, da Silveira TR, Geyer G, Grigoletti-Scholl J. Congenital hepatic fibrosis: a family study. J Pediatr Gastroenterol Nutr 1984;3:626–629

4. Desmet VJ. Congenital diseases of intrahepatic ducts: variations in the theme of "ductal plate malformation." Hepatology 1992;16:1069–1083

5. Jorgensen M. The ductal plate malformation. Acta Pathol Microbiol Scand 1977;(suppl A):257

6. Caroli J, Soupault R, Kossakowski J et al. La dilatation polykystique congenitale des voies biliaires intra-hepatiques: essai de classification. Semin Hop Paris 1958;14:496

7. Kerr DN, Okonkwo S, Choa RG. Congenital hepatic fibrosis: the long term prognosis. Gut 1978;19:514–520

8. Fiorillo A, Migliorati R, Vajro P, Caldore M, Vecchione R. Congenital hepatic fibrosis with gastrointestinal bleeding in early infancy. Clin Pediatr 1982;21:183–185

9. Odievre M, Chaumont P, Montagne JP, Alagille D. Anomalies of the intrahepatic portal venous system in congenital hepatic fibrosis. Radiology 1977;122:427–430

10. Murray-Lyon IM, Shilkin KB, Laws JW et al. Non-obstructive dilatation of the intrahepatic biliary tree with cholangitis. Q J Med 1972;41:477

11. Alvarez F, Hadchouel M, Bernard O. Latent chronic cholangitis in congenital hepatic fibrosis. Eur J Pediatr 1982;139:203–205

12. Howlett SA, Shulman ST, Ayoub EM et al. Cholangitis complicating congenital hepatic fibrosis. Am J Dig Dis 1975;20:790–795

13. Murray-Lyon IM, Shilkin KB, Laws JW et al. Non-obstructive dilatation of the intrahepatic biliary tree with cholangitis. Q J Med 1972;164:477

14. Naveh Y, Roguin N, Ludatscher R et al. Congenital hepatic fibrosis with congenital heart disease. A family study with ultrastructural features of the liver. Gut 1980;21:799–807

15. King K, Genta RM, Giannella RA, Weesner RE. Congenital hepatic fibrosis and cerebral aneurysm in a 32-year-old woman. J Pediatr Gastroenterol Nutr 1986;5:481–484

16. Lam SK, Wong KP, Chan PK et al. Fatal cholangitis after endoscopic retrograde cholangiopancreatography in congenital hepatic fibrosis. Aust NZ J Surg 1978;48:199–202

56

HEPATOBLASTOMA AND HEPATOCELLULAR CARCINOMA

JOHN M. MARIS

Malignancies arising within the liver are uncommon in childhood. However, malignant hepatic tumors are an important part of the differential diagnosis of abdominal distention or a right upper quadrant mass. The two most common pediatric hepatic neoplasms, hepatoblastoma and hepatocellular carcinoma, are discussed with an emphasis on differentiating these malignant lesions from benign processes. This is often possible with a thorough history, physical examination, and limited ancillary tests. The primary practitioner is essential in determining the likelihood of malignancy, so that appropriate referral may be made.

PATHOPHYSIOLOGY

Epidemiology

Hepatic malignancies account for less than 2% of all childhood cancer, with an annual incidence of 1.6 per one million children in the United States.[1] Hepatoblastoma and hepatocellular carcinoma constitute the vast majority of all primary hepatic malignancies of childhood. Thirty cases of hepatoblastoma and 22 cases of hepatocellular carcinoma among 5,570 entrants in the Children's Hospital of Philadelphia-based Greater Delaware Valley Tumor Registry were seen between 1970 and 1995 (0.9%). Like many childhood cancers, there is a slight male preponderance. Although most series report a male-to-female ratio of 1.4 to 1.7:1, in our experience

the disparity was greater (2.4:1). Hepatoblastoma is occasionally seen in familial clusters, segregating as an autosomal dominant trait.[2–4] The incidence of malignant hepatic tumors is increased in Asian and African children relative to those in North America, most likely due to an increase in environmental exposure to hepatocellular carcinoma potentiating agents.[5]

Associated Conditions

Hepatoblastoma and Wilms' tumor (both pediatric embryonal cancers) are both associated with the Beckwith-Wiedemann somatic overgrowth syndrome[6–8] and hemihypertrophy.[9] A common molecular genetic abnormality that links these diverse conditions is hemizygous deletion of the distal short arm of chromosome 11. This finding is present in the germline of patients with the Beckwith-Wiedemann syndrome and is detectable in a subset of hepatoblastomas and Wilms' tumors.[10,11] There is also a strong association of hepatoblastoma with the familial adenomatous polyposis (FAP) syndrome.[12–15] Indeed, the gene primarily responsible for the FAP syndrome has been found to be homozygously inactivated in some sporadic hepatoblastomas.[16] There have also been reports of hepatoblastoma in patients with dysplastic kidneys,[17] Meckel's diverticulum[18] and maternal use of alcohol[19] and oral contraceptives.[20]

Hepatocellular carcinoma is more likely to occur in a liver that has suffered hepatocellular injury.[21] There is a strong association with chronic hepatitis B infection, similar to the adult population.[22–26] This is somewhat surprising, since the reported latency for the development of hepatocellular carcinoma in adults is in excess of 20 years. However, the documentation of hepatocellular carcinoma within 7 years of perinatal transmission of hepatitis B virus suggests a much shorter latency in children.[27–29] Several inborn errors of metabolism are known to cause hepatocellular injury and greatly increase the risk of hepatocellular carcinoma. In one series, 37% of children with the chronic form of tyrosinemia who survived beyond 2 years of age developed hepatocellular carcinoma.[30] Other metabolic diseases in which there is a higher than expected rate of hepatocellular carcinoma include type 1 glycogen storage disease (glucose-6-phosphatase deficiency) and the homozygous ZZ phenotype of alpha-1-antitrypsin disease. In addition, biliary cirrhosis due to extrahepatic biliary atresia has been associated with hepatocellular carcinoma whereas noncirrhotic forms of chronic cholestasis do not seem to predispose to hepatic tumors.

Pathology

Although the tumors can be quite large, hepatoblastomas are typically unifocal and confined to one lobe of the liver. There are two major histologic subsets of hepatoblastoma (Table 56-1). Epithelial hepatoblastomas are composed of immature fetal and/or embryonal cells, suggesting that the malignant clone arose from an undifferentiated hepatoblast. A mixed hepatoblastoma has abnormal mesenchymal architecture admixed with the fetal and/or embryonal cells. The malignant fetal or embryonal cells are recognized microscopically as being smaller than normal hepatocytes and extramedullary hematopoiesis is common. Tumors composed mainly of a fetal component are associated with a more favorable prognosis.[31] However, the difference between histologic subtypes is small and overridden by the stage at diagnosis, diminishing the prognostic significance of histology alone.[32,33]

The pathologic appearance of hepatocellular carcinoma presenting in childhood is similar to that in adult patients. The tumors are often multicentric and hemorrhagic, making initial resection difficult. In general, hepatocellular carcinoma cells are much larger than normal hepatocytes and have pleomorphic nuclei. Typically, there are large numbers of tumor giant cells, and extramedullary hematopoiesis is not observed. In children, there is often a lack of background cirrhosis, which is almost universally seen in adult patients. Although the histopathologic distinction between hepatocellular carcinoma and hepatoblastoma is usually straightforward, this may be difficult when the specimen is limited to a core biopsy.

A variant of hepatocellular carcinoma is the fibrolamellar carcinoma. This tumor is unique to adolescence and early adulthood, occurs in noncirrhotic livers, and has a more favorable prognosis.[34] Fibrolamellar carcinoma is distinguished by deeply eosinophilic hepatocytes with a dense fibrous stroma, but it is sometimes difficult to differentiate from focal nodular hyperplasia.

CLINICAL PRESENTATION

Hepatoblastoma classically presents as an asymptomatic right upper quadrant mass in an otherwise well child less than 2 years of age. The vast majority of cases occur before age 5. Most patients are brought to medical attention due to generalized abdominal enlargement or a solid abdominal mass, often noted by a caretaker. Associated symptoms, such as weight loss, anorexia, vomiting, abdominal pain, and fever, are uncommon and, when present, are suggestive of advanced disease. Jaundice is rare.

A unique and almost pathognomonic feature of children with newly diagnosed hepatoblastoma is severe osteopenia. Presenting symptoms and signs may include irritability, refusal to walk, back pain, and pathologic fractures. Vertebral body compression fractures may be evident on lateral chest radiography. The etiology of this association is not directly related to liver dysfunction and remains obscure.

Hepatocellular carcinoma usually occurs in an older child, often with a history of an underlying condition, such as chronic hepatitis B infection or hereditary tyrosinemia. The median age of diagnosis in two pediatric series was 12 years.[35,36] Most patients present with generalized abdominal distention and/or a right upper quadrant mass. However, in contradistinction to hepatoblastoma, most patients with hepatocellular carcinoma also have abdominal pain, emesis, weight loss, fever, or other constitutional symptoms, usually of relatively short (1- to 2-month) duration. Acute hemmorrhagic abdominal crisis is the initial presentation in a small percentage of patients and may be fatal. Patients with the fibrolamellar

TABLE 56-1. Histopathologic Classification of Primary Hepatic Malignancies of Childhood

Hepatoblastoma

Epithelial
    Embryonal
    Fetal
Mixed epithelial and mesenchymal

Hepatocellular carcinoma

Adult type
Fibrolamellar carcinoma

variant of hepatocellular carcinoma typically present between 10 and 20 years of age, often with chronic (1 year) and insidious symptoms of abdominal pain and swelling.

DIAGNOSIS

Differential Diagnosis

The differential diagnosis of a right upper quadrant mass is large and includes both malignant and benign conditions. The diagnostic possibilities can be substantially narrowed on the basis of the age and clinical appearance of the patient along with historical and physical examination data. The differential diagnosis of a right upper quadrant mass discovered in a child is presented in Table 56-2. Only intrinsic hepatic lesions will be dealt with further.

The age of the patient with a primary hepatic mass is the first important consideration. Since malignant conditions are rare in infancy, a hepatic mass in a child less than 12 months of age is much more likely due to a congenital vascular or hamartomatous anomaly than to a malignant tumor. However, hepatoblastoma often occurs during infancy, and congenital hepatoblastoma has been described.[7,37] The second consideration is the clinical status of the patients. A child with a well appearance is much more likely to have a vascular anomaly or hepatoblastoma than hepatocellular carcinoma.

Of all primary hepatic tumors at any age or clinical presentation, approximately two-thirds are subsequently

TABLE 56-2. Differential Diagnosis of Nonhepatic Right Upper Quadrant Masses in Children

Organ	Malignant	Benign
Adrenal	Neuroblastoma Adrenal carcinoma Pheochromocytoma	Adenoma Hemorrhage
Gallbladder	Leiomyosarcoma	Hydrops/obstruction Choledochal cyst
Gastrointestinal tract	Non-Hodgkin's lymphoma Desmoplastic small cell tumor Leiomyosarcoma	Intussusception Intestinal duplication Mesenteric cyst
Kidney	Wilms' tumor Renal cell carcinoma Mesoblastic nephroma	Hydronephrosis Cystic kidney disease
Retroperitoneum	Lymphoma Rhabdomyosarcoma Neuroblastoma Germ cell tumor	Lymphangioma Aortic aneurysm

TABLE 56-3. Primary Hepatic Tumors in Children

Malignant	Benign
Hepatoblastoma	Hemangioendothelioma
Hepatocellular carcinoma	Hemangioma
Rhabdomyosarcoma	Mesenchymal hamartoma
Angiosarcoma	Simple cyst
Mesenchymal hamartoma	Adenoma
Carcinoid (apudoma)	
Leiomyosarcoma	
Malignant teratoma	
Primary lymphoma	

proved to be malignant. Benign lesions of the liver are usually vascular in nature and are more likely to be discovered during the first 12 months of life (Table 56-3). Although hepatoblastoma and hepatocellular carcinoma constitute most malignant hepatic neoplasms in children, other less common malignancies do occur (Table 56-3). As discussed below, measurement of serum alphafetoprotein (AFP) provides the simplest and most efficient means of differentiating a primary hepatic neoplasm from most other entities.

Evaluation

Initial diagnostic evaluations should be directed toward defining the likelihood of malignant disease, extent of disease and potential for primary resectability. Although laboratory evaluations may be helpful, diagnostic imaging studies are necessary to narrow the differential diagnosis.

Many vascular lesions can be documented with great certainty using real time Doppler ultrasonography. Magnetic resonance imaging (MRI) with intravenous contrast may also be useful. However, if a solid intrahepatic neoplasm is strongly suggested, abdominal computed tomography (CT) will provide the most complete diagnostic evaluation (Fig. 56-1). Furthermore, CT is useful in documenting pulmonary metastases that may be missed by routine chest radiography.

Staging

A complete radiologic staging evaluation for a suspected hepatic malignancy includes an abdominal and chest CT with intravenous contrast. It is unusual with current CT technology that other imaging tests, such as a celiac arteriogram or Doppler ultrasonography, would be necessary to define intrahepatic involvement. Since metastases outside the pulmonary bed are rare in children with pri-

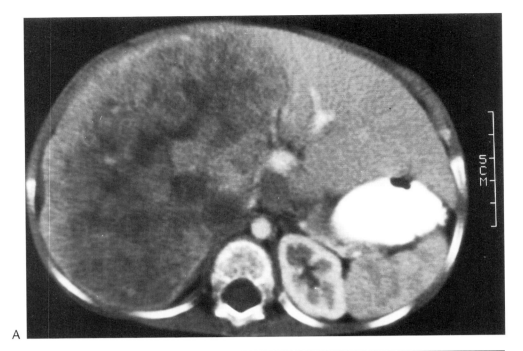

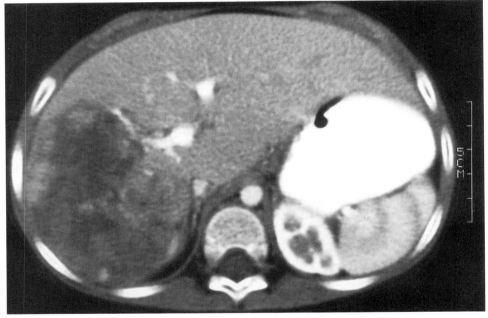

FIGURE 56-1. Abdominal computed tomography scans of a 3-year-old boy with hepatoblastoma at diagnosis (*A*) and following two cycles of combination chemotherapy (*B*). The neoadjuvant chemotherapy converted the unresectable mass in *A* to one that was subsequently completely removed.

mary hepatic malignancies, bone marrow aspirates and biopsies as well as bone scintigraphy should be performed only in the presence of appropriate clinical findings such as extremity pain or pancytopenia.

Most currently used staging systems for malignant hepatic tumors are surgicopathologic (Table 56-4). This system has been useful in predicting outcome in the past

(Fig. 56-2) but was devised at a time when effective chemotherapy was unavailable. A simplified staging system based on clinical and radiographic material is needed, as most patients are currently being treated with preoperative chemotherapy. For future chemotherapeutic trials, stratification of therapy may be based largely on the extent of disease (localized versus multifocal versus

TABLE 56-4. Children's Cancer Group Staging System for Primary Malignant Hepatic Tumor

Stage	Description
I	Complete resection
	A. Favorable histology
	B. Unfavorable histology
II	Microscopic residual disease
	A. Intrahepatic residual tumor
	B. Extrahepatic residual tumor
III	Gross residual disease
	A. Complete resection, regional nodes positive
	B. Incomplete resection
IV	Metastatic disease
	A. Primary tumor completely excised
	B. Primary tumor not completely excised

metastatic), rather than on traditional surgicopathologic staging.

LABORATORY EVALUATION

All children with a suspected liver tumor should be screened with a complete blood count (CBC) and a panel of liver function and enzymatic tests. A CBC may reveal thrombocytopenia in a cavernous hemangioma (Kasabach-Merritt syndrome). Conversely, thrombo-

cytosis is often associated with hepatoblastoma. Pancytopenia may identify the rare patient with malignant disease and overt bone marrow metastases. A prothrombin time (PT) should be measured to assess liver synthetic function. It is rare that there is significant elevation of liver transaminases or bilirubin with primary hepatic malignancies. However, if hepatocellular carcinoma is subsequently confirmed, laboratory investigation for underlying viral and metabolic disease is warranted.

AFP is a serum glycoprotein produced in abundance by fetal liver cells and yolk sac tissue. Relative to normal adult values, serum AFP levels are substantially elevated at the time of birth and fall to less than 10 ng/mL by 8 months of age.[38] AFP has a biologic half-life of 5 to 7 days. Most primary hepatic malignancies produce substantial quantities of AFP, providing a useful diagnostic marker. This is true even in an infant, in whom a rising or stable AFP would be distinctly abnormal. Although the initial serum value of AFP is not prognostically important,[33] the rate of fall following primary chemotherapy may be of prognostic value. In addition, serum AFP values are useful during and after therapy to monitor disease status. Values should reach normal levels 6 to 8 weeks after a complete resection. An elevated AFP following previous normalization is highly suggestive of disease recurrence.

A small percentage of hepatoblastomas secrete the beta-subunit of human chorionic gonadotropin (beta-HCG). These rare patients are usually boys who may present with precocious puberty.

TREATMENT

Surgical Management

In the past, complete surgical resection was considered essential for the successful treatment of either hepatoblastoma or hepatocellular carcinoma. Aggressive surgical management with initial en bloc removal of large tumors was often attempted. However, this was associated with high morbidity due to the large size and friable nature of many hepatic tumors. The exquisite sensitivity of hepatic neoplasms as a whole to cisplatin-based chemotherapy has therefore changed the timing of surgery in many instances.[39,40] Indeed, there is one case report of a large hepatoblastoma disappearing completely with intra-arterial infusions of multiagent chemotherapy resulting in long-term remission without surgery.[41] In addition, pulmonary metastases may disappear completely with chemotherapy.[40] Taken together with anecdotal reports of cure without surgery, it is now generally agreed that preoperative chemotherapy is the treatment of choice, unless a relatively small tumor, clearly localized within one lobe of the liver, is identified. Since only 20% of patients will fit this criterion, the majority of newly diagnosed patients with hepatic malignancies will receive preoperative chemotherapy. As demonstrated in

FIGURE 56-2. Surgicopathologic staging of pediatric hepatic tumors predicts survival. Kaplan–Meier overall survival estimates in 61 children with either hepatoblastoma or hepatocellular carcinoma stratified by surgicopathologic staging. (From Evans et al.,[44] with permission.)

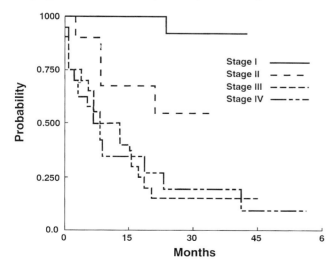

Figure 56-1 this approach cannot only often convert an unresectable tumor to one that is resectable, but also seems to decreased the friability of the tumor, thereby decreasing the surgical morbidity.[46] Pathologic confirmation of the diagnosis before initiation of therapy, preferably by open biopsy at a tertiary referral center, is essential.

Chemotherapy

Chemotherapeutic approaches to the management of children with primary hepatic malignancies can be defined as either adjuvant (after surgery) or neoadjuvant (before and after surgery). No patient is treated with surgery alone, as chemotherapy has been clearly demonstrated to improve survival.[43,44] Several different chemotherapeutic regimens have been used to treat hepatoblastoma and hepatocellular carcinoma. Most large pediatric oncology cooperative groups are now treating these two entities in a uniform fashion.

Liver Transplantation

Orthotopic liver transplantation may have a role in the management of children with primary hepatic malignancies that remain unresectable following chemotherapy. Results in children have been mixed, with survival of 50% to 90% for hepatoblastoma and 20% to 30% for hepatocellular carcinoma in several small, heterogeneous series.[42,44] These patients must be carefully selected since hepatic transplantation will have no effect on metastatic disease. Minimum criteria include the patient's having failed (tumor remains unresectable) conventional multiagent chemotherapy and no evidence of metastatic disease following a thorough evaluation.

Radiation Therapy

Currently, radiation therapy has a limited role in the management of hepatic malignancies of childhood. Although this modality could theoretically be used in patients who have microscopic residual disease following resection, the interference with liver regeneration when radiation is given postoperatively has limited its applicability. Moreover, liver regeneration alters hepatic anatomy quickly and unpredictably, making radiation field planning difficult.

Survival

Because of the rarity of hepatic malignancies in childhood, the heterogeneity of the tumors themselves, and the various chemotherapeutic regimens with which they are treated, it is difficult to ascertain accurate current survival estimates. However, it is clear that significant improvement has been made in the treatment of hepatoblastoma (Fig. 56-3), with overall survival estimates of nearly two-thirds and as much as 90% in stage I, favorable histology patients. Much of the improved survival is due to neoadjuvant chemotherapy converting previously unresectable tumors to those that can be removed. Hepatocellular carcinoma remains a more difficult condition to treat successfully. Newer therapeutic strategies may be necessary to achieve further improvement in survival.

REFERRAL PATTERN

All patients with a suspected liver tumor should be referred to a tertiary care facility experienced with both the surgical and medical management of these rare con-

FIGURE 56-3. Improved survival with platinum-based chemotherapy. Kaplan-Meier event-free survival estimates in 60 children with hepatoblastoma treated with VCR/ CDDP/5-FU. Most children with stage III and IV disease were given neoadjuvant chemotherapy. Note the improved survival compared to Figure 56-2 (chemotherapy did not include CDDP), especially in the patients with stage III disease. (From Douglass et al.,[43] with permission.)

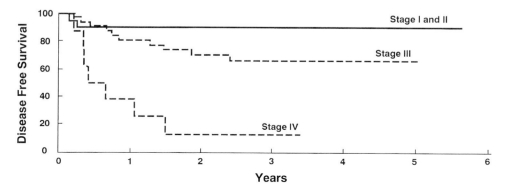

ditions. Differentiation between the benign and malignant conditions often requires multidisciplinary evaluation and treatment planning. Biopsy should take place in a facility experienced in processing these rare specimens so that appropriate diagnostic and therapeutic decisions may be made. If a primary hepatic malignancy is confirmed, the primary care provider will play an integral role in the long-term management of these patients. This will include evaluation of toxicity during initial management and surveillance for recurrent disease and/or late effects of treatment during long-term follow-up.

REFERENCES

1. Young JL, Miller RW: Incidence of malignant tumors in U.S. children. J Pediatr 1975;86:254–258

2. Fraumeni JF, Rosen PJ, Hull EW et al: Hepatoblastoma in infant sisters. Cancer 1969;24:1086–1090

3. Napoli VM, Campbell WGJ: Hepatoblastoma in infant sister and brother. Cancer 1977;39:2647–2650

4. Surendran N, Radhakrishna K, Chellam VG: Hepatoblastoma in siblings. J Pediatr Surg 1989;24:1169–1171

5. Lanzkowsky P: Manual of Pediatric Hematology and Oncology. 2nd Ed. New York: Churchill Livingstone, 1995

6. Wilfong AA, Parke JT, McCrary JAD: Opsoclonus-myoclonus with Beckwith-Wiedemann syndrome and hepatoblastoma. Pediatr Neurol 1992;8:77–79

7. Orozco-Florian R, McBride JA, Favara BE et al: Congenital hepatoblastoma and Beckwith-Wiedemann syndrome: a case study including DNA ploidy profiles of tumor and adrenal cytomegaly. Pediatr Pathol 1991;11:131–142

8. Martelli C, Blandamura S, Massaro S et al: A case study of Beckwith-Wiedemann syndrome associated with hepatoblastoma. Clin Exp Obstet Gynecol 1993;20:82–87

9. Geiser C, Baez A, Schindler A, Shih V: Epithelial hepatoblastoma associated with congenital hemihypertrophy and cystathioninuria: presentation of case. Pediatrics 1970;46:66–73

10. Koufos A, Grundy P, Morgan K et al: Familial Wiedemann-Beckwith syndrome and a second Wilms tumor locus both map to 11p15.5. Am J Hum Genet 1989;44:711–719

11. Koufos A, Hansen MF, Copeland NG et al: Loss of heterozygosity in three embryonal tumours suggests a common pathogenetic mechanism. Nature 1985;316:330–334

12. Bernstein IT, Bulow S, Mauritzen K. Hepatoblastoma in two cousins in a family with adenomatous polyposis. Report of two cases. Dis Colon Rectum 1992;35:373–374

13. Giardiello FM, Offerhaus GJ, Krush AJ et al: Risk of hepatoblastoma in familial adenomatous polyposis. J Pediatr 1991;119:766–768

14. Hughes LJ, Michels VV: Risk of hepatoblastoma in familial adenomatous polyposis. Am J Med Genet 1992;43:1023–1025

15. Shneider BL, Haque S, van Hoff J et al: Familial adenomatous polyposis following liver transplantation for a virilizing hepatoblastoma. J Pediatr Gastroenterol Nutr 1992;15:198–201

16. Kurahashi H, Takami K, Oue T et al: Biallelic inactivation of the APC gene in hepatoblastoma. Cancer Res 1995;55:5007–5011

17. Khosla A: Hepatoblastoma and congenital dysplastic kidney. J Pediatr Surg 1990;25:924

18. Greenberg M, Filler RM: Hepatic tumors. In: Pizzo PA, Poplack DG, eds. Principles and Practice of Pediatric Oncology. 2nd ed. Philadelphia: JB Lippincott 1994:717–732

19. Khan A, Bader JL, Hoy GR, Sinks LF: Hepatoblastoma in child with fetal alcohol syndrome. Lancet 1979;1:1403–1404

20. Otten J, Smets R, De Jager RN et al: Hepatoblastoma in an infant after contraceptive intake during pregnancy. N Engl J Med 1977;297:222

21. Esquivel CO, Gutierrez C, Cox KL et al: Hepatocellular carcinoma and liver cell dysplasia in children with chronic liver disease. J Pediatr Surg 1994;29:1465–1469

22. Wu TC, Tong MJ, Hwang B et al: Primary hepatocellular carcinoma and hepatitis B infection during childhood. Hepatology 1987;7:46–48

23. Pontisso P, Morsica G, Ruvoletto MG et al: Latent hepatitis B virus infection in childhood hepatocellular carcinoma. Analysis by polymerase chain reaction. Cancer 1992;69:2731–2735

24. Di Bisceglie AM, Order SE, Klein JL et al. The role of chronic viral hepatitis in hepatocellular carcinoma in the United States. Am J Gastroenterol 1991;86:335–338

25. Chen DS: From hepatitis to hepatoma: lessons from type B viral hepatitis. Science 1993;262:369–370

26. Chang MH, Chen PJ, Chen JY et al. Hepatitis B virus integration in hepatitis B virus-related hepatocellular carcinoma in childhood. Hepatology 1991;13:316–320

27. Harvey VJ, Woodfield DG, Probert JC: Maternal transmission of hepatocellular carcinoma. Cancer 1984;54:1360–1363

28. Beasley RP, Shiao IS, Wu TC Hwang LY: Hepatoma in an HBsAg carrier—seven years after perinatal infection. J Pediatr 1982;101:83–84

29. Shimoda T, Uchida T, Miyata H et al: A 6-year-old boy having hepatocellular carcinoma associated with hepatitis B surface antigenemia. Am J Clin Pathol 1980;74:827–831

30. Weinberg AG, Mize CE, Worthen HG: The occurrence of hepatoma in the chronic form of hereditary tyrosinemia. J Pediatr 1976;88:434–438

31. Lack EE, Neave C, Vawter GF: Hepatoblastoma. A clinical and pathologic study of 54 cases. Am J Surg Pathol 1982;66:693–705

32. Conran RM, Hitchcock CL, Waclawiw MA et al. Hepatoblastoma: the prognostic significance of histologic type. Pediatr Pathol 1992;12:167–183

33. von Schweinitz D, Wischmeyer P, Leuschner I et al: Clinicopathological criteria with prognostic relevance in hepatoblastoma. Eur J Cancer 1994;30A:1052–1058

34. Craig JR, Peters RL, Edmondson HA, Omata M: Fibrolamellar carcinoma of the liver: a tumor of adolescents and young

adults with distinctive clinicopathologic features. Cancer 1980;46:372–379

35. Lack EE, Neave C, Vawter GF: Hepatocellular carcinoma. Review of 32 cases of childhood and adolescence. Cancer 1983;52:1510–1515

36. Giacomantonio M, Ein SH, Mancer K, Stephens CA: Thirty years of experience with pediatric primary malignant liver tumors. J Pediatr Surg 1984;19:523–526

37. Marakchi Z, Chaouachi B, Kaabar N et al: Congenital hepatoblastoma: a case report. Tunisie Med 1992;70:499–502

38. Wu JT, Book L, Sudar K: Serum alpha fetoprotein (AFP) levels in normal infants. Pediatr Res 1981;15:50–52

39. Ninane J, Perilongo G, Stalens JP et al: Effectiveness and toxicity of cisplatin and doxorubicin (PLADO) in childhood hepatoblastoma and hepatocellular carcinoma: a SIOP pilot study. Med Pediatr Oncol 1991;19:199–203

40. Filler RM, Ehrlich PF, Greenberg ML, Babyn PS: Preoperative chemotherapy in hepatoblastoma. Surgery 1991;110: 591–596

41. Yokomori K, Hori T, Asoh S et al: Complete disappearance of unresectable hepatoblastoma by continuous infusion therapy through hepatic artery. J Pediatr Surg 1991;26:844–846

42. Reynolds M, Douglass EC, Finegold M et al: Chemotherapy can convert unresectable hepatoblastoma. J Pediatr Surg 1992;27:1080–1083

43. Douglass EC, Reynolds M, Finegold M et al: Cisplatin, vincristine, and fluorouracil therapy for hepatoblastoma: a Pediatric Oncology Group Study. J Clin Oncol 1993;11:96–99

44. Evans AE, Land VJ, Newton WA et al: Combination chemotherapy (vincristine, adriamycin, cyclophosphamide, and 5-fluorouracil) in the treatment of children with malignant hepatoma. Cancer 1982;50:821–826

45. Black CT, Cangir A, Choroszy M, Andrassy RJ: Marked response to preoperative high-dose cisplatinum in children with unresectable hepatoblastoma. J Pediatr Surg 1991;26: 1070–1073

46. Ortega JA, Douglass E, Feusner J et al: A randomized trial of cisplatin (DDP)/vincristine (VCR)/5-fluorouracil (5FU) vs. DDP/doxorubicin (DOX) I.V. continuous infusion for the treatment of hepatoblastoma (HB). Results from the pediatric intergroup hepatoma study (CCG-8881/POG-8945). Proc Am Soc Clin Oncol. Dallas, TX 1994; Abs 1421

47. Koneru B, Flye MW, Busuttil RW et al: Liver transplantation for hepatoblastoma. The American experience. Ann Surg 1991;213:118–121

48. Tagge EP, Tagge DU, Reyes J et al: Resection, including transplantation, for hepatoblastoma and hepatocellular carcinoma: impact on survival. J Pediatr Surg 1992;27:292–296

49. Lockwood L, Heney D, Giles GR et al: Cisplatin-resistant metastatic hepatoblastoma: complete response to carboplatin, etoposide, and liver transplantation. Med Pediatr Oncol 1993;21:517–520

50. Stringer MD, Hennayake S, Howard ER et al: Improved outcome for children with hepatoblastoma. Br J Surg 1995; 82:386–391

57

GALACTOSEMIA

JAMES B. GIBSON

When many primary care practitioners hear the term *galactosemia* they think of only one of the three disorders of galactose catabolism that have been called by this name. The three disorders correspond to deficiencies in the three enzymes in the usual catabolic pathway: the kinase, transferase, and epimerase.[1] It is transferase deficiency that is most commonly called galactosemia or hereditary galactosemia. This chapter deals primarily with transferase deficiency, with the other two disorders mentioned briefly for the sake of completeness.

PATHOPHYSIOLOGY

Galactose is presented to the liver and the rest of the body in several ways. The majority of ingested galactose is found as a component of lactose in milks. Catalyzed by lactase, the disaccharide is split into glucose and galactose at the intestinal microvillous border, and the monosaccharides are absorbed into the bloodstream. The liver clears the galactose from the portal system, beginning the intrahepatic phase of galactose utilization. The other two mechanisms by which galactose may be presented to the body are as a free sugar found in many fruits and vegetables[2] and as a bound sugar residue in glycoproteins or complex carbohydrates such as raffinose and stachyose.[3] The digestion of the latter carbohydrate compounds in man is controversial. Bacterial action in the intestinal tract may be responsible for the limited digestion that occurs.

Galactose is an essential molecule for humans, as it is necessary in the post-translational modification of peptides that occurs in the Golgi apparatus. Proteins with galactose residues are found on cell surfaces as antigens, receptors, and, in some cases, the presence of the carbohydrate is essential for the functioning of certain enzymes. As a result, there is an obligatory turnover of galactose as the body recycles these macromolecular components.

The Major Catabolic Pathway

The first step of the major hepatic catabolic pathway for galactose is phosphorylation by galactose kinase (EC 2.7.1.6) producing galactose-1-phosphate. The second step of the pathway is the transfer of galactose from the phosphate residue to a uridine diphosphate (UDP) moiety as an exchange between galactose-1-phosphate and UDP-glucose, catalyzed by galactose-1-phosphate uridyltransferase (EC 2.7.7.10) to produce UDP-galactose and glucose-1-phosphate. The final step of this pathway is the conversion of UDP-galactose to UDP-glucose by epimerazation at the C-4, catalyzed by galactose-4-epimerase (EC 5.1.3.2). Thus, dietary galactose can directly contribute to the pool of UDP-glucose for glycogen synthesis as well as be used for galactosylation reactions (Table 57-1; Fig. 57-1).

The Minor Pathways

In addition, minor catabolic pathways account for some of the distinctive products seen in the disorders of galactose metabolism (Fig. 57-1). Galactose can be reduced to galactitol, its sugar alcohol, in an irreversible step by aldose reductase. A minor pathway for the oxidation of galactose

TABLE 57-1. Enzymes of the Major Catabolic Pathway

	Kinase	Transferase	Epimerase
Chromosome	17q21–22	g13	1p34
Protein structure	Dimer	Dimer	Dimer
Molecular weight	2×25–27 kD	2×44–45 kD	70 kD
Substrates	Galactose, ATP	Gal-1P, UDP-glucose	UDP-galactose or UDP-glucose
Cofactor	None	None	NAD^+
Products	Galactose-1-phosphate, ADP	Glucose-1-phosphate, UDP-galactose	UDP-glucose or UDP-galactose

occurs via a shunt to galactonate, subsequently to xylulose phosphate, and then into the pentose phosphate pathway.[1] A uridine diphosphate glucose pyrophosphorylase exists whose primary purpose is the synthesis of UDP-glucose from UTP and glucose-1-phosphate. However, it can react with galactose to form UDP-galactose. As a reversible reaction, the pyrophosphorylase can form galactose-1-phosphate from UDP-galactose and potentially contribute to the pool of this toxic metabolite,[4] even in the absence of galactose flux through galactokinase.

Kinase Deficiency

In galactokinase deficiency, the toxic metabolite is postulated to be the sugar alcohol. Galactitol accumulation in the lens causes swelling and cataract formation, the

hallmark of the disorder (Table 57-2). Several children have been reported with other symptoms that cannot be clearly attributed to accumulation of galactitol. Screening detects the elevated galactose concentration and the diagnosis is confirmed by enzyme analysis. Treatment entails the exclusion of galactose from the diet. Cataract removal may be needed to retain vision.

Epimerase Deficiency

In this disorder, the body is unable to form UDP-galactose from the nucleotide and glucose. The production via the galactose catabolic pathway must not be sufficient because clinical manifestations (Table 57-2) may be seen. However, only a very few patients have been documented to have complete epimerase deficiencies. Most

FIGURE 57-1. Galactose metabolic pathway. The major catabolic path and several of the minor paths are depicted. Xylulose can be further metabolized. UDP-glucose is the substrate for glycogen synthesis. The recycling of cellular components is suggested by the single arrow from glycoproteins and glycolipids to galactose, which then repeats the catabolic pathway. UDP, uridine diphosphate.

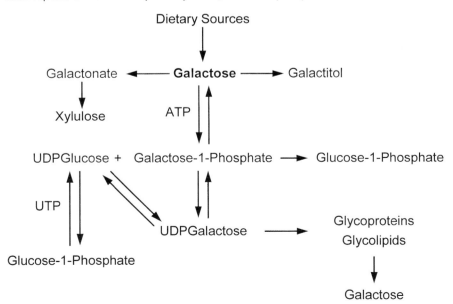

TABLE 57-2. Summary of the Disorders of Galactose Metabolism

	Kinase	Transferase	Epimerase
Inheritance	Autosomal recessive	Autosomal recessive	Autosomal recessive
Frequency	<1:40,000	1:18,000-1:180,000; generally 1:40,000	Severe: very rare peripheral: 1:20–30,000
Acute clinical effects			
Eyes	Cataracts	Cataracts	Unknown
Liver/GI tract	Generally none	Acute hepatotoxicity, vomiting, diarrhea, cirrhosis, ascites	Acute hepatotoxicity syndrome–like transferase defect
Renal	Generally none	Tubular dysfunction	Similar to transferase defect
Other		Cerebral edema, failure to thrive, sepsis, hemolytic anemia	
Major chronic effects	Recurrence of cataracts	Ovarian failure, developmental delays, late neurologic syndrome	Developmental delays
Laboratory findings			
Specific	Galactitol, galactose, kinase deficiency	Galactose-1-phosphate, galactitol, transferase deficiency	UDP-Glu:UDP-gal ratio, epimerase deficiency
General	Galactosuria	Hyperbilirubinemia ALT, AST, prolonged PT/PTT, aminoaciduria, galactosuria	Aminoaciduria, galactosuria
Treatment	Galactose exclusion	Galactose exclusion	Small amounts of galactose required
Prenatal diagnosis	Possible	Possible	Possible

have the so-called peripheral epimerase defect, which appears to be limited to blood cells and has little or no long term consequence. Routine screening may not detect these patients. A diet with a minimal essential amount of galactose has been postulated for treatment.

GENETIC/STRUCTURE/FUNCTION RELATIONSHIPS OF THE TRANSFERASE

Transferase deficiency galactosemia is known worldwide with varying incidence.[1] Overall, 1:40,000 to 1:65,000 whites in the United States have less than 2% of normal transferase activity and would be considered to have the classic form of galactosemia, an autosomal recessive disorder. The transferase is encoded by a single gene with several highly conserved domains.[5] The resultant protein is an 88-kD dimer with bound divalent metal ions. Enzymatic activity is present only in the dimeric state.

The presence of several polymorphisms and low activity mutations adds complexity to the genetics. Before mutational analysis was possible, isoelectric focusing demonstrated that the transferase enzyme had several genetically determined isoforms,[6] some of which were associated with lower activity in vitro. Clinical disease is generally associated only with in vitro activity less than 15% of normal. Variant galactosemia (2 to 10% of normal activity) involving combinations of mutations and polymorphisms is about 10 times more common than classical disease.[1] Individuals with 25% or more activity

have no neonatal disease manifestations. As adults they may have an increased risk of earlier onset of cataracts and earlier age of menopause.[7]

More recently, the DNA sequence mutations responsible for a number of the variant isoforms and phenotypes of transferase galactosemia have been described.[5,8,9] The most common polymorphism is the Duarte allele, an asparagine-to-aspartic acid change at position (N314D),[8] which is found in 4 to 14% of the population.[10] Each Duarte allele is associated with approximately 40 to 60% of the activity of the normal allele. Compound heterozygotes of Duarte and alleles which yield no enzymatic activity may represent 1 : 4,000 of the general population. There may be a need to treat these patients, especially as infants, because the metabolites believed to cause toxicity can accumulate in this population.[11]

A common glutamine-to-arginine mutation (Q188R) that has no in vivo transferase activity has been found in more than 66% of the mutant alleles in whites with classic galactosemia.[5] In African Americans however, the most common mutation is S135L.[9] Homozygotes for S135L have nearly absent transferase activity in their erythrocytes but 8 to 14% of normal activity may remain in hepatic tissues.[1,9] This unique property of the transferase may account for a number of the observations about the improvement in galactose tolerance reported in the older literature as retrospective analysis has shown that a significant number of those earliest recognized patients were African Americans.

TOXICITY

Transferase deficiency has two major disease states with corresponding pathophysiology: (1) an acute (untreated) toxicity that responds to treatment, and (2) a long-term pathology despite the institution of treatment. Acute toxicity results from elevated galactitol and galactose-1-phosphate concentrations, low ATP concentrations from phosphate trapping as galactose-1-phosphate, and possibly disordered NAD/NADH[+] levels as inhibition of other cellular processes occurs when metabolites accumulate. The organ systems most commonly affected in the acute toxic state are the eye, liver, and brain.[1] The pathology in the eye is most clearly related to the activity of aldose reductase, with the trapping of galactitol and osmotic swelling within the lens, resulting in cataract formation. The acute results of deranged galactose metabolism within the liver are hepatic dysfunction, organ enlargement, and cerebral edema. Subacutely, with inability to use the calories from galactose and the hepatic dysfunction, failure to thrive results. Many of the acute, central nervous system (CNS) findings are logically related to alterations in osmolality as the result of galactitol accumulation and altered cerebral blood flow. Alterations in neuronal ATP concentrations has also been postulated.[1] Additionally, the acutely toxic galactosemic infant is at high risk of *Escherichia coli* sepsis, perhaps as a result of altered leukocyte bactericidal function.[12]

Chronic galactosemia manifestations are diet independent. Toxicity may be a result of chronically elevated cellular galactose-1-phosphate concentrations.[4,13] Despite the most rigorous galactose-free diet, galactosemic patients produce measurable quantities of galactitol and galactose-1-phosphate.[13] Isotope dilution studies have proven that normal and galactosemic individuals produce 0.5 to 1 mg of galactose/kg body mass/hr.[14] This endogenous production may be more important than the small amount of free galactose from exogenous sources in the chronic pathology of "treated" galactosemia.

There is also evidence that galactosylation is altered in galactosemic cell lines and in vivo.[15,16] The direct association of the altered galactosylation of proteins with the diet-independent disease characteristics has not yet been proven. Galactitol alone cannot explain the chronic disease since patients with kinase deficiency do not have a predominance of extraocular manifestations.[1] The alternative hypothesis that diet-independent disease manifestations may be the result of intra-uterine toxicity cannot be proven or disproven.

CLINICAL PRESENTATION

Transferase deficiency galactosemia has two presentations: (1) as an acute toxicity syndrome with generally overt manifestations, and (2) as a chronic partially treat-

ment-independent disorder whose course is dependent on the amount of residual activity, sex of patient, and perhaps, the interaction of other gene products (Table 57-2).

The complete "acute toxicity" syndrome is rarely seen today in populations that have rapid, effective newborn screening. The classic presentation is an infant with jaundice, hepatic dysfunction and hepatomegaly, an unconjugated hyperbilirubinemia, vomiting, diarrhea, galactosuria, possible glucosuria, failure to thrive, cerebral edema and/or sepsis.[1] *E. coli* infections in untreated neonatal galactosemic patients are common.[12] Cataracts may be present at birth or develop in early infancy. They may be visible only upon slit-lamp examination of the infant. Some infants will manifest only feeding intolerance and a moderate hyperbilirubinemia during the first weeks of life despite absence of transferase activity. The diagnostic differential, in the absence of cataracts, includes many disorders that result in neonatal hepatic dysfunction, such as hepatitis, biliary atresia, hereditary fructose intolerance, tyrosinemia (α-1-antitrypsin deficiency), and cystic fibrosis among others.

A modified version of acute toxicity occurs when an older patient ingests large quantities of galactose. Those patients may experience abdominal cramping, nausea, bloating and malaise. Mild to moderate elevations in liver function tests have been seen. With repeated exposure to gram quantities of galactose, these patients can develop cataracts as children, adolescents, or even adults.

Some patients will present with psychomotor retardation and possibly cataracts at several years of age. A careful evaluation of the history may find partial avoidance of lactose-containing formula and self-selection of milk-free products.

The chronic disease state includes some non-life-threatening complications. One of the first that may be recognized is altered articulation termed verbal dyspraxia as a result of impaired motor planning of the speech musculature.[17,18] Other late developmental and CNS complications include delayed cognitive development, an increased risk of retardation, possibly with progressive intellectual deficits,[19,20] and in the third to fourth decade, a cerebellar ataxia disorder.[21] Behavioral disorders, short attention spans and psychological problems are common.[22] MRI changes such as mild atrophy and multiple white matter lesions have been reported in a significant fraction of patients examined.[23]

Bone mass is lower in galactosemic children and growth may be less than expected by mean parental centiles.[24] These complications may be diet dependent as the major sources of calcium in the diet are removed with therapy.

Ovarian pathology that presents as hypergonadotrophic hypogonadism is found in at least 85% of all transferase-deficient females. The manifestations range from an absence of pubertal changes to irregular menses to premature ovarian failure. The ovarian dysfunction may be detectable within months of birth if the FSH and LH levels do not fall as in normal infants. As a result of this widespread diet-independent complication, there have been very few pregnancies in galactosemic women reported in the literature.[25]

DIAGNOSIS

Prior to the advent of newborn screening programs for galactosemia, all infants who were diagnosed with one of these disorders were detected on the basis of clinical presentation. This resulted in underdetection and exposed subsequent siblings to preventable morbidity from acute intoxication. Certainly infants with sepsis may not have the underlying diagnosis considered and, with commercial lactose-free formula, other affected infants would escape clinical detection. A few of those infants might be detected later when they were ingesting milk products, but it is only during infancy when milk products and consequently galactose ingestion constitutes such a large part of the caloric intake.

Screening

Newborn screening programs for galactosemia have been in existence since the 1960s. Not all states or industrialized countries currently screen for disorders of galactose metabolism.[26] One of the arguments used to justify not screening is that infants may have life-threatening signs at 3 to 7 days of age, and before the screening test results are available to the practitioner.

There are several tests used for screening for galactosemia: a bacterial metabolite inhibition assay similar to that used for phenylketonuria (PKU), detection of blood galactose or galactose-1-phosphate, qualitative detection of the transferase, and the detection of galactose in the urine as a non-glucose reducing substance. The latter is a very insensitive screen because, for the most part, infants and children with galactosemia who are not receiving galactose will have negative urinary reducing substances. A positive urinary screen requires high circulating galactose levels that will not be present in those fed lactose-free diets or who are not receiving enteral nutrition. Many states use combinations of two screening systems in efforts to detect affected individuals who are not receiving galactose.[26]

The definitive diagnosis for each of the disorders of galactose metabolism is by enzymatic assay which can be performed using washed erythrocytes. As these assays rely on native erythrocytes, transfusion of a young child may delay the diagnosis for up to 120 days until the patient has turned over all the donor cells. Additional information is obtained by performing isoelectric focusing of the transferase enzyme[6] which helps characterize the lower activity phenotypes such as Duarte.

Other tests that will establish the diagnosis include assays for the presence of the sugar alcohol and for elevations of erythrocyte galactose-1-phosphate.[4,13] Even in the child with significant transferase deficiency who has not received any galactose, the excretion of urinary galactitol and the erythrocyte galactose-1-phosphate will be elevated beyond the normal range.[4,13] The source of the galactose is the endogenous production of the sugar and recycling of complex macromolecules with galactose moieties.

Some older children, adolescents, and adults who were not screened as newborns will present later in life with signs or symptoms compatible with galactosemia. Speech delays, especially verbal dyspraxia, in a preschool-age to school-age child, and premature ovarian failure are examples of presenting complaints that should prompt testing for transferase deficiency. In rare cases[1] (personal observation), the history will raise a suspicion. Older children may self-select against lactose-containing products because such foods make them feel bad. A review of infant feeding may find refusal of breast milk or of lactose/galactose-containing formula, "colic," or poor weight gain until a substitute formula was begun.

TREATMENT

Acute toxicity, or untreated galactosemia, is a potentially life-threatening disorder. The first step in treatment is considering galactosemia as part of the differential diagnosis. As soon as that possibility is considered, all galactose-containing substances must be stopped until a definitive assay has been done.[1] A lactose-free, galactose restricted diet is the mainstay of specific therapy.[2] Signs of GI distress such as vomiting and diarrhea may resolve as quickly as the first few feeds of galactose-free formula. Supportive therapies for any other complications must also be initiated. In those infants who present with a septic appearance, antibiotic therapy is imperative. Cerebral edema may require measures to reduce intracranial pressure. However, without removing the source of the majority of the toxic metabolites, the acute symptoms will continue.

For infants, there are adequate nutritional substitutes available as lactose-free/galactose-free formula. The introduction of solid foods presents a separate problem. Many commercially prepared foods have milk solids, milk protein, or lactose as ingredients. In general, substitutes can be found which do not have the potential for containing lactose or galactose. Fruits and vegetables are the second area of concern for parents. Most fruits and vegetables contain some detectable galactose at some stage of commercial use.[2] The amount of galactose ranges up to 40 mg/100 g wet weight for tomato, as an example. Tomato-based products that are the result of removal of water, like sauces, will contain even higher quantities per unit mass. The role of hidden dietary galactose in the form of complex sugars that may be fermentable by the intestinal flora is unproven.[3] Small amounts of ingested galactose in the range of 1 mg/kg/day would add very little free galactose to the body pool (see Toxicity above) and would not be expected to increase the amount of galactitol excreted or the erythrocyte galactose-1-phosphate level. The relative contributions of endogenous production vs. cryptic exogenous galactose remain enigmatic.

Development delays require evaluation and intervention. Verbal dyspraxia responds very well to long-term speech therapy. In non-infants, calcium supplementation may be necessary to help normalize bone density and linear growth. Dietary analysis will help to prevent other deficiencies. A multivitamin taken on a daily basis will help offset the lack of vitamin D from fortified milk. Compliance with nutritional therapy is generally assessed by monitoring erythrocyte galactose-1-phosphate concentrations[1,11,13,18,20] and a review of dietary records. Urinary galactitol excretion may prove equally valuable.

REFERRAL PATTERN

All families with a galactosemic member need to have genetic counseling because the recurrence risk is 25% in future pregnancies. Counseling about the potential for the diet-independent complications is also essential so that the families will help anticipate complications and be acceptive of therapy. Speech therapy at an early age is essential to normal language production. Referral for ovarian dysfunction or failure of pubertal changes may be needed. Cataract regression should be monitored by slit-lamp evaluations, a technique not available in most generalist offices. As most of the laboratory testing described above is performed only at reference laboratories, specimens may need to be shipped to monitor the compliance with dietary interventions. The interpretation of genotype-phenotype correlations is best left to biochemical geneticists who have expertise in this disorder.

REFERENCES

1. Segal S, Berry GT. Disorders of galactose metabolism. In: Scriver CH, Beaudet AL, Sly WS, Valle D, Eds. The Metabolic and Molecular Bases of Inherited Diseases. New York: McGraw-Hill, 1995:967–1000

2. Gross KC, Acosta PB. Fruits and vegetables are a source of galactose: Implications in planning the diets of patients with galactosemia. J Inher Metab Dis 1991;14:253–258

3. Weismann UN, Rosé-Beutler B, Schlüchter R. Leguminosae in the diet: the raffinose-stachyose question. Eur J Pediatr 1995;154(suppl 2):S93–S96

4. Gitzelmann R. Galactose-1-phosphate in the pathophysiology of galactosemia. Eur J Pediatr 1995;154(suppl 2): S45–S49

5. Elsas LJ, Fridovich-Keil JL, Leslie ND. Galactosemia: a molecular approach to the enigma. Int Pediatr 1993;8:101–109

6. Kelley RI, Harris H, Mellman WJ. Characterization of normal and abnormal variants of galactose-1-phosphate uridyltransferase (EC 2.7.7.12) by isoelectric focusing. Hum Genet 1983;63:274–279

7. Elsas LJ, Dembure PP, Langley S et al. A common mutation associated with the Duarte galactosemia allele. Am J Hum Genet 1994;54:1030–1036

8. Cramer DW, Harlow BL, Barbieri RL, Ng WG. Galactose-1-phosphate uridyl transferase activity associated with age at menopause and reproductive history. Fertil Steril 1989; 51:609–615

9. Lai K, Langley SD, Singh RH et al. A prevalent mutation for galactosemia among black Americans. J Pediatr 1996; 128:89–95

10. Mellman WJ, Tedesco TA, Feigl P. Estimation of the gene frequency of the Duarte variant of galactose-1-phosphate uridyl transferase. Ann Hum Genet 1968;32:1–8

11. Gitzelmann R, Bosshard NU. Partial deficiency of galactose-1-phosphate uridyltransferase. Eur J Pediatr 1995;154 (suppl 2): S40–S44

12. Levy HL, Sepe SJ, Shih VE et al. Sepsis due to *Escherichia coli* in neonates with galactosemia. N Engl J Med 1977;297: 823–825

13. Gitzelmann R, Hansen RG, Steinmann B. Biogenesis of galactose a possible mechanism of self-intoxication. In: Hommes F, Van den Berg G, Eds. Normal and pathological development of energy metabolism. London: Academic Press, 1975;25–37

14. Berry GT, Nissim I, Lin Z et al. Endogenous synthesis of galactose in normal men and patients with hereditary galactosemia. Lancet 1995;346:1073–1074

15. Ornstein KS, McGurie EJ, Berry GT et al. Abnormal galactosylation of complex carbohydrates in cultured fibroblasts from patients with galactose-1-phosphate uridyltransferase deficiency. Pediatr Res 1992; 31:508–511

16. Petry K, Greinix HT, Nudelman E et al. Characterization of a novel biochemical abnormality in galactosemia: deficiency of glycolipids containing galactose or N-acetylgalactosamine and accumulation of precursors in brain and lymphocytes. Biochem Med Mol Biol 1991;46:93–104

17. Nelson CD, Waggoner DD, Donnell GN et al. Verbal dyspraxia in treated galactosemia. Pediatrics 1991;88:346–350

18. Waisbren SE, Norman TR, Schnell RR, Levy HL. Speech and language deficits in early-treated children with galactosemia. J Pediatr 1983;102:75–77

19. Waggoner DD, Buist NMR, Donnell GN. Long-term prognosis in galactosemia: Results of a survey of 350 cases. J Inher Metab Dis 1990;13: 802–818

20. Schweitzer S, Shin Y, Jakob C, Brodehl J. Long-term out-

come in 134 patients with galactosaemia. Eur J Pediatr 1993; 152:36–43

21. Lo W, Packman S, Nash S et al. Curious neurological sequelae in galactosemia. Pediatrics 1984;73:309–312

22. Komrower GM, Lee DH. Long term follow-up of galactosemia. Arch Dis Child 1970;45:367–369

23. Nelson MD, Wolff JA, Cross CA et al. Galactosemia: evaluation with MR imaging. Radiology 1992;184:255–261

24. Kaufmann FR, Loro ML, Azen C et al. Effect of hypogonadism and deficient calcium intake on bone density in patients with galactosemia. J Pediatr 1993;123:365–370

25. Gibson JB. Gonadal function in galactosemics and galactose-intoxicated animals. Eur J Pediatr 154 (suppl 2) 1995; S14–S20

26. Committee on Genetics. Newborn Screening Fact Sheets. Pediatrics 1996; 98:473–501

58

LIVER TRANSPLANTATION

KARAN MCBRIDE
ERIC S. MALLER

Liver transplantation has become the accepted method of treatment for end-stage liver failure. The practice of orthotopic liver transplantation began in 1963 and has progressively become a reliable life-saving technique in children over the past 8 to 10 years. A major advance in transplantation success came in 1980 with the introduction of cyclosporine as an effective immunosuppressive medication. In 1995 most centers were reporting 5-year survival of 80% to 90% in children post liver transplant.[1,2] Liver transplantation offers escape from end-stage liver failure in exchange for a life of chronic immunosuppression with its many potential complications. These children are susceptible to all the usual benign childhood infections; however, their ability to combat even minor infections may be compromised by long-term immunosuppression. In addition, they must face the potential complications of organ rejection, opportunistic infections, and early and late postsurgical complications. Management of this patient population requires vigilance and aggressive investigation of problems as they arise. This chapter is intended to outline some of the most common post-transplant problems and an approach to their diagnosis and management.

INDICATIONS FOR TRANSPLANT

The most common indication for liver transplantation in the pediatric age group is biliary atresia with chronic liver failure status post hepatoportoenterostomy (Kasai procedure). The next most common indication is the inherited metabolic disease (e.g., alpha-1-antitrypsin de-

ficiency).[2] Chronic liver disease secondary to chronic active hepatitis with cirrhosis and acute liver failure are also common reasons for liver transplantation in this population.

Acute Liver Failure

Acute liver failure is defined as rapid onset of hepatic synthetic dysfunction in an individual who was previously free of liver disease. Characteristically the dysfunction develops within 6 months from the onset of the illness.[3] The cause of the failure is identified in only 60% to 80% of cases. The most common causes of acute liver failure include viral hepatitis and drug- or toxin-induced hepatic injury. The majority of cases in which there is no serologic evidence of hepatitis A or B will have no identifiable cause (Fig. 58-1).

METHODS OF LIVER TRANSPLANTATION

Two options exist for liver transplantation in children; a full-sized cadaveric transplant from a similar-size donor; a reduced-size graft from a living related adult donor or from an adult cadaveric donor. The transplant procedure involves four main anastomoses between the donor organ and recipient vessels and ducts. These include the portal venous and hepatic arterial anastomoses (usually done end to end and sometimes requiring interposition grafts to more proximal inferior mesenteric venous or suprarenal aortic sites, respectively). The hepatic venous

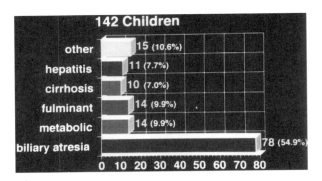

FIGURE 58-1. Indications for liver transplantation in children; total number of children equals 142. (From Cox et al.,[12] with permission.)

outflow is accomplished either as a donor hepatic vein to intact recipient IVC anastomosis for a reduced-size graft or as donor to recipient supra- and infrahepatic IVC anastomoses. The biliary anastomosis in children is usually carried out as a donor bile duct to recipient Roux-en-Y jejunal limb connection or rarely, as in the adult whole liver transplant, as a direct donor to recipient end-to-end bile duct connection[1] (Fig. 58-2). Post-transplant, any of these anastomotic sites may develop complications. Thrombosis of the hepatic artery or portal vein can develop and may manifest only as a rising bilirubin or hepatic transaminase but may be clinically silent otherwise. The bile duct anastomosis, whether a duct-to-duct or duct-to-Roux jejunal limb connection, may develop leaks or strictures, especially if the essential hepatic arterial flow is compromised by a thrombosis. This leakage can result in bile peritonitis or sepsis.

IMMUNOSUPPRESSIVE MEDICATIONS

Post-transplant, all children require immunosuppression (Table 58-1). The mainstay of immunosuppression used for solid organ transplantation is usually cyclosporin A (Cy-A) or tacrolimus (FK506), both potent T-cell function inhibitors. Most patients require adjuvant therapy with prednisone and/or azathioprine. Most programs use either triple drug therapy (Cy-A + prednisone + azathioprine) or double drug therapy (Cy-A + prednisone or FK506 + prednisone).[4] More recently, some programs have used mycophenolate mofetil (MMF) in place of azathioprine as initial therapy. The medications usually begin at high doses post-transplant, especially the prednisone, and are weaned over months if the patient is doing well. The side effects of the medications can be significant and are mostly dose related.

Starting doses of cyclosporine have been within the range of 6 mg/kg/day in two divided doses orally. A new microemulsion form, Neoral (Sandoz Pharmaceuticals), has all but replaced the standard formulation of cyclospo-

rine and often allows decreased dosing to achieve the same trough drug level in blood. Doses of standard cyclosporine or Neoral may vary widely, particularly in young infants due in part to decreased absorption caused by the presence of the Roux-en-Y jejunal limb which excludes a significant segment of bowel from the absorptive path.[5] The ultimate dose is determined from following trough (i.e., predose) blood levels. Cyclosporine absorption is dependent on good bile flow, as it is highly lipid soluble. Any impairment in bile flow (i.e., biliary duct stricture or organ rejection) or alteration in gut dynamics (i.e., diarrhea) can diminish CyA absorption and therefore serum drug levels, particularly with the standard, nonmicroemulsion formulation. Drug levels are checked regularly to ensure therapeutic and avoid toxic levels. The major side effects of CyA are nephrotoxicity, hypertension, gingival hyperplasia, hirsutism, tremor, seizures (>20% of children), and hypomagnesemia secondary to magnesium wasting in the urine. As with all immunosuppressant drugs used over an extended period, there is also a risk of lymphoma with long-term immunosuppression.[6]

Tacrolimus (FK506), a macrolide lactone, is another highly potent T-cell inhibitor used for both primary antirejection therapy and as rescue therapy for chronic rejection. It appears to inhibit both the proliferation and generation of cytotoxic T lymphocytes and also inhibits T-cell dependent antibody responses. FK506 is at least 100 times more potent than cyclosporine (on a per weight basis) at inhibiting in vitro proliferation of mixed lymphocyte cultures, and 10 times more potent for prolongation of allograft survival in animal models.[6] The side effects are similar to those of CyA: nephrotoxicity, hypertension, impaired glucose metabolism, and neurotoxicity manifesting as tremor, headache, seizures, and dizziness.[7]

Prednisone (orally) or methylprednisone (IV) is given in a widely varying dose, depending on the time out from transplant or on the time proximity to an acute episode of rejection. Average doses upon hospital discharge range from 0.3 mg/kg/day up to 1.0 mg/kg/day. Adult or large pediatric patients usually are prescribed 20 g/day PO. The side effects of steroids are well known and include hypertension, weight gain, fluid retention, glucose intolerance, and aseptic necrosis of bones (i.e., femoral heads or vertebral bodies). Decreased bone density and chronic growth failure are problems of particular concern in the pediatric population.

Azathioprine is an antimetabolite which inhibits cell division. It is usually given in a dose of 1 to 2 mg/kg/day as a single dose. The major side effect is bone marrow suppression which is assessed by monitoring peripheral blood counts.

POSTOPERATIVE MANAGEMENT

Owing to the significant immunosuppression, the post-transplant patient is susceptible to opportunistic infections and therefore will receive prophylactic antimicro-

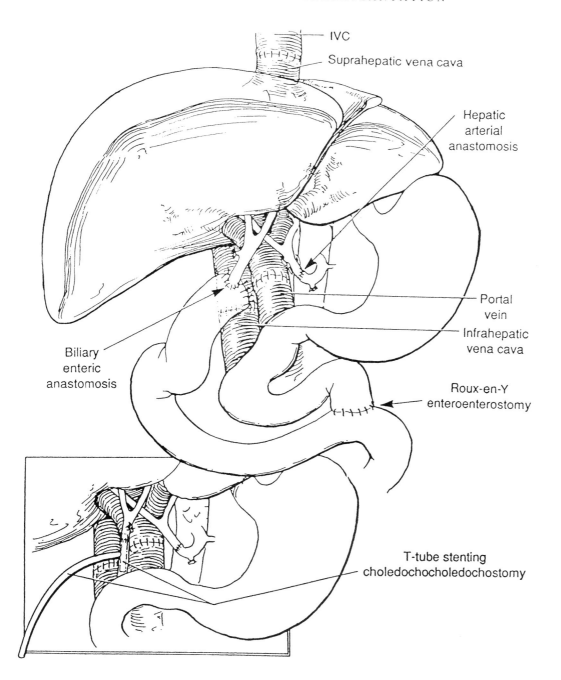

IVC
Suprahepatic vena cava
Hepatic arterial anastomosis
Portal vein
Infrahepatic vena cava
Biliary enteric anastomosis
Roux-en-Y enteroenterostomy
T-tube stenting choledochocholedochostomy

FIGURE 58-2. Anastomoses in liver transplantation. (From Mallen, Hoffman,[1] with permission.)

bial agents. Because *Pneumocystis carinii* pneumonia is a major threat, especially during the first year post-transplant, when levels of immunosuppression are at the highest, these patients are maintained on trimethoprim-sulfamethoxazole at one-half therapeutic doses, dosed either daily or three times per week.[4]

Cytomegalovirus (CMV) infection can also be devastating to the post-transplant patient especially in the case of a CMV-negative recipient of a liver from a CMV-positive donor, which is often the scenario when a small CMV-negative infant receives a portion of a CMV-positive adult donor liver. The highest incidence of primary infection occurs during the first 1 to 6 months post-transplant; therefore, CMV prophylaxis with either high-dose oral acyclovir or daily intravenous gancyclovir (in the CMV-negative recipient of a CMV-positive donor liver, at a dose of 6 mg/kg/day) is used for usually 120 days postoperatively.[8]

TABLE 58-1. Immunosuppressive Medications Used in Liver Transplantation

Medication	Activity	Usual Dose	Side Effects
Cyclosporin A	T-cell inhibitor by blocking cytokine production	6 mg/kg/day divided bid orally, titrated by serum levels	Nephrotoxicity, hypertension, gingival hyperplasia, hirsutism, glucose intolerance
Tacrolimus (FK506)	T-cell inhibitor by blocking cytokine production	0.05–0.15 mg/kg/dose bid titrated by serum levels	
Prednisone	Reversibly blocks T cells and antigen-presenting cells	0.3–1.0 mg/kg/day	Hypertension, weight gain, glucose intolerance
Azathioprine	Inhibits purine synthesis and therefore cell division	1–2 mg/kg/day	Myelosuppression, pancreatitis
Mycophenolate mofetil	Inhibits formation of guanine and blocks T-cell proliferation	600 mg/m^2/day optimal dosing not established in children	Leukopenia, esophagitis, gastritis

Post-transplant children should receive all the usual childhood immunizations except live virus vaccines. They should not receive the live oral polio vaccine (OPV) or the measles, mumps, and rubella (MMR) vaccine post-transplant. They also should not be given the new varicella vaccine. They may be given the killed-virus vaccines, such as diphtheria, pertussis, and tetanus (DPT), the polysaccharide vaccines such as *Haemophilus influenzae* (Hib), Pneumovax and influenza vaccine.[1] Post-transplant patients may also receive inactivated polio vaccine (IPV), as well as the hepatitis B vaccine.

POST-TRANSPLANT COMPLICATIONS

Hypertension

Hypertension is present in 60% to 85% of patients post-transplant, with the common factor the use of CyA or tacrolimus and steroids. Studies reveal that the severity of the hypertension is generally CyA and steroid dependent. The hypertensive effect of CyA appears to be multifactorial and includes afferent vasoconstriction (resulting in a prerenal-like effect on the nephron with subsequent increased reabsorption of sodium chloride and extracellular fluid), magnesium wasting, and local effects of the drug on the endothelium. Adrenergic tone is usually low or normal in post-transplant patients and is not a likely contributor. The hypertension secondary to CyA is very difficult to treat with antihypertensive therapy and the reduction of steroid and CyA doses to the lowest possible level without provoking rejection remains the most effective therapy. However, given the need for optimal immunosuppression, the first line of medical therapy is the use of angiotensin-converting enzyme (ACE) inhibitors (e.g., enalapril) or calcium channel blocking agents (nifedipine) alone or with a loop diuretic such as furosemide. Beta-blockers constitute second-line therapy.[9]

Renal Insufficiency

Renal insufficiency (as measured by decreased glomerular filtration rate or creatinine clearance) is also a common occurrence. It is already known that intrinsic glomerular abnormalities occur commonly in association with liver cirrhosis regardless of the etiology of the liver disease. It is therefore important to recognize that some degree of decreased renal function may exist prior to transplantation in these patients, including that associated with the patient's previous disorder leading to the transplant, such as nephropathy associated with Wilson's disease, alpha-1-antitrypsin deficiency, tyrosinemia, congenital hepatic fibrosis with polycystic renal disease and hepatitis B, among others. Whether this affects the further development of renal insufficiency post-transplant has not been established. Post-transplant renal insufficiency may be acute or chronic depending on the onset. The incidence of acute renal insufficiency (ARI) post-transplant is 20% to 73% with acute tubular necrosis involved in one-half of cases (e.g., secondary to sepsis, volume depletion, drugs). Cyclosporine or FK506 toxicity is the second most common cause of ARI. The mechanism of injury associated with these medications appears to be intense renal vascular constriction that decreases effective renal plasma flow and therefore glomerular filtration rate. Dose adjustments in drug-related acute renal insufficiency result in recovery and improvement in most cases.[9]

Chronic Nephropathy

Chronic nephropathy is also observed post transplant and is linked to more permanent cyclosporine toxicity. In chronic nephropathy due to cyclosporine use, renal arteriolar changes are observed and are associated with interstitial fibrosis and tubular atrophy. This damage is irreversible even with the withdrawal of cyclosporine. The greatest decline in renal function appears to occur during the first 18 months post-transplant, however GFR appears to stabilize secondary to glomerular hypertrophy despite ongoing chronic damage.[9] Long-term data regarding chronic renal toxicity of tacrolimus are not yet as extensive, particularly in children.

Infections

Infectious complications are the leading cause of early and late mortality in transplanted patients, with the highest risk occurring during the first 6 months after transplant. Chronic immunosuppression predisposes transplanted children to numerous infectious complications. In general the onset and types of infections follow patterns that relate to the amount and type of immunosuppression being used and the time since the transplant procedure (Fig. 58-3). Decreased T-cell function contributes to primary infection or reactivation of latent infections by intracellular pathogens, that is, viruses of the herpes family (CMV, EBV, herpes simplex, and varicella zoster), also *Listeria*, fungi, *Toxoplasma*, *Pneumocystis carinii* [PCP] and hepatitis viruses B and C[8] (Fig. 58-3).

PNEUMOCYSTIS CARINII

PCP can occur at any time but is most common in months 2 to 6 post-transplant.[1] It usually presents as shortness of breath and cough with dyspnea out of pro-portion to radiographic findings. If this pathogen is suspected, urgent bronchoscopy for bronchioalveolar lavage is indicated in order to examine silver stained washings for the organism. Urgent treatment with parenteral trimethoprim-sulfamethoxazole or pentamidine is indicated when the organism is found or strongly suspected, even with negative lung washings.

CMV

CMV infection occurs post-transplant either as a primary infection in the host from a CMV-positive donor organ, as reactivation of latent infection as a consequence of immunosuppression, or as superinfection of an already seropositive host with a different strain of CMV that had infected the donor organ. Azathioprine and OKT3 have the highest risk for reactivating CMV disease. CMV infections may present with fevers, malaise, and myalgias that present as a flu-like syndrome. In 30% of febrile patients with CMV infections, pulmonary symptoms will develop that may progress to acute respiratory distress syndrome (ARDS).[10] The patient may also develop ulcerations of the GI mucosa and develop GI bleeding, sometimes massive. Therapy in these cases includes decreasing the patients' immunosuppression to allow their immune system to combat the viral infection. Intravenous gancyclovir is begun if CMV is strongly suspected

FIGURE 58-3. Timetable for infection in the transplant patient. (From Maller, Hoffman,[1] with permission.)

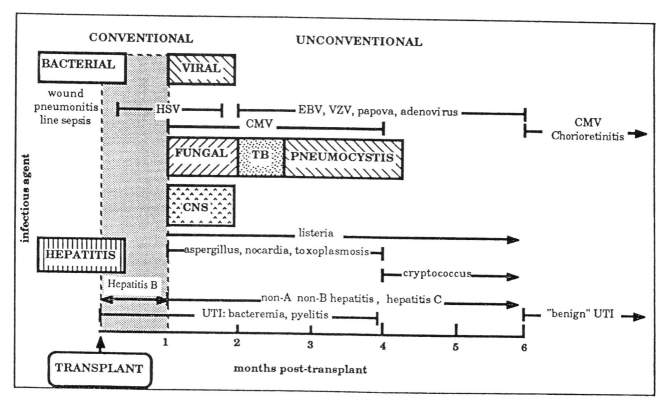

or is isolated. Isolation of the virus is most often by detection of the antigen in urine, stool, or blood (buffy coat), or tissue immunoperoxidase staining with confirming by isolation of the virus by viral culture.[11]

HERPES SIMPLEX VIRUS

Herpes simplex virus (HSV) presenting as oral or genital lesions and confirmed by Tzanck cell preparation should be treated with oral acyclovir. If the lesions are extensive or the patient has systemic symptoms, the patient may require intravenous acyclovir treatment (750 to 1,500 mg/m²/day divided TID) with a possible reduction or temporary cessation of immunosuppression.

VARICELLA

Varicella infection in transplanted patients places them at risk for disseminated disease and requires that they receive intravenous acyclovir therapy (500 mg/m²/day divided TID). Patients who have been exposed to varicella should receive varicella-zoster immunoglobulin (VZIG) intramuscularly within 72 hours of exposure.

EBV

Epstein-Barr virus seropositivity has been linked to post-transplant lymphoproliferative disease (LPD) with an incidence as high as 20% in some series. This may present with tonsillar hypertrophy and upper airway obstruction (from enlargement of Waldeyer's ring), GI bleeding or obstruction secondary to abdominal lymphoid tissue enlargement, splenomegaly, or peripheral lymph node enlargement. Therapy includes decreasing or even temporarily stopping the patient's immunosuppressive therapy.[1] Intravenous acyclovir is usually begun despite lack of definitive evidence of its in vivo efficacy in this setting. Cytoreductive chemotherapy may be used in selected cases in which tissue analysis demonstrates monoclonality of the lymphoid proliferative tissue and malignant changes on histology.

GASTROINTESTINAL

Transplanted patients may also develop a variety of GI complications that can be secondary to infection, immunosuppressive medications, or post-surgical complications. Intestinal obstruction from post-surgical adhesions or from intraintestinal lymphatic hypertrophy secondary to lymphoproliferative disease (LPD) may occur. Often enlarged lymph nodes may provide leading points for intussusception or cause frank intraluminal obstruction. Perforation and GI bleeding may occur secondary to necrotic lymph nodes in LPD, gastroduodenal ulcers, or even small bowel ulcerations due to CMV infection. Peritonitis may occur secondary to any of the aforementioned problems or because of a bile leak caused by an anastomotic breakdown or bile duct ischemia after he-

patic artery thrombosis with perforation. Post-transplant patients may also develop pancreatitis as a complication of taking azathioprine.

NEUROLOGIC

Neurologic symptoms are relatively common post-transplant and are predominantly either secondary to side effects of the immunosuppressive medications or due to CNS infection. Symptoms of tremor, headache, dizziness, or seizures may indicate high levels of CyA or FK506 or may be the only signs of a bacterial or fungal CNS infection. Steroid therapy in these patients may mask the usual clinical signs of meningismus and thus this finding may prove to be unreliable for assessment for meningitis. Complete neurologic evaluation, computed tomographic (CT) scan of the head, and lumbar puncture with cerebrospinal fluid (CSF) sent for bacterial and fungal stains, culture, and rapid antigen assay are indicated when the patient has the onset of new neurologic signs or symptoms not otherwise explained by drug effects.

CLINICAL PRESENTATION/DIAGNOSIS

Assessment of the post-transplant patient is challenging because many of the classic signs of a particular pathologic process (i.e., meningismus in CNS infection or rebound tenderness in an intra-abdominal process) may be absent due to the patient's immunosuppression. Therefore, all new signs and symptoms, regardless of how apparently benign, must be considered for investigation and involvement of the graft assessed by measuring the patient's liver function tests.

Fever is one of the most common reasons for a pediatric liver transplant patient to present for evaluation. A fever could represent a spectrum of disease which extends from a simple viral infection to acute organ rejection or hepatic artery thrombosis. Therefore, if the patient does not have an obviously toxic appearance and is hemodynamically stable, the most important step in the initial evaluation will be to determine the involvement of the graft by monitoring serum aminotransferases and to obtain a blood culture. If the aminotransferases are at their baseline, there is unlikely to be a graft-threatening process; the continuation of an investigation of an "immunosuppressed patient with a fever" can be instituted (i.e., urine culture, urinalysis, complete blood cell count with differential). If the aminotransferases are elevated, then plans for transfer to a transplant center need to be initiated (Table 58-2).

In the transplant patient with elevated aminotransferases and a fever, an ultrasound examination with Doppler flow study is necessary to rule out thrombosis of the hepatic artery to the graft. Arterial thrombosis can

TABLE 58-2. Approach to the Management of the Febrile Liver Transplant Patient

Clinical Finding	Pathogen	Evaluation	Treatment
Initial febrile episode without source	Gram-bacilli *Staphylococcus*, *Streptococcus*	Bacterial/fungal cultures of blood wounds, drains, T-tube urine, and sputum	Antibiotics (cefuroxime plus piperacillin); avoid aminoglycosides if possible
Intra-abdominal infection: cholangitis, peritonitis, or abscess	Gram-bacilli *Staphylococcus*, *Streptococcus* anaerobes	Bacterial/fungal cultures of blood, wounds, drains, and T tube	Antibiotics, surgical drainage
Wound infection	Gram-bacilli *Staphylococcus*, *Streptococcus*	Bacterial/fungal cultures of blood, wounds	Antibiotics, wound debridement
Pneumonia	Gram-bacilli *Staphylococcus*, fungus (*Aspergillus*), virus (CMV), *Pneumocystis carinii*	Chest radiographs, bacterial and fungal cultures of blood and sputum, bronchoscopy, or lung biopsy if routine cultures are negative	Antibiotics, amphotericin B if fungal infection diagnosed, trimethoprim-sulfa for *P. carinii*, gancyclovir for CMV
Oral mucositis	Herpes simplex virus, fungus (*Candida*)	Viral/fungal cultures	Acyclovir for herpes, oral Nystatin or clotrimazole for *Candida*
Persistent fever, no identifiable source	Fungus (*Candida*), virus (CMV), lymphoproliferative disease	Fungal/viral cultures of blood, urine, oral cavity; fungal cultures of wound and drains	Empiric amphotericin B if fungus is isolated from three or more separate sites
Liver graft dysfunction	Virus (CMV), rejection	Liver biopsy, culture	Gancyclovir for CMV

(Adapted from Colonna et al.,[13] with permission.)

lead to bile duct anastomotic breakdown in the early post-transplant period with subsequent bile leakage and even loss of the graft if the thrombus is extensive. The ultrasound examination will also indicate whether there is any portal venous thrombosis or any biliary dilation showing obstruction of the bile ducts. Both would require intervention; however, they would not imminently threaten the graft as much as arterial thrombosis would. If the ultrasound is normal and there is no obvious source for the fever and elevated liver function tests (LFTs), a liver biopsy would be necessary to rule out rejection or viral hepatitis.

If the transplant patient appears hemodynamically unstable, the patient needs to be stabilized in the usual fashion with aggressive attention to the key parameters: airway, breathing, and circulation. In the process of assessing the patient, blood cultures need to be drawn immediately (if possible) and empirical coverage for infection started as soon as possible with intravenous antibiotics, since the immunosuppression of the transplant patient may predispose to life-threatening sepsis. In pediatric patients, the administration of stress-dose steroids is advocated only in the critical setting or with evidence of cardiovascular compromise.

If the patient presents with cough, tachypnea, or dyspnea the essential initial evaluation would include meticulous physical examination, pulse oximetry monitoring and chest radiography. If the patient is hypoxic with mild or no changes on chest radiography, viral, fungal, or PCP infection becomes highly suspect. Again, the initial workup would include blood culture for bacteria, fungus, and blood for CMV antigen detection (buffy coat). Urine can be sent for rapid CMV assay and CMV culture. In all cases of evaluating the sick transplanted patient, a set of LFTs and a complete blood count (CBC) with differential should be included in the initial laboratory studies. A prothrombin time (PT) and partial thromboplastin time (PTT) with or without a screen for disseminated intravascular coagulation (DIC) may be helpful in assessing the degree of hepatic dysfunction and differentiating that from the effects on the graft of sepsis.

A transplant patient presenting with vomiting or severe abdominal complaints may have a broad spectrum of pathology ranging from a viral illness to intestinal obstruction, or even a visceral perforation masked by steroid treatment. Supine and upright radiographs of the abdomen are recommended in order to rule out evidence of obstruction (dilated loops with air-fluid levels), perforation (free air) or ileus (possible peritonitis). If patients have no evidence of serious abdominal pathology (i.e., benign examination, normal LFTs, amylase, lipase, and abdominal radiographs) but show evidence of a gastroenteritis with persistent vomiting and diarrhea, they may require hospital admission for intravenous administration of their immunosuppressive medications, since they may not be able to maintain therapeutic levels of CyA or tacrolimus in the presence of vomiting and diarrhea.

If the patient presents with evidence of gastrointestinal bleeding (hematemesis, coffee-ground emesis, melena, or hematochezia), he or she should be managed as would any other patient with bleeding from the gastrointestinal tract. This includes large-bore IV access with fluid resuscitation, nasogastric tube placement with lavage, type, and cross-match for red blood cells (RBCs), laboratory evaluation of hemoglobin and coagulation status, and frequent monitoring of vital signs. In addition, cultures of body fluids and GI tract biopsies, if obtained as part of diagnostic endoscopy, for CMV should be considered. The patient will require hospital admission and eventual transfer to a transplant center.

LABORATORY EVALUATION

As previously outlined all transplant patients presenting for evaluation of a complaint (e.g., fever, upper respiratory infection, vomiting/diarrhea or abdominal pain) should have LFTs drawn to evaluate the involvement of the graft in the present process. The remainder of the necessary evaluation, including radiographic investigation and ultrasound exam of the graft may be indicated in relation to the patient's symptoms and signs on examination, once the results of the initial hemogram and aminotransferases are known.

REFERRAL PATTERNS

The encounter with the ill liver transplant recipient may provoke anxiety for the physician unfamiliar with this patient population. As a general principle, unless the patient's presentation is clearly minor, the transplant center should be contacted at the time of evaluation as a source of information and assistance. Any critically ill patient should be treated with the same life-saving interventions that a nontransplanted patient would re-

ceive. The well-being of the patient will always take precedence over that of the allograft.

REFERENCES

1. Maller E, Hoffman M. Transplantation emergencies. In: Fleisher G, Ludwig S, Eds. Texbook of Pediatric Emergency Medicine. Baltimore: Williams & Wilkins, 1993:1417–1427
2. Revell SP, Friend PJ, Noble-Jamieson G et al. Liver transplantation in children. Transplantation Reviews 1992;6: 1–9
3. Lake JR. Changing indication for liver transplantation. Gastroenterol Clin North Am 1993;22:213–229
4. Zetterman R, McCahland T. Long-term followup of the orthotopic liver transplant patient. Semin Liver Dis 1995;15: 173–180
5. Whitington PF, Edmond JC, Whitington SH et al. Small-bowel length and the dose of Cyclosporine in children after liver transplantation. N Engl J Med 1990;322:733–738
6. Bumgardener GL, Roberts JP. New immunosuppressive agents. Gastroenterol Clin North Am 1993;22:213–229
7. Klintman G. A review of FK506. Transplant Rev 1994;8: 53–63
8. Dominquez EA. Long-term infectious complications of liver transplantation. Semin Liver Dis 1995;15:133–138
9. Monsour HP, Wood RP, Dyer CH et al. Renal insufficiency and hypertension as long-term complications in liver transplantation. Semin Liver Dis 1995;15:123–132
10. Singh N, Dummer S, Kusne S et al. Infections with CMV and other herpesviruses in 121 liver transplant recipients. J Infect Dis 1988;158:124–131
11. Rubin RH. Infectious disease problems. In: Maddrey WC, Ed. Transplantation of the Liver. New York: Elsevier, 1988: 279
12. Cox KL, Lawrence-Mujasaki LS, Garcia-Kennedy R, et al. An increased incidence of Epstein-Barr virus (EBV) infection and lymphoproliferative disorder (LPD) in young children on FK506 after liver transplantation. Transplantation 1995;59:524
13. Colonna J, Winston D, Bull J et al. Infectious complications in liver transplantation. Arch Surg 1988;123:360

59

PANCREATITIS

JANE M. GOULD
KURT A. BROWN

Pancreatitis is defined as inflammation of the pancreas resulting in acinar cell injury caused by the destructive effects of pancreatic enzymes. It is a relatively infrequent illness in pediatrics, affecting males and females equally and involving all ages. The etiology of pancreatitis in pediatrics is diverse in nature, with an equally unpredictable clinical course and prognosis. The diagnosis requires a high index of suspicion and should be considered in all children that present with abdominal pain and elevation of pancreatic enzymes. The disease is classified into acute and chronic forms or single and recurring episodes, respectively.

PATHOPHYSIOLOGY

Four basic alterations occur in the pancreas during episodes of pancreatitis regardless of whether the illness is acute or chronic: (1) proteolytic destruction of pancreatic tissue; (2) necroses of blood vessels with subsequent hemorrhage; (3) necroses of fat by lipolytic enzymes; and (4) associated inflammatory reaction.[1] These derangements occur to varying degrees from mild disease causing peripancreatic fat necrosis and interstitial edema to the more severe form that produces peri- and intrapancreatic fat necroses, parenchymal necrosis, and hemorrhage.[2] Pancreatic involvement may be localized or diffuse and may produce impairment of both the exocrine and endocrine functions of the gland. Many investigators believe that trypsin plays a key role in the pathogenesis of pancreatitis. Trypsin activates most proenzymes that

take part in the process of autodigestion. Trypsin also converts prekallikrein to kallikrein which directly activates the kinin system and indirectly causes abnormalities in clotting and the complement system. These substances contribute to local inflammation, thrombosis, hemorrhage, and tissue damage seen in the pancreas.[1]

ACUTE PANCREATITIS

Four major predisposing factors for acute pancreatitis were described by Durie[2]: (1) mechanical/structural causes; (2) metabolic/toxic; (3) systemic diseases; and (4) idiopathic. The mechanical or structural etiologies that cause pancreatitis include obstruction of the common bile duct promoting bile reflux into the pancreatic duct causing local inflammation (gallstones, biliary sludge, or strictures), outflow obstruction caused by sphincter of Oddi dysfunction, congenital anomalies of the pancreas and/or biliary tree (pancreas divisum, choledochal cyst, annular pancreas), and pancreatic tumors. It is estimated that obstruction from congenital or acquired anomalies accounts for approximately 10% of all cases.[3] Reflux of duodenal contents initiated by passage of a stone, parasites (ascaris), Crohn's disease of the duodenum, or as a complication of endoscopic retrograde cholangiopancreatography (ERCP) can cause pancreatitis by irritation from intestinal enterokinase and active pancreatic proteases that activate proenzymes within the pancreas. Blunt or penetrating abdominal trauma is believed to cause acute pancreatitis secondary to disruption of the pancreatic ducts, impairment of the vascular supply, and compression injury to the pancreas; 10% to 15% of all childhood cases are believed to be caused by trauma.[3]

Second, the metabolic and toxic causes include the hyperlipidemias (especially types I, IIa, IV, and V) which can cause both acute and chronic disease although the exact mechanism is unknown.[2,3] Patients with acute pancreatitis secondary to hyperlipidemia often have normal serum amylase and lipase levels.[4] Cystic fibrosis promotes viscous secretions within the pancreatic ducts causing protein precipitation and pancreatic duct obstruction. Approximately 15% of cystic fibrosis patients are known to retain sufficient pancreatic function for digestion; however, they are susceptible to recurrent attacks of acute pancreatitis.[5] Malnutrition can lead to atrophied acini with increased levels of pancreatic enzymes. The acinar cells are believed to be susceptible to injury following hormonal stimuli induced by refeeding; thus, aggressive refeeding can induce acute pancreatitis. This phenomenon has been seen in patients with anorexia nervosa.[6]

Many drugs and toxins have a direct or indirect effect on the pancreas[2,7] (Table 59-1). Acute pancreatitis can occur following renal transplantation. Hypothermia has

TABLE 59-1. Drugs and Toxin-Induced Pancreatitis

Therapeutic agents

Definite cause-and-effect relationship
   Chlorthiazides
   Estrogen
   Furosemide
   L-Asparaginase
   6-Mercaptopurine
   Sulfonamides
   Tetracyclines
   Valproate

Possible cause-and-effect relationship
   Azathioprine
   Corticosteroids
   Methyldopa
   Metronidazole
   Nonsteroidal anti-inflammatory drugs
   Nitrofurantoin
   Pentamidine

Nontherapeutic agents (poisons, drugs of abuse, or overdoses)
   Acetaminophen overdose
   Amphetamines
   Ethyl alcohol
   Heroin
   Iatrogenic hypercalcemia
   Methyl alcohol
   Organophosphate insecticides

(Modified from Miller et al,[11] with permission)

TABLE 59-2. Etiology of Acute Pancreatitis

Etiology	Percentage
Idiopathic	25
Multisystem disease	35
Reye's syndrome	
Sepsis/shock	
Hemolytic uremic syndrome	
Viral infection	
Systemic lupus erythematosus	
Traumatic	15
Structural	10
Biliary (cyst, stone, stricture)	
Pancreas divisum	
Metabolic	10
Hyperlipidemia (I, IIa, IV)	
Cystic fibrosis	
Hypercalcemia (TPN induced)	
Drugs	3
Familial	2

(Modified from Weizman and Durie,[3] with permission.)

been seen in adults as a cause of acute pancreatitis but is not commonly seen in the pediatric population. Diabetes mellitus as a cause of acute pancreatitis has been reported in patients with severe diabetic ketoacidosis.[8]

Third, many systemic diseases are associated with acute pancreatitis. Infectious disorders causing acute pancreatitis include mumps (70% of patients with mumps parotitis have elevated amylase and lipase levels, but pancreatitis rarely occurs)[9]; coxsackievirus B; Epstein-Barr virus; hepatitis A and B (necropsy studies in fatal hepatitis contain evidence of acute pancreatitis in 10% to 40% of cases and hyperamylasemia is found in 30% of patients with nonfatal hepatitis[10]); congenital rubella, echovirus, rubeola, influenza A and B, varicella, and human immunodeficiency virus (HIV) (pancreatitis has been reported to develop in 17% of pediatric patients with acquired immunodeficiency syndrome [AIDS], and this may be related to exposure to pentamidine isethionate)[11] (Table 59-2). Severe hemorrhagic pancreatitis is a frequent complication of Reye's syndrome, which is closely associated with influenza B and varicella infections. Other more unusual infectious causes include ascaris lumbricoides secondary to worms invading the ampulla of Vater, *Mycoplasma*, leptospirosis, *Salmonella typhi* (there have been several cases of pancreatitis following typhoid fever), and the verocytotoxin producing *Escherichia coli* O157, the etiologic agent of hemolytic uremic syndrome (HUS).[3] Acute pancreatitis has been reported to occur in association with collagen vascular diseases (e.g., systemic lupus erythematosis [SLE], rheumatoid arthritis, polyarteritis nodosa, and Behçet's syndrome), as well as inflammatory bowel disease. However, these patients are commonly taking medications known to cause pancreatitis, which makes establishing the true cause for the pancreatitis difficult. In addition, any situation that causes shock could potentially cause pancreatitis because of decreased blood flow with resultant hypoxia.[3]

Lastly, up to 25% of patients with acute pancreatitis may have no known precipitating factor. Idiopathic acute pancreatitis is a diagnosis of exclusion. Unfortunately, recurring attacks are a consistent finding in these patients.[3]

CHRONIC PANCREATITIS

Chronic pancreatitis is defined clinically as recurring or persisting abdominal pain with the development of pancreatic exocrine or endocrine insufficiency. As in acute pancreatitis, the mechanisms of disease induction are not fully understood. There are two major morphologic forms of chronic pancreatitis: calcific and obstructive. The obstructive form is more rare in childhood and is secondary to obstruction of the main pancreatic duct or one of its branches by fibrosis, tumor, or a congenital anomaly. Histologically, the pancreatic parenchyma is characterized by either diffuse or focal infiltration and replacement by fibrous tissue. The etiologies include trauma, ductal strictures, compression by pseudocyst formation, congenital anomalies, choledochal cysts, sphincter of Oddi dysfunction, renal disease, sclerosing cholangitis, and idiopathic fibrosing pancreatitis.

Calcific pancreatitis is the most common form of chronic pancreatitis in adults but is rare in childhood. The histology is generally patchy. Duct lesions are often severe and contain protein plugs that evolve over several years with eventual calcification. The pathophysiology of these protein plugs involves the reduction of two pancreatic proteins (pancreatic stone protein [PSP] and pancreatic thread protein [PTP]) with calcium deposits. The etiology of calcific chronic pancreatitis includes juvenile tropical pancreatitis; hereditary pancreatitis; hypercalcemia; hypertriglyceridemia; and cystic fibrosis (both the familial and idiopathic forms). Hereditary pancreatitis is the most common form of chronic calcific pancreatitis in childhood, characterized by autosomal dominant inheritance with variable penetrance. The pathology may involve the precipitation of pancreatic proteins: PSP and PTP within ducts or a primary defect of ductal fluid secretion. The pancreas ultimately becomes a shrunken, fibrotic gland with extensive acinar atrophy containing small proteinaceous plugs and calculi within the ducts. The islet cells remain normal.

Juvenile tropical pancreatitis (JTP) has several synonyms, such as nutritional pancreatitis, tropical pancreatitis, Afro-Asian pancreatitis, or fibrocalculous pancreatic diabetes. It is characterized by recurrent abdominal pain, pancreatic calculi, and diabetes. In addition, there may be signs of long-standing malnutrition such as emaciation, bilateral parotid gland enlargement, and nail and skin changes.[12] The cause of this form of pancreatitis is believed to be related to protein malnutrition; its prevalence is almost restricted to latitude 30 degrees north and south of the equator.[12] However, in India and Africa, the prevalence of JTP does not correlate well with the prevalence of kwashiorkor.[13,14] Another theory has linked JTP to cassava ingestion, which contains cyanide glycosides and is high in carbohydrates, which can result in protein plugs because of the inadequate pancreatic secretion.[15,16] The histology is similar to that of other forms of chronic pancreatitis.

CLINICAL PRESENTATION

Most children with acute pancreatitis present with sudden abdominal pain that progresses in severity over a few hours.[3,17,18] In 30% of patients, pain first develops in the epigastric region but other sites of pain include right upper quadrant of the abdomen and the periumbilical area.[3] Radiation of the pain to the back has been noted in 8% to 30% of cases.[3,17] Eating has been found to aggravate the pain in most patients.[3] Other frequent symptoms include anorexia, nausea, and persistent vomiting (bilious in 10% of cases).[3]

The most frequent finding on presentation is epigastric tenderness associated with intestinal ileus.[3] One-third of patients present with guarding,[17] which, when present, localizes to the epigastrium or the upper part of the abdomen.[3] Low-grade fever may be present.[3,18] In hemorrhagic pancreatitis, patients may demonstrate the Grey Turner sign, a bluish discoloration of the flanks secondary to blood within fascial planes. Other signs and symptoms include the Cullen sign, a bluish discoloration of the periumbilical area, pleural effusions, ascites, shock, icterus, melena, hematemesis, abdominal mass, and coma.[2] The clinical course for acute pancreatitis is extremely variable.[3]

In chronic pancreatitis, approximately one-half of patients present initially with episodes of acute pancreatitis, the other half present with an insidious, unrelenting form of abdominal pain while a small percentage of patients will have no pain at all.[2] Symptoms usually begin by 10 to 12 years of age. By the age of 20 years, 75% of patients are symptomatic.[2] Females and males are affected equally. Spontaneous resolution of each independent episode occurs over a period of 4 to 8 days; between episodes, patients are well. Recurrences may occur monthly or only twice a year.[20] The diagnosis of chronic pancreatitis should be considered in patients who present with the signs and symptoms of diabetes mellitus, malabsorption, or obstructive jaundice. However, symptoms of nutrient malabsorption do not become clinically apparent until 97% to 98% of the exocrine pancreas is destroyed.[21] Patients with hereditary pancreatitis are more likely to develop steatorrhea than are patients with idiopathic relapsing pancreatitis.[20] In general, the symptoms of abdominal pain abate with the development of the calcifications and destruction of both the exocrine and endocrine functions of the gland.[22]

Accurate mortality data in children do not exist. In adults, the overall mortality rate per attack is approximately 9%.[19] In hemorrhagic and/or necrotic pancreatitis the mortality ranges from 15% to 50%.[19] Most children who experienced a fatal outcome after acute pancreatitis had a multisystem disorder, with Reye's syndrome accounting for most cases.[3]

DIAGNOSIS

The diagnosis of both acute and chronic pancreatitis, regardless of etiology, rests upon a compilation of a careful history, clinical features, supportive laboratory tests, and imaging techniques. A thorough medical history, including a family history, is mandatory in order to determine the etiology. Serum amylase, although not specific for pancreatitis, is the most frequently ordered test.[23] Of note, 33% to 45% of serum amylase is of pancreatic origin, the remainder is produced in the lungs, fallopian tubes, and the salivary glands.[24] Elevated levels can be found in other conditions, such as acute appendicitis, perforated viscus, intestinal obstruction, acute cholecystitis, mesenteric ischemia, cystic fibrosis, diabetic ketoacidosis, and pregnancy.[2,24] In a large proportion of children with both clinical and sonographic evidence of acute pancreatitis, serum amylase level is normal. Amylase has a short half-life; therefore, large quantities must continue to enter the bloodstream or the level will equilibrate quickly.[2] When abnormal, serum amylase levels are elevated within hours of the onset of acute pancreatitis and, in uncomplicated cases, may remain elevated for 3 to 5 days. The degree of elevation does not correlate with clinical severity or with the etiology for the pancreatitis.[25] It has been estimated that up to 40% of cases of acute pancreatitis in children could be missed if the diagnosis relied solely on amylase levels.[3] Hypertriglyceridemia is known to produce false-negative amylase levels. Occasionally, an elevated serum amylase may be caused by renal dysfunction resulting in poor clearance of normal serum amylase or from macroamylasemia which results from the development of a large amylase macromolecule that is unable to be filtered by the kidney. The measurement of isoamylases has superior sensitivity and specificity when studied in adults.[26]

The second most commonly used test is serum lipase. Like amylase, other sources of lipases exist (i.e., saliva, gastric, and breast milk).[2] It is unclear how much these sources contribute. Animal studies have shown that serum lipase is primarily pancreatic in origin.[27] It is still debated whether lipase levels remain elevated longer than amylase levels.[2] A serum lipase level greater than 3 times normal has been associated with better diagnostic accuracy than has serum amylase in differentiating nonpancreatic abdominal pain from acute pancreatitis.[28]

Immunoassay techniques with excellent sensitivity and specificity exist for measuring levels of other proteases, such as trypsin(ogen). Studies have shown that the trypsin(ogen) assay detects pancreatic inflammation with greater sensitivity in children than does serum amylase.[3] Trypsinogen rises earlier in acute pancreatitis than amylase and remains elevated during the first five days.[3] However, the test is labor intensive and expensive. The laboratory indicators of severe disease include hyperglycemia, hypocalcemia, hypoxemia, hypoproteinemia, an elevated blood-urea nitrogen (BUN), leukocytosis, and a decreased hematocrit.

In chronic pancreatitis, amylase, lipase, and protease concentrations may be normal. When long-standing chronic pancreatitis results in pancreatic insufficiency, levels of pancreatic enzymes, such as trypsinogen, lipase, and pancreatic isoamylase, may be decreased. Since pancreatic failure causes deficiencies in fat-soluble vitamins, laboratory analysis may reveal decreased carotene levels, prolonged prothrombin time, decreased vitamin D and E levels, and decreased essential fatty acids. Direct function testing of the pancreas may be necessary if the indirect tests of pancreatic function are normal and the patient is still suspected of having chronic pancreatitis.[21] (See Chapter 78 for further information.)

In addition to laboratory tests, several imaging techniques exist to aid in the diagnosis of acute pancreatitis. Plain films of the abdomen should be obtained in all patients who present with an acute abdomen to exclude other abdominal disasters. Plain film findings that suggest acute pancreatitis include the sentinel loop (caused by distention of a small intestine loop near the pancreas); paralytic ileus, which may involve the entire small intestine; the "cutoff" sign of the colon (which is the absence of colonic gas distal to the transverse colon); and pancreatic calcification, which is diagnostic of chronic pancreatitis. A routine chest film should be obtained to rule out diaphragmatic involvement or pulmonary complications, such as pleural effusions or adult respiratory disease syndrome. Contrast studies of the upper gastrointestinal (GI) tract do not usually help in establishing the diagnosis. One may see the inverted "3" sign or Frostberg sign in the duodenum near the ampulla of Vater also where the middle apex of the "3" represents the origin of the pancreatic duct and the curves of the "3" indicate swelling of the pancreatic head. The "Poppel sign" defines a widening of the duodenal loop with prominence of the duodenal mucosal folds and the sphincter of Oddi. A mass effect on the stomach or midtransverse colon may occur secondary to a pseudocyst.

Abdominal ultrasound, the most commonly used technique, has been found to be the most useful of all radiologic tests.[3,17] It can establish the diagnosis of both acute and chronic pancreatitis, identify the cause of the inflammation (stones or congenital abnormalities), and determine complications (pseudocysts or abscesses). When further anatomic definition is required, a computed tomography (CT) scan should be performed. It is useful in assessing the abdomen after trauma and in evaluating for the complications of pancreatitis (cysts, abscesses, or duct enlargement).

ERCP has been used primarily in adults to evaluate the pancreatobiliary tree for acquired or structural lesions. It is becoming an important modality in pediatrics for both the diagnosis and treatment of the complications of pancreatitis, including drainage of pseudocysts, removal of ductal stones, sphincterotomy, stent placement across strictures, and for anatomic definition prior to surgery.[29,30] The evaluation of recurrent pancreatitis is the most frequent indication for ERCP.[29] The morbidity is a mild self-limiting pancreatitis that occurs in 1% to 3% of cases, with mortality within the range of 0.4% to 1.2%.[29]

TREATMENT

Treatment for acute pancreatitis is primarily supportive, with the goal of relief from symptoms and complications. Whenever an etiology for the pancreatitis exists, treatment should be directed to the etiologic cause. General principles of supportive therapy include removing the precipitating cause, achieving adequate hydration, reducing pancreatic secretions, relieving pain, and correcting the systemic abnormalities. Since shock is the main cause of death in acute pancreatitis, the patient's vital signs, urine output, and central venous pressure should be monitored, corrected, and stabilized. Electrolyte abnormalities, including calcium and magnesium and fluid imbalances, should be closely followed. Most centers recommend that a nasogastric tube be placed to decrease the amount of gastric acid entering the duodenum, which in turn reduces the hormonal stimulation of the pancreas; gastric losses (fluid and electrolytes) should be replaced. The major complications of fluid therapy in cases of severe pancreatitis are pulmonary edema and congestive heart failure. The cause is not always known, but in some cases may be secondary to fluid overload which usually occurs within 3 to 7 days after the onset of the pancreatitis. An estimated 2% to 17% of patients with acute pancreatitis will develop renal failure; therefore, potassium should not be added to intravenous fluids until a stable urine output has been established.[31]

Antacids or H_2-histamine blockers may also help reduce duodenal acid, as well as help prevent stress gastri-

tis. The patient should not be refed until the abdominal pain and ileus have resolved and the serum amylase level has returned to normal.[31] Patients should be started on total parenteral nutrition. The initial diet upon refeeding should only be carbohydrates, as this causes less hormonal stimulation of the pancreas.[31] Fats and proteins are subsequently introduced. Pain control should be achieved with meperidine HCl (Demerol) or nalbuphine (Nubane). Morphine sulfate should be avoided, as it can cause sphincter of Oddi spasm. If the patient has persistent abdominal pain and elevation of the serum amylase for two or more weeks, a pseudocyst should be suspected.[31] An abdominal ultrasound is recommended every 3 to 4 days to monitor for this complication.[2] Inhibitors of pancreatic enzymes, such as aprotinin (Trasylol) and ε-aminocaproic acid (EACA), or suppressors of secretion, such as anticholinergic drugs, glucagon, somatostatin, calcitonin, and tranquilizers, have not consistently shown any benefit.[2,3,31]

Malabsorption secondary to pancreatic exocrine failure and diabetes mellitus need to be managed by oral pancreatic enzymes and insulin replacement, respectively. Nutritional support is essential in order to avoid growth failure; this may require total parenteral nutrition or tube feedings. A high energy diet supplemented with adequate amounts of fat and fat-soluble vitamins is recommended. Some patients will have chronic pain requiring the long-term use of narcotics.

Pseudocyst

A common complication following an episode of acute or chronic pancreatitis is the formation of a pseudocyst. Data show that the prevalence of pseudocysts after an acute attack ranges from 16% to 50%.[32,33] Extrahepatic cysts usually occur after an episode of acute pancreatitis. These cysts are usually postnecrotic, developing within 2 weeks, and do not communicate with the pancreatic duct. By contrast, chronic pancreatic cysts are intrapancreatic, communicate with the pancreatic duct, and may cause stricture of the pancreatic duct.[34,35] Most pseudocysts spontaneously resolve; almost always, those that persist for greater than 6 weeks require surgical intervention. If diseased, the pancreatic duct will also require surgical intervention.[34] Persistent cysts can cause other complications, including rupture, hemorrhage, or infection. Ruptured cysts can cause a severe, often life-threatening, chemical peritonitis. GI bleeding may result if a cyst drains into the duodenum through the pancreatic duct.

REFERRAL PATTERN

A pediatric gastroenterologist should be consulted during episodes of severe acute pancreatitis with complications, for recurrent pancreatitis of unknown etiology, and for all cases of chronic pancreatitis. A surgical or interventional radiology consultation will be necessary in all patients who have developed a persistent pseudocyst for either diagnostic or therapeutic procedures.

REFERENCES

1. Robbins S, Cotran R, Kumar V, Eds. Pathologic Basis of Disease. 3rd Ed, Philadelphia: WB Saunders, 1984:960

2. Durie P. Pancreatitis. In: Walker W, Durie P, Hamilton J et al, Eds. Pediatric Gastrointestinal Disease. Philadelphia: BC Decker, 1991:1209

3. Weizman Z, Durie P. Acute pancreatitis in childhood. J Pediatr 1988;113:24–29

4. Cameron J, Crisler C, Margolis S et al. Acute pancreatitis with hyperlipidemia. Surgery 1971;70:53–61

5. Durie P, Forstner G. Pathophysiology of the exocrine pancreas in cystic fibrosis. J R Soc Med 1989;18:2–10

6. Rampling D. Acute pancreatitis in anorexia nervosa. Med J Aust 1982;2:194–195

7. Mallory A, Kern F. Drug-induced pancreatitis: a critical review. Gastroenterology 1980;78:813–820

8. Schindler AM, Kowlessar M. Prolonged abdominal pain in a diabetic child. Hosp Pract 1988;23(3):134–136

9. Feldstein J, Johnson F, Kallick C et al: Acute hemorrhagic pancreatitis and pseudocyst due to mumps. Ann Surg 1974; 180:85–88

10. Rosenblum J. Pancreatitis. In: Feigin R, Cherry J, Eds. Textbook of Pediatric Infectious Diseases, 2nd Ed. Philadelphia: WB Saunders, 1987:750

11. Miller T, Winter H, Luginbuhi L et al. Pancreatitis in pediatric human immunodeficiency virus infection. J Pediatr 1992; 120:223–227

12. Pitchumoni C. Juvenile tropical pancreatitis. In: Walker W, Durie P, Hamilton J, et al, Eds. Pediatric Gastrointestinal Disease. Philadelphia: BC Decker, 1991:1236

13. Pitchumoni C. "Tropical" or "nutritional pancreatitis"—an update. In: Gyr K, Singer M, Sarles H, Eds. Pancreatitis—Concepts and Classification. Amsterdam: Elsevier Science, 1984:359

14. Pitchumoni C. Special problems in tropical pancreatitis. Clin Gastroenterol 1984;3:941–959

15. Shaper A. Chronic pancreatic disease and protein malnutrition. Lancet 1960;1:1223–1224

16. Nwokolo C, Oli J. Pathogenesis of juvenile tropical pancreatitis syndrome. Lancet 1980;1:456–459

17. Haddock G, Coupar G Youngson G et al. Acute pancreatitis in children: a 15-year review. J Pediatr Surg 1994;29: 719–722

18. Nguyen T, Abramowsky C, Ashenburg C, Rothstein F. Clinicopathologic studies in childhood pancreatitis. Hum Pathol 1988;19:343–349

19. Durr H. Acute pancreatitis. In: Howat H, Sarles H, Eds. The Exocrine Pancreas. London: WB Saunders, 1969:352

20. Perrault J. Hereditary pancreatitis. Gastroenterol Clin North Am 1994;4:743–751

21. Gaskin K, Durie P, Lee L et al. Colipase and lipase secretion in childhood onset pancreatic insufficiency. Gastroenterology 1984;86:1–7

22. Grendell J, Cello J. Chronic pancreatitis. In: Sleisenger M, Fordtran J, Eds. Gastrointestinal Disease, 4th Ed. Philadelphia: WB Saunders, 1989;1842

23. Mossa A. Diagnostic tests and procedures in acute pancreatitis. N Engl J Med 1984;311:639–643

24. Pieper-Bigelow C, Strocchi A, Levitt M. Where does serum amylase come from and where does it go? Gastroenterol Clin North Am 1990;19:793–810

25. Pezzilli R, Billi P, Migliolli M, Gullo L. Serum amylase and lipase concentrations and lipase/amylase ratio in assessment of etiology and severity of acute pancreatitis. Dig Dis Sci 1993;38:1265–1269

26. Steinberg W, Goldstein S, Davis N et al. Diagnostic assays of acute pancreatitis. Ann Intern Med 1985;102:576–580

27. Jacobs R. The origins of canine serum amylases and lipase. Vet Pathol 1989;26:525–527

28. Gumaste V, Roditis N, Mehta D, Dave P. Serum lipase levels in nonpancreatic abdominal pain versus acute pancreatitis. Am J Gastroenterol 1993;88:2051–2055

29. Allendorf M, Werlin S, Geenen J et al. Endoscopic retrograde cholangiopancreatography in children. J Pediatr 1987; 110:206–211

30. Kozarek R, Christie D, Barclay G. Endoscopic therapy of pancreatitis in the pediatric population. Gastrointest Endosc 1993;39:665–669

31. Cox K. Pancreatic diseases. In: Burg F, Ingelfinger J, Wald E, Eds. Current Pediatric Therapy. Vol 14. Philadelphia: WB Saunders, 1993;227

32. O'Malley V, Cannon J, Postier J. Pancreatic pseudocysts: cause, therapy, and results. Am J Surg 1985;150:680–682

33. Siegelman S. CT of fluid collections associated with pancreatitis. AJR 1980;134:1121–1132

34. Grace P, Williamson R. Modern management of pancreatic pseudocysts. Br J Surg 1993;80:573–581

35. D'Egidio A, Schein M. Pancreatic pseudocysts: a proposed classification and its management implication. Br J Surg 1992;78:981–984

60

TYROSINEMIA

BARBARA A. HABER

Tyrosinemia type I, also known as hepatorenal tyrosinemia, is an inborn error of metabolism that affects the liver, kidney, and nervous system.[1] Until recently, most patients died by early childhood. However, liver and renal transplantation have improved the outcome significantly.[2,3]

PATHOPHYSIOLOGY

Hereditary tyrosinemia type I is an autosomal recessive disorder characterized by progressive hepatocellular necrosis and cirrhosis, with varying degrees of renal and neurologic involvement. It is a result of a deficiency of fumarylacetoacetate hydrolase (FAH), the last enzyme in the degradation of tyrosine.[4] FAH is a 419-amino acid protein that exists as a cytosolic homodimer in liver.[5] Although predominantly a liver enzyme, FAH activity is also found in kidney, lymphocytes, erythrocytes, fibroblasts, oligodendrocytes, and chorionic tissue.[3] The FAH CDNA has been mapped to the human chromosome 15q23–q25. Seven separate disease-inducing mutations of the gene have been described.[5–9]

Deficiency of FAH leads to organ damage because of the accumulation of toxic metabolites.[10] This is best documented for neurologic crises, in which patients present with symptoms indistinguishable from acute intermittent porphyria. The constellation of symptoms is due to increased levels of circulating succinylacetone, which is a potent inhibitor of the delta-aminolevulinic acid dehydratase, a key enzyme in porphyrin synthesis. Inhibition of the enzyme leads to the accumulation of delta-amino-

levulinic acid and, as a consequence, neurologic crises.[11] The hepatocellular damage, although still not completely understood, has also been attributed to damage from circulating toxins. The toxins most commonly implicated are maleyl- and fumarylacetoacetate.[10,12,13] Recent cell culture studies have supported this notion.[12,13]

CLINICAL PRESENTATION

Both an acute and a chronic form of tyrosinemia type I are classically described. The acute form of the disease is characterized by signs of severe liver failure with ascites, coagulopathy and hypoglycemia.[10,14,15] Affected infants have a cabbage-like odor during liver crises and often die within the first year. The chronic form is milder and liver function less abnormal. In both clinical forms, the risk of hepatocellular carcinoma is increased, and carcinoma has been estimated to develop in up to 37% of patients surviving beyond 2 years of age.[16] The distinction between the two forms is based on vague clinical criteria, which are currently being revised. Both forms of the disease can occur within the same kindred. This heterogeneity of the disease is attributed to FAH activity found in regenerating liver nodules due to a spontaneous reverse mutation.[8,17]

Genetics

Tyrosinemia type I is an autosomal recessive disease that affects both sexes equally. There is a high prevalence of the trait in the Lac-St. Jean region of Quebec. The

427

prevalence in Quebec is 8 per 100,000 and in the Lac-St. Jean region is 1:14.[18,19] A high incidence is also found in Scandinavia (1:120,000 in Sweden and 1:100,000 in Norway).[20] Heterozygotes have no clinical manifestations of disease, and their FAH enzyme levels are half-normal in fibroblasts and lymphocytes.

Liver

Liver crises typically present during the first 2 years of life and decrease in frequency thereafter. The episodes are often precipitated by an intercurrent viral infection and a catabolic state that leads to liver decompensation associated with a rapidly enlarging liver, ascites, anasarca, and a hemorrhagic diathesis. Jaundice is usually a terminal event.[21,22]

The laboratory findings are particularly characteristic in tyrosinemia. During liver crises, the transaminase levels are initially less than twice normal, and the prothrombin time (PT) and partial thromboplastin time (PTT) are exceedingly prolonged.[18,22,23] The coagulopathy is generally unresponsive to oral or parenteral vitamin K but may be corrected with FFP. Most factor levels (II, VII, IX, X, XI, XII) are less than 15% of normal, yet factors V and VIII are either normal or close to normal.[22] The serum amino acids, tyrosine, methionine, and phenylalanine, are elevated. At baseline, the transaminases, bilirubin, albumin, and gamma-glutamyltransferase, are normal to slightly abnormal. Lastly, alpha-fetoprotein (AFD) fluctuates widely and is often elevated in a range suggestive of malignancy. The urine amino acids are consistent with Fanconi syndrome.

Physical examination findings result from the cirrhotic liver disease and renal dysfunction. Hepatosplenomegaly is found in 70% of patients. Spider hemangiomas, clubbing, and rickets occur as nonspecific consequences of cirrhotic liver disease and kidney disease.[21]

Neurologic

Neurologic crises, like the liver crises, are often precipitated by a catabolic state.[11] The typical course of the neurologic crises is as follows. A prodrome of irritability and mild lethargy is followed by increasing pain, especially over the lower extremities. The patient in this state often adopts an opisthotonic posturing. The crisis may also be associated with weakness or paralysis. Those patients who have frequent bouts may develop chronic weakness. Oral anesthesia may also develop and be associated with severe bruxism and oral lacerations. Autonomic dysfunction during these periods impacts a number of other physiologic systems and leads to problems including electrolyte imbalance, hypertension, tachycardia, and intestinal ileus. The attacks last 1 to 7 days.

Neurologic crises can lead to death, especially if paralysis with respiratory insufficiency is a component. Interestingly, the neurologic crises often occur without decompensation of the liver.[11,21]

Kidney

Renal dysfunction to some degree is a constant finding in tyrosinemia type I.[22] The proximal renal tubular defects include glucosuria, amino aciduria, tubular acidosis, and hypophosphatemic rickets. Glomerular filtration rate is generally decreased. Nephromegaly is common as is some degree of fibrosis on biopsy. The severity of dysfunction increases during periods of decompensation.

Other Organ Systems

Pancreatic involvement leading to IDDM has been reported, although pancreatic islet cell hypertrophy seen histologically is usually without clinical significance.[21] Hypertrophic cardiomyopathy has also been reported.[24]

DIAGNOSIS

Tyrosinemia should be suspected in any infant or child with evidence of hepatocellular necrosis, cirrhosis, or decreased hepatic synthetic function (especially those with altered coagulation). If an isolated high tyrosine level is detected, the diagnoses to be considered include tyrosinemia type I, neonatal tyrosinemia, and tyrosinemia type II.[1] If an elevated tyrosine is found along with a number of other amino acids such as phenylalanine and methionine, the differential is broadened to include many neonatal liver diseases. Even the combination of elevated tyrosine and renal tubular dysfunction is not specific, since diseases such as galactosemia, hereditary fructose intolerance, Wilson's disease, certain lactic acidoses, and glycogen storage disease type I can have similar liver and kidney abnormalities.[3] Therefore, the clinician must establish the diagnosis by assaying for the specific metabolic byproduct, succinylacetone, and for the enzyme FAH. However, it must be cautioned that both tests can be subject to false negatives and positives.

Deficiency of FAH is obligatory for the diagnosis.[3] Enzymatic activity can be determined in easily accessible tissues such as lymphocytes, fibroblasts, and erythrocytes. However, because genetic variants of FAH exist that result in low enzymatic activity without apparent disease, the enzyme determination should be combined with succinylacetone measurements or enzyme determinations of the parents. The carrier state can be detected on cultured fibroblasts, and the activity of the carrier is usually half-normal. If succinylacetone determination is used, the most sensitive fluid to assay is urine, not blood. However, even this urine test can produce false-negative results. In one study, 3 of 35 patients had no elevation of succinylacetone on the first determination. The initial low levels may have been due to fluctuations that are commonly found in this disease.

Prenatal diagnosis of tyrosinemia can be made (1) from determination of succinylacetone in amniotic fluid, (2) by FAH assay of cultured amniotic fluid cells, and (3) by direct FAH determination of chorionic villus biopsy obtained at 10 weeks gestation. The succinylacetone level in the amniotic fluid supernatant is increased 3- to 30-fold higher than in normal pregnancies.[3,25]

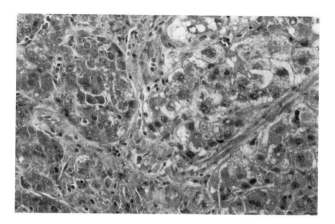

FIGURE 60-2. Hematoxylin & eosin stain of a liver section obtained from a child transplanted for tyrosinemia type I. Typical micronodular cirrhosis, cholestasis, iron deposition, and fatty changes are visualized (40×).

LABORATORY EVALUATION

Serologic Tests

Normocytic anemia and leukocytosis are commonly present, and the platelet count may be increased. In the acute form, during the first month of life, when jaundice, ascites, anasarca, and a bleeding diathesis are typically found, the laboratory findings are notable for hypoalbuminemia, prolonged PT, and marked hyperbilirubinemia, despite only mildly abnormal aminotransferases. The alpha fetoprotein is increased in a range suggestive of malignancy. Plasma tyrosine and methionine are increased, especially in the acute form; other amino acids may be increased as well. The amino acids excreted in excessive amounts, in decreasing order, are tyrosine (64 to 150 times normal), proline (10 to 125 times normal), threonine (10 to 37 times normal) alanine (9 to 30 times normal), glycine (8 to 20 times normal), phenylalanine (8 to 16 times normal), alpha-aminobutyric acid (7 to 30 times nor-

mal), and isoleucine, serine, leucine aspartic acid, and methionine.

Liver

The liver is minimally to moderately enlarged and pale with macronodular cirrhosis (Fig. 60-1). Histologically, micronodules are seen with bile duct proliferation, fibrous septa, fat deposition, pseudoacinar formation, iron accumulation, and giant cell transformation (Fig. 60-2). As the disease progresses, the liver shrinks, the macronodules become more prominent, and the risk of hepatocellular carcinoma increases. Premalignant cells are difficult to determine, as there is considerable cellular disarray as part of the usual pathology in this disease and the alpha fetoprotein, which is used as a marker for malignancy in other liver disease, is often markedly elevated and therefore not helpful.

Kidneys

The kidney disease associated with tyrosonemia type I is characterized by Fanconi's syndrome (glucosuria, amino aciduria, tubular acidosis) and hypophosphatemic rickets. Some patients with long-standing kidney disease develop renal failure. The kidney pathology includes nephromegaly with histologic changes of glycogen accumulation in the collecting tubules, nephrocalcinosis, irregular dilations of the proximal tubules and vacuolization of tubular epithelial cells. Approximately 30% will have mild to moderate glomerulosclerosis.[3,25,26]

FIGURE 60-1. Characteristic CT scan demonstrating macronocules found in tyrosinemia type I.

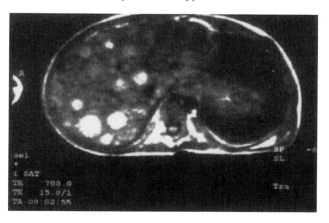

Pancreas

Hyperplasia and hypertrophy of the islets of Langerhans have been reported, however, this is rarely associated with any clinically significant glucose problems.[21]

Peripheral Neuropathy

Peripheral nerve damage can be found after paralytic crises. The typical changes include axonal degeneration and secondary demyelination. These changes are similar to those found in acute intermittent porphyria and most likely have a similar pathogenesis.[11]

TREATMENT

Until recently, dietary restriction of phenylalanine and tyrosine was the only available treatment for tyrosinemia.[1] The principle of this therapy was to limit precursor amino acid intake to the minimum needed to provide growth. However, because of the lack of a large clinical trial and the variable presentation of this disease, the benefit from such dietary intervention has never been formally proved for tyrosinemic liver disease.

In fact, there is evidence of prenatal liver dysfunction in tyrosinemia, even though fetal amino acid levels are maintained at physiologic levels by placental exchange.

The renal tubular dysfunction is improved by dietary manipulation. In sum, dietary therapy improves renal tubular function and probably slows but does not prevent the progression of liver disease.

Management of the Neonate

Once the diagnosis of tyrosinemia type I is made, the neonate is started on a diet void of phenylalanine and tyrosine. The highly restricted diet is continued for 1 to 2 days; then, based on the clinical response and the plasma tyrosine levels, tyrosine and phenylalanine are reintroduced at low levels. Typically, amino acid levels normalize along with other liver enzyme determinations in days to weeks after initiation of therapy.[21,27]

Management of Acute Liver Disease

Infections are a frequent precipitant of liver crises and should be treated aggressively. All infections warrant hospitalization. Therapy is aimed at nutrition to minimize catabolism by providing sufficient caloric intake by mouth, gavage, or total parenteral nutrition. Reduction or cessation of phenylalanine and tyrosine may be needed for 24 to 48 hours. Supplemental glucose to induce an anabolic state can be useful. Most acute crises resolve over a few weeks without the need for transplantation.

Management of Chronic Liver Disease

TRANSPLANTATION

Liver transplantation is the most effective and definitive treatment for children with this disorder. Survival rates for patients with metabolic diseases are within the range of 90%. The timing of transplantation is crucial. The major issues to be weighed include risk of malignant transformation, liver failure, and quality of life, balanced against the problems associated with transplantation. The liver transplantation is effective not only for the liver disease, but also for the kidney disease.

Normalization of renal tubular and glomerular function has been documented; however, in some cases, the kidney dysfunction is so significant that a combined liver/kidney transplant is needed. Low levels of urine succinylacetone are detected post isolated liver transplantation, probably from kidney production, as the serum levels are undetectable.[2,28,29]

NTBC

NTBC is an inhibitor of 4-hydroxyphenylpyruvate dioxygenase, an enzyme just prior to FAH in the degradation of tyrosine. Nine patients who were recently treated normalized their liver enzymes, succinylacetone, coagulation profile, and alpha-fetoprotein. Neurologic crises, fulminant liver failure, and renal tubulopathy can be reversed in some cases within hours of NTBC administration. However, administration probably does not impact on the risk of hepatocellular carcinoma (HCC). Pharmacokinetic and dose response information is currently being gathered. Because NTBC can be effective for all aspects of this disease except for the malignant transformation, it is now recommended that NTBC be used as the first line treatment. Children are screened for hepatocellular carcinoma while being provided a chance to grow. If needed, liver transplantation is offered. The most likely indications for liver transplantation are either concerns regarding malignancy or progressive liver disease.[6,30,31]

GENE THERAPY

Gene therapy is not yet feasible therapy for tyrosinemia type I. In most metabolic disorders, gene therapy will be highly effective treatment. The therapy is generally aimed at converting a sufficient number of cells to overcome the blocked enzymatic step. However, in tyrosinemia type I the disease results from production of toxic intermediates. Therefore, unless 100% of the cells are genetically corrected, toxic intermediates that lead to hepatocellular carcinoma, neurologic crises, and other clinical aspects of this disease will still be produced.

Management of Neurologic Crises

During the acute phase of neurologic crisis, analgesia is provided for the severe pain. A high level of carbohydrate is needed, since glucose inhibits the enzyme delta-aminolevulinate synthase, reducing the production of delta-aminolevulinic acid. It is important to provide symptomatic relief for the hypertension, hyponatremia, hypokalemia, and hypophosphatemia that may accompany crises.[21]

Management of Renal Involvement

Renal proximal tubular defects with glucosuria, aminoaciduria, tubular acidosis, and hypophosphatemic rickets may be present. The dysfunction usually responds at least partially to dietary therapy. Rickets is the main clinical sign of tubular dysfunction in tyrosinemia and is due to urinary phosphate loss coupled with impaired hepatic hydroxylation of vitamin D.[32]

REFERENCES

1. Goldsmith LA, Laberge C. Tyrosinemia and related disorders. In: The Metabolic Basis of Inherited Disease. Scriver CR, Beaudet AL, Sly WS, Valle D, Eds. New York: McGraw-Hill, 1989:547–562

2. Paradis K, Weber A, Seidman EG. Liver transplantation for hereditary tyrosinemia: the Quebec experience. Am J Hum Genet 1990;47:338–342

3. Kvittingen E. Hereditary tyrosinemia type I—an overview. Scand J Clin Lab Invest 1986;46:s27–34

4. Linblad B, Lindstedt S, Steen G. On the enzymatic defects in hereditary tyrosinemia. Proc Natl Acad Sci USA 1977; 74:4641–4645

5. Phaneuf D, LaBelle Y, Berube D et al. Cloning and expression of the cDNA encoding human fumarylacetoacetate hydrolase, the enzyme deficient in hereditary tyrosinemia: assignment of the gene to chromosome 15. Am J Hum Genet 1991;48:525–535

6. Grompe M, Al-Dhalimy M. Mutations of the fumarylacetoacetate hydrolase gene in four patients with tyrosinemia type I. Hum Mutat 1993;2:85–93

7. Grompe M, St. Louis M, Devers S et al. A single mutation of the fumarylacetate hydrolase gene in French Canadians with hereditary tyrosinemia type I. N Engl J Med 1994;331: 353–357

8. Phaneuf D, Lambert M, Laframboise R et al. Type I hereditary tyrosinemia: evidence for molecular heterogeneity and identification of a causal mutation in a French Canadian patient. J Clin Invest 1992;90:1185–1192

9. LaBelle Y, Phaneuf D, Leclerc B et al: Characterization of

the human fumarylacetoacetate hydrolase gene and identification of a missense mutation abolishing enzymatic activity. Hum Mol Genet 1993;2:941–946

10. Hoffman J, Dixit V, O'Shea K. Expression of thrombospondin in the adult nervous system. J Comp Neurol 1994;340: 126–139

11. Mitchell G, Larochelle J, Lambert M et al. Neurological crises in hereditary tyrosinemia. N Engl J Med 1990;322: 432–437

12. Ruppert S, Kelsey G, Schedl A et al. Deficiency of an enzyme of tyrosine metabolism underlies altered gene expression in newborn liver of lethal albino mice. Genes Dev 1992;6: 1430–1443

13. Ruppert S, Boshart M, Bosch FX et al. Two genetically defined trans-acting loci coordinately regulate overlapping sets of liver-specific genes. Cell 1990;61:895–904

14. Ward JM. Morphology of foci of altered hepatocytes and naturally-occurring hepatocellular tumors in F344 rats. Virchows Arch 1981;390:339–345

15. Van Sponsen F, Thomasse Y, Smit G et al. Hereditary tyrosinemia type 1: a new classification with difference in prognosis on dietary treatment. Hepatology 1994;20:1187–1191

16. Weinberg A, Mize C, Worthen H. The occurrence of hepatoma in the chronic form of hereditary tyrosinemia. J Pediatr 1976;88:434–438

17. Kvittingen E, Rootwelt H, Brandtzaeg P et al. Hereditary tyrosinemia type I: self-induced correction of the fumarylacetoacetase defect. J Clin Invest 1993;91:1816–1821

18. Bergeron P, Laberge C, Grenier A. Hereditary tyrosinemia in the province of Quebec: prevalence at birth and geographic distribution. Clin Genet 1974;5:157

19. De Braeleleer M, Larochelle J. Genetic epidemiology of hereditary tyrosinemia in Quebec and Saguenay-Lac St-Jean. Am J Hum Genet 1990;47:302–307

20. Salo M, Laine J, Holmberg C. Hereditary tyrosinemia type 1 (HT1) in Finnish population. First International Symposium on Hereditary Tyrosinemia 1994;October 15–17

21. Paradis K, Mitchell G, Russo P. Tyrosinemia. In: Suchy A, Ed. Liver Disease in Children. Philadelphia: Mosby, 1994:803–818

22. Forget S, Merouani A, Lafortune M et al. Renal involvement in tyrosinemia. Gastroenterology 1994;106:A893

23. Kvittingen E, Halvorsen S, Jellum E. Deficient fumarylacetoacetate fumarylhydrolase activity in lymphocytes and fibroblasts from patients with hereditary tyrosinemia. Pediatr Res 1983;14:541

24. Gentz J, Jagenburg R, Zetterstrom R. Tyrosinemia: an inborn error of tyrosine metabolism with cirrhosis of the liver and multiple renal tubular defects (de Toni-Debre-Fanconi syndrome). J Pediatr 1965;66:670–696

25. Jakobs C, Stellaard F, Kvittingen E et al. First trimester prenatal diagnosis of tyrosinemia type 1 by amniotic fluid succinylacetone determination. Prenat Diagn 1990;10:133–134

26. Laine J, Salo M, Krogerus L et al. The nephropathy of type 1 tryosinemia after liver transplantation. Pediatr Res 1995; 37:640–645

27. Larochelle J, Prive L, Belanger M. Hereditary tyrosinemia.

1. clinical and biological study of 62 cases. Pediatrie 1996; 28:5–18

28. Luks FI, St.-Vil D, Hancock BJ et al. Surgical and metabolic aspects of liver transplantation for tyrosinemia. Transplantation 1993;56:1376–1380

29. Freese DK, Tuchman M, Schwartzenberg SJ et al. Early liver transplantation is indicated for tyrosinemia type 1. J Pediatr Gastroenterol Nutr 1991;13:10–15

30. Lindstedt S, Holme E, Lock E et al. Treatment of hereditary tyrosinemia type I by inhibition of 4-hydroxyphenylpyruvate dioxygenase. Lancet 1992;340:813–817

31. Schirmacher P, Held WA, Yang D et al. Reactivation of insulin-like growth factor II during hepatocarcinogenesis in transgenic mice suggests a role in malignant growth. Cancer Res 1995;52:2549–2556

32. Shoemaker L, Strife CF, Balistreri WF. Rapid improvement in the renal tubular dysfunction associated with tyrosinemia following hepatic replacement. Pediatrics 1992;89:251–255

61

VASCULAR DISORDERS OF THE LIVER

DOUGLAS C. B. REDD
KENNETH E. FELLOWS

The liver is a highly vascular organ served by three separate vascular systems: hepatic arteries, portal veins, and hepatic veins. The chances for either congenital or acquired abnormalities are large. The diagnosis and treatment of these many possible lesions require perseverance. With the exception of postorthotopic liver transplantation (OLT) vascular complications, the manifestations of hepatic vascular abnormalities are usually hemodynamic, with little impact on hepatic function.

CONGENITAL HEPATIC VASCULAR ABNORMALITIES

Hepatic Hemangioendotheliomas

These characteristically benign tumors of infancy can result in a fatal outcome, due to either spontaneous hemorrhage or congestive heart failure, which may develop in approximately 10 to 30% of cases. Hemangioendotheliomas are immature variants of hemangiomas that occur more commonly as cutaneous lesions in the newborn. Like cutaneous hemangiomas, these usually multiple nodular hepatic tumors have a growth phase lasting from birth through 12 to 18 months; this is followed by an involutional stage lasting several months to years. The diagnosis is usually suggested by ultrasound imaging (Fig. 61-1A) and confirmed by three-phase computed tomographic (CT) scanning[1] (Fig. 61-1B).

Although diffuse involvement of the liver rarely affects liver function, high flow with arteriovenous shunting may result in congestive heart failure. Medical therapy for this complication may include digitalization, diuretics, and steroids.[2] Failure of conservative medical therapy to control heart failure may lead to the use of interferon-alpha (IFN-alpha),[3] or even chemotherapeutic agents.[4] Medically refractory heart failure generally requires arterial embolization of hepatic artery branches and collaterals to the liver[2] (Fig. 61-1C & D). Medical therapy should be aimed only at controlling congestive heart failure long enough to allow sufficient growth of the child over the first 12 to 18 months of life, since the natural history of hemangioendotheliomas is spontaneous involution after this interval (Fig. 61-2).

For the most refractory cases, surgical management, with either resection (if a suitable liver segment is uninvolved) or hepatic transplantation, may be necessary. Hepatic irradiation has been effective in promoting involution of these vascular lesions but is not recommended because of the long-term risks of secondary malignancy.

A confounding factor in this disease is that congenital arteriovenous malformations (AVMs) of the liver may simulate hemangioendotheliomas, by presenting as vascular masses causing congestive heart failure.[2] Since AVMs are developmental abnormalities of vascular tissue, not vascular tumors with a predictable life cycle, they will not involute, nor do they respond to steroids, alpha-interferon, or other antimetabolic drugs that are effective in treating hemangioendotheliomas. Additionally, AVMs will persist throughout life, and may even enlarge as the child ages. Differentiation between he-

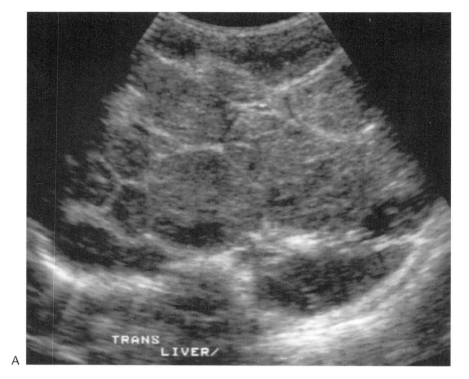

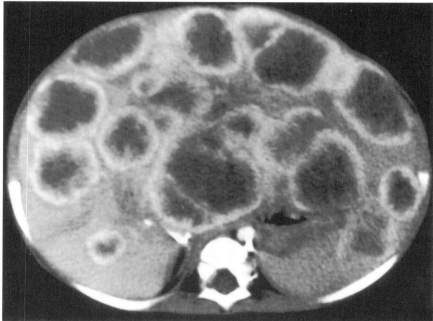

FIGURE 61-1. *(A)* Ultrasound imaging in a 13-month-old child with hemangioendo-theliomas shows multiple rounded mass lesions of heterogeneous echogenicity in-volving both right and left hepatic lobes. *(B)* Contrast-enhanced CT shows hepato-megaly in this same child with multiple lesions that are hypodense centrally with intense peripheral enhancement on dynamic imaging following bolus contrast injec-tion. Centripetal enhancement caused these lesions to become isodense on delayed imaging.

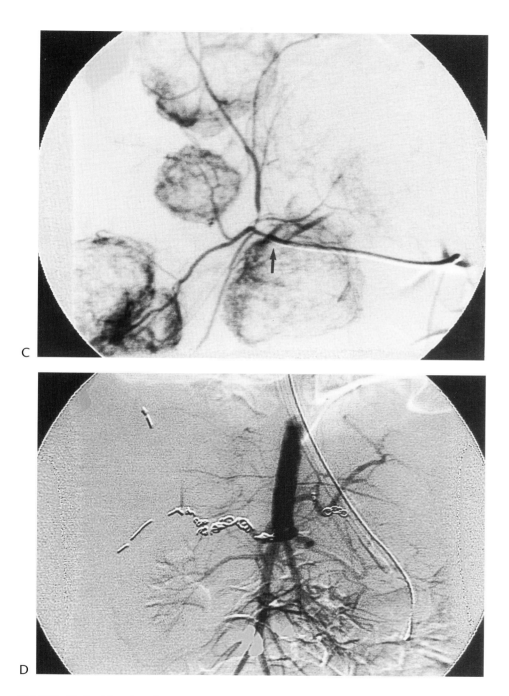

FIGURE 61-1. *(Continued)* *(C)* Arteriography and embolization were performed in this same child after failure of conservative therapies. Selective catheter placement distally within the right hepatic artery (arrow) shows multiple, rounded, hypervascular lesions. *(D)* Abdominal arteriogram performed following embolization of the right and left hepatic arteries shows subtraction artifacts from multiple coils together with arterial devascularization of the liver.

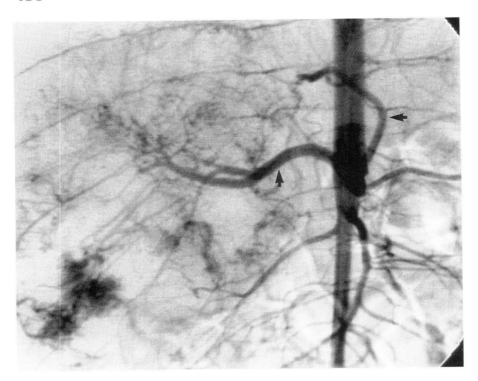

FIGURE 61-2. Abdominal arteriogram performed in a 13-month-old child with hepatomegaly shows enlarged right and left hepatic arteries (arrows) as well as reduction in caliber of the abdominal aorta distal to the level of the celiac axis. Spontaneous resolution of this hemangioendothelioma occurred over the ensuing 6 months.

mangioendotheliomas and AVMs of the liver in infants is therefore important for proper patient management (see next section).

ARTERIOVENOUS MALFORMATION

Congenitally abnormal connections between the arterial and venous vascular systems of the liver may occur in a variety of forms. Commonest are large (usually lobar), complex vascular malformations involving high flow between branches of the hepatic arteries and hepatic veins; torrential flow may lead to congestive heart failure and thereby simulate hemangioendotheliomas; however, the latter are usually multiple, nodular, and diffusely disseminated throughout both lobes of the liver. Differentiation usually can be accomplished by arteriography, or possibly by magnetic resonance imaging (MRI), using angiographic criteria. Because AVMs are often lobar, they can usually be surgically excised. Preoperative embolization may facilitate surgical management by decreasing the vascularity of these lesions allowing operative management with lower morbidity.[2]

Hepatic artery to portal vein fistulas may also occur and usually result in portal hypertension from excessive flow through this arterioportal shunt.[5] Diagnosis is often established by Doppler ultrasonography[6]; verification and treatment can be accomplished by arteriography and portal venography.[2] Management may include either surgical ligation or transcatheter embolization.[7]

The rarest of hepatic vascular malformations are portohepatic venous (or portocaval) fistulas. Although flow is usually not excessive enough to produce congestive heart failure, these congenital portosystemic shunts can lead to hyperammonemia[8] and hepatic encephalopathy. These anomalies are often discovered incidentally during ultrasound examination in infants. A number have been shown to be transient in nature, disappearing by mid-infancy or early childhood.[8] The diagnosis is confirmed by Doppler ultrasound and can also be demonstrated by spiral CT or MRI (Fig. 61-3A & B).

ACQUIRED HEPATIC VASCULAR ABNORMALITIES

Cavernous Transformation of the Portal Vein

The commonest cause of portal hypertension in infants and children, cavernous transformation of the portal vein, is a process of prehepatic obstruction resulting from

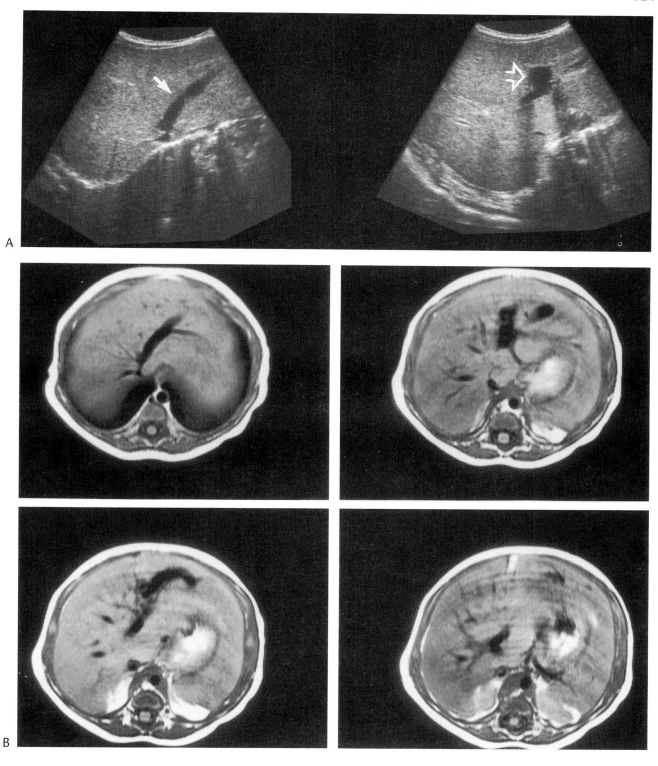

FIGURE 61-3. *(A)* A 6-week-old child with prolonged neonatal jaundice was evaluated by abdominal ultrasound. Diagnosis of portohepatic venous fistula was suggested due to enlargement of both the left hepatic vein (solid arrow) and the proximal left portal vein (open arrow). *(B)* This diagnosis was confirmed by magnetic resonance imaging with multiple axial images revealing an intrahepatic connection within the left lobe of the liver between the left branch of the portal vein and left hepatic vein.

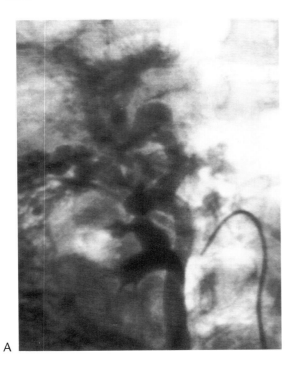
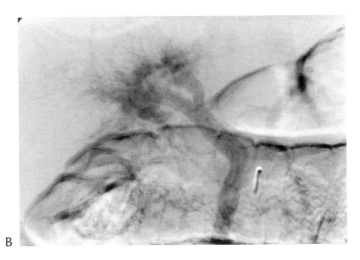

A   B

FIGURE 61-4. *(A)* Cavernous transformation of the portal vein is demonstrated in this visceral arteriogram performed to further evaluate upper gastrointestinal hemorrhage in a young child. On the portal venous phase of this superior mesenteric arterial injection, large periportal collaterals reconstitute the main portal vein with hepatopetal flow noted into the liver. Selective splenic arterial injection (not shown) demonstrated occlusion of the splenic vein, which drained via short gastric collaterals. *(B)* Cavernous transformation of the intrahepatic portal veins is demonstrated in this visceral arteriogram in which the extrahepatic portal vein and the proximal branches of the right and left main portal veins remain patent.

thrombosis of the portal vein, with subsequent development of hepatopetal venous collaterals extending into the hepatic hilum, which feed the intrahepatic portal venous circulation (Fig. 61-4A & B). The condition is rarely found in newborns, with suggested causes including umbilical venous catheterization, sepsis, dehydration, omphalitis, and clotting abnormalities.[9] Congenital origins have not been excluded, as may be suggested by the association between cavernous transformation and such anomalies as esophageal atresia, duodenal atresia, and Turner's syndrome.[9]

The presenting symptom in cavernous transformation of the portal vein is usually upper gastrointestinal variceal bleeding. Although there are innumerable periportal venous collaterals, these are insufficient to decompress the mesenteric venous system adequately; thus, hepatofugal collaterals develop to the systemic venous circulation, with the largest collateral the left gastric (coronary) vein draining into the azygous venous system through gastroesophageal varices.

Cavernous transformation is therefore characterized by portal hypertension due to "prehepatic" obstruction

with normal liver function and no intrinsic liver disease. Because of the involvement of the extrahepatic portal vein, this prehepatic obstruction cannot be relieved by the transjugular intrahepatic portocaval shunt (TIPS) procedure; instead, operative intervention may be required with the creation of a surgical portosystemic shunt or even OLT, wherein the donor portal vein is anastomosed to the recipient superior mesenteric vein.

This diagnosis is almost always established by ultrasound examination. Definitive anatomy of the residual portal vein and collaterals is obtained by superior mesenteric arterial portography. In addition to gastroesophageal varices, portal venography may demonstrate other hepatofugal collaterals including spontaneous splenorenal collaterals or through the inferior mesenteric vein into hemorrhoidal veins.[9]

Budd-Chiari Syndrome

Obstruction to hepatic venous outflow at the level of large hepatic veins or the inferior vena cava (IVC) results in the Budd-Chiari syndrome. The disease is un-

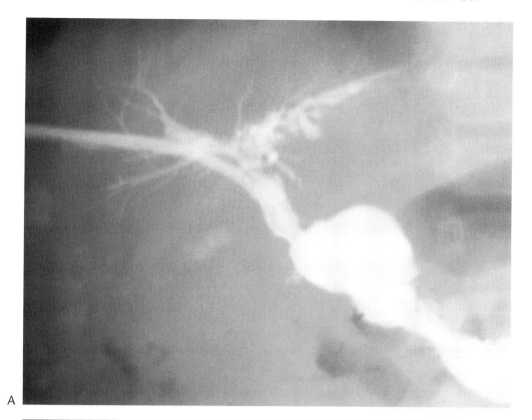

A

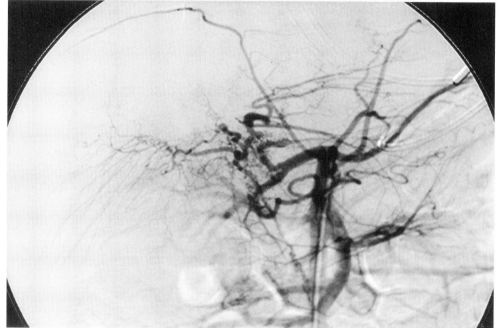

B

FIGURE 61-5. *(A)* Percutaneous transhepatic cholangiogram was performed to evaluate recurrent cholangitis in an 8-month-old child transplanted at age 2 months for biliary atresia. Internal/external biliary drainage was performed. Diffuse irregularity, with pseudodiverticula, is present in the left bile duct. *(B)* Doppler ultrasound showed pulsatile arterial flow within the intrahepatic arterial branches in this child. Visceral arteriography was ultimately performed at age 13 months, showing the intrahepatic arterial branches to fill through diffuse perihilar collaterals.

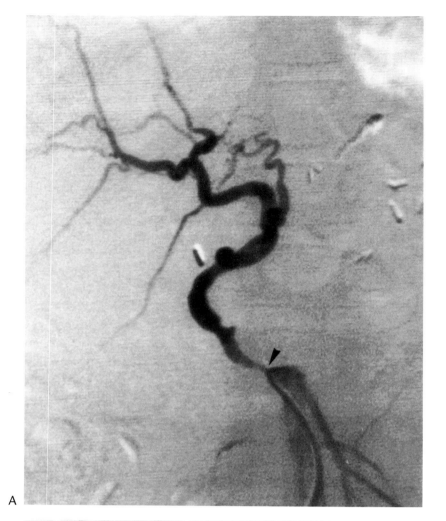

A

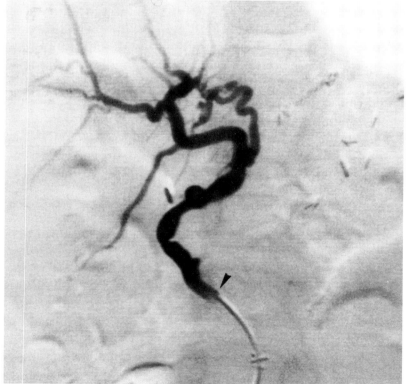

B

FIGURE 61-6. *(A)* Following orthotopic liver transplantation, hepatic arterial thrombosis was noted in this 7-year-old girl. Diagnostic arteriography confirmed findings of hepatic arterial stenosis suggested on Doppler ultrasound. Anastomotic narrowing of the hepatic artery (arrowhead) is present with proximal luminal irregularity suggesting thrombosis. *(B)* Thrombolysis was performed via an intra-arterial infusion of urokinase, which achieved a decrease in luminal narrowing. As a final intervention, balloon angioplasty was performed to treat the anastomotic narrowing of the hepatic artery.

common at all ages and is especially rare in children. Whatever the cause of major hepatic vein and/or IVC obstruction, the clinical features of Budd-Chiari syndrome include intractable ascites, abdominal pain, and hepatomegaly.[10] Originally thought to be an endophlebitis of the hepatic venous ostia, Budd-Chiari is known to have many causes, including hepatic venous or caval thrombosis in patients with polycythemia vera or coagulation abnormalities, direct tumor extension or extrinsic tumoral compression, and obstructing membranes (usually noted in Asian and South African populations).[10]

The diagnosis of Budd-Chiari syndrome may be made by real-time Doppler ultrasonography, which demonstrates abnormal hepatic vein and inferior vena caval flow patterns with decreased velocity; echogenic obstructing membranes may be shown as well.[10] The diagnosis can be difficult to establish in children; MR angiography or percutaneous venography may be necessary to establish this diagnosis.[11] Diagnostic catheter studies require the retrograde catheterization of the hepatic veins for hepatic venography and manometry; absence of the main hepatic veins, or small hepatic veins with a "spiderweb" pattern of collaterals on a wedged injection is diagnostic of Budd-Chiari. Inferior vena cavography and free hepatic vein injections are more helpful in showing the number and level of the obstructions and in planning therapy.

Obstructing membranes at hepatic vein ostia and in the IVC respond well to balloon catheter dilation but may require repeat dilatations or eventual insertion of endoluminal vascular stents.[12,13] Thrombosis can be treated by thrombolysis if recent, or by dilation/stenting if chronic and organized.[12] Some cases may be so extensive and refractory to medical or transcatheter therapies that liver transplantation is the only practical alternative.[12]

Obstruction of small hepatic veins at the central and sublobular levels, whether due to alkaloids (Senecio and Jamaican bush tea), hepatic irradiation, or chemotherapy, is usually termed hepatic veno-occlusive disease[14] and should be considered separately from Budd-Chiari syndrome, as there are vastly different diagnostic and therapeutic implications.

Postoperative Liver Transplantation

The most common postoperative vascular complication following OLT in infants and children is stenosis or thrombosis of the hepatic artery.[15] Hepatic arterial ischemia is particularly critical for the bile ducts, which receive end-arterial supply with poor collateral flow; significant postoperative hepatic artery obstruction usually results in biliary scarring and stenosis, which may ultimately require repeat transplantation. Routine postoperative evaluation of hepatic arterial patency is usually made by ultrasound, which is reliable in most cases. However, because intra- and extra-hepatic arterial collaterals can mask significant hepatic arterial obstruction, arteriography is sometimes required for complete evaluation (Fig. 61-5A & B). When hepatic artery thrombosis occurs in

FIGURE 61-7. *(A)* Percutaneous transhepatic catheterization of the portal vein was performed in this 4-year-old child who presented with gastrointestinal (GI) hemorrhage following OLT. An anastomotic hibistenosis was shown. *(B)* Visceral arteriogram showing extrahepatic portal vein obstruction with prominent varices involving the Roux-en-Y loop is noted in another child with history of OLT. This patient also presented with a history of GI hemorrhage.

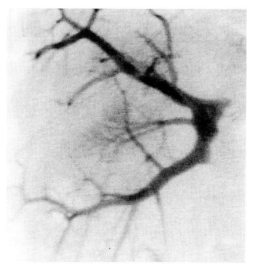

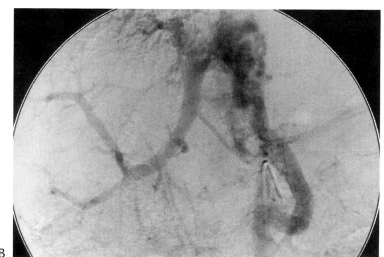

A   B

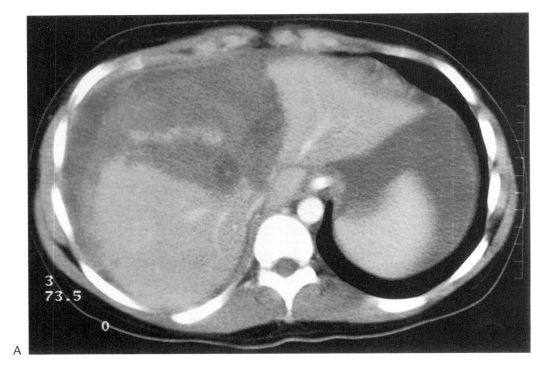

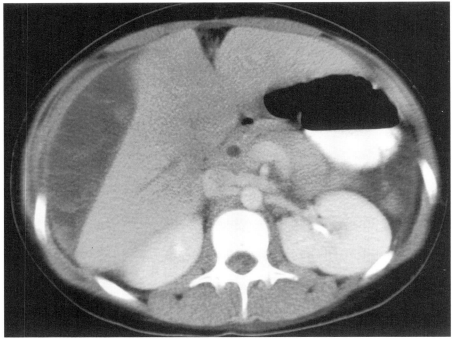

FIGURE 61-8. *(A & B)* Hepatic laceration with subcapsular hematoma and hemoperitoneum is noted in this 14-year-old girl following blunt abdominal trauma. The child recovered uneventfully without surgical intervention.

the recent post-operative period, immediate reoperation is usually indicated. If this complication is discovered at a time remote from surgery, thrombolysis of the thrombosed hepatic artery and balloon dilation of any hepatic artery stenosis may be possible (Fig. 61-6A & B).

Postoperative portal vein stenosis and thrombosis occur in less than 5% of children after liver transplantation.[15] The diagnosis is almost always made by ultrasonic examination. Percutaneous transhepatic (retrograde) portal vein catheterization (Fig. 61-7A & B) permits balloon dilation (and stenting, if necessary) of portal vein stenoses. Transcatheter thrombolysis by this approach can also be performed, when necessary, to treat portal or mesenteric venous thrombosis.

Children who have had repeated liver transplantation procedures may develop a Budd-Chiari syndrome caused by outflow obstruction due to stenosis of the suprahepatic inferior vena cava or the hepatic vein anastomoses. Balloon dilation of these postoperative stenoses must often be done on repeat occasions,[16] and either endovascular stenting or surgical revision, possibly by a transthoracic right atrial approach, may ultimately be required to relieve the hepatic venous obstruction.

Post-Trauma

Hepatic lacerations, when large, may cause such severe hemorrhage that imaging studies are rarely requested as the patient's clinical status requires immediate operative exploration. Smaller hepatic lacerations often cause intraparenchymal or subcapsular bleeding, a finding demonstrable either on CT scan (Fig. 61-8A & B) or ultrasound examination. Arteriography in these patients is usually indicated only when chronic peritoneal hemorrhage results in persistent right upper quadrant pain or when an ongoing transfusional requirement necessitates embolization of the bleeding peripheral hepatic arteries.[17]

Hemobilia is a rare, and often occult, source of GI bleeding that follows traumatic or percutaneous invasive procedures.[18] In children, the most frequent cause is blunt abdominal trauma that may antedate clinical symptoms by weeks or months.[19] Discovery of the source invariably requires arteriography for diagnosis. This is often accompanied by therapeutic transcatheter embolization as definitive treatment for the process.

REFERENCES

1. Mahboubi S, Sunaryo FP, Glassman MS, Patel K. Computed tomography, management, and follow-up in infantile hemangioendothelioma of the liver in infants and children. J Comput Tomogr 1987;11:370–375

2. Fellows KE, Hoffer FA, Markowitz RI, O'Neill J Jr. Multiple collaterals to hepatic infantile hemangioendotheliomas and arteriovenous malformations: effect of embolization [see comments]. Radiology 1991;181:813–818

3. Hatley RM, Sabio H, Howell CG et al. Successful management of an infant with a giant hemangioma of the retroperi-toneum and Kasabach-Merritt syndrome with alpha-interferon. J Pediatr Surg 1993;28:1356–1357

4. Hurvitz CH, Alkalay AL, Sloninsky L et al. Cyclophospha-mide therapy in life-threatening vascular tumors. J Pediatr 1986;109:360–363.

5. Heaton ND, Davenport M, Karani J et al. Congenital hepa-toportal arteriovenous fistula [see comments]. [Review.] Surgery 1995;117:170–174

6. Shapiro RS, Winsberg F, Stancato-Pasik A, Sterling KM. Color Doppler sonography of vascular malformations of the liver. Ultrasound Med 1993;12:343–348

7. Routh WD, Keller FS, Cain WS, Royal SA, Transcatheter embolization of a high-flow congenital intrahepatic arterial-portal venous malformation in an infant. J Pediatr Surg 1992; 27:511–514

8. Kitagawa S, Gleason W Jr, Northrup H et al. Symptomatic hyperammonemia caused by a congenital portosystemic shunt. [Review.] J Pediatr 1992;121: 917–919

9. Brunelle F, Pariente D, Charmont P. Liver Disease in Children. An Atlas of Angiography and Cholangiography. London: Springer-Verlag, 1993

10. Stanley P. Budd-Chiari syndrome [see comments]. [Review.] Radiology 1989;170(3 pt 1):625–627

11. Kane R, Eustace S. Diagnosis of Budd-Chiari syndrome: comparison between sonography and MR angiography. Radiology 1995;195:117–121

12. Veubraux A, Scott J, Mitchell S, Osterman F. Interventional management of Budd-Chiari syndrome. Semin Intervent Radiol 1994;11:312–320

13. Blum U, Rossle M, Haag K et al. Budd-Chiari syndrome: technical, hemodynamic, and clinical results of treatment with transjugular intrahepatic portosystemic shunt. Radiology 1995;197:805–811

14. Shulman HM, Hinterberger W. Hepatic veno-occlusive disease—liver toxicity syndrome after bone marrow transplantation. [Review.] Bone Marrow Transplant 1992;10:197–214

15. Zajko A, Bron K, Orons P. Vascular complications in liver transplant recipients: angiographic diagnosis and treatment. Semin Intervent Radiology 1992;9:270–282

16. Johnson JL, Fellows KE, Murphy JD. Transhepatic central venous access for cardiac catheterization and radiologic intervention. Cathet Cardiovasc Diagn 1995;35:168–171

17. Schwartz RA, Teitelbaum GP, Katz MD, Pentecost, MJ. Effectiveness of transcatheter embolization in the control of hepatic vascular injuries. J Vasc Intervent Radiol 1993;4: 359–365

18. Czerniak A, Thompson JN, Hemingway AP et al. Hemobilia. A disease in evolution. Arch Surg 1988;123:718–721

19. MacGillivray DC, Valentine RJ. Nonoperative management of blunt pediatric liver injury—late complications: case report. [Review.] Trauma 1989;29:251–254

62

VIRAL HEPATITIS

WILLIAM J. WENNER
DAVID A. PICCOLI

The liver is often the target of viral infection. Seven heterotropic viruses that predominantly affect the liver have been identified: hepatitis A, B, C, D, E, F(?), and G(?) (Table 62-1). With regard to the nonheterotropic viruses, liver involvement is just one of multiply involved organ systems. These viruses include cytomegalovirus (CMV), Epstein-Barr virus (EBV), herpes simplex virus (HSV), varicella zoster virus (VZV), adenovirus, enterovirus, echovirus, coxsackievirus, rubella, human immunodeficiency virus (HIV), mumps, Marlburg, Lassa fever, reovirus, Rift Valley fever, and others.

PATHOPHYSIOLOGY

Heterotropic viruses, particularly hepatitis B virus, (HBV), are rarely cytopathic, as they do not directly destroy the hepatocyte. In the small minority of patients who have fulminant hepatic failure, a cytopathic effect can occur. Cellular damage is produced through a multifaceted inflammatory response consistent with chronic infection. Severe pathologic lesions demonstrate panlobular infiltration with a predominance of mononuclear cells and hepatocyte necrosis. Usually these lesions have multiple foci. Hepatitis C virus (HCV) often shows biliary ductular damage and steatosis in addition to lymphocyte aggregates and/or follicles.

CLINICAL PRESENTATION

Jaundice is the most common clinical symptom that occurs in children presenting to a physician with viral hepatitis. Other common signs and symptoms include an enlarged liver or spleen, anorexia, and lethargy. Unexplained fever, upper respiratory symptoms, or gastrointestinal symptoms may also be noted (Table 62-2). Occasionally, the first hint of a viral hepatitis may be the presence of an asymptomatic transaminase elevation. To a varied degree, certain clinical features can help identify the specific etiology (Table 62-3). Most investigators believe that asymptomatic patients are no less infectious than symptomatic patients.

DIAGNOSIS

As the presentation is protean, it must be considered to be diagnosed. The diagnosis is made through serologic confirmation of infection. The tests may detect acute antibody response, late-phase antibody response, virus, or nucleic acids (Table 62-4). The child who presents with signs of hepatic inflammation must be evaluated for functional status of the liver. In addition to serum transaminases, bilirubin, glucose, and complete blood count (CBC), prothrombin time (PT) is an important indicator of liver function, as an elevated PT that is unresponsive to vitamin K indicates liver failure.

Heterotropic Viruses

HEPATITIS A VIRUS

Hepatitis A virus (HAV) infections are generally asymptomatic in 85% of children less than 2 years of age; between 2 and 4 years, 50% are asymptomatic, and only

TABLE 62-1. Viral Physiology

	Type	Genome	Envelope	Transcription	Misc
HAV	Picornavirus	ssRNA	Unenveloped	+ sense	
HBV	Hepadnavirus	ds/ss DNA	Enveloped	− sense	
HCV	Flavivirus	ssRNA	Enveloped	+ sense	
HDV	Viroid (needs HBV)	ssRNA	Enveloped with HBSag	− sense	
HEV	Calicivirus ?	ssRNA	Unenveloped	+ sense	Rare in U.S.
HGV	Flavivirus	ssRNA	?	?	

TABLE 62-2. Clinical Features of Viral Hepatitis

	Incubation	Prodrome	Icteric Phase	LFT Elevation
HAV	28 days (14–35)	1–7 days	<14 days	2–3 wk
HBV	75 days (30–180)	≤60 days	>14 days	Months
HCV	56 days (14–180)	?14 days?	>14 days	Fluctuation (indefinitely)
HEV	42 days	?5–30 days?	0–15 days?	14 days?

TABLE 62-3. Clinical Forms of Viral Hepatitis

	Acute Hepatitis	Fulminant Failure	Chronic Carrier	Cirrhosis	Hepatic Cancer
HAV	Common	Very rare	No	No	No
HBV	Common	Yes	Yes	Yes	Yes
HCV	Yes	Very rare	Yes	Common	Yes
HDV	Yes	Yes	Yes	Yes	Yes
HEV	Yes	Common	No	No	No
HGV	Yes	?	Yes	?Yes	??

TABLE 62-4. Serology of Hepatitis

	Acute Antibody	Late Antibody	Virus	Nucleic Acid
HAV	HAV IgM	HAV IgG or total antibody	Not used	Not used
HBV	HBV core IgM	HBV core IgG AB, HBsAg HBV surface AB HBV e AB	HBV DNA HBeAg	
HCV	No response	HCV ELISA HCV RIBA	Not identified	HCV PCR
HDV	Not used	HDV AB	HDV Ag	Not used
HEV	HEV IgM	HEV IgG	Not used	HEV PCR
HGV	?	?	?	HGV PCR

TABLE 62-5. Serologic Diagnosis[a]

	HAV IGM	HAV Total	IgM HBcAb	HBsAg	HBsAb	HCV Ab	HCV PCR	Interpretation
1	+	+	−	−	−	−	−	Acute HAV
2	−	+	−	−	−	−	−	Resolved HAV
3	−	−	+	−	−	−	−	Chronic HBV
4	−	−	+	+	−	−	−	Acute/chronic HBV
5	−	−	−	+	−	−	−	Incubation/chronic
6	−	−	+	−	+	−	−	Recovering from acute
7	−	−	−	−	+	−	−	Resolved/immunized HBV
8	−	+	+	+	−	−	−	History of HAV, acute/chronic HBV
9	−	−	−	−	−	+	−	Resolved/chronic HCV
10	−	−	−	−	−	+	+	Chronic HCV

[a] Frequently received laboratory results and interpretation.

20% of children 5 years and older are asymptomatic. HAV is a common illness often spread among people who have poor hygiene. It has a swift onset (usually with fever, anorexia, headache, and jaundice) and patients often remember precisely when they "became ill." The fever of HAV is greater than 39°C in more than 50% of patients but usually resolves prior to jaundice and before the patient seeks medical attention. Diarrhea is observed in one-half of infected children but is more infrequent in adults. Leukopenia, hepatomegaly, and splenomegaly are common findings.

HAV is highly contagious and is typically spread by the fecal-oral route. The incubation period is usually 15 to 40 days. Children under age 2 years rarely exhibit clinical manifestations. Institutionalized patients are at increased risk of infection. Extrahepatic manifestations are very rare in HAV although an associated meningoencephalitis has been reported. While HAV is almost always self-limited, in rare cases, acute liver failure can occur.

The initial response to HAV infection is the production of neutralizing antibody, IgM (Table 62-5). More than 99% of infected patients have serologic evidence of this antibody at presentation. HAV IgM peaks in the first month of clinical illness and becomes undetectable within 6 to 12 months. Therefore, a positive HAV IgM is the diagnostic test of an acute infection. Total HAV antibody testing is also available; it detects both IgG and IgM. A positive total test indicates an infection but does not allow the physician to determine whether it is an acute infection or a previous infection. Neither test is influenced by immunoglobulin in normal doses.

HEPATITIS B VIRUS

While the spread of HBV is usually considered to occur from parenteral transmission, this virus has been detected in all body fluids (except stool), and nonparenteral spread can occur through the exchange of many body fluids. Perinatal transmission, from mothers to their offspring, represents another important mode of viral spread and can still occur even when the parents are asymptomatic. While it has been observed that the proportion of symptomatic cases increases with age, the definitive proportions have not been determined.

The onset of HBV is more insidious than that of HAV. The incubation period is usually 50 to 180 days. Symptoms of HBV are variable and may either resemble those of the common "flu" or in some cases present as fulminant liver failure. The clinical features of HBV are often thought to occur in three distinct phases: prodromal, symptomatic, and convalescent. The prodromal phase usually precedes the symptomatic phase by 2 weeks and is typically manifested by complaints of constitutional symptoms, such as nausea, myalgia, fever, anorexia, and rash. The symptomatic phase is generally documented by jaundice and "liver pain" with pruritus; however, anicteric hepatitis can also occur. The convalescent phase may last weeks or months.

Angioedema, transient arthralgia of the large and small joints, glomerulonephritis, serum sickness-like illness, polyarteritis nodosa, and an urticaria type rash may be associated with the prodrome of HBV or may occur as a complication of the disease. A rare but specific rash, Gianotti-Crosti disease, is associated with childhood HBV infection. The rash is a popular acrodermatitis visible on the extremities. It most commonly occurs in children less than 5 years of age and is hypothesized to be due to vascular immune complex deposition. It is generally followed by an anicteric hepatitis.

The serologic diagnosis of HBV is complex. Reports of varied mutations and carrier states support the impression of complexity. (See Table 62-6 for definition of hepatitis B nomenclature.) However, by remembering the sequence of the infection, the diagnosis of most cases

TABLE 62-6. Hepatitis B Virus Nomenclature

HBV	Description
HBVsAg	Surface antigen (outer shell—product of active replication)
HBVsAb	Surface antibody
HBVcAg	Core antigen (inner core—product of active replication)
HBVcAb	Core antibody
HBVeAg	E antigen (precore product—indicates active replication)
HBVeAb	E antibody
HBV DNA	DNA (genome of HBV—quantitates active replication)

need not be complex (Table 62-5). The first product of the infected cell is the virus particle, core antigen. This product is not detected by currently available serology but can be found in liver tissue. The first detectable serologic defense product is HBVcAb IgM antibody to hepatitis B core antigen (HBcAg). IgM HBcAb disappears in 6 months to 2 years. Close to the appearance of core antibody is the appearance of the second product of the infected cell, the viral envelope—surface antigen (HBsAg) which is detectable by serologic testing. Subsequently, the second immunologic defense product is produced, HBV surface antibody (HBsAb). Its presence indicates pending or actual resolution of the infection in the majority of patients or can indicate a history of immunization to HBV.

Chronic hepatitis B frequently occurs and is defined by the continued presence of hepatitis B surface antigen (HBsAg) or by evidence of markers of active viral replication (HBeAg in serum, HBV DNA in serum or liver, HBcAg in liver). Chronic disease can be manifested by chronic liver disease (elevated serum transaminases and/or abnormal liver histology) or the healthy "carrier" state (evidence of active viral replication without serum or liver evidence of clinical disease). The carrier state is frequently defined by the serologic marker, HBVAg. A large number of chronic carriers to HBV have had no prior knowledge of having hepatitis other than testing positive for HBsAg. Further evaluation should always be performed in these patients. Generally, younger patients are more likely to develop a chronic infection. Approximately, 10 to 15% of patients who are chronic carriers will spontaneously recover.

HEPATITIS C VIRUS

HCV is one of the most common forms of viral hepatitis in the United States. Active forms of HCV present asymptomatically in all age groups. HCV is often diagnosed in the evaluation of unexplained elevated serum transaminases. HCV can be transmitted by blood products, maternal-fetal transmission, or sexual contact; however, in many cases, no specific etiology is found. It has been suggested that greater than 90% of infected patients develop a chronic persistent infection. HCV is endemic in some populations; in the United States, more than one-half of infected patients have no known predisposing etiologic factors. In transfusion-associated HCV infection, only 30% of recipients had a bilirubin greater than 2.5 mg/dl. None had a protracted or severe illness. By contrast, 70% of community-acquired cases that required hospitalization were jaundiced. This reinforces the idea that HCV can present as a clinical hepatitis, indistinguishable from HAV or HBV on the basis of symptoms.

The clinical symptoms of HCV are similar to those of nonspecific viral hepatitis (not of HAV and HBV). While most affected patients develop fever, nausea, abdominal pain, and fatigue, most remain anicteric. Serum transaminases tend to fluctuate widely and at times are normal, even in the presence of active disease. Nonhepatic manifestations include serum sickness and vasculitis.

First described in 1989, HCV is diagnosed by the detection of HCV antibody (Table 62-5). Early tests had variable sensitivity and specificity but newer generations of antibody tests have resulted in significant improvement. Antibody production occurs late in the infection. Anti-HCV by EIA-2 does not appear until week 12 following a contaminated transfusion. Viral nucleic acid in the serum can be detected by polymerase chain reaction (PCR) testing as early as 2 weeks after a transfusion. Little is known about the sequence of non-transfusion–associated HCV infection. Both antibody and PCR testing should be performed in the initial evaluation of suspected HCV.

HEPATITIS D VIRUS

Hepatitis D virus (HDV), or hepatitis delta virus, can only cause clinical symptoms when associated as a co-infection with HBV. This virus acts like a parasite of HBV, using ithe basic components of hepatitis B for its replication. HDV can infect not only individuals with active HBV but also chronic carriers of hepatitis B. Because of these features, the epidemiology of HDV is exactly the same as that for HBV. Clinically, patients with HBV and HDV co-infection develop severe clinical symptoms. The acute features of HDV are similar to those of HBV; however, the mortality rate is 10 to 20 times higher. A rapidly progressive cirrhosis develops in patients who have chronic HDV.

Acute HDV infection occurs in two forms. The first form, co-infection, indicates the development of a simultaneous infection with HBV and HDV. By contrast, superinfection relates to patients who develop an HDV infection after previously having a chronic HBV infection. Patients with superinfection often manifest a more severe clinical course often leading to chronic illness.

HEPATITIS E VIRUS

Hepatitis E virus (HEV) is very rare in developed countries, but it is the cause of "endemic non-A, non-B" virus on the Indian subcontinent, Asia, and Africa. It is transmitted through the fecal-oral route, does not appear to cause chronic disease, and has a very high fatality rate during pregnancy. The incubation period is 35 to 50 days, with adolescents and young adults the most likely to become infected. Clinically, the symptoms of HEV resemble those of HAV. The development of fulminant hepatitis may occur in up to 20% of patients. Currently, the diagnosis of HEV is based on the presence of IgM and IgA antibodies.

Nonheterotropic Viruses

CYTOMEGALOVIRUS AND EPSTEIN-BARR VIRUS

While CMV and EBV are usually mentioned when discussing liver disease unrelated to the hepatic viruses, all human herpes viruses have been etiologically linked to liver disease, particularly in neonates. In older children, the herpes viruses generally cause liver disease in immunocompromised hosts. In neonates, CMV causes a chronic hepatitis with progressively elevated transaminases and has been associated with encephalitis, chorioretinitis, nephritis, and aplastic anemia. EBV is typically associated with a transient hepatitis.

TREATMENT

Immunization

The most effective treatment available is prevention (Table 62-7). Active immunization, with long-term immunity, is available for both HAV and HBV. Adverse effects are extremely rare, with effective protection afforded in 94 to 100% of cases. Universal immunization against HBV is now recommended by both the American Academy of Pediatrics and the Immunization Practices Advisory Committee of the Centers for Disease Control. Passive immunization with immunoglobulin therapy is also appropriate for both HAV and HBV. Immunoglobulin therapy is effective in up to 75% cases of HAV and in 95% of neonates, when combined with active immunization, if given in an appropriate interval following exposure. There is a specific HBV immunoglobulin. It contains up to 10,000 times the HBs antibody as immunoglobulin. Peak levels of circulating anti-HBs are seen in 3 to 7 days after intramuscular injection. It has a half-life of 17.5 to 25 days.

Therapy for Perinatal Infection

A child born to a mother who is positive for HBVsAg and HBVeAg has a greater than 80% chance of becoming a chronic carrier of HBV. Perinatal transfer of HBV is a major cause of chronic HBV. Prophylaxis can prevent 90% of perinatal transmission. Specific doses and schedules are updated and improved continuously. For the current approach to therapy is referred to the most recent recommendations of the Advisory Committee on Immunization Practices (ACIP), found in the Morbidity and Mortality Weekly Report published by the Centers for Disease Control and Prevention (CDC), the Red Book: Report of the Committee on Infectious Diseases, the Physicians' Desk Reference (PDR), or other current reference.

THERAPY FOR ACUTE AND CHRONIC INFECTIONS

Multiple modalities have been used to treat viral hepatitis. Most have varied success. Interferon-alpha (IFN-alpha) is the only approved treatment for chronic hepatitis in the United States. The success rate, defined as either normalization of transaminases, loss of viral replication markers, or improvement in histologic disease, varies with the virus, subtype, and other factors. The

TABLE 62-7. Therapy

	Immunization	Immunoglobulin	Immune Enhancing	Transplantion
HAV	Yes	Yes—pre/post exposure	No	Yes
HBV	Yes	Yes—post exposure	Yes	Yes
HCV	None	No proven efficacy	Yes	Yes
HDV	Yes—for HBV	No proven efficacy	Treat HBV	Yes
HEV	None	No data	No	Yes
HGV	None	No data	No	Yes

pediatric use of interferon is documented but like many pediatric therapies is not approved by the Food and Drug Administration (FDA). Many questions remain regarding indications, duration, dosage, and outcome. Replacement therapy with liver transplantation is occasionally required for all forms of viral hepatitis. Required in irreversible liver failure, transplantation is often complicated by recurrence of the hepatitis.

REFERRAL PATTERN

The diagnosis of acute viral hepatitis is usually the appropriate responsibility of the primary physician. Close monitoring for changes in liver status is mandatory. After resolution of the acute phase, the patient should be monitored for development of a chronic infection. If chronic infection is noted, the patient warrants referral for evaluation of suitability for interferon therapy and development of a plan to monitor the subsequent course.

REFERENCES

Koff RS. Viral hepatitis. In: Walker W, Durie P, Hamilton J et al., Eds. Pediatric Gastrointestinal Disease. Philadelphia: BC Decker, 1991:857–873

Balistreri WF. Acute and chronic viral hepatitis. In: Suchy FJ, Ed. Liver Diseases in Children. St. Louis: CV Mosby, 1993: 460–509

Hadler SC, Webster HM, Erben SS et al. Hepatitis A in day care centers: a community wide assessment. N Engl J Med 1980;302:1222–1227

Centers for Disease Control. Hepatitis B virus: a comprehensive strategy for eliminating transmission in the United States through universal childhood vaccination: recommendations of the Immunization Practice Advisory Committee (ACIP). MMWR 1991;40:1–25

Committee on Infectious Diseases. Universal hepatitis B immunization. Pediatrics 1992;89:795–899

Lemon SM. Type A viral hepatitis. N Engl J Med 1985;313: 1059–1067

Alter MJ, Ahtone J, Weisfuse I et al. Hepatitis B virus transmission between heterosexuals. JAMA 1986;256:1307–1310

Bortolotti F, Calzia R, Cadrobbi P et al. Liver cirrhosis associated with chronic hepatitis B infection in childhood. J Pediatr 1986;108:224–227

Purcell RH, Gerin JL. Hepatitis delta virus. In: Fields BN, Knipe DM, Eds. Virology. 2nd Ed. New York: Raven Press, 1990: 2275–2287

Stevens CE, Taylor PE, Pindyck J et al. Epidemiology of hepatitis C virus: a preliminary study in volunteer blood donors. JAMA 1990;263:49–53

Inone Y, Miyamura T, Unayama T et al. Maternal transfer of HCV. Nature 1991;353:609

63

WILSON'S DISEASE

MARK J. INTEGLIA
RANDI G. PLESKOW
RICHARD J. GRAND

Wilson's disease, a rare autosomal recessive disorder of copper metabolism, was first described in 1912 by Kinnear Wilson.[1] The American neurologist considered it a degenerative disorder of the central nervous system (CNS) associated with cirrhosis. We now know that this disorder is characterized by excessive accumulation of copper in the CNS, liver, kidneys, cornea, skeletal system, and other organs. With a prevalence of 1 in 30,000 and carrier frequency of 1 in 90, Wilson's disease may not be diagnosed until adulthood although manifestations may be seen in childhood.[2]

PATHOPHYSIOLOGY

Wilson's disease has been recognized as a distinct entity for more than 70 years, yet despite this, the mechanism of the biochemical defect remains to be defined. Studies using genetic linkage have localized the Wilson's disease locus to chromosome 13, and the gene has been sequenced and mapped; the defective protein is a P-type ATPase. An abnormality in serum ceruloplasmin levels is a nearly constant feature of Wilson's disease. Ceruloplasmin is a copper-containing alpha-2-globulin and its gene is located on chromosome 3; it has an unclear role in the pathogenesis of Wilson's disease. The derangement in organ function occurs secondary to abnormal copper deposition due to inadequate biliary excretion.[3] Copper, an essential trace element in a number of en-

zyme systems, is found in dietary sources of liver, kidney, shellfish, chocolate, dried beans, peas, and unprocessed wheat. In Wilson's disease, copper accumulation first occurs abnormally in the liver early in life. After the first to second decades of life, copper is released from the liver as the storage capacity is exceeded.[2] This excessive amount of copper is then deposited into other tissues. The average American diet consists of 1.0 mg of copper per day,[4,5] of which approximately 50% is unabsorbed and passed in the feces,[6] while 30% is lost through the skin.[7] The remaining 20% is normally excreted with bile by the biliary system into the feces. It is here the abnormality arises with an inability to excrete this remaining 0.2 mg of copper.[3,4,8,9] Noteworthy is that copper accumulation is not secondary to increased absorption from the gastrointestinal (GI) tract.

CLINICAL PRESENTATION

The clinical manifestations (Table 63-1) are related to deposition of copper in specific organs, most commonly the liver and CNS. Presentation is variable in children, with disease rarely present before 4 to 5 years of age. It is common in children for hepatic manifestations to precede the neurologic manifestations by many years. Primary hepatic manifestations are most often seen first in the second decade of life, with the remainder of patients presenting later with primarily neurologic or psychiatric findings.[2]

451

TABLE 63-1. Clinical Manifestations of Wilson's Disease

Liver
    Acute hepatitis
    Chronic active hepatitis
    Cirrhosis
    Fulminant hepatic failure
Central nervous system
    Neurologic
    Psychiatric
Ophthalmologic
    Kayser-Fleischer rings
    Sunflower cataracts
Other
    Renal
    Skeletal
    Cardiac
    Hemolytic anemia
    Cholelithiasis

Hepatic Manifestations

All patients with Wilson's disease have hepatic involvement. Hepatic features may vary, however, and clinical manifestations can mimic both acute and chronic liver disease. Forms of presentation of Wilson's disease include "acute hepatitis," chronic active hepatitis, cirrhosis, or fulminant hepatic failure. After an episode of "acute hepatitis," the patient may either appear to recover and then may be thought (erroneously) to have had a self-limited illness, or the patient may progress to fulminant hepatic failure. If the patient recovers, time may pass before the patient re-presents with liver or CNS disease. Patients with a presentation similar to that of chronic active hepatitis may have more insidious abdominal pain, fatigue, abdominal distension, hepatomegaly, splenomegaly, and jaundice. Patients with cirrhosis may demonstrate similar features as well as palmar erythema, spider nevi, hematemesis, and digital clubbing.

Fulminant hepatic failure is evident when the young patient exhibits hypoalbuminemia, coagulopathy, jaundice, and encephalopathy.[10] In the absence of a positive family history for neurologic, hepatic, or Wilson's disease, it becomes very difficult to distinguish fulminant hepatic failure of other causes from severe Wilson's disease. Thus, any child or adolescent with hepatic failure should be considered to have Wilson's disease until proved otherwise. The clinical presentation of chronic hepatitis may also progress within weeks to hepatic failure, ascites, renal insufficiency, and ultimately, death.[11] Young patients presenting with fulminant failure have a poor outcome, even if a diagnosis of Wilson's disease is made. Appropriate intervention with D-penicillamine may do little to halt the progression of hepatic necrosis for the patient who presents in hepatic failure; however, vigorous treatment should be instituted.

Chronic liver dysfunction can be seen in older patients who may demonstrate evidence of portal hypertension, cirrhosis, and other stigmata of liver disease; jaundice may or may not be present. Hepatocellular carcinoma in patients with Wilson's disease has been reported.[12] Presentation with histologic and clinical manifestations similar to chronic active hepatitis can even be seen in young patients. The classic features of Wilson's disease, such as Kayser-Fleischer rings, neurologic dysfunction, and altered serum ceruloplasmin levels, may not be present in these patients.

CNS Manifestations

CNS pathology typically involves the basal ganglia and can be quite extensive with a wide presentation of neurologic symptoms. Children may manifest evidence of neurologic disease as early as 6 years of age, but the typical presentation is in the second to third decade of life. Neurologic dysfunction is slow in progression, warranting a high clinical suspicion. Kayser-Fleischer rings are typically associated with the onset of neurologic findings. Motor system involvement predominates, with the sensory system virtually spared. Common symptoms include dystonia, incoordination, tremor, and difficulty with fine motor tasks. Without proper treatment and intervention, the patient may experience rigidity, drooling, dysarthria, mask-like facies, and gait disturbances. Intellect is unchanged, and the older patient is at risk of being diagnosed with a pure psychiatric disorder. This stage of disease may also resemble other conditions, such as multiple sclerosis or disorders of the basal ganglia.

Psychiatric Manifestations

Psychiatric manifestations may be evident at home, at school, or in the playground. Behaviors that may be observed include compulsivity, aggressiveness, impulsivity, depression, phobias, and declining performance in the classroom.[13] From this description of possible clinical symptoms, it is easy to understand how children may be inappropriately diagnosed with other psychiatric ailments. As in all patients with chronic illness, appropriate psychiatric evaluation should be made to differentiate symptoms that occur secondary to ongoing copper deposition from nonorganic psychological stress. As imagined, this can be very difficult.

Ophthalmologic Manifestations

The presence of ophthalmologic findings in patients suspected to have Wilson's disease may be helpful in the diagnosis prior to laboratory testing. Kayser-Fleischer rings consist of copper granules, deposited primarily in the stromal layer, with color change visible only in Descemet's membrane. Vision is not impaired due to copper deposition in the cornea. These rings have been described as a golden brown, brownish green, greenish yellow, bronze, or tannish green discoloration located in the limbic region of the cornea. Although visualization with the naked eye is possible, slit-lamp evaluation is mandatory. Owing to dependence on solvent flow and evaporation of tears from the cornea, copper is first seen in the superior and inferior areas of the limbus. Later, copper deposition is seen laterally to complete the ring. With appropriate therapy, these rings should fade and disappear.

When neurologic symptoms due to Wilson's disease are evident, Kayser-Fleischer rings are virtually always found. These may also be seen when only hepatic manifestations are present, but this is much less common.[14] Kayser-Fleischer rings are not specific for Wilson's disease, as they have been described in patients with chronic active hepatitis, cryptogenic cirrhosis, and primary biliary cirrhosis and in children with long-standing intrahepatic cholestasis.[15]

Other ophthalmologic findings in Wilson's disease include sunflower cataracts. These cataracts accompany Kayser-Fleischer rings and, when viewed with an ophthalmoscope, appear as golden discs in the anterior capsule of the lens. As with Kayser-Fleischer rings, sunflower cataracts typically resolve with therapy and usually do not impair visual function.

Renal Manifestations

Renal complications of Wilson's disease are expressed as disorders of proximal tubular function. This is exhibited as aminoaciduria, glycosuria, increased excretion of uric acid, and calcium, as well as decreased filtration rate.[16] Despite an acidification defect secondary to distal tubular dysfunction, patients with Wilson's disease are able to maintain normal or near-normal plasma pH values. Urolithiasis is precipitated by hypercalciuria and poor urine acidification. Therapy with copper chelating agents can improve renal function.

Skeletal Manifestations

Skeletal abnormalities induced by altered copper metabolism include osteoporosis, osteomalacia, rickets, spontaneous fractures, osteoarthritis, and osteochondritis dissecans.[17] Bone demineralization secondary to renal complications is most commonly seen. Radiographs add little to the evaluation, as abnormalities are infrequently seen in the pediatric population.

Other Manifestations

Cardiac manifestations have been seen in patients with Wilson's disease. Abnormalities in rhythm, electrocardiograms (ECGs), and autonomic tone have been de-scribed.[16] Autopsy findings have included cardiac hypertrophy, small vessel disease, and focal inflammation.[16]

Hemolysis is a known complication of Wilson's disease. Red blood cell destruction may be due to oxidative injury of the cell membrane from excess copper. Anemia may be the initial presentation of Wilson's disease. Cholelithiasis can occur either from hemolysis and/or cirrhosis.

DIAGNOSIS

The diagnosis of Wilson's disease may be difficult to verify, as no single test is confirmatory. If the classic triad of hepatic disease, neurologic manifestations, and Kayser-Fleischer rings is present, the diagnosis is more easily made. The classic triad rarely occurs; thus, the astute physician must have knowledge of the disease and a high clinical suspicion. A careful clinical history, family history, physical examination, and specific laboratory evaluations will provide the key to rapid diagnosis and required therapy. The differential diagnosis of liver involvement includes chronic autoimmune hepatitis, other forms of chronic hepatitis, and cryptogenic cirrhosis. Neurologic manifestations may mimic multiple sclerosis and a variety of psychiatric disorders.

LABORATORY TESTS

An initial screening complete blood count (CBC) performed in an ill child may display evidence of a hemolytic process. Liver function tests may be only mildly elevated or may indicate active hepatic inflammation with evidence of cholestasis, as demonstrated by an elevated total bilirubin. Serum uric acid and phosphate may be low, due to renal losses. Once the suspicion of Wilson's disease is raised, a 24-hour urine collection should be started to quantitate urine copper. A serum specimen should also be sent to determine the ceruloplasmin and copper levels.

Urine collections should be performed using a copper-free container. Normally, 24-hour copper excretion will be less than 40 μg in unaffected patients. Patients with Wilson's disease will have urinary copper excretion greater than 100 μg/day. This study is not specific for Wilson's disease, however, as elevated values for 24-hour urine collections for copper can be seen in chronic active hepatitis, primary biliary cirrhosis, fulminant hepatic failure, and cholestatic syndromes.[15] Other instances leading to difficult interpretation include those who are heterozygote carriers for Wilson's disease and the pre-symptomatic affected patient. Once the diagnosis is established, urinary copper excretion is a good study to follow during treatment.

Serum ceruloplasmin is decreased in the majority of asymptomatic patients with Wilson's disease as well as those with active hepatic disease. With the appropriate clinical presentation, the finding of a ceruloplasmin level of less than 20 mg/dl is suggestive of Wilson's disease. Levels may be increased during episodes of acute and chronic hepatitis, as ceruloplasmin may act as an acute-phase reactant. Decreased values may be seen in a number of conditions, including malnutrition, protein-losing enteropathy, nephrotic syndromes, severe hepatic insufficiency,[2] and hereditary hypoceruloplasminemia.[18] Normal neonates are found to have low values for ceruloplasmin relative to older children.

Slit-lamp evaluation for the presence of Kayser-Fleischer rings is required. These may be seen in more than one-half of patients with hepatic manifestations and in greater than 90% with neurologic findings. The absence of Kayser-Fleischer rings in a patient with neurologic or psychiatric findings essentially excludes the diagnosis of Wilson's disease. As Kayser-Fleischer rings may be seen in other conditions, they are not specific for Wilson's disease.

Liver biopsy remains the gold standard in the diagnosis of Wilson's disease. Quantitative hepatic content is crucial as part of this study. While normal hepatic copper content is less than 50 μg dry weight of liver, patients with Wilson's disease will have values of greater than 250 μg dry weight. An elevated hepatic copper content within the context of the appropriate clinical setting confirms the diagnosis of Wilson's disease. Elevated levels of hepatic copper may be seen in patients with other liver diseases, such as chronic autoimmune hepatitis. Negative stains for copper on liver biopsy never rule out Wilson's disease, as stored copper may be heterogeneously distributed. Histologic findings typically consist of steatosis and inflammation with or without fibrosis. Electron microscopy may be helpful as ultrastructural mitochondrial changes characteristic of Wilson's disease may be seen.

Computed tomography (CT) may be a useful study in both asymptomatic and symptomatic patients with Wilson's disease. Ventricular dilatation, cortical atrophy, brain stem atrophy, basal ganglia hypodensity, and posterior fossa atrophy are possible findings.[19] Changes seen on CT are secondary to damage by copper deposition. Extent of CT involvement does not give prognostic information, as patients with rather extensive disease may respond nicely to therapy. Magnetic resonance imaging (MRI) tends to be more sensitive and can further delineate CNS involvement.

Screening of relatives of patients with Wilson's disease should be performed. Screening should occur after age 3 to 5 years unless hepatomegaly or LFT derangements are seen earlier. All of the following should be accomplished: careful physical examination, determination of 24-hour urine copper excretion, levels of serum transaminases, ceruloplasmin, copper and haptoglobin, and slit lamp examination. If one of the above is abnormal, a liver biopsy should be obtained for histology, electron microscopy, and quantitative hepatic copper content.

TREATMENT

Once the diagnosis of Wilson's disease is made, therapy is essential to avoid a fatal outcome. Therapy first became available in 1951 with the introduction of 2,3-dimercaptopropanol (British Anti-Lewisite [BAL]), an agent that had to be given as daily intramuscular injections. In 1956, D-penicillamine was introduced as an effective form of therapy.[20] Sternlieb and Scheinberg[21] later showed that treatment of asymptomatic affected patients could prevent CNS and liver injury.

D-Penicillamine

D-Penicillamine, a copper chelating agent, is a sulfur-containing metabolite of penicillin. Initial starting doses should be small and gradually increased to 20 mg/kg body weight per day. Dose should not exceed 1 g/day (unless justified by the clinical status of the patient) and should be given in four divided doses. Dosing is at either 1 hour before meals or 2 hours after mealtime, as penicillamine is better absorbed in the absence of food. Appropriate supplementation with pyridoxine should be instituted as D-penicillamine may interfere with B_6 metabolism. Significant clinical improvement is seen within weeks with return to baseline in months, although this is not always the rule. If little improvement is seen, the dose of D-penicillamine may be increased to 1.5 to 2.0 g/day. One should always consider poor compliance if symptoms persist. Generally, symptoms improve first, followed by the disappearance or fading of Kayser-Fleischer rings, if present. Liver function tests will show improvement within several months, and hepatic copper content decreases subsequently. Liver pathology shows improvement with decreasing inflammation and necrosis. Urinary copper excretion will commonly be greater than 1,000 μg/day initially, decreasing after months of treatment. Patient compliance may be ascertained by the use of 24-hour urinary copper collections. Another method to evaluate compliance involves obtaining spot determinations of serum ceruloplasmin and serum copper to assess the amount of free copper. The ceruloplasmin value (in μg/dl) is multiplied by a factor of 3 and subtracted from the serum copper value. If the remaining number is greater than 20, the patient has not been compliant.

Side effects from D-penicillamine include fever, rash, leukopenia, thrombocytopenia, and lymphadenopathy.[21] These findings may occur within weeks of initiating therapy in as many as 20% of patients. Other significant drug complications include proteinuria, lupus-like syndrome, Goodpasture's syndrome, and pemphigoid of the mouth.[15] Significant reactions should be treated with cessation of therapy. Pretreatment with steroids should be instituted 2 to 3 days prior to reintroducing D-penicillamine. The dose of D-penicillamine should be lowered initially when treatment is resumed. Prednisone may be discontinued once therapy is well tolerated.

There has been concern for worsening neurologic symptoms secondary to the introduction of D-penicillamine. This may be due to large amounts of copper released from the liver and deposited in the CNS at the onset of therapy. Starting with a smaller dose and gradually increasing medication may perhaps preclude this occurrence. Concern for this possible complication has led to searches for other therapeutic modalities. Renal failure makes treatment with D-penicillamine difficult. Pregnancy is not a contraindication to the use of D-penicillamine.

Patients who abruptly stop therapy may be at risk of massive copper release and subsequent deposition. This has been hypothesized in cases where death has occurred within one year after drug cessation. The proposed mechanism by Scheinberg and colleagues is complexing of D-penicillamine with copper to form a nontoxic moiety. This complex may suddenly disassociate when therapy is discontinued leading to massive copper release.

Trientine

Triethylene tetramine dihydrochloride (Trientine) was introduced in 1969 as an alternative to D-penicillamine.[22] Copper chelation is as effective as with D-penicillamine. Once placed on Trientine, patients should experience reversal of prior side effects from D-penicillamine. Dosage is 1 to 1.5 g/day in divided doses given 1 hour before meals or 2 hours after eating. The dose for younger children is 20 mg/kg of body weight given daily.[23]

Zinc

Zinc is a known antagonist of copper absorption used as primary and adjunctive therapy for Wilson's disease. An appropriate dose for children is 25 mg per dose, given three times per day, and at least 1 hour after ingestion of food. Urinary copper reflects total body copper burden and should be less than 125 μg per 24-hour collection.

Other Therapies

Dietary copper sources (e.g., animal liver, kidney, shellfish, chocolate, dried beans, peas, and unprocessed wheat) should be restricted. Ammonium tetrathiomolybdate is a recently introduced therapy that acts by complexing ingested copper and preventing absorption. This agent will also complex with copper and albumin in the blood, preventing uptake. Orthotopic liver transplantation is now an accepted form of therapy with specific indications; it is indicated for patients with Wilson's disease with fulminant hepatic failure, decompensated cirrhosis with end-stage liver disease, and worsening disease despite intensive therapy. The outcome in these patients has been favorable; a recent review showed a 77% survival rate at 2.7 years after transplantation.[24] Neurologic symptoms have been shown to improve after transplantation, and further copper chelation is unnecessary.

REFERRAL PATTERN

Once the diagnosis of Wilson's disease is suspected, time is of the essence, as therapy can be life-saving. Laboratory evaluation for Wilson's disease should be initiated locally only if results can be obtained in an expedient manner. Otherwise, the patient should be referred immediately to a pediatric gastroenterologist for evaluation and workup.

Follow-up evaluation after the diagnosis has been made must occur in a coordinated fashion between primary care provider and subspecialist. Monitoring of therapy should include liver function tests, 24-hour urinary copper quantitation, serum ceruloplasmin, serum copper, and periodic ophthalmologic examinations. One would expect liver function tests to decline to normal values over the first year of therapy. Urinary copper values may initially fall within the range of 1 to 3 mg/day, but over months to years of therapy will typically come to lie within 300 to 800 μg/day. Values of less than 300 μg/day should raise concerns about poor compliance. For example, sudden elevations in urinary copper values could reflect a pattern of discontinuation of medicines followed by recent reinitiation of therapy close to the time of each appointment. Kayser-Fleischer rings, if present, should fade with therapy.

REFERENCES

1. Wilson SAK. Progressive lenticular degeneration: a familial nervous disease associated with cirrhosis of the liver. Brain 1912;34:295–509

2. Scheinberg IH, Sternlieb I. Wilson's Disease. Philadelphia: WB Saunders, 1984

3. Frommer DJ. Defective biliary excretion of copper in Wilson's disease. Gut 1974;15:125–129

4. Hill GM, Brewer GJ, Prasad AS et al. Treatment of Wilson's disease with zinc. I. Oral zinc therapy regimens. Hepatology 1987;7:522–528

5. Holden JM, Wolf WR, Mertz W. Zinc and copper in self selected diets. J Am Diet Assoc 1979;75:23–28

6. Strickland GT, Becker WM, Leu ML. Absorption of copper

in homozygotes and heterozygotes for Wilson's disease and controls: isotope tracer studies with [67]copper-[64]copper. Clin Sci 1972;43:617–625

7. Jacob RA, Sandstead HH, Munoz JM, et al. Whole body surface loss of trace metals in normal males. Am J Clin Nutr 1981;34:1379–1383

8. Sternlieb I, Scheinberg IH. Radiocopper in diagnosing liver disease. Semin Nucl Med 1972;2:176–188

9. Gibbs K, Walshe JM. Biliary excretion of copper in Wilson's disease. Lancet 1980;2:538–539

10. Doering EG III, Savage RA, Dittmer TE. Hemolysis, coagulation defects and fulminant hepatic failure as a presentation of Wilson's disease. Am J Dis Child 1979;133:440–441

11. Adler R, Matinovski V, Heuser ET et al. Fulminant hepatitis: a presentation of Wilson's disease. Am J Dis Child 1977; 131:870–872

12. Terao H, Itakura H, Nakota K et al. An autopsy case of hepatocellular carcinoma in Wilson's disease. Acta Hepatol Jpn 1982;23:439–445

13. Goldstein NP, Ewert MA, Randall RV, Gross JB. Psychiatric aspects of Wilson's disease (hepatolenticular degeneration). Results of psychometric tests during long-term therapy. Am J Psychiatry 1968;124:1555–1561

14. Werlin SL, Grand RJ, Perman JA, Watkins JB. Diagnostic dilemmas of Wilson's disease: diagnosis and treatment. Pediatrics 1978;62:47–51

15. Pleskow RG, Grand RJ. Wilson's disease. In: Walker WA, Durie PR, Hamilton JR et al, Eds. Pediatric Gastrointestinal Disease: Pathophysiology, Diagnosis, Management. 2nd Ed. St Louis: Mosby-Year Book, 1996:1233–1246

16. Sokol RJ. Wilson's disease and Indian childhood cirrhosis. In: Suchy FJ, Ed. Liver Disease in Children. St Louis: Mosby-Year Book, 1994:747–764

17. Mindelzun R, Elkin M, Scheinberg IH, Sternlieb I. Skeletal changes in Wilson's disease. A radiological study. Radiology 1970;94:127–132

18. Edwards CQ, Williams DM, Cartwright GE. Hereditary hypoceruloplasminemia. Clin Genet 1979;15:311–316

19. Williams FJB, Walshe JM. Wilson's disease. An analysis of the cranial computerized tomographic appearances found in 60 patients and the changes in response to treatment with chelating agents. Brain 1981;104:735–752

20. Walshe JM. Penicillamine, a new oral therapy for Wilson's disease. Am J Med 1956;21:487–495

21. Sternlieb I, Scheinberg IH. Penicillamine therapy in hepatolenticular degeneration. JAMA 1964;189:748–754

22. Walshe JM. Management of penicillamine nephropathy in Wilson's disease: a new chelating agent. Lancet 1969;2: 1401–1402

23. Trientine for Wilson's disease. Med Lett Drug Ther 1986; 28:67

24. Schilsky ML, Scheinberg IH, Sternlieb I. Hepatic transplantation for Wilson's disease: indications and outcome. Hepatology 1992;16:50A

64

CONTRAST STUDIES

FREDERICK R. LONG

GENERAL INDICATIONS

Gastrointestinal (GI) contrast studies provide important information that may not be obtained by endoscopy or other imaging modalities. They are ideal for demonstrating bowel obstructions secondary to masses, strictures, adhesions, or volvulus; for identifying the location of bowel perforations or fistulas; for characterizing mucosal or intraluminal abnormalities such as ulceration and polyps; and for evaluating postoperative anatomy and complications. Table 64-1 groups the more common pathologic entities that are well demonstrated by contrast studies according to major GI symptoms.

Contrast Media

Barium is the intraluminal contrast agent of choice because it is inexpensive and produces the highest-quality images owing to its high attenuation of X-rays and good mucosal coating properties. Water-soluble contrast agents are used instead of barium in the following circumstances: (1) risk of barium leakage because barium acts as a foreign body and incites an inflammatory response, (2) if endoscopy or computed tomography (CT) is planned immediately following a barium study because barium is an opaque medium and causes CT streak artifacts, and (3) if there is risk of barium inspissation, as in patients with cystic fibrosis. The newer and more expensive low-osmolality, near-isotonic water-soluble contrast agents produce adequate images and are used when there is risk of aspiration or when performing studies on infants, who are the most sensitive to fluid shifts.[1]

Single Versus Double Contrast

In pediatrics, single-contrast rather than double-contrast studies (using air and high-density barium) are usually perfomed. Single-contrast studies do not require the same degree of patient cooperation, are better tolerated, and are best at demonstrating the most common pathologic conditions encountered. For example, "rule out malrotation," which is more readily diagnosed by single-contrast technique, is one of the most common reasons for performing a pediatric upper GI examination. On the other hand, peptic ulcer disease, which may be better visualized by double-contrast technique, is uncommon in children less than 10 years old.[2]

MAJOR INDICATIONS BY SYMPTOMS

Dysphagia

Dysphagia, which is defined as difficulty with swallowing, is broadly interpreted in this section to include painful swallowing, stridor, and choking from reflux or aspiration. The evaluation usually commences with a video swallowing study for swallowing dysfunction or with an esophagram for evaluation of motility disorders, tracheoesophageal fistulas, inflammatory disease, gastroesophageal reflux, hiatal hernia, or intrinsic and extrinsic obstructing lesions. Intrinsic obstructions may be the result of foreign bodies, congenital stenoses, or inflammatory strictures secondary to caustic ingestion or gastroesophageal reflux. Extrinsic obstructing lesions include vascular rings and mediastinal masses. The major limita-

457

TABLE 64-1. Choice of Contrast Study Based on Major Indication

Major Indication	Esophagram	UGI	SBFT	Enema
Dysphagia				
Vascular ring	X			
Aspiration	X			
Tracheoesophageal fistula	X			
Esophageal stricture	X			
Vomiting				
Gastric volvulus		X		
Malrotation		X		X
Duodenal hematoma		X		
Superior mesenteric artery syndrome		X		
Hirschsprung's disease				X
Intussusception				X
Meconium ileus				X
Distal atresia/volvulus				X
Abdominal pain				
Bezoar		X		
Malrotation		X		X
Peptic ulcer disease		X[a]		
Inflammatory bowel disease		X	X	X
Rectal bleeding				
Intussusception				X
Colitis				X[a]
Polyps			X	X[a]

Abbreviations: UGI, upper gastrointestinal contrast examination; SBFT, small bowel follow-through.

[a] Double-contrast examination preferred if appropriate age.

tion of the esophagram is its inability to detect mild to moderate esophagitis, which is usually caused by gastroesophageal reflux.[3]

A common indication for an esophagram is to evaluate a child with a suspected vascular ring, in whom the radiographic findings are usually characteristic. A less common indication is in the child with paroxysmal choking or recurrent pneumonia for a suspected "H type" tracheoesophageal fistula. This anomaly is rare and may not always be identified on a routine study unless special techniques are used, such as studying the patient in the prone position or obtaining distended views of the esophagus by direct injection of barium.[3]

Vomiting

Vomiting is a common symptom with a large number of potential causes. Contrast studies are indicated when bowel obstruction is suspected on the basis of history or plain radiographs. In infants with recurrent vomiting suggestive of benign gastroesophageal reflux, an upper GI examination is not routinely needed. When the pattern of reflux is atypical or does not respond to the usual

medical management, an upper GI is recommended to exclude an underlying obstructing condition or structural anomaly (Fig. 64-1).[4]

Aside from hypertrophic pyloric stenosis, gastric outlet obstructions as a cause of vomiting are rare and include gastric volvulus, complications of ulcers, eosinophilic gastritis, leiomyomas, duplication cysts, and pyloric or prepyloric congenital webs or atresias, all of which can be demonstrated on upper GI examination. Hypertrophic pyloric stenosis can be well demonstrated by upper GI, but if the diagnosis is strongly suspected by history, ultrasound is the usual initial study, as it directly images the hypertrophied musculature and avoids radiation exposure.[5]

Obstructing lesions of the duodenum or small bowel are well demonstrated on contrast examinations and include malrotation with Ladd's bands or midgut volvulus (see the section *Specific Diseases*, below), hematoma secondary to trauma or vasculitis (Fig. 64-2), superior mesenteric artery syndrome, and adhesions or strictures.[3] Congenital duodenal atresias or webs or jejunal atresias are usually found on plain film evaluation due to a characteristic "double bubble" appearance or proximal bowel distention with air-fluid levels. Further radiographic evaluation with contrast studies is usually not necessary.[6]

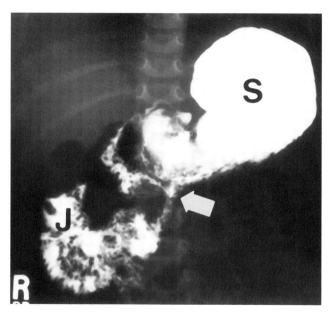

FIGURE 64-1. Three-year-old girl with persistent abdominal pain and nonbilious vomiting. Image obtained at upper GI examination depicts the duodenojejunal junction (arrow) to be low and midline, indicative of malrotation, with the jejunum (J) in the right upper quadrant. At surgery, the mesenteric base was narrow with a tight isthmus and dilated veins suggestive of intermittent volvulus. S, stomach.

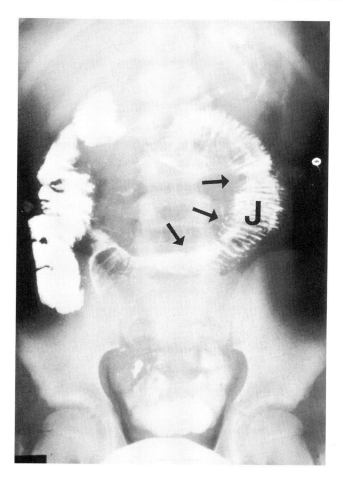

FIGURE 64-2. Twelve-year-old boy with severe abdominal pain and vomiting. Delayed image obtained at upper GI examination and small bowel follow-through demonstrates a long segment of fold thickening (arrows) involving the jejunum (J). At surgery, this segment was resected and represented an organizing submucosal hematoma from suspected nonaccidental trauma.

If a distal bowel obstruction (distal ileum or colon) is suspected on the basis of multiple distended or fluid-filled bowel loops on abdominal radiographs, a contrast enema is the preferred initial study. This approach allows one to exclude a colonic etiology (Fig. 64-3) and to possibly define more clearly the level of obstruction if free reflux of barium into the distal ileum is obtained. Contrast medium from above in cases of suspected distal small bowel obstruction may require much more time to reach the level of obstruction and may be difficult to interpret. An upper GI and small bowel follow-through can always be subsequently performed after contrast evacuation if the enema is nondiagnostic. A contrast enema is particularly useful in neonatal obstructions, when Hirschsprung's disease (see the section *Specific Diseases*, below), ileal atresia, meconium ileus, colonic atresia, or complications secondary to malrotation frequently present.[3]

Abdominal Pain

Contrast studies are usually employed for chronic or recurrent abdominal pain to exclude an underlying obstructing lesion (Fig. 64-4) or inflammatory bowel or peptic ulcer disease. The etiology of acute pain will often be diagnosed by other imaging modalities; for example, ultrasound is now preferred instead of barium enema in the diagnosis of atypical appendicitis, followed by CT in complicated cases.[7]

In the evaluation of peptic ulcer disease, upper endoscopy is frequently employed in diagnosis because of its sensitivity in identifying mucosal disease and ease in obtaining biopsy specimens. Barium studies are limited

FIGURE 64-3. Seven-year-old boy with sudden abdominal pain and vomiting. Image obtained at barium enema examination depicts an obstruction in the transverse colon. At the site of obstruction, the barium column ends in a ''beak'' indicative of volvulus (arrows). At surgery, the patient had malrotation with volvulus of the transverse colon. C, colon.

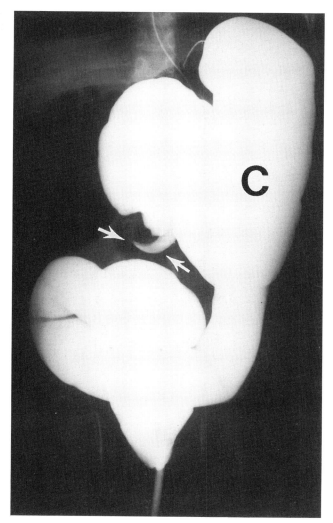

in detecting subtle mucosal disease, particularly of the esophagus, but will demonstrate more advanced changes. Upper GI studies in children report varying ulcer detection rates of 14% to 50% for gastric ulcer and 50% to 89% for duodenal ulcer.[2,8]

Gastrointestinal Bleeding

Endoscopy plays a major role in the diagnosis of GI bleeding in which ulcerative or inflammatory conditions predominate. Contrast studies play a complementary role, particularly in the diagnosis of polyps (Fig. 64-5). In lower GI bleeding, contrast studies are indicated if intussusception is suspected, as the diagnosis can easily be excluded and effective treatment provided if intussusception is found (see the section *Specific Diseases*, below).

FIGURE 64-4. Ten-year-old boy with a 1-month history of abdominal pain and blood in the stool. Image obtained at double-contrast barium enema examination demonstrates an obstruction of the barium column at the transverse colon by an intraluminal mass (arrowheads). The mass represented an ileocolic intussusception secondary to involvement of the ileum with Burkitt's lymphoma. C, colon.

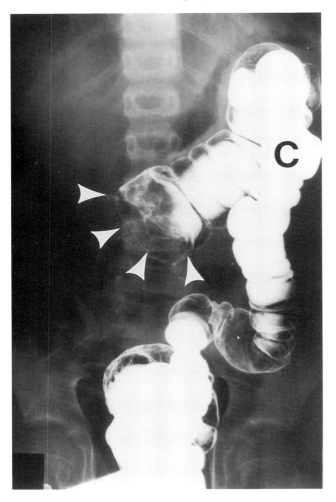

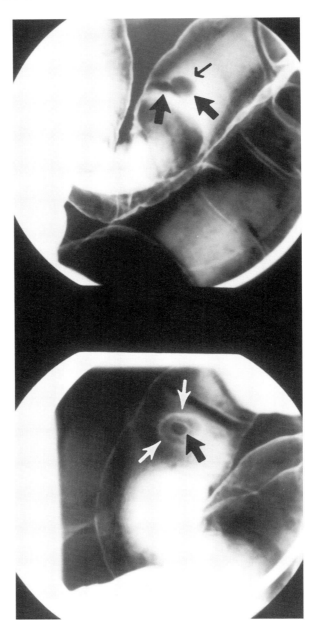

FIGURE 64-5. Four-year-old boy with painless rectal bleeding. Two images obtained from a double-contrast barium enema examination demonstrate a pedunculated polyp in the sigmoid colon. On the upper image, a prone view shows the polyp (arrows) as a filling defect in a pool of barium. On the lower image, the stalk of the polyp (black arrow) and the head of the polyp (white arrows) are seen on end, coated by a thin ring of barium.

Malabsorption

The causes of malabsorption, of which cystic fibrosis and celiac disease are most common, are usually diagnosed clinically and by laboratory studies. Contrast examinations may suggest malabsorption if there is flocculation and segmentation of the barium column, dilated loops

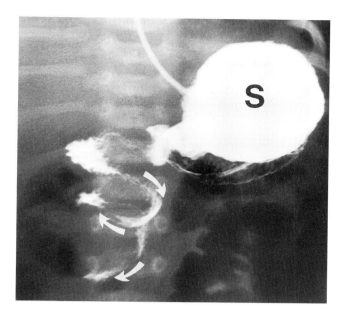

FIGURE 64-6. Thirteen-year-old girl with bilious vomiting. Image obtained at upper GI examination reveals a corkscrew configuration (arrows) of the duodenum and jejunum. Midgut volvulus without ischemia was found at surgery. S, stomach. (From Long et al,[10] with permission.)

of small bowel, or thickening of mucosal folds. Unfortunately, the findings are nonspecific and can be seen in the absence of malabsorption.[9]

SPECIFIC DISEASES

Malrotation

"Malrotation" encompasses both an abnormality of rotation or position of the bowel and an abnormality of fixation, which predispose the midgut to twist or volvulate around its vascular pedicle (Fig. 64-6), with potentially life-threatening consequences, namely infarction of the midgut. Malrotation is well known for presenting with a wide variety of symptoms, including bilious or nonbilious vomiting, intermittent abdominal pain, malabsorption, and failure to thrive.[10] Symptoms may result from obstructing Ladd's bands or volvulus, which may be intermittent. Children most commonly develop symptoms in the first year of life, but symptoms including life-threatening volvulus may occur at any age, including adulthood. Thus, clinicians must always consider the possibility of malrotation in a child with GI complaints.[10]

The radiographic diagnosis of malrotation is usually straightforward, but in approximately 16% of cases, it may be difficult, requiring a radiologist with experience

and specialized training.[11] Both the duodenum and colon are usually abnormally positioned in the patient with malrotation, thus, an upper GI study or barium enema can be performed to make the diagnosis. Presently in the United States, the upper GI examination has become the favored first study because the cecum can normally be mobile in up to 15% of all age groups, causing confusion with malrotation, and the cecum may be in a normal position in the right lower quadrant in 5% to 10% of children with malrotation.[10] The upper GI study, however, is technically more difficult to perform and requires a clear delineation of the duodenal sweep and identification of the duodenojejunal junction, the site of insertion of the ligament of Treitz, which represents a key landmark for normal fixation of the proximal midgut. Unfortunately, normal variants of the duodenum may occasionally be difficult to distinguish from malrotation.[11]

It is recognized that on rare occasions the upper GI examination can be "normal" in the face of malrotation. This may occur in the unusual case of isolated colonic malrotation (with normal rotation/fixation of the duodenum), which may result in symptoms related to distal bowel obstruction secondary to adhesive bands or distal volvulus. It may also be related to an abnormally fixed duodenum and jejunum approximating a "normal position" by chance.[11] The routine addition of a small bowel follow-through to the upper GI study to increase sensitivity in detecting malrotation by identifying an abnormal position of the cecum is not recommended.[11] The cost (length of the examination, additional charge, and additional radiation exposure) would greatly exceed the very small increased diagnostic yield. In addition, the rate of misdiagnoses might actually increase because normal cecal mobility, as stated earlier, can be misinterpreted as malrotation. However, it should be emphasized that one should not hesitate to perform a barium enema or repeat the upper GI examination in a patient who has had a normal upper GI study but in whom there is still a high index of suspicion for malrotation.[10,11]

Inflammatory Bowel Disease

The two most common types of inflammatory bowel disease, ulcerative colitis and Crohn's disease, have similar radiographic appearances to those seen in adults.[12] Crohn's disease is characterized by transmural inflammation, in contrast to the more limited mucosal and possible submucosal involvement of ulcerative colitis. In ulcerative colitis, the mucosa initially has a granular appearance, which may progress to ulceration that may deepen to track in the submucosa, forming "collar button" ulcers. In Crohn's disease, the earliest lesions are "aphthous erosions," which may deepen to form linear ulcers that penetrate the full thickness of the bowel wall to form fistulous tracts.[13] The most frequent radiographic signs of Crohn's disease, which reflect transmural inflam-

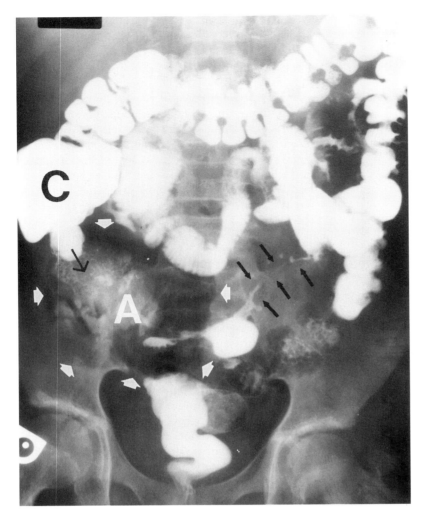

FIGURE 64-7. Fourteen-year-old girl with Crohn's disease. A delayed image obtained following a barium enema and small bowel follow-through demonstrates an air-filled abscess cavity (A, outlined by white arrows) containing extravasated barium from a cecal (C) perforation. Note the narrowed segment of ileum (black arrows).

mation, are thickened folds, which may be nodular and irregular, and luminal narrowing.[12] Deep ulceration and irregular fold thickening may result in a "cobblestone" appearance. The end stages of both diseases may have similar appearances secondary to fibrosis or pseudopolyp formation.[12,13]

In contrast to ulcerative colitis, Crohn's disease may have "skip areas" of involvement that asymmetrically involve the bowel wall. In addition, Crohn's disease often involves both the small and large bowel, whereas ulcerative colitis is limited to the colon. Crohn's disease is estimated to be ileocolonic in 73% of cases, with terminal ileal involvement in over 80%.[14] The differential diagnosis of terminal ileal disease includes tuberculosis, amebiasis, and *Yersinia* infection. Rarely, the terminal ileum may be normal in the presence of small bowel disease. Proximal small bowel disease, including of the duodenum, may be more common (approximately 30%) than is generally appreciated, according to endoscopic biopsy studies.[14]

Gastrointestinal contrast studies are employed to initially evaluate the anatomic extent of disease, which

in the absence of surgery changes little over time. The radiographic detection rate for Crohn's disease is reported to be approximately 90%.[13] Detection may be increased by performing a "preoral pneumocolon" or enterolysis in select cases.[13] Routine radiologic follow-up studies are not necessary. However, they are indicated in the evaluation of suspected complications (Fig. 64-7), such as obstruction, fistula formation, and abscess, as well as for suspected postoperative recurrence.[14]

Hirschsprung's Disease

Although usually a disease of infancy (25% of neonatal obstructions), Hirschsprung's disease may occasionally be found in older children with long-standing constipation.[14] In infants, a contrast enema is usually the first study obtained, as it helps to differentiate among various causes of "failure to pass meconium."[3] The radiographic diagnosis centers on the detection of a "transition zone" between small or normal caliber distal bowel and more dilated proximal bowel, which reflects the failure of relaxation of the aganglionic segment.[14] Occasionally, functional immaturity of the colon may mimic a transition zone. The transition zone may be gradual or abrupt, and it is not always seen, particularly in the first weeks of life and in patients with total colonic or "ultrashort" segment aganglionosis.[3] The identification of irregular contractions (Fig. 64-8) in the aganglionic segment is another reliable sign, which is not as frequently seen.[15] The radiographic detection of Hirschsprung's disease has a sensitivity reported of approximately 55% to 70% and a high specificity (near 100%) if irregular contractions or a transition zone is identified.[15] The retention of barium after 24 or 48 hours on a delayed radiograph is a nonspecific finding that has not been clearly defined as a diagnostic tool (a false-positive rate reported of 27% and false-negative rate of 42%).[15]

Intussusception

Intestinal intussusception is the most common abdominal emergency in young children (less than 2 years old). When intussusception is suspected, after surgical consultation, a liquid or air enema is indicated for diagnosis

and treatment except in cases of bowel perforation, peritonitis, and septic shock. Bowel perforation during attempted reduction is estimated to occur in less than 1% of cases.[16]

Air contrast enemas or pneumatic reduction techniques have become popular and are now the method of choice in many large pediatric centers. Pneumatic reduction techniques have recently been demonstrated to be more effective, faster, and safer than hydrostatic techniques. The enhanced margin of safety is due to smaller and less complicated perforations with air if they should occur. Success rates of 75% to 95% are now reported using continuous monitoring of insufflated pressure.[16]

CONCLUSION

Gastrointestinal contrast studies still play a major role in the diagnosis of GI disease and have not been replaced by more technologically advanced and expensive modalities. The quality of fluoroscopic contrast examinations is very operator dependent, requiring experience and special expertise. In the hands of an experienced radiologist, they remain a formidable diagnostic technique.

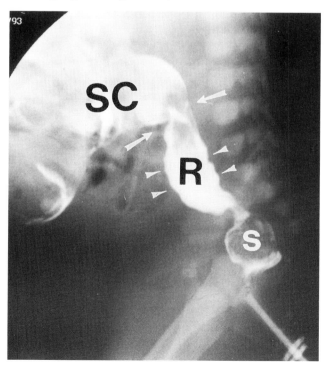

FIGURE 64-8. Three-week-old boy with Hirschsprung's disease. Lateral image obtained at barium enema examination after initial filling of the rectum (R) and sigmoid colon (SC). There is a transition zone (arrows) between dilated proximal sigmoid colon and the narrowed distal aganglionic rectum. Note the irregular contractions (arrowheads) of the aganglionic segment. S, stool.

REFERENCES

1. Cohen MD. Choosing contrast media for the evaluation of the gastrointestinal tract of neonates and infants. Radiology 1987;162:447–456
2. Drumm B, Rhoads JM, Stringer DA et al. Peptic ulcer disease in children: etiology, clinical findings, and clinical course. Pediatrics 1988;82:410–414
3. Stringer DA. Pediatric Gastrointestinal Imaging. Toronto: BC Decker, 1989
4. Miller JH, Gelfand MJ. Pediatric Nuclear Medicine. Philadelphia: WB Saunders, 1994
5. Hernanz-Schulman M, Sells LL, Ambrosino MM et al. Hypertrophic pyloric stenosis in the infant without a palpable olive: accuracy of sonographic diagnosis. Radiology 1994; 193:771–776
6. Schnaufer L: Duodenal atresia, stenosis and annular pancreas. In: Welch KJ, Randolph JG, Ravitch MM et al, Eds. Pediatric Surgery. Chicago: Year Book Medical Publishers, 1986
7. Franken EA, Kao SS, Smith WL, Sato Y. Imaging of the acute abdomen in infants and children. ASR 1989;153: 921–928
8. Nord K, Rossi TM, Lebenthal E. Peptic ulcer in children. Am J Gastroenterol 1981;75:153–157
9. Weizman Z, Stringer DA, Durie P. Radiologic manifestations of malabsorption: a nonspecific finding. Pediatrics 1984;74: 530–533
10. Long FR, Kramer SS, Markowitz RI, Taylor GE. Radiographic patterns of intestinal malrotation in children. Radiographics 1996;16:547–560

11. Long FR, Kramer SS, Markowitz RI et al. Intestinal malrotation in children: tutorial on radiographic diagnosis in difficult cases. Radiology 1996;198:775–780

12. Stringer DA. Imaging inflammatory bowel disease in the pediatric patient. Radiol Clin North Am 1987;25:93–113

13. Glick SN. Crohn's disease of the small intestine. Radiol Clin North Am 1987;25:25–45

14. Roy CC, Silverman A, Alagille D. Pediatric Clinical Gastroenterology. 4th Ed. St. Louis: Mosby-Year Book, 1995

15. Rosenfield NS, Ablow RC, Markowitz RI et al. Hirschsprung disease: accuracy of the barium enema examination. Radiology 1984;150:393–400

16. Shiels WE. Childhood intussusception: management perspectives in 1995. J Pediatr Gastroenterol Nutr 1995;21:15–17

65

ABDOMINAL ULTRASOUND

RICHARD D. BELLAH

Technologic advancements in high-resolution ultrasonography have opened opportunities to the pediatric sonographer for more careful assessment of the pediatric gastrointestinal (GI) tract. The lack of significant gas or fat, as well as the small size of most pediatric patients, also facilitates better resolution of the alimentary canal (and wall), from esophagus to rectum. Knowledge of the sonographic appearance of the normal bowel wall is basic for understanding and diagnosing maladies that afflict the pediatric GI tract.

NORMAL BOWEL WALL

The normal bowel wall has five layers: mucosa, muscularis mucosae, submucosa, lamina propria, and serosa. Under optimal (often experimental) conditions, these five layers can be clearly resolved sonographically as alternating layers of echogenic (hypoechoic, hyperechoic) tissue. The superficial mucosal layer is echogenic compared to the muscularis mucosae. The submucosa is echogenic compared to the muscularis mucosae, and the lamina propria is hypoechoic relative to the mucosa and serosa. The ability of the sonographer to distinguish these layers depends on the frequency of the transducer, the acoustic window, and the proximity of the probe to the structure being examined (Fig. 65-1). In most clinical settings, these five layers are difficult to resolve separately. Hence, the bowel wall may simply appear with a hyperechoic inner wall and a hypoechoic outer wall, like the distal esophagus (Fig. 65-2), or as a target, like the gastric antrum.[1] The presence of intra- or extraluminal

fluid (ascites) helps one to more clearly evaluate the outer wall of the bowel and its overall thickness. It is apparent that sonography does have distinct advantages over barium studies, which provide only limited information about the mucosal surface of the bowel.

Clinical applications of sonography to the pediatric GI tract usually involve the evaluation of the infant or child with vomiting (obstruction), GI bleeding, abdominal pain, or mass. In most instances, the pathology that exists, whether it involves the stomach, small bowel, or colon, manifests itself sonographically as bowel wall thickening. The principal questions that investigators should ask themselves when faced with these clinical concerns are (1) is this a normal-appearing bowel wall, (2) is this bowel wall abnormally thickened in a way that might account for this patient's symptomatology, and (3) which layers of bowel wall are abnormally involved?

ESOPHAGUS

Gastroesophageal Reflux

Sonography can provide morphologic information about the gastroesophageal junction (including length of the abdominal esophagus) that has some relevance in gastroesophageal reflux studies.[2] Sonography can detect gastroesophageal reflux in some infants when the lower esophageal sphincter opens and gastric fluid enters the distal esophagus. Practically speaking, however, this evaluation can be time-consuming and requires careful technique if

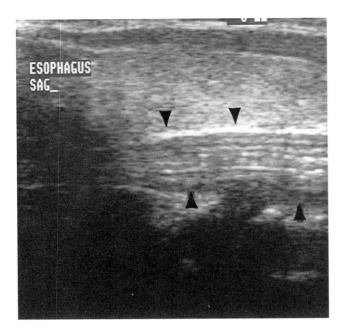

FIGURE 65-1. Normal cervical esophagus. High-resolution ultrasound sagittal view of cervical esophagus (arrows) shows alternating bands of hyper- and hypoechogenicity corresponding to bowel wall layers.

useful functional data about the gastroesophageal junction are to be obtained.

Gastroesophageal Varices

Formed from the coronary vein, esophageal varices appear sonographically as tortuous vessels near the (gastroesophageal) junction. One may identify either varices or thickening of the lesser omentum (without visualization of vessels) (Fig. 65-3) as evidence of portosystemic collateral formation in portal hypertension.[3]

STOMACH

Hypertrophic Pyloric Stenosis

Since the first description of hypertrophic pyloric stenosis (HPS) with sonography in 1977, sonography has been the preferred method for evaluating the infant (typically 3 to 8 weeks) with nonbilious projectile vomiting. In experienced hands, the examination can be done quickly and with accuracy approaching 100%. With a high-frequency transducer (7.5 megahertz, 10 megahertz), the sonographer examines the infant in the supine and/or right decubitus position; the latter position helps to distend the gastric antrum with fluid. Although some may feed water during the examination when HPS exists, a moderate amount of retained fluid is often already present within the stomach. Technical problems arise when there is (1) a tense crying infant difficult to examine, (2) gas artifact, or (3) overdistention of the stomach with fluid, causing the pylorus to orient itself more posteriorly. Sonographic findings of "classic" HPS include elongation of the pyloric channel by 17 mm or greater and thickening of the pyloric muscle.[4] Thickening of the pyloric muscle is most reliable if the diameter is 4 mm or greater (Fig. 65-4). One needs to be aware, however, that the size of the muscle mass may vary according to infant age; that is, in younger infants (3 weeks) muscle thickening may be between 3 and 4 mm. In some instances, sonography can be used to follow the evolution of HPS if the diagnosis is suspected and initial measurements do not meet suggested criteria. Pyloro-

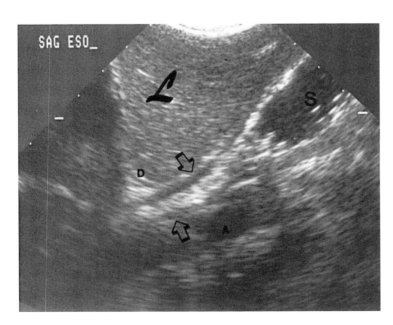

FIGURE 65-2. Normal gastroesophageal junction. Transabdominal ultrasound sagittal view of the esophagus near the gastroesophageal junction shows hypoechoic (outer) smooth muscular layers (arrows) surrounding the hyperechoic (inner) mucosa. L, liver; S, stomach; D, diaphragm; A, aorta.

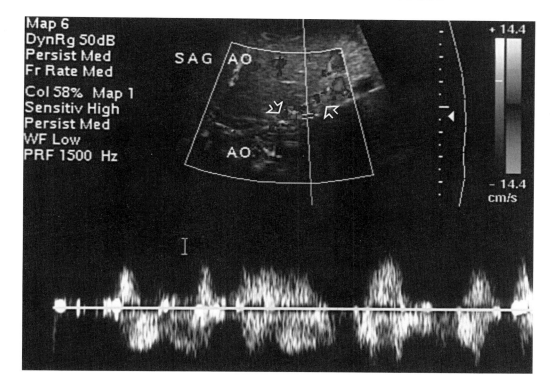

FIGURE 65-3. Omental varices (portal hypertension). Pulsed wave Doppler ultrasound (and color flow Doppler ultrasound) near the esophageal hiatus shows thickening of the lesser omentum (arrows). The spectral Doppler waveform shows a complex venous pattern consistent with collateral venous (variceal) blood flow. Ao, aorta.

spasm that causes contraction and pseudothickening of the pyloric muscle does not result in muscle thickening of any significant degree and should be distinguishable from HPS. Following surgery, sonography should not be used to assess incomplete pyloromyotomy, as it may take 4 to 6 weeks for the muscle mass of HPS to recede.

Gastritis

Gastritis and peptic ulcer disease are relatively rare in children. Abnormal sonographic findings may be found incidentally during an examination for abdominal pain, hematemesis, or vomiting, even in an infant. Gastritis may be idiopathic, associated with stress or medication (steroids), or be immune-related (eosinophilic gastritis) (Fig. 65-5). Sonographic findings in gastritis include variable thickening of the gastric mucosa and submucosa (between 4 and 7 mm) and elongation of the antropyloric channel.[5] Thickening may be focal or diffuse. Ulcers are not easily identifiable on sonography in children.

Other Conditions

Other pediatric conditions that may cause gastric wall thickening and smooth, lobulated, or redundant folds include Ménétrier's disease, a protein-losing enteropathy

frequently associated with cytomegalovirus (CMV) infection (Fig. 65-6); chronic granulomatous disease of childhood (circumferential antral thickening); and prostaglandin-induced foveolar hyperplasia.

Benign gastric neoplasms (polyps, leiomyoma, teratoma) are rare in children. Malignant non-Hodgkin's lymphoma occasionally involves the stomach, producing diffuse gastric wall thickening due to tumor infiltration. At sonography, the tumor appears diffusely hypoechoic but is not always distinguishable from inflammatory (non-neoplastic) conditions affecting the stomach. Clinical correlation is usually necessary.

SMALL BOWEL

Aside from the proximal portion of the duodenum and the distal ileum, the small bowel is generally difficult to assess sonographically unless it is pathologically affected. Positive contrast studies, like barium upper GI series or computed tomography, are far more effective in allowing one to evaluate the small bowel. If gas does not obscure the sound beam, and if intraluminal fluid accumulation caused by intestinal obstruction exists or extraluminal fluid caused by ascites is present, the sonographer may

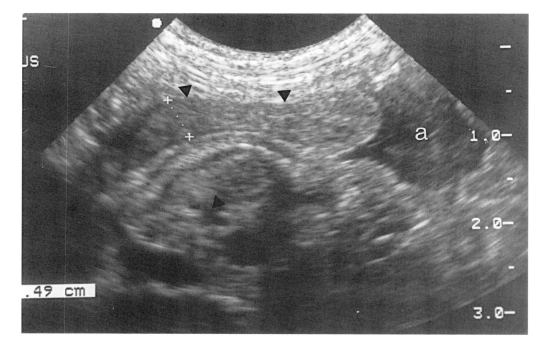

FIGURE 65-4. Hypertrophic pyloric stenosis. Sagittal (magnified) view of the right upper quadrant shows a thickened pyloric muscle (arrowheads) and elongation of the pyloric channel. The hypoechoic muscle layer (cursors [+]) is thickened greater than 4 mm. Residual fluid is seen within the gastric antrum (a).

be able to visualize the wall of the small bowel. Small bowel wall generally has a "target-like" appearance with a hyperechoic inner mucosa and hypoechoic outer lamina propria (Fig. 65-7). Wall thickness normally ranges between 2 and 5 mm, depending on the amount of intraluminal fluid that may be present. The bowel wall may be thickened either segmentally (Crohn's disease, ischemia) or diffusely (lymphangiectasia) (Fig. 65-8).

Midgut Malrotation

Rotational anomalies of the midgut are associated with shortening of the mesenteric attachment. This may predispose the midgut to ischemia from intestinal volvulus, which can be either acute or intermittent (chronic). Midgut malrotation complicated by acute volvulus is a surgical emergency. In the absence of volvulus, peritoneal bands (Ladd's bands) due to midgut malrotation can also produce obstruction from extrinsic compression of the duodenum. In the child with bilious vomiting, the upper GI series remains the examination of choice in most institutions for determining the location of the ligament of Treitz. However, one should be aware that sonography has been used to demonstrate duodenal obstruction due to acute midgut volvulus by showing dilation and hyperperistalsis of the duodenum and a "whirlpooling" of the superior mesenteric vein (SMV) around the axis of the superior mesenteric artery (SMA). Inversion of the normal SMA-SMV relationship (SMV

to the left of the lateral margin of the SMA) is an important sonographic finding that is an accurate indicator of malrotation[7] (Fig. 65-9); a normal SMA-SMV relationship does not necessarily exclude malrotation, however. Knowledge of these findings is important because they may be found incidentally or in the child with emesis who undergoes abdominal sonography.

Intussusception

Despite the frequency with which the diagnosis of intussusception is considered, imaging protocols for diagnosis and reduction, at present, are somewhat controversial. Most radiologists use either air or barium for diagnosing and reducing ileocolic intussusceptions (the most common form). Sonography can readily diagnose intussusception and has also been used to monitor its hydrostatic reduction. The typical sonographic appearance of an intussusception is a "target, donut, or pseudokidney" formed by the multilayered central echoes (intussusceptum) surrounded by the peripheral hypoechoic intussuscipiens (Fig. 65-10). If a lead point is present, it may occasionally be detected with sonography as a discrete soft tissue mass within the inner loop.[8]

Ileitis

Inflammatory bowel disease due to Crohn's disease commonly presents as crampy abdominal pain, diarrhea, and weight loss in children 10 years of age or older. Inflamma-

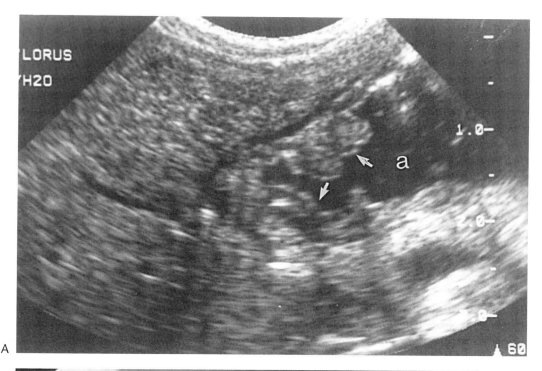

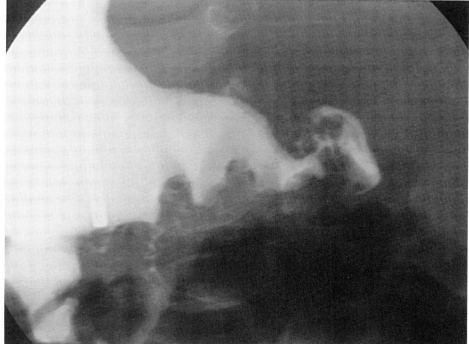

FIGURE 65-5. Eosinophilic gastritis. *(A)* Sagittal (magnified) ultrasound view of the right upper quadrant shows lobulated thickening of the gastric antral mucosa and submucosa (arrows) deep to the normal hypoechoic muscularis. Retained fluid is seen within the gastric antrum (a). *(B)* Upper GI shows markedly thickened, irregular folds within the gastric antrum with narrowing of the gastric antrum and partial gastric outlet obstruction.

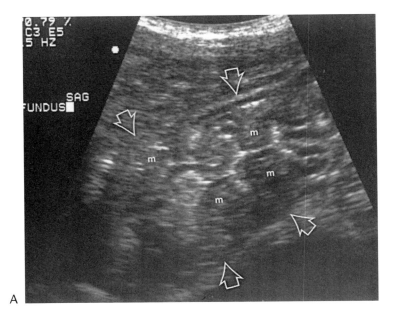

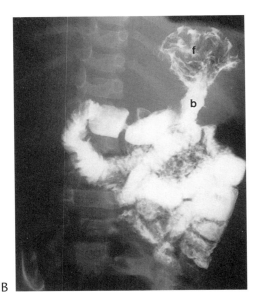

FIGURE 65-6. Ménétrier's disease (hypertrophic gastropathy). *(A)* Sagittal (magnified) ultrasound shows a "pseudokidney" appearance of the gastric fundus (arrows) and markedly thickened gastric mucosa (m). *(B)* Upper GI examination shows marked thickening of rugae in the gastric fundus (f) and circumferential narrowing of the gastric body (b).

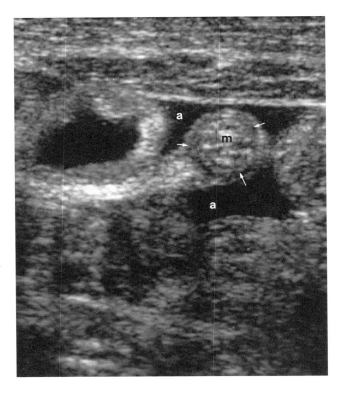

FIGURE 65-7. Normal small bowel. Transabdominal ultrasound (high-resolution transverse view) in a patient with ascites (a) shows target-like appearance of a normal small bowel loop suspended on its mesentery. Hypoechoic muscular layers (arrows) are seen surrounding hyperechoic mucosa (m).

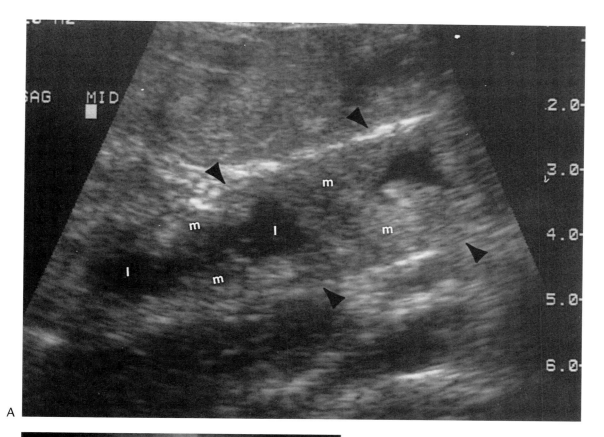

A

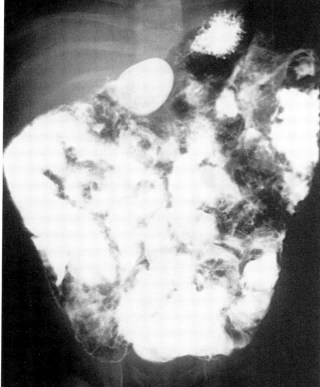

B

FIGURE 65-8. Intestinal lymphangiectasia. *(A)* Sagittal (magnified) ultrasound view of a loop of small bowel (arrowheads) shows irregular, nodular thickening of the small bowel mucosa (m). Retained fluid is seen within the bowel lumen (l). *(B)* Barium upper GI with small bowel series shows diffuse nodular thickening of the small bowel mucosa.

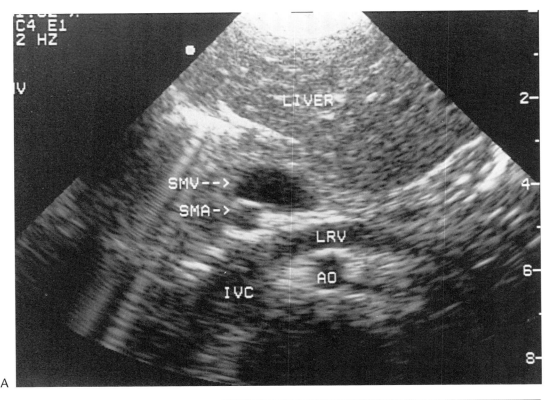

A

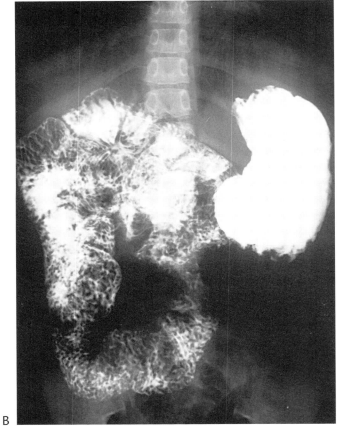

B

FIGURE 65-9. Intestinal malrotation (without volvulus). *(A)* Transabdominal ultrasound (magnified transverse view) shows the superior mesenteric artery (SMA) to the right of the superior mesenteric vein (SMV). LRV, left renal vein; IVC, inferior vena cava; AO, aorta. *(B)* Upper GI examination shows malfixation of the small intestine with proximal small bowel to the right of the spine and absence of the ligament of Treitz.

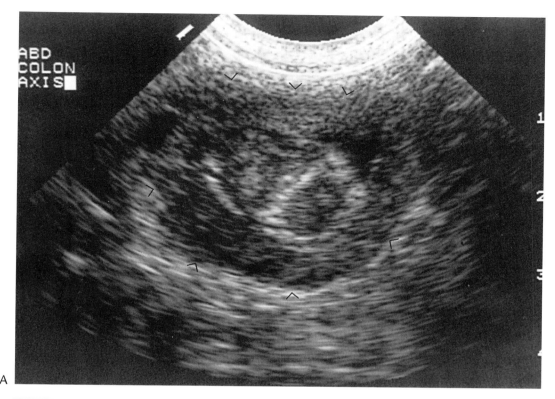

A

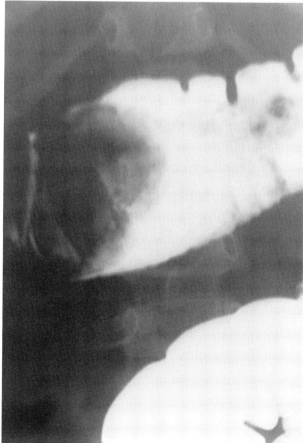

B

FIGURE 65-10. Intussusception (ileo-colic). (A) Transabdominal ultrasound (transverse magnified view) shows target-like (arrowheads) appearance of intussusception. (B) Barium enema shows intussusception (indenting the column of contrast) in the transverse colon.

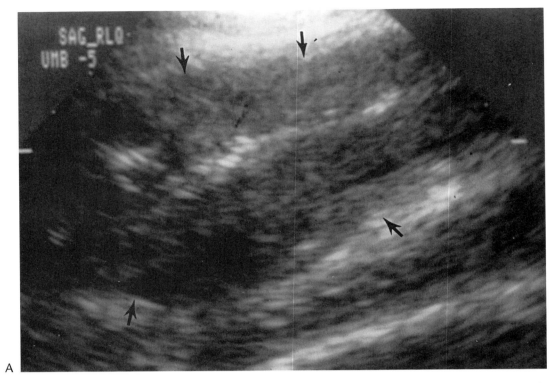

A

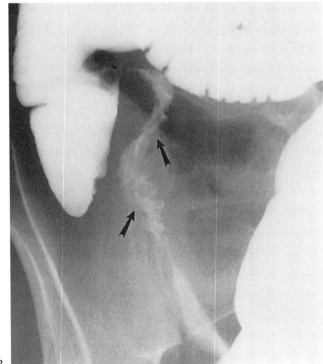

B

FIGURE 65-11. Crohn's disease. (A) Transabdominal ultrasound (sagittal view) of the right lower quadrant shows a "pseudokidney" due to transmural thickening of the bowel wall (arrows). (B) Barium enema (with reflux into the terminal ileum—arrows) shows mucosal irregularity and ulceration with circumferential narrowing of the terminal ileum.

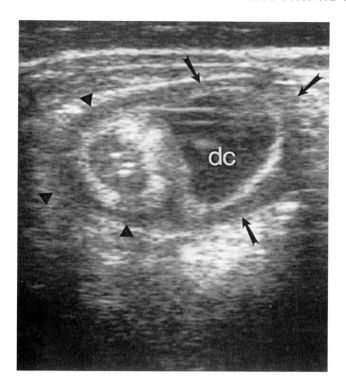

FIGURE 65-12. Enteric duplication cyst. High-resolution ultrasound (transverse view) through the right lower quadrant shows a duplication cyst (dc) with bowel wall features (hyperechoic mucosal layer surrounded by hypoechoic smooth muscle layer—arrows) similar to the normal contiguous ileum (arrowheads).

tory bowel disease can also occasionally mimic chronic appendicitis. Barium upper GI with small bowel series remains the primary study of choice for demonstrating extent of disease, but at times abdominal sonography may be the initial study in any young patient presenting with abdominopelvic pain. Sonography of inflammatory bowel disease shows circumferential thickening of the bowel wall with a thin echogenic lumen (Fig. 65-11). Adjacent enlarged lymph nodes may also be present. Extramural complications include mesenteric abscess phlegmon formation and ureteral obstruction.[9] Conditions that may also cause thickening of the terminal ileum include *Yersinia, Mycobacterium tuberculosis, Campylobacter,* and *Salmonella* enterocolitis.

Enteric Duplication Cyst

Enteric duplication cyst may cause small bowel obstruction or intestinal bleeding or may present as an asymptomatic mass in an infant or child. Occasionally, duplication cysts may be detected on prenatal sonography. Although they may occur anywhere along the GI tract, enteric duplication cysts are most commonly located at or near the ileocecal valve. Small bowel obstruction may

be the result of either mass effect by the cyst on the bowel lumen or of intussusception when it acts as a lead point. The cyst is anechoic unless containing mucus or blood. The wall is usually 2 to 4 mm thick and is often multilayered, with an echogenic inner mucosal lining and hypoechoic outer smooth muscle lining similar to the sonographic appearance of the normal bowel wall (Fig. 65-12). These wall characteristics help differentiate duplication cysts from other cystic abdominal masses, such as mesenteric or ovarian cysts.[10]

Hematoma

Small bowel hematoma may be secondary to either trauma (duodenal hematoma) or bleeding diathesis (drugs, leukemia, Henoch-Schönlein purpura). A duodenal hematoma may appear sonographically as a focal area of bowel thickening at the site of shearing injury between the spine and superior mesenteric artery (Fig. 65-13). The appearance of the hematoma changes with time as the clot liquefies and retracts.[11] Henoch-Schönlein purpura is an acute inflammatory condition of unknown etiology that principally affects the small blood vessels of the skin, joints, gut, and/or kidney. Abdominal pain is a frequent manifestation that often precedes the appearance of a rash. Localized submucosal edema or hemorrhage may be severe enough to cause small bowel obstruction or small bowel intussusception. Sonographic findings of the bowel wall are nonspecific for bowel wall thickening, which can be focal or diffuse. Serial sonographic examination may demonstrate improvement in bowel thickening over the patient's clinical course.[12]

COLON

The colon is often difficult to assess in its entirety with sonography because of the amount of gas and echogenic fecal debris. When intraluminal fluid is present, the haustra are usually seen well enough to allow proper recognition of the bowel as being large bowel. The wall of the cecum and rectum can be assessed when intraluminal fluid exists; the transverse colon is more difficult to evaluate because it is air-filled with the patient in the supine position. Conditions that involve the colon for which sonography has been utilized include anorectal malformations and colitides.

Anorectal Malformations (Imperforate Anus)

The surgical approach for imperforate anus is determined by the level of the hindgut pouch. If the pouch lies above or at the levator sling, a colostomy is done, followed at

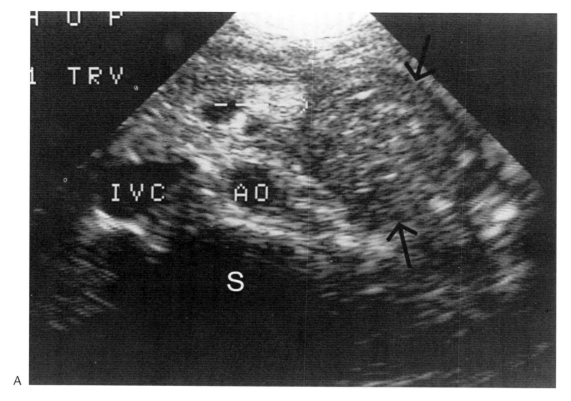

A

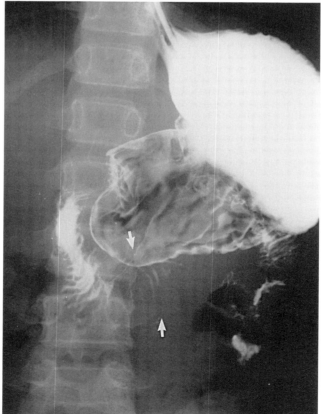

B

FIGURE 65-13. Duodenal hematoma. *(A)* Transabdominal ultrasound (transverse view) shows a rounded echogenic retroperitoneal mass (arrows) just left of the spine (S). IVC, inferior vena cava; AO, aorta. *(B)* Upper GI examination shows stretching of the column of contrast (arrows) around the submucosal hematoma and obstruction in transverse portion of duodenum.

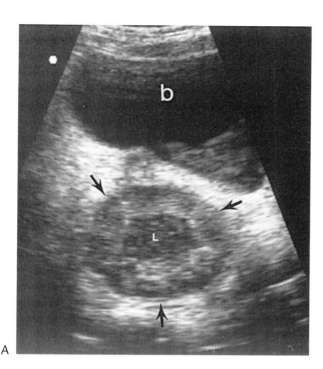
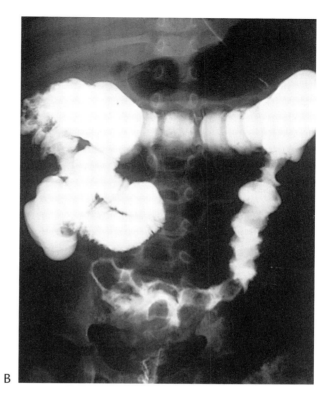

FIGURE 65-14. *Escherichia coli* colitis (hemolytic uremic syndrome). *(A)* Transpelvic ultrasound (transverse view) through the bladder (b) shows thickening of the wall of the rectum (arrows) and echogenic fluid within the lumen (L). *(B)* Barium enema shows thumbprinting of the rectosigmoid and descending colon due to mucosal and submucosal edema and hemorrhage.

a later date by a colon pull-through. If the pouch lies below the sling, a primary perineal approach or anoplasty is undertaken. The imaging method by which the level of the pouch is determined varies from center to center and includes "invertogram" radiography, contrast pouch injection under fluoroscopy, and perineal sonography. In the last instance, sonography is used to measure the distance between the pouch and the perineum (1.0 cm or less is low, 1.5 cm or greater is high).[13] Other signs of high lesions include bladder air or intraluminal (meconium) calcifications.

Colitis

The colitides (Crohn's ileocolitis, ulcerative colitis, infectious colitis, hemolytic uremic syndrome, Behçet's disease, pseudomembranous colitis) have similar nonspecific apearances on sonography.[14] Unlike the common viral gastroenteritis, in which the bowel loops are usually distended with fluid and thin-walled, the various colitides typically display diffuse thickening of mucosa and submucosa and large amounts of complex intraluminal fluid (Fig. 65-14). Typhlitis is a localized inflammation of the right colon that afflicts neutropenic patients and can mimic appendicitis. Sonography may demonstrate localized bowel mucosal edema or hemorrhage with thickened, echogenic mucosa, and occasionally pericecal fluid.[15]

APPENDIX

The normal appendix can be identified infrequently at sonography as a compressible tubular structure (6 mm or less in diameter) with a hypoechoic outer wall and an echogenic inner lining, with or without luminal fluid. The tip may appear slightly bulbous.

Appendicitis

In most cases, the diagnosis of appendicitis should rest with clinical examination by an experienced clinician or surgeon. In cases where there is uncertainty, sonography with graded compression of the right lower quadrant has proved useful, with sensitivity, accuracy, and specificity reportedly above 90%.[16] Having the patient localize the point of maximal tenderness is often helpful for the so-

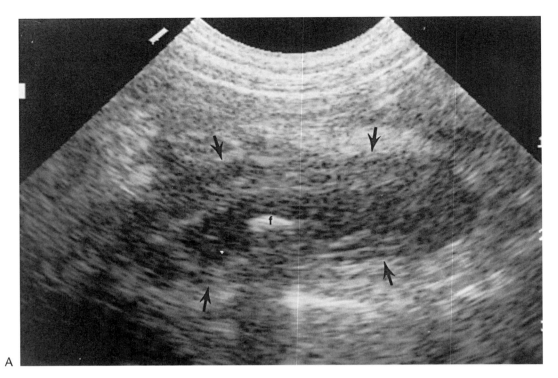

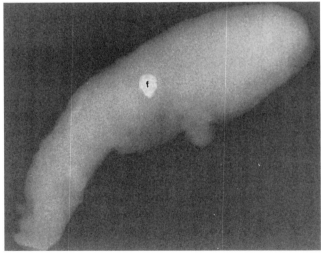

FIGURE 65-15. Appendicitis. *(A)* transabdominal ultrasound (magnified sagittal view) through the right lower quadrant shows a thickened appendix (arrows). A shadowing echogenic fecalith (f) is seen within the lumen. *(B)* Radiograph of appendix after removal shows calcified fecalith (f) in the midportion of the appendix (corresponding to the preoperative sonogram).

nographer. The abnormal appendix should appear as a *noncompressible*, blind-ending tubular structure or as a target (on transverse images). The lumen often contains hypoechoic fluid, which is surrounded by an echogenic mucosal layer and peripheral hypoechoic muscle layer. The diameter of an abnormal appendix is 7 mm or greater. Intraluminal echogenic foci (shadowing) may be due to gas or appendicolith (Fig. 65-15). Echogenic periappendiceal inflammation of the mesentery is often apparent. Sonographic findings of perforation include loculated abscess/pericecal fluid and lack of visualization of the echogenic mucosal layer (suggesting ulceration).[17] In cases where children are referred with abdominal pain for suspected appendicitis, most will have no apparent cause or some other diagnosis, while about one-quarter will have appendicitis.[16]

REFERENCES

1. Lorentzen T, Nolsoe CP, Khattar SC et al. Gastric and duodenal wall thickening on abdominal sonography. J Ultrasound Med 1993;12:633–637

2. Gomes H, Lallemand A, Lallemand P. Use of the gastroesophageal junction. Pediatr Radiol 1993;23:94

3. Patriquin H, Tessier G, Grignon A, Boisvert J. Lesser omental thickness in children: baseline for detection of portal hypertension. AJR 1985;145:693–696

4. O'Haller J, Cohen H. Hypertrophic pyloric stenosis: diagnosis using ultrasound. Radiology 1986;164:131–134

5. Hayden C, Swischuk L, Rytting J. Gastric ulcer disease in infants: ultrasound findings. Radiology 1987;164:131–134

6. Kopen P, McAlister W. Upper GI and US examination of gastric antral involvement in chronic granulomatous disease. Pediatr Radiol 1984;14:91–93

7. Loyer E, Eggli K. Sonographic evaluation of superior mesenteric vascular relationship in malrotation. Pediatr Radiol 1989;19:173–175

8. Swischuk L, Hayden C, Boulden T. Intussusception: indications for sonography and an explanation of the donut and pseudokidney signs. Pediatr Radiol 1985;15:388–391

9. Dinkel E, Dittrich M, Peters H, Baumann W. Realtime US in Crohn's disease: characteristic features and clinical implications Pediatr Radiol 1986;16:8–12

10. Barr L, Hayden CK Jr, Stansberry SD, Swischuk LE. Enteric duplication cysts in children: are their sonographic wall characteristics diagnostic? Pediatr Radiol 1990;20:326–328

11. Hernanz-Schulman M, Genieser NB, Ambrosino M. Sonographic diagnosis of intramural duodenal hematoma. J Ultrasound Med 1989;8:273–276

12. Martinez-Frontanillo LA, Silvermen L, Meaghen DP Jr. Intussusception in Henoch-Schönlein purpura: diagnosis with ultrasound. J Pediatr Surg 1988;23:375–376

13. Schuster S, Teele R. An analysis of ultrasound scanning as a guide in determination of "high" or "low" imperforate anus. J Pediatr Surg 1979;14:798–800

14. Stringer DA, Cleghorn GJ, Durie PR et al. Behçet's syndrome involving the gastrointestinal tract: a diagnostic dilemma in childhood. Pediatr Radiol 1986;16:131–134

15. Alexander JE. Williamson SL, Seibert JJ et al. The ultrasonographic diagnosis of typhlitis (neutropenic colitis). Pediatr Radiol 1988;18:200–204

16. Siegel MJ, Carel C, Surratt S. Ultrasonography of acute abdominal pain in children. JAMA 1991;266:1987–1989

17. Borushok K, Jeffry RB Jr, Laing FC, Townand RR. Sonographic diagnosis of perforation in patients with acute appendicitis. AJR 1990;154:275–278

66

ABDOMINAL COMPUTED TOMOGRAPHY

JOHN J. NICOTRA
SANDRA S. KRAMER

In the 10 years following the advent of computed tomography (CT) in the early 1970s, CT played a limited role in the evaluation of disorders of the pediatric abdomen. The inherent advantages of CT over conventional radiographs, the cross-sectional tomographic display and the ability to discriminate between tissues of similar radiographic density, were recognized early, but CT was primarily reserved for children with potential tumors. The examinations were long and complicated, and the image quality was poor. In the early 1980s, modern CT scanners became available with hardware and software improvements that included 2- to 3-second scan times, improved spatial resolution, and lower radiation dose. These advances enabled CT to reach its full potential in depicting cross-sectional anatomy and pathology in children, unobscured by overlying structures. New applications to nonmalignant diseases became possible: trauma, postoperative problems, abscess formation, complications of inflammatory bowel disease, and so on. More recent improvements in technology, such as faster scan times, better spatial and contrast resolution, and spiral techniques, have continued to increase the diagnostic power of CT. New capabilities have also emerged: two-dimensional images reconstructed in coronal and sagittal planes, three-dimensional images, CT angiography, and imaging of organs in different phases of blood flow (e.g., arterial and venous) using intravenously injected contrast media.

Although CT is an invaluable diagnostic tool in the proper clinical setting, it should not be employed without an appropriate indication. To promote the most effective use of CT, this chapter will briefly cover a few fundamental concepts, including the role of CT relative to other imaging techniques, preparation for and basic aspects of the examination, and practical applications in pediatric disease.

ROLE OF CT COMPARED TO OTHER MODALITIES

The screening for abdominal pathology usually begins with readily available and time-honored x-ray examinations, such as plain radiographs and fluoroscopy (barium studies), which can answer many diagnostic questions simply and inexpensively for clinicians and radiologists alike. When additional information is needed, more advanced imaging techniques can be employed.

Ultrasound is frequently the next imaging modality used as an abdominal "screening tool"; it has become the imaging technique of choice for detection of cholelithiasis and biliary dilation and for screening evaluations of the appendix and vascular structures. The advantages of ultrasound include its ready availability, lack of ionizing radiation, low cost, and easy portability, enabling examinations to be performed even at the bedside. It is often limited by the presence of bowel gas, making it difficult to evaluate the retroperitoneum, mesentery, and bowel. The examination is also "operator dependent," meaning that the images obtained depend on the ability and experience of the examiner, and interpretation of the study by others is difficult.

CT is next in the hierarchy of imaging examinations and may be employed instead of or after an ultrasound examination, depending on the clinical problem.

Magnetic resonance imaging (MRI) may be used as an alternative or additional cross-sectional imaging tool to evaluate certain problems, such as liver masses and vascular tumors, and to provide vascular "road maps." The advantage of MRI lies in its exquisite depiction of differences in soft tissues, lack of artifacts from adjacent bowel or bone, absence of ionizing radiation, and visualization of vascular structures without the use of intravenous contrast. Factors limiting its more extensive use include cost, long imaging times, lower spatial resolution, and degradation of images by motion artifact. Peristaltic motion of the bowel and lack of a good intraluminal contrast agent have prevented satisfactory bowel imaging with MRI. Critically ill patients present a special problem, since they are relatively inaccessible in the MRI scanner and require specialized monitoring devices because of the strong magnetic fields used to obtain images.

THE CT EXAMINATION

Obtaining diagnostic CT images is the responsibility of the supervising radiologist. It requires attention to detail and is a team effort involving the radiologist, technologist, and nursing staff. Safe and effective sedation is necessary in young children to eliminate confusing or nondiagnostic images caused by motion artifact. The relative lack of innate contrast differences within and between organs and the paucity of intra-abdominal and retroperitoneal fat to outline structures necessitate the use of intravenous contrast material in almost every case. The importance of adequate bowel opacification using dilute, water-soluble contrast cannot be overemphasized, since it will eliminate many difficulties in differentiating nonopacified bowel from pathologic conditions, especially when searching for intra-abdominal infection or adenopathy.

Table 66-1 shows general guidelines used in the Department of Radiology at the Children's Hospital of Philadelphia. The actual technical features of CT scanning vary according to the individual clinical question, the age of the patient, and the type of CT scanner used. It is important to remember that each CT examination must be tailored to the individual patient and the clinical question at hand; therefore, goals must be clearly defined before the study is undertaken.

The ready availability and the wealth of information

TABLE 66-1. Preparation Guidelines for Pediatric Abdominal CT Imaging

NPO status
   Newborn to 2 yr: 2 hr
   >2 yr: 4 hr
Sedation: carefully monitored
   <18 mo: chloral hydrate, 60–75 mg/kg PO
   >18 mo: phenobarbital, 2–6 mg/kg IV
Oral contrast
   Dilute (2%) Gastrografin: volume given based on patient
      weight
Intravenous (IV) contrast
   2 ml/kg iohexol 300 or its equivalent

potentially derived from a CT examination must be weighed against the ionizing radiation involved and the use of intravenous contrast and sedation often required to obtain optimal images in infants and children. An important role of the radiologist is to minimize radiation exposure and to suggest other imaging modalities, such as ultrasound or MRI, when they may provide similar or superior information in a given clinical setting.

CLINICAL CT APPLICATIONS

Rather than providing an exhaustive review of disease processes, this section will highlight important diagnostic contributions of CT in the pediatric gastrointestinal tract. A discussion of lesions of adrenal or genitourinary origin will not be included.

Masses and Neoplasms

The evaluation of intra-abdominal masses and neoplasms was the original and remains an important application of body CT in children. CT can depict the site of origin and extent of the mass, characteristic imaging features, and the presence of local or metastatic spread. Both benign and malignant processes can be accurately assessed and then re-evaluated after therapy to determine interval change. Although certain lesions may have a very characteristic, almost pathognomonic appearance, other masses may share features with both benign and malignant processes. CT does not replace histopathology; in most cases, the final diagnosis rests on the tissue sample.

Infantile hemangioendotheliomas of the liver can cause hepatic enlargement in the neonate. They may be single or multifocal and exhibit a characteristic pattern of enhancement (Fig. 66-1). These lesions are quite vascular, with high blood flow, so that the caliber of the aorta may diminish below the origin of the celiac axis, the source of the hepatic arterial supply. In extreme ex-

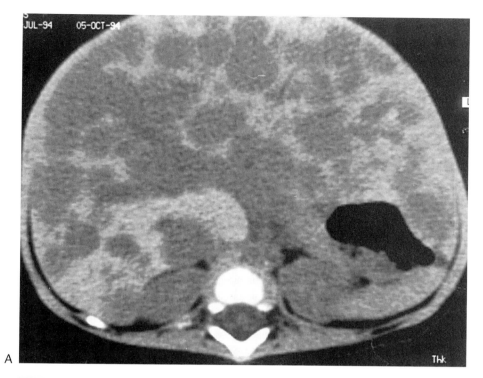

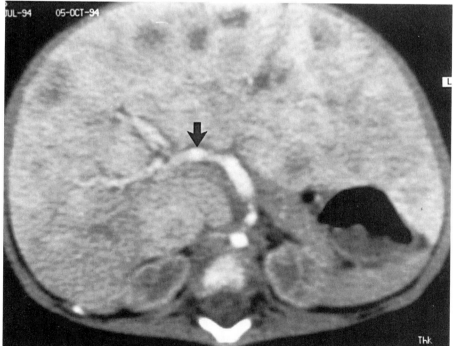

FIGURE 66-1. Multiple infantile hemangioendotheliomas. *(A)* Unenhanced image through the abdomen reveals multiple low-density lesions involving the liver of this newborn. *(B)* Contrast-enhanced CT image shows peripheral enhancement of the hepatic lesions that later became isodense with the remainder of the liver. The hepatic artery is enlarged (arrow) due to the increased arterial blood supply to the lesions.

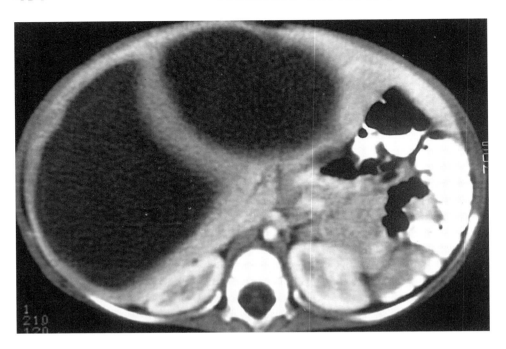

FIGURE 66-2. Mesenchymal hamartoma of the liver. Enhanced CT scan of the liver portrays cystic mass with enhancing septa.

amples, hemangioendotheliomas of the liver may cause high-output congestive heart failure.[1]

Mesenchymal hamartoma is a rare benign tumor in which the normal components of the liver are organized in an abnormal way. It often presents in the neonatal period as a hepatic mass consisting of multiple cysts with internal septa; the lesion may grow in size over time as fluid accumulates in the cysts[2] (Fig. 66-2). Other benign lesions of the liver include adenomas, focal nodular hyperplasia, and simple cysts.[3]

In the pediatric population, primary malignant tumors are less frequent than metastatic disease.[4] Common neoplasms that metastasize to the liver include neuroblastoma, Wilms' tumor, and lymphoma. Large adjacent tumors may impress and displace the liver; in these cases, it can be difficult to differentiate local invasion from mere contiguity.

Malignant primary liver lesions in the pediatric population include hepatoblastoma (Fig. 66-3) and, in older children, hepatocellular carcinoma.[5,6] Both lesions present as solid masses with variable enhancement as well as cystic or necrotic components. Unlike benign tumors of the liver, they have a propensity to invade hepatic and portal veins and surrounding structures as well as spread to lymph nodes and distant organs.

Primary tumors of the other solid abdominal organs such as the spleen and pancreas are uncommon in childhood. Tumors of the bowel and mesentery are also rare.[7]

Lymphoma is one of the more common neoplasms to involve the abdomen in the pediatric population. Retroperitoneal lymphadenopathy is the usual presentation,

but involvement of the solid intra-abdominal organs may also occur (Fig. 66-4). Lymphoma can also have a number of unusual manifestations, including involvement of the bowel that can mimic Crohn's disease (Fig. 66-5).

Infection and Inflammation

Abscesses typically are low-density, well-defined fluid collections, with enhancing rims, that may contain internal septations (Fig. 66-6) and have a local mass effect. Abscesses can be single or multiple; they are usually bacterial in origin, although amebic, hydatid, or fungal lesions can occur. They may develop anywhere in the abdomen, including the solid organs, peritoneal space, and extraperitoneal soft tissues. Although uncommon, gas bubbles within the lesion are a diagnostic feature. Immunocompromised patients, especially those with neutropenia, are at risk to develop fungal microabscesses, and multiple small, low-density foci within the liver, spleen, and kidneys are suggestive of this diagnosis[8] (Fig. 66-7).

Appendicitis and its complications are a common indication for abdominal imaging. Uncomplicated appendicitis is usually best evaluated using ultrasound, but findings that can be detected on CT include appendicoliths, edema of the fat adjacent to the cecum and appendix, and thickening of adjacent bowel indicating local inflammation. Complicated appendicitis, such as missed perforation and periappendiceal abscess (Fig. 66-8), or complications following appendectomy are often better delineated by CT. Abscesses related to appendicitis may occur anywhere within the abdomen and pelvis, includ-

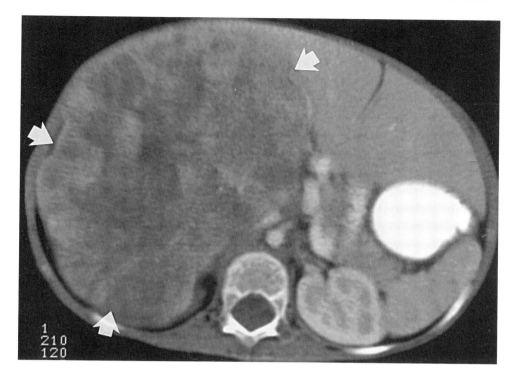

FIGURE 66-3. Hepatoblastoma. Contrast-enhanced CT image demonstrates a large heterogeneously enhancing mass (arrows) involving the right lobe of the liver.

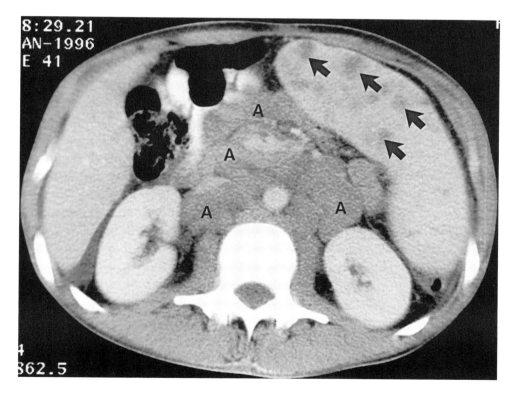

FIGURE 66-4. Splenic involvement in lymphoma. Contrast-enhanced CT scan reveals retroperitoneal adenopathy (A) and an enlarged spleen with multiple low-density lesions (arrows) caused by surgically proven lymphoma.

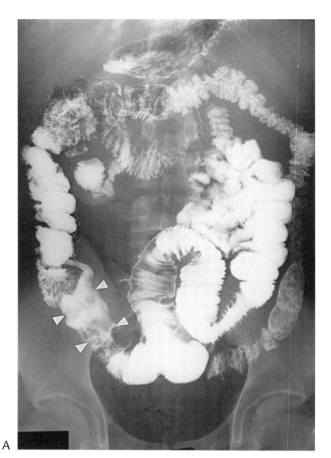

A

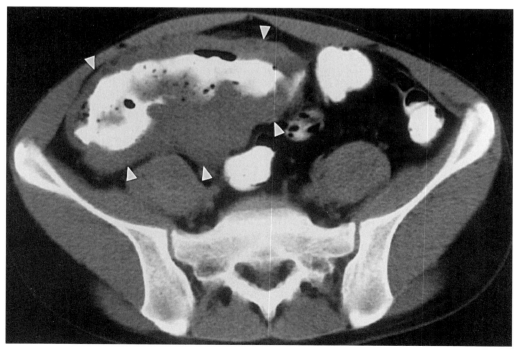

B

FIGURE 66-5. Small bowel lymphoma. *(A)* Small bowel barium examination shows a dilated, irregular, and nodular segment of terminal ileum (arrowheads). *(B)* CT scan reveals a contrast-filled loop of distal small bowel with an irregularly thickened bowel wall (arrowheads) and an ulcer crater.

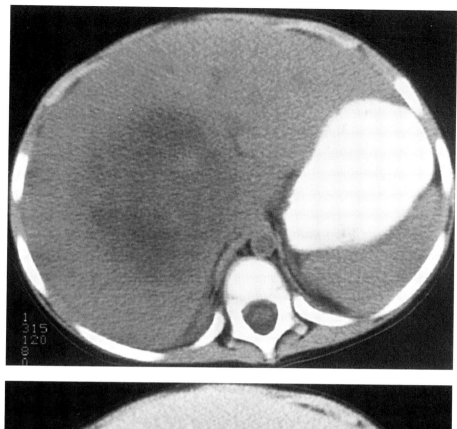

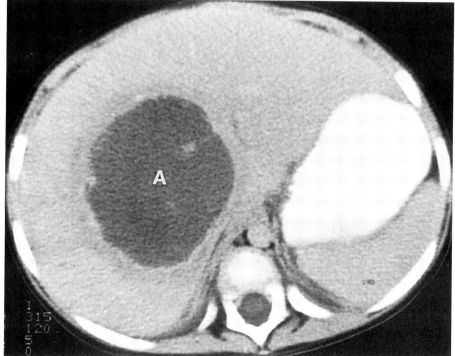

FIGURE 66-6. Hepatic abscess. *(A)* CT image without intravenous contrast shows an ill-defined hepatic focus of low density. *(B)* Contrast-enhanced CT scan demonstrates an enhancing rim surrounding the nonenhancing low-density lesion, proven to be an amebic abscess (A).

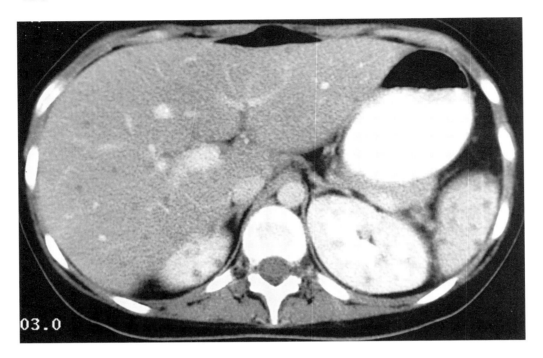

FIGURE 66-7. Fungal microabscesses. Contrast-enhanced CT scan reveals multiple tiny, low-density lesions scattered throughout the liver, spleen, and kidneys due to fungal microabscesses in this patient with acute myeloid leukemia and neutropenia.

ing the paracolic gutters, dependent portions of the pelvis (cul-de-sac), the subphrenic or subhepatic spaces, and even the lesser sac, regions that may be inaccessible to ultrasound examination because of overlying bowel gas. Since fluid-filled, nonopacified bowel loops can have a similar CT appearance, the importance of oral contrast preparation to ensure adequate bowel opacification cannot be overemphasized. Other findings in complicated appendicitis include peritoneal enhancement suggesting peritonitis, free intraperitoneal air, and extraluminal bowel contrast indicating bowel perforation.

The earliest mucosal changes of Crohn's disease cannot be appreciated by CT techniques and are best imaged with conventional single- or double-contrast barium studies. However, CT has an important role to play in evaluating mural changes of bowel wall thickening in both large and small bowel (Fig. 66-9) and extraluminal abnormalities, including mesenteric fibrofatty proliferation, mesenteric adenopathy, fistulas, edematous mesenteric and intra-abdominal fat, and phlegmon and abscess formation.[9] CT can also prove helpful in evaluating other forms of inflammatory bowel disease such as ulcerative colitis and pseudomembranous colitis.[9,10]

Typhlitis or neutropenic colitis occurs in patients with severe neutropenia, usually as a complication of leukemia. The cecum is most commonly affected, but the remainder of the colon as well as the distal ileum may also be involved. CT findings include diffuse or focal colonic wall thickening (usually involving the cecum, frequently with layers of alternating density) (Fig. 66-10), pneumatosis, and inflammatory changes involving the surrounding fat and soft tissues. Clinical improvement and the return of adequately functioning neutrophils coincide with a decrease in cecal wall thickening on CT.[11]

Sonography is the initial imaging modality of choice for evaluation of acute pancreatitis, and in uncomplicated pancreatitis, further imaging may not be necessary. CT changes in typical acute pancreatitis may vary from a normal-appearing pancreas to a diffusely enlarged pancreas exhibiting a heterogeneous enhancement pattern. However, CT may prove very effective in imaging complications of acute pancreatitis such as pancreatic necrosis, phlegmon (Fig. 66-11), abscess, pseudoaneurysms, and pseudocyst formation.[12]

Chronic pancreatitis is often less clinically obvious than acute pancreatitis, and imaging may provide important clues to the diagnosis. Findings noted in chronic pancreatitis on CT examination include pancreatic duct dilation (Fig. 66-12), abnormal parenchymal texture, pancreatic calcifications, and gland atrophy.[12]

Trauma

Abdominal CT examinations have made an important contribution to the evaluation and management of blunt abdominal trauma in children. CT provides a rapid overall assessment of the abdominal and pelvic contents in hemodynamically stable patients. Several studies have

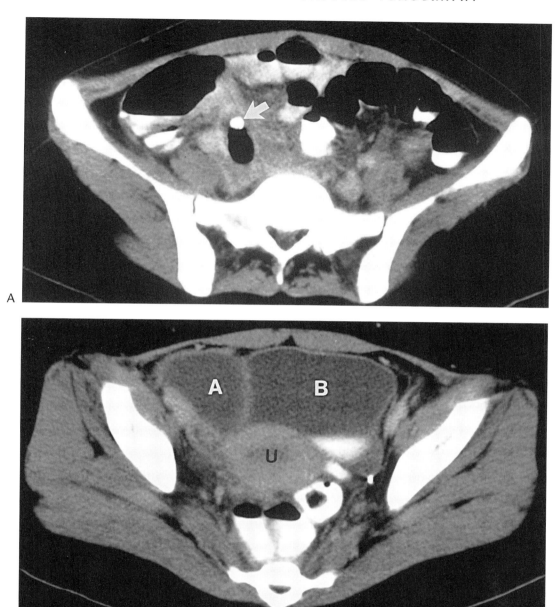

FIGURE 66-8. Complicated appendicitis. *(A)* CT image in a patient with right lower quadrant pain reveals an appendicolith (arrow). *(B)* A scan through the pelvis depicts a fluid collection with enhancing margins representing a pelvic abscess (A) from a perforated appendix, adjacent to the bladder (B). U, uterus.

documented the superiority of CT over other imaging modalities for the evaluation of the traumatized child.[13,14] CT is relatively contraindicated for hemodynamically unstable patients; in this setting, stabilizing the patient and prompt surgical exploration may be required to evaluate injuries and prevent further morbidity or even mortality.

Careful patient monitoring is necessary, even though studies can be completed rapidly on modern CT scan-

ners. Adequate evaluation requires intravenous contrast administration; preliminary unenhanced scans are not usually necessary. Although slightly controversial, we have found water-soluble contrast bowel preparation to be quite helpful; a nasogastric tube is often placed to facilitate the administration of bowel contrast. Complete evaluation in abdominal trauma includes imaging of the pelvis for the presence of fluid or blood, injury to the pelvic organs, and pelvic fractures. The lower lung zones

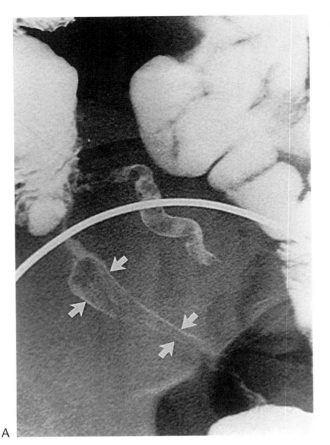

A

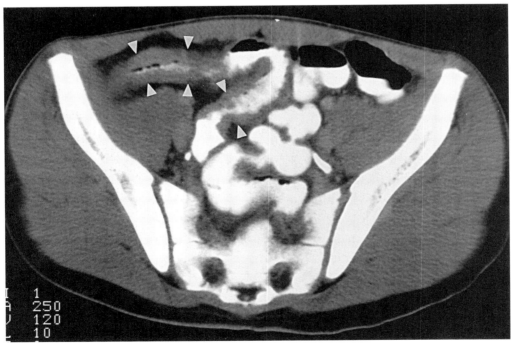

B

FIGURE 66-9. Crohn's disease. *(A)* Fluoroscopic spot film from a barium small bowel follow-through examination reveals a markedly narrowed segment of terminal ileum (arrows). *(B)* CT scan through the same region demonstrates the thickened wall as well as the narrow lumen of the terminal ileum (arrowheads).

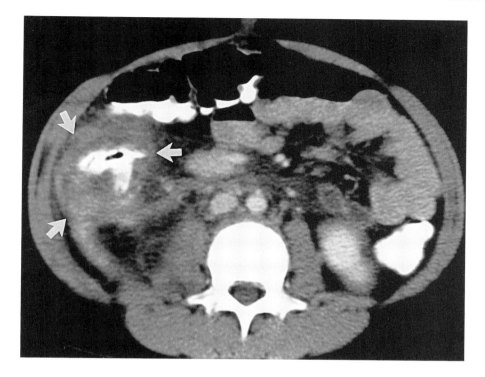

FIGURE 66-10. Neutropenic colitis (typhlitis). A patient with acute myeloid leukemia and neutropenia has a layered, thick-walled cecum (arrows) and inflammatory changes in the surrounding intraperitoneal fat.

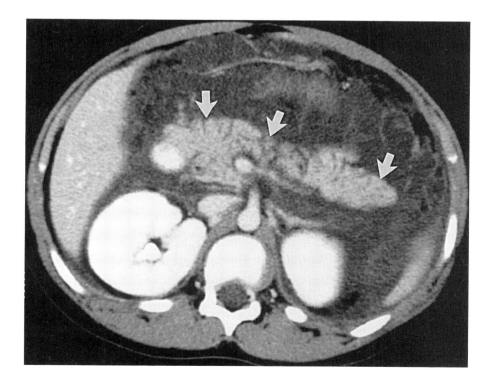

FIGURE 66-11. Acute pancreatitis. Contrast-enhanced CT scan in a patient with severe epigastric pain shows an enlarged pancreas (arrows) surrounded by phlegmon.

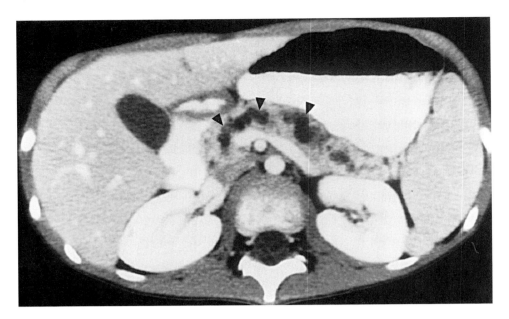

FIGURE 66-12. Chronic pancreatitis. A patient with recurrent episodes of epigastric pain has a dilated pancreatic duct (arrowheads) surrounded by an atrophic pancreas on contrast-enhanced CT examination.

should be scrutinized for abnormalities unsuspected on plain films, such as lung contusion, pneumothorax, and pleural effusion.

The liver is the most commonly injured organ. Hepatic parenchymal injuries vary in severity from small self-contained hepatic lacerations to extensive fractures with clinically significant symptoms indicating massive hemorrhage. Hepatic lacerations on enhanced CT scans appear as linear, round, or stellate regions of hypoattenuation (Fig. 66-13) with or without evidence of fluid (hemoperitoneum) in the peritoneal space. Hepatic lacerations may also extend into vascular structures such as

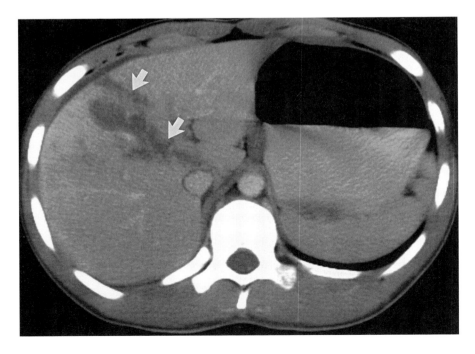

FIGURE 66-13. Hepatic laceration. A low-density linear defect due to a hepatic laceration (arrows) was found in a patient with blunt abdominal trauma.

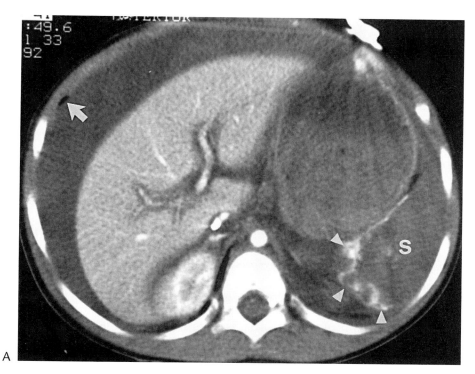

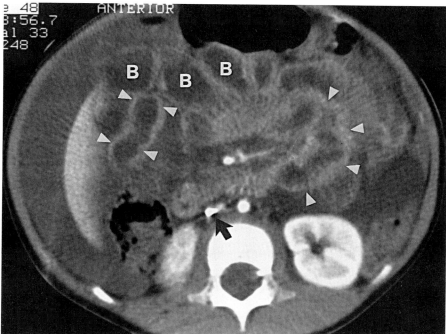

FIGURE 66-14. Abdominal trauma. *(A)* Contrast-enhanced CT scan in a patient with hypovolemic shock after a motor vehicle accident reveals a large amount of free intraperitoneal fluid adjacent to the liver with a tiny free air collection (arrow), no enhancement of the spleen (S), and extravasation of intravascular contrast (arrowheads) from an avulsed splenic vascular pedicle. *(B)* At a lower level, a large amount of free intraperitoneal fluid, a collapsed inferior vena cava (arrow), and multiple dilated, fluid-filled loops of small bowel (B) with enhancement of the bowel wall (arrowheads) are seen. These findings have been described in the literature as indicating intravascular collapse and a poor prognosis.

the inferior vena cava and portal and hepatic veins. Injuries to the biliary system can result in hematobilia or bilomas from bile duct laceration or even free intraperitoneal leakage of bile. Blood may also dissect underneath the hepatic capsule, producing a lenticular-shaped hypodense fluid collection called a subcapsular hematoma. Statistically, trauma to the right lobe of the liver is more frequent, but injuries to the left lobe are more likely to be associated with pancreatic or duodenal lesions.

The spleen is the second most commonly injured abdominal organ. Splenic contusions appear as low-density intraparenchymal regions, whereas splenic lacerations have a similar appearance to those in the liver. More severe injuries to the spleen include fragmentation and the rare fracture that extends into the splenic hilum and interrupts the blood supply to the entire organ (Fig. 66-14A). Splenic injuries are also associated with injuries to adjacent organs such as the left lung, left kidney, and tail of the pancreas.

Accidental or nonaccidental trauma is the most common cause of acute pancreatitis in children. In the setting of blunt abdominal trauma, CT may be used to evaluate the pancreas along with other abdominal organs. In addition to those previously described in acute pancreatitis (see the section *Infection and Inflammation*, above), CT findings may include laceration or fracture of the pancreas, peripancreatic fluid, and defective enhancement of the gland due to disruption of the blood supply.

Injuries to the bowel and mesentery, although less common, may also be detected on CT. The duodenum and proximal jejunum are the portions of the bowel most frequently injured by blunt trauma. Bowel wall hematoma appears as an irregular narrowing of the bowel lumen or a focal hypodense mass or thickening within the wall. Free intraperitoneal fluid without a source (e.g., solid organ laceration) or a focal fluid collection in the mesentery may be the only subtle clues to an injury to the bowel or mesentery, and intraperitoneal lavage may be required to exclude this type of injury.[15] Free intraperitoneal air (Fig. 66-14A) or air within the adjacent retroperitoneum may rarely be seen.

The "hypoperfusion complex"[16,17] occasionally seen on trauma CT examinations has been described as due to systemic shock and is associated with a poor prognosis. Findings include a small inferior vena cava from intravascular volume depletion, increased enhancement of the intraperitoneal organs, and dilated, fluid-filled loops of bowel with intense enhancement of the bowel wall ("shock bowel") (Fig. 66-14B).

Miscellaneous

Many diffuse processes involving the liver can be detected with CT including low density or attenuation in the liver due to fatty replacement or infiltration, increased hepatic attenuation (seen in primary or secondary iron overload states and glycogen storage disease), and cirrhosis with portal hypertension and varices.

Biliary tract abnormalities are usually first screened by ultrasound examinations. Ultrasound depicts mild intra- or extrahepatic dilation that may be undetectable on CT. A nuclear medicine ^{99m}Tc–diisopropyl iminodiacetic acid scan is often the next examination performed to evaluate biliary excretion. However, CT may be helpful in depicting the cause and level of obstruction as well as providing an overall survey of the entire biliary system.

CONCLUSION

CT has many distinct advantages for use in pediatric abdominal imaging. Understanding its role in the imaging hierarchy, basic aspects of CT technique (especially the importance of bowel opacification and intravenous contrast enhancement), and its unique clinical applications is important for its most effective use.

REFERENCES

1. Mahboubi S, Sunaryo FP, Glassman MS, Patel K. Computed tomography in the management and follow-up of infantile hemangioendothelioma of the liver in infants and children. J Comput Tomogr 1987;11:370–375

2. Stanley P, Hall TR, Wooley MM et al. Mesenchymal hamartomas of the liver in childhood: sonographic and CT findings. AJR 1986;147:1035–1039

3. Boechat MI, Kangarloo H, Gilsanz V. Hepatic masses in children. Semin Roentgenol 1988;23:185–193

4. Babyn P, Stringer DA: Computed tomography. In: Walker WA, Durie PR, Hamilton JR et al, Eds. Pediatric Gastrointestinal Disease: Pathophysiology, Diagnosis, Management. Vol. 2. Philadelphia: BC Decker, 1991:1484

5. Boechat MI, Kangarloo H, Ortega J et al. Primary liver tumors in children: comparison of CT and MR imaging. Radiology 1988;169:727–732

6. Dachman AH, Pakter RL, Ros PR et al. Hepatoblastoma: radiologic-pathologic correlation in 50 cases. Radiology 1987;164:15–19

7. Ruess L, Frazier AA, Sivit CJ. CT of the mesentery, omentum, and peritoneum in children. Radiographics 1995;15: 89–104

8. Francis IR, Glazer GM, Amendola MA, Trenkner SW. Hepatic abscesses in the immunocompromised patient: role of CT in detection, diagnosis, management, and follow-up. Gastrointest Radiol 1986;11:257–262

9. Jabra AA, Fishman EK, Taylor GA. CT findings in inflammatory bowel disease in children. AJR 1994;162:975–979

10. Philpotts LE, Heiken JP, Wescott MA, Gore RM. Colitis: use of CT findings in differential diagnosis. Radiology 1994; 190:445–449

11. Frick MP, Maile CW, Crass JR et al. Computed tomography of neutropenic colitis. AJR 1984;143:763–765

12. Thoeni RF, Blankenberg F. Pancreatic imaging: computed tomography and magnetic resonance imaging. Radiol Clin North Am 1993;31:1085–1113

13. Brick SH, Taylor GA, Potter BM, Eichelberger MR. Hepatic and splenic injury in children: role of CT in the decision for laparotomy. Radiology 1987;165:643–646

14. Roberts JL, Dalen K, Bosanko CM, Jafir SZH. CT in abdominal and pelvic trauma. Radiographics 1993;13:735–752

15. Sivit CJ, Eichelberger MR, Taylor GA. CT in children with rupture of the bowel caused by blunt trauma: diagnostic efficacy and comparison with hypoperfusion complex. AJR 1994;163:1195–1198

16. Sivit CJ, Taylor GA, Bulas DI et al. Posttraumatic shock in children: CT findings associated with hemodynamic instability. Radiology 1992;182:723–726

17. Taylor GA, Fallat ME, Eichelberger MR. Hypovolemic shock in children: abdominal CT manifestations. Radiology 1987;164:479–481

67

NUCLEAR MEDICINE

SYDNEY HEYMAN

Radionuclide imaging is extremely useful in assessing the gastrointestinal (GI) system in children. Nuclear medicine radiography provides a noninvasive technique to monitor enteric motility, hepatic function, biliary excretion, and GI bleeding. This chapter provides detail on specific radionuclide tests.

GASTROESOPHAGEAL SCINTIGRAPHY (LIQUID-SOLID EMPTYING SCAN)

The uses of gastroesophageal radionuclide imaging include assessing esophageal motility, gastroesophageal reflux, delayed gastric emptying, and primary and secondary aspiration.

Esophageal Transit

Esophageal motor function may be studied using manometry or cine-esophagography. Since the latter imparts a high radiation dose, esophageal manometry is generally used to record intraluminal pressures, giving a measure of esophageal motility. There appears to be a correlation between esophageal motor activity and transit when manometry is performed concurrently with an analysis of esophageal transit.[1,2]

Gastroesophageal scintigraphy utilizes a small volume of milk feeding (or other liquid) tagged with 50 to 100 μCi of technetium ^{99m}Tc–sulfur colloid. A swallowed bolus, 1 to 10 ml depending on the age of the patient, is acquired on the computer at a frame rate of 0.4 second for 150 seconds. Time activity curves are generated from regions of interest over the upper, middle, and lower thirds of the esophagus, with a fourth region around the stomach. The transit time is expressed as the time of initial entry into the esophagus until total clearance occurs into the stomach. Abnormal transit has been observed in conditions such as achalasia, scleroderma, esophageal stricture, esophagitis, and status post surgery for tracheoesophageal fistula. The transit of the swallowed bolus may also be represented as a functional image, or bolus transport diagram. This gives a good visual display of the bolus transit.[3] Esophageal transit is usually evaluated as part of a radionuclide study for GI motility, without increasing the radioactive dose.

Gastroesophageal Reflux

Gastroesophageal scintigraphy has been adapted for use in infants and children.[4] It is best performed at the time of a scheduled feeding. ^{99m}Tc–sulfur colloid in a dose ranging from 200 μCi to 1 mCi is added to the patient's usual milk or formula feeding. After the initial swallow is evaluated, the remainder of the feeding is consumed. The infant is then placed supine on the table, and anterior images are obtained at 5-second intervals for 60 minutes. At this stage, anterior and posterior static images of the lung field are obtained, looking for evidence of aspiration. Five-second images are acquired during the second hour, followed by repeat images of the lung fields. Further delayed images may be obtained when aspiration is suspected.

The study is reviewed frame by frame using high contrast. The number of episodes of reflux, those reaching the upper esophagus, and the clearance rate are noted. These may be represented graphically by drawing time activity curves from regions of interest drawn over the entire esophagus and the upper esophagus (Fig. 67-1).

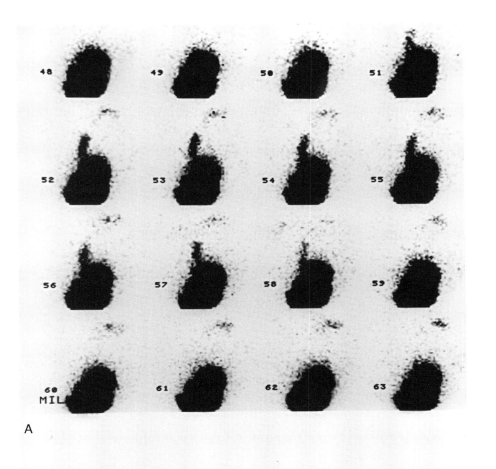

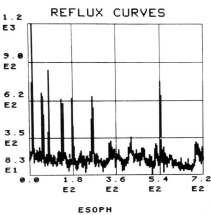

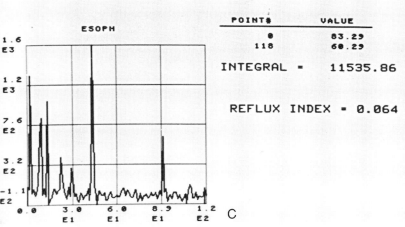

POINT$	VALUE
0	83.29
118	60.29

INTEGRAL = 11535.86

REFLUX INDEX = 0.064

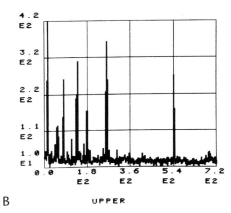

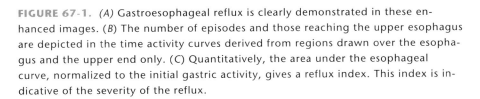

FIGURE 67-1. (A) Gastroesophageal reflux is clearly demonstrated in these enhanced images. (B) The number of episodes and those reaching the upper esophagus are depicted in the time activity curves derived from regions drawn over the esophagus and the upper end only. (C) Quantitatively, the area under the esophageal curve, normalized to the initial gastric activity, gives a reflux index. This index is indicative of the severity of the reflux.

Reflux indices have been described to quantitate reflux. These are all dependent on the number of episodes, the volume (activity) refluxed, and the clearance rate from the esophagus.

Studies comparing scintigraphy with pH monitoring for the evaluation of gastroesophageal reflux, performed in a sequential manner, have shown discordance. Some investigators have favored scintigraphy, while others regard it as inferior to pH monitoring. A partial explanation may be the nonstandardization of both techniques. In a few studies, both were compared simultaneously, and scintigraphy was found to be superior. More recent comparisons on a peak by peak basis, during the postprandial period, showed a much higher sensitivity for scintigraphy.[5]

A possible limitation of scintigraphy is the limited observation period, particularly the absence of monitoring during the night. However, as previously mentioned, the results of scintigraphy compare favorably with 24-hour pH monitoring. In a study using an independent standard for reflux, namely esophagitis, the sensitivity of scintigraphy was 79%, and that of the pH probe 73%.[6] It is true that it is not possible to distinguish normal from pathologic reflux, even though the intensity of reflux is statistically associated with a higher complication rate. For ethical reasons, reflux indices cannot be obtained in normal infants. It is questionable whether any recording technique can make this distinction, and the finding has to be interpreted in the context of the clinical presentation.

Gastric Emptying

The rate of gastric emptying is very dependent on the test meal. Liquids, solids, and indigestible solids all empty at different rates. Caloric content (rather than the meal size) and increased osmolality delay the emptying. However, osmolar loads were not found to exert a significant effect in premature infants and normal newborns within limits.[7] Cow's milk empties at a slower rate than human milk, and whey-based formulas empty more rapidly than casein-based milk formulas, even when there are no differences in osmolality, caloric value, or fat content.[8,9]

In infants, milk or formula is used to assess gastric emptying. In practice, most patients are on modified schedules so we use the usual feeding or any modification requested by the referring physician. The study is usually performed in conjunction with the reflux study. If gastric emptying alone is of interest, the dose of ^{99m}Tc–sulfur colloid may be reduced to 100 μCi. After consuming the feeding, the patient is placed supine beneath the camera, and sequential images are obtained for the next hour. We have shown that anterior imaging alone is satisfactory, since attenuation in small patients does not have a significant effect. A time activity curve derived from a region of interest placed around the stomach is decay corrected. If the gastric residual is abnormally high, it is important to acquire images for a further 60 minutes. We

do this routinely, since images are taken over the lung fields up to 120 minutes, looking for aspiration. Patients showing delayed emptying at 60 minutes often empty at an increased rate during the second hour so that the residual is normal at 120 minutes. In such instances, the gastric emptying is regarded as normal. We do not alter the patient's position after 60 minutes when emptying is slow, as has been suggested. The shape of the gastric curve, not only the residual counts at the end point, is important, as discussed below.

Milk usually empties in a monoexponential fashion. Since healthy infants are not studied, the normal range has been difficult to establish. An early study in normal infants showed that milk emptied with a $t^{1/2}$ of 87 $\pm$ 29 minutes. A diphasic pattern was observed in a smaller number, which was attributed to swallowed air.[10] Each laboratory needs to establish its normal range. We have used this study as a guide and established a normal residual of 48 to 70% at 60 minutes and 24 to 48% at 120 minutes. The rate of emptying may be more rapid in older children, although the composition of the meal may play a role.[11] As mentioned, the emptying pattern is important. For example, intermittent emptying (periods of delay followed by episodes of rapid emptying) may occur with intermittent gastric outlet obstruction.

In older children, techniques used for measuring solid, liquid, or combined emptying in adults are applicable. The solid meal is usually an egg sandwich, again labeled with ^{99m}Tc–sulfur colloid (250 to 300 μCi). If the liquid phase is labeled, 50μCi indium In 111 DTPA is added to water. The meal is scaled according to patient size based on the adult meal of four eggs and 500 ml of water. Since the liquid usually empties more readily than the solid, we have chosen to label only the solid phase in the interest of reducing the radiation dose to the patient. However, the liquid is part of the standard meal. Rarely, in selected cases, the liquid emptying is evaluated separately.

The meal is consumed in about 5 minutes, and the patient is placed supine beneath the camera. Thirty-second anterior images are obtained every 10 minutes. Between images, the patient sits upright. Imaging is continued for 120 minutes. At the end of this time, a decay-corrected time activity curve is obtained from the stomach region. As in the case of infants, normal gastric emptying values have not been established for older children. Figure 67-2 details values reported for young adult volunteers[12] using anterior imaging.[13]

Aspiration

Pulmonary aspiration after reflux has been detected less frequently than expected given the clinical presentation. The sensitivity was reportedly increased by giving patients a small volume of milk at night with a slightly higher concentration of the radiopharmaceutical.[14] We have tailored the study depending on whether the pa-

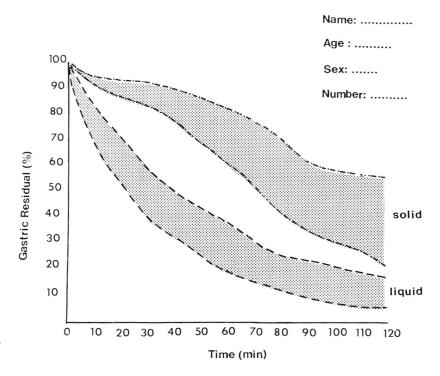

GASTRIC EMPTYING

Name: ....

Age : ....

Sex: ....

Number: ....

solid

liquid

FIGURE 67-2. These curves show the gastric residual over time after a solid and liquid meal as a percentage of the initial activity. The data were derived from young normal volunteers. Imaging was in the anterior projection only.

tient is thought to aspirate during swallowing or whether the aspiration of oral contents is due to a neuromuscular incoordination. In the first instance, the patient is offered a liquid bolus (10 to 15 ml) and swallows with the back to the collimator. Sequential images are taken over the next 2 to 3 minutes. When aspiration occurs, it is seen as the abnormal appearance of activity in the airway (Fig. 67-3). In the latter group we introduced the "salivagram."[15] A small drop (100 μl) is placed on the tongue and posterior images obtained for 60 minutes. In abnormal cases, aspiration of saliva is clearly documented (Fig. 67-4). This study is indicated for patients with incoordination or absence of a swallowing reflex who have recurrent episodes of aspiration pneumonia even though they are tube fed.

GASTROINTESTINAL BLEEDING

The role of nuclear medicine in the evaluation of patients with GI bleeding has been limited to the demonstration of a Meckel's diverticulum and the localization of an actively bleeding site.

Meckel's Scan

A Meckel's scan is indicated in the workup for rectal bleeding, after excluding a surgical abdomen. The nuclear medicine study should be performed before any

contrast studies with barium or should be postponed until barium has been cleared from the abdomen, since barium attenuates the 140-kev photon emitted by ^{99m}Tc–pertechnetate. This radiopharmaceutical is actively taken up by gastric mucosa, probably in the surface mucus secreting cells, which is the rationale for its use. It has been estimated that while only 30 to 50% of diverticula have ectopic gastric mucosa, it is present in nearly all those responsible for rectal bleeding. Pharmacologic intervention has been advocated to improve the sensitivity of the study. Pentagastrin given subcutaneously 20 minutes before the pertechnetate has been shown to enhance gastric uptake. Cimetidine, an H_2 receptor antagonist, also enhances localization, probably by inhibiting the intraluminal release of the pertechnetate.[16]

The patient should not have been fed for 2 to 4 hours. Anterior imaging proceeds for 30 minutes with the patient in the supine position. This is followed by anterior and right lateral static images. The study is not complete until images with an empty bladder are obtained. Typically, a positive study demonstrates an abnormal focus in the right lower quadrant, appearing at the time of stomach uptake (Fig. 67-5). However, a Meckel's diverticulum may be seen almost anywhere in the abdomen. False-negative studies may occur when the diverticulum is closely applied to an area of normal accumulation of the radiopharmaceutical, such as the bladder, or when there is only a minimal amount of gastric mucosa (Table 67-1). False-positive studies may occur but can be mini-

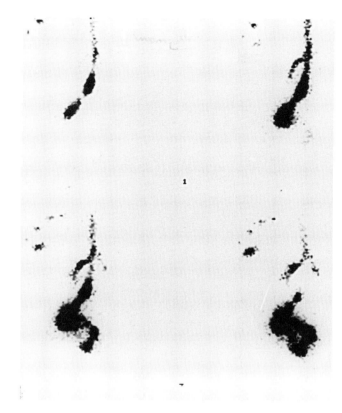

FIGURE 67-3. While seated with her back to the collimator, this 7-year-old girl swallowed a 10-ml bolus labeled with 300 μCi of sulfur colloid. The image reveals bilateral pulmonary aspiration as well as activity in the tracheostomy site.

FIGURE 67-4. This is an example of a positive salivagram. Approximately 100 μl of labeled sulfur colloid (300 μCi) was placed on the tongue and allowed to mix with oral secretions. There is aspiration into both lungs.

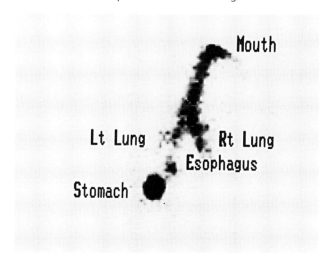

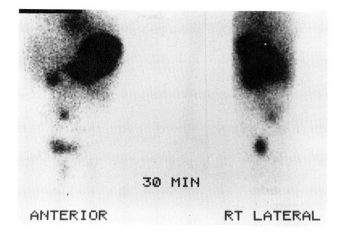

30 MIN

ANTERIOR   RT LATERAL

FIGURE 67-5. Following premedication with pentagastrin, an abnormal focus was seen above the bladder, to the right of the midline and anteriorly, due to a Meckel's diverticulum. The patient is a 9-month-old boy who presented with a large, painless rectal bleed.

mized with good imaging technique (Table 67-2). In surgically proven cases, the sensitivity of the test has been found to be 85% with a specificity of 95%. Using clinical criteria as well, the accuracy is about 98%.[17]

Gastrointestinal Bleeding (Other Sites)

For the localization of a bleeding focus in the bowel, two techniques are generally available. One utilizes ^{99m}Tc–sulfur colloid injected intravenously. This agent is rapidly cleared by the liver and spleen and only appears in the bowel if there is active bleeding. It is a very sensitive technique but has the disadvantage that patients must be bleeding at the time of injection.

A second technique utilizing ^{99m}Tc labeled red blood cells is generally preferred. Two to three milliliters of the patient's blood is labeled with a radiopharmaceutical by an in vitro kit, giving a high labeling efficiency. The blood is reinjected, and 15-second images are obtained in the anterior projection. If the patient is not bleeding

TABLE 67-1. False-Positive Meckel's Scan

1. Ectopic gastric mucosa (duplications)
2. Urinary tract (ectopic kidney, extrarenal pelvis, reflux)
3. Inflammatory foci (appendicitis, abscess, inflamed bowel, ulcer)
4. Surgical condition (intussusception, volvulus)
5. Uterine blush
6. Anterior meningomyelocele
7. Vascular tumors (arteriovenous malformation, hemangioma)
8. Solid tumors (rhabdomyosarcoma)

TABLE 67-2. False-Negative Meckel's Scan

1. No gastric mucosa present
2. Hyperperistalsis (causing washout of excreted activity)
3. Insufficient or hypofunctioning gastric mucosa
4. Overlying structures (bladder, kidneys)
5. Poor technique
6. Active bleeding (causing dilution of material)
7. Mucosal ischemia or necrosis

at the time of injection, the imaging period may be extended for an hour or more. Playing back the contrasted images in cine mode is a useful way to detect and localize the bleeding site (Fig. 67-6). Bringing the patient back for delayed imaging has limited value. If interval bleeding has occurred, it will be recognized, but the origin cannot be determined. Delayed imaging is only useful if active bleeding recurs while under the gamma camera. The diagnosis of an active bleed requires movement of the focus of increased activity. A focal increase that does not move over time may be due to abnormal vessels or vascular lesions.

HEPATOBILIARY SCINTIGRAPHY (DISIDA SCAN)

Hepatobiliary scintigraphy is most frequently performed in the evaluation of neonatal hyperbilirubinemia. The differential diagnosis of persistent, primarily conjugated jaundice in the newborn is extensive and includes various infections, anatomic abnormalities, metabolic disease, and genetic causes.

Hepatobiliary scintigraphy is also useful in assessing liver function, gallbladder disease, and post liver transplant or hepatobiliary surgery.

Neonatal Jaundice

With regard to biliary obstruction in neonates, it may be difficult to distinguish biliary atresia from severe intrahepatic cholestasis. The urgency in making this distinction is reflected in the results of surgical intervention. In infants with biliary atresia, sustained bile flow is significantly greater after portal enterostomy in infants operated on before 60 days of age (91%), compared with those operated on after 3 months (17%).[18] While abdominal ultrasound may show dilated intrahepatic ducts

FIGURE 67-6. Following a liver transplant, rectal bleeding was noted in this 5-year-old boy. A scan to delineate the bleeding site performed with ^{99m}Tc labeled red blood cells was positive in the distal small bowel.

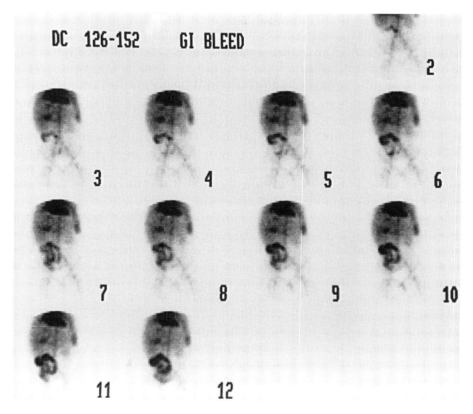

(associated with common bile duct obstruction due to stones or stricture or a choledochal cyst), the features of biliary atresia and neonatal hepatitis are not specific. Hepatobiliary imaging is extremely useful in these cases, since biliary excretion into the bowel excludes biliary atresia.

Imaging is usually performed with ^{99m}Tc–diisopropyl iminodiacetic acid (DISIDA) or ^{99m}Tc–methylbromo iminodiacetic acid (Mebrofenin). These radiopharmaceuticals are lipophilic and are transported to the liver, bound to albumin, and actively taken up by the hepatocytes. Although they are not conjugated, they are excreted into the bile canaliculi following the same anionic pathway as bilirubin. Pretreatment with phenobarbital (5 mg/kg daily in divided doses given orally for 5 days) may increase the specificity of the study. Images are obtained for 1 hour. If there is no evidence of excretion, further views are obtained 4 to 6 hours and even up to 24 hours after injection if necessary. Based on the presence or absence of radioactivity in the bowel, biliary atresia is diagnosed with a sensitivity of 97%, a specificity of 82%, and an accuracy of 91%.[19]

The DISIDA scan relies on the ability of the liver to actively extract the radionuclide from the bloodstream. In individuals with liver disease, pharmaceutical uptake may be poor. Hepatocyte function is relatively preserved in the first 2 to 3 months of life in patients with biliary atresia; thus, the lack of biliary excretion in these infants will suggest a greater likelihood of biliary atresia. In infants with neonatal hepatitis, there is a variable degree of hepatocyte dysfunction, manifesting as impaired uptake by the liver, which often makes biliary excretion difficult to demonstrate. Evidence of excretion into the bowel may occur, although it may be considerably delayed.

Cholecystitis

Hepatobiliary imaging is useful for evaluating patients with right upper quadrant pain. Acute cholecystitis is reliably excluded by demonstrating normal filling of the gallbladder. Functional abnormalities associated with pain, such as spasm of Oddi's sphincter or the cystic duct syndrome, can be excluded by quantitating the gallbladder contraction in response to sincalide, a synthetic cholecystokinin. The normal gallbladder has an "ejection fraction" of greater than about 37%.

Occasionally, the administration of cholecystokinin, which causes gallbladder contraction, can be used as an adjunct to the DISIDA scan in an attempt to reduce the patient's pain and to demonstrate adequate gallbladder emptying.

Postsurgical Biliary Disease

Biliary scintigraphy is useful for demonstrating obstruction or leaks after hepatobiliary surgery. The findings in liver transplant rejection are not specific. These findings are similar to biliary infection or other causes of cholestasis. A normal study excludes rejection with a high degree of confidence. Sequential studies are also useful for monitoring the effect of therapy for infection or rejection. Quantitative techniques, such as deconvolutional analysis, add objectivity to the visual interpretation of the images.

REFERENCES

1. Holloway RH, Orenstein SR. Gastroesophageal disease in adults and children. Baillieres Clin Gastroenterol 1991;5: 337–370

2. Richter JE, Blackwell JN, Wu WC et al. Relationship of radionuclide liquid bolus transport and esophageal manometry. J Lab Clin Med 1987;109:217–224

3. Svedburg JB. The bolus transport diagram: a functional display method applied to oesophageal studies. Clin Phys Physiol Meas 1982;3:267–272

4. Heyman S, Kirkpatrick JA, Winter HS, Treves S. An improved method for the diagnosis of gastroesophageal reflux and aspiration in children (milk scan). Radiology 1979;131: 479–482

5. Piepsz A. Recent advances in pediatric nuclear medicine. Semin Nucl Med 1995;25(2):165–182

6. Ham HR, DiLorenzo C, Cadranel S et al. Gastroesophageal scintiscanning in children: a retrospective study on 500 examinations. J Nucl Med 1987;28:715–720

7. Siegel M, Lebenthal E, Topper W et al. Gastric emptying in prematures of isocaloric feedings with different osmolalities. Pediatr Res 1982;16:448–451

8. Cavell B. Gastric emptying in preterm infants. Acta Pediatr Scand 1979;68:725–730

9. Fried MD, Khoshoo V, Secker DJ et al. Decrease in gastric emptying time and episodes of regurgitation in children with spastic quadriplegia fed a whey based formula. J Pediatr 1992; 120:569–572

10. Signer E, Fridrich R. Gastric emptying in newborns and young infants. Acta Pediatr Scand 1975;64:525–530

11. DiLorenzo C, Piepsz A, Ham H, Cadranel S. Gastric emptying with gastroesophageal reflux. Arch Dis Child 1987;62: 449–453

12. Malmud LS, Fisher RS, Knight LC, Rock E. Scintigraphic evaluation of gastric emptying. Semin Nucl Med 1982;11 (1):116–125

13. Hollemeier AC, McCallum R, Gryoboski J. Delayed gastric emptying in infants with gastroesophageal reflux. J Pediatr 1981;98:190–193

14. Orellana P, Olea E, Pino C et al. Detection of pulmonary aspiration in children with gastroesophageal reflux, abstract. J Nucl Med 1985;26:P10

15. Heyman S, Respondek M. Detection of pulmonary aspiration in children by radionuclide "salivagram." J Nucl Med 1989; 30:697–699

16. Datz FL, Christian PE, Hutson WR et al. Physiological and pharmacological interventions in radionuclide imaging of

the gastrointestinal tract. Semin Nucl Med 1991;21: 140–152

17. Sfakianakis GN, Conway JJ. Detection of ectopic gastric mucosa in Meckel's diverticulum and in other aberrations by scintigraphy 11: indications and methods — a 10 year experience. J Nucl Med 1981;22:732–738

18. Kasai M, Suzuki K, Ohashi E et al. Technique and results of operative management of biliary atresia. World J Surg 1978;2:571–580

19. Gerhold JP, Klingensmith WC III, Kuni CC et al. Diagnosis of biliary atresia with radionuclide hepatobiliary imaging. Radiology 1983;146:499–504

68

MAGNETIC RESONANCE IMAGING

JAMES S. MEYER
ANNE M. HUBBARD

In this chapter, we review the technical aspects and diagnostic capabilities of magnetic resonance imaging (MRI), briefly compare MRI with computed tomography (CT), and propose how MRI can be used, both now and in the future, for the evaluation of the gastrointestinal (GI) system in children.

The first human magnetic resonance image was obtained in 1977, and by the mid-1980s, MRI had gained acceptance as a valuable clinical imaging examination.[1] MRI has become the diagnostic imaging study of choice for the evaluation of many disease processes, especially in the central nervous and musculoskeletal systems. Motion artifact and the lack of a suitable oral contrast agent, however, have limited the use of MRI in the GI system. Presently, advances in MRI and contrast technology are expanding the indications for the use of MRI. Familiarity with the strengths and weaknesses, as well as current and potential clinical applications, will enhance the physician's ability to use this technology for the diagnosis and management of children with GI disease.

TECHNICAL ASPECTS

MRI uses radio waves in conjunction with an external magnetic field and computer manipulation to provide images of virtually any part of the body.[2] The resulting magnetic resonance image depends on the magnetic field strength, pulse sequence used, intrinsic characteristics of the tissue imaged,[3] and patient motion. Both high (1.5 T) and low (less than 0.5 T) field strength scanners are used for clinical MRI.

Numerous pulse sequences are available and provide tissue-specific information such as T_1 and T_2 relaxation times, density of mobile protons, and blood flow.[3] Patient motion decreases image quality, and various techniques have been developed to minimize the artifact caused by physiologic activities such as respiration and vascular pulsation.

Though physiologic motion (including peristalsis) can lessen image quality, gross patient movement can make images interpretable. At our institution, all children are evaluated by the MRI staff prior to the examination. Most children older than 6 years of age are able to cooperate and are told that they must remain stationary while the examination is being performed. Younger children usually require medication for conscious sedation.[4] General anesthesia is rarely required to obtain an examination of diagnostic quality.

MRI examinations of the abdomen are usually composed of multiple sets of pulse sequences with each sequence resulting in a corresponding set of images. These pulse sequences can be performed in any imaging plane, and specific sequences are optimized to accentuate different tissue characteristics such as T_1 and T_2 relaxation times, proton density, blood flow, and magnetic susceptibility. A single sequence can last from 15 seconds to more than 10 minutes. Each MRI examination is tailored to the specific clinical problem being evaluated, and a complete examination may be performed in as little as 15 minutes or may last longer than 2 hours. Magnetic resonance angiography (MRA), post–gadolinium injection T_1-weighted, or other sequences may also be performed to help answer specific clinical questions.

A typical MRI examination of the abdomen will include T_1 and T_2-weighted sequences (Fig. 68-1). T_1-weighted sequences yield excellent anatomic information and detail. T_2-weighted sequences are particularly useful for showing areas of disease, which often have high signal intensity due to the presence of increased fluid. MRA sequences (Fig. 68-2) are sensitive to flow, which is high signal intensity, and these sequences can be reconstructed and presented as three-dimensional maximal intensity projection images (Fig. 68-3B). Though contrast injection is not needed to visualize most blood vessels, images obtained after intravenous injection of gadolinium chelates (Fig. 68-4) can make some lesions more conspicuous and clarify whether areas of abnormality are due to soft tissue or fluid-filled structures. Other specific sequences can be done to evaluate the presence of fat or hemosiderin.

MRI VERSUS CT

Unlike CT and plain radiography, MRI does not use ionizing radiation. Since variations of T_1 and T_2 relaxation times are much greater than variations in soft tissue density, MRI provides much better soft tissue contrast than CT.[3] The image resolution of CT, however, is greater than that for MRI. The improved resolution of CT is even more significant when patient motion, a major factor in children, is considered. As noted previously, MRI is quite sensitive to patient motion (Fig. 68-5A). Though CT images are also degraded by motion, a single CT image can be acquired in less than 1 second, and an entire CT scan of the abdomen using spiral technique can be acquired in less than 30 seconds. As a result, sedation that would be necessary for an MRI is often not required for a CT scan of the abdomen. Additionally, peristalsis causes no significant image degradation on CT scans. Recent MRI techniques, employing pulse sequences during which multiple images can be obtained during a single breath-hold (Fig. 68-5B), minimize motion but are only possible in extremely cooperative patients. New developments in echo planar MRI, which acquires a multisection study of the upper abdomen in 2 seconds, are likely to further enhance the effectiveness of MRI in evaluating the GI tract.[5]

Abdominal MRI images can be acquired in any plane. CT images are acquired axially. While CT images can be reconstructed in other planes, the directly acquired MRI image usually has better resolution and is of higher quality than a comparably reconstructed CT image. This multiplanar capability, along with the ability to visualize blood vessels without contrast injection, gives MRI a great advantage over CT for the evaluation of vascular relationships and encasement.

When intravenous contrast is administered for MRI, the distribution of the gadolinium chelates is similar to that of iodinated contrast used for CT. Lower volumes of contrast, however, are used for MRI, and the gadolinium chelates have a larger margin of safety than the contrast used in CT[3] Oral contrast is used to distinguish bowel from other fluid collections and to improve the visualization of bowel lesions on CT scans. No generally accepted oral contrast agent is currently available for MRI. Clinical studies with materials as diverse as manganese chloride, carbon dioxide, and baby formulas, however, have been performed in an attempt to fill this void in abdominal MRI.[6]

CLINICAL APPLICATIONS

We do not believe that MRI, in its present form, is an appropriate screening study for the examination of the abdomen. Rather, we recommend MRI as a problem-solving technique to further evaluate abdominal abnormalities found by other imaging studies, usually CT or ultrasonography. Occasionally, we use MRI rather than CT in a child with an allergy to iodinated contrast. In the following sections, we will discuss clinical applications of MRI to the GI system.

Abdominal Masses

A child with a suspected abdominal mass will usually undergo ultrasonography to confirm the presence of the mass and determine the organ of origin. When a solid tumor is found or an abnormality is inadequately demonstrated by ultrasonography, additional cross-sectional imaging will be performed. We usually perform CT as the next imaging study because of the advantages of oral contrast and negligible motion artifact; however, others prefer MRI. MRI should be used if clinically important questions regarding organ of origin, lesion characterization, vascular encasement, or spinal involvement remain after the performance of a CT scan.

Liver

Abdominal MRI has been most successful and generally accepted in the evaluation of the liver. Clinical application in children is generally limited to the evaluation of tumors and vascular flow.

In children with hepatic tumors (Fig. 68-6), MRI can define liver anatomy and help plan surgical resection.[7,8] MRI characteristics, however, do not always differentiate benign from malignant lesions.[9] Nonetheless, an MRI showing the classic appearance of a benign lesion can guide patient management by avoiding unnecessary biopsy and reassuring both the parents and physicians.

MRI, especially with MRA sequences, is excellent for the noninvasive evaluation of vascular abnormalities

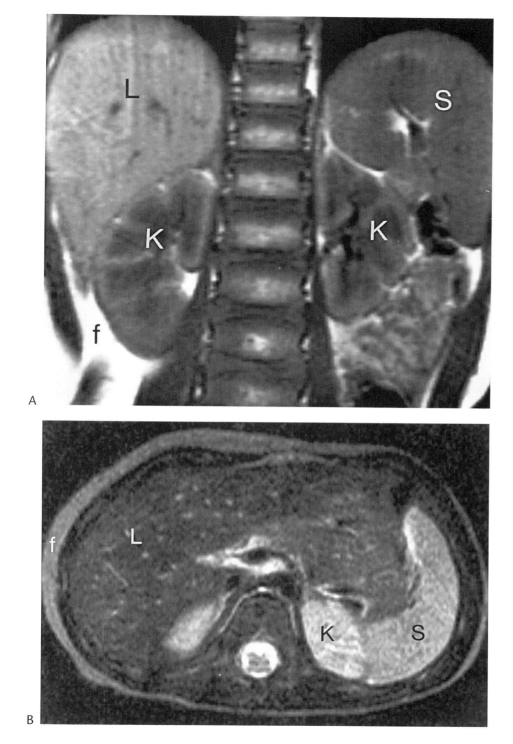

FIGURE 68-1. Coronal T_1-weighted *(A)* and axial T_2-weighted *(B)* images in normal patients. Normal liver (L) is brighter than spleen (S) on T_1-weighted sequences; spleen is brighter than liver on T_2-weighted sequences. K, kidneys; f, fat.

such as thrombosis or cavernous transformation of the portal vein, portal hypertension, and congenital anomalies.[7] Abnormalities may be suspected from the findings on routine MRI and confirmed by MRA without contrast injection. For instance, an area of intermediate signal within a vessel on a T_1-weighted sequence (Fig. 68-7A) suggests the presence of a blood clot. An MRA sequence (Fig. 68-7B) can confirm this by showing the absence of blood flow in the area of abnormality. MRA sequences also can be used to confirm the blood flow in collateral vessels and to detect reversal of flow in the portal vein as an indication of portal hypertension.

An additional application for MRI in the liver is the evaluation of fatty infiltration. Hepatic fatty infiltration may be suspected from the low attenuation of the liver on CT scan or increased liver echogenicity on ultrasonography. The diagnosis of diffuse fatty infiltration is usually apparent. Focal fatty infiltration, however, may simulate a tumor, and in these patients MRI may provide the correct diagnosis.

MRI has been suggested as the imaging study of choice for children prior to liver transplantation.[10] We and others[11] feel that MRI should be reserved only for preoperative patients in whom vascular structures are not adequately defined by ultrasonography. Following transplantation, ultrasonography is the primary imaging study to confirm vascular patency, detect biliary dilation, and determine the presence of perihepatic fluid collections. Though MRI may rarely be used to evaluate vascular patency, contrast angiography is required when there is a strong suspicion of hepatic artery occlusion.[2]

Biliary System

Currently, MRI plays no role in the direct visualization of the biliary system in children. Though gallbladder wall disease and gallstones may be seen on MRI,[12] ultrasonography and CT are better for demonstrating these abnormalities. Advances in contrast chemistry are being directed toward the development of gadolinium-based contrast agents to enhance visualization of the biliary tree on MRI. The availability of such compounds, combined with ultrafast MRI pulse sequences displayed as maximal intensity projections, could result in high-quality three-dimensional images of the biliary system. Then MRI may become a significant imaging modality for the evaluation of the biliary system.[12]

Pancreas

MRI has been shown to be useful for the evaluation of a variety of pancreatic diseases in adults.[13] In children, MRI has a very limited role. In children with Schwachman's syndrome, MRI can confirm fatty infiltration of the pancreas.[14] For pancreatitis, MRI has no clear

FIGURE 68-2. Axial two-dimensional MRA image shows high signal intensity representing flowing blood in patent umbilical vein (arrow) and collaterals (arrowheads) in a 7-year-old girl with portal hypertension. p, portal vein; a, aorta; curved arrow, inferior vena cava.

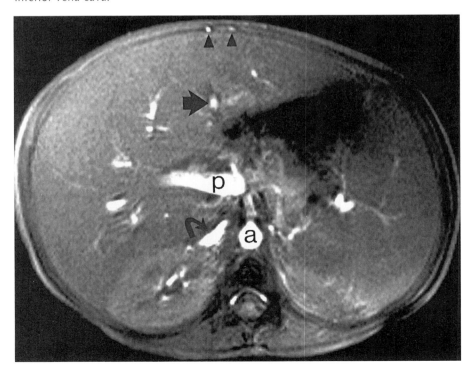

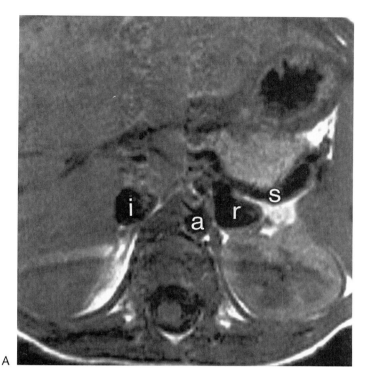

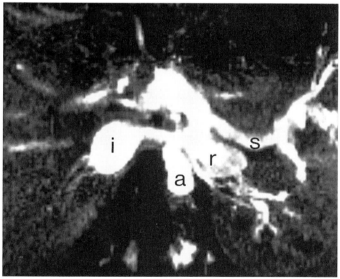

FIGURE 68-3. Axial T$_1$-weighted image *(A)* and three-dimensional maximal intensity projection MRA image *(B)* show connection between splenic (s) and left renal (r) veins in a 1-year-old boy with spontaneous porto-systemic shunt. i, inferior vena cava; a, aorta.

advantage over CT, and its routine use is not recommended.[15] MRI, however, may be useful for the localization of islet cell tumors, which tend to be small and can be difficult to locate by any modality. MRI, when optimized, is superior to CT and transabdominal ultrasonography for the detection of these tumors.[13]

Spleen

Splenomegaly and focal splenic lesions such as abscesses, tumors, vascular malformations, and cysts can be demonstrated by MRI.[16] Nonetheless, MRI is not generally used as a primary imaging modality for the spleen but rather as a complement to CT and ultrasonography. The mul-

tiplanar capability and potential for tissue characterization inherent in MRI, however, may make it useful as a problem-solving tool. Current research into reticuloendothelial system–specific contrast agents may give MRI the ability to provide not only anatomic but also physiologic information and make MRI the imaging study of choice for the spleen in the future.[17]

Bowel

Physiologic and gross motion artifacts and the absence of a suitable oral contrast agent have limited the use of MRI in the evaluation of the bowel. Intravenous gado-

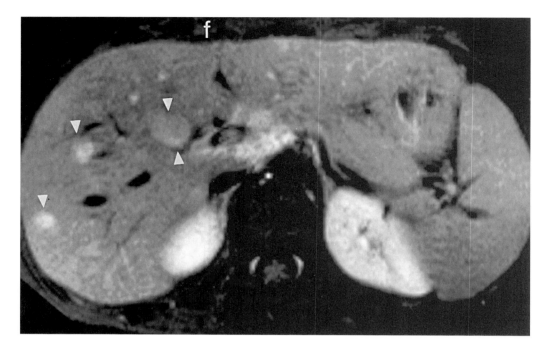

FIGURE 68-4. Axial T$_1$-weighted image with fat suppression shows multiple enhancing areas (arrowheads) after gadolinium-DTPA injection in a 9-year-old girl with cat-scratch fever. Note the lack of signal from the subcutaneous fatty tissue (f) due to fat suppression.

linium administration combined with recent advances of breath-hold and fat suppression sequences has improved the capability of MRI to demonstrate disease and increased the utilization of MRI for evaluation of bowel disease, especially in adults. Polyps, duplication cysts, Meckel's diverticula, malignant tumors, inflammatory bowel disease, and appendicitis have all been demonstrated on MRI.[18] At the present time we do not use MRI for these purposes, but we remain open to its potential for the future. Development of a generally accepted oral contrast agent will likely further increase the use of MRI in the GI tract.

FIGURE 68-5. (*A*) Coronal T$_1$-weighted spin echo image degraded by motion artifact in a 13-year-old boy. (*B*) Coronal T$_1$-weighted breath-hold image in an adult.

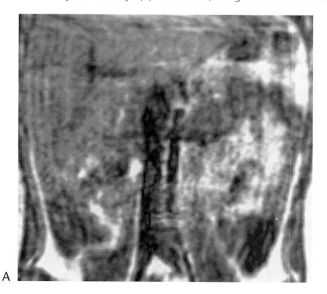

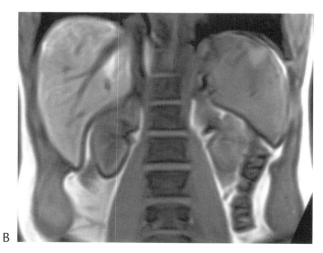

A   B

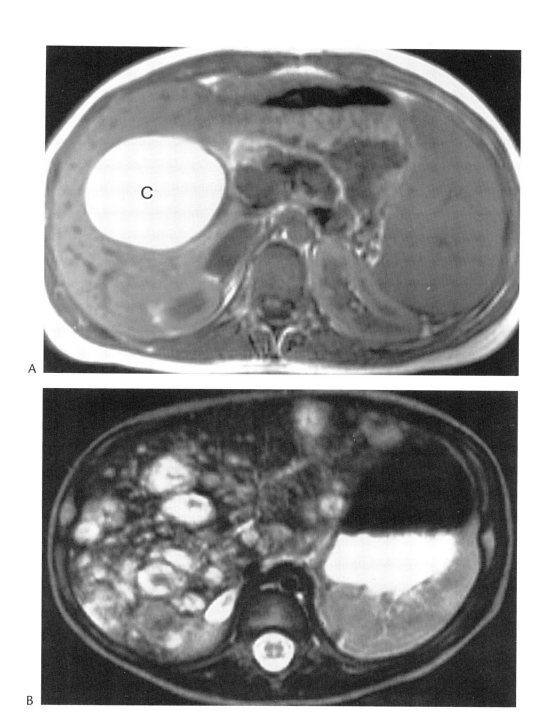

FIGURE 68-6. (A) Axial T$_1$-weighted image shows large mass in a 17-year-old girl with benign intrahepatic cyst (C). (B) Axial T$_2$-weighted image shows multiple high-intensity masses, some with central areas of thrombosis, in a 1-month-old boy with hemangioendothelioma.

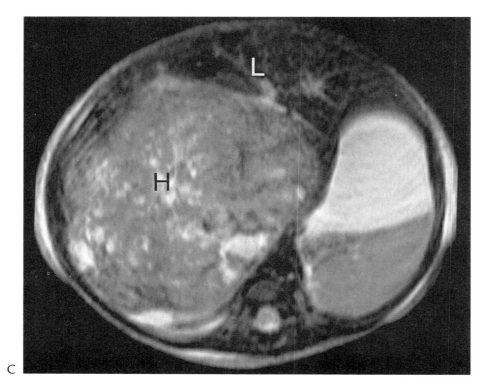

FIGURE 68-6. *(Continued)* (*C*) Axial T$_2$-weighted image shows a large mass in a 1-year-old boy with hepatoblastoma (H). L, normal liver.

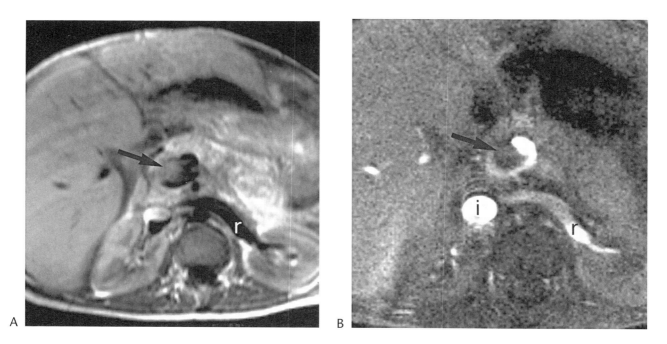

FIGURE 68-7. *(A)* Axial T$_1$-weighted image in a 15-year-old boy shows an intermediate-signal clot (arrow) in portal vein. *(B)* Axial MRA sequence shows bright signal representing blood flowing around the clot (arrow). i, inferior vena cava; r, left renal vein.

CONCLUSION

Currently, MRI is best used to clarify abnormalities demonstrated on CT and ultrasonography. MRI can be particularly valuable for the demonstration of hepatic and other abdominal vascular abnormalities, showing the origin and extent of abdominal tumors and defining and characterizing hepatic masses. MRI should also be considered the primary modality for the localization of islet cell tumors. Technical advances in MRI, however, are occurring rapidly, and it is reasonable to expect that in the future there will be more widespread clinical application for MRI in evaluation of GI disease in children.

REFERENCES

1. Seibert JA. One hundred years of medical diagnostic imaging technology. Health Phys 1995;69:695–720

2. Meyer JS, Fellows KE. Vascular imaging in children. Semin Pediatr Surg 1994;3:79–86

3. Edelman RR, Warach S. Magnetic resonance imaging. N Engl J Med 1993;328:708–716

4. Hubbard AM, Markowitz RI, Kimmel B et al. Sedation for pediatric patients undergoing CT and MRI. J Comput Assist Tomogr 1992;16:3–6

5. Edelman RR, Wielopolski P, Schmitt F. Echo-planar MR imaging. Radiology 1994;192:600–612

6. Rijcken P, Davis MA, Ros PR. Intraluminal contrast agents for MR imaging of the abdomen and pelvis. J Magn Reson Imaging 1994;4:291–300

7. Hubbard AM, Meyer JS, Mahboubi S. Diagnosis of liver disease in children: value of MR angiography. AJR 1992;159:617–621

8. Boechat MI, Kangarloo H. MR imaging of the abdomen in children. AJR 1989;152:1245–1250

9. deLange EE. Cross-sectional imaging of the liver. Baillieres Clin Gastroenterol 1995;9:97–120

10. Bissett GS III, Strife JL, Balistreri WF. Evaluation of children for liver transplantation: value of MR imaging and sonography. AJR 1990;155:351–356

11. Bowen AD, Applegate GR, Kanal E. Sonography vs MR imaging in children who are candidates for liver transplantation. AJR 1992;158:692–693

12. Brink JA, Borrello JA. MR imaging of the biliary system. Magn Reson Imaging Clin North Am 1995;3:143–160

13. Mitchell DG. MR imaging of the pancreas. Magn Reson Imaging North Am 1995;3:51–71

14. Bom EP, van der Sande FM, Tjon A et al. Schwachman syndrome: CT and MR diagnosis. J Comput Assist Tomogr 1993;17:474–476

15. Cohen MD: Gastrointestinal system. In: Cohen MD, Edwards MK, Eds. Magnetic Resonance Imaging of Children. Philadelphia: BC Decker, 1990;632

16. Siegel MJ. MR imaging of the pediatric abdomen. Magn Reson Imaging North Am 1995;3:161–182

17. Torres GM, Terry NL, Mergo PJ, Ros PR. MR imaging of the spleen. Magn Reson Imaging Clin N Am 1995;3:39–50

18. Kettritz U, Shoenut JP, Semelka RC. MR imaging of the gastrointestinal tract. Magn Reson Imaging Clin N Am 1995;3:87–98

69

ANGIOGRAPHY AND INTERVENTIONAL PROCEDURES

DOUGLAS C. B. REDD
KENNETH E. FELLOWS

Angiography is an inclusive term, usually implying the use of catheters and contrast material to visualize the arterial, venous, or lymphatic vessels of the body. In pediatric gastrointestinal (GI) diseases, arteriography and venography are useful in certain clinical situations, especially when other "noninvasive" imaging studies have failed to provide a definitive diagnosis. These catheter-based techniques also have the advantage of allowing transcatheter therapies, or "interventions," such as embolization for GI bleeding or transjugular intrahepatic portocaval shunting (TIPS) for nonoperative management of portal hypertension or refractory ascites.

Nonvascular diagnostic and interventional procedures have also become common in children. For example, percutaneous transhepatic cholangiography (PTC) not only allows exquisite visualization of the biliary system, but also permits intrabiliary access for dilation of biliary strictures or removal of retained stones. Percutaneously inserted catheters placed under fluoroscopic, ultrasound, or computed tomographic (CT) guidance allow minimally invasive access for enteral feeding and drainage of parenchymal or peritoneal cysts and intra-abdominal abscesses. Using these same techniques, transcutaneous and transvenous biopsy can be performed with low morbidity, even in the coagulopathic patient. This chapter will review these diagnostic and interventional procedures, explaining for each the indications, risks, and alternatives.

VASCULAR DIAGNOSTIC AND INTERVENTIONAL PROCEDURES

Arteriography and Embolization

ABDOMINAL ARTERIOGRAPHY

There is no minimum age or size limit for abdominal arteriography; this study can be performed safely in newborns, infants, older children, and adolescents when properly sized catheters and other instruments are used by skilled and experienced physicians.

The best approach to the abdominal aorta and its branch vessels in the child is invariably from the femoral artery. Depending on the type of examination and operator preference, arteriography can be done under either general anesthesia or conscious sedation using local anesthesia. Abdominal arteriography not requiring concomitant interventional therapy usually takes 1 to 2 hours and can be done on an outpatient basis. The addition of procedural intervention typically prolongs the study and increases the periprocedural risks for which hospitalization is often warranted.

The single greatest risk of arteriography in the infant and small child is femoral artery (puncture site) thrombosis.[1,2] This complication occurs in less than 1% to 2% of patients (almost always in infants and smaller children) and has been reduced considerably by the use of 3 and 4 Fr catheters together with the immediate institution of systemic thrombolysis when the leg is pulseless after the procedure.[3] In children less than 5 years of age in whom there are no contraindications, anticoagulation is usually recommended at the outset of the procedure to minimize thrombotic complications. Transcatheter interventions, such as embolization, carry the risk of is-chemic injury from inadvertent migration of embolic material (nontarget embolization).[4] Dissection and arte-rial perforation by catheters or guidewires are distinctly rare complications when currently available catheter technologies are used; when these complications do occur, they can lead to significant intraperitoneal or ret-roperitoneal hemorrhage, necessitating prompt surgical repair. Much more common during arteriography is the occurrence of vasospasm, which both prolongs the exam-ination and may require the use of vasodilators. Allergic and anaphylactic reactions to intra-arterial injection of iodinated contrast media are very rare in the child and are even less common than similar injections into the venous circulation.

GASTROINTESTINAL

The exact site or source of bleeding in the GI tract needs to be established only when hemorrhage is large or so persistent that surgical intervention is being considered. Arteriography is usually the last resort after conservative therapies have failed to control hemorrhage and when endoscopy, nuclear medicine, or other tests fail to pre-cisely localize the bleeding site. Such severe GI bleeding is much less common in children than in adults, the most frequent causes in children being stress or peptic ulcer disease, typhlitis, inflammatory bowel disease, vascular malformations, and clotting disorders.[5]

In our experience, very brisk arterial bleeding must exist for arteriography to unequivocally demonstrate the bleeding source; this means that vigorous resuscitation, including ongoing transfusion, is required to keep up with the GI blood losses (Fig. 69-1). Arteriography may, however, demonstrate a vascular malformation or other abnormality as the cause.[6] When a precise site is identi-fied, embolization may be the treatment of choice as long as it can be performed peripherally (close to the hemor-rhage) such that normal tissues are not jeopardized by ischemia.

ARTERIAL PORTOGRAPHY

Ultrasound imaging is the primary screening modality used to evaluate for changes associated with portal hyper-tension. Magnetic resonance imaging (MRI) is also use-ful and can demonstrate variceal collaterals. In children suspected of having portal hypertension, the most com-prehensive physiologic imaging of the portal venous sys-tem is by "arterial portography" in which a bolus of iodi-nated contrast is injected into either the splenic or superior mesenteric artery with delayed imaging followed into the (portal) venous phase. Arterial portography is usually reserved for those patients in whom anatomic

definition is not provided by less invasive examinations; it is most often requested either to verify the presence of cavernous transformation of the portal vein (the most common cause of portal hypertension in children) or to document the extent of gastroesophageal varices. Arte-rial portography is also valuable following pediatric liver transplantation to exclude stenosis of the portal venous anastomosis and to evaluate for other causes of postoper-ative portal hypertension. When the portal vein is pat-ent, and varices are present, arterial portography can be combined with measurements of the free and wedged hepatic vein pressures to approximate the portal venous pressure and portosystemic gradient.

Optimal visualization of the portal venous system may require that the examination be performed under general anesthesia, during which respirations may be suspended. Direct opacification of the portal venous system may be obtained percutaneously, via either transhepatic porto-graphy or direct splenoportography. These methods carry a slightly higher procedural risk but are still safe enough to be performed on an outpatient basis.

LIVER TRANSPLANTATION

Normal hepatic arterial blood flow is critical to the long-term success of orthotopic liver transplantation; unfortu-nately, postoperative hepatic arterial stenosis and throm-bosis are more common in infants and children than in adults, largely because of the smaller size of the arteries involved. As even mildly diminished hepatic arterial per-fusion can lead to biliary ductal ischemia and subsequent biliary stricture formation, the hepatic arteries require frequent monitoring, which is usually accomplished by Doppler ultrasonography in the postoperative period. If there is any question about the integrity of the hepatic artery, or if the clinical and Doppler ultrasound findings are disparate, arteriography is indicated.[7]

Other common postoperative vascular complications following orthotopic liver transplantation may require alternative means of evaluation, such as venography via a transfemoral or transjugular route (Fig. 69-2). Transhe-patic access may also be necessary to treat strictures of the hepatic and portal veins (Fig. 69-3).

PREOPERATIVE HEPATIC ARTERIOGRAPHY

Magnetic resonance arteriography (MRA) is a variation on standard body MRI techniques that allows visualiza-tion of vascular structures without requiring the injection of contrast material. This modality has generally replaced diagnostic arteriography in the preoperative evaluation of children who have hepatoblastoma and other liver malignancies, hepatic vascular malformations, or other indications for partial hepatectomy. The variable arterial and venous supply of the liver can usually be sufficiently predicted by MRA, ultrasound, and other studies that arteriography is seldom required. Use of arteriography is usually limited to children who require preoperative embolization to facilitate a safer surgical procedure.

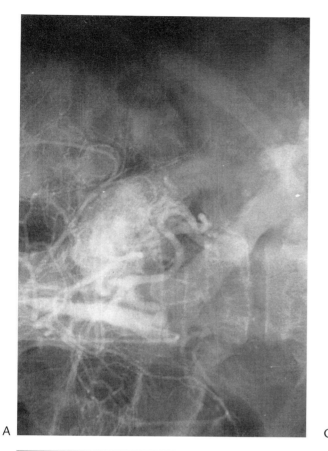

A

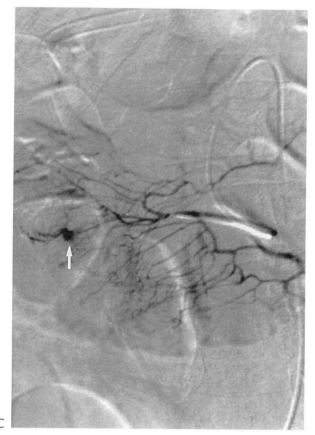

C

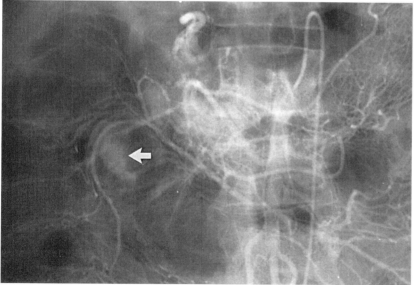

B

FIGURE 69-1. *(A)* Visceral arteriogram in a patient with Osler-Weber-Rendu disease who presents with acute upper GI bleeding. An area of hypervascularity supplied by arteries from the inferior pancreaticoduodenal arcade shows early arterioportal shunting during superior mesenteric arterial injection. *(B)* An image obtained during the late arterial phase shows pooling of contrast in the jejunum (arrow). *(C)* Subselective imaging in the same patient demonstrates active hemorrhage into the jejunum (arrow).

Inferior Vena Cavography, Hepatic Venography, and TIPS

The systemic venous system (hepatic veins and inferior vena cava) and the portal venous system both may be involved in GI diseases. Catheter approaches to these systems, whether for pressure monitoring, diagnostic imaging, or intervention (e.g., transvenous biopsy, variceal embolization, and TIPS), are quite different. Systemic veins can be easily catheterized from the femoral (most common), internal jugular, and axillary venous approach. The risks of diagnostic venography are low when compared to arteriography; these represent mostly allergic contrast reactions. Postcatheterization thrombosis at

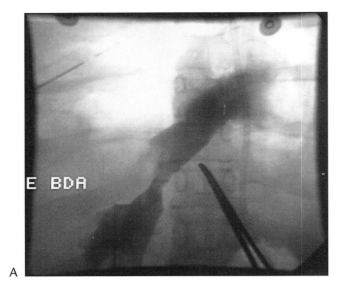

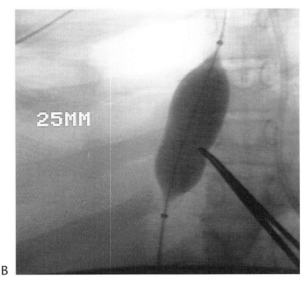

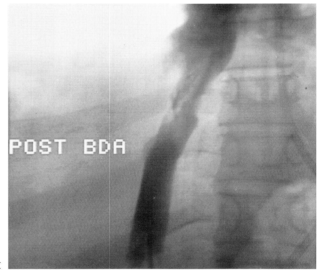

FIGURE 69-2. *(A)* Postoperative stenosis in a child following orthotopic liver transplantation involving the retrohepatic inferior vena cava diagnosed by contrast venography using a transfemoral approach. *(B)* and *(C)* Balloon dilation of the lesion is followed by significant improvement in luminal diameter with commensurate reduction in pressure gradient measured across this stenosis.

the venous puncture site is rare beyond infancy and is usually clinically inconsequential. Systemic venous access usually requires only conscious sedation using local anesthesia at the puncture site and is commonly performed on an outpatient basis.

TRANSHEPATIC PORTOGRAPHY

Transhepatic portography is the only nonsurgical means of catheterization of the portal system and is achieved by a needle puncture of an intrahepatic branch of the portal system, which can be approached either in a retrograde manner through a hepatic vein or by direct percutaneous transhepatic puncture, using an intercostal or subcostal approach,[8] often with ultrasound guidance. In children, either method is usually performed under general anesthesia. Following transhepatic catheterization, branches of the portal and mesenteric veins may easily be selected. Transhepatic portography allows exquisite portal venography and precise measurements of portal

venous pressures and gradients. It also facilitates catheter-based interventions, such as embolization of varices and balloon dilation or stenting of portal venous strictures (Fig. 69-4), as well as access for thrombolysis of portal or mesenteric venous thrombosis. Percutaneous transhepatic entry via puncture of the liver capsule carries a higher risk of bleeding, both intra- and postprocedurally, especially if the patient's clotting factors are not optimal. To increase safety of this procedure, the catheter tract may be embolized with gelatin sponge, coils, or other embolic materials on withdrawal of the catheter at the completion of the study. Using these guidelines and techniques, we have had no instances of bleeding in over 25 pediatric patients in whom we have performed transhepatic access.

If direct transhepatic catheterization is not required, indirect measurement of portal pressure can be obtained by hepatic vein wedge measurements, in which a catheter is passed, via either a superior or inferior vena caval

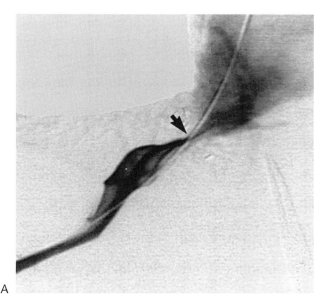

A

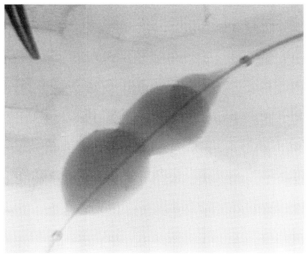

B

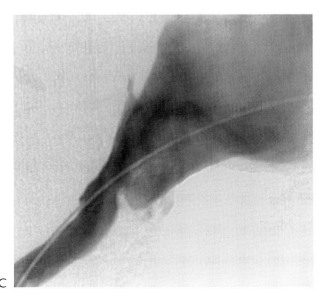

C

FIGURE 69-3. *(A)* Postoperative hepatic vein stenosis following orthotopic liver transplantation in a child with a reduced-size grate (left lateral segment) with hepatocellular dysfunction. Following percutaneous transhepatic access, a catheter and guidewire have been advanced across the hepatic vein stenosis (arrow) into the right atrium. *(B)* and *(C)* Balloon dilation of the stenosis is followed by modest improvement in luminal diameter of the hepatic vein. Technical failure and early restenosis appear to be due to elastic recoil of the surrounding scar tissues.

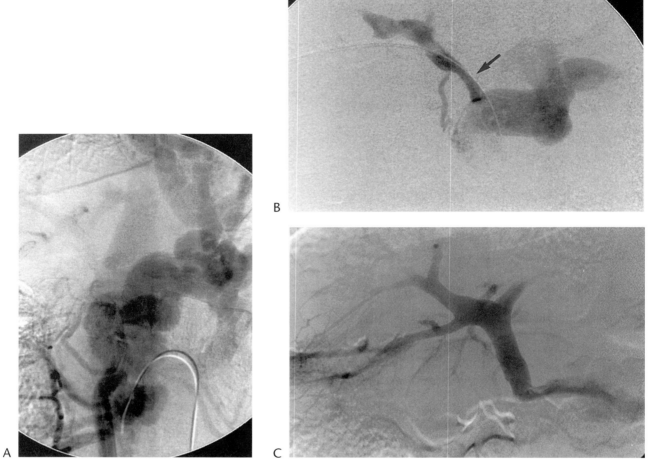

FIGURE 69-4. *(A)* Visceral arteriography was performed in an 18-year-old woman with remote history of radiation following right upper quadrant surgery. She presented with splenomegaly, hypersplenism, and varices on upper endoscopy. An image from the portal venous phase of a superior mesenteric artery injection shows a massively enlarged coronary vein filling gastroesophageal varices with only minimal hepatopetal flow into the portal vein. *(B)* Percutaneous transhepatic access of the portal system was performed and shows a significant stenosis of the proximal extrahepatic portal vein (arrow), again with filling of the coronary vein. *(C)* Following balloon dilation of the extrahepatic portal vein stenosis, there was a significant increase in hepatopetal portal venous flow with diminished variceal filling. Postprocedurally, the patient's spleen size decreased, and hypersplenism resolved.

approach, into a hepatic vein branch and "wedged" as distally as possible. In this manner, the catheter records hepatic sinusoidal pressure, which is an indirect measure of the portal venous pressure.

SPLENOPORTOGRAPHY

Splenoportography is a means of visualizing the portal venous system by a direct injection of contrast into the splenic pulp through a needle or sheath. Opacification of the splenic vein, portal vein, and gastroesophageal varices is usually good, unless there is massive splenomegaly or severely elevated portal venous pressures. Splenoportography can usually be done under conscious sedation with local anesthesia; normal clotting factors are a prerequisite. To increase procedural safety and decrease risk of bleeding, the needle or sheath tract can be embolized at the end of the study. Because these veins can now be more safely visualized with spiral CT and MRA techniques, splenoportography is seldom indicated in contemporary pediatric diagnosis.

TIPS

TIPS is a percutaneous catheter-based procedure that creates an intrahepatic portosystemic shunt by the insertion of a transparenchymal expandable metallic stent between a branch of the portal vein and the hepatic veins (Fig. 69-5).[9] Developed in adults over the past 10 years, TIPS is beginning to find a useful role in the management of certain diseases of childhood (e.g., palliation of recurrent variceal bleeding or refractory ascites in children with portal hypertension and in some cases of Budd-Chiari syndrome). Because the procedure can be relatively long and involved, general anesthesia in children is recommended, but not absolutely essential.

Briefly, the sequential steps for percutaneous creation of a portosystemic shunt involve first the retrograde catheterization of a hepatic vein (usually via the right internal jugular approach) with a sheath positioned within the hepatic vein; next, with a Colapinto needle, a puncture is made into the hepatic parenchyma to locate an intrahepatic branch of the portal venous system. This is followed by threading a guidewire from the hepatic vein into the portal vein to facilitate dilation of the hepatic parenchymal tract between the hepatic and portal venous branches (Fig. 69-5A). The TIPS is finished with deployment of a metallic stent to create a persistent shunt that decompresses the portal venous system into the systemic venous circulation. In this manner, portal hypertension can be controlled. Embolization of undesirable gastroesophageal varices may also be done at the

FIGURE 69-5. *(A)* During the TIPS procedure, the internal jugular vein is accessed, allowing the hepatic veins to be catheterized in a retrograde manner. In this example, a right hepatic vein has been entered. After puncture of an intrahepatic branch of the right portal vein, a guidewire is passed through the portal vein into a mesenteric vein. A vascular sheath is advanced into the hepatic parenchymal tract (arrow). *(B)* Transhepatic portography performed after a catheter has been inserted into the splenic vein demonstrates an enlarged coronary vein with filling of larger gastroesophageal varices in this child with cystic fibrosis, portal hypertension, and acute upper GI hemorrhage.

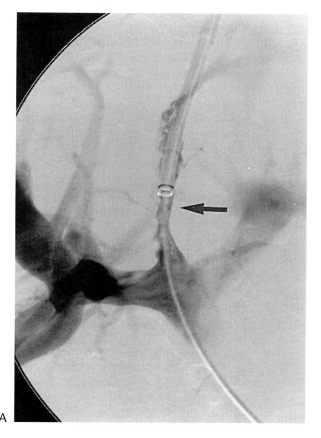

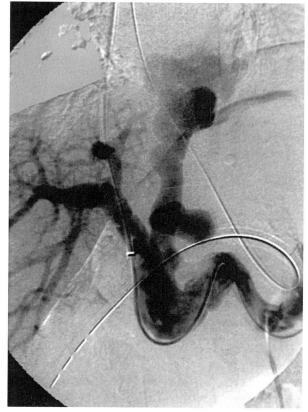

A

B

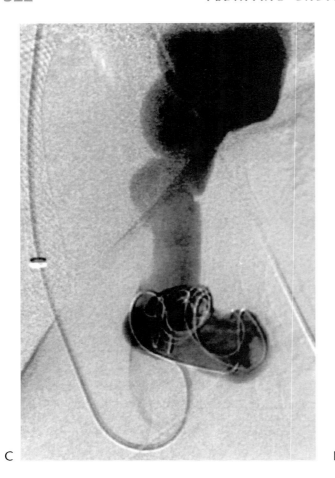

C

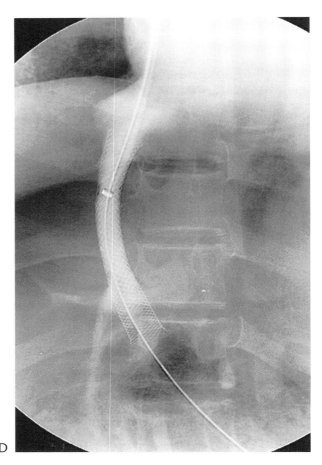

D

FIGURE 69-5. *(Continued)* *(C)* After placement of a metallic stent in this same patient between intrahepatic branches of the right portal and right hepatic veins, persistent variceal bleeding required coil embolization of the coronary vein. *(D)* Final TIPS venogram shows positioning of a metallic stent with contrast draining through a right hepatic vein into the right atrium.

time of TIPS while the catheter is in the portal venous system (Fig. 69-5C).

Eventual narrowing over subsequent months usually affects shunt function, with recurrence of portal hypertension. Follow-up monitoring is essential, and repeat interventions (dilation and/or stenting) may be needed to maintain satisfactory decompression of portal hypertension.[10] Results reported in adults show that procedural mortality is low (0.6% to 4.3%) with a highly variable 30-day mortality (0% to 40%) that reflects the clinical status of the patient pre-TIPS.[11] Procedural complications can include perforation of the liver capsule, hepatic artery, right atrium, and main (extrahepatic) portal vein puncture. Postshunt encephalopathy in adults is observed in approximately 20% of patients.[10] In children, the experience is small, but both the severe complication rates and the incidence of postshunt encephalopathy appear to be lower.[12]

NONVASCULAR DIAGNOSTIC AND INTERVENTIONAL PROCEDURES

Percutaneous Transhepatic Cholangiography

PTC offers, with low morbidity, precise visualization of the intra- and extrahepatic biliary tree via direct injection of iodinated contrast through a small-caliber needle. Contrast is slowly injected into the bile ducts, and fluoroscopic films are taken in multiple projections. With proper technique, this procedure is safe, reliable, and diagnostically accurate in infants and children. When the intrahepatic bile ducts are dilated, success approaches 100%; when ductal dilation is absent, success rates are considerably lower (50% to 75%). Indications for PTC include suspected obstruction of the intra- or extrahepatic biliary tree or when further investigation of dilated ducts detected on ultrasound or CT is required. Contraindications to PTC are obvious parenchymal disease of the liver with nondilated bile ducts or uncorrectable coagulopathy. Preparation of the patient with suspected biliary obstruction includes antibiotic prophylaxis, especially if biliary drainage is to follow PTC. As in adults, complications of PTC occur infrequently but include hemorrhage, pneumothorax, cholangitis, bile peritonitis, and sepsis.

PTC in children typically requires only conscious sedation, though selected patients may require general anesthesia. Initial duct puncture using a fine needle (21 to 25 gauge) may be optimized by ultrasound guidance. A right transcostal or subxiphoid midline approach is used for right or left duct puncture, respectively. In the absence of biliary ductal dilation (e.g., primary sclerosing cholangitis or biliary atresia), direct cholangiography may be performed by percutaneous puncture of the gallbladder when it is present. In this technique, the gallbladder is punctured with a small-gauge needle under ultrasound control using a transhepatic approach. Contrast is then slowly injected to opacify the cystic duct and extrahepatic biliary tree; with dependent positioning or distal obstruction, the intrahepatic biliary tree may also be visualized. This examination frequently may be performed with conscious sedation and local anesthesia. As with PTC, complications include bile peritonitis, infection, and intraperitoneal bleed.

Percutaneous Biliary Drainage

Transhepatic biliary drainage may be performed after PTC if external drainage or other intervention is required. Indications include removal of retained stones in the common bile duct and intrahepatic ducts following surgery (e.g., sickle cell anemia) or to provide biliary drainage in the child with obstructive jaundice or cholangitis. Preprocedural antibiotics are mandatory and should be started 24 hours (if possible) prior to the procedure. Complications include intrahepatic hematoma, hemobilia, postprocedural pain, cholangitis, and rarely contrast reaction.

Cyst and Abscess Drainage

Hepatic and splenic cysts may be either congenital (possessing an epithelial lining) or post-traumatic (without epithelial lining; the fluid remnant of a large hematoma). When large (over 3 to 4 cm in diameter), they represent a risk for traumatic rupture and subsequent hemorrhage. Needle aspiration and sclerosis may offer a nonoperative approach for management.

Pancreatic pseudocysts are probably less common in children than in adults, but in both age groups, treatment may be either by percutaneous techniques[13] or by surgery. Small and moderate-sized cysts may be cured by needle aspiration alone; large cysts may require catheter placement for long-term drainage. In addition to conventional transabdominal drainage, it is possible to use transhepatic and transgastric routes to drain pancreatic pseudocysts. In most cases, pseudocyst drainage procedures are low risk and can be done under conscious sedation with local anesthesia.

The most common peritoneal abscesses requiring percutaneous drainage are postappendiceal rupture. Patients with intra-abdominal and perirectal abscesses that represent complications of inflammatory bowel disease may also benefit from percutaneous intervention. Percutaneous abscess drainage achieves success similar to surgical abscess drainage and in most cases with lower morbidity, mortality, and cost.[14] The decision whether to use interventional or surgical techniques for drainage depends on many factors. Multiple, separate abscesses and multiloculated collections respond less favorably to percutaneous intervention and may require surgical drainage for optimal management. For percutaneous catheter placement, a safe approach is required that does not transgress bowel, vascular structures, or solid organs. Percutaneous abscess drainage can almost always be done with sedation and local anesthesia; however, an exception to this may be the perirectal abscess, which requires general anesthesia for adequate treatment in the child, whether interventional or surgical approaches are used. Puncture itself can be guided by either CT or ultrasound, and a catheter of appropriate size introduced (8 Fr to 14 Fr) for management of the process that is present. Appropriate antibiotic therapy and aggressive nutritional support are required for successful abscess therapy.

Indications for percutaneous aspiration or drainage include the determination of fluid characteristics within any abnormal collection, treatment or palliation of sepsis, and to minimize mass effect or symptoms. Absolute contraindication to percutaneous abscess drainage exists only when a safe route to the collection is not present. While the GI tract (especially the colon) should be avoided, reports indicate that nontraditional drainage routes appear safe in expert hands.[15] Correctable abnormalities, including coagulopathy, electrolyte imbalance, fluid deficit, and respiratory compromise, should be addressed to minimize morbidity and mortality; frequently, however, abscess drainage is the single most effective therapy for consequent multisystem failure.

Large superficial collections may be safely entered in a single pass using a direct trocar technique. Smaller or deeper collections may be punctured using the Seldinger technique, which involves using standard angiographic needles, guidewires, fascial dilators, and catheters to obtain optimal position within the fluid collection. This technique provides greater control and accuracy compared to that offered by direct trocar technique. Sump (double lumen) and gravity (single lumen) drainage catheters may be used, ranging in size from 8 Fr to 24

Fr, depending on the characteristics of the fluid aspirated and the clinical setting. Drainage catheter output should decrease progressively over several days, depending on cavity size and nature of the fluid collection; any sudden decrease or cessation of drainage may mean the tube is obstructed or malpositioned, while any sudden increase or change in character of fluid suggests fistulous communication to the bowel. Approximately 2 days following initial drainage, contrast is injected to define the size and extent of the cavity and to determine the presence of communications with the alimentary, biliary, or genitourinary tract. Repeat CT scan may be required to assess for adequacy of drainage. Based on abatement of clinical symptoms and radiographic documentation of resolution of the abscess, the catheter may be removed.

REFERENCES

1. Wursten HU, Stricker H, Salzmann C et al. Peripheral arterial complications of various catheter angiography methods. Helvetica Chir Acta 1990;57:193–197

2. Gutschi S, Koter H, Justich E. Iatrogenic vascular injuries in childhood. Zentralbl Chir 1984;109:854–858

3. Wessel D, Keane J, Fellows K et al. Fibrinolytic therapy for femoral arterial thrombosis after cardiac catheterization in infants and children. Am J Cardiol 1986;58:347–351

4. Fellows K, Hoffer F, Markowitz R, O'Neill J. Multiple collaterals to hepatic infantile hemangioendotheliomas and arteriovenous malformations: influence on embolization. Radiology 1991;181:813–818

5. Meyerovitz M, Fellows K. Angiography in gastrointestinal bleeding in children. Am J Roentgenol 1984;143:833–835

6. Kandarpa K, Fellows K, Eraklis A, Flores A. Solitary ileal AVM: preoperative localization by coil embolization. Am J Roentgenol 1986;146:787–788

7. Zajko A, Bron K, Orons P. Vascular complications in liver transplant recipients: angiographic diagnosis and treatment. Semin Intervent Radiol 1992;9:270–282

8. Lois J, Hartzman S, McGlade C et al. Budd-Chiari syndrome: treatment with percutaneous transhepatic recanalization and dilation. Radiology 1989;170:791–793

9. Lakin P, Saxon R, Barton R. TIPS: indications and techniques. Semin Intervent Radiol 1995;12:347–354

10. Barton R, Rösch J, Saxon R et al. TIPS: short- and long-term results: a survey of 1750 patients. Semin Intervent Radiol 1995;12:364–367

11. Coldwell DM, Ring EJ, Rees CR et al. Multicenter investigation of the role of transjugular intrahepatic portosystemic shunt in management of portal hypertension. Radiology 1995;196:335–340

12. Redd D, Kaye R, Burrows P et al. Pediatric transjugular intrahepatic portosystemic shunt: a multi-institutional collaborative experience. International Pediatric Radiology Third Conjoin Meeting, Boston, MA, 1996:67–68

13. Corbally M, Blake N, Guiney E. Management of pancreatic pseudocyst in childhood: an increasing role for percutaneous external drainage. J Coll Surg Edinb 1992;37:169–171

14. vanSonnenberg E, D'Agostino H, Casola G et al. Percutaneous abscess drainage: current concepts. Radiology 1991;181:617–626

15. Ho C, Taylor B. Transgastric drainage of pancreatic pseudocyst. AJR 1984;143:623–625

70

PLAIN ABDOMINAL RADIOGRAPHY

M. PATRICIA HARTY
JAMES S. MEYER

Plain film radiography is a fundamental tool in the evaluation of the child with abdominal pain. Even with the availability of more advanced imaging modalities, the initial plain radiograph may provide all the information essential to diagnosis. Accurate interpretation requires familiarity with the normal appearance of the abdomen and recognition of subtle signs of pathology.[1]

The abdominal film is often the initial diagnostic step in the evaluation of the acute abdomen. It reveals evidence of bowel obstruction, perforation, and calcifications. Early imaging studies during the investigation of an abdominal mass or inflammatory bowel disease include plain radiographs. They are used to help direct management of chronic conditions and search for extraintestinal causes of abdominal pain such as renal colic and basilar pneumonia. Abdominal radiographs are also obtained prior to contrast studies.

RADIOGRAPHIC TECHNIQUE

Most abdominal radiographic examinations include supine anteroposterior (AP) and erect films. The erect film permits detection of air-fluid levels and is more sensitive than supine views for free intraperitoneal air. When a child cannot be imaged upright, a left lateral decubitus view is the most useful alternative, since free air will be visible over the liver. Right-side down decubitus views are not recommended, as superimposed large and small bowel loops make evaluation of free air more difficult. Occasionally, cross-table lateral films are obtained in ex-

tremely unstable children. However, these views may cause limited radiation exposure to nearby patients and hospital personnel and may be difficult to interpret, since distended bowel loops may obscure free air.[1]

Differentiation of small and large bowel on standard views can be difficult in children and impossible in neonates. A prone cross-table lateral view is often helpful in these patients. In prone patients, gas in the sigmoid rises into the rectum. This confirms the presence of air in the colon and excludes obstruction. Inverted lateral views are occasionally ordered in children with imperforate anus. However, these films may be misleading, since meconium obscuring the distal rectum may give a false impression of high imperforate anus. A single AP view may be all that is required in evaluating the fecal load in a constipated child or in a child with cystic fibrosis. Surveillance for bowel obstruction in postoperative patients often requires only a single supine view. However, it is necessary to be aware of the signs of free air on a supine film.

INTRAPERITONEAL EVALUATION

In the adult and older child, intra-abdominal fat delineates the solid organs, the flank stripes, and psoas margins. Bowel gas in adults is found predominantly in the stomach and colon.[2] There is less intra-abdominal fat in the young child and infant, and gas may be found throughout the small bowel as well as in the stomach and colon.

Bowel Gas Pattern

The bowel gas pattern usually provides the most information about the peritoneal contents on the plain film. In normally rotated bowel, the colon frames the margins of the abdominal cavity, with small bowel lying centrally and the stomach in the left upper quadrant. The position of the stomach in the left upper quadrant indicates normal abdominal situs. The bowel gas pattern may be altered following nephrectomy or partial hepatectomy. The splenic flexure of the colon will be displaced into the left upper quadrant in children without spleens. In supine films, the gastric fundus is often fluid filled, and air is visualized primarily in the antrum and body. The stomach lies in a more horizontal position in young infants, gradually acquiring the adult J-shaped configuration as the child grows.[3] Since infants and small children frequently cry during imaging, the stomach is often distended secondary to air swallowing. Gastric distention will also be found in hypertrophic pyloric stenosis (Fig. 70-1), gastric outlet obstruction, and proximal duodenal obstruction. A mottled gastric shadow that does not change on supine and erect views may indicate a bezoar.

Focal bowel dilation (sentinel loop) may be seen in an area of inflammation.[4] Dilation of several small bowel loops in the mid-abdomen or left upper quadrant may be found in pancreatitis (Fig. 70-2), and dilated loops in the right lower quadrant are often seen in appendicitis.

FIGURE 70-1. The stomach is distended and a large air-fluid level is seen in this 5-week-old male infant with nonbilious projectile vomiting.

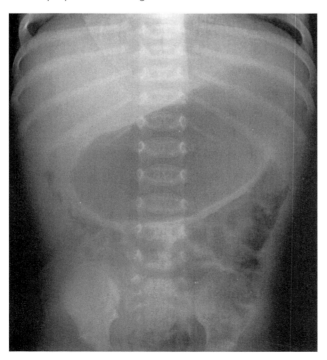

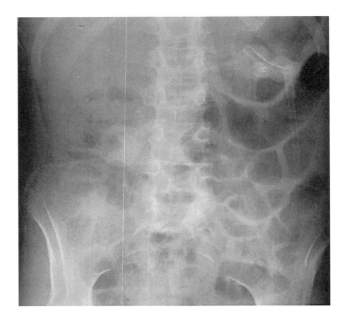

FIGURE 70-2. Focal dilation of small bowel loops in the left upper quadrant is present in this 16-year-old girl with acute pancreatitis.

Abrupt termination of the colonic gas column in the region of the proximal descending colon (colon cutoff sign) may be seen in pancreatitis.[4,5]

Both mechanical obstruction and adynamic ileus result in bowel dilation. Paralytic ileus usually causes diffuse distention of large and small bowel. Air-fluid levels are seen in erect and decubitus films in both conditions. Air-fluid levels at different heights in the same loop of bowel due to peristalsis are often associated with mechanical obstruction, while air-fluid levels at the same height are commonly associated with paralytic ileus. Fluid levels in both large and small bowel may indicate gastroenteritis. Classically, meconium ileus presents with distended loops of bowel without air-fluid levels, since meconium is viscous and does not layer. The increased viscosity of meconium also contributes to the typical mottled "soap bubble" appearance of meconium and air (Fig. 70-3).

Bowel dilation occurs proximal to an obstruction, and the length of dilated bowel can indicate the point of obstruction. There are multiple causes, both congenital and acquired, of bowel obstruction in the newborn and child.

Duodenal atresia usually involves the descending duodenum in the region of the ampulla of Vater and presents as the "double bubble." The larger of the two bubbles is the distended stomach (Fig. 70-4). The smaller bubble is the distended duodenal bulb proximal to a complete obstruction.[6] Ileal and jejunal atresias are less common. Colonic atresia is rare; however, when dilated loops fill the abdomen, suggesting a distal point of obstruction, a contrast enema is the next step in the evaluation (Fig. 70-5).

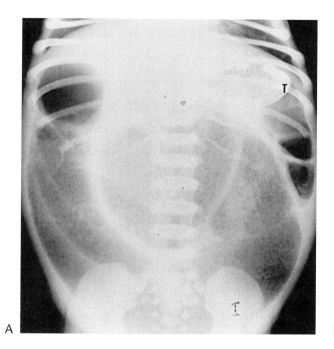
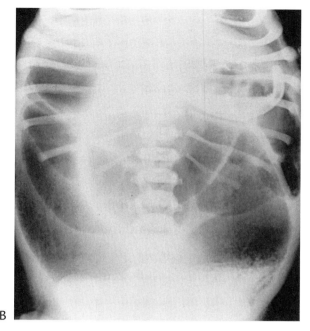

A   B

FIGURE 70-3. Radiographs taken in supine *(A)* and *(B)* erect positions show dilated bowel loops of different caliber with a mottled or "soap bubble" appearance. Only a single air-fluid level is found in this infant with cystic fibrosis and meconium ileus.

FIGURE 70-4. The double bubble of gastric and duodenal bulb distention is seen in this newborn infant with Down's syndrome and duodenal atresia.

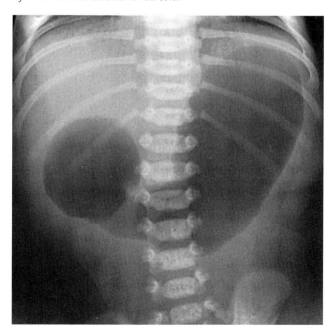

Hirschsprung's disease is the differential diagnosis for distal obstruction in the infant and chronic constipation in an older child. Distended loops of colon filled with fecal residue may be seen in Hirschsprung's disease; however, these findings are often not apparent in the newborn. Cross-table prone lateral films may demonstrate the narrow rectal contour or transition zone characteristic of Hirschsprung's disease, although a contrast enema is necessary for further evaluation (Fig. 70-6).

A narrow lumen may be a manifestation of severe wall edema, stricture, or a constricting mass. Edema may be due to trauma, severe inflammatory bowel disease, or inflammation (Fig. 70-7).

The mucosal pattern of the bowel may contribute additional information. Thickened bowel wall may indicate intramural edema or hemorrhage, as in Henoch-Schönlein purpura. Well-defined mucosal impressions on the colon wall ("thumbprinting") are seen in the colon if there is extensive hemorrhage or edema (Fig. 70-8). Wall edema in the small bowel has been called "pinky printing" and has been likened to a "stack of coins."

Gasless Abdomen

A gasless abdomen may indicate gastroenteritis, bowel infarction, or an acute abdomen. In addition, infants with swallowing disorders, pharmacologically paralyzed infants, and vomiting children may have a gasless abdomen.[1,7]

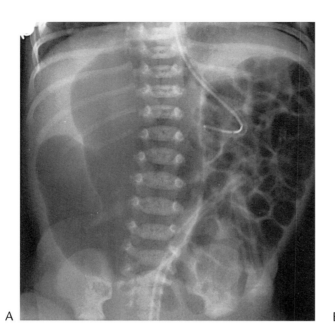
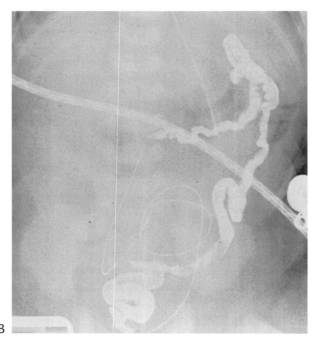

A   B

FIGURE 70-5. *(A)* Abdominal radiograph in a newborn infant shows a nasogastric tube in the stomach. Multiple small-caliber loops of bowel are present on the left side of the abdomen, and a large-caliber dilated loop is seen on the right. *(B)* Barium enema reveals a microcolon that terminates in the mid transverse colon. Transverse colon atresia with dilated proximal colon was found at surgery.

Pneumatosis Intestinalis

Pneumatosis intestinalis is indicated by small round or curvilinear lucencies paralleling the bowel wall. This finding indicates loss of integrity of the bowel wall. Necrotizing enterocolitis (NEC) is a common cause in infants (Fig. 70-9). Pneumatosis may also occur in Hirschsprung's disease and ischemia associated with volvulus. Occasionally, benign pneumatosis cystoides intestinalis is incidentally found in children with cystic fibrosis and in children treated with immunosuppressive therapy or steroids.[8]

Extraluminal Gas

Possible locations of extraintestinal gas include the peritoneum ("free air"), biliary and portal systems, and localized gas collections in abscesses and tumors. Small volumes of free air are best seen on erect or left lateral decubitus films. When children are unstable and only supine films can be performed, we must search for signs of free air on the supine film. Air rises to the least dependent position in the peritoneum. The falciform ligament may be seen as a radiopaque vertical line in the right upper quadrant. It is surrounded by free air on both sides as it extends from the anterior wall of the peritoneum to the liver. An oval lucency will be seen in the mid-abdomen with a large amount of free air. This finding as well as the visible falciform ligament has been called the "football" sign.[1] Gastric air may delineate the inferior margin of the left hemidiaphragm, but complete visualization of the caudal surface of the diaphragm indicates free air. This finding has been called the "continuous diaphragm" sign. When extraluminal gas is present, both the mucosal and serosal surfaces of gas-filled bowel loops are outlined by air (Rigler's sign). The triangle sign refers to a small triangle of extraluminal gas lying between two adjacent loops of bowel and the wall of the peritoneal cavity.[9] This may be seen on both supine and cross-table views. Free air may also be seen beneath the anterior margin of the liver as a curvilinear lucency separate from the hepatic flexure[1] (Fig. 70-10).

Branching lucent channels overlying the liver suggest portal venous gas, which is frequently associated with pneumatosis in infants with necrotizing enterocolitis (Fig. 70-11). Air in the biliary tree may be seen with cholangitis or in children who have undergone a biliary diversion procedure.

Calcifications

The abdominal plain film may demonstrate calcifications. Renal calculi are one of the most common types of calcifications in children. They may overlie the renal pelvis, the ureter, or the bladder. Adrenal calcifications include small, dense, irregular opacities associated with prior adrenal hemorrhage and tumoral calcifications. Psammomatous or fine, diffuse, sandlike calcifications are found in up to 50% of neuroblastomas[10] (Fig. 70-12). Calcification in renal tumors is not as common as in adrenal malignancies. Occasionally, there may be rim calcification in Wilms' tumors. Although cholelithiasis is less common in children than in adults, other calcifications may overlie the liver such as vascular and tumor calcifications, granulomas, peritoneal calcifications, and intrahepatic calculi, as in Caroli's disease.[11]

Granulomas are often multiple. They are well-defined densities, 2 to 3 mm in diameter, and may be seen in the spleen as well as in the liver. Calcification may occasionally be found in hepatoblastomas and hemangioendotheliomas. Irregular pancreatic calcifications extending across the midline may be seen in chronic pancreatitis.[12] Ovarian teratomas may also contain well-defined calcifications.

Calcification in the infant's peritoneal cavity suggests meconium peritonitis. Calcified meconium may be seen in the scrotum in infants with a patent processus vaginalis.

Solid Organs

The location of bowel loops reflects the size and location of the solid organs. In the upper abdomen, gas-filled bowel adjacent to the medial margin of the right hepatic lobe indicates hepatic size and position. The liver edge may extend down to the iliac crest in normal infants and young children. If the lungs are hyperinflated, the liver may extend even more caudad. Further displacement of bowel loops may indicate hepatosplenomegaly, a horizontal liver, or a hepatic mass. As well as displaced bowel loops, there may be an associated soft tissue mass with nephromegaly, renal masses, and adrenal masses. Elevation of the bowel loops with associated soft tissue density in the chest may indicate a diaphragmatic hernia or eventration. In these patients, ultrasound or magnetic resonance imaging is helpful. A pancreatic mass or pseudocyst may cause inferior displacement of the transverse colon, and pelvic masses may displace bowel loops superiorly out of the pelvis. A distended bladder may have the same effect, and occasionally a large pelvic "mass" can disappear on a post-void film.

The bowel must be scrutinized for ingested material. Coins and other metal objects are easily seen; however, ingested lead flakes may be mistaken for the residua of a recent barium study. In spite of current regulations regarding lead paint, it continues to be a source of poisoning in small children, and any intraluminal small, irregular, dense particles must be interpreted as lead or heavy metal unless a history of a recent barium study is available (Fig. 70-13).

Intraperitoneal Extraintestinal Spaces

Interpretation of the abdominal film also includes evaluation of intraperitoneal extraintestinal spaces and structures. Fluid, air, masses, and collections may lie in the peritoneal cavity. Small volumes of free fluid lie in the most dependent parts of the peritoneum, deep in the pelvis and along the paracolic gutters. Fluid may obscure the borders of the bladder with triangular densities, or "dog ears," along the superolateral margins of the bladder. This finding is not readily seen in infants but may be found in older children.[8] As fluid extends up the paracolic gutters, it can separate the ascending colon from the flank stripe as well as obscure the lower margin of the liver. Occasionally, fluid may be seen lateral to the liver (Hellmer's sign).[13] A "ground-glass" appearance throughout the abdomen is the classic description of a large volume of ascites. Gas-filled bowel loops floating centrally in the abdomen may also be seen with a large amount of free fluid.[13]

Abscesses and masses in the peritoneal cavity tend to

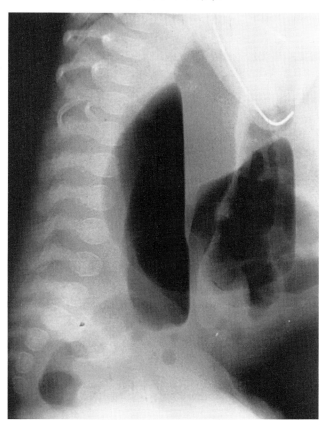

FIGURE 70-6. A lateral radiograph in a 3-day-old infant with signs of obstruction shows rectal gas; however, the rectal gas shadow is narrow. Hirschsprung's disease was confirmed on barium enema and biopsy.

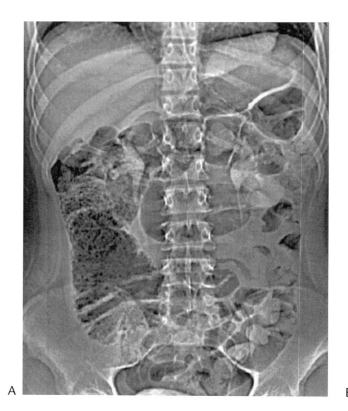
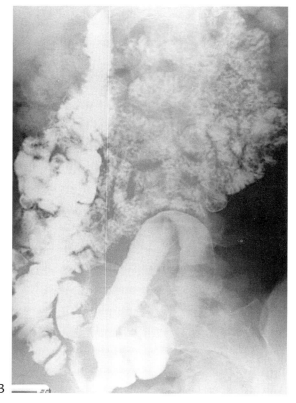

FIGURE 70-7. *(A)* Abdominal radiograph shows a narrow featureless loop of bowel in the left lower quadrant in a 14-year-old boy with a lap seat belt injury. *(B)* Small bowel follow-through reveals marked bowel wall thickening consistent with mural hematoma.

displace bowel loops. Appendiceal abscesses may exert mass effect on the cecum. Collections in the lesser sac may displace the stomach. Gas collections in unusual locations or a gas collection that does not change configuration between supine and erect films suggests an abscess. Subphrenic abscesses may displace the liver or spleen inferiorly and the stomach medially. These processes are often associated with ipsilateral pleural effusions and atelectasis.[8]

EXTRAPERITONEAL EVALUATION

Evaluation of extraperitoneal structures is an integral component of the abdominal plain film interpretation. Pneumonia in the lung bases may present as acute abdominal pain. This may be visible only on the corner of the film (Fig. 70-14). Properitoneal fat stripes define the lateral margins of the peritoneal cavity. Adjacent inflammation, such as appendicitis, may obscure the fat stripe. Psoas margins may be seen if there is sufficient intra-abdominal fat to define the muscle edges. An inflammatory process adjacent to the psoas muscle may obscure the shadow; however, this is not a reliable sign in children. Abdominal wall masses and inflammatory processes be-

come visible on the plain radiograph when they displace bowel or obliterate landmarks such as the flank stripes. Superficial masses, such as umbilical hernias, are usually distinguished from intra-abdominal masses by well-defined margins (Fig. 70-15).

It is important to evaluate the skeletal structures on the abdominal film. Ribs must be checked for fractures contributing to abdominal pain. Fractures related to non-accidental trauma may be seen (Fig. 70-16). A subtle vertebral curve concave to the right may be associated with appendicitis. Primary bone tumors may present with abdominal or pelvic pain and be visible on radiographs as subtle calcification or displaced fat planes. Congenital anomalies such as scimitar sacrum may be associated with anterior sacral meningoceles.

COMMON ABDOMINAL ABNORMALITIES

Necrotizing Enterocolitis

NEC is a frequent diagnostic concern in the neonatal intensive care unit. Many etiologic factors have been proposed including prematurity, hypoxia, perinatal

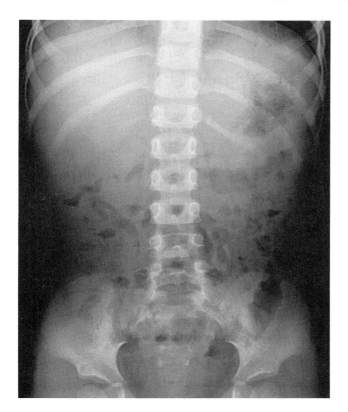

FIGURE 70-8. Abdominal radiograph in a child with hemolytic uremic syndrome shows a straightened transverse and descending colon with extensive mucosal edema thumbprinting.

FIGURE 70-10. A curvilinear gas collection under the right hepatic lobe indicates free intraperitoneal air in this child with a bowel perforation.

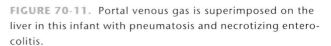

FIGURE 70-11. Portal venous gas is superimposed on the liver in this infant with pneumatosis and necrotizing enterocolitis.

FIGURE 70-9. Pneumatosis in the wall of the rectum in a preterm infant with necrotizing enterocolitis.

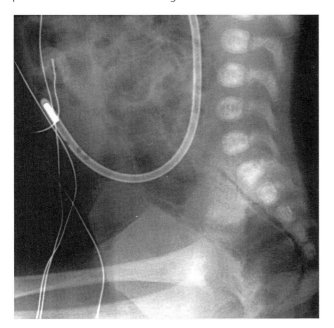

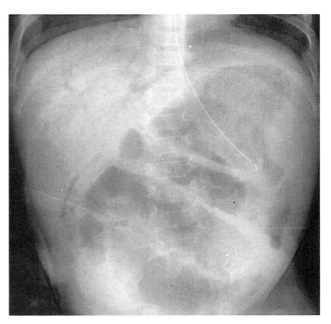

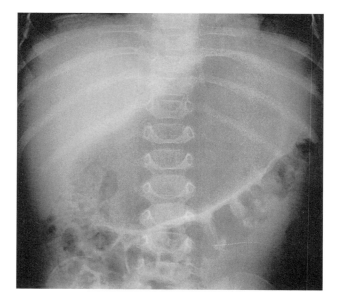

FIGURE 70-12. Abdominal radiograph in an infant with diarrhea shows fine sandlike or psammomatous calcifications in the left upper quadrant. Calcifications are subtle but can be seen through the gastric air bubble. Subsequent computed tomography scan revealed a large retroperitoneal neuroblastoma.

FIGURE 70-13. Dense particulate matter is seen in the colon consistent with heavy-metal ingestion, in this case lead. If there is concern for chronic lead ingestion, images of the fastest-growing areas such as knees and wrists may be obtained. Sclerotic lead lines may also be seen along the iliac crests and proximal femurs on the abdominal radiograph.

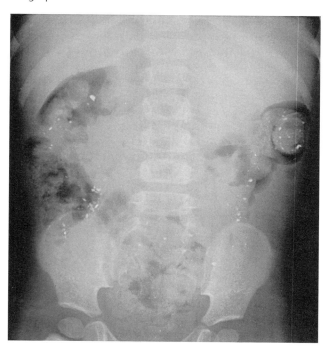

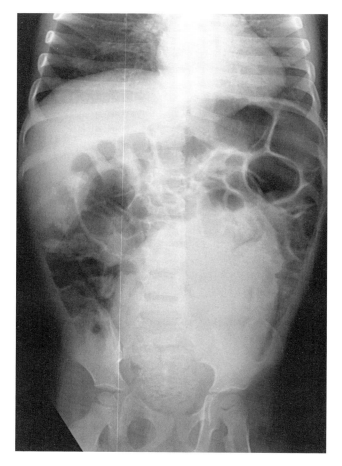

FIGURE 70-14. This scout radiograph obtained prior to a BE in a child with abdominal pain, suspected of having an intussusception, revealed a left lower lobe pneumonia.

FIGURE 70-15. Abdominal film in a vomiting child shows a soft tissue mass that corresponded to the small umbilical hernia.

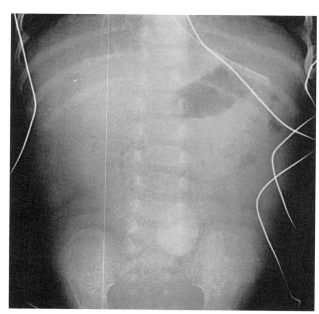

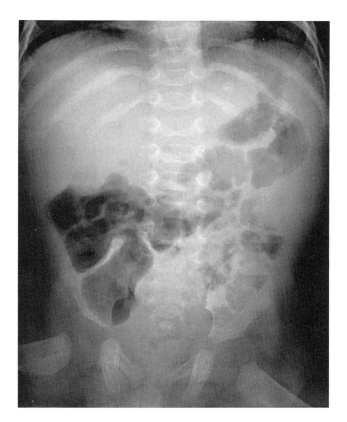

FIGURE 70-16. The abdominal film on a skeletal survey performed for suspected abuse shows healing right eleventh and twelfth rib fractures overlying the liver. An adrenal calcification is seen in the left upper quadrant. Multiple fractures at different stages of healing were found on the extremity films, confirming the suspicion of nonaccidental trauma.

stress, umbilical venous catheterization, infection, and carbohydrate malabsorption.[6,14] Plain films aid in the diagnosis and help to direct the management of NEC. Clinical indicators of NEC include abdominal distention, bloody diarrhea, and metabolic acidosis.[14] Abdominal radiographs are usually obtained as the early signs of NEC become apparent. The earliest sign of NEC visible on the plain radiograph is bowel dilation. The dilation usually involves the small bowel, followed by the large bowel, and bowel loops may appear straightened.[15] Dilated bowel loops that do not change in configuration on sequential films suggest wall edema. A persistent segment of dilated bowel when surrounding loops have decompressed has been described as an indicator of wall necrosis.[16]

As NEC progresses, bowel dilation may be followed by pneumatosis intestinalis, transient portal venous air, and if perforation occurs, signs of free intraperitoneal air. Intramural pneumatosis is visible as curvilinear or round lucencies along the bowel wall. It may be seen throughout the bowel down to the rectum, although NEC appears to involve predominantly the ileocecal region.[17] Pneumatosis must be distinguished from intraluminal gas surrounding meconium, which may have a similar appearance. Linear lucencies following the path of the portal vasculature are frequently seen with pneumatosis. This is a serious but not necessarily an ominous finding in NEC.[14]

The most important role of the plain film in the management of the infant with NEC is demonstrating signs of bowel perforation. Small amounts of free air are best seen over the right hepatic lobe on left lateral decubitus films. On a supine film, a large volume of free air in the peritoneal cavity outlines the caudal surface of the diaphragm, the continuous diaphragm sign. The falciform ligament, outlined by air on both sides, may be seen in the right upper quadrant parallel to the spine (Fig. 70-17). Rigler's sign and the triangle sign both indicate air outside the bowel lumen. When two loops of distended bowel abut, both sides of bowel wall may be visualized, and this may be mistaken for pneumoperitoneum. In these cases, cross-table views are helpful.

Approximately 20% to 25% of infants with NEC develop strictures, primarily in the colon. Symptoms may manifest weeks to months after the clinical episode with subtle signs of obstruction.[16] Contrast studies are indicated to define the location of the stricture.

Malrotation with Volvulus

Midgut volvulus is one of the most disastrous entities encountered in the practice of pediatrics. Volvulus is a consequence of malrotation, the abnormal rotation and fixation of the bowel.[18] Normally, the base of the small bowel mesentery extends from the ligament of Treitz in the left upper quadrant to the cecum in the right lower quadrant. With an anomalously positioned duodenojejunal junction, the narrow mesenteric base predisposes the small bowel to volvulus. During midgut volvulus, obstruction typically occurs in the descending duodenum distal to the ampulla of Vater, resulting in the characteristic finding of bile in the vomitus.

The plain films in malrotation may show the small bowel gas pattern lying predominantly on the right, and the cecal gas shadow may not be apparent in the right lower quadrant.[19] With volvulus, the initial plain film may show dilation of the stomach and descending duodenum, with gastric and duodenal air-fluid levels on the decubitus view (Fig. 70-18). The appearance of the double bubble differs from that seen in duodenal atresia, since the duodenal bubble is elongated corresponding to the bulb and descending duodenum. There may be a paucity of gas in the distal bowel. However, the plain film is often nonspecific, and a completely normal film

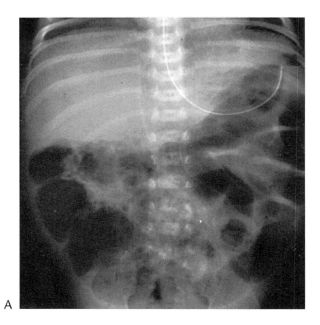
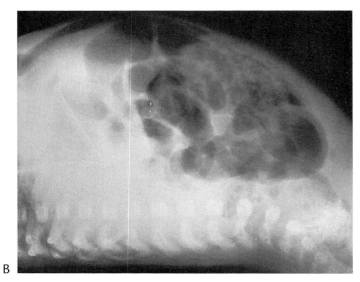

A   B

FIGURE 70-17. *(A)* Radiograph in a supine preterm infant with necrotizing enterocolitis shows a vertical linear density parallel with the spine overlying the liver consistent with the falciform ligament, indicating free air. There is also a diffuse lucency in the mid-epigastric area demarcating the caudal surface of the diaphragm, the continuous diaphragm sign. *(B)* Free air is seen over the liver on the cross-table lateral film.

FIGURE 70-18. Left lateral decubitus view in an infant with bilious vomiting shows a dilated loop with an air-fluid level that corresponded to the obstructed descending duodenum on an upper GI contrast study.

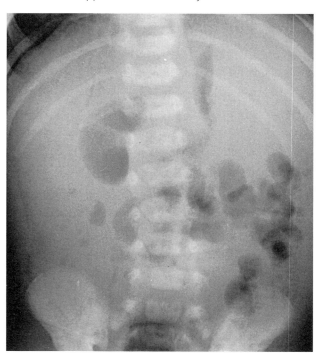

cannot exclude volvulus. Any infant or child with a history of bilious vomiting suspected of having malrotation must receive a contrast examination to determine the position of the ligament of Treitz, whether or not there is radiographic evidence of proximal duodenal obstruction.

Appendicitis

Appendicitis is one of the most common causes of abdominal pain requiring laparotomy in children.[2] Abdominal radiographs are frequently unnecessary, since the clinical findings are often diagnostic. The presence of a calcified appendicolith on the plain film in association with the appropriate clinical setting virtually confirms the diagnosis of appendicitis (Fig. 70-19).[2] The diagnosis may be difficult, however, especially in young children, necessitating further diagnostic evaluation. Abdominal radiographic findings tend to correspond to the degree of inflammation. Early films show diminished or absent bowel gas, coinciding with nausea and vomiting. As inflammation progresses, signs of early obstruction develop with right lower quadrant sentinel loops, splinting with lumbar scoliosis convex to the left. The right psoas margin may be obscured.[20]

In young children presenting with perforated appendix, there may be a mass in the right lower quadrant or evidence of an abscess such as a loculated air collection or a mottled gas pattern in the right paracolic gutter (Fig. 70-20).

Intussusception

Intussusception is one of the most common causes of abdominal pain in early childhood. Clinical features include intermittent bouts of severe abdominal pain, vomiting, and bloody stools. Intussusception occurs most often in infants and children between the ages of 5 months and 4 years, with the highest incidence between 5 and 9 months. The overall incidence of lead points is less than 10%, with a higher number of lead points found in young infants and children older than 3 years of age.[14] Lead points include Meckel's diverticulum, polyp, hypertrophied lymphoid patches,

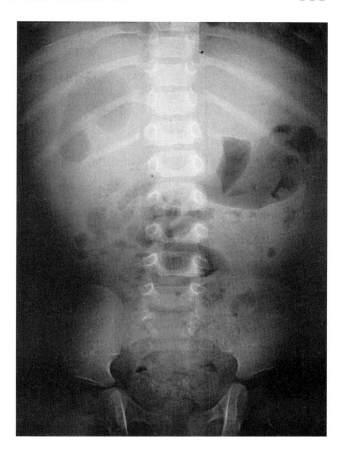

FIGURE 70-20. Supine abdominal film reveals an unusual gas collection in the right upper quadrant overlying the liver that remained in the same position on the decubitus film. This gas shadow proved to be air within a right paracolic abscess, and a perforated appendix was found at surgery.

FIGURE 70-19. An appendicolith overlies the right iliac bone, confirming the clinical impression of appendicitis. No further imaging was required, and appendicitis was confirmed at surgery.

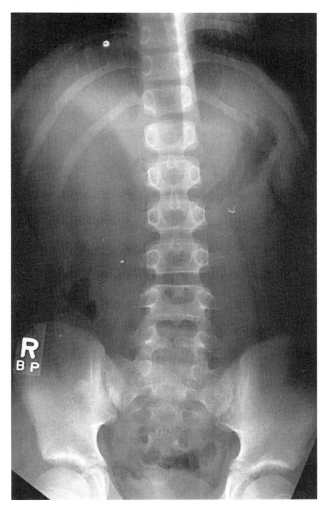

cysts, and lymphoma. Intussusception also occurs in children who have undergone surgery in the preceding 2 to 4 days.

The plain abdominal radiograph has recently been shown to be unhelpful in diagnosing intussusception, and an abdominal radiograph is unlikely to influence the decision for a diagnostic enema if the clinical suspicion is high.[21] The classic signs of intussusception on plain film include sparse large bowel gas with a paucity of gas or a soft tissue mass in the area of the intussusception (Fig. 70-21). The majority of intussusceptions are ileocolic, and the intussusception is usually found along the course of the ascending colon. However, during reduction, the intussusceptum may be encountered as far distal as the sigmoid. It is important to search for radiographic signs of bowel infarction and perforation, and erect or decubitus views are mandatory prior to any attempt of reduction. Any evidence of perforation, infarcted bowel, or free air is a contraindication to hydrostatic or pneumatic reduction.

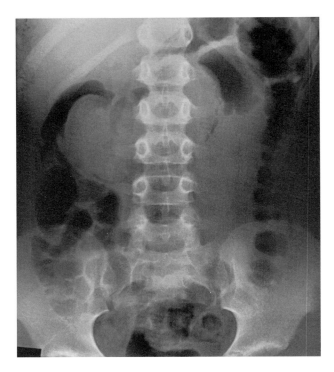

FIGURE 70-21. Abdominal radiograph shows an intussusception mass in the right upper quadrant with distal colonic gas defining the intussusceptum. The intussusception was reduced during barium enema.

REFERENCES

1. Ominsky SH, Margulis AR. Abdominal scout film assessment. In: Gastroenterology. 4th Ed. Philadelphia: WB Saunders, 1985:445–455

2. Babyn P, Stringer DA. Radiography: plain film. In: Pediatric Gastrointestinal Disease: Pathophysiology, Diagnosis, Management. Philadelphia: BC Decker, 1991:1403–1418

3. Franken EA. Gastrointestinal Imaging in Pediatrics. 2nd Ed. Philadelphia: Harper & Row, 1982:110

4. Swischuk LE. Emergency Radiology of the Acutely Ill or Injured Child. 2nd Ed. Baltimore: Williams & Wilkins, 1986:161

5. Eisenberg RL. Gastrointestinal Radiology: A Pattern Approach. 2nd Ed. Philadelphia: JB Lippincott, 1990:341

6. Kirks DR. Practical Pediatric Imaging: Diagnostic Radiology of Infants and Children. Boston: Little, Brown, 1984: 569–579, 658

7. Franken EA. Gastrointestinal Imaging in Pediatrics. 2nd Ed. Philadelphia: Harper & Row, 1982:358–360

8. Swischuk LE. Emergency Radiology of the Acutely Ill or Injured Child, 2nd Ed. Baltimore: Williams & Wilkins, 1986:171–185

9. Kirks DR. Practical Pediatric Imaging: Diagnostic Radiology of Infants and Children. Boston: Little, Brown, 1984:547

10. Silverman FN, Ed. Caffey's Pediatric X-Ray Diagnosis: An Integrated Imaging Approach. 8th Ed. Chicago: Year Book Medical Publishers, 1985:1734

11. Franken EA. Gastrointestinal Imaging in Pediatrics. 2nd Ed. Philadelphia: Harper & Row, 1982:446

12. Silverman FN, Ed. Caffey's Pediatric X-Ray Diagnosis: An Integrated Imaging Approach. 8th Ed. Chicago: Year Book Medical Publishers 1985:1396

13. Franken EA. Gastrointestinal Imaging in Pediatrics. 2nd Ed. Philadelphia: Harper & Row, 1982:411–413

14. Silverman FN, Ed. Caffey's Pediatric X-Ray Diagnosis: An Integrated Imaging Approach, 8th Ed. Chicago: Year Book Medical Publishers, 1985:1501–1513

15. Franken EA. Gastrointestinal Imaging in Pediatrics. 2nd Ed. Philadelphia: Harper & Row, 1982:328

16. Daneman A, Woodward S, de Silva M. The radiology of neonatal necrotizing enterocolitis (NEC). Pediatr Radiol 1978;7:70–77

17. Frey EE, Smith W, Franken EA, Wintermeyer KA. Analysis of bowel perforation in necrotizing enterocolitis. Pediatr Radiol 1987;17:380–382

18. Long FR, Kramer SS, Markowitz RI et al. Intestinal malrotation in children: tutorial on radiographic diagnosis in difficult cases. Radiology 1996;198:775–780

19. Yanez R, Spitz L. Intestinal malrotation presenting outside the neonatal period. Arch Dis Child 1986;61:682–685

20. Singleton EB, Wagner ML. The acute abdomen in the pediatric age group. Semin Roentgenol 1973;8:339–356

21. Sargent MA, Babyn P, Alton DJ. Plain abdominal radiography in suspected intussusception: a reassessment. Pediatr Radiol 1994;24:17–20

71

UPPER ENDOSCOPY

KAREN LIQUORNIK
CHRIS A. LIACOURAS

Esophagogastroduodenoscopy (EGD) has become an invaluable tool in helping with the diagnosis and treatment of myriad pediatric gastrointestinal (GI) disorders. The development of the endoscope has improved not just the approach to treatment but also the understanding of pathophysiology of disorders in the upper GI tract. Upper endoscopy is now an integral part of the practice of pediatric gastroenterology.

INDICATIONS

Upper GI Bleeding

Upper GI bleeding should be suspected in any patients who demonstrate melena, hematemesis, or occult blood in their stools. In contrast, hematochezia usually indicates a lower GI source, although occasionally bright red blood from the rectum may be a sign of rapid, brisk upper GI bleeding. The search for the cause of GI bleeding is the reason for 30% of all upper endoscopies.[1] EGD is superior to barium studies in determining the source of bleeding because of the ability to directly visualize the GI mucosa. In addition, if an abnormality is found during EGD, therapy can often be administered via the endoscope. In 10 to 20% of cases, endoscopy does not reveal a source of bleeding.[2] EGD should be performed under a controlled setting within 24 hours of bleeding. Prior to endoscopy, the patient should be hemodynamically stabilized with intravenous fluids and blood products as needed. Nasogastric lavage often provides additional information.

Recurrent Abdominal Pain

Recurrent abdominal pain is the most common indication for an upper endoscopy in pediatrics.[3] Patients who localize their pain to the epigastric region, who complain of nausea, vomiting, and diarrhea, who display weight loss or failure to thrive, or who experience persistent pain often are candidates for upper endoscopy. Possible causes of these symptoms include esophagitis, gastritis, ulceration, *Helicobacter pylori*, eosinophilic enteritis, celiac disease, or inflammatory bowel disease.

Dysphagia

Patients with dysphagia or odynophagia symptoms should first be evaluated by barium study followed by upper endoscopy. EGD is almost always indicated in these patients for several reasons: (1) if an esophageal stricture, web, or ring is demonstrated by x-ray study, endoscopy provides therapy (dilation) and tissue analysis for diagnosis; and (2) when no structural lesions are demonstrated by radiographic study, EGD can provide visual or histologic diagnosis of the cause for the patient's symptoms (esophagitis, Barrett's esophagus, radiolucent foreign body). Occasionally, small webs or diverticula that were not seen on barium studies can be appreciated by EGD.[4] In immunocompromised patients who have dysphagia, endoscopy is performed to identify any infectious agents, such as cytomegalovirus (intracellular inclusions on histopathology), herpes simplex, or fungal (*Candida*) infection.

Abnormal Radiograph Study

Patients who have had abnormal barium studies including gastritis, duodenitis, esophagitis, ulcer, or filling defect should undergo EGD not only to obtain a tissue diagnosis but also to complete an in-depth visual evaluation.

Persistent Vomiting

An EGD should be done in patients with persistent vomiting after a metabolic, infectious, neurologic, and anatomic workup has been completed. Possible causes include gastritis, duodenitis, ulceration, reflux esophagitis, or *H. pylori*. In addition, a normal endoscopy is also helpful, as other non-GI causes of vomiting, such as renal and central nervous system disease or drug use, should subsequently be considered.

Malabsorption

Patients with failure to thrive or diarrhea may have a variety of disorders ranging from celiac disease, inflammatory bowel disease, allergic enteritis, post-viral enteropathy, or sucrase-isomaltase disaccharidase. All of these disorders require endoscopy for diagnosis.

Caustic Ingestions

When a strong acid or alkali is ingested, damage to the upper GI tract mucosa can occur. Endoscopy should be performed within 12 to 24 hours of the ingestion. EGD aids in determining the presence or absence of mucosal damage, the extent of the damage, and the specific area of damage. Burns in the esophageal or gastric mucosa typically appear as a gray-white eschar at the areas of contact. Edema may be visualized early, while strictures are a late finding. See Chapter 5 for further information on treatment of caustic ingestions.

Surveillance

Patients with specific GI conditions require follow-up endoscopy to assess the progression of the specific disease. Patients with chronic esophagitis require routine assessment for Barrett's esophagus, while patients with polyposis syndromes or ureterosigmoidostomies require cancer surveillance. In addition, some children warrant repeat EGD to assess their improvement on treatment.

Therapy

Upper endoscopy has become a superior tool for the treatment of a large number of GI disorders.[5,6] Table 71-1 depicts the most common therapies that can be performed by EGD.

TABLE 71-1. Therapeutic Uses for Upper Endoscopy

Foreign body ingestion[5,6]
Esophageal or duodenal strictures
Esophageal varices (sclerotherapy)
Placement of percutaneous endoscopic gastric and jejunal tubes
Electrocautery (ulcer, arteriovenous malformation)
Therapeutic endoscopic retrograde cholangiopancreatography
Polypectomy

Endoscopic Retrograde Cholangiopancreatography

Endoscopic retrograde cholangiopancreatography (ERCP) is now available in most pediatric tertiary care centers for the diagnosis and treatment of recurrent or chronic pancreatitis, obstructive jaundice, and cholangitis. ERCP is performed by cannulating the ampulla of Vater with a side-viewing scope after entering the duodenum. After cannulation, a radiopaque dye is injected, and the pancreatic duct and extrahepatic biliary duct system are visualized under fluoroscopy. Findings can range from a normal ductal pattern to focal areas of obstruction, areas of pancreatic duct narrowing (e.g., typical for chronic pancreatitis), filling defects (e.g., stone), and intrahepatic biliary duct narrowing (e.g., primary sclerosing cholangitis).

PREPARATION

Diet

Infants less than 6 months old should be fasted for 4 to 6 hours prior to endoscopy. Older children should be fasted for 6 to 8 hours prior to the procedure.

Sedation

In the past, most endoscopies were performed under general anesthesia; however, a study in 1994 showed that in a properly equipped endoscopy suite with experienced personnel, the procedure can be performed safely, effectively, and at a substantially lower cost with conscious sedation than under general anesthesia.[7] A variety of medications can be used for conscious sedation. The combination of midazolam (an anxiolytic and amnestic agent) and meperidine or fentanyl (analgesics) is most commonly used. A recent study compared the use of midazolam and meperidine to midazolam and fentanyl and showed that while both combinations were safe and effective, the use of fentanyl resulted in a quicker recovery time and the need for less midazolam.[8,9] Another study of 40 pediatric patients undergoing endoscopy found that the addition of midazolam to meperidine alone enhanced the sedation and provided amnesia to the patients without increased complications. Often, parents remain in the endoscopy suite while the child is being sedated to help alleviate the youngster's fears. A topical anesthetic is also used to anesthetize the pharynx to decrease gagging and choking.

General anesthesia is indicated in children with known respiratory compromise, neurologically impaired children with decreased muscle tone, children who previously failed intravenous sedation, children with cyanotic congenital cardiac disease, and most patients who require a therapeutic EGD.

Monitoring

Before, during, and after sedation, patients are monitored by pulse oximetry and by cardiorespiratory monitor.[10] A secure line for intravenous medications is necessary until the patient has recovered. In addition, oxygen, suction, and a resuscitation cart should be available if needed.

CONTRAINDICATIONS

Absolute contraindications to EGD include shock, perforation, and cervical spine injury. Patients with respiratory distress should be monitored by an anesthesiologist. A patient with thrombocytopenia, anemia, or a coagulopathy should be given blood products prior to or during the endoscopy. Endoscopy is not contraindicated in patients with heart disease or prosthetic devices such as central nervous system shunts or heart valves.

COMPLICATIONS

When performed in the proper setting and by an experienced pediatric endoscopist, upper endoscopy in pediatrics is extremely safe.[11] Morbidity has been reported to be less than 2%, while mortality is less than 0.001%. In one large prospective study involving 2,046 endoscopies, the overall complication rate was found to be 1.7%.[12] Minor complications such as postprocedural vomiting, abdominal distention, sore throat, nausea, and intravenous phlebitis occur in up to 10% of patients. Major complications such as infection, bleeding (less than 0.0001%), perforation (0.001%), broken teeth (less than 0.01%), and side effects from sedation or drug allergy (less than 0.1%) are very rare. The risk of major complication increases when the patient is critically ill (e.g., bleeding from a perforated ulcer or varix).

Complications secondary to ERCP include all the above complications. In addition, pancreatitis and cho-

langitis have been reported to occur in 3% of pediatric patients. One study of 39 children who had ERCPs performed reported a rate of 10% for pancreatitis, but these were all mild cases that resolved with supportive short-term measures.[13] Esophageal dilation can also cause pneumothorax, while percutaneous gastrostomy placement can cause the formation of fistulous tracts and puncture of abdominal organs.

ENDOSCOPY SUITE

Equipment

There are many different types of endoscopes, which vary in length, diameter, and components (fiberoptic versus video). Presently, the smallest endoscope is 5.3 mm in diameter and is used in neonates and premature infants (2.5 kg). The largest endoscopes have therapeutic uses for which an array of equipment, including retrieval devices for foreign objects, sclerotherapy needles and banding, cautery, and dilators, can be used.

Procedure

After sedation, the patient is placed in the left lateral position, and the endoscope is passed through the pharynx into the upper esophagus. It is then advanced along the greater curvature through the pylorus and into the proximal duodenum. After the mucosa is examined, biopsies and cultures can be taken, and the endoscope is then withdrawn into the stomach. The examiner may then retroflex the endoscope to obtain a view of the cardia and fundus. Upon removal, the endoscopist empties the stomach of introduced air to ease comfort and to avoid respiratory compromise from gastric distention. During the procedure, other diagnostic tests may be obtained, such as biopsies for intestinal disaccharidases, small bowel aspirates for parasites and bacterial overgrowth, biopsies for H. pylori, and esophageal brushings for infections.

Personnel

Endoscopy requires experienced nursing assistance. It is helpful if nurses have previous pediatric experience, as the preparation of the pediatric patient is typically more difficult than performing the actual procedure. The personnel should be well trained in patient care, resuscitation, and the endoscopy equipment. Two dedicated support personnel (at least one nurse) must be present for proper monitoring of the patient and for technical assistance for the physician.

CONCLUSION

Upper endoscopy has become an invaluable tool for the practice of pediatric gastroenterology. Although the procedures may be performed similarly in both adults and children, the preparation, sedation, indications, and interpretations of pediatric endoscopy require specially trained physicians experienced in pediatric care and knowledgeable about pediatric disease.

REFERENCES

1. Kohli Y, Fuse Y, Kodawa T et al. Upper gastrointestinal endoscopy in pediatric patients. Gastrointest Endosc 1981; 23: 1294–1301

2. Prolla JC, Diehl AS, Benvenuti GA et al. Upper gastrointestinal fiberoptic endoscopy in pediatric patients. Gastrointest Endosc 1983; 29: 279–281

3. Ament ME, Christie DL. Upper gastrointestinal fiberoptic endoscopy in pediatric patients. Gastroenterology 1977; 72: 1244–1248

4. Berggreen PJ, Harrison ME, Sanowski RA et al. Techniques and complications of esophageal foreign body extraction in children and adults. Gastrointest Endosc 1993; 39: 626–630

5. Blair SR, Graeber GM, Cruzzavala JL et al. Current management of esophageal impactions. Chest 1993; 104: 1205–1209

6. Dajani AS, Biso AL, Chung KJ et al. Prevention of bacterial endocarditis: recommendations by the American Heart Association. JAMA 1990; 264:2919

7. Squires RH, Morriss F, Schluterman S et al. Efficacy, safety, and cost of intravenous sedation versus general anesthesia in children undergoing endoscopic procedures. Gastrointest Endosc 1995; 41: 99–104

8. Chuang E, Wenner WJ, Piccoli DA et al. Intravenous sedation in pediatric upper gastrointestinal endoscopy. Gastrointest Endosc 1995; 42:156–160

9. O'Mara R, Nahata MC, Murray RD et al. Sedation with meperidine and midazolam in pediatric patients undergoing endoscopy. Eur J Clin Pharmacol 1994; 47: 319–323

10. Bendig DW. Pulse oximetry and upper intestinal endoscopy in infants and children. J Pediatr Gastroenterol Nutr 1991; 12: 39–43

11. Ament ME. Prospective study of risks of complications in 6,424 procedures in pediatric gastroenterology. Pediatr Res 1981; 15:524

12. O'Connor HJ, Axon AR. Gastrointestinal endoscopy: infection and disinfection. Gut 1983; 24: 1067–1077

13. Allendorph M, Werlin SL, Greenan JE. Endoscopic retrograde cholangiopancreatography in children. J Pediatr 1987; 110: 206–211

72

COLONOSCOPY

ROBERT H. SQUIRES, JR.

Over the last 25 years, the advances in endoscopy equipment, patient monitoring and sedation, and physician and nursing experience have enabled the pediatric gastroenterologist to identify and characterize important disease processes within the colon of infants and children.[1–3] Once limited to indirect examination of the colonic mucosa by contrast radiography, physicians can use flexible colonoscopy for direct inspection and histologic confirmation of mucosal abnormalities as well as for therapeutic opportunities. Considerable differences exist between pediatric and adult patients and their diseases. Factors unique to children (e.g., physical, psychological, developmental) make colonoscopy particularly challenging.

INDICATIONS

The decision to utilize colonoscopy to evaluate signs or symptoms should be made by a physician familiar with the patient, pediatric diseases, and the capabilities and limitations of the procedure in children.[4] The procedure is most useful when it leads to an alteration in diagnosis, prognosis, or therapy. Now that colonoscopy can be performed in any age child, the emphasis must be placed on when the procedure is indicated and safe (Table 72-1).

Colonoscopy is generally indicated to evaluate patients with suspected inflammatory bowel disease, unexplained hematochezia or iron deficiency anemia, or clinically significant diarrhea. Cancer surveillance is an uncommon indication for colonoscopy in children, but it may be considered for children in known risk groups.

These include patients with long-standing ulcerative colitis, Crohn's colitis, an inherited polypoid syndrome known to be at risk for neoplastic change, or ureteral implantation into the sigmoid. Colonoscopy may also be useful to evaluate an anatomic abnormality found with a barium enema such as a filling defect or stricture.

Colonoscopy is generally not indicated for acute, self-limited diarrhea, constipation and encopresis, or intestinal bleeding with a demonstrated upper intestinal source. Chronic or recurrent abdominal pain without other signs or symptoms (e.g., weight loss, anorexia, perianal disease) is not an indication for colonoscopy. The procedure is contraindicated in patients with fulminant colitis or toxic megacolon, suspected perforated viscus, or a recent intestinal resection.

PATIENT PREPARATION

Preparation of the young patient and the family for the procedure is essential to obtain optimal results. The procedure is explained in detail to the parents, as they provide a great source of comfort and reassurance to the child if they are knowledgeable of the logistics and expected benefits of the procedure. To communicate with the child, the physician must appreciate the child's cognitive and psychological development and identify tools to ease anxiety, provide reassurance, and establish rapport with the patient. A sketch of the procedure is useful to some patients. Children respond favorably to the knowledge that they will have a photograph of the findings at colonoscopy.

TABLE 72-1.   Indications for Pediatric Colonoscopy

Diagnostic colonoscopy with biopsy—generally indicated
   Unexplained iron deficiency anemia
   Unexplained melena
   Hematochezia
   Clinically significant diarrhea of unexplained origin
   Evaluate inflammatory bowel disease
   Evaluate a radiographic abnormality likely to be clinically significant
   Intraoperative identification of a lesion that is not apparent at surgery
   To obtain ileal or colonic tissue for diagnosis
Diagnostic colonoscopy—generally not indicated
   Acute self-limited diarrhea
   Gastrointestinal bleeding with demonstrated upper intestinal source
   Chronic, stable irritable bowel syndrome
   Chronic nonspecific abdominal pain unassociated with significant morbidity
   Constipation with or without encopresis
   Inflammatory bowel disease responding to therapy
Sequential or periodic diagnostic colonoscopy and biopsy—generally indicated
   Surveillance for dysplasia/malignancy
   Patients at increased risk for colonic malignancy
      Ureterosigmoidostomy
      Long-standing universal inflammatory bowel disease
      Polyposis syndromes
   Surveillance for rejection or other complications following intestinal transplantation
Diagnostic colonoscopy—contraindicated
   Fulminant colitis/toxic megacolon
   Suspected perforated viscus
   Recent intestinal resection

Adequate bowel preparation is critical to ensure satisfactory visualization of the colonic mucosa.[5-7] A number of regimens are available, which can usually be broadly classified as a lavage method or a clear liquid–cathartic method (Table 72-2).

The lavage method is useful in pediatric patients to prepare for surgery or colonoscopy or to treat severe constipation. The advantage of the lavage regimen is that the patient can eat a regular diet until the lavage is started and avoid a prolonged period of clear liquids. One protocol for using a lavage solution is as follows: After a 2- to 4-hour fast, metoclopramide (0.1 mg/kg, maximum 10 mg) is given by mouth 20 minutes before the lavage fluid and can be repeated every 4 hours to minimize gastric bloating and nausea. A commercially available balanced oral electrolyte solution is taken by mouth in aliquots of 5 to 10 ml/kg (maximum 250 ml) as quickly as possible (avoid sips) every 10 minutes until the rectal effluent becomes clear. The solution may be more palatable if chilled; however, nothing should be added to the

solution to improve its taste (e.g., ice, flavoring). Usually, no more than 4 L is necessary to adequately prepare the patient for colonoscopy. If the child is unable to drink the designated amount in the first 30 minutes, success with this method is unlikely without placement of a nasogastric tube. With a nasogastric tube in place, the infusion rate can range from 25 to 40 ml/kg/hr. For children less than 12 months of age, the infusion should begin at 25 ml/kg/hr and may be increased if the infusion is tolerated and stool effluent is not clear within 4 hours. Higher rates allow for more rapid clearing of stool but may be associated with side effects. If significant abdominal pain or vomiting occurs, the patient should be examined and the infusion rate reduced or stopped. Contraindications for using the lavage method include gastrointestinal (GI) obstruction, gastric retention, bowel perforation, or toxic megacolon. Adverse reactions

TABLE 72-2.   Colonoscopy Bowel Preparation Protocol

Lavage method—by mouth
   Regular diet until the afternoon prior to the procedure
   Fast for 2–4 hr
   Lavage solution is best chilled, but do not add ice or flavorings
   Give metoclopramide (0.1 mg/kg, maximum 10 mg) 20 min before lavage
   Give 5–10 ml/kg up to 250 ml of lavage fluid every 10 min
   Continue the lavage fluid until the rectal effluent is clear
   Use nasogastric tube method if patient is unable to take the expected amount during the first 30 min
   Metoclopramide may be repeated every 4 h
   Notify physician for:
      Rectal effluent not clear after 4 L of fluid
      Vomiting
      Abdominal pain
      No stool produced after the first hour
Lavage method—by nasogastric tube
   Regular diet until the afternoon prior to the procedure
   Special precautions for patients unable to tolerate a prolonged fast
   Fast for 2–4 hr
   Use 8 Fr soft nasogastric tube
   Fluid may be at room temperature
   Give metoclopramide as for oral lavage method
   Infuse solution at a rate of 25–40 ml/kg/hr until rectal effluent is clear
   Children less than 12 mo—begin infusion at 25 ml/kg/hr
   Notify physician for problems similar to oral lavage method
Clear liquid–cathartic method
   Clear liquid diet 48 h prior to the procedure
   Give magnesium citrate (1 oz/yr of age, up to 10 oz) the afternoon before the procedure
   Give bisacodyl or glycerin suppository the evening prior to the procedure
   Avoid giving an enema or suppository on the day of the procedure

experienced by some patients include nausea, vomiting, intestinal cramps, abdominal distention, perianal irritation, and a mild metabolic acidosis with prolonged irrigation.

Alternatively, children are offered a clear liquid diet 48 hours prior to the procedure and receive magnesium citrate (1 ounce per year of age up to 10 ounces) the afternoon before the procedure and a bisacodyl or glycerin suppository later that evening. An enema or suppository should be avoided on the day of the procedure, as visible and histologic mucosal inflammation caused by rectal medications can confound the interpretation of findings.

For infants under a year of age, the protocol for bowel preparation must be individualized to avoid excessive catharsis, dehydration, or a prolonged fast.

On the day of the procedure, the risks and benefits of the colonoscopy are reviewed with the family with ample time for questions and concerns. After informed consent is obtained, the child and selected family members are brought to the endoscopy suite, where an intravenous line is secured and monitoring equipment is applied. Parents are allowed to be with the child to provide comfort and reassurance as sedation medications are started.[8] Once the early effects of sedation are apparent, the family returns to the waiting room until after the procedure.

EQUIPMENT

The fiberoptic colonoscope, which brings the image along thousands of fine fibers to a hand-held eyepiece, has been largely replaced by video technology. With a video colonoscope, the image is captured by a tiny computer chip at the tip of the instrument and transported to a video screen where the endoscopist and other personnel in the room can see the image. Fiberoptic technology is still found in smaller endoscopes (less than 8.3 mm in external diameter as of this writing), since the size of the video chip is not yet adaptable to the smaller-sized instrument.

Video colonoscopes are available in sizes that range from 11.3 to 13.7 mm in diameter and 133 to 164 cm in length. The working channel through which accessories can be passed (e.g., biopsy and retrieving forceps, snares, baskets) can range from 2.8 to 4.2 mm. The field of view and angulation capabilities are similar for all colonoscopes. The larger channel allows for better suction and larger accessories to be used. The size and character of the endoscope are selected to be appropriate for the age and size of the patient. For infants and toddlers, a pediatric video upper GI endoscope (external diameter = 9.7 mm) or the smaller fiberoptic endoscope is used. Endoscopes used to examine the upper GI tract are less stiff and have a smaller suction channel than the colono-

scope, which makes them technically more difficult to use.

TECHNIQUE

Conscious sedation is most commonly used for colonoscopy, providing maximal patient comfort while allowing the patient to communicate with the physician.[9] When pain or discomfort is voiced or observed, a change in the technique or position can relieve symptoms. This interaction between the patient and physician is lost if the patient is under general anesthesia, and significant tension may be placed on the bowel unexpectedly, which increases the risk of colonic perforation.

After adequate sedation is achieved, the child is positioned on the left side. The physician advances the colonoscope quickly but gently to the terminal ileum or the area of concern while abiding by a few principles. These principles include minimizing pain and discomfort, always keeping the lumen of the bowel in sight, knowing the location of the tip of the colonoscope, and keeping the endoscope "straight" with avoidance of loops. To adhere to these principles, a number of different maneuvers are used separately or in combination. Transillumination of the bowel will aid in the location of the tip of the endoscope. If the tip of the scope is in the left lower quadrant and an excessive length of the endoscope is within the colon, one should suspect a loop has been created. Increased tension on the sigmoid colon or the presence of a large loop can result in sufficient discomfort to the patient and make the procedure impossible to complete. If a loop develops within the sigmoid or other segment of colon, the endoscope can be flexed to "hook" around a fold to anchor the proximal tip while the insertion tube is drawn back and torqued in a clockwise fashion. This maneuver can straighten the sigmoid loop. Another useful tool is to "telescope" the bowel on the endoscope by advancing and withdrawing in a repetitious manner. Suction of air and fluid from the colon can advance the tip of the scope. Repositioning the patient to be supine or on the right side may also help. Gentle but firm pressure on the abdomen at the apex of a palpable loop while the insertion tube is withdrawn can straighten the loop and advance the tip. Intubation of the terminal ileum is difficult when the ileocecal valve is tucked behind a fold. Special techniques used to enter the terminal ileum include suctioning air and fluid to partially collapse the cecum and open the valve, placing the patient in the prone position to bring the ileocecal valve into alignment with the endoscope, or retroflexing the tip and withdrawing the colonoscope a few centimeters to better visualize and approach the terminal ileum. The colonoscope must be as straight as possible, without loops, to enter the terminal ileum. The mucosal pattern of the colon is best evaluated as the instrument is slowly withdrawn. Biopsy samples are obtained in areas where the mucosa appears abnormal and also in areas appearing normal, as the ability to predict underlying histopathology based solely on visual endoscopic findings is imperfect.[10]

RISKS AND COMPLICATIONS

Potential risks and complications of colonoscopy include perforation, bleeding, infection, and difficulty with sedation. A higher dose of analgesic and amnesic medication is often required for colonoscopy when compared to upper endoscopy, for colon procedures are likely to produce more intense pain and require longer procedure time.[11] The narrow margin between inadequate sedation and oversedation in children mandates that a vigilant and experienced pediatric endoscopy team carefully observe and monitor the patient.

Bowel perforation and hemorrhage are serious but rare complications of colonoscopy. Colonic perforation during diagnostic colonoscopy occurs with an estimated frequency of 0.2% to 0.8%.[12–14] As might be expected, the frequency is higher with therapeutic colonoscopy procedures but still is a modest 0.5% to 3.0%. Mortality is low (0.14% to 0.65%). Although perforations occur most commonly in the rectosigmoid, they can occur anywhere along the colon.[15] Injuries may result from mechanical

TABLE 72-3. Risk Categories for Development of Endocarditis Following Endoscopy

High-risk cardiac lesions
    Prosthetic cardiac valves (bioprosthetic and homograft)
    Previous bacterial endocarditis
    Most congenital cardiac malformations
    Rheumatic and other acquired valvular dysfunction
    Hypertrophic cardiomyopathy
    Mitral valve prolapse with valvular regurgitation

High-risk endoscopy procedures
    Sclerotherapy for esophageal varices
    Esophageal dilation

Low-risk cardiac lesions
    Isolated secundum atrial septal defect
    Surgical repair without residual beyond 6 months of secundum atrial septal defect, ventricular septal defect, patent ductus arteriosus
    Physiologic, functional, or innocent murmur
    Previous Kawasaki syndrome without valvular dysfunction
    Cardiac pacemaker
    Mitral valve prolapse without valvular regurgitation

Low-risk endoscopy procedures
    Endoscopy with or without GI biopsy

TABLE 72-4. Infections Transmitted by Colonoscopy

Pseudomonas aeruginosa	Salmonella goerlitz
Enterobacter aerogenes	Salmonella newport
Salmonella oslo	Citrobacter freundii
Staphylococcus epidermidis	

forces (e.g., forceful insertion, laceration, forceps biopsy), pneumatic pressures, and therapeutic procedures (e.g., polypectomy, electrocautery, dilation of stricture). Patients with connective tissue disorders (e.g., Ehlers-Danlos syndrome) may be more susceptible to perforation.[16] Management of colonic perforation varies with each clinical circumstance and may involve conservative nonoperative therapy or surgery.[12] Intestinal bleeding following diagnostic or therapeutic colonoscopy is reported, but significant hemorrhage requiring a transfusion is rare in children.[2]

Infectious complications following flexible colonoscopy may result from bacteremia following instrumentation or by direct introduction of pathogens by a contaminated endoscope.[17–19] Bacteremia following colonoscopy with or without biopsy is estimated to occur in 3% to 4% of patients.[20] Because of these low rates of bacteremia, recommendations from the American Heart Association for prophylactic antibiotics in susceptible patients have changed in recent years.[21] Current guidelines recommend antibiotic prophylaxis only for those patients at high risk for developing endocarditis and who undergo a procedure with a high risk for bacteremia (Table 72-3). Prophylactic antibiotics are optional for patients with a "high-risk" cardiac lesion who undergo "low-risk" procedures. For patients with "low-risk" heart lesions, antibiotic prophylaxis is not recommended. Despite these recommendations, antibiotic prophylaxis is often used inappropriately.[22,23] Pathogens transmitted to the patient by contaminated endoscopes are listed in Table 72-4.[17] The sources for infection are improper cleaning techniques and an inability to adequately decontaminate the endoscope due to its complex design.

APPLICATIONS FOR COLONOSCOPY

Rectal Bleeding

Colonoscopy has revolutionized the evaluation of children with rectal bleeding.[24,25] Certainly, not every child with hematochezia requires colonoscopy. A comprehensive history and physical examination can identify important clues to the diagnosis such as recent exposure to antibiotics to suggest Clostridium difficile–associated colitis, perianal streptococcal cellulitis, or an anal fissure.

Stool studies should include a smear for polymorphonuclear leukocytes, cultures, and special assays (e.g., C. *difficile* toxin, ova and parasite examination) to identify an infectious cause for the blood in the stool. For the pediatric patient with persistent or recurrent hematochezia and no identifiable cause, however, colonoscopy or flexible sigmoidoscopy is the procedure of choice to search for mucosal changes or other lesions associated with bleeding.

Colitis is characterized endoscopically by obscuration of submucosal vessels, mucosal friability, and ulceration. Colitis may be uniform or patchy, mild or intense, and involve all or part of the colon.[26] Endoscopic inspection of the colonic mucosa may suggest a specific diagnosis. For example, the presence of pseudomembranes, although rarely reported with cytomegalovirus[27] or chemical injury,[28] is visually distinctive and virtually diagnostic of C. *difficile*–associated colitis, and biopsy is not essential.[29] Other forms of colitis have nonspecific endoscopic findings, and a mucosal biopsy will help characterize the inflammation as infectious, allergic, or consistent with inflammatory bowel disease.[10,30–33]

Other conditions associated with rectal bleeding in which colonoscopy aids in the diagnosis or treatment include polyps, foreign body, internal trauma from abuse, arteriovenous malformations, varices, and anastomotic ulcers.[34–37]

Therapeutic Colonoscopy

Juvenile hamartomatous or "inflammatory" polyps are common in children. Autoamputation without recurrence is the natural history for these polyps, but adenomatous change in the polyps has been described, which adds to the importance of removal and histologic examination.[38] Hereditary polyposis syndromes are also confirmed following colonoscopy and polypectomy.[39] The procedure is to secure a wire snare over the polyp and then tighten the loop around the base like a noose. Electrosurgical current is passed through the wire to desiccate the stalk and coagulate vessels feeding the polyp. The wire loop is then closed around the stalk to mechanically cut and cauterize the tissue.

Strictures or stenotic lesions of the colon can result from Crohn's disease, epidermolysis bullosa, or necrotizing enterocolitis or following colonic resection and anastomosis. The traditional method of treatment for these lesions is surgical exploration with resection or stricturoplasty. Recently, balloon dilators have been designed to pass through the colonoscope and provide an opportunity to dilate the lesions without surgery.[40]

Specialized instruments are needed to treat vascular lesions such as angiodysplasia, hemorrhoids, varices, or hemangiomas. Heater probe, bipolar electrocoagulation, and laser therapy have all been used successfully in the colon.[41–44]

Chronic Diarrhea

Chronic nonbloody diarrhea is an uncommon indication for colonoscopy. A microscopic colitis has been described in five children presenting with chronic diarrhea, abdominal pain, anorexia, and weight loss.[32] Although the mucosa appears endoscopically normal, mucosal biopsies showed evidence of a mixed inflammatory infiltrate in the lamina propria associated with intraepithelial polymorphonuclear cells and lymphocytes and edema. Treatment with sulfasalazine resulted in clinical and histologic improvement. Atypical presentations of conditions such as inflammatory bowel disease and pseudomembranous colitis may also be diagnosed by colonoscopy and biopsy.

Cancer Surveillance

The development of colon cancer in children is rare but does occur as a consequence of chronic universal ulcerative colitis, Crohn's colitis, an inheritable polypoid syndrome, or ureterosigmoidostomy. The time to initiate surveillance colonoscopy in children with these disorders is unclear. In ulcerative colitis, the time interval since diagnosis, not severity or duration of symptoms, seems to be the most predictive risk factor for development of carcinoma.[45,46] Patients with ulcerative colitis who also have primary sclerosing cholangitis are an identifiable subgroup who are at increased risk for colonic neoplasia.[47] The cumulative cancer risk for patients with universal ulcerative colitis increases by 0.5 to 1.0% per year after 8 to 10 years of disease, the time point at which many surveillance programs of scheduled colonoscopy procedures begin.[48] Recent data suggest that patients with Crohn's colitis are also at increased risk for carcinoma, particularly those with rectal strictures or total colonic involvement. Some experts have recommended surveillance colonoscopy at a frequency similar to that for patients with ulcerative colitis.[49–51] For children of patients with inheritable polyposis syndromes, surveillance colonoscopy to identify the presence of adenomatous polyps is recommended to begin at 11 years of age.[52] Once the patient is recognized to have inherited the condition, the role of serial colonoscopy is unclear, as sampling error may not detect high-grade dysplasia or carcinoma. Adenocarcinoma at the site of ureterosigmoidostomies develops between 10 and 46 years following the initial procedure.[53] Although established guidelines are not available for surveillance endoscopy for these patients, it is reasonable to initiate a yearly sigmoidoscopy 7 to 8 years following the surgical procedure.

REFERENCES

1. Hassall E, Barclay GN, Ament ME. Colonoscopy in childhood. Pediatrics 1984; 73: 594–599
2. Steffen RM, Wyllie R, Sivak MV et al. Colonoscopy in the pediatric patient. J Pediatr 1989; 115: 507–513

3. Fox VL: Colonoscopy. In: Walker WA, Durie PR, Hamilton JR et al, Eds. Pediatric Gastrointestinal Disease. 2nd Ed. St. Louis: Mosby, 1996: 1533–1541

4. Squires RH, Colletti RB. Indications for pediatric gastrointestinal endoscopy: a medical position statement of the North American Society for Pediatric Gastroenterology and Nutrition. J Pediatr Gastroenterol Nutr 1996;23(2):107–110

5. Tuggle DW, Hoelzer DJ, Tunell WP, Smith EI. The safety and cost-effectiveness of polyethylene glycol electrolyte solution bowel preparation in infants and children. J Pediatr Surg 1987; 22: 513–515

6. Vanner SJ, MacDonald PH, Paterson WG et al. A randomized prospective trial comparing oral sodium phosphate with standard polyethylene glycol-based lavage solution (Golytely) in the preparation of patients for colonoscopy. Am J Gastroenterol 1990; 85: 422–427

7. Millar AJW, Rode H, Buchler J, Cywes S. Whole-gut lavage in children using an iso-osmolar solution containing polyethylene glycol (Golytely). J Pediatr Surg 1988; 23: 822–824

8. Bauchner H. Procedures, pain, and parents. Pediatrics 1991; 87: 563–565

9. Kauffman RE, and the Committee on Drugs A. Guidelines for monitoring and management of pediatric patients during and after sedation for diagnostic and therapeutic procedures. Pediatrics 1992; 89: 1110–1115

10. Heyman MB, Perman JA, Ferrell LD, Thaler MM. Chronic nonspecific inflammatory bowel disease of the cecum and proximal colon in children with grossly normal-appearing colonic mucosa: diagnosis by colonoscopic biopsies. Pediatrics 1987; 80: 255–261

11. Squires RH, Morriss F, Schluterman S et al. Efficacy, safety, and cost of intravenous sedation versus general anesthesia in children undergoing endoscopic procedures. Gastrointest Endosc 1995; 41: 99–104

12. Kavin H, Sinicrope F, Esker AH. Management of perforation of the colon at colonoscopy. Am J Gastroenterol 1992; 87: 161–167

13. Kozarek RA, Earnest DL, Silverstein ME, Smith RG. Air-pressure-induced colon injury during diagnostic colonoscopy. Gastroenterology 1980; 78:7–14

14. Carpio G, Albu E, Gumbs MA, Gerst PH. Management of colonic perforation after colonoscopy: report of three cases. Dis Colon Rectum 1989; 32: 624–626

15. Foliente RL, Chang AC, Youssef AI et al. Endoscopic cecal perforation: mechanisms of injury. Am J Gastroenterol 1996; 91: 705–708

16. Nardone DA, Reuler JB, Girard DE. Gastrointestinal complications of Ehlers-Danlos syndrome. N Engl J Med 1979; 300: 863

17. Spach DH, Silverstein FE, Stamm WE. Transmission of infection by gastrointestinal endoscopy and bronchoscopy. Ann Intern Med 1993; 118: 117–128

18. Schembre D, Bjorkman DJ. Review article: endoscopy-related infections. Aliment Pharmacol Ther 1993; 7: 347–355

19. Zuckerman GR, O'Brien J, Halsted R. Antibiotic prophylaxis in patients with infectious risk factors undergoing gastrointestinal endoscopic procedures. Gastrointest Endosc 1994; 40: 538–543

20. Botoman VA, Surawicz CM. Bacteremia with gastrointestinal endoscopic procedures. Gastrointest Endosc 1986; 32: 342–346

21. Dajani AS, Bisno AL, Chung KJ et al. Prevention of bacterial endocarditis: recommendations by the American Heart Association. JAMA 199; 264: 2919–2920

22. Mogadam M, Malhotra SK, Jackson RA. Pre-endoscopic antibiotics for the prevention of bacterial endocarditis: do we use them appropriately? Am J Gastroenterol 1994; 89: 832–834

23. Meyer GW. Antibiotic prophylaxis for gastrointestinal procedures: who needs it? Gastrointest Endosc 1994; 40: 645–646

24. Chong SKF, Blackshaw AJ, Morson BC et al. Prospective study of colitis in infancy and early childhood. J Pediatr Gastroenterol Nutr 1986; 5: 352–358

25. Holgersen LO, Mossberg SM. Colonoscopy for rectal bleeding in childhood. J Pediatr Surg 1978; 13:83–85

26. Surawicz CM. Diagnosing colitis: biopsy is best. Gastroenterology 1987; 92: 538–540

27. Franco J, Massey BT, Komorowski R. Cytomegalovirus infection causing pseudomembranous colitis. Am J Gastroenterol 1994; 89: 2246–2248

28. Jonas G, Mahoney A, Murray J, Gertler S. Chemical colitis due to endoscope cleaning solutions: a mimic of pseudomembranous colitis. Gastroenterology 1988; 95: 1403–1408

29. Fekety R, Shah AB. Diagnosis and treatment of *Clostridium difficile* colitis. JAMA 1993; 269: 71–75

30. Surawicz CM, Haggitt RC, Husseman M, McFarland LV. Mucosal biopsy diagnosis of colitis: acute self-limited colitis and idiopathic inflammatory bowel disease. Gastroenterology 1994; 107: 755–763

31. Nostrant TT, Kumar NB, Appelman HD. Histopathology differentiates acute self-limited colitis from ulcerative colitis. Gastroenterology 1987; 92:318–328

32. Machida HM, Catto-Smith AG, Gall CG et al. Allergic colitis in infancy: clinical and pathologic aspects. J Pediatr Gastroenterol Nutr 1994; 19: 22–26

33. Odze RD, Wershil BK, Leichtner AM, Antonioli DA. Allergic colitis in infants. J Pediatr 1995; 126:163–170

34. Schrock TR. Colonoscopic diagnosis and treatment of lower gastrointestinal bleeding. Surg Clin North Am 1989; 69: 1309–1325

35. Sondheimer JM, Sokol RJ, Narkewicz MR, Tyson RW. Anastomotic ulceration: a late complication of ileocolonic anastomosis. J Pediatr 1995; 127: 225–230

36. Johansen K, Bardin J, Orloff MJ. Massive bleeding from hemorrhoidal varices in portal hypertension. JAMA 1980; 244: 2084–2085

37. Cynamon HA, Milov DE, Andres JM. Diagnosis and management of colonic polyps in children. J Pediatr 1989; 114: 593–596

38. Heiss KF, Schaffner D, Ricketts RR, Winn K. Malignant risk in juvenile polyposis coli: increasing documentation in the pediatric age group. J Pediatr Surg 1993; 28: 1188–1193

39. Rustgi AK. Hereditary gastrointestinal polyposis and nonpolyposis syndromes. N Engl J Med 1994; 331: 1694–1702

40. Kingsley AN. Colonic strictures: management by endoscopic balloon dilatation. Contemp Surg 1991; 38: 50–53

41. Rutgeerts P, Van Gompel F, Gegoes K et al. Long term results of treatment of vascular malformations of the gastrointestinal tract by neodymium YAG laser photocoagulation. Gut 1985; 26: 586–590

42. Noronha P, Leist M. Endoscopic laser therapy for gastrointestinal bleeding from congenital vascular lesions. J Pediatr Gastroenterol Nutr 1988; 7: 375–378

43. Hutcheon DF, Kabelin J, Buldley GB. Effect of therapy on bleeding rates in gastrointestinal angiodysplasia. Am Surg 1987; 53: 6–13

44. Jensen DM, Machicado GA. Endoscopic diagnosis and treatment of bleeding colonic angiomas and radiation telangiectasia. Perspect Colon Rectal Surg 1989; 2: 99–103

45. Greenstein AJ, Sachar DB, Smith H et al. Cancer in universal and left-sided ulcerative colitis: factors determining risk. Gastroenterology 1979; 77: 290–294

46. Ekbom A, Helmick C, Zack M, Adami HO. Ulcerative colitis and colorectal cancer. N Engl J Med 1990; 323: 1228–1233

47. Brentnall TA, Haggitt RC, Raminovitch PS et al. Risk and natural history of colonic neoplasia in patients with primary sclerosing cholangitis and ulcerative colitis. Gastroenterology 1996; 110: 331–338

48. Nugent FW, Haggitt RC, Gilpin PA. Cancer surveillance in ulcerative colitis. Gastroenterology 1991; 100: 1241–1248

49. Sachar DB. Cancer in Crohn's disease: dispelling the myths. Gut 1994; 35: 1507–1508

50. Nidias G, Eisner T, Katz S et al. Crohn's disease and colorectal carcinoma: rectal cancer complicating longstanding active perianal disease. Am J Gastroenterol 1995; 90: 216–219

51. Gillen CD, Walmsley RS, Prior P et al. Ulcerative colitis and Crohn's disease: a comparison of the colorectal cancer risk in extensive colitis. Gut 1994; 35: 1590–1592

52. Petersen GM, Slack J, Nakamura Y. Screening guidelines and premorbid diagnosis of familial adenomatous polyposis using linkage. Gastroenterology 1991; 100: 1658–1664

53. Eraklis AJ, Folkman MJ. Adenocarcinoma at the site of ureterosigmoidostomies for extrophy of the bladder. J Pediatr Surg 1978; 13: 730–734

73

ESOPHAGEAL pH MONITORING

STEPHEN E. SHAFFER

The technique of intraesophageal pH assessment has played an important role in our understanding of the pathophysiology and clinical management of gastroesophageal reflux (GER) since it was first described in the late 1950s by Tuttle and Grossman.[1] Technologic advances allowing for the miniaturization of the pH recording apparatus as well as a need to improve upon the sensitivity and specificity of earlier short-term methods eventually led to the concept of prolonged esophageal pH monitoring (EpHM), first introduced over 25 years ago. Today, EpHM is recognized by most pediatric gastroenterologists as the gold standard for diagnosing and quantifying GER in infants and children. Its utility in assessing GER is often misunderstood though, and thus the aim of this chapter is to focus on several key elements of EpHM that relate to its use as an important clinical diagnostic tool.

INDICATIONS

For the majority of otherwise healthy infants in whom a history of effortless regurgitation beginning before 6 months of age can be elicited, no further diagnostic testing should be required to establish the diagnosis of functional GER. In patients who exhibit an atypical history of reflux (e.g., onset beyond 6 months, projectile emesis), or when there is concern of pathogenic GER (see Ch. 25), evaluation with an upper gastrointestinal series and endoscopy should suffice in diagnosing GER and identifying associated esophagitis. Information obtained by EpHM would not be expected to result in an alteration in

diagnosis, treatment, or prognosis in these more obvious clinical scenarios. However, EpHM may be quite useful in situations where occult pathogenic reflux is suspected or as a means of establishing a temporal relationship between acid GER and a particular nongastrointestinal symptom. EpHM also has an established role, albeit more academic, in documenting GER in patients who fail to respond to standard medical therapy or to track reflux following treatment by medical or surgical means.

Subclinical GER

The identification of subclinical GER in patients with chronic, unexplained pulmonary symptoms or chest pain has become one of the primary indications for EpHM. In adults, EpHM has confirmed a high incidence of abnormal GER in patients with chronic hoarseness, a manifestation commonly referred to as reflux laryngitis.[2] Recurrent laryngeal symptoms in children have also been associated with increased acid reflux time and a higher frequency of proximal esophageal reflux episodes as determined by dual-channel monitoring.[3] EpHM may be used to diagnose other respiratory problems associated with reflux including chronic cough (particularly nocturnal), nonallergic asthma, and recurrent pneumonia. The use of EpHM in the evaluation of infantile apnea is common, yet its impact on establishing a causal role for GER and on outcome remains controversial. It should be reserved for cases where GER is a suspected but clinically inapparent cause for obstructive, and not central, apnea.[4] EpHM should always be performed with simultaneous pneumocardiography and oxygen saturation monitoring in the evaluation of infantile apnea. Recently, ambulatory EpHM, sometimes with simultaneous esophageal manometry, has been utilized in the evaluation of non-cardiac chest pain in adult and pediatric patients without other typical reflux symptoms. In general, however, inferring a causal relationship between such symptoms and GER is usually quite difficult given the limitations of EpHM. Often, more important information regarding the role of acid reflux in producing chest or respiratory symptoms is gained by gauging the overall response to medical therapy for GER.

Post-medical Therapy

The use of EpHM as a research tool in the evaluation of the medical treatment of GER is usually less relevant from a practical clinical standpoint. Efficacy of a given therapeutic regimen is often based solely on demonstrating a statistically significant improvement in EpHM criteria. Less emphasis is placed on clinical-based outcomes, as the signs and symptoms of GER may persist after a given intervention despite improved EpHM data. Correlating symptom responses with pH data is essential if meaningful comparisons of treatment protocols for GER are desired.

Pre- and Postsurgical Evaluation

Another common practice is the use of EpHM in documenting significant GER prior to a surgical antireflux procedure or in assessing the response to a given therapy. Despite the claim that a variety of pH monitoring criteria seem to predict a favorable response to antireflux surgery, most surgeons and gastroenterologists rely on additional factors when judging failure of medical therapy. More importantly, EpHM, by demonstrating the absence of pathologic GER, may serve to exclude potential candidates for fundoplication when the causal role of reflux in the intractable symptoms is questionable. In the patient with persistent or recurrent symptoms following an antireflux procedure, EpHM is also valuable in differentiating problems attributable to postoperative complications or outright failure of the surgery in controlling GER.

CONTRAINDICATIONS

Contraindications for EpHM are few and generally relate to the physical tolerance of the pH electrode in the nasopharynx and esophageal body. Occasionally, small infants will suffer respiratory compromise by its presence in the nose. Others may be provoked into uncontrolled gagging or retching by the electrode placement, thus making interpretation of the EpHM study difficult if not impossible. Lastly, EpHM would not be indicated in patients who are known to be achlorhydric, as gastric acid production is necessary for meaningful data to be recorded.

TECHNIQUE

The techniques and conditions for recording esophageal pH vary considerably and may significantly affect the interpretation of the data. Details of the methodology that are clinically relevant are presented below.

Devices

The monitoring apparatus consists of an esophageal pH electrode, reference electrode, and a data recording device. The "probe" is typically a soft, thin wire or plastic tube assembly (up to about an 8 Fr size) with a pH electrode at or near the distal tip. Most probes contain a monopolar glass electrode with an external reference electrode, usually a disposable electrocardiographic skin patch. Such cutaneous reference electrodes are a source of artifact due to poor skin adhesion, not infrequently resulting in large sections of absent pH data. In an attempt to overcome this, glass electrodes are also available with internal referencing electrodes, but they have the disadvantage of a larger diameter size, which makes transnasal passage more difficult, especially in children. The antimony electrode is another commercially available form of pH probe. It is a less expensive alternative but suffers from a much shorter usable life and has a longer response time compared with glass electrodes. Newer ion-sensitive field effect transistor (ISFET) pH electrodes offer excellent response characteristics and a small size allowing for multichannel probe construction. Prior to placement, the pH electrode must be calibrated using suitable neutral and acid buffers or, in the case of antimony electrodes, buffer solutions provided by the manufacturer.

Modern pH recording devices are now available as portable, battery powered, digital data loggers, replacing the more cumbersome pH meter and strip chart recorder, which prevented studies from being performed in an ambulatory setting. The pH and reference electrode are attached to the portable data logger, which samples pH information every 5 to 10 seconds and stores it in digital format. Some ambulatory devices also allow the real-time data to be transmitted from the patient's location to the hospital or laboratory. The ability to record information from one or several event markers is a feature found on most data loggers. Events such as meal times, body position, state of arousal, and various symptoms can be logged and transposed onto the pH record, providing information essential to the interpretation of the study. Pediatric EpHM requires careful parental or adult observation and data recording to obtain the most information possible from a study. At the completion of the study, the logger's digital pH data are usually transferred to a computer for analysis, printout of the record, and long-term storage.

Placement

Accurate placement of the pH electrode within the esophagus is necessary to obtain comparable, standardized information regarding GER. The method for placement of the probe in children has evolved from the practice in adults of locating the electrode 5 cm above the upper border of the lower esophageal sphincter (LES). This corresponds to approximately 87% of the distance from the nares to the LES. The most precise technique for determining this is accomplished by directly measuring the distance utilizing esophageal manometry. Although some centers still use manometrically determined placement, it is not widely available, is time-consuming, and generally requires intravenous sedation of the pediatric patient. Newer commercially available pH probes have a single, built-in pressure sensor that can define the LES location by a simple pull-through technique performed at the time of the pH probe placement.

Fluoroscopically guided electrode placement is an acceptable alternative to manometry. Locating the electrode at the level of the right atrium has been shown to correspond to placement at the standard 87% of the nares-to-LES distance.[5] Radiographic positioning is unreliable, however, in the presence of hiatal hernia or other alterations in esophageal anatomy. Numerous formulas have been devised to estimate esophageal length based on manometric data in children. All are versions of the basic calculation published by Strobel et al.[6]: nares to LES (cm) = 5 + 0.252 × height (cm). Using the drop in pH associated with passage of the electrode into the gastric lumen is unacceptable for accurate placement.

Variables Affecting pH Results

Various conditions of the EpHM study including its duration, meal composition and timing, body position, activity, and concurrent medication usage can greatly affect the data and their interpretation. Despite several conflicting claims that techniques of short-duration monitoring are equally sensitive in diagnosing pathologic GER, prolonged EpHM (e.g., 16 to 24 hours) continues to be the method of choice, as it offers improved specificity and reproducibility. Prolonged studies would also be expected to be more sensitive in attempts to correlate relatively infrequent symptoms with acid reflux. For studies performed in older children, meals should approximate their usual dietary habits. Acidic foods and beverages are restricted for many adult protocols because of their ability to drop esophageal pH transiently during consumption. Certain foods that tend to buffer gastric

acid, such as dairy products, are often prohibited. This, however, creates a significant problem for infants and children whose diet is limited to a "milk"-based formulation. Many pediatric gastroenterologists use acidic apple juice feedings to circumvent this difficulty and increase sensitivity to postprandial reflux. The obvious disadvantage to this approach is that clear liquid feedings are not handled by the stomach in the same fashion as more nutritionally complex infant formulas. Protein hydrolyzed formulas that have been acidified have been proposed as a more physiologic alternative to apple juice for EpHM,[7] although questions remain regarding their comparability to neutral formula feedings. The timing and duration of meals and snacks are also regulated to ensure the study includes adequate postprandial and fasting information.

Attention must be paid to the level of physical exercise and the amount of time spent in the recumbent position, as both may enhance reflux. In the infant or nonambulatory patient, body positioning must attempt to simulate a realistic setting depending on the issues that are to be resolved by the study. Typically, prone positioning will significantly diminish GER episodes compared with supine positioning in the majority of infants.

Acid neutralizing or blocking medications should be discontinued several days before conducting the study. Prokinetic therapy may be continued or stopped, again dependent on the ultimate question being addressed by EpHM.

INTERPRETATION

Following completion of the EpHM study, the downloaded data are usually analyzed by a computer software program that reports a variety of reflux criteria and scores (Fig. 73-1). The program also generates a hard copy of the study displaying the pH and event marker data over time (Fig. 73-2). GER episodes are recorded when the intraesophageal pH falls below 4, a level chosen by most investigators for physiologic and clinically relevant purposes. The amount of time recorded below this cutoff point, referred to as the reflux index, is the most frequently used reflux criterion. It is easily calculated by analysis programs and expressed as an absolute value (minutes per 24 hours) or percentage of time. Measurement of the frequency or number of reflux episodes is more complex, dependent on a calculation that utilizes a definition of the time parameters of an episode. For a reflux episode to be counted, the pH must fall below the level of 4 for a minimum amount of time, generally between 10 and 15 seconds, and then rise above 4, again for a specified minimum duration.

Meticulous review of the pH record and, if necessary,

```
                    *** Continuous Esophageal pH Monitoring ***

   Patient Name:           ******* *******
   Patient Number:         *******
   Test Started:           14:06  02/28/94  (Day 0)
   Analysis Duration:                (Hour : Minute / Day)
                           14:06 / 0  -  09:53 / 1


   Johnson+DeMeester pH Threshold:  4.0   (Acid Episodes <4.0)

   Upright:        113 episodes of reflux during 9 hours 6 minutes
                   3 episodes lasted over 5 minutes.
                   The longest episode occurred at 03:44 / 1
                     and lasted 10 minutes.
                   There was a total of 76 minutes of reflux
                     (14% of the time).


   Supine:         202 episodes of reflux during 10 hours 41 minutes.
                   15 episodes lasted over 5 minutes.
                   The longest episode occurred at 21:06 / 0
                     and lasted 81 minutes.
                   There was a total of 306 minutes of reflux
                     (48% of the time).


   Total:          315 episodes of reflux during 19 hours 47 minutes.
                   18 episodes lasted over 5 minutes.
                   The longest episode occurred at 21:06 / 0
                     and lasted 81 minutes.
                   There was a total of 382 minutes of reflux
                     (32% of the time).


   Johnson+DeMeester Table:  (During 19 hours 47 minutes)
```

--Parameter--	Value	Normal	Score
% time reflux upright	14.0	<6.3	6.9
% time reflux supine	48.0	<1.2	103.2
% time reflux total	32.0	<4.2	23.1
Episodes > 5 min.	18.	<3	15.0
Longest episode (min.)	81.0	<9.2	29.7
Total episodes	315.	<50	20.9
Composite Score (Normal < 22)			198.8

FIGURE 73-1. Example of computer-generated EpHM analysis that includes separate reporting of data from upright and supine positioning as well as a Johnson and DeMeester composite score.

scoring episodes by hand are thus essential for proper interpretation. For these reasons, many investigators regard frequency-dependent pH criteria as having limited usefulness. The mean acid clearance time represents the average duration of a reflux episode and is calculated by dividing the reflux index (total time pH less than 4) by the number of episodes. This variable is a reflection of the esophageal clearance capacity, but its utility is also limited, as it is derived from the calculation of the number of episodes. Several other EpHM criteria that assess esophageal clearance are often reported and include the number of episodes greater than 5 minutes, the percentage of episodes greater than 5 minutes, and the duration of the longest episode. Most centers continue to use all or a combination of these six criteria to establish a diagnosis of pathologic GER. A minimum of two abnormal criteria of the six is needed to make a positive diagnosis.[8] Adherence to the practice of basing diagnosis on only one criterion should be avoided.

One must also consider which portion of the pH tracing should be evaluated. The first and most common method involves the use of the entire pH recording including mealtimes (unless the patient is drinking a standard acid meal). Other methods score reflux differently, separating the 2-hour postprandial period from the preprandial period or "fasting" period (beyond 2 hours post-

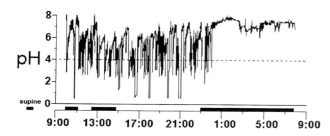

FIGURE 73-2. An example of an abnormal 24-hour esophageal pH recording. The pH is on the vertical axis, while the time of day is on the horizontal axis. Reflux episodes are indicated when the pH falls below 4. Frequent reflux episodes in this patient are noted exclusively during daytime waking hours, with none occurring during sleep.

TABLE 73-1. Reported Limits of Normal for Prolonged EpHM Criteria in Infants and Children

Criteria	Infants <1 yr[9] (n = 509)	Infants & Children[8] (summary of 7 studies)
Reflux index (%) (time pH <4)	10[a]	6[b]
Frequency of reflux (episodes/hr)	3	1.5
No. episodes >5 min (no./hr monitored)	0.35	0.30
Percent episodes >5 min	12	12
Longest episode (min)	41	20
Mean acid clearance time (min)	—	4

[a] 95th percentile.

[b] Mean + 2 standard deviations.

(Data from Vandenplas et al.[9] and Boyle.[8])

prandially). Some investigators concentrate on reflux occurring during sleep. Each system has the advantage of potentially identifying different patterns of GER. Drawbacks, particularly for the latter two methods, stem from a general lack of normative data from carefully chosen pediatric control populations. More complex systems aimed at generating a single "reflux score" from the six criteria have been devised, such as the Johnson and DeMeester score. However, they are no better at discriminating normal from abnormal GER when compared to the more simplified system as described above.

With the large number of methodologic and interpretive considerations involved in EpHM, it comes as no surprise to see a similar variability in the reporting of normative data. In the absence of a consensus approach, each center would ideally establish its own reference standards from control studies. As this is impractical for most clinicians, we must thus rely on existing published data from other centers, provided the studies are performed under comparable conditions. The most meaningful information on norms for EpHM in infants and children has come from Boyle,[8] who presented summary values based on several different published reports. Vandenplas et al.[9] reported values based on a large series performed in asymptomatic infants (Table 73-1). This latter study also characterized the temporal changes in the reflux index, revealing a decrease in physiologic GER by the age of 7 to 8 months to near adult levels by 1 year of age. In addition, Vandenplas et al.,[9] among others, have shown that data for the reflux index and other measured pH parameters do not fit a normal (gaussian) distribution, and the previous practice of reporting normative values in terms of mean plus 2 standard deviations is thus no longer appropriate. The use of nonparametric statistical methods to derive normal ranges for the various EpHM criteria from percentiles (e.g., 95th percentile) is therefore more accurate.

EpHM should be able to demonstrate a temporal cor-

relation between acid reflux and a wide variety of classic and nongastrointestinal reflux symptoms (Fig. 73-3). Practical experience, however, would seem to indicate otherwise, as the average patient or parent often fails to use event markers appropriately. The yield of EpHM in the role of symptom association may be further enhanced by using more objective measures such as pneumocardiography in the evaluation of obstructive apnea or video monitoring. Cautious interpretation of multichannel studies is needed though, as the limited response time of most EpHM equipment does not permit the accurate resolution of two events occurring close together in time.

FIGURE 73-3. A 1-hour segment of an esophageal pH recording that demonstrates the use of event markers in an attempt to associate symptoms with acid reflux. The vertical bars indicate the time of onset of the particular symptom.

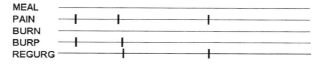

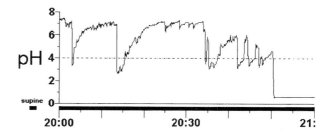

For symptoms such as cough, chest pain, or infant irritability, visual inspection of the pH record may readily suggest an association between it and GER.

To produce a quantitative measure of symptom association with GER, many investigators use a symptom index determined by the following equation[10]:

$$\frac{\text{Number of reflux-related symptom episodes}}{\text{Total number of symptom episodes}} \times 100\%$$

High values (i.e., greater than 75%) seem to suggest a positive correlation and low values (i.e., less than 25%) a negative correlation between reflux and the inciting symptom.[10] The low range of a positive symptom index has not been established, and such a system has not been validated in pediatric patients. Finally, as EpHM may provide information only about the temporal relationship between reflux and a particular symptom, consideration must be given to provocative tests such as the modified Bernstein test to better demonstrate causality.

SUMMARY

There is no doubt that the advent of prolonged esophageal pH monitoring has significantly advanced our knowledge of the pathophysiology of gastroesophageal reflux and has afforded the opportunity to study many different clinical settings and symptoms in which the role of reflux was previously unsuspected or unclear. However, the emphasis often placed on the objective quantification of GER provided by EpHM in lieu of clinical judgment suggests a relative lack of understanding of this technique's true capabilities and limitations. EpHM is most useful in situations where occult pathogenic reflux is suspected or as a means of establishing a temporal relationship between acid GER and a particular symptom. It provides little additional information in uncomplicated functional GER or in patients with documented reflux esophagitis.

REFERENCES

1. Tuttle SG, Grossman MI. Detection of gastroesophageal reflux by simultaneous measurement of intraluminal pressure and pH. Proc Soc Exp Biol 1958;98:225–227

2. Wiener GJ, Koulman JA, Wu WC et al. Chronic hoarseness secondary to gastroesophageal reflux disease: documentation with 24-h ambulatory pH monitoring. Am J Gastroenterol 1989;12:1503–1508

3. Contencin P, Narcy P. Gastropharyngeal reflux in infants and children. Arch Otolaryngol Head Neck Surg 1992;118:1028–1030

4. Colletti RB, Christie DL, Orenstein SR. Statement of the North American Society for Pediatric Gastroenterology and Nutrition (NASPGN): indications for pediatric esophageal pH monitoring. J Pediatr Gastroenterol Nutr 1995;21:253–262

5. Putnam PE, Orenstein SR. Determining esophageal length from crown-rump length. J Pediatr Gastroenterol Nutr 1991;13:354–359

6. Strobel CT, Byrne WJ, Ament ME, Eula AR. Correlation of esophageal lengths in children with height: application to the Tuttle test without prior esophageal manometry. J Pediatr 1979;94:81–84

7. Sutphen JL, Villard DL. pH-adjusted formula and gastroesophageal reflux. J Pediatr Gastroenterol Nutr 1991;12:48–51

8. Boyle JT. Gastroesophageal reflux in the pediatric patient. Gastroenterol Clin North Am 1989;18:315–337

9. Vandenplas Y, Goyvaerts H, Helven R, Sacre L. Gastroesophageal reflux, as measured by 24-hour pH monitoring, in 509 healthy infants screened for risk of sudden infant death syndrome. Pediatrics 1991;88:834–840

10. Wiener GJ, Richter JE, Copper JB et al. The symptom index: a clinically important parameter of ambulatory 24-hour esophageal pH monitoring. Am J Gastroenterol 1988;83:358–361

74

MANOMETRY

DELMA L. BROUSSARD

There are many gastrointestinal (GI) symptoms such as heartburn, difficulty swallowing, abdominal or chest pain, vomiting, diarrhea, and constipation that are commonly attributed to abnormal GI motility. A number of procedures have been developed to evaluate GI movements. This chapter will review the technique of GI manometry in different segments of the gut.

EQUIPMENT

Multisensor manometry catheters measure the strength of luminal contractions of the bowel wall, in addition to their duration, velocity, and direction. There are two types of catheter systems, a water perfused catheter and a catheter that contains microtransducers within the wall of the tube. In both systems, the catheter must be flexible and small enough to ensure patient comfort, as well as ease of intubation of the gut lumen.

The water perfused system is the most widely used apparatus because of its low cost and durability. This manometry system relies on the continuous infusion of a catheter, with side-hole recording ports, with distilled water by a low-compliance pump. A luminal contraction causes compression of the water-filled catheter side hole, which causes an increase in pressure within the lumen of the catheter, which is then sensed by a pressure transducer. The accuracy of the infusion catheter system is directly related to the infusion rate and inversely related to the compliance (measurement of the ease with which the system senses a change in pressure) of the catheter system.[1] Therefore, accurate recording requires a high

enough rate of infusion and low enough compliance that a contraction does not block the recording port. The compliance of the manometry catheter is inversely related to the luminal diameter and the thickness and stiffness of the catheter wall and directly related to the catheter length.[2] As a result, these catheters are made using relatively elastic polyvinyl chloride, in addition to being thick-walled with the smallest internal diameter and the shortest length possible. Multiple small, single catheters with side holes placed circumferentially for recording are fused together longitudinally to make a multilumen catheter (Fig. 74-1). A pneumohydraulic capillary infusion system allows a low capillary infusion rate (0.5 ml/min or lower), which decreases the risk of aspiration, and large intraluminal fluid volumes, which may induce secondary peristalsis.[1,2] The catheter is connected to external pressure transducers and a recording device, either a chart polygraph or a computer polygraph.

A solid-state catheter embedded with microtransducers has the advantage of generally being smaller than the perfused catheter and decreases the risk of aspiration in studies of the upper GI tract. The catheter is connected directly to a computer polygraph or a small digitrapper, which gives the flexibility of performing a study at any bedside. Catheters embedded with three microtransducers spaced 5 cm apart, are used in our laboratory for esophageal manometry with an outer diameter of 4 mm and pH sensor at the distal end. For antroduodenal manometry, we use catheters with four microtransducer sensors each that are either 5 or 8 cm apart, also with an outer diameter of 4 mm (Fig. 74-1). The anorectal manometry catheter has four solid-state pressure transducers spaced 1 cm apart and a distal latex balloon.

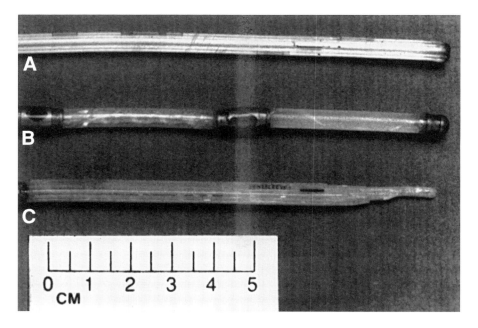

FIGURE 74-1. Manometry catheters. *(A)* Infused catheter with radially placed side recording ports. *(B)* Solid state antroduodenal manometry catheter with pressure transducers within the catheter. *(C)* Dent sleeve infused manometry catheter for measuring the esophageal sphincter.

ESOPHAGEAL MANOMETRY

Esophageal manometry is commonly used to evaluate primary esophageal motor dysfunction or dysfunction in association with a systemic disorder, chest pain, lower esophageal sphincter pressure (LES) prior to antireflux surgery, or the position of the LES.[3] During the procedure, changes in pharyngeal and esophageal pressures associated with swallowing are recorded. A normal swallow starts with relaxation of the upper esophageal sphincter, which allows passage of a bolus into the esophageal body. The bolus must then be propelled down the esophagus by coordinated contractions of the smooth muscle of the esophageal body. LES relaxation enables the bolus to enter the stomach. Esophageal manometry has proved to be a safe and technically easy procedure to perform in the pediatric population, including premature infants.[4–6] The primary limitations for the procedure include lack of cooperation and patient discomfort.

Prior to each use, a manometry system must be calibrated according to manufacturer's instructions. In the pneumohydraulic infusion system, it is especially important to remove any bubbles from the catheters, as they will increase compliance. All medications that affect GI motility should have been discontinued. The patient is not permitted anything by mouth for 4 to 8 hours prior to the procedure, and written consent is obtained. It may be necessary to give a small amount of sedation such as chloral hydrate[7] or midazolam[8] to get an accurate study.

Lubricating the manometry tube and spraying the pharynx with lidocaine can also decrease the discomfort.

The catheter is passed through the nares (or orally) with the aid of wet or dry swallows until the most proximal recording channel is in the stomach. Gastric pressure waves can be recognized as low-amplitude (5 to 10 mmHg) waves, whose amplitudes are increased by inspirations and unaffected by swallowing. At the start of the study using a water perfused system, the patient should be in a supine position such that the pressure transducers are at the level of the esophagus to minimize pressure artifact from the hydrostatic force of the water column. This is not a factor when using the solid-state catheter system.

There are two methods of measuring the LES, the rapid[9] and station pull-through techniques. In the rapid pull-through technique, the catheter is withdrawn continuously (0.5 cm to 1.0 cm/s) through the LES while the patient ceases respirations. This technique is difficult for the majority of the pediatric population; therefore, the preferred method is the station pull-through. In the station pull-through technique, the catheter is slowly (0.5 to 1.0 cm in 20-second intervals) withdrawn until there is a rise in the baseline pressure of the proximal channel. This will correspond to the LES pressure and is verified by observing relaxation with swallowing. The catheter is withdrawn at 0.5- to 1.0-cm intervals until all recording ports are through the LES. The elevated LES pressure should appear at each recording site in sequence, at the distances between the ports. The maximum LES pressure is a combination of the tonic sphincter contraction and phasic diaphragmatic contractions in response to respiration. The LES pressure at each site may vary for each channel because of the differences in radial orientation of the side holes in the perfused catheter system and the asymmetry of the LES. Therefore, the basal LES pressure is determined by calculating the mean of the midpoint of the amplitude of the mid-expiratory pressure at each recording site, using the gastric pressure as the reference point. If an infused catheter is used, the asymmetry of the LES can be overcome by using a system with a side hole that opens into a sleeve that forces the water to exit distally at the end of the sleeve (a Dent sleeve).[10] This modification enables continuous measurement of the LES, as a change in pressure anywhere along the sleeve will be sensed by the transducer. The microtransducer catheter records pressure changes circumferentially so that the measurement of the LES is not a problem. Normal LES location from the nares in infants and adults is about 20 cm and 40 cm, respectively.[11,12] Small pediatric series have reported normal values of basal LES pressure to be from 13 to 27 mmHg.[13]

After the LES has been identified, the catheter is repositioned so that the distal recording channel is within the LES, and the catheter is fixed with tape. The patient should be instructed to swallow two to three times to check the position of the catheter and the recording scales adjusted so that maximal pressures remain within the scale. The esophageal body location is confirmed by negative baseline pressure (intrathoracic pressures) and positive pressure waves with swallowing. Having the patient take sips of water through a straw enables the observance of peristaltic contractions and spontaneous contractions in the esophageal body, as well as LES relaxation (Fig. 74-2). The catheter can be pulled further into the esophageal body at 1-cm intervals so that the most distal channel is above the LES to further assess contractions within the esophageal body. The amplitude, duration, and velocity of esophageal body contractions should be recorded. Further withdrawal of the tube until the most proximal channel demonstrates another high-pressure zone will identify the upper esophageal sphincter (UES). This area can be confirmed by observing relaxation in response to swallows. If using a water infusion catheter, turn off the water for the proximal channel to prevent aspiration. Continued withdrawal of the catheter will demonstrate the high pressure of the pharynx at the most proximal recording site, while the middle channel will be recording the UES. Peak pharyngeal contraction pressures occur during the trough of UES relaxation.

ANTRODUODENAL MANOMETRY

Antroduodenal manometry measures antral and duodenal pressures. It is most helpful in cases of suspected neuromuscular disorders of the stomach and small bowel if routine studies are nondiagnostic[14] (see Ch. 40 for re-

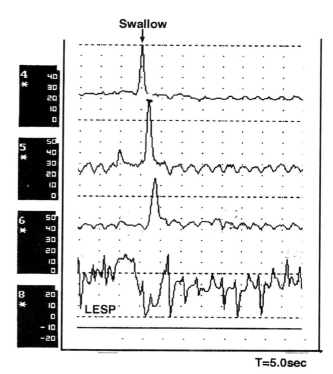

FIGURE 74-2. Normal esophageal manometry with peristalsis within the esophageal body and decrease of the lower esophageal sphincter pressure (LESP) following initiation of a swallow.

view of clinical motility disorders of the small intestine and stomach). Antroduodenal manometry is not widely utilized in the pediatric population because of the technical difficulties in placing the catheter transpylorically, lack of commercially available small tubes for infants, and recording artifact with activity. Either an infusion system or a microtransducer catheter system can be used. One advantage to using the infused system if the catheter is made with access to the central lumen is that the center lumen can be used as a feeding port during the study with minimal disturbance of the tube position. However, catheters embedded with miniature transducers are very well tolerated because of their small size and flexibility. Depending on the type of catheter and the time allowed for placement, the antroduodenal catheter can be placed endoscopically, allowed to pass on its own with or without a dose of a prokinetic agent, or fluoroscopically placed using a guidewire. The location of each of the recording ports should be confirmed by x-ray prior to recording, although some authors have reported using waveforms to determine the location of each of the recording ports.[15]

Two main motility patterns of the stomach and small intestine are investigated. During fasting, nonruminants exhibit cyclic bands of contractile activity within the small intestine. These repetitive contractions, known as the migrating motor complex (MMC), often start in the gastroduodenal region and are propagated a variable distance down the small intestine[16] (Fig. 74-3). It has been postulated that the MMC sweeps residual products of digestion toward the colon, a "housekeeper" function.[17] These phasic contractions occur about every 90 to 110 minutes in the adult preprandial period and every 50 to 100 minutes in infants.[18,19] After nutrients are introduced into the lumen, the fed pattern occurs, which consists of diffuse contractions throughout the stomach and small intestine (Fig. 74-4). Therefore, a study of the small bowel should be long enough to observe sufficient numbers of MMC cycles in addition to the fed pattern following a standardized meal.

We use solid-state catheters placed under endoscopic guidance directly into the duodenum, with the most proximal sensor in the antrum. Because of the sedation during the endoscopy, patients are studied overnight to ensure a study independent of pharmacologic effects. When patients can tolerate feeds, a standard caloric meal is given. The subsequent fasting periods are used to observe MMCs. There are several phases of the MMC. Phase I is quiescent. Phase II consists of clusters of irregular contractions. Phase III is characterized by groups of maximal amplitude and spike frequency contractions, which migrate down the intestine in a sequential order. Phase III is a recognizable pattern by which pharmacologic agents and normal motility are measured. A neurogenic abnormality will show a poorly coordinated MMC, while a myogenic process will show low-amplitude contractions.

ANORECTAL MANOMETRY

The internal and external rectal sphincters are tonically contracted in their resting state.[19] Normal defecation involves an increase in rectal pressure with a simultaneous decrease in pressure in the anal canal. With rectal distention, there is relaxation of the internal anal sphincter and contraction of the external anal sphincter—the rectoanal reflex.[21] Anorectal manometry investigates the rectoanal reflex by distending the rectum with a balloon.[20]

There are several techniques for anorectal manometry in the literature.[8,11,22] Prior to the procedure, the patient receives an enema to clear the rectum of stool. The balloon and catheter are inserted into the rectum until all the recording ports are beyond the internal sphincter. The catheter is slowly withdrawn in 0.5- to 1.0-cm increments until the internal and external anal sphincters are located. Cooperative patients can voluntarily contract the external anal sphincter to aid in its identification. Following localization of the internal anal sphincter, the balloon is reinserted until the recording ports are within the sphincter zones. Subsequent inflation of the balloon with incremental volumes of air is utilized to determine the sensory threshold for rectal distention (in older children) and the threshold of the rectoanal inhibitory reflex. There is a normal rectoanal reflex in functional constipation, but the reflex is absent in Hirschsprung's disease. Anorectal manometry has been performed successfully on premature infants, as well as older children.

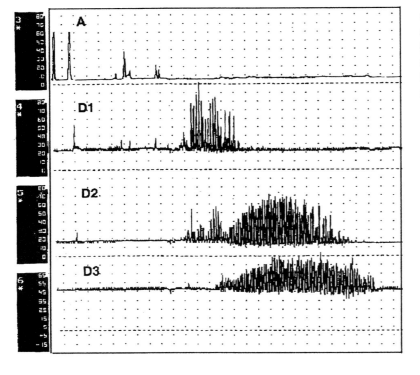

FIGURE 74-3. Antroduodenal manometric study of an MMC, which begins in the antrum (site 3) and propagates through the upper small intestine (sites 4 to 6). The antral recording shows the characteristic 3/min contraction rate. A, antrum; D1-2, duodenum.

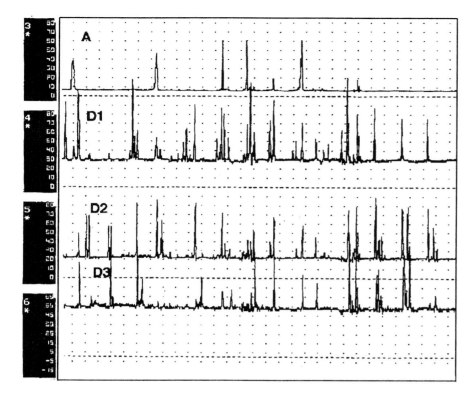

FIGURE 74-4. Antrum and duodenal tracing of the fed pattern with generalized contractions in all areas. A, antrum; D1-2, duodenum.

However, falsely abnormal results may occur if the balloon is not inflated adequately, if there is retained fecal material, or if the catheter slips out of the sphincter zone.[23,24]

REFERENCES

1. Dodds WJ. Instrumentation and methods for intraluminal esophageal manometry. Arch Intern Med 1976;136:515–523

2. Arndorfer RC, Stef JJ, Dodds WJ et al. Improved infusion system for intraluminal esophageal manometry. Gastroenterology 1977;73:23–27

3. Cohen S. Motor disorders of the esophagus, review. N Engl J Med 1979;301:184–192

4. Gryboski JD. The swallowing mechanisms of the neonate: I. Esophageal and gastric motility. Pediatrics 1965;35:445–452

5. Newell SJ, Sarkar PK, Durbin GM. Maturation of the lower esophageal sphincter in the preterm baby. Gut 1988;29:167–172

6. Werlin SL, Dodds WJ, Hogan WJ, Arndorfer RC. The use of esophageal manometry in children. Wis Med J 1979;78:25–27

7. Vanderhoof JA, Rapoport PJ, Paxson CLJ. Manometric diagnosis of lower esophageal sphincter incompetence in infants: use of a small, single lumen perfused catheter. Pediatrics 1978;62:805–808

8. Werlin SL, Brown CW. Gastrointestinal motility. In: Wyllie R, Hyams JS, Eds. Pediatric Gastrointestinal Disease. Philadelphia: WB Saunders, 1993:1016–1026

9. Dodds WJ, Hogan WJ, Stef JJ et al. A rapid pull-through technique for measuring lower esophageal sphincter pressure. Gastroenterology 1975;68:437–443

10. Dent J. A new technique for continuous sphincter pressure measurement. Gastroenterology 1976;71:263–267

11. Scott B. Motility studies. In: Walker-Smith WA, Durie PR, Hamilton JR, Walkins JB, Eds. Pediatric Gastrointestinal Diseases. Philadelphia: BC Decker, 1991:1324–1330

12. Clouse RE. Motor disorders. In: Sleisenger MH, Fordtran JS, Eds. Gastrointestinal Disease. 4th Ed. Philadelphia: WB Saunders, 1989:561–562

13. Hillemeier A, et al. Esophageal and gastric motor abnormalities in gastroesophageal reflux during infancy. Gastroenterology 1983;84:741–746

14. Mearin F, Malagelada JR. Gastrointestinal manometry: A practical tool or research technique? J Clin Gastroenterol 1993;16:281–291

15. Berseth CL. Neonatal small intestinal motility: motor responses to feeding in term and preterm infants. J Pediatr 1990;117:777–782

16. Code CF, Marlett JA. The interdigestive myoelectric complexes of the stomach and small bowel of dogs. J Physiol (Lond) 1975;246:289–309

17. Code CF, Schlegel J. The gastrointestinal interdigestive

housekeeper: Motor correlates of the interdigestive myoelectric complex of the dog. In: Daniel EE, Gilbert JAL, Schofield B et al, Eds. Proceedings of the IV International Symposium on GI Motility. Vancouver: Mitchell Press, 1973: 631–634

18. Kerlin P, Phillips S. Variability of motility of the ileum and jejunum in healthy humans. Gastroenterology 1982;82: 694–700
19. Berseth CL. Gestational evolution of small intestine motility in preterm and term infants. J Pediatr 1989;115:646–651
20. Schuster MM, Hendrix TR, Medeloff AI. The internal anal sphincter response: manometric studies on its normal physiology, neural pathways, and alteration in bowel disorders. J Clin Invest 1963;42:196–207
21. Denny-Brown D, Robertson GE. An investigation of the nervous control of defaecation. Brain 1935;58:256–310
22. Rosenberg AJ, Vela AR. A new simplified technique for pediatric anorectal manometry. Pediatrics 1983;71:240–245
23. Ito Y, Donahoe PK, Hendren WH. Maturation of the rectoanal response in premature and perinatal infants. Pediatr Surg 1977;12:477–482
24. Bowes KL, Kling S. Anorectal manometry in premature infants. J Pediatr Surg 1979;14:533–535

75

PERCUTANEOUS LIVER BIOPSY

ELIZABETH B. RAND

Collection of a liver biopsy sample is often a necessary step in the evaluation of children with liver diseases or with systemic illnesses involving the liver. Increasing use of percutaneous techniques for liver biopsy collection means that crucial diagnostic information can be obtained safely without open abdominal surgery. This chapter discusses the indications for liver biopsy in the evaluation of children with liver disease, indications for and contraindications to a percutaneous approach, the methodology of performing a percutaneous liver biopsy, and the potential complications of this approach and suggests some alternative routes for liver biopsy when the percutaneous approach is not recommended.

INDICATIONS FOR PERCUTANEOUS LIVER BIOPSY

Although many common pediatric liver disorders may be adequately evaluated and diagnosed with indirect liver testing, liver biopsy remains a necessary part of a complete evaluation in a significant number of cases. General indications for percutaneous liver biopsy fall into several categories. Liver tissue may be used for diagnosis of an intrinsic liver disorder, to evaluate progression of disease or response to therapy in a known liver disorder, or to diagnose or evaluate change in a metabolic disorder, toxic injury, secondary liver injury, or hepatic infections. Focal liver tumors are not well suited for percutaneous liver biopsy because of an increased risk of hemorrhage; however, infiltrative processes may be diagnosed and monitored by this route. Liver tissue can be examined

by light or electron microscopy, specially stained for abnormal deposits or sequestered metabolites, analyzed for specific enzyme activities, or subjected to bacterial, viral, or fungal culture.

It is important to carefully consider the differential diagnosis prior to the liver biopsy so that tissue can be collected in an appropriate manner for all relevant special tests. If multiple analyses will be required, several needle passes may be necessary to collect adequate tissue by the percutaneous route. Table 75-1 lists various general indications for liver biopsy and specific disorders that may be diagnosed in this fashion. Percutaneous liver biopsy has been performed successfully in children for at least 50 years, with early English language reports dating back to the 1940s.[1,2] There are several clear advantages to the percutaneous versus the surgical approach including decreased morbidity, shorter hospital stay (or outpatient biopsy in selected cases), lack of need for general anesthesia, decreased recovery time, and reduced costs. Generally speaking, the percutaneous route should be considered in every child with an indication for liver biopsy and an alternative route selected for those children with a specific contraindication to percutaneous biopsy.

CONTRAINDICATIONS TO PERCUTANEOUS LIVER BIOPSY

Any condition that increases the complication risk to the patient from a percutaneous route of biopsy should be considered a relative contraindication. It is important

TABLE 75-1.   Indications for Percutaneous Liver Biopsy

Evaluation of general hepatic abnormalities

Neonatal cholestasis/hepatitis

Cholestasis

Hepatitis/elevated liver enzymes

Hepatosplenomegaly

Diagnosis/Evaluation of progression of specific hepatic disorders

Biliary atresia

Giant cell hepatitis

Viral hepatitis (all types)

Fibrosis/cirrhosis (of any cause)

Alpha-1-antitrypsin deficiency

Ductal plate abnormalities

Cholangitis (particularly in the setting of fever, elevated enzymes, and/or cholestasis following a Kasai procedure)

Alagille syndrome

Sclerosing cholangitis

Byler's syndrome

Persistent familial intrahepatic cholestasis

Evaluation of metabolic disorders

Disorders of carbohydrate metabolism
  Glycogen storage diseases
  Galactosemia
  Hereditary fructose intolerance

Disorders of amino acid metabolism
  Tyrosinemia

Disorders of lipid metabolism (inborn errors of fatty acid oxidation)
  Medium-chain acyl-CoA dehydrogenase deficiency (MCAD)
  Long-chain acyl-CoA dehydrogenase deficiency (LCAD)

Disorders of lysosomal storage
  Gaucher's disease
  Niemann-Pick disease
  Wolman's disease
  Cholesterol ester storage disease

Urea cycle defects

Peroxisomal disorders

Wilson's disease

Zellweger syndrome

Ivemark syndrome

Evaluation of liver disease associated with extrahepatic/systemic diseases

Graft-versus-host disease

Langerhans' cell histiocytosis

Erythrophagocytic syndrome

Amyloidosis

Sarcoidosis

Granulomatous diseases

Infectious processes

Inflammatory bowel disease

Toxin/drug exposures

Evaluation of liver disease associated with liver transplantation

Acute or chronic allograft rejection

Infectious processes

Lymphoproliferative disease

Vascular insufficiency

---

to note that although many of these conditions may also increase the risk of liver biopsy done by an open, laparoscopic, or transjugular route, these alternative methods may allow for compensating measures (e.g., direct visualization, suturing of biopsy site) to reduce complication risks. The most important potential complication from a percutaneous liver biopsy is hemorrhage. Factors that would be expected to increase the risk of hepatic bleeding are common in patients with indications for liver biopsy, for example, coagulopathy, thrombocytopenia, and ascites. Coagulopathy and thrombocytopenia can often be corrected by administration of fresh frozen plasma (FFP) and platelet transfusions and generally need be considered only relative contraindications.[3] A mildly elevated prothrombin time (PT) or decreased platelet count may not require correction.[3,4] Massive ascites may prevent tamponade of the hepatic needle puncture site and should be treated medically or by paracentesis prior to percutaneous biopsy. Solid or cystic lesions within the liver should not be biopsied blindly by the percutaneous route because of the increased risk of hemorrhagic complications, especially if the lesion is malignant.[4] Cystic or fluid-filled lesions are particularly suspect for bleeding and possible infection; these are best approached by interventional radiologic techniques or open surgical exploration. Table 75-2 lists relative and absolute contraindications to percutaneous liver biopsy.

METHOD OF PERCUTANEOUS LIVER BIOPSY

Percutaneous liver biopsy should only be performed by individuals specifically trained in usage of this technique along with appropriate monitoring and management of the potential complications. The procedure should only be undertaken in a hospital setting where surgical sup-

TABLE 75-2. Contraindications to Percutaneous Liver Biopsy

Relative contraindications
  Moderate coagulopathy
  Right pulmonary effusion or infection
  Ascites
  Need for large amounts of tissue
Absolute contraindications
  Severe, uncorrectable coagulopathy
  Hepatic malignancy
  Vascular lesion
  Lack of experienced operator

port is available should laparotomy be necessary for treatment of complications.

Preprocedure Studies

Once the need for a liver biopsy is established, various laboratory and radiologic studies are generally required prior to the procedure to determine if the percutaneous route is appropriate. A complete blood count should be performed to document the baseline hemoglobin and hematocrit. A platelet count should be included along with measurement of the PT and partial thromboplastin time to determine if thrombocytopenia or coagulopathy exists. Measurement of the bleeding time may be indicated in patients with a history of unanticipated bleeding complications or of recent use of medications that may alter platelet function. If the platelet count is less than 50,000/mm^3, an infusion of platelets should be administered just prior to the liver biopsy, and similarly, an infusion of FFP should be administered to patients with PT elevated over 1.5 seconds above the upper limit of normal. FFP infusions are best administered at a dose of 10 to 15 ml/kg starting 30 minutes prior to the biopsy and continuing over the next 2 hours. It is not necessary to complete the infusion and repeat the PT measurement, as this causes delay and decline of the protective effects of the FFP.[3] A blood sample for type and crossmatch is not routinely performed at all centers but should certainly be considered for neonates or for patients requiring correction of coagulopathy or platelet count.

Radiologic evaluation of pediatric patients with liver disease generally includes an abdominal ultrasound, which will document liver size and position and the presence or absence of ascites or overlying bowel loops. Although some experienced individuals select the biopsy site by physical examination alone (marking the biopsy site at the point of maximal dullness on percussion), many choose to use ultrasonography marking just prior to the procedure. This is especially useful when localization of the liver by physical examination is difficult, for example, in obese patients, those with small livers, or

those with prior abdominal surgeries who may have fixed bowel loops overlying the biopsy site.

Patient Preparation

Pediatric patients should have abstained from food and liquids for 4 hours prior to liver biopsy because of the sedation administered. Percutaneous liver biopsy should be carried out in a hospital setting (inpatient or outpatient for selected patients) with cardiorespiratory monitoring including pulse, respiratory rate, blood pressure, and pulse oximetry. Supplemental oxygen should be immediately available, as should life support equipment. As mentioned above, the procedure should only be done where surgical support is available should laparotomy be needed to treat a massive hepatic hemorrhage or other complication. An intravenous line is placed for administration of fluids and medications (though some use the rectal route for sedation). A combination of several agents selected to provide both analgesia and amnesia is useful for sedation in the pediatric age group; many use a narcotic for pain relief together with midazolam for its anxiolytic and amnestic effects. The child should be placed in a supine position on a flat procedure table or bed without a pillow. The right arm should be positioned with the right hand above the head and restrained by an assistant; additional restraints may be necessary.

Performing the Biopsy

Percutaneous liver biopsy can be performed via an anterior abdominal, right lateral abdominal, or right lateral intercostal approach. The intercostal approach (generally in the 10th intercostal space) is the most common in older children and adults, but small infants with large abdominal livers may be better approached subdiaphragmatically. As discussed above, the site is selected in advance by physical examination with or without ultrasonography. The biopsy site is cleansed with antibacterial soap as for a surgical procedure and sterilely draped. A local anesthetic (generally lidocaine 1%) is administered as a subcutaneous wheal at the selected site, and then additional anesthetic is infiltrated along the expected biopsy needle route to the liver capsule. If the site is intercostal, the subcostal vessels and nerves must be avoided. Once the local anesthetic is administered, a small (approximately 3 mm) incision is made in the skin at the site to allow passage of the biopsy needle. This is important, as the needle itself is not sharp enough to cleanly penetrate the skin and will drag if a large enough entrance is not prepared. Numerous styles of biopsy needles are available (Menghini, Klatskin, Jamshidi, Tru-cut, ASAP); however, they fall into two main categories.

The Menghini needle is the prototype for the Klatskin and Jamshidi needles, and all consist basically of a hollow beveled needle with a syringe that is filled with sterile nonbacteriostatic saline.[5,6] The needle is advanced through the chest or abdominal wall parallel to the table angled cephalad toward the xiphoid process until a sudden decrease of resistance signifies penetration into the peritoneal cavity. The needle is flushed with a small amount of saline, and the position against the liver capsule may be checked by allowing the needle to move with respirations. If positioned correctly, the needle tip will move downward (toward the patient's feet) with inspiration, causing the syringe top to move upward (toward the head). Once the position is confirmed, the biopsy pass must be made swiftly to minimize risk of laceration by the intrahepatic needle. The plunger is retracted with one hand to provide suction, and the needle is abruptly thrust 2 to 3 cm (marked by the thumb and forefinger of the other hand on the needle shaft) into the liver and then completely withdrawn, all while maintaining suction. The dwell time within the liver should be no more than 1 second to minimize the risk of hepatic laceration. With a Menghini needle, the suction will cause the liver core to reflux into the saline-filled syringe as soon as it is withdrawn. If a Klatskin or Jamshidi needle is used, the specimen will be retained in the needle lumen and must be flushed out of the biopsy needle with a small amount of saline.

The Tru-cut and ASAP needles do not use suction to collect the core and are considerably sharper than the Menghini style needles. The placement of these needles is identical to that described above. Each needle has its own type of either manual or automatic firing mechanism with an internal needle and outer sheath such that the specimen is cored out of the liver rather than drawn into the needle by suction. These cutting needles are more likely to result in collection of an adequate specimen in the case of fibrotic or cirrhotic livers, which will tend to result in fragmented specimens when using the suction technique. Because of the sharper needle and longer dwell times needed to operate some of the Tru-cut and ASAP needles, their use may be associated with an increased risk for hepatic laceration and hemorrhage.[7]

Handling of Liver Tissue

The biopsy specimen should be immediately evaluated for adequacy so that additional passes can be made using the same needle if necessary. The specimen can be divided for various uses, and it is crucial to have appropriate fixatives, culture media, liquid nitrogen, or other special processing needs available. The biopsy should always be handled in a sterile fashion and with universal precautions.

Postprocedure Patient Care

Following confirmation of collection of adequate tissue, the biopsy site can be dressed with a bandage. If an abdominal approach was used, pressure should be applied to the site with a fingertip for 5 minutes. A pressure dressing may be placed over an abdominal puncture site; however, the minimal benefit to be derived from this is offset by constriction of respirations in small children and infants. The patient should be positioned with the biopsy site down for 4 hours to allow the liver to fall against the internal abdominal wall and thereby tamponade the hepatic puncture site. For agitated pediatric patients, it is more advisable to allow the patient to sit in the parent's lap rather than enforce a right decubitus position, as vigorous crying will cause more hepatic motion than a quiet upright posture. Careful cardiorespiratory monitoring should be continued after the procedure with ascertainment of vital signs every 15 minutes for 1 hour, every 30 minutes for 2 hours, and hourly for 3 hours. If the patient is admitted, the checks should continue every 4 hours for 24 hours. Outpatient liver biopsies are performed in carefully selected children at some large centers, with discharge at 6 to 8 hours postbiopsy.[3] Hemoglobin levels are checked at 6 and 24 hours for inpatients and at 2 and 6 hours for outpatients. Vital sign checks are especially important in the pediatric population, in whom overt clinical signs of the progression

TABLE 75-3. Complications of Percutaneous Liver Biopsy

Complications of sedation
   Allergic reaction
   Respiratory depression
   Nausea/emesis
   Fever
Minor complications
   Irritation at biopsy site
   Muscular pain/dyspnea
      Intercostal
      Diaphragmatic
   Pain due to subcapsular hematoma
   Skin hematoma
   Pneumothorax (small) with or without subcutaneous emphysema
   Insufficient tissue recovered
Major complications
   Hepatic bleeding
      Laceration
      Puncture
   Pneumothorax
   Hemothorax
   Bacteremia
   Liver abscess
   Bile leak
   Ascitic fluid leak
   Hemobilia
   Gallbladder puncture
   Intestinal puncture
   Death

to shock occur later than in adults. Tachycardia or hypotension following biopsy should be considered to represent significant hemorrhage until proved otherwise.

POTENTIAL COMPLICATIONS OF PERCUTANEOUS LIVER BIOPSY

The rates of significant morbidity or mortality associated with percutaneous liver biopsy are quite low for both children and adults. A list of potential complications is provided in Table 75-3. Minor complications such as muscular pain at the biopsy site or diaphragmatic pain referred to the right shoulder are not uncommon but are transient and easily controlled with nonsteroidal anti-inflammatory agents. Complications related to sedation (respiratory depression, nausea, emesis) are also transient and may be avoided by using minimal doses of medications. Allergic reactions to medications occur (particularly hives in response to narcotics) and are generally easily treated with intravenous diphenhydramine.

Significant bleeding requiring transfusion is the most common major complication of percutaneous liver biopsy, occurring in 1.1% to 2.8% of pediatric patients in various large studies.[3–10] Bleeding and even death may occur in any patient, and the risk does not correlate with coagulation profile, number of needle passes, or the ultimate liver diagnosis.[4,10] There is an increased risk of bleeding in patients with cancer and those who have undergone bone marrow transplantation.[7,10] Other significant complications include pneumothorax, hemothorax, bile leak, hemobilia, and puncture of the gallbladder or intestine.

ALTERNATIVE ROUTES OF LIVER BIOPSY

Laparoscopic and transjugular liver biopsy techniques are increasingly available through surgical and interventional radiology departments, respectively. When the percutaneous technique is contraindicated, these alternatives may be considered. Laparoscopic biopsy is performed by an abdominal approach and allows direct visualization of the hepatic biopsy site and control of bleeding. This technique may be especially useful for sampling heterogeneous areas of the liver or focal lesions under direct vision. The transjugular approach has been used in adults, particularly for patients with ascites or coagulopathy, with the advantage that hepatic bleeding occurs into the vascular space and so blood loss is limited.

REFERENCES

1. Gillman T, Gillman J. A modified liver aspiration biopsy apparatus and technique with special reference to its clinical applications as assessed by 500 biopsies. S Afr J Med Sci 1945;10:53–58
2. Meneghallo J, Espinoza J, Coronel L. Value of biopsy of the liver in nutritional dystrophy: Evaluation of treatment with choline dried stomach. Am J Dis Child 1949;78:141–151
3. Gonzalez-Vallina R, Alonso EM, Rand E et al. Outpatient percutaneous liver biopsy in children. J Pediatr Gastroenterol Nutr 1993;17:370–375
4. McVay PA, Toy PTCY. Lack of increased bleeding after liver biopsy in patients with mild hemostatic abnormalities. Am J Clin Pathol 1990;94:747–753
5. Menghini G. One-second needle biopsy of the liver. Gastroenterology 1958;35:190–199
6. Hong R, Schubert WK. Menghini needle biopsy of the liver. Am J Dis Child 1960; 100:92–116
7. Piccinino F, Sagnelli E, Pasquale G, Giusti G. Complications following percutaneous liver biopsy: a multicentre retrospective study on 68,276 biopsies. J Hepatol 1986;2:165–173
8. Walker WA, Krivit W, Sharp HL. Needle biopsy of the liver in infancy and childhood. Pediatrics 1967;40:946–950
9. Lichtman S, Guzman C, Moore D et al. Morbidity after percutaneous liver biopsy. Arch Dis Child 1987;62:901–904
10. Cohen MB, A-Kader HH, Lambers D, Heubi JE. Complications of percutaneous liver biopsy in children. Gastroenterology 1992;102:629–632

76

BREATH TESTING

DAVID A. PICCOLI

Many volatile compounds are excreted in expired air. Breath tests are used to detect these molecules. If the metabolism of a given substrate is known, breath tests provide a prediction about the adequacy of its absorption by measuring expiration of an end product of degradation of the substrate. In clinical practice, the most common breath tests are used to measure carbohydrate absorption. Hydrogen breath tests can be used to measure the absorption of either simple or complex sugars. The results can provide information about isolated defects in the absorption of individual sugars (e.g., inborn errors of transport proteins or disaccharidases) or global defects in carbohydrate metabolism (e.g., celiac disease). Carbohydrate breath tests can also be used to detect small bowel bacterial overgrowth and to estimate transit time to the colon. Breath tests have obvious advantages for the care of infants and children. They are noninvasive, painless, well tolerated, reliable, and widely available. In addition to absorption testing, breath tests can be employed to measure hepatic function, pancreatic function, and intermediary metabolism.

BREATH TEST STRATEGIES

There are several strategies for breath tests. The simplest of these is used in carbohydrate, or sugar, breath tests. Metabolism of sugars by humans results in carbon dioxide production. Bacteria in the bowel will ferment sugars, producing hydrogen, methane, carbon dioxide, and low-molecular-weight acids such as acetate, propionate, and butyrate. Although most of the gases produced in the colon are passed as flatus, some of the hydrogen and methane produced in the bowel are absorbed into the bloodstream and exhaled in expired breath. The generation (and exhalation) of hydrogen during a sugar breath test indicates that the human did not fully absorb the sugar, allowing bacterial fermentation of the residual in the colon. These gases, particularly hydrogen, can be detected by readily available diagnostic equipment. Many different carbohydrate substrates can be administered, although the test is most commonly used to detect lactose intolerance. Studies using monosaccharides test only for absorptive capacity, as monosaccharide uptake requires adequate bowel surface area and the specific sugar transporter. Disaccharide absorption requires the additional step of hydrolysis (digestion) prior to transport into the enterocyte. The hydrogen breath test is inexpensive, noninvasive, and reliable. The substrate is not labeled in any way, no radioactivity is involved, and the technology is simple and relatively inexpensive.

A second strategy for breath tests also involves bacterial metabolism, although this group of breath tests is designed to detect the presence of certain bacteria in the bowel. An example is the urea breath test used to detect *Helicobacter pylori* infection in the stomach. Urea is cleaved by *H. pylori* but not by humans. *H. pylori* in the stomach produces carbon dioxide almost immediately after ingestion of urea. To distinguish this carbon dioxide from carbon dioxide produced by normal human metabolism, the urea carbon must be labeled. There are two groups of labeling isotopes: stable (nonradioactive) isotopes (e.g., ^{13}C) and radioactive isotopes (e.g., ^{14}C). The radioactive isotopes are more easily detected in small quantities in expired air, but radioactive labels are generally not used in pediatric diagnostic testing. The technology to detect radioactive carbon in carbon dioxide is widely available. The detection of stable isotopes is much more technically difficult. It may require larger quantities of expensive isotope and generally requires sophisticated (and expensive) mass spectrometry for detection. This technique detects an increase in the ratio of the stable ^{13}C isotope to the normal ^{12}C in expired air if *H. pylori* metabolizes the labeled urea. This type of breath testing is noninvasive and safe but more expensive because of the cost of the labeled substrate and the diagnostic machinery. Consequently, the availability of these studies is limited.

A third strategy for breath testing involves the detection of labeled carbon dioxide released by normal human metabolism. This can be applied to normal hepatic or pancreatic function. For example, the terminal carbon of a fatty acid molecule can be labeled with a stable or radioactive isotope. By creating labeled triglycerides synthesized from labeled fatty acids, the absorption and metabolism of ingested fats can be evaluated. As in the previous strategy, the detection of labeled carbon dioxide is more difficult than of hydrogen, but it can easily be accomplished in a laboratory dedicated to this purpose. Similar studies of protein metabolism and body composition can be performed using stable isotopes of nitrogen and deuterium. This third group of breath tests are more commonly used for clinical research than for patient care.

MONOSACCHARIDES AND MONOSACCHARIDE ABSORPTION

The most important naturally occurring monosaccharides are glucose and fructose. They occur as free sugars (as in fruits) and as the hydrolysis products of disaccharides (e.g., sucrose) and larger carbohydrates. Galactose (derived from the hydrolysis of the disaccharide lactose) and mannose are also monosaccharides. These sugars have six carbons and are termed hexoses. Xylose is a five-carbon sugar, or pentose. It is used diagnostically to evaluate small bowel absorptive integrity, but it is not metabolized significantly by humans. Sorbitol is a sugar alcohol. It is used as a sweetener in candies, medicines, some sugar-free gums, and diabetic foods and drinks. Sorbitol is not absorbed in the intestine, and it is therefore metabolized by colonic bacteria. Sorbitol ingestion causes a syndrome indistinguishable from carbohydrate malabsorption in some people.

Glucose and galactose are actively transported into the enterocyte by the glucose-galactose transporter. This pump has the highest affinity for these two sugars but will transport other hexoses and pentoses. Fructose is transported by a different transporter via passive diffu-

sion. An inborn error of metabolism resulting in an absence of the glucose-galactose transporter is seen in humans as a profound early-onset severe diarrhea. Breath testing is the most reliable screening study for the identification of this profound disorder, which is easily treated with a carbohydrate-free formula supplemented with fructose (which is absorbed by a separate transport mechanism). Genetic testing for confirmation is now available. The absorption of monosaccharides also requires adequate surface area of the small intestine. The intestinal folds, the villi, and the microvilli increase the surface area of the intestine by 400-fold, and any disorder that damages this surface results in diminished absorptive capacity and abnormal carbohydrate absorption. Celiac disease, allergic enteropathy, Crohn's disease, viral and bacterial enteritis, and radiation enteritis are examples of the many disorders that diminish surface area. Short bowel syndromes also have diminished surface area due to diminished bowel length, although the villi and microvilli are generally normal. The diminished surface area may affect the absorption of disaccharides more than of monosaccharides because of the significant concentration of these enzymes at the mature enterocyte surface. Monosaccharide absorption is also affected by abnormalities of transit if substrate does not spend adequate time at the intestinal surface. Bacterial overgrowth of the small intestine results in early presentation of substrate to bacteria and is commonly associated with rapid transit and damage to the enterocyte surface. Breath testing can determine the malabsorption of monosaccharides and provide information that will be useful to help diagnose more complicated disorders. By combining different breath tests, the etiology of malabsorption can commonly be determined noninvasively, or essential information can be obtained to guide a subsequent invasive evaluation.

DISACCHARIDES AND DISACCHARIDE ABSORPTION

The most commonly occurring disaccharides are composed of two hexose molecules. Sucrose (table sugar) is composed of glucose and fructose. It is produced from sugar beets and sugar cane. It is hydrolyzed by sucrase-isomaltase (also called sucrase, saccharase, or invertase) at the brush border of the enterocyte. A deficiency of this enzyme is the most common primary inherited disorder of disaccharide absorption. Maltose is composed of two molecules of glucose, and it is an important component of starch. It is cleaved by maltase. Lactose (milk sugar) is composed of glucose and galactose. It is hydrolyzed by the enzyme lactase. Lactose malabsorption is the most important clinical problem of carbohydrate malabsorption, and most breath testing is used to detect this entity (see the section Detection of Lactose Malabsorption, below).

BREATH HYDROGEN MEASUREMENTS IN HEALTH AND MALABSORPTION

A fasted individual will normally expire small quantities of hydrogen due to the residual food and fiber in the colon and to some extent from the bacterial metabolism of gut glycoproteins. Levels may be slightly higher in the morning as a result of hypoventilation overnight and decreased colonic motility during sleep. In a fasted individual, the levels of breath hydrogen will typically fall throughout the day. Following the administration of a carbohydrate load, the levels of hydrogen will increase if the substrate is not absorbed in the small intestine. If the carbohydrate is totally absorbed in the small bowel, there will be no change in colonic fermentation or the level of expired hydrogen (Fig. 76-1A). An increase of 20 ppm of hydrogen during the course of a test signifies significant malabsorption of substrate (Fig. 76-1B).

DETECTION OF LACTOSE MALABSORPTION

Lactose malabsorption is the most common and clinically important carbohydrate absorption abnormality. Patients with lactose malabsorption may have a variety of complaints and in some cases may be totally asymptomatic (Table 76-1). There are three clinical situations that result in lactose intolerance. Congenital lactase deficiency is a severe, but quite rare, autosomal recessive inborn error. It presents clinically in the first days of life as profound watery diarrhea in any infant on a lactose-containing formula or breast milk. The diarrhea resolves totally with any lactose-free formula. Acquired or post-enteritis secondary lactase deficiency is the most common cause of lactose intolerance in infancy and childhood. It occurs when there is temporary, reversible damage to the villous and microvillous surface. This may occur during any bacterial, viral, or parasitic infection involving the small intestine. Damage to the villous surface may also occur in any form of enteritis, or bowel inflammation, including celiac disease, inflammatory bowel disease, radiation damage, allergic inflammation, and other conditions. This is termed secondary lactose intolerance, as lactose absorption will return to normal if the primary condition is resolved. In infants, the resolution of "postenteritis" lactose intolerance may be quite prolonged. The third form of lactose intolerance is genetically determined late-onset lactase deficiency. The incidence of late-onset lactose malabsorption is lowest in populations of Northern European descent, at 1 to 15%. Oriental adults have a greater than 90% incidence of lactose intolerance. Native Americans and Black Americans have a 70% to 85% incidence, and Mediterranean and Middle Eastern adults have a 60% incidence of lactose malabsorption.

FIGURE 76-1. (A) The baseline is elevated at time 0, prior to administration of carbohydrate substrate. There is an initial early rise in hydrogen concentration in the expired air, peaking at 30 minutes, and signifying bacterial metabolism of substrate in the proximal small bowel. Malabsorbed substrate passes through the small intestine and is then metabolized in the colon, resulting in a second peak at 90 minutes. This pattern is consistent with small bowel bacterial overgrowth.

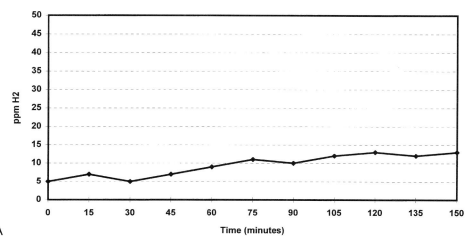

Normal Breath Hydrogen Test

A

Abnormal Breath Hydrogen Test

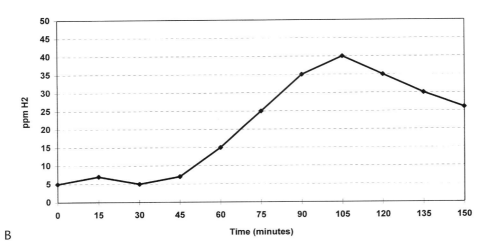

B

Small Bowel Overgrowth

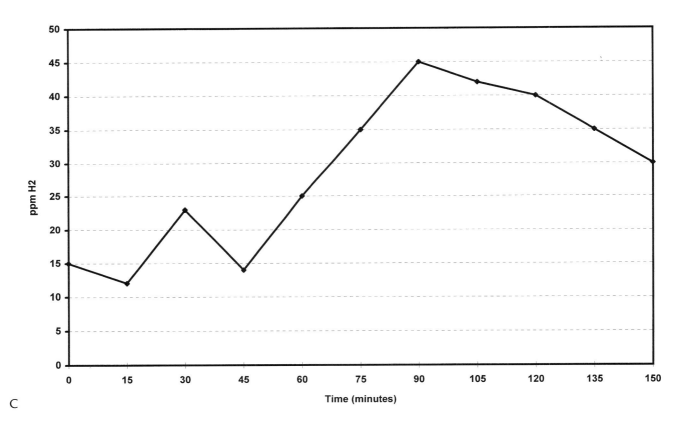

C

FIGURE 76-1. *(Continued)* *(B)* After administration of carbohydrate substrate at time 0, there is a rise in expired hydrogen concentration, peaking at 105 minutes, signifying sugar malabsorption and subsequent bacterial metabolism in the colon. This pattern is consistent with lactase deficiency. *(C)* After administration of carbohydrate substrate at time 0, there is only minimal rise in the concentration of hydrogen over the next 150 minutes, signifying that the sugar was absorbed in the small intestine without spillover into the colon. This is a normal breath test.

TABLE 76-1. Indications for Breath
Hydrogen Testing

Chronic abdominal pain

Chronic diarrhea

Flatulence

Evaluation for bacterial overgrowth

Screening for generalized malabsorption

Lactose malabsorption should be suspected based on clinical information that a patient has problems with abdominal pain, distention, flatulence, or episodic diarrhea (Table 76-1). Lactose presented to colonic bacteria will be metabolized to several gases and to low-molecular-weight osmotically active particles. These contribute to increased colonic water content and increased motility. Sugar malabsorption in infants is suspected when the stool pH is low and the water content high. The stool Clinitest can detect malabsorbed reducing sugars in the stool. A milk challenge test can be performed in a fasted patient, who is then observed for the onset of symptoms. Unfortunately, symptom production may be delayed for hours, and both false-positive and false-negative results occur. Lactase deficiency can be determined invasively by the direct enzymatic measurement of surface lactase activity from endoscopically obtained small bowel biopsies.[1] Biopsies can also be obtained blindly via a spring-loaded capsule positioned fluoroscopically. Tissue obtained by either technique can readily be used to assay a number of disaccharidases, but monosaccharide transport cannot be estimated in this fashion. Histologic evaluation of the tissue, however, is often useful for determining the primary cause of the deficiency, such as inflammation or atrophy (Table 76-2).

LACTOSE BREATH HYDROGEN TEST FOR LACTOSE MALABSORPTION

The lactose breath hydrogen test is a reliable, safe, noninvasive test to diagnose lactose malabsorption. It can be performed blind to the patient if necessary. The pa-

TABLE 76-2. Diagnosis of Lactose Intolerance

Clinical information

Successful lactose elimination diet

Milk challenge test with observation for symptoms

Blood glucose curve following lactose administration

Lactose breath hydrogen test

Direct enzyme analysis of biopsy specimens

tient must be fasted for 8 to 12 hours prior to the study, depending on age. The baseline hydrogen excretion is measured until it has fallen below 10 ppm. Lactose is administered at 2 g/kg PO, up to a maximum of 50 g, in a solution of water and flavoring. Some authors recommend a maximum dose of 25 g, which should cause fewer symptoms if the patient is severely intolerant. Administration of the lactose in a milk solution results in slower gastric emptying, variable transit, and a longer duration until the peak is identified and therefore is not generally advised. An 8-ounce dose of milk contains 12 g of lactose. If a patient is studied for presumed lactose intolerance causing pain, it is important to note that a standard diagnostic challenge test may contain the equivalent of 1 quart of milk, which is well above the daily amount ingested by many patients. In these patients, a physiologic dose of 0.5 g/kg may provide useful and relevant information.

During the test, the end-expired air is carefully obtained by an experienced technician every 15 minutes for 150 to 210 minutes. Each sample of expired air is assayed by a desktop analyzer for hydrogen concentration. It is important for the technician to carefully collect at end expiration, where the hydrogen and carbon dioxide concentrations are most elevated. Experienced technicians can perform this collection satisfactorily, even in young infants with high respiratory rates, large dead space ventilation, and small tidal volumes. Many techniques are now available to aid in collection, some of which have relatively sophisticated techniques to optimize sample collection. Diagnostic equipment is available to measure the carbon dioxide and methane in expired samples, which can be used as correction factors for the collection, but in general this adds to the expense and is not necessary. The change in hydrogen concentration from the lowest baseline levels is recorded and plotted. If the peak level is more than 20 ppm above baseline, significant lactose has been malabsorbed and metabolized.[2] In some cases, a rise of 10 ppm above baseline is significant, but in general, values in this range are borderline, and clinical correlation is necessary.[3] It is advisable for the technician to record symptoms before, during, and following the test. Patients may be instructed to record symptoms for the subsequent 24-hour period. The characteristics of pain caused by the test should be compared to the patient's original symptoms. Occasionally, the breath test will be negative by hydrogen analysis, but the patient will have characteristic symptoms. Consideration must be given to a possible placebo effect of the test, to totally unrelated symptoms, or to the possibility that the patient is lactose intolerant but does not make significant quantities of hydrogen. In the last case, the ability to produce hydrogen can be determined by a lactulose breath test. Since humans do not absorb lactulose, hydrogen should be produced during a lactulose study. Some patients have flora that do not make hydro-

TABLE 76-3. Abnormal Breath Hydrogen Test Results

Early hydrogen peak
    Bacterial overgrowth
    Proximal-to-distal enteric fistulas
    Dumping syndrome
    Markedly increased transit time
    Short bowel syndrome

Double peak
    Bacterial overgrowth
    Blind loop

Single peak
    Lactase deficiency
        Congenital
        Acquired
      Late-onset

Delayed or missed peak
    Gastroparesis
    Profoundly delayed transit
    Intestinal obstruction
    Intestinal pseudo-obstruction

gen in response to a carbohydrate load. More commonly, recent antibiotic administration will suppress bacterial counts and metabolism, resulting in only low levels of hydrogen production. In cases where artifact cannot be excluded, the direct determination of enzyme activity will be diagnostic.

A patient with lactose malabsorption will typically produce hydrogen at about 90 to 180 minutes after the administration of substrate. This time lag is due to gastric emptying and small bowel transit prior to bacterial metabolism in the colon. The time course of single and double peaks provides a clue to the pathophysiologic process causing carbohydrate malabsorption and should be analyzed carefully with respect to the patient's age, anatomy, and clinical presentation (Table 76-3).

INTESTINAL BACTERIAL OVERGROWTH

Some patients will produce hydrogen within 15 to 30 minutes of lactose administration. This is due to either bacterial metabolism in the proximal bowel, markedly short gut, rapid transit as seen in gastric dumping syndromes, or proximal-to-distal enteric fistulas. In duodenal or small bowel overgrowth syndromes, there is characteristically a double peak configuration to the hydrogen curve.[4] When lactose or lactulose is presented to the duodenal bacteria, hydrogen is produced early in the test, and then the residual substrate is passed through the intestine to the colon, where colonic fermentation results in a second peak (Fig. 76-1C).[5]

When bacterial overgrowth is present in the proximal small intestine, a high fasting baseline hydrogen level may be persistently recorded.[6] This is presumably the consequence of bacterial fermentation of intestinal surface glycoproteins. If bacterial overgrowth is suggested by the lactose (or the lactulose) breath test, confirmation by direct intubation of the duodenum may be helpful in identifying the type and antibiotic sensitivity of the causative organisms.

An occasional patient will produce hydrogen only very late in the course of the test or after the test has been completed. Severe prolongation of transit time, as seen in gastroparesis and intestinal pseudo-obstruction, may result in false-negative results. The lactose breath test can also be falsely negative if a dose is calculated incorrectly, if there is only partial administration, or if the child vomits at the beginning of the study.

HYDROGEN NONPRODUCERS

A different form of artifact occurs in patients whose flora do not generate hydrogen during metabolism of carbohydrates, which may occur in 2 to 9% of patients. It is more common if the stool pH is low, which inhibits hydrogen production, or if the patient has been on recent antibiotics. Broad-spectrum antibiotics have an effect against the hydrogen-producing bacteria of the colon. This effect is reversible in most children after about 2 weeks, and therefore testing should be postponed if a child is on antibiotics. If a lack of hydrogen production is seen during a lactose breath test, a lactulose breath test is indicated. Lactulose is a disaccharide of galactose and fructose. Humans do not metabolize lactulose, and ingestion will result in carbohydrate malabsorption symptoms. Lactulose syrup is used therapeutically for constipation in children and adults and for the suppression of ammonia absorption from the gut (by increasing transit speed and by decreasing gut pH, which increases ammonia trapping and elimination in the stool) in patients with chronic liver disease and encephalopathy. Lactulose is used for diagnostic breath tests to verify the ability of enteral bacteria to make hydrogen, to determine transit time to the colon, and to estimate oral-cecal transit time. Since lactulose is not absorbed by humans, it is presented to the colonic bacteria, where fermentation normally occurs. The hydrogen production at this point gives an estimate of transit time to the colon. A color marker that will be visible in stool can be given concomitantly with the substrate to estimate mouth-anus transit time. One important use of the lactulose breath test is to verify the ability of gut bacteria to produce hydrogen. If the colonic bacteria have been suppressed by antibiotic administration or if the flora do not produce significant quantities of hydrogen, the lactose breath test will appear (falsely) to be negative (but symptoms may occur). The artifact can be identified definitively by a lactulose breath test that fails to produce hydrogen. In patients who produce no hydrogen, results cannot be interpreted reliably. In small bowel bacterial overgrowth, presentation of the lactulose to duodenal bacteria will result in an early peak of hydrogen followed by a second (colonic) peak (see below).

OTHER CARBOHYDRATE SUBSTRATES

Other carbohydrates can easily be substituted for lactose to seek specific information about absorption and digestion (Table 76-4). Sucrose, at a dose of 2 g/kg, can be used to screen for sucrase-isomaltase deficiency.[7] As in the lactose breath test, any cause of generalized mucosal damage will cause sucrose malabsorption, and therefore some measure of normal intestinal integrity (e.g., lactose breath test, xylose absorption test) is required to support the diagnosis of sucrase-isomaltase deficiency. This diagnosis must be confirmed by enzymatic assay of the disaccharidase and normal intestinal histology. The congenital defect in glucose absorption due to the glucose-galactose transporter is best diagnosed by a glucose breath hydrogen test, using glucose as a substrate at a dose of 1 g/kg. Although the direct transporter assay is not available clinically, the genetic defect has been identified and can be used for verification. Fructose malabsorption may be diminished in some children, and a fructose breath test at a dose of 1 g/kg may reproduce symptoms and demonstrate malabsorption.[8] Sorbitol is quite common in the pediatric diet, and its ingestion has been reported to cause chronic abdominal pain. Sensitivity can be reproduced by a sorbitol absorption test.[9] The absorption of other polysaccharides and oligosaccharides can be assayed in a similar fashion in children with unusual symptoms of carbohydrate malabsorption and negative screening tests.

SUMMARY

Breath hydrogen tests play a primary role in the evaluation of children with abdominal pain, diarrhea, or suspected small bowel damage. They are safe, noninvasive, and well tolerated. Although lactose testing is most commonly used, other substrates can yield valuable information about specific carbohydrate malabsorption. Breath test technology has improved recently, and its application to problems of specific enteric infections and intermediary metabolism will augment the more invasive clinical diagnostic studies currently available in pediatrics.

TABLE 76-4. Uses for Carbohydrate Breath Hydrogen Testing

Glucose malabsorption

Fructose malabsorption

Sucrose malabsorption

Lactose malabsorption

Other carbohydrate tolerances

Sorbitol tolerance

Bacterial overgrowth

Oral-cecal and mouth-anus transit studies

Screening test for small intestinal damage

REFERENCES

1. Hyams JS, Stafford RJ, Grand RJ, Watkins JB. Correlation of lactose breath hydrogen test, intestinal morphology, and lactase activity in young children. J Pediatr 1980;97:609–612

2. Solomons NW, Barillas C. The cut-off criterion for a positive hydrogen breath test in children: a reappraisal. J Pediatr Gastroenterol Nutr 1987;6:995–996

3. Barr RG, Watkins JB, Perman JA. Mucosal function and breath hydrogen excretion: comparative studies in the clinical evaluation of children with nonspecific abdominal complaints. Pediatrics 1981;68:526–533

4. Davidson GP, Robb TA, Kirubakaran CP. Bacterial contamination of the small intestine as an important cause of chronic diarrhea and abdominal pain: diagnosis by breath hydrogen test. Pediatrics 1984;74:229–235

5. Rhodes JM, Middelton P, Jewell DP. The lactulose hydrogen breath test as a diagnostic test for small-bowel overgrowth. Scand J Gastroenterol 1979;14:333–336

6. Perman JA, Modler S, Barr RG, Rosenthal P. Fasting breath hydrogen concentration: normal values and clinical application. Gastroenterology 1984;87:1358–1363

7. Perman JA, Barr RG, Watkins JB. Sucrose malabsorption in children: noninvasive diagnosis by interval breath hydrogen determination. J Pediatr 1978;93:17–22

8. Kneepens CM, Vonk RJ, Fernandes J. Incomplete intestinal absorption of fructose. Arch Dis Child 1984;59:735–738

9. Hyams JS. Sorbitol intolerance: an unappreciated cause of functional gastrointestinal complaints. J Pediatr 1983;84:30–33

77

LIVER FUNCTION TESTS

ERIC S. MALLER

Although the term *liver function tests* is in common usage, most of the laboratory tests clinicians use routinely in the assessment of children with liver disease do not measure the function of the liver. Tests to evaluate liver disease can be divided into five categories (Table 77-1).

The measurement of multiple laboratory tests plays a central role in the diagnosis and management of liver disease in children. In some situations, abnormal laboratory tests may be the only indication of liver dysfunction. In contrast, the pattern of abnormalities in laboratory tests may be helpful in diagnosing whether the patient's liver dysfunction falls into a predominantly cholestatic or biliary obstructive versus hepatocellular injury pattern. Lastly, changes in laboratory tests over time aid in following the course and response to treatment of liver disease.

TESTS OF BIOCHEMICAL ACTIVITY

Tests of Hepatocellular Injury

ALANINE AMINOTRANSFERASE AND ASPARTATE AMINOTRANSFERASE

Alanine aminotransferase (ALT) and aspartate aminotransferase (AST) are the most common serum tests used to assess hepatocellular injury. They are sensitive tests of hepatocyte necrosis.[1] AST is not as specific as ALT for liver dysfunction. It is present in high concentrations in many other tissues including liver, heart muscle, skeletal muscle, kidney, pancreas, and red cells. Hemolysis from any cause (including rough handling of a blood

specimen secondary to a difficult venipuncture in a small infant through a small-bore needle) can easily produce artificial elevations. The presence of acute rhabdomyolysis during a systemic viral illness or in subclinical myopathy can also produce mild elevations in AST.[2] Elevated serum lactate dehydrogenase (hemolysis, myopathy) and creatine kinase or aldolase (muscle disease) can be used to differentiate these problems. ALT is more specific for the presence of liver disease and tends to rise and fall together with AST but may be increased alone in hepatocellular disease. Significant liver disease may be present even when AST and ALT are normal. Measurements of aminotransferases in serum are of most value in detecting hepatocellular damage and in monitoring the patient's clinical progress. The trends in the values of the aminotransferases may be of value; rapidly falling aminotransferase levels together with a rising bilirubin, particularly with prolongation of the prothrombin time (PT), may suggest submassive hepatic necrosis and a very poor outcome.[3]

Tests of Cholestasis

ALKALINE PHOSPHATASE

Serum alkaline phosphatase is a group of isoenzymes that hydrolyze organic phosphate esters at alkaline pH, generating inorganic phosphate and an organic radical.[4] Elevated serum alkaline phosphatase activity represents cholestatic conditions in adults, both intrahepatic and extrahepatic. Biliary obstruction results in a greater than twice normal rise in serum alkaline phosphatase activity

TABLE 77-1. Laboratory Tests to Assess Liver Dysfunction

Tests of Biochemical Activity

Hepatic injury
    Alanine aminotransferase (ALT)
    Aspartate aminotransferase (AST)
    Lactate dehydrogenase (LDH)

Cholestasis
    Gamma-glutamyltranspeptidase (GGTP)
    Alkaline phosphatase (AP)
    5'-Nucleotidase (5'-NT)
    Bilirubin (total, conjugated, unconjugated, delta)
    Urinary urobilinogen
    Serum and urine bile acids

Tests of Synthetic Function

Albumin, globulin

Prothrombin time (PT)

Ammonia (NH$_3$)

Plasma amino acids

Radiographic Imaging Studies

^{99m}Tc–diisopropyl iminodiacetic acid (^{99m}Tc–DISIDA) scan

Abdominal ultrasound, computed tomography (CT) scan, magnetic resonance imaging (MRI)

Percutaneous transhepatic cholangiogram (PTC)

Endoscopic retrograde cholangiopancreatography (ERCP)

Technetium (Tc) 99m sulfur colloid scan

Histology

Percutaneous/intraoperative liver biopsy

Other Serum Tests

Alpha-1-antitrypsin (Pi typing)

Ceruloplasmin

Viral hepatitis antibodies

Autoantibodies

---

in over 90% of adult patients and greater than four times normal in over 75% of patients. Alkaline phosphatase is found in other tissues including bone (osteoblasts), small intestine (brush border), and kidney (proximal tubule). Serum alkaline phosphatase is not particularly useful for assessing liver disease in children. The main source of an elevated alkaline phosphatase level in children is derived from bone activity secondary to active epiphyseal plates.[5] When liver disease is suspected, another enzyme (gamma-glutamyltranspeptidase (GGTP) or 5'-nucleotidase) should be used to confirm cholestasis. The measured activity of alkaline phosphatase may be spuriously low owing to zinc deficiency states (e.g., Crohn's disease).

GAMMA-GLUTAMYLTRANSPEPTIDASE

GGTP is one of the most sensitive indicators of hepatobiliary disease.[6] GGTP is a microsomal enzyme whose activity is detected in serum and that is found in the liver in the epithelium of the small bile ductules and hepatocytes. Activity is highest in concentration in the renal tubules but also is found in high amounts in the pancreas, spleen, brain, breast, and small intestine. GGTP does not rise in patients with bone disease or in children with active bone growth, unlike alkaline phosphatase. Elevations are seen in adults with chronic alcoholism, pancreatic disease, myocardial infarction, renal failure, chronic obstructive pulmonary disease, and diabetes.[7] GGTP activity is inducible by certain drugs (anticonvulsants, warfarin). These rises may be accentuated by alcohol.[8] Newborns have very high levels of GGTP, up to five to eight times the upper limit of normal for adults.[9]

5'-NUCLEOTIDASE

5'-Nucleotidase catalyzes the hydrolysis of nucleotides in which the phosphate group is attached to the 5' position of a pentose sugar moiety such as adenosine-5'-phosphate and inosine-5'-phosphate. 5'-Nucleotidase is specific for hepatobiliary disease when it is elevated in the nonpregnant patient. Pregnancy causes an increase in its measured serum value.

BILIRUBIN

Bilirubin is a yellow tetrapyrrole pigment formed from the degradation of the heme moiety, found in largest amounts in hemoglobin in the red cells of the blood. Heme is also found in myoglobin and several enzymes including catalase, peroxidases, and the cytochromes. About 75% of the daily production of bilirubin in the adult comes from the breakdown of senescent red cells in the reticuloendothelial system of the bone marrow, liver, and spleen. Newly formed unconjugated bilirubin is carried from its site of production in the plasma to the liver bound to albumin because of its low aqueous solubility. In the liver, unconjugated bilirubin is then covalently bound, or conjugated, with one or two moieties of glucuronic acid to produce water-soluble, conjugated bilirubin in two forms: bilirubin mono- and diglucuronide. A fourth form of bilirubin, delta-bilirubin, occurs in the serum when abnormally elevated bilirubin glucuronides become covalently bound to albumin.

Many clinical laboratories now measure and report separate true values for conjugated, unconjugated, and total bilirubin, with delta-bilirubin being calculated as the difference when the directly measured conjugated and unconjugated fractions are subtracted from the total. Bilirubin in the serum of normal patients is almost all unconjugated. Normal total serum bilirubin levels are less than 1.0 mg/dl. Increased serum bilirubin reflects increased production (as in hemolysis), reduced hepatic uptake (as in parenchymal liver disease) and/or decreased conjugation (as in Gilbert's disease), or decreased biliary excretion (as in bile duct obstruction). Unconjugated hyperbilirubinemia is usually due to hemolysis or to Gilbert's disease. Conjugated hyperbilirubinemia (greater than 2.0 mg/dl conjugated bilirubin or conjugated bilirubin greater than 15% of the total bilirubin) indicates hepatobiliary disease and is always pathologic. (See Chapter 8 for differential diagnosis.)

URINARY UROBILINOGEN

Urobilinogen is formed from the degradation of conjugated bilirubin by bacteria in the intestinal lumen. Up to 20% is reabsorbed into the portal circulation and undergoes enterohepatic circulation. In hepatic dysfunction, urobilinogen escapes hepatic uptake and biliary-enteric excretion, and thus more appears in the urine. In complete biliary obstruction, urinary urobilinogen falls almost to zero as less bilirubin enters the intestine to be converted to urobilinogen.

SERUM AND URINE BILE ACIDS

The level of bile acids in the blood at any given time represents a balance of input (absorption from the intestine) and removal (uptake by the hepatocyte). It is useful as an indicator of the integrity of the enterohepatic circulation but is not particularly useful in pediatric liver disease except in the diagnosis of rare inborn errors of bile acid synthesis.[10]

TESTS OF LIVER SYNTHETIC FUNCTION

Albumin and Other Serum Proteins

Albumin is the principal serum protein. It is synthesized only in the rough endoplasmic reticulum of hepatocytes at a rate of 150 mg/kg/day and has a half-life in the serum of approximately 20 days. Albumin maintains intravascular colloid osmotic pressure and serves as a carrier for many compounds in serum including bilirubin, inorganic ions such as calcium, and many drugs. Decreases in the serum level may result from decreased production (liver) or increased loss (kidneys, intestine). Albumin concentration in serum has therefore been used as a major indicator of the residual synthetic capacity of the injured or dysfunctional liver. Nonhepatic causes of hypoalbuminemia include poor nutrition and excessive losses from the urine, as in nephrosis, or from the gut in the case of various protein-losing enteropathies.

Serum Globulins

Serum globulins are usually calculated clinically by the difference in the measured amounts of total proteins in serum minus the albumin concentration. Measurements of total serum globulins are often elevated in chronic liver disease (cirrhosis due to any cause) and chronic autoimmune hepatitis.

Abnormalities of Coagulation

The liver plays three roles in the control of coagulation: (1) the production partly or exclusively of all coagulation factors with the exception of von Willebrand's[1] factor; (2) the production and breakdown of factors integral to fibrinolysis such as plasminogen and plasminogen activator; and (3) the clearance of activated clotting factors from the circulation.[11] Synthesis of factors II, VII, IX, and X is dependent on an adequate supply of vitamin K, a fat-soluble vitamin that may be deficiently absorbed in patients with cholestatic liver disease.

Prothrombin Time

PT is a measure of the time it takes for prothrombin (factor II) to be converted into thrombin in the presence of tissue extract (thromboplastin), calcium ions, and activated clotting factors V, VII, and X. Prolongation of greater than 2 seconds from control is considered pathologic; values greater than 3 seconds above control indicate a risk for bleeding.[12] This reaction evaluates the extrinsic pathway of coagulation and is prolonged when factors I, II, V, VII, and X are deficient either individually or in combination.

Vitamin K deficiency must be excluded. The exclusion of vitamin K deficiency can be accomplished by giving vitamin K_1 (phytomenadione), 1 mg/yr of age (maximum initial dose 5 mg Im or IV), with a minimum of 1 mg in a full-term infant, at least 4 to 6 hours before the PT is measured.

Partial Thromboplastin Time

Partial thromboplastin time (PTT) measures the generation of thrombin but by the intrinsic pathway, which uses all of the coagulation factors including factors IX (vitamin K dependent) and VIII (with the exception of factor VII). Caution should be used in interpreting the significance of a prolonged PT or PTT in patients with liver disease because nonhepatic factors other than vitamin K deficiency may affect the PT and PTT. These include consumption of clotting factors, as occurs in disseminated intravascular coagulation.

Ammonia

The concentration of ammonia in the blood is regulated by the balance of its production and clearance. Production occurs mainly in the large intestine by the action of bacterial urease on dietary protein and amino acids. Clearance of ammonia occurs in the liver by its transformation of ammonia into urea via the urea cycle and into glutamine by transamination of alpha-ketoglutarate to glutamate and hence to glutamine. The liver ordinarily removes 80% of the portal venous ammonia in a single pass. In chronic liver disease states, disturbed urea cycle function due to parenchymal liver cell destruction and shunting of portal venous blood due to extra- and intra-hepatic portal-systemic shunts permit large amounts of ammonia and other putative toxins to bypass the liver and reach the central nervous system.[13] Rises in fasting serum ammonia levels may portend the onset of hepatic encephalopathy. However, the level of encephalopathy and serum ammonia levels have a poor correlation.[14] Patients with advanced cirrhosis may have normal levels of fasting ammonia.

Plasma and Urine Amino Acids

Several inborn errors of intermediary metabolism manifest themselves as hepatomegaly with or without evidence of hepatocellular injury or cholestasis. These include hereditary tyrosinemia, the various urea cycle enzyme defects, specific disorders of amino acid transport that affect the urea cycle, and several specific disorders of organic acid metabolism.[15] Elevations of blood methionine, phenylalanine, and tyrosine may also occur in patients with significant hepatocellular disease of any cause as well as in the specific inherited disorders of hereditary galactosemia, hereditary fructose intolerance, and Wilson's disease. These inherited disorders may also be associated with a nonspecific aminoaciduria characteristic of the renal Fanconi's syndrome. In the defects of ureagenesis, there are variable hepatomegaly and aminotransferase elevation and specific (but also often variable) elevations of the amino acid intermediates of the urea cycle, depending on the specific defect involved. Of the several defects in organic acid metabolism, the most common is methylmalonic acidemia caused by several specific enzymatic defects. Hepatomegaly and hyperammonemia may be seen during episodes of acute metabolic decompensation.

REFERENCES

1. Ellis G, Goldberg D, Spooner FM. Serum enzyme tests in diseases of the liver and biliary tree. Am J Clin Pathol 1978; 70:248–258

2. Treem WR. Persistent elevation of transaminases as the presenting finding in an adolescent with an unsuspected muscle glycogenosis. Clin Pediatr 1987;26:605–607

3. Chopra S, Griffin PH. Laboratory tests and diagnostic procedures in evaluation of liver disease. Am J Med 1985;79: 221–230

4. Gutman AB. Serum alkaline phosphatase activity in disease of the skeletal and hepatobilliary systems. Am J Med 1959; 27:875–901

5. Clarke LC, Beck E. Plasma "alkaline" phosphatase activity: I. Normative data for growing children. J Pediatr 1950;36: 335–341

6. Whitfield JB, Pounder RE, Neale G et al. Serum Gamma-glutamyl transpeptidase activity in liver disease. Gut 1972; 13:702–708

7. Goldberg DM, Martin JV. Role of gamma-glutamyl transpeptidase activity in the diagnosis of hepatobiliary disease. Digestion 1975;12:232–246

8. Rosalki SB, Tarlow D, Rau D. Plasma gamma-glutamyl transpeptidase elevation in patients receiving enzyme-inducing drugs. Lancet 1971;2:376–377

9. Priolisi A, Didata M, Fazio M, Gioeli RA. Variations of the serum gamma-glutamyl transpeptidase activity in full-term and pre-term babies during their first two weeks of life. Minerva Pediatr 1980;32:291–296

10. Heubi J. Serum bile acids as markers of liver disease in childhood. J Pediatr Gastroenterol Nutr 1982;1:457–458

11. Aledort LM: Blood clotting abnormalities in liver diseases. In: Popper H, Schaffner F, Eds. Progress in Liver Diseases. Vol. 5. New York: Gruine & Stratton, 1976:350

12. Spector I, Corn M. Laboratory tests of hemostasis: the relation to hemorrhage in liver disease. Arch Intern Med 1967; 119:577–582

13. Treem WR. Hepatic failure. In: Walker WA, Durie PR, Hamilton JR, et al, Eds. Pediatric Gastrointestinal Disease: Pathophysiology, Diagnosis and Management. Vol 1. Philadelphia: BC Decker, 1990:158

14. Conn HO, Lieberthal MM. Blood ammonia determination. In: Conn HO, Lieberthal MM, Eds. The hepatic coma syndromes and lactulose. Baltimore: Williams & Wilkins, 1978: 73–76

15. Berry GT. Disorders of amino acid metabolism. In: Walker WA, Durie PR, Hamilton JR, Walker-Smith et al, Eds. Pediatric Gastrointestinal Disease: Pathophysiology, Diagnosis and Management. Vol 2. Philadelphia: BC Decker, 1990: 943

78

LABORATORY TESTING

INTESTINAL TESTING

DONNA ZEITER

When a gastrointestinal (GI) disorder is suspected, non-invasive testing can often provide clues to the type of disorder present including its location and etiology. Table 78-1 lists the noninvasive tests that are helpful when evaluating GI disease.

MUCOSAL MALABSORPTION

Blood Chemistries

Serum levels of sodium, chloride, potassium, and bicarbonate may be decreased through increased stool losses. Low albumin and total protein may reflect either stool protein losses or malnutrition.[1]

Complete Blood Cell Count

A complete blood count may demonstrate hypochromic microcytic anemia (iron deficiency) or megaloblastic anemia (vitamin B_{12} and folate deficiencies).

D-Xylose Absorption Test

The D-xylose absorption test is a simple, minimally invasive test of mucosal absorptive capacity. Intestinal absorption of D-xylose is passive and independent of bile salt pools, exocrine pancreatic secretions, and villous brush border enzymes; however, it is dependent on intact microvillous absorptive surface area. Once ingested, half of the D-xylose is absorbed and metabolized in the liver, while the other half is excreted in the urine. While an abnormal test is not diagnostic for a specific disease entity, a normal test is highly predictive of a normal jejunal mucosal biopsy.

To perform a D-xylose test, the patient should be NPO for 8 hours prior to the study. The patient is given an oral dose of 10% D-xylose, 14.5 g/m² (maximum dose of 25 g). A serum D-xylose level is obtained 1 hour after ingestion of the dose. A serum level less than 30 mg/dl suggests that the total absorptive surface area of the jejunum is decreased.[1] False low values occur when the patient has a delay in gastric emptying, rapid intestinal transit, small bowel overgrowth, or ascites.[2]

CARBOHYDRATE MALABSORPTION

Stool pH

The presence of acidic stool defined as stool with a pH below 5.5 indicates the presence of carbohydrate malabsorption and fermentation of colonic fatty acids. This test is performed by dipping nitrazine pH paper into a liquid stool specimen.

Stool Reducing Substances

The presence of a significant amount of carbohydrate in the stool points toward a defect in duodenal-jejunal absorption. To detect reducing sugars, the test is per-

TABLE 78-1. Summary of Intestinal Testing

Disorder	Testing
Mucosal Malabsorption	Complete blood cell count
	Electrolytes
	D-Xylose test
	Upper endoscopy with biopsy
Carbohydrate Malabsorption	Stool pH
	Stool reducing substances
	Stool osmolality and electrolytes
	Breath hydrogen tests
	Mucosal biopsy for histology and disaccharidase testing
Protein Malabsorption	Serum total protein and albumin
	Prothrombin time
	Urinalysis
	Sweat chloride test
	Test of pancreatic function
	Bentiromide test
	72-hour fecal fat
	Pancreatic stimulation test
	Fecal alpha-1-antitrypsin (protein-losing enteropathy)
Fat Malabsorption	Fat-soluble vitamin levels
	Serum carotene
	Prothrombin time
	Sudan red III stain
	Steatocrit
	72-hour fecal fat collection
	Sweat chloride test
	Tests of pancreatic function
	Bentiromide test
	Pancreatic stimulation test

formed by placing a small volume of stool in a test tube with 2 volumes of water. Subsequently, 15 drops of this suspension is placed into a second test tube containing a Clinitest tablet. The color of the suspension is compared to a color chart provided.[3] To detect nonreducing sugars (i.e., sucrose), a small volume of stool is placed in a test tube with 2 volumes of 1 N HCl. Subsequently, 15 drops of this suspension is placed into a second test tube containing a Clinitest tablet. The color of the suspension is again compared to the color chart provided.[3] The presence of greater than 0.5% reducing substances is considered abnormal and supports the diagnosis of carbohydrate malabsorption.[3]

Stool Electrolytes and Osmolality

Carbohydrate malabsorption leads to the production of osmotically active particles as a result of colonic bacterial metabolism of undigested sugars. This osmotic diarrhea may be detected by obtaining stool for fecal osmolality, fecal sodium, and potassium levels. The fecal osmotic gap may be calculated using the following formula:

[measured fecal osmolality in mOsm/kg H_2O (normal 290)] − [(stool Na^+ in mEq/L) + (stool K^+ in mEq/L) × 2] = osmotic gap (normal < 50 mEq/L)

In carbohydrate malabsorption, the osmotic gap is greater than 50 mEq/L; however, an osmotic gap of 100 mEq/L is often used to differentiate between a secretory and an osmotic diarrhea. The pitfalls of this test are that stool osmolarity increases after stool excretion secondary to continued bacterial fermentation. Also, healthy children often ingest many nonabsorbable sugars.

Breath Hydrogen Testing

Breath hydrogen testing determines the malabsorption of a specific ingested carbohydrate (lactose, sucrose), which may be primary (absence of the enzyme) or secondary (villous destruction). See Chapter 76 for further description.

Disaccharidase Testing

Biopsies of the small intestine may be obtained endoscopically to quantitatively measure specific disaccharidase activities.

PROTEIN MALABSORPTION

Protein absorption is primarily dependent on pancreatic exocrine function and thus is usually found in association with fat malabsorption. Other intestinal causes of hypoalbuminemia and hypoproteinemia include a congenital enterokinase deficiency (rare) resulting in primary protein malabsorption and protein-losing enteropathy secondary to intestinal lymphangiectasia, damaged villi, or severe heart disease.

Screening tests for active protein loss from the serum into the bowel include fecal alpha-1-antitrypsin, blood chemistries, and urinalysis.

Fecal Alpha-1-Antitrypsin

Fecal alpha-1-antitrypsin is an excellent marker of protein loss because it is a serum protein of approximately the same molecular weight as albumin and the protein is not present in foods (the protein, a serum protease, is resistant to proteolysis within the GI tract).[1] The test is performed by obtaining a random stool specimen. While the test does not require immediate freezing, approximately 7% of alpha-1-antitrypsin activity is lost over 72 hours when the specimen is kept at or above 37°C; therefore, specimens should be kept between −20°C and +4°C.[4,5] Fecal alpha-1-antitrypsin cannot be interpreted in patients less than 1 week of age because meconium contains higher levels of alpha-1-antitrypsin than does normal stool.[6] Patients with Pi ZZ alpha-1-antitrypsin deficiency may have elevated stool levels of alpha-1-antitrypsin for reasons currently not well understood.[7] Mean levels of fecal alpha-1-antitrypsin in normal individuals are somewhat variable; however, levels of 0.8 mg/g of stool and 0.98 ± 0.17 mg/g of stool have been documented in the literature.[8,9] In a study by Thomas and Sinatra,[8] 36 out of 37 patients with documented disease processes leading to protein-losing enteropathy were found to have fecal alpha-1-antitrypsin greater than 2.6 mg/g of stool.

Blood Chemistries

Serum blood testing measures serum total protein, albumin, and prealbumin. Patients with intestinal malabsorption secondary to an inflamed intestinal mucosa often have decreased levels.

Urinalysis

Urinalysis is important to rule out renal protein loss.

FAT MALABSORPTION

Stool analysis for fat malabsorption is extremely helpful when performed properly, as normal fat absorption can only occur when the liver, pancreas, and intestines all work together for proper micelle formation, fat digestion, and intestinal absorption.

Serum Carotene

Serum carotene is not a truly reliable screening test for fat malabsorption; however, it continues to be useful, as dietary carotene is the only human source of carotene. Serum carotene level is dependent on normal fat malabsorption. Low levels may indicate fat malabsorption or inadequate intake.[10] The pitfalls of this test are that carotene is not stored in the body, and if the diet is deficient in carotene, serum levels can decrease within 3 to 4 weeks. Therefore, low levels may occur in normal individuals when dietary intake is inadequate.[10] The normal serum carotene level is greater than 100 IU/dl.[11]

Fat-Soluble Vitamin Levels—Serum

Serum levels for vitamins A, 25-hydroxy D, E, and K (prothrombin time) can be useful in assessing fat malabsorption, as these fat-soluble vitamins require proper fat digestion and absorption to achieve normal levels.

Sudan Red III Stain—Fecal

The fecal Sudan stain is a good initial screening method for detection of fat malabsorption. This test indicates the qualitative presence of triglycerides. When assessing neutral fat analysis, the test is performed by placing a small amount of stool on a microscope slide. Two drops of 95% ethanol and 2 drops of Sudan III stain are then added. Neutral fat will appear as orange droplets. To assess free fatty acids, a small amount of stool is placed on a microscope slide, and 2 drops of 36% acetic acid and 2 drops of Sudan III stain are added to the preparation. Free fatty acids will appear as orange droplets. When performing a rectal examination to obtain stool for the smear, avoid using petroleum jelly because this may show a false orange appearance. Moderate steatorrhea is suspected if there are up to 100 fat droplets per high-power field with a diameter of 4 to 8 μm. Severe steatorrhea is suspected if there are greater than 100 fat droplets per high-power field with a diameter of 6 to 75 μm.[12]

72-Hour Fecal Fat Collection

The 72-hour fecal fat collection test provides a quantitative evaluation of both triglycerides and free fatty acids and involves both documenting a diet history to ensure adequate fat intake over the period of the stool collection and collection of all stools over a 3-day period. To perform the test, 3 days prior to the stool collection, the patient is started on a stable diet containing adequate fat to establish a dietary equilibrium. A diet is considered adequate if it contains approximately 35% of calories from fat. After equilibrium is established, for 3 days all stools, including oil mixed with stool, must be collected into preweighed containers. The containers are stored in the freezer between collecting specimens.[1] Once obtained, the stool is transported on ice and analyzed quantitatively for fat. The results are expressed as total grams of fat and grams of fat per 24 hours.[13]

Problems occur when patients fail to provide and document an adequate fat intake in their diet, fail to provide an equilibrating period, fail to freeze the specimens, or fail to collect all stools. Steatorrhea is defined when stool fat is greater than 7% of recorded dietary fat in children over 6 months of age. For infants less than 6 months, normal stool fat output may reach 15%.[1]

Classic Steatocrit

The classic steatocrit test is a semiquantitative screening test for fat malabsorption initially described by Phuapradit et al. in 1981.[14] To perform the test, 0.5 g of feces is obtained. The stool is vortexed vigorously with 2 volumes of water. Subsequently, 70 μl of this homogenate is placed into a heparinized hematocrit tube, which is sealed and centrifuged for 15 minutes at 12,000 rpm. The homogenate will form three different layers: a lower layer of nonfat fecal solids (S); an intermediate layer, which is liquid; and an upper fatty layer (F).[14] The steatocrit is expressed as follows:

$$\text{Steatocrit} = \frac{F \times 100}{S + F}$$

If the steatocrit is greater than 2.1%, the steatocrit determination has between 79 and 98% sensitivity and 97% specificity for detection of steatorrhea of greater than 10 g/day.[15]

Acid Steatocrit

Recently, Tran et al.[16] introduced acidification as a means of improving the liberation of fat during performance of the steatocrit. The test is performed similarly to the classic steatocrit except before placing homogenate into the capillary tube, the specimen is acidified with 5 N perchloric acid by adding a volume one-fifth the volume of the homogenate. It is then vortexed for 30 seconds.[16] The reported normal range is 2.8 to 4.8%.[16] The correlation between fecal fat content and acid steatocrit is more significant with the acidification. Many pediatric studies have demonstrated adequate sensitivities and specificity of the classic steatocrit as compared to the gold standard of 72-hour fecal fat collections. However, there have also been studies disputing the test's reliability.[17] Thus, although this test does not replace the quantitative fecal fat collection, it is an inexpensive, quick, and reliable tool for the screening of patients with moderate to severe fat malabsorption.

REFERENCES

1. Wyllie R, Hyams J. Pediatric Gastrointestinal Disease: Pathophysiology, Diagnosis, Management. Philadelphia: W.B Saunders, 1993:514–527, 537–538

2. Peled Y, Doron O, Lauffer H et al. d-Xylose absorption test: urine or blood? Dig Dis Sci 1991; 36: 188–192

3. Johnson KB, Ed. The Harriet Lane Handbook. 13th Ed. Chicago: Year Book Medical Publishers, 1993:176

4. Florent C, L'Hirondel C, Desmazures C et al. Intestinal clearance of alpha 1-antitrypsin: a sensitive method for the detection of protein-losing enteropathy. Gastroenterology 1981; 81: 777–780

5. Bernir JJ, Demazures C, Florent C et al. Diagnosis of protein losing enteropathy by gastrointestinal clearance of α1-antitrypsin. Lancet 1078; 2: 763–764

6. Ryley HC, Lynne N, Brogan T et al. Plasma proteins in meconium from normal infants and from babies with cystic fibrosis. Arch Dis Child 1974; 49: 901–904

7. Grill B, Tinghitella T, Hillemeier A et al. Increased intestinal clearance of alpha 1-antitrypsin in patients with alpha 1-antitrypsin deficiency. J Pediatr Gastroenterol Nutr 1983; 2: 95–98

8. Thomas DW, Sinatra FR. Random fecal alpha-1-antitrypsin concentration in children with gastrointestinal disease. Gastroenterology 1981; 80: 776–782

9. Crossley JR, Elliot RB. Simple method for diagnosing protein losing enteropathy. Br Med Jr 1977; 1: 428–429

10. Onstad GR, Zoeve L. Carotene absorption: a screening test for steatorrhea. JAMA 1972; 221: 677–679

11. Greenberger NJ, Isselbacher KJ. Disorders of absorption. In: Harrison's Principles of Internal Medicine. 11th Ed. New York: McGraw-Hill, 1987

12. Drummy G, Benson J, Jones C. Microscopical examination of the stool for steatorrhea. N Engl J Med 1961; 264: 85–87

13. Van de Kamer J, Huinink H, Weyers H. Rapid method for determination of fat in feces. J Biol Chem 1949;177: 349–355

14. Phuapradit P, Narang A, Mendonca P, et al. The steatocrit: a simple method for estimating stool fat content in newborn infants. Arch Dis Child 1981; 56: 725–727

15. Sugai E, Guillermo S, Vazquez H et al. Steatocrit: a reliable semiquantitative method for detection of steatorrhea. J Clin Gastroenterol 1994; 19: 206–209

16. Tran M, Forget P, Van den Neucker A et al. The acid steatocrit: a much improved method. J Pediatr Gastroenterol Nutr 1994; 19: 299–303

17. Walters M, Kelleher J, Gilber J, Littlewood J. Clinical monitoring of steatorrhea in cystic fibrosis. Arch Dis Child 1990; 65: 99–102

PANCREATIC FUNCTION TESTS

CHRIS A. LIACOURAS

SERUM AMYLASE

Serum amylase is a nonspecific enzyme that when elevated often represents acute pancreatitis. Levels increase with 3 hours of pancreatic inflammation and may persist for 2 to 4 days. Serum amylase can also be elevated in patients with perforated gastric or duodenal ulcers, post abdominal surgery, secondary to pancreatic duct obstruction, or with alcohol poisoning. Amylase levels can also indicate salivary gland inflammation, macroamylasemia, acute cholecystitis, ruptured tubal pregnancy, mesenteric thrombosis, or carcinoma of the lung.

SERUM LIPASE

Elevated serum lipase levels usually represent pancreatitis. Abnormal lipase measurements occur in acute pancreatitis but may remain elevated as long as 14 days after the initial insult. Lipase levels are normal in mumps.

PROTHROMBIN TIME

Prothrombin time (PT) is synthesized in the liver and is vitamin K dependent. Because vitamin K is fat soluble, PT can be used as an indicator of fat-soluble vitamin absorption. However, the sensitivity and specificity of this test are low secondary to the production of vitamin K by colonic bacteria.

STOOL FECAL FAT SMEAR

The stool fecal fat smear test is a rapid analysis that determines the presence of fat droplets in the stool. The test is sensitive, as most individuals with fat malabsorption have positive smears; however, its specificity is poor, as the amount of fat present in the smear is diet dependent. A low diet will produce a false-negative result despite true fat malabsorption.

FECAL CHYMOTRYPSIN

The fecal chymotrypsin test can differentiate between pancreatic sufficient and insufficient patients. Patients receiving pancreatic enzymes should discontinue them at least 3 to 5 days prior to the test.

SERUM CATIONIC TRYPSINOGEN

The serum catronic trypsinogen test can be used as a sensitive diagnostic screening test, especially in infants. Immunoreactive trypsinogen determinations of dried blood spots are currently used as screening for cystic fibrosis. Serum trypsinogen levels are elevated manyfold in infants with cystic fibrosis. These values rapidly decline during the first 5 to 7 years of life in pancreatic insufficient patients.

72-HOUR FECAL FAT STUDY

While the 72-hour fecal fat study is very difficult to perform properly, it is an extremely valuable test, as a normal study shows that all GI organ systems are functioning properly (intestinal uptake, hepatic bile salt production, and pancreatic enzyme excretion). Patients must be on at least 2 g/kg/day of fat for at least 3 days prior to the test (3 g/kg is better). All dietary intake should be rigorously monitored and analyzed by a dietician. All stool must be collected into preweighed containers and must be kept frozen to prevent fat degradation. Formulas high in MCT oil can cause an artifact in the quantitative fat calculation. During the period of collection, the stools must be stored in the refrigerator. The coefficient of fat absorption is determined by measuring grams of fecal fat excreted in 72 hours divided by grams of fat intake during the same time interval (multiplied by 100 to obtain percent).

Steatorrhea is used to define malabsorption when the amount of fat excreted in the stool over a period of 72 hours exceeds 7% (adults) of ingested fat. Due to the physiologic immaturity of the pancreatic and biliary secretions, the normal absorption of fat varies with age: premature infants, 60% to 70%; full-term newborn infants, 80% to 85%; 10 months to 3 years, 85% to 93%; and older than 3 years, 93% or greater.

DIRECT HORMONAL STIMULATION PANCREATIC FUNCTION TEST

The direct hormonal stimulation pancreatic function test allows both the collection and quantification of pancreatic enzyme secretion, including trypsin, chymotrypsin, amylase, and lipase, and the analysis of the pancreatic fluid for electrolytes. This technique allows quantitative assessment of pancreatic function. It has also been shown to be useful for the longitudinal follow-up of children with cystic fibrosis and pancreatic function abnormalities. The procedure involves fluoroscopic placement of the double-lumen pancreatic tube and the collection of pancreatic fluid after hormonal stimulus with cholecystokinin and secretin. Patients should be fasting for this study, and pancreatic enzymes should be stopped at least 48 hours prior to the study. Specific values of the enzymes lipase, amylase, colipase, trypsin, and chymotrypsin have been established for timed, size adjusted collections.

BENTIROMIDE TEST

Bentiromide (Chymex) is a synthetic peptide that contains para-aminobenzoic acid (PABA) linked to a benzoyl-tyrosine. It is nontoxic, and the linkage is cleaved only by chymotrypsin (a pancreatic enzyme). Unconjugated PABA is readily absorbed through the intestine and can be assayed via the bloodstream or urine.

The adult dose (greater than 12 years) is 500 mg orally, the school-age dose is 14 mg/kg, and the toddler dose (0 to 4 years) is 30 mg/kg after a fast. Following the oral dose, a light meal and fluids are given. A serum level can be obtained 2 hours postdose; urinary excretion can also be documented. Less than 50% urine recovery of PABA is abnormal, while 50% to 60% recovery is borderline. The serum level should generally be 4 to 6 ng/ml. False-positive results can occur in patients with flat villous lesions because of decreased intestinal PABA absorption.

REFERENCES

1. Couper R, Durie PR. Pancreatic function tests. In: Walker et al, Eds. Paediatric Gastrointestinal Disease. Philadelphia: BC Decker, 1991: 1341–1353

2. Gowenlock AH. Tests of exocrine pancreatic function. Ann Clin Biochem 1977; 14: 61–89

3. Durie PR. Pancreatic function tests. Med Clin North Am 1988; 20: 3842–3845

4. Dockter G, Nacu I, Kohlberger E. Determination of protease-cleaved P-aminobenzoic acid (PABA) in serum after oral administration of N-benzoyl-l-tyrosyl-p-aminobenzoic acid (PABA-peptide) in children. Eur J Pediatr 1981; 135: 277–279

5. Shwachman H, Dooley RR. Tests of exocrine functions of the pancreas in childhood. Pediatr Clin North Am 1955; 2: 201–271

6. Lebenthal E, Lee PC. Development of functional response in human exocrine pancreas. Pediatrics 1980; 66: 556–560

METABOLIC TESTING

MICHAEL J. PALMIERI
ROBERT M. COHN

Many inborn errors of metabolism present with features suggestive of septicemia, while others, constituting the largest subgroup of patients with inborn errors, present with some mix of neurologic findings including seizures, abnormal movements, developmental delay, and coma. While it is less common for an infant or child with an inherited disorder to present only with GI signs and symptoms, it is essential for the gastroenterologist to recognize that a patient with GI manifestations in association with neurologic features, hyperammonemia, or metabolic acidosis could be suffering from an inherited metabolic defect. In this section, we will consider the laboratory tests that are useful in the diagnostic evaluation of a patient suspected of having an inborn error who has significant hepato- or splenomegaly, hyperammonemia, metabolic acidosis, or hypoglycemia or who evidences liver failure. Taken together, a purely GI presentation for an inborn error is decidedly unusual, but GI manifestations as one facet of the clinical picture of some inborn errors are fairly common.

CLINICAL PATTERNS

Hepatomegaly and associated liver dysfunction presenting in the neonatal period are often characteristic of galactosemia; however, liver dysfunction presenting later in the first year may indicate hereditary fructose intolerance (after introduction of fruits and vegetables), tyrosinemia type I, alpha-1-antitrypsin deficiency, or certain of the respiratory chain disorders. In an older child (greater than 4 years of age) who presents with liver dysfunction, Wilson's disease should be considered. Complicating the evaluation of patients with liver failure is the occurrence of mellituria, hypertyrosinemia, and hypermethioninemia (Tables 78-2 and 78-3). Other patients will come to attention because of cholestatic jaundice with an elevated plasma conjugated bilirubin. Still other considera-

tions are peroxisomal disorders (with associated striking physical findings), Niemann-Pick disease type II, and bile acid synthetic defects (Table 78-4).

Some of these same diseases can cause hepatomegaly unassociated with liver dysfunction. In that case, a firm consistency to the liver may indicate galactosemia, tyrosinemia, glycogen storage disease (GSD) type IV (brancher deficiency), alpha-1-antitrypsin deficiency, or Wilson's disease. When the consistency of the enlarged liver is normal, and particularly if there is associated splenomegaly and evidence of involvement of other organs, the lysosomal disorders become important considerations. This is a rather broad differential diagnosis, and the lysosomal disorders that fall within this category are included in Table 79-2.

When hepatomegaly is associated with hypoglycemia, the gluconeogenic defects may be to blame (GSD-I, glucose-6-phosphatase, fructose-1,6-bisphosphatase, phosphenolpyruvate carboxykinase). Hepatomegaly without hypoglycemia is found in GSD VI (phosphorylase and phosphorylase *b* kinase) and several lipid disorders including cholesteryl ester storage disease and Tangier's disease. The porphyrias are listed in Table 78-5, distinguishing those presenting with abdominal pain from those where abdominal pain does not occur.

SPECIMEN REQUIREMENTS

For a laboratory to perform a clinically rewarding analysis on a submitted specimen, that specimen must be collected without contamination and stored under the appropriate conditions. For most organic acidurias, a random urine collection is usually sufficient to provide a diagnosis, although a 24-hour collection eliminates any artifact attributable to diurnal variations in excretion of some compounds. A urine specimen should be collected without preservative and subsequently frozen. Most

TABLE 78-2. Metabolic Disorders

	Clinical Features	Laboratory Tests
Galactosemia (galactose-1-phosphate uridylyltransferase deficiency)	Clinical deteriorations associated with milk feeding; vomitng FTT, ↑ bilirubin, cataracts Hepatomegaly Renal Fanconi's syndrome with *Escherichia coli* sepsis	Urine for reducing substances and galactitol; RBC enzyme analysis Clinical deterioration may occur before results of state screening tests are available
Hereditary fructose intolerance (fructose-1,6-bisphosphate aldolase deficiency)	Infant grows normally until fructose or sucrose introduced into diet (3–6 mo of age) FTT, hypoglycemia after dietary challenge, hepatomegaly, liver dysfunction, hypophosphatasia Voluntary avoidance of sweets by older children	Carbohydrate analysis using gas chromatography
Tyrosinemia (fumarylacetoacetate hydrolase deficiency)	FTT, hepatomegaly, liver failure, vomiting, cabbage-like odor	Plasma amino acid quantitation: ↑ tyrosine & methionine Presence of succinylacetone by gas chromatography/mass spectrometry is diagnostic
GSD Ia (glucose-6-phosphatase deficiency)	FTT, hepatomegaly, hypoglycemia Lactic acidosis Hyperuricemia, hypertriglyceridemia, xanthomas	IV glucagon fails to elicit rise in blood glucose Enzyme assay
GSD Ib (translocase deficiency)	Clinically like GSD Ia with neutropenic episodes	Enzyme assay in fresh liver: ↑ activity when homogenate treated with deoxycholate, pointing to a defect in membrane translocase
GSD III (amylo-1,6-glucosidase [debrancher])	Hepatomegaly; ± cardiomegaly	Glucagon increases glucose after a meal but not after fasting Limit dextran on liver biopsy Enzyme assay
GSD IV (amylo-1:3,1:6-transglucosidase [brancher])	Hepatosplenomegaly, cirrhosis, liver failure	Glycogen resembles amylopectin Enzyme assay Prenatal possible

Abbreviations: FTT, failure to thrive; RBC, red blood cell; GSD, glycogen storage disease.

aminoacidopathies are readily diagnosed in plasma isolated from heparinized blood.

In certain instances, it may be necessary to perform enzyme assays on white blood cells as a surrogate for disorders affecting liver and other organs. To be sure, some defects must be diagnosed using a sample from the affected target organ, and it behooves the clinician to find out from the reference laboratory the specimen requirements. Along with the specimen, clinicians should supply a description of the patient's clinical features and a list of any medications that the patient is currently or has recently received. The drug history is particularly important because many drugs affect the accuracy of the testing.

In the past, simple spot tests for ketones, phenylalanine metabolites, and methylmalonic acid were in vogue. But today, most metabolic diagnostic laboratories will evaluate specimens by quantitation of amino and organic acids, foregoing the simpler and less accurate tests. Still, the Clinitest for reducing substances, the nitroprusside for sulfhydryl-containing compounds, and the sulfite oxidase test have a niche in many metabolic protocols.

Some disorders of intermediary metabolism fail to disclose abnormalities in urine or plasma during periods when the patient is clinically well. Accordingly, it is vital to collect specimens when the patient is experiencing clinical symptoms, before or concurrent with the institution of therapy. If the patient suffers an acute attack of a catastophic illness, a specimen for electrolytes (including Ca), arterial blood gases, ammonia, and glucose should be obtained. In the presence of an anion gap, gas chromatographic–mass spectrometric analysis of urine for organic acids becomes a high priority.

TABLE 78-3. Other Metabolic Disorders

	Clinical Features	Laboratory Tests
I-cell disease (deficiency of mannose-6-phosphate receptor: zip code for lysosomes)	Hepatosplenomegaly; mental retardation Gingival hyperplasia Hernias	↑ Lysosomal enzymes in plasma
Mucopolysaccharidoses	Hepatosplenomegaly; mental retardation Coarsened features, dysostosis multiplex, eye findings	↑ Urinary glycosaminoglycans Specific enzyme assays
Zellweger syndrome	Hepatomegaly; high forehead, upslanting palpebral fissures Abnormal ears, cataracts & corneal clouding Deafness	↑ Plasma VLCFA, phytanic acid, pipecolic acid; bile acid intermediates; ↓ plasmalogens
Wilson's disease	Three modes of presentation: hepatic, neurologic, or psychiatric Kayser-Fleischer rings	↑ Urinary copper further augmented by penicillamine ↑ Liver copper
Urea cycle defects (multiple enzyme defects)	Hyperammonemia; coma Other neurologic features	Amino acid quantitation Specific liver enzyme assays
Organic acidurias	Metabolic acidosis with secondary hyperammonemia	Organic acid identification by gas chromatography/mass spectrometry

TABLE 78-4. Hepatomegaly with Prominent Liver Dysfunction

	Clinical Features	Laboratory Tests
GSD VI (liver phosphorylase ± activating systems)	Hepatomegaly sometimes massive	Blood glucose fails to rise after epinephrine or glucagon Enzyme assay of liver phosphorylase
GSD IX (liver phosphorylase kinase deficiency)	Marked hepatomegaly that decreases in size with increasing age	Blood glucose rises after epinephrine or glucose, thus distinguishing GSD IX from GSD VI
Niemann-Pick disease, types A & B (I) (sphingomyelinase deficiency)	Hepatosplenomegaly; progressive neurologic deterioration; cherry-red spot (50%)	Enzyme assay
Gaucher's disease type II (glucocerebrosidase deficiency)	Hepatosplenomegaly; progressive neurologic deterioration; congenital ichthyosis	Enzyme assay
GM$_1$ gangliosidosis (β-galactosidase deficiency)	Hepatosplenomegaly; progressive neurologic deterioration; gingival hypertrophy; cherry-red spot (50%) Dysostosis multiplex	Enzyme assay
Farber's disease type I (lysosomal acid ceramidase deficiency)	Hepatomegaly (50%); progressive psychomotor impairment; joint swelling; hoarseness; fever; dysphagia; vomiting	Enzyme assay
Wolman's disease (lysosomal acid lipase deficiency)	Hepatosplenomegaly; vomiting; diarrhea; steatorrhea; abdominal distention Adrenal calcifications	Enzyme assay Vacuolated lymphocytes

Abbreviation: GSD, glycogen storage disease.

TABLE 78-5. Porphyrias

	Clinical Features	Laboratory Tests
Recurrent abdominal pain		
AIP (porphobilinogen deaminase deficiency)	Abdominal pain but no rigidity, nausea, vomiting Hyperkinesia, tachycardia, seizures Neuropsychiatric findings	↑ ALA & porphobilinogen in urine during latent and acute phases
Variegate porphyria (protoporphyria oxidase deficiency)	Neurovisceral findings similar to AIP Skin manifestations in 80% of cases—fragility, scarring	During attack, ALA & porphobilinogen in urine ↑ Urinary and fecal porphyrins
Hereditary coproporphyria (deficiency of coproporphyrin oxidase)	Neurovisceral findings similar to AIP Skin manifestations in 30% of cases	↑ Urinary and fecal coproporphyrins During acute attack, ALA & porphobilinogen in urine
No abdominal pain		
Porphyria cutanea tarda 　Familial: uroporphyrinogen decarboxylase deficiency 　Sporadic: environmental exposure	Skin—photosensitivity, fragility, vesicles, poor wound healing Liver disease in some patients	↑ Urinary uroporphyrin Fecal isocoproporphyrin is diagnostic

Abbreviations: AIP, acute intermittent porphyria; ALA, delta-aminolevulinic acid.

Lysosomal Enzymes

Isolation of white blood cells for lysosomal enzyme assays is done by the method of Skoog and Beck, one which is rapid and reproducible and yields a total white cell population. Whole blood is mixed with dextran and the red cells allowed to settle at room temperature. After collection of the white-red cell pellet by low-speed centrifugation and subsequent lysing with water of the residual red cells, the white blood cells are layered with a 2 to 3 mm column of water and frozen at −40°C. Most of the lysosomal enzymes are stable in this form for many months.

Fluorogenic substrates and in some cases radioactively labeled substrates are employed for the enzymatic diagnosis of the lysosomal enzyme disorders. While the majority of these diagnoses can be made in white blood cells, some disorders such as Hunter's syndrome and Sanfilippo's syndrome type B are more easily diagnosed in plasma or serum. Inclusion cell (I-cell) disease is assayed initially in serum, and in contrast to the other lysosomal disorders where a deficiency of enzyme activity is required for a definitive diagnosis, elevations of 5- to 20-fold of many lysosomal enzymes are associated with this disorder. Confirmation is done in white blood cells or cultured skin fibroblasts, assaying for the activity of *N*-acetylglucosamine-1-phosphotransferase. Commercially available substrates can now be used for the reliable analysis of phosphotransferase activity.

Mucopolysaccharidosis Disorders

Analysis of the enzymes deficient in the mucopolysaccharidoses is more complex, and few artificial substrates are available, thus making assay of these enzymes tedious, time-consuming, and expensive. To facilitate the diagnosis of one of these disorders, we initially screen urine from a 12- to 24-hour collection by an electrophoretic technique that separates the sulfates of heparan, dermatan, chondroitin, and keratan. Using a qualitative approach based on the intensity of the alcian blue stain of the various mucopolysaccharides and the clinical history of the patient, we are able, in most cases, to determine which enzyme to assay. Since patients with Sanfilippo's syndrome may not excrete any excess heparan sulfate, diagnosis of this disease might be missed if mucopolysacchariduria were the only criterion. Of course, the clinical history and the presence of severe mental retardation help focus the clinician and the laboratory's decision as to which enzyme to assay.

Organic Acids

Analysis of organic acids in urine is performed using gas chromatography–mass spectrometry of the trimethylsilyl derivatives. An aliquot of urine equivalent to a known quantity of creatinine and to which is added an internal standard, undecenoic acid, is treated with methoxyamine to block the keto groups, thus preventing keto-enol tautomerization of the keto acids and facilitating the interpretation of the spectral data. After acidification and saturation with sodium chloride, the urine is extracted successively three times with ethyl acetate, dried, and treated with methanol-methylene chloride to remove all traces of water. The partially purified organic acids are then derivatized with BSTFA/TMCS and analyzed by gas chromatography–mass spectrometry. Separation and quantitation of the organic acids is achieved on a 5%

phenyl methyl siloxane capillary column, and spectral data are compared to the spectra of known organic acids.

A dramatic innovation in screening of newborns is tandem mass spectrometry. This powerful technique can identify many of the organic acidemias simply by analysis of the carnitine esters in blood, making early identification of some of these life-threatening disorders possible. Unfortunately, even this method has limitations in detecting metabolites in older children, when concentrations of the offending metabolites may not be prominent enough to trigger recognition.

Amino Acids

Amino acids are analyzed in plasma, urine, and cerebrospinal fluid on a Beckman Amino Acid Analyzer equipped with a triketohydrindene-post-column detection system. Diagnosis of most metabolic disorders such as urea cycle defects, maple syrup urine disease, phenylketonuria, and tyrosinemia is easily made in plasma, while secondary renal tubule disorders galactosemia, hereditary fructose intolerance, Wilson's disease, cystinosis, and tyrosinemia are detected in urine. Preparation of specimens for amino acid analysis is quite simple in contrast to the analysis of urine organic acids and requires an initial deproteinization, centrifugation, and pH adjustment with buffer. Up to 40 amino acids can be separated and quantitated in plasma using an ion exchange resin. Urine, on the other hand, contains a variety of salts and, in many cases, antibiotics, which interfere with the resolution of amino acids in the region of the branched-chain acids, cystine, and phenylalanine, making both quantitation and separation more difficult.

D-Xylose

Malabsorption problems are routinely screened in plasma 1 hour after a D-xylose load. For this analysis, a Somogyi filtrate 2 of plasma is prepared followed by derivatization and subsequent analysis by gas chromatography. Identification of D-xylose is performed by comparison to a known standard of trimethylsilyl-D-xylose, and quantitation is accomplished by the introduction into the specimen of known quantities of two internal standards, ribitol and perseitol. While this method is not absolute in defining the malabsorptive state, it allows the clinician to decide whether further testing is required.

Disaccharidase Deficiency

The diagnosis of disaccharidase deficiency can be made on duodenal biopsies. Our method involves incubation of a sonicate of the biopsy with the appropriate substrate (lactose, maltose, sucrose, or isomaltose) and subsequently measuring the release of the liberated glucose by the tris-glucose oxidase method.

REFERENCES

1. Skoog WA, Beck WS. Studies on the fibrinogen, dextran and phytohemagglutinin methods of isolating leukocytes. Blood 1956; 11:346–454

2. Somogyi M. Determination of blood sugar. J Biol Chem 1945; 160:69–73

SUGGESTED READINGS

Cohn RM, Roth KS. Biochemistry and Disease: Bridging Basic Science and Clinical Practice. Baltimore: Williams & Wilkins, 1996.

Fernandes J, Saudubray JM, Van den Berghe G, Eds. Inborn Metabolic Diseases. Berlin, Springer-Verlag, 1995.

Scriver CR, Beaudet AL, Sly WS, Vallee D, Eds. The Metabolic and Molecular Basis of Inherited Disease. 7th Ed. New York: McGraw-Hill, 1995.

79

GASTROINTESTINAL MICROBIOLOGY TESTING

KARIN L. MCGOWAN

The infectious causes of diarrhea and gastroenteritis have increased significantly over the past decade and now include a wide spectrum of bacteria, viruses, and parasites. While there are a number of new proposed agents of diarrhea whose pathogenesis has yet to be defined, this chapter deals only with the laboratory diagnosis of the bacteria and some parasites that are presently recognized as definitive causes of diarrhea.

LABORATORY DIAGNOSIS OF BACTERIAL DIARRHEA

The bacteria that cause infectious gastrointestinal (GI) disease are listed in Table 79-1. Because the etiologic agent of infectious diarrhea may be influenced by many factors such as age, hospitalization, geographic location, travel history, immune status of the host, history of antibiotic use and/or cancer chemotherapy, or recent ingestion of water or certain food products, input from the clinician is critical to help maximize laboratory results.[1] Faced with declining resources and increased costs, no laboratory can afford to test for all of the pathogens listed in Table 79-1. How far a specimen is evaluated and which laboratory methods are employed are frequently driven by additional patient information provided to the laboratory.[2] Methods employed for the laboratory diagnosis of bacterial and parasitic diarrhea include direct detection, culture, and toxin detection. While molecular methods such as polymerase chain reaction (PCR) and use of DNA probes are appearing in the literature, they

are presently a research methodology and are not available in most routine or reference laboratories. In addition, with both probe and PCR technology, the organisms are not available for antibiotic susceptibility testing, which may be a disadvantage.

SPECIMEN SELECTION, COLLECTION, AND TRANSPORT

Traditionally, multiple specimens have always been submitted for bacterial and parasitic analysis. During most episodes of acute infectious diarrhea, regardless of the immune status of the host, bacterial pathogens are present in stool in the highest quantities during the early stage of the illness. For this reason, a single, adequately collected and transported stool specimen should be sufficient for ruling out bacterial pathogens if collected early. If collected later in the course of illness, then two to three specimens may be required. If patients are taking antibiotics or antidiarrheal agents at the time of specimen collection, then culture results will be adversely affected, and no good rule applies. In patients with acquired immunodeficiency syndrome (AIDS) multiple specimens may be required to successfully recover enteric pathogens, particularly mycobacteria. Studies have shown that even in immunocompromised hosts, stool is superior to intestinal biopsy specimens for culturing enteric pathogens.[3] Because parasites are excreted in varying numbers at different stages of their life cycle, at least three stool specimens taken 2 to 3 days apart should

TABLE 79-1. Bacterial Causes of Infectious Gastrointestinal Disease

Aeromonas hydrophila

Campylobacter species (*C. jejuni, C. coli,* and other species)

Clostridium difficile

Escherichia coli (enterotoxigenic [ETEC], enterohemorrhagic [EHEC], enteropathogenic [EPEC], enteroinvasive [EIEC], enteroadherent [EAEC])

Mycobacterium avium-intracellulare (MAC)

Plesiomonas shigelloides

Salmonella species

Shigella species

Streptococcus, group A

Vibrio cholerae and *Vibrio parahaemolyticus*

Yersinia enterocolitica

be submitted for parasite testing. See Table 79-2 for specific specimen collection guidelines.

A number of general guidelines should be considered when collecting specimens:

1. Stool specimens are superior to rectal swabs for isolation of bacteria. In addition, gross examination of stool allows the laboratory to select areas for culture that are most likely to harbor organisms.

2. Stool must be transported rapidly. If more than a 2-hour delay will occur before culturing, then the specimen should be placed in an enteric transport medium.

3. If a rectal swab must be collected, feces should be evident on the swab, and it should be placed in a transport medium or container that prevents drying. A dry rectal swab is worthless.

4. The following substances and medications can interfere with the laboratory detection of parasites, particularly protozoa: antibiotics, antimalarial agents, barium, bismuth, nonabsorbable antidiarrheal products, and mineral oil. Parasites may not be visible for up to several weeks after administration of any of these products (2 weeks after antibiotics; 7 to 10 days following barium).

5. Stool collected for bacterial culture or parasitology should not be contaminated with water or urine.

6. Unless fresh stool can be examined for parasites within 1 hour of collection, it is recommended that stool preservative collection vials be used. There are a number of commercial systems available with a variety of preservative choices; in general, all do the job sufficiently.

DIRECT DETECTION FROM FECAL MATERIAL OF AGENTS OF GASTROENTERITIS

Because of the complexity and cost to analyze fecal specimens for all of the agents listed in Table 79-1, a number of procedures are available for use as screening tests for specific pathogens or for use to determine if further testing is necessary.

Wet Mount

The direct wet mount is a simple procedure that provides a quick answer when positive. It is excellent for examining small bowel aspirates to detect motile trophozoites of *Giardia lamblia, Entamoeba histolytica,* and *Dientamoeba fragilis* and the larvae of *Strongyloides.* With stool specimens, however, direct wet mount reveals such a small percentage of positive results that the test is not recommended for routine use.[4]

Fecal Leukocytes and Lactoferrin

The fecal leukocyte assay is a simple, rapid, and inexpensive procedure that when used properly is an excellent screen for stool specimens. This test distinguishes between inflammatory and noninflammatory diarrhea.[5] A positive result rules out noninvasive agents such as *Vibrio* spp., enterotoxigenic *Escherichia coli,* and all protozoa except *E. histolytica;* thus a result would eliminate the need to perform tests aimed at detecting these organisms. Tests for fecal lactoferrin are more sensitive than stained smears for fecal leukocytes because lactoferrin remains stable after freezing, refrigeration, and delayed transport of stool, situations that frequently lead to morphologic loss of leukocytes.[6]

Gram Stain and Phase Microscopy

Gram stain of feces is not helpful except in a few very specific circumstances. Many white blood cells plus sheets of gram-positive cocci or large numbers of yeast is indicative of staphylococcal or candidal infection.[7] Many comma-shaped, thin, gram-negative rods can be indicative of *Campylobacter* or *Vibrio* infection, but in general, most gram-negative enteric pathogens are not distinguishable by this stain. The diagnosis of both *Campylobacter jejuni* and *Vibrio cholerae* can be made presumptively when stool is examined directly by phase-contrast microscopy. Unfortunately, this is impractical in most office and hospital settings.

Rapid Tests for *Giardia lamblia* and *Cryptosporidium parvum*

Fluorescent antibody (direct or indirect) or enzyme immunoassay monoclonal kits are now available for detection of cysts or antigens from *G. lamblia* or *C. parvum.* For *G. lamblia,* test sensitivity ranges from 91% to 100% and specificity from 94% to 100%, depending on kit manufacturer.[8,9] For *C. parvum,* test sensitivity and specificity both range from 93% to 100%.[8,10] Because these two organisms account for most cases of parasitic infec-

TABLE 79-2. Specimen Collection Guidelines

Specimen: Procedure	Collection Guidelines
Stool: bacterial culture, white blood cells, & EHEC	Place stool directly into a sterile, leakproof, widemouthed container. Transport within 1 hr, or transfer to an ETS. Store at 4°C for <24 hr, at room temperature for ETS.
Rectal swab: bacterial culture	Insert swab approximately 1 inch past anal sphincter, then gently rotate swab. Feces should be evident. If perianal rash is present, culture skin surface separately for group A streptococcus.
Small bowel aspirate: bacterial culture	Place directly into a sterile, leakproof, widemouthed container. Transport within 1 hr, or transfer to an ETS. Store at room temperature.
Gastric biopsy: *Helicobacter pylori* culture	Because organism is unevenly distributed, obtain multiple biopsies, including one each from the gastric antrum and corpus. Tissue must be kept moist through use of a transport medium or physiologic saline. Store at room temperature. If being placed directly into rapid urea agar, place biopsy pieces below surface of medium.
Stool: *C. difficile* or *E. coli* toxin analysis	Place stool directly into a sterile, leakproof, widemouthed container. Transport within 1 hr, or transfer to an ETS. Store at 4°C for <48 hr; freeze at −70°C if delayed. Minimum of 5 ml needed for adequate testing. Toxin shed unevenly; multiple specimens preferred.
Stool: acid-fast smear & culture	Place stool directly into a sterile, leakproof, widemouthed container. Transport within 1 hr, or refrigerate at 4°C. Do not use waxed containers, which cause false-positive smears. Do not use ETS. Avoid contamination with tap water or urine. Swabs unacceptable.
Tissue/biopsy: acid-fast smear & culture	Aseptically collect as much tissue as possible, and place in a sterile container without fixative, preservative, formalin, or saline. Transport within 1 hr, or refrigerate at 4°C.
Blood: acid-fast smear & culture	Isolator lysis-centrifugation collection or the radiometric Bactec 13A blood bottle preferred. Two separate blood cultures are adequate. Transport Bactec bottles within a few hours; keep at room temperature. Isolator bottles can be delayed as long as 24 hr at room temperature.
Stool: ova & parasites	Place stool directly into a sterile, leakproof, widemouthed container. If specimen is not examined microscopically within 60 min, stool preservative collection vials must be used. At least 3 specimens taken 2–3 days apart should be submitted. Stool or vials should be kept at room temperature.
Small bowel/duodenal drainage: ova & parasites	Submit immediately to the laboratory in sterile tube containing no preservatives. Rapid transport (<2 hr) is critical for analysis; 0.5 ml minimum. If specimen is not examined microscopically within 2 hr, preservative collection vials or formalin should be used.
Perianal: pinworm analysis	Stool unacceptable for pinworm analysis. Scotch tape preparation or sticky paddles (available commercially) specimen of choice. Obtain in the morning before patient bathes or defecates. Transport at room temperature.

Abbreviations: EHEC, enterohemorrhagic *Escherichia coli*; ETS, enteric transport system.
(Data from Baron et al.,[7] Garcia and Bruckner,[8] and Murray et al.[18])

tions acquired in the United States, use of such tests is appropriate screening rather than ordering complete ova and parasite workups.

CULTURE FOR ISOLATION OF BACTERIAL AGENTS

Stool and Rectal Cultures

Stool cultures are indicated when blood is present on gross examination, when fecal leukocytes or lactoferrin is present on microscopic examination, when significant diarrhea occurs in an immunocompromised host, or in any child ill enough to require hospitalization. In addition, cultures should be performed in outbreak situations in day-care centers, hospitals, or extended-care facilities,

where only symptomatic patients should be screened.[1,2] Good laboratory practice dictates that all stool specimens be cultured for *Salmonella*, *Shigella*, *Campylobacter*, and with pediatric patients, *Yersinia enterocolitica*. Individuals living along the Gulf of Mexico should be routinely screened for *Vibrio* spp. Because it is now associated with both bloody and nonbloody diarrhea, many states require that *E. coli* O157:H7 be part of routine testing. A wide variety of *E. coli* are now associated with GI disease, but with the exception of enterohemorrhagic *E. coli* (EHEC), routine testing is either impractical or not yet available. Patients who have a history of international travel or of ingestion of raw seafood should be examined for *Vibrio* spp. and *Plesiomonas*. *Aeromonas* spp. are associated with consumption of contaminated water; they should be tested for in the summer months when incidence is highest and only after routine pathogens have been eliminated as possible causes. Stools from patients who have received antibiotics or cancer chemotherapy within the past 4 weeks should be examined for *Clostridium difficile* toxins A and B. Such patients rarely have other enteric pathogens present.[11]

Until the onset of human immunodeficiency virus (HIV), fecal and GI specimens were rarely analyzed for mycobacteria. The frequent isolation of highly drug-resistant *Mycobacterium avium-intracellulare* (MAC) from patients with HIV has now made culturing GI specimens standard practice. Stool is an excellent specimen for diagnosing MAC infections. In addition, a biopsy with acid-fast bacterial smear and culture should be performed on any area of the GI tract or liver suspected of being infected. In patients suspected of having disseminated MAC, blood culture using lysis centrifugation is the best specimen; two blood cultures are adequate to make the diagnosis.[12]

Small Bowel Aspirate Cultures

As a result of a variety of factors including anatomic alterations, intestinal pseudo-obstruction, altered intestinal communication, and changes in motility, bacterial overgrowth syndrome in the small bowel may occur. Numerous diagnostic procedures can be used to diagnose bacterial overgrowth syndrome, but one of the simplest is to *quantitatively* culture small bowel aspirate material for aerobic and microaerophilic bacteria. Because calibrated loops must be used to plate the specimen and the results listed as colony-forming units (CFU) per milliliter, the laboratory should be notified when such data are needed. Total counts of 10^4 CFU/ml or greater are indicative of bacterial overgrowth.[13] Precise identification of isolates and susceptibility testing of isolates are not necessary. Refer to Table 79-2 for specimen guidelines.

LABORATORY DETECTION OF TOXIN-MEDIATED GASTROENTERITIS

Clostridium difficile

Current methods for the laboratory diagnosis of *C. difficile* include culture, detection of toxin B through cytotoxicity testing, detection of toxin A through immunoassays, detection of a *C. difficile* – associated protein using a latex test, and PCR. While culture is the most sensitive method and is helpful for establishing strain prevalence and type, it is problematic in that it detects nontoxigenic strains as well as toxigenic. This requires that all isolates obtained by culture be further tested for their ability to produce toxins, a process that can take as long as 5 days.[14] In addition, toxin testing is preferred over culture because as many as 20% of patients receiving antibiotics

will be asymptomatic carriers of the organism. Toxin is detected in the feces of approximately 30% of patients with antibiotic-associated diarrhea and 100% of patients with pseudomembranous colitis.[11] *C. difficile* cytotoxicity detection is considered the gold standard for detection of toxin B and is considered the most specific laboratory method for diagnosing disease. This is a problem for some laboratories because it requires maintenance of cell lines or routine purchase of commercial lines available in microtiter format and the test requires a 48-hour turnaround time.

Because it is more straightforward and can give same-day results, many laboratories use an immunoassay for detection of the enterotoxin, toxin A or toxin B. Such tests are available in commercial kit form and are more rapidly performed than culture or cytotoxicity testing. Immunoassays have a rapid turn-around time, but their sensitivity (71% to 94%) and specificity (92% to 100%) vary considerably depending on the kit manufacturer.[15] Because of relatively poor predictive values obtained with immunoassay testing, an alternative method should probably be used to confirm positive immunoassay results. For many laboratories, this is impractical. A significant problem with the immunoassay format is the number of "indeterminant" results obtained with such testing. With some kits, this can be as high as 15% of all samples tested. Specimens yielding indeterminant results must be retested, and the initial result is clinically useless to the physician.

Latex agglutination tests detect glutamate dehydrogenase a metabolic enzyme of *C. difficile*. The detected enzyme is nontoxic, nonvirulent, not related to either toxin A or B, and produced by nontoxigenic strains of *C. difficile* as well as other anaerobic bacteria. The test is rapid (minutes), simple to perform, and requires few reagents. The specificity values of the test range from 85% to 95% but sensitivity has been reported as low as 68%.[16] For that reason, many consider it unacceptable as a single choice for diagnostic testing. Because the test does not detect toxin, positive latex results should be confirmed by toxin assay. PCR has been used to distinguish toxigenic from nontoxigenic strains of *C. difficile* and for direct detection of the organism in human feces.[17] It has been demonstrated to be a useful tool for both purposes; however, in its present format, it is too costly and cumbersome to be practical for most clinical laboratories.

The role of *C. difficile* as a cause of diarrheal disease in neonates and young children (2 years or less) is confusing and controversial. The organism has been shown to be normal GI flora in children less than a year of age, and toxins will be detectable but not necessarily associated with disease. Conversely, chronic diarrhea and failure-to-thrive syndrome from *C. difficile* have clearly been proved in this group. In young children, diagnosis should be based on positive toxin results *plus* strong clinical and/or endoscopic findings.[11] Prompt recognition is helped by a history of antibiotic use and the presence of liquid diarrhea.

Escherichia coli (Shiga Toxin and Verotoxin Producing)

The EHEC produce a cytotoxin that affects Vero cells and resembles the cytotoxin of *Shigella dysenteriae*. Because EHEC infection in children can lead to life-threatening illness such as hemolytic uremic syndrome and because these strains are also associated with hemorrhagic colitis, laboratory diagnosis of EHEC is critical. The serotype 0157:H7 accounts for the majority of EHEC that have been isolated to date in the United States. This particular serotype does not ferment d-sorbitol in the first 24 hours, and for this reason, the organism can be cultured on sorbitol MacConkey agar and detected by most laboratories.[7,18] There are, however, a total of 64 serotypes of EHEC, and recent outbreaks involving serotypes other than 0157:H7 have led many to conclude that detection of Verotoxin (VT) from stool is the preferred method, since the toxin is identical in all 64 serotypes. VT can be detected from bacterial broth, bacterial colonies, or directly from filtered stool extract, which is inoculated onto Vero cell lines and then confirmed using neutralizing antibody to VT1 or VT2. A commercially manufactured enzyme immunoassay test for direct detection of VT from stool is now also available (Meridian). The test is easily and rapidly performed (2 hours), is extremely sensitive, and eliminates the need to maintain Vero cell lines.

REFERENCES

1. Guerrant RL, Bobak DA. Bacterial and protozoal gastroenteritis. N Engl J Med 1991;325:327–340

2. Gilligan PH. Diarrheal disease and DRGs. Clin Microbiol News 1986;8:1–4

3. Liesenfeld O, Schneider T, Schmidt W et al. Culture of intestinal biopsy specimens and stool culture for detection of bacterial enteropathogens in patients infected with human immunodeficiency virus. J Clin Microbiol 1995;33:745–747

4. Estevez EG, Levine JA. Examination of preserved stool specimens for parasites: lack of value of the direct wet mount. J Clin Microbiol 1985;22:666–667

5. Siegel D, Cohen PT, Neighbor M et al. Predictive value of stool examination in acute diarrhea. Arch Pathol Lab Med 1987;111:715–718

6. Guerrant RL, Araujo V, Soares E et al. Measurement of fecal lactoferrin as a marker of fecal leukocytes. J Clin Microbiol 1992;30:1238–1242

7. Baron EJ, Peterson LR, Finegold SM. Bailey and Scott's Diagnostic Microbiology. 9th Ed. St. Louis: Mosby, 1994

8. Garcia LS, Bruckner DA. Diagnostic Medical Parasitology, 2nd Ed. Washington, DC: American Society for Microbiology Press, 1993

9. Janoff EN, Craft JC, Pickering LK et al. Diagnosis of *Giardia lamblia* infections by detection of parasite-specific antigens. J Clin Microbiol 1989;27:431–435

10. Kehl KS, Cicirello H, Havens PL. Comparison of four different methods for detection of *Cryptosporidium* species. J Clin Microbiol 1995;33:416–418

11. Bartlett JG. *Clostridium difficile*: history of its role as an enteric pathogen and the current state of knowledge about the organism. Clin Infect Dis 1994; 18(Suppl): S265–S272

12. Desforges JF. *Mycobacterium avium* complex infection in the acquired immunodeficiency syndrome. N Engl J Med 1991; 324:1332–1338

13. King CE: Bacterial overgrowth syndromes. In: Berk JE, Ed. Gastroenterology. 4th Ed. Philadelphia: WB Saunders, 1985

14. Lyerly DM, Krivan HC, Wilkins TD. *Clostridium difficile*: its disease and toxins. Clin Microbiol Rev 1988;1:1–18

15. Whittier S, Shapiro DS, Kelly WF et al. Evaluation of four commercially available enzyme immunoassays for laboratory diagnosis of *Clostridium difficile*–associated diseases. J Clin Microbiol 1993;31:2861–2865

16. Lyerly DM. *Clostridium difficile* testing. Clin Microbiol News 1995;17:17–22

17. Gumerlock PH, Tang YJ, Meyers FJ, Silva J. Use of the polymerase chain reaction for the specific and direct detection of *Clostridium difficile* in human feces. Rev Infect Dis 1991;13:1053–1060

18. Murray PR, Baron EJ, Pfaller MA et al. Manual of Clinical Microbiology. 6th Ed. Washington, DC: American Society for Microbiology Press, 1995

80

ANTHROPOMETRIC ASSESSMENT OF NUTRITIONAL STATUS

BABETTE ZEMEL

Monitoring growth and physical development can be the simplest, most effective means of assessing the nutritional status and overall health of a child. Children with a wide range of chronic diseases or health conditions affecting nutrient intake or absorption are at high risk of malnutrition, as described in Chapter 11. Altered nutrient requirements associated with inflammation, high cell turnover, drug-nutrient interactions, and reduced physical activity also can affect nutritional status. Children with gastrointestinal disorders are at especially increased risk of malnutrition. For these patients, accurate measurements of growth and body composition to assess nutritional status are an important component of routine clinical care. Comparisons with national reference norms for growth and nutritional status provide a means for interpreting these measurements to characterize the presence and severity of malnutrition. Monitoring changes in growth and body composition in individual patients is important for detection and treatment of nutritional problems.

Physical development can also be affected by nutritional status but is often overlooked as an indicator of malnutrition. Obese children are more likely to mature early, whereas delayed maturation is frequently associated with chronic undernutrition. Monitoring physical development in terms of skeletal and sexual maturation is necessary in assessing the severity of malnutrition, as well as in interpreting measures of growth and body com-

position in children with significantly advanced or delayed development.

REFERENCE CHARTS

Reference charts are the primary tool in assessing whether indicators of growth and nutritional status are within normal ranges. However, the reference charts for growth and nutritional status based on normal, healthy children show a wide range of variability, reflecting both genetic and environmental influences in body size and shape. A single evaluation of growth and nutritional status will identify only those children with severe problems outside the normal reference ranges (below the 5th or above the 95th percentile). Adjusting for genetic potential with the use of mid-parental height corrections[1] assists in correctly identifying the child whose growth status is outside the reference range. Tracking the growth of an individual patient over time relative to reference charts is more telling, especially when initial growth status is within the reference range but growth increments are insufficient to maintain previous status. During periods of rapid growth (infancy and adolescence), crossing percentiles on the reference charts can easily occur, since these charts are derived from cross-sectional data and do not reflect the longitudinal growth of individuals.

During adolescence, incremental charts for stature for early, average, and late-maturing children aid in assessing whether growth increments are appropriate.

TECHNIQUES FOR ANTHROPOMETRIC ASSESSMENT OF NUTRITIONAL STATUS

An anthropometric evaluation is a rapid, inexpensive, noninvasive means of characterizing both short- and long-term nutritional status. It should be conducted in conjunction with an overall assessment of nutritional status including a medical and dietary history, physical examination for clinical signs of malnutrition, and laboratory tests. A well-trained anthropometrist and suitable equipment are essential for obtaining accurate, reproducible measurements. Standardized anthropometric techniques have been published[2,3] and are summarized below, with special consideration of children who are at risk for both overnutrition and undernutrition. It should be realized that there is no single measure that sufficiently fully characterizes nutritional status; numerous measurements are ideal, because each one contains different kinds of information about nutritional status, as detailed below.

Measurement of Growth

WEIGHT

Weight should be measured at each office visit. Excess weight can be caused by excess fat or edema, ascites, or organomegaly. Excessive weight gain over a short period of time is more likely to be a gain in water rather than fat. Depending on the time interval, monitoring fatness by arm circumference and skinfold thickness measures (see the section *Anthropometric Assessment of Body Composition* below) provides a means for distinguishing between excess fat and excess water gain.

Weight should be measured with children wearing an examination gown or lightweight clothing and without shoes. Infants should be weighed without clothing or diapers. A digital electronic scale or beam balance scale is ideal and should be set to zero between readings. Children should be weighed to the nearest 0.1 kg and infants to the nearest 0.01 kg. Reference data for weight[4,5] and weight gain[6–8] for infants, children, and adolescents are available.

LENGTH (STATURE)

Length and stature are influenced by heredity, nutritional status, and overall health. Following periods of illness or malnutrition when linear growth is suppressed, a period of catch-up or compensatory growth may occur where rapid gains are observed. Under many circum-

stances, full catch-up growth does not occur. Consequently, length, stature, or other measures of linear growth provide an index of both current and previous nutritional status. Adjustment for the genetic potential for growth should be made when parents are very tall or short in stature.[1] However, parent-specific adjustments should not be used for children of underprivileged families from lesser-developed countries because it is likely that the parents have not reached their full genetic potential for growth.

Because of the potential for measurement error due to positioning and cooperation of the child, it is particularly important that great care be taken in length and stature measurements so that they provide meaningful information. During periods of rapid growth such as infancy and adolescence, significant gains in length or stature can occur in a week. During mid-childhood, increases in stature can be difficult to detect in less than a 6-month interval. These can be important considerations in interpreting sequential measurements in an office setting.

Children below the age of 2 years should be measured for length at each office visit. Standing height or stature should be measured starting at age 2 years. Children greater than 2 years of age may be measured in a supine position if they are unable to stand erect unsupported. Supine length measurements in older children are approximately 2 cm greater than stature measurements due to the effects of gravity.[9] Supine length can be adjusted accordingly, and the estimated stature can be plotted on the growth chart.

For both length and stature measurements, it is essential that the measuring devices are sturdy and maintain a stable 90-degree angle at the head and feet. For infants, an infantometer or inflexible length board with a fixed headboard and movable footboard is required. For stature measurements, the ideal device is a stadiometer with a head paddle that is firmly perpendicular to the back of the stadiometer but glides smoothly. If a stadiometer is not available, a tape measure affixed to a wall or door frame can be used along with a head paddle that gives a 90-degree angle to the wall during stature measurements. Both length and stature should be measured in triplicate to the nearest 0.1 cm. The three readings should be in agreement within 0.5 cm of each other; if not, additional measurements should be taken. The average of the three measurements should be used.

To measure supine length, two people are required to hold and position the child correctly. One person (the parent can assist) holds the head firmly to the top of the board with the Frankfurt plane perpendicular to the floor. The Frankfurt plane is an imaginary line from the upper margin of the auditory meatus to the lower margin of the orbit. The torso should rest flat on the length board with the midline centered on the board. The legs should be extended gently but firmly with the feet together and flexed at a 90-degree angle by the footboard at the time of measurement. For stature, the child should be relaxed with arms at the side and the heels together. The heels, buttocks, shoulders, and head should be touching the back of the stadiometer. For very obese children, this may not be possible, and the child should be positioned so that the spine is in alignment with the child standing as erect as possible. The head should be held in the Frankfurt plane at the time of measurement.

Excellent reference data are available for evaluating stature and increments in growth for infants, children, and adolescents. Poor linear growth status or failure to achieve adequate increments in length or stature can be indicative of underlying nutritional problems. For example, losses in growth status have been observed in children with Crohn's disease prior to the onset of clinical symptoms.

WEIGHT-FOR-HEIGHT MEASURES

Weight-for-height measures are useful tools for assessing weight adjusted for length or height. As discussed in Chapter 11, weight and length (stature) are used in clas- sifying the presence and severity of stunting and wasting in children under 5 years of age. For older children, per- cent of ideal body weight can be used. This is calculated as follows: The child's height for age is plotted on the growth chart. A horizontal line is drawn from the child's height to the 50th percentile height curve. The 50th percentile weight corresponding to that point is used as the ideal body weight. Percent of ideal body weight is calculated as the measured weight divided by the ideal body weight times 100. Some children with nutritional problems are able to maintain adequate ideal body weight while gradual stunting in height occurs, as in the case of children with cystic fibrosis. Percent of ideal body weight is also used in the classification of overnutrition (110% to 120%, overweight; greater than 120%, obese) and undernutrition (80% to 90%, mildly malnourished; 70% to 80%, moderately malnourished; less than 70%, severely malnourished).

Another frequently used weight-for-height measure is the body mass index. This is calculated as weight in kilo- grams divided by the square of stature in meters. The

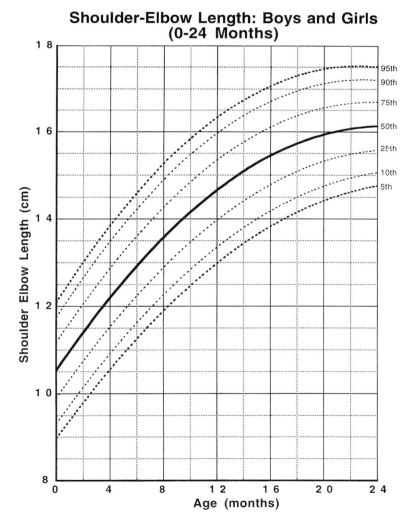

FIGURE 80-1. Shoulder-elbow length for boys and girls ages birth to 24 months. (From Stall- ings and Zemel,[13] with permission.)

body mass index changes through the course of growth and development, so age- and sex-specific reference charts are used for nutritional assessment. The 85th and 95th percentiles have been used to classify overweight and obesity.[10,11] Because the body mass index is a composite measure of muscle, fat, and bone, the combined use of body mass index and the triceps skinfold (see below) is useful in distinguishing between excess fat and high lean body mass.

HEAD CIRCUMFERENCE

During the first 3 years of life, brain growth is most rapid, and head circumference is a good indicator of this aspect of growth. With severe malnutrition, growth of the brain can be compromised, so it is important to include this measure routinely in the assessment of nutritional status for children below 3 years of age and for older children with severe stunting. Head circumference is a poor indicator of nutritional status in children with micro- or mac-

rocephalus or central nervous system damage of non-nutritional etiology.

Head circumference should be measured to the nearest 0.1 cm. Hair clips and plaits should be removed for an accurate measurement. A flexible, nonstretchable measuring tape should be used. The tape is placed above the supraorbital ridge and around the occiput and positioned evenly on both sides. Slight repositioning of the tape is necessary to identify the maximum circumference. The tape should be tightened firmly about the head and three measurements taken and the mean recorded. Reference data for head circumference are given in Roche et al.[12]

ALTERNATIVE MEASURES OF LINEAR GROWTH ASSESSMENT

Length and stature measurements are not always possible, as in the case of children who are immobile or have body shape abnormalities. Upper arm length and lower leg length are alternative measures that provide upper

FIGURE 80-2. Knee-heel length for boys and girls ages birth to 24 months. (From Stallings and Zemel,[13] with permission.)

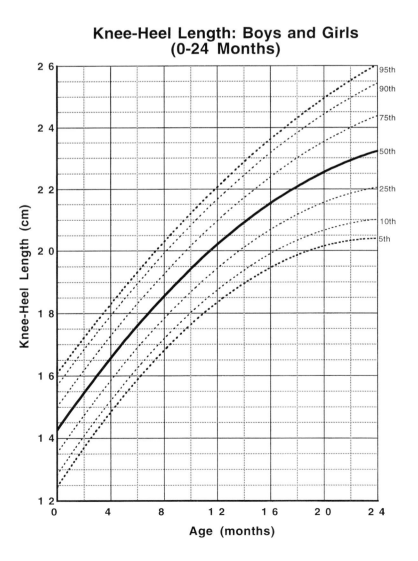

Upper Arm Length: Boys 3-18 Years

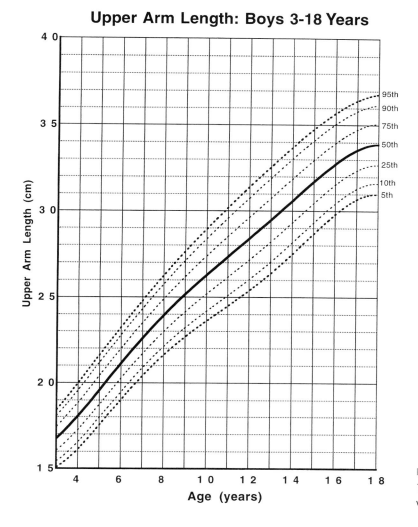

FIGURE 80-3. Upper arm length for boys 3 to 18 years of age. (From Stallings and Zemel,[13] with permission.)

and lower body measures of linear growth. Growth charts for upper arm and lower leg length (Figs. 80-1 through 80-6) provide a reference for interpretation of these measurements.[13] As with length or stature measures, these linear growth measures can be used to aid in the interpretation of weight measurements to determine whether a child is wasted or stunted.

Sliding calipers (0 to 200 mm) are used for measuring upper arm and lower leg length in young infants. For older infants and children, an anthropometer is used. In infants (0 to 24 months), upper arm length is measured as shoulder-elbow length. The measurement is taken from the superior lateral surface of the acromion to the inferior surface of the elbow with the arm flexed at a 90-degree angle. In children 2 to 18 years, upper arm length is measured from the superior lateral surface of the acromion to the radiale (tip of the radius) with the arm relaxed at the side. In infants (0 to 24 months), lower leg length is measured as knee-heel length. The infant should be lying on the back with the leg flexed to 90 degrees at the hip, knee, and ankle. The measurement is made from the heel to the superior surface of the knee.

For children ages 3 to 18 years, the lower leg length measure is taken with the patient sitting in a relaxed position and the right leg crossed over the left. The measurement is taken from the lower border of the medial malleolus (sphyrion) to the medial tip of the tibia. The right side should be measured unless there is unilateral involvement affecting the right side. The least affected side should be measured, and the side that is measured should be noted. All measurements are taken in triplicate to the nearest 0.1 cm and repeated every 3 months.

Anthropometric Assessment of Body Composition

Measures of lean and fat tissues of the body at sites known to be sensitive to nutrition and health are extremely useful because (1) they are an index of energy and protein reserves in the body and (2) they help distinguish between excess fat and excess water. Upper arm anthropometry, which involves the measurement of arm circumference and skinfold thickness over the triceps muscle, is used to this end. Excellent reference data are available for these measures for their interpretation in assessing nutritional status.

MID UPPER ARM CIRCUMFERENCE

The mid upper arm circumference is sensitive to current nutritional status and is often used in nutrition surveys because of its ease of measurement and prognostic value. It is measured to the nearest 0.1 cm using a flexible, nonstretchable tape. The length of the upper arm must first be measured and the midpoint located. With the arm flexed to a 90-degree angle at the elbow, the midpoint is located halfway between the lateral tip of the acromion and the olecranon. Once identified, the midpoint should be marked (with a washable ink pen). For measuring arm circumference, the arm should be extended downward at the side in a fully relaxed position. Gently shaking the arm usually ensures that it is relaxed. Infants may be held by their parent provided they are in an upright position. The tape is placed gently around the arm at the midpoint, and care should be taken so

that there is no pinching or gaping of the tape as it encircles the arm. The tape should be perpendicular to the long axis of the arm and three measurements taken and the mean recorded. Excellent reference data for mid upper arm circumference are available.[14]

TRICEPS SKINFOLD THICKNESS

Measurement of the subcutaneous fat gives an indication of whole body fat stores, and the triceps skinfold is particularly sensitive to changes in nutritional status. In normally growing infants and children, overall body fatness increases markedly during infancy such that the percentage of body weight that is fat reaches a peak between 6 and 18 months of age.[15] Percent body fat then declines during childhood, although the total amount of fat increases slowly. It is common for boys to undergo a prepubescent increase in fatness and then experience a decline in fatness following the onset of puberty. Girls experience rapid increases in fatness with the onset of puberty. Because of the sex- and puberty-related differences in fatness, it is important to use the reference data[14] as a

FIGURE 80-4. Upper arm length for girls 3 to 16 years of age. (From Stallings and Zemel,[13] with permission.)

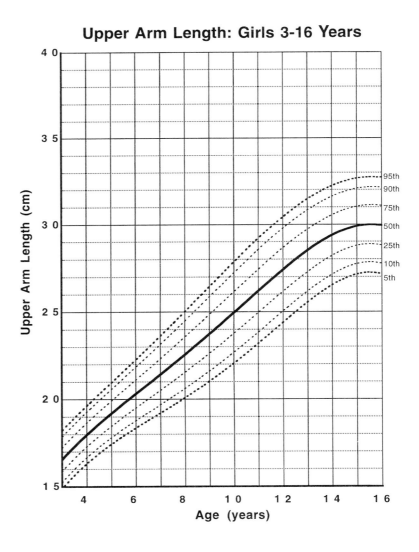

Lower Leg Length: Boys 3-18 Years

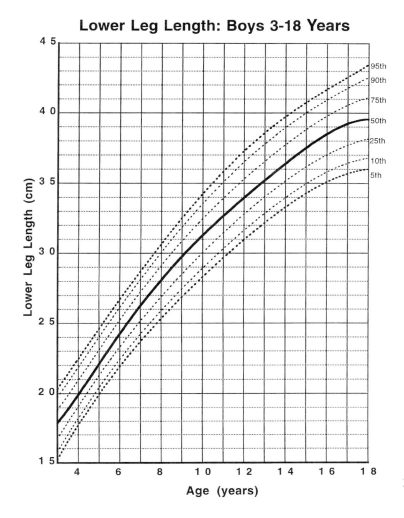

FIGURE 80-5. Lower leg length for boys 3 to 18 years of age. (From Stallings and Zemel,[13] with permission.)

guide and adjust for delayed puberty when necessary in interpreting skinfold thickness data.

The triceps skinfold thickness is measured at the level of the midpoint of the upper right arm over the center of the triceps muscle on the back of the arm. The patient should be upright with the arm at the side and fully relaxed. If this positioning is not possible, then the position should be noted for purposes of comparison with future measurements. The fold of fat and skin is lifted away from the underlying muscle just above the midpoint and held in position so that the calipers can be placed just below the fingertips. While the skinfold is held in position, the handles of the calipers are released and the reading is taken after 4 seconds. The calipers are then opened and removed and the fold released. These steps are repeated twice and the average of the three readings recorded.

SUBSCAPULAR SKINFOLD THICKNESS

The subscapular skinfold is less sensitive to short-term nutritional changes and thereby is an indicator of long-term nutritional status. It is a measure of truncal fat and,

when combined with the triceps skinfold, is useful in assessing fat distribution and total body fat. The subscapular skinfold is measured 1 cm below the tip of the scapula at a 45-degree downward angle following the natural contour of the body. The patient should be upright with the arms down and fully relaxed. If this positioning is not possible, an alternate position should be noted for comparative purposes with future measurements. As with the triceps skinfold measurement, the fold is lifted and held in place while the calipers are placed just below the fingertips. The reading is taken 4 seconds after releasing the handles of the calipers. The calipers should be opened and removed before releasing the skinfold. The measurement should be taken in triplicate and the mean recorded. National reference data are available.[16,17]

CALCULATIONS OF BODY COMPOSITION

Measurement of the upper arm is extremely useful because estimates of upper arm muscle area and upper arm fat area can be computed, as shown in Table 80-1. These estimates of muscle and fat are important for several reasons. First, they correlate highly with total body measures

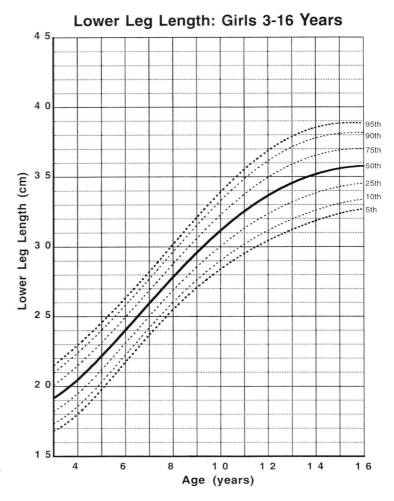

Lower Leg Length: Girls 3-16 Years

FIGURE 80-6. Lower leg length for girls 3 to 16 years of age. (From Stallings and Zemel,[13] with permission.)

of lean tissue and fatness. Secondly, they are indicative of protein and energy reserves in the body and thus are indicative of nutritional adequacy. Finally, excellent reference data are available for interpretation of these measures.[14]

In older children (8 years and older), body composition (percent body fat and fat-free mass) can be predicted from the triceps and subscapular skinfold thicknesses, provided puberty stage is assessed. The equations (Table 80-2) used to predict body composition are specific to puberty status, gender, race, and obesity. They correlate highly with body composition measured by stable isotopes in normal children,[18] as well as children with chronic diseases such as cystic fibrosis and cerebral palsy.

TABLE 80-1. Computation of the Muscle Area and Fat Area of the Upper Arm

---

Upper arm muscle area (mm²) = [armcirc − (triceps × π)]²/(4 × π), where π = 3.14

Upper arm fat area = upper arm area − upper arm muscle area, where upper arm area = armcirc²/(4 × π)

The major limitation of this approach is that reference data for body composition based on a nationally representative sample are not available. However, the sum of triceps and subscapular skinfolds is an excellent indicator of overall body fatness. Race-, age-, and gender-specific reference data for the sum of skinfolds are available.[16]

Assessment of Sexual and Skeletal Maturation

Delayed or advanced sexual and skeletal maturation can be due to underlying medical conditions, but undernutrition or overnutrition can be contributory factors. In children at risk for malnutrition, evaluation of maturation is important for overall nutritional assessment and for interpretation of other growth and body composition measures. Pubertal maturation should be noted as part of the physical examination and scored according to the Tanner stages (I to V) for breast and pubic hair growth in girls and for genital and pubic hair growth in boys.[19] Menarcheal status should also be noted.

Skeletal maturation is used as an indicator of biologic age to classify children as advanced, normal, or delayed

TABLE 80-2. Anthropometric Equations for Prediction of Percent Fat (ages 8–18 yr)

White males:
Prepubescent:	1.21 (triceps + subscapular) − 0.008 (triceps + subscapular)^2 − 1.7
Pubescent:	1.21 (triceps + subscapular) − 0.008 (triceps + subscapular)^2 − 3.4
Postpubescent:	1.21 (triceps + subscapular) − 0.008 (triceps + subscapular)^2 − 5.5

Black males:
Prepubescent:	1.21 (triceps + subscapular) − 0.008 (triceps + subscapular)^2 − 3.2
Pubescent:	1.21 (triceps + subscapular) − 0.008 (triceps + subscapular)^2 − 5.2
Postpubescent:	1.21 (triceps + subscapular) − 0.008 (triceps + subscapular)^2 − 6.8

All females:	1.33 (triceps + subscapular) − 0.013 (triceps + subscapular)^2 − 2.5

Obese:

If (triceps + subscapular) greater than 35 mm:
Males:	0.783 (triceps + subscapular) + 1.6
Females:	0.546 (triceps + subscapular) + 9.7

(From Slaughter et al,[18] with permission.)

in their skeletal development. In children with unusual growth patterns, this is important information for the interpretation of growth measurements. Skeletal age can also be used as an indicator of growth potential and in the prediction of adult height. However, delayed bone age can be an indicator of impaired skeletal growth rather than growth potential, especially in children with chronic diseases or treated with immunosuppressive drugs or corticosteroids. Skeletal maturation is assessed by a hand-wrist radiograph and scored according to the standards of Greulich and Pyle[20] or Tanner et al.[21]

SUMMARY

Growth, maturation, and body composition are important components in the clinical care of children with gastrointestinal and nutritional disorders. They provide information about current and previous nutritional status and are useful in detection, monitoring, and treatment of ongoing health and nutritional problems.

REFERENCES

1. Himes JH, Roche AF, Thissen D, Moore WM. Parent-specific adjustments for evaluation of recumbent length and stature of children. Pediatrics 1985;75:2304–2313
2. Lohman TG, Roche AF, Martorell R. Anthropometric standardization reference manual. Champaign, IL: Human Kinetics Books, 1988
3. Cameron N: The methods of auxological anthropology. In: Falkner F, Tanner JM, Eds. Human Growth: A Comprehensive Treatise. 2nd Ed. Vol. 3. New York: Plenum, 1986
4. Hamill PVV, Drizd TA, Johnson CL et al. Physical growth: national center for health statistics percentiles. Am J Clin Nutr 1979;32:607–629
5. Casey PH, Kraemer HC, Bernbaum J et al. Growth status and growth rates of a varied sample of low birth weight, preterm infants: a longitudinal cohort from birth to three years of age. J Pediatr 1991;119:599–605
6. Guo S, Roche AF, Fomon SF et al. Reference data on gains in weight and length during the first two years of life. J Pediatr 1991;119:355–362
7. Roche AF, Himes JH. Incremental growth charts. Am J Clin Nutr 1980;33:2041–2052
8. Tanner JM, Davis PSW. Clinical longitudinal standards for height and height velocity for North American children. J Pediatr 1985;107:3317–3329
9. Roche AF, Davila GH. Differences between recumbent length and stature within individuals. Growth 1974;38:313
10. Must A, Dallal GE, Dietz WH. Reference data for obesity: 85th and 95th percentiles of body mass index (wt/ht^2) and triceps skinfold thickness. Am J Clin Nutr 1991;53:839–846
11. Must A, Dallal GE, Dietz WH. Reference data for obesity: 85th and 95th percentiles of body mass index (wt/ht^2)—a correction. Am J Clin Nutr 1991;54:773
12. Roche AF, Mukherjee D, Guo S, Moore WM. Head circumference reference data: birth to 18 years. Pediatrics 1987;79:706–712
13. Stallings V, Zemel B: Nutritional assessment of the disabled child. In: Sullivan P, Rosenbloom L, Eds. Clinics in Developmental Medicine: Feeding the Disabled Child. London: MacKeith, 1996:62–76
14. Frisancho AR. New norms of upper limb fat and muscle areas for assessment of nutritional status. Am J Clin Nutr 1981;34:2540–2545
15. Fomon SJ, Haschke F, Ziegler EE, Nelson SE. Body composition of reference children from birth to age 10 years. Am J Clin Nutr 1982;35:1169–1175
16. Frisancho AR. Anthropometric standards for the assessment of growth and nutritional status. Ann Arbor: University of Michigan Press, 1990
17. Johnson CL, Fulwood R, Abraham S, Bryner JD. Basic data of anthropometric measurements and angular measurements

of the hip and knee joints for selected age groups 1–74 years of age: United States 1971–75. DHHS Publication No. (PHS) 81–1669. Vital and Health Statistics Series 11, No. 219. Hyattsville, MD: National Center for Health Statistics 1981

18. Slaughter MH, Lohman TG, Boileau RA et al. Skinfold equations for estimation of body fatness in children and youth. Hum Biol 1988;60:5709–5723

19. Tanner JM. Growth at Adolescence. 2nd Ed. Oxford: Blackwell Scientific Publications, 1962

20. Greulich WW, Pyle SI. Radiographic Atlas of the Skeletal Development of the Hand and Wrist. 2nd Ed. Palo Alto: Stanford University Press, 1959

21. Tanner JM, Whitehouse RH, Cameron N et al. Assessment of skeletal maturity and prediction of adult height (TW2). 2nd Ed. London: Academic Press, 1983

81

RESTING ENERGY EXPENDITURE

VIRGINIA A. STALLINGS

Energy balance problems are common in clinical pediatrics, both in the inpatient and outpatient settings, and are encompassed in the diagnoses failure to thrive, undernutrition, wasting, nutritional stunting, overweight, and obesity. Energy balance is the result of the total energy (calories) obtained from food and other nutrient sources (i.e., total parenteral nutrition, tube feedings) compared to the total energy requirement for all physiologic activities (basal or resting metabolic needs, thermic effect of food, physical activities, growth, and disease effects). To maintain energy balance in children with gastrointestinal (GI) diseases, energy intake must be balanced against calories lost through malabsorption, severe emesis, excessive urination, or loss through other bodily fluids.

The definition of energy balance, as stated by the World Health Organization (WHO), is "the level of energy intake that will balance energy expenditure when the individual has a body size and composition, and a level of physical activity consistent with long-term good health. In children . . . the energy requirement includes the energy needs associated with the deposition of tissues (growth) . . . at rates consistent with good health."[1] So, for infants, children, and adolescents, the goal is to provide energy to achieve normal growth (sustain the individual patient's genetic potential) and normal body composition (optimal proportions of muscle, bone, and fat) and to maintain normal patterns of activities of daily living, including play activities. Negative energy balance (semistarvation) causes an alteration of all of these desirable goals and leads to abnormal patterns of growth and body composition and decreased physical activity. Persistent excess positive energy balance also fails to meet these goals and results in more rapid growth rates, abnormal body composition (excess adiposity or obesity), and decreased physical activity.

PREDICTING ENERGY NEEDS

Various sources in the literature provide values of predicted total daily energy needs for groups of healthy, normally growing children. The Recommended Dietary Allowances (RDA) are the standards for the United States[2] (Table 81-1), while the Recommended Nutrient Intakes for Canadians are the criteria for Canada.[3] In the practice of clinical medicine, the medical team needs to know the energy requirement of an individual patient who has a medically significant illness, which often causes an abnormal pattern of body composition, growth, and physical activity. The estimate of the energy requirement is translated into the appropriate number of calories from food, tube feeding, or intravenous nutritional support. Many common pediatric GI diseases (e.g., inflammatory bowel disease, cystic fibrosis, liver disease) have a direct impact on energy expenditure due to associated malabsorption, inflammation, chronic infection, or changes in body composition. Because these types of factors affect energy expenditure, the energy needs of children with illnesses are very difficult to predict accurately from standard dietary recommendations developed from studying requirements of healthy children.

For many years, the only alternative to the population-based recommendations (the RDA approach) for energy intake was to use one of the various mathematical formu-

TABLE 81-1. Energy Intake Recommendations from the Recommended Dietary Allowances (10th Edition) with Median Heights and Weights[2]

Category	Age (yr)	Weight (kg)	Height (cm)	REE[a] (kcal/day)	Average Energy Allowance (kcal)		
					Multiples of REE	Per kg	Per day
Infants	0.0–0.5	6	60	320	2.03	108	650
	0.5–1.0	9	71	500	1.70	98	850
Children	1–3	13	90	740	1.76	102	1,300
	4–6	20	112	950	1.89	90	1,800
	7–10	28	132	1,130	1.77	70	2,000
Males	11–14	45	157	1,440	1.70	55	2,500
	15–18	66	176	1,760	1.67	45	3,000
	19–24	72	177	1,780	1.67	40	2,900
Females	11–14	46	157	1,310	1.67	47	2,200
	15–18	55	163	1,370	1.60	40	2,200
	19–24	58	164	1,350	1.60	38	2,200

[a] *Abbreviation*: REE, resting energy expenditure.

(From National Academy of Sciences. Recommended Dietary Allowances. Washington, DC: National Academy Press, 1989:24–38.)

las to predict the basal metabolic rate or resting energy expenditure (REE) and then predict the total daily energy needs of a patient by adjusting the REE with sets of physical activity and illness factors reflecting the patient's condition. The most commonly known method in estimating REE requirements is the pair of Harris and Benedict equations for adults,[4] which use the patient's gender, age, height, and weight to estimate the REE. This formula was derived mostly from adult measurements and is not recommended for use in the pediatric age group. More recently, WHO created new REE prediction equa-

tions that are designed for use in infants, children, and adolescents (Table 81-2). These equations use the patient's age group, gender, and body weight to predict REE and are the formulas used in clinical practice in many pediatric care settings.

A more detailed evaluation of the WHO data resulted in the Schofield equations,[5] which provide predictive equations for REE using either weight alone or weight and height (Table 81-3), age group, and gender. Significant limitations of these three sets of predictive equa-

TABLE 81-2. WHO Equations for Predicting Resting Energy Expenditure from Body Weight (W), Gender, and Age Group[1]

Age Range (yr)	Kcal/day
Males	
0–3	60.9 W − 54
3–10	22.7 W + 495
10–18	17.5 W + 651
18–30	15.3 W + 679
Females	
0–3	61.0 W − 51
3–10	22.5 W + 499
10–18	12.2 W + 746
18–30	14.7 W + 496

(From FAO/WHO/UNU Expert Consultation. Energy and Protein Requirements. Geneva: World Health Organization, 1985:71–112.)

TABLE 81-3. Schofield Equations for Predicting Resting Energy Expenditure from Body Weight (W), Height (H), Gender, and Age Group[5]

Age Range (yr)	Kcal/day
Males	
0–3	0.167W + 1517.4H − 617.6
3–10	19.59W + 130.3H + 414.9
10–18	16.25W + 137.2H + 515.5
18–30	15.057W + 10.04H + 705.8
Females	
0–3	16.252W + 1023.2H − 413.5
3–10	16.969W + 161.8H + 371.2
10–18	8.365W + 465.H + 200.0
18–30	13.623W + 283.0H + 98.2

(From Schofield WN. Predicting basal metabolic rate: new standards and review of previous work. Hum Nutr Clin Nutr 1985;39[Suppl 1]:5–41.)

tions in clinical practice have been demonstrated. Kaplan et al.[6] showed that wide variability occurs when measuring the REE in children with illnesses compared to the predicted REE from pediatric-oriented WHO, Schofield weight, or Schofield weight and height equations. The equations, even the one using both the weight and height information with gender and age, often were unable to predict accurately the measured REE in children with a variety of common clinical pediatric diagnoses resulting in failure to thrive or obesity.

In summary, the energy needs of pediatric patients are difficult to predict because of the variations in metabolic demands of illness, alterations in growth and body composition, and the poor predictive power of available equations developed from measurements of healthy children. The actual measurement of REE is the best available method to accurately determine the individual patient's caloric needs for use in clinical care to promote weight gain or loss or to provide for weight maintenance.

REE MEASUREMENT BY INDIRECT CALORIMETRY

The study of energy metabolism in clinical settings has been made possible in recent years by the advances in the construction and availability of the open-circuit ventilated-hood indirect calorimeters. Whereas direct calorimetry consists of measurements of the heat dissipated by the body as the by-product of all metabolic processes (not used in clinical medicine), the indirect calorimeter or metabolic cart measures a patient's oxygen consumption and carbon dioxide production. These values are used to calculate the REE, which is expressed as kilocalories per day. The metabolic cart provides minute-by-minute values that are averaged over the testing interval to provide the final REE value.

The REE measurement should be conducted under standardized conditions to ensure the accuracy of the data and clinical interpretation. The optimal REE measurement is conducted in a supine, resting, awake patient in the early morning (7 A.M. to 10 A.M.), after a night of restful sleep and overnight or age- or disease-appropriate fast. The test should be performed prior to any physical activity, and the patient should not be given any metabolically active medications known to change the heart rate (e.g., bronchodilators). The protocol includes a fast to prevent exposure to all calories (PO or IV) for 8 to 12 hours. If this is not possible because of the patient's age or clinical condition (e.g., hypoglycemia), the fast should be shortened, or minimal calories provided (with low-concentration dextrose–containing IV fluids). Most patients requiring IV fluids can tolerate the use of nondextrose (noncaloric) fluids such as half-normal saline for 6 to 12 hours before and during the REE measurement. In infants, the age-appropriate fast is usually between 3 and 6 hours. Noncaloric, noncaffeinated oral fluids may be provided during the pre-REE fast.

Because spontaneous physical activity must be restricted during the REE measurement, cooperation of the patient is important. Developmentally normal children older than 5 years usually do well while watching VCR movies on TV. Younger children, who may not be able to cooperate for the duration of the testing experience, may be sedated with a short-acting oral agent, such as chloral hydrate, given about 30 minutes prior to the test. The lightly sleeping patient will have a slightly reduced (approximately 10%) REE, compared to a resting, awake child.

The usual clinical REE lasts 40 to 60 minutes, with the first 10 minutes omitted from data analysis to account for patient equilibration. Tests lasting only 10 to 20 minutes may not allow the pediatric patient to completely adjust to the testing conditions and may provide results that are artificially high. If the child has a brief period of movement that temporarily raises the REE, the minutes associated with the movement episode should be removed from the data set used to calculate the final REE value. REE varies over the course of the day owing to known diurnal variations in energy expenditure and the effects of food ingestion and physical activity. Changes in the protocol allowing food intake or variations in time of day will artificially increase the REE compared to an early morning, fasted study and should be avoided when possible.

Another factor to consider is body temperature. Elevated body temperature is a common symptom in children with a variety of illnesses and causes a predictable increase in REE. Each degree centigrade elevation increases REE by 13% (7.2% in Fahrenheit scale). If a patient has a temperature of 40°C rather than 38°C at the time of the REE assessment, the REE will be elevated about 26% owing to the abnormal body temperature. If possible, REE should be measured during periods of normal body temperature to avoid the elevation related to temporary increases in temperature.

CLINICAL USE OF REE

The use of indirect calorimetry and REE measurements in clinical medicine evolved from the determination of metabolic rate for the diagnosis of thyroid disease prior to the availability of blood levels for thyroid hormone. REE measured by the modern metabolic cart according to the described protocol will determine if the patient is hypermetabolic, hypometabolic, or eumetabolic compared to predicted values for age, gender, and size (WHO or Schofield equations). The etiology of the altered metabolic state is varied and in pediatric clinical nutrition practice is rarely a classic endocrine cause.

Today, REE is measured to determine the total caloric needs of an individual patient to achieve a specific clinical goal (weight maintenance, loss, or gain). REE represents a large portion of the energy needed each day. The

TABLE 81-4. Approximate Energy Expenditure for Various Activities in Relation to Resting Needs for Males and Females of Average Size[2]

Activity Category[a]	Representative Value for Activity Factor per Unit of Time Activity
Resting Sleeping, reclining	REE × 1.0
Very light Seated and standing activities, painting trades, driving, laboratory work, typing, sewing, ironing, cooking, playing cards, playing a musical instrument	REE × 1.5
Light Walking on a level surface at 2.5 to 3.0 mph, garage work, electrical trades, carpentry, restaurant trades, housecleaning, child care, golf, sailing, table tennis	REE × 2.5
Moderate Walking 3.5 to 4.0 mph, weeding and hoeing, carrying a load, cycling, skiing, tennis, dancing	REE × 5.0
Heavy Walking with load uphill, tree felling, heavy manual digging, basketball, climbing, football, soccer	REE × 7.0

[a] When reported as multiples of basal needs, the expenditures of males and females are similar.

(From National Academy of Sciences. Recommended Dietary Allowances. Washington, DC: National Academy Press, 1989:24–38.)

additional energy needed for normal growth and physical activity (everything except quietly resting supine), to adjust for malabsorption, or to support therapeutic growth acceleration must be added to the REE to determine the total energy expenditure (TEE). Table 81-4 shows the physical activity and normal growth factors for healthy, normally active children.[2]

The physical activity/growth factors for infants and children range from 1.70 to 2.03 × REE based on the age and gender group. Children who are significantly ill or hospitalized have less spontaneous physical activity, and a factor of 1.3 to 1.5 × REE is a better estimate of the energy needs above REE. An additional correction factor for disease severity is used to adjust REE in some settings. For example, in the care of children with cystic fibrosis, the REE is adjusted for degree of pulmonary disease.[6]

Often in children with GI diseases, the actual amount of fat or total calories lost in the usual stool output has been quantified by a 72-hour stool collection, so an additional correction factor may be used to improve the accuracy of the total energy needs. Since most of the calories lost in stool come from the unabsorbed fat component (compared with the total stool calories lost from fat, carbohydrate, and protein), the analysis for stool fat calories is as clinically useful as bomb calorimetric analysis for total calories lost in the stool. The energy lost in the stool is compared to the total dietary fat intake, and a coefficient of fat absorption is calculated. The energy intake recommendation is then corrected for the degree of malabsorption. For example, if the energy intake recommendation is for 1,200 kcal/day based on REE and physical activity and growth correction factors, and the patient is known to have a persistent coefficient of fat absorption of 80% (i.e., a loss of 20% of the fat energy in the stool), the dietary intake recommendation should be adjusted as follows: 1,200 kcal/day × 1.2 (20% fat loss) = 1,440 kcal/day energy intake goal. These are approximate corrections, so the factor is not routinely adjusted for the normal stool fat losses of 5% to 7% in healthy adults.

The last consideration in using REE to determine the total daily energy requirement is to add a factor that adjusts for "catch-up" growth when clinically indicated. As previously discussed, the REE is adjusted by a factor (1.70 to 2.07 × REE) that provides adequate energy for the usual amount of weight gain and physical activity in healthy, active children. In patients with significant failure to thrive, the clinical goal may be to increase the rate of weight gain above the normal rate (often called catch-up growth), and this requires additional calories (as well as other nutrients). A general approach is to use the approximate relationship that 1 kg of weight gain (or loss) requires an excess (or deficiency) of 7,700 calories. In pounds, the relationship is 1 pound to 3,500 calories. If the 1-kg weight gain is planned to occur over 1 month, then 7,700 kcal ÷ 30 days = 257 kcal/day additional calories to be added to the previously calculated total caloric intake goal. If the 1-kg weight gain is to be achieved over 14 days, then 513 kcal/day (7,700 kcal ÷ 14 days) is added to the total caloric intake goal.

EXAMPLE OF CALCULATION FOR DAILY ENERGY NEEDS FROM REE

A 15-kg, 5-year-old girl is hospitalized with complications of chronic diarrhea, and an REE is measured to determine metabolic rate and to serve as the basis to determine the total daily energy need.

Measured REE:

950 kcal/day

Activity factor:

1.3 (bed rest) × 950 kcal/day = 1,235 kcal/day

Weight gain goal:

257 kcal/day (1 kg over 1 mo) + 1,235 = 1,492 kcal/day

Stool fat losses:

1.15 (15% kcal loss) × 1,492 = 1,716 kcal/day

Total caloric needs:

1,716 kcal/day, 114 kcal/kg/day

Comparison to WHO prediction:

(22.5 × 15 [weight, kg]) + 499 = 836 kcal/day

% predicted WHO:

950 (measured REE)/836 (predicted REE) = 114% predicted

Assessment:

Mildly increased metabolic rate (range 90 to 110% predicted)

REFERENCES

1. FAO/WHO/UNU Expert Consultation. Energy and Protein Requirements. Geneva: World Health Organization, 1985: 71–112

2. National Academy of Sciences. Recommended Dietary Allowances. Washington, DC: National Academy Press, 1989: 24–38

3. Health and Welfare Canada. Recommended Nutrient Intakes for Canadians. Ottawa: Minister of National Health and Welfare, 1983:17–27

4. Harris JA, Benedict FG. A Biometric Study of Basal Metabolism in Man. Publication No. 279. Washington, DC: Carnegie Institution, 1919

5. Schofield WN. Predicting basal metabolic rate: new standards and review of previous work. Hum Nutr Clin Nutr 1985; 39(Suppl 1):5–41

6. Kaplan AS, Zemel BS, Neiswender KM, Stallings VA. Resting energy expenditure in clinical pediatrics: measured versus predicted equations. J Pediatr 1995;127:200–205

7. Ramsey BW, Farrell PM, Pencharz P. Nutritional assessment and management in cystic fibrosis: a consensus report. Am J Clin Nutr 1992;55:108–116

82

BONE DENSITOMETRY

VIRGINIA A. STALLINGS

Osteoporosis is a significant cause of morbidity, mortality, and health care expenditure and has become the focus of increased attention in the general public and in the medical community. Bone mass accounts for up to 80% of the variance in skeletal strength and thus is the most important factor in preventing fracture. Since most of the bone mass accumulation occurs during childhood and adolescence, increasing attention is focused on the components of bone health during the pediatric years. Achieving the maximum peak bone mass during childhood is predicted to be one of the more effective methods of primary prevention of adult osteoporosis. Physicians caring for children will contribute to improved bone health of both children and future adults by encouraging an optimal dietary intake of calcium and vitamin D and an optimal pattern of physical activity. In addition, physicians should be particularly concerned about the bone mass status of children at high risk for mineralization abnormalities. Many of the risk factors for poor mineralization such as chronic diarrhea, lactose intolerance, poor dietary intake, fat-soluble vitamin malabsorption, decreased physical activity, and oral corticosteroid medication are common in clinical gastroenterology. Recent reviews of the issue present a compelling argument that bone mineral issues must be a part of pediatric health care.[1-3]

Bone mass is estimated from indirect, noninvasive measurements of bone mineral content or bone mineral density (g/cm^2) in different regions of the skeleton or the whole body. Several methods have been used, including single photon absorptiometry, dual photon absorptiometry, quantitative computed tomography, and dual-energy x-ray absorptiometry (DXA). DXA is available in an increasing number of clinical settings and has several advantages for use in pediatric care. The precision of the measurement is excellent, 1% to 2%, and the radiation dose is small, less than 3 mrem (about 1/20 of a chest x-ray). The most commonly performed scan is at the anteroposterior lumbar spine site, which can be completed within about 2 minutes.

CLINICAL INDICATIONS FOR DXA

In most children and adolescents, traditional age-appropriate nutritional and physical activity guidance is all that is needed to ensure good bone health. Total calcium and vitamin D intake from food and supplements should be evaluated and compared to the recommendations (recommended dietary allowances [RDA])[4] for the patient's appropriate age and gender group (Tables 82-1, 82-2, and 82-3). Calcium intake in children who are lactose intolerant or dairy product refusers should be carefully evaluated with a 3-day diet record analyzed by a software program for calcium intake. A more specific calcium intake questionnaire may be used to determine the child's customary dietary intake. Since dietary vitamin D is provided almost exclusively from vitamin D fortified dairy products, the child who is routinely ingesting an unusual or noncommercial (non–vitamin D fortified) source of milk (e.g., goat's milk; fresh, noncommercial cow's milk) should be evaluated carefully to confirm that the sunlight exposure and other dietary vitamin D sources are adequate to ensure optimal vitamin D status during all seasons. This is particularly important in children with darkly pigmented skin. Most one-a-day type vitamin and mineral supplements for children contain

TABLE 82-1. Recommended Dietary Allowances for Vitamin D, Calcium, Phosphorus, and Magnesium for Adults and Children

Category	Age (yr) or Condition	Vitamin D[a] (IU)	Calcium (mg)	Phosphorus (mg)	Magnesium (mg)
Infants	0.0–0.5	300	400	300	40
	0.5–1.0	400	500	500	60
Children	1–3	400	800	800	80
	4–6	400	800	800	80
	7–10	400	800	800	170
Males	11–14	400	1,200	1,200	270
	15–18	400	1,200	1,200	350
	19–24	400	1,200	1,200	350
	25–50	200	800	800	350
	51+	200	800	800	350
Females	11–14	400	1,200	1,200	280
	15–18	400	1,200	1,200	300
	19–24	400	1,200	1,200	280
	25–50	200	800	800	280
	51+	200	800	800	280
Pregnant		400	1,200	1,200	320
Lactating	1st 6 mo	400	1,200	1,200	355
	2nd 6 mo	405	1,200	1,200	340

[a] As cholecalciferol, 10 μg of cholecalciferol = 400 IU of vitamin D.

the RDA for vitamin D but contain no or minimal calcium. Calcium supplements should be evaluated for elemental calcium content (Table 82-4) rather than the compound content (i.e., elemental calcium versus calcium carbonate) to ensure accurate comparison to the RDA, which is expressed as elemental calcium. Healthy children with normal intake of calcium and vitamin D do not require monitoring of bone density unless there is a strong family history of osteoporosis.

Children who have chronic illness that includes unusual intestinal or renal calcium losses are at higher risk for bone density abnormalities. These patients should have their dietary intake (food and supplements) carefully evaluated as described above. In addition, serum vitamin D levels should be checked, treated if abnormal, supplemented, and rechecked to confirm normalization of the serum level. Since serum calcium levels usually are well maintained, the decision to supplement the calcium intake depends more on the evaluation of the usual dietary intake and quantification of the chronic gastrointestinal (GI) or renal losses. Gastrointestinal fat malabsorption increases the risk for low bone density through two mechanisms: (1) direct loss of fat-soluble vitamins, including vitamin D, and consequently low calcium absorption, and (2) binding of intestinal calcium to the unabsorbed fat, resulting in excessive fecal loss of calcium.

The other common risk factor for low bone mass development in children and adolescents with chronic disease is the use of medications known to negatively affect bone mineralization and growth. Oral corticosteroid medication is used frequently in pediatric care for a variety of GI and other diseases and is known to impair normal bone metabolism and growth in children and adults. Other medications (Table 82-5) such as furosemide, methotrexate, phenytoin, and phenobarbital also negatively affect calcium and/or vitamin D metabolism and thus may result in suboptimal bone mass development. The exact clinical impact of these drugs on bone mineralization during childhood and the impact on bone health in adulthood are unclear and the subject of ongoing clinical investigation. Pathologic vertebral fractures and other bone fractures with minimal trauma are seen in children on oral corticosteroids.[5] Patients with conditions requiring the medications discussed above, those with pathologic fractures, and those with an unusual fracture history (multiple fractures, fracture with minimal trauma) should have a baseline bone mass status evaluated by DXA and have follow-up evaluations to determine the success of intervention or the progression of the disease if the initial scan shows an abnormal pattern of mineralization. Children who have a baseline DXA scan that is normal and continue to require the risk-associated medication should be re-evaluated at intervals of 1 to 2 years.

Other nongastrointestinal disorders can impair calcium absorption or metabolism and increase the risk of osteoporosis. Renal disease, as previously mentioned, can increase risk due to the tubular disorders that result in calcium loss, secondary hyperparathyroidism, and chronic metabolic acidosis. Endocrine disorders with as-

TABLE 82-2. Dietary Sources of Calcium

Food	Serving Size	Calcium (mg)
Milk and milk products		
Milk (e.g., skim, whole)	8 oz	300
Ice cream, vanilla	8 oz	208
Ice milk, vanilla	8 oz	283
Nonfat dry milk	1 tbs	57
Yogurt, whole milk	8 oz	275
Yogurt, skim with nonfat milk solids	8 oz	452
Cheese		
American	1 oz	195
Cheddar	1 oz	211
Cottage, creamed	8 oz	211
Cottage, low-fat dry	8 oz	138
Cream cheese	1 oz	23
Parmesan, grated	1 tbs	69
Swiss	1 oz	259
Fish/seafood		
Mussels (meat only)	3½ oz	88
Oysters	5–8 medium	94
Salmon, canned with bones	3½ oz	198
Sardines, canned with bones	3½ oz	449
Shrimp	3½ oz	63
Fruit		
Figs, dried	5 medium	126
Orange	1 medium	65
Prunes, dried	10 large	51
Nuts/seeds		
Almonds or hazelnuts	12–15	38
Sesame seeds	1 oz	28
Sunflower seeds	1 oz	34
Vegetables		
Bean curd (tofu)	3½ oz	128
Beans, garbanzo	½ cup	80
Beans, pinto	½ cup	135
Beans, red kidney	½ cup	110
Broccoli, cooked	⅔ cup	88
Chard, cooked[a]	½ cup	61
Collard greens, cooked[a]	½ cup	152
Fennel, raw	3½ oz	100
Kale, cooked	½ cup	134
Lettuce, romaine	3½ oz	68
Mustard greens, cooked[a]	½ cup	145
Rutabaga, cooked	½ cup	59
Seaweed, agar, raw	3½ oz	567
Seaweed, kelp, raw	3½ oz	1,093
Squash, acorn	½ medium, baked	62

[a] Foods high in oxalic acid, which hinders absorption
(Data from U.S. Department of Agriculture, Human Nutrition Information Service.)

TABLE 82-3. Food Sources of Calcium Providing the Calcium Equivalent of 1 (8 oz) Cup of Milk

¾ cup yogurt,[a] plain or flavored
⅞ cup yogurt,[a] fruited
1½ oz cheddar cheese
2 cups cottage cheese
⅘ cup almonds
2½ oz sardines

[a] Dried milk solids added.

sociated risk for low bone mass include hyperthyroidism, Cushing's disease, hyperparathyroidism, rickets, and hypogonadism. Also at risk are children and adolescents with anorexia nervosa and young women athletes with secondary amenorrhea. One recent report showed a surprising long-term (5-year) loss of bone mass in children who survived severe burn injury.[6] Children and adolescents with these diagnoses should have a baseline DXA evaluation for bone mass and follow-up examinations as indicated by the level of mineralization abnormality, ongoing nature and severity of the illness, and other associated risk factors such as calcium and vitamin D intake and level of physical activity.

INTERPRETATION AND TREATMENT

In most settings, the DXA scan of the anteroposterior view of the lumbar vertebrae (L1–4 or L2–4) will be used for clinical interpretation and compared to healthy children of the same gender and chronologic age by year. The report includes information such as bone area (cm^2), bone mineral content (g), and bone mineral density (g/cm^2) for each vertebral body and the mean of all four.

TABLE 82-4. Elemental Calcium Content of Calcium Salts

Supplement	Percent Calcium	Ca^{++} in 1000-mg Dose	mEq Ca^{++}/g
Calcium acetate	25	250	12.6
Calcium carbonate	40	400	20
Calcium citrate	21	210	12
Calcium glubionate	6.5	65	3.3
Calcium gluconate	9.3	90	4.6
Calcium lactate	13	130	9.2

(Adapted from Facts and Comparisons, Inc., January 1996.)

TABLE 82-5. Medications Affecting Calcium

Medication	Effect
Antacids containing aluminum	
Maalox, Mylanta, Amphojel, and others	Increased calcium excretion
Antibiotics	
Tetracycline	Decreased absorption of calcium
Erythromycin	
Isoniazid (used to treat tuberculosis)	
Anticoagulants	
Heparin	Increased calcium secretion
Cholesterol-reducing drugs	
Cholestyramine	Increased calcium excretion
Diuretics	
Furosemide	Increased calcium excretion in urine
Thiazide group	Decreased calcium excretion in urine
Hormone preparations	
Corticosteroids	Increased trabecular bone loss
Thyroid hormone	Increased bone loss

The z score (standard deviation score) for the patient is given, which allows comparison with the reference database. A z score of zero is the mean (similar to the 50th percentile on a growth chart) for the reference data, with $+1$, $+2$ and -1, -2 representing ± 1 and 2 standard deviations of the reference mean. The results are also reported as the percent predicted comparing the patient to the reference database for bone mineral density for that age and gender group.

Since DXA measurements are new to clinical pediatrics, the approach to interpretation of the scans is evolving. In general, a DXA result that shows the patient with a z score of greater than -2 (2 standard deviations below the mean) for age and gender is clinically significant and should be considered for treatment. In some high-risk settings, such as GI conditions that include continued symptoms of malabsorption, poor oral intake, and/or decreased physical activity and require continued oral steroids, intervention may be considered in patients with a z score of less than -1. Clinical judgment based on all of the interrelated factors is important in deciding on an approach to therapy and monitoring of the patient with reduced bone mineral density.

The approach to treatment of low bone mineral density also is evolving. The etiology of low bone density is multifactorial, and, in general, each of these potential contributory factors should be considered in the therapeutic approach. Calcium intake is a major modifiable determinant in bone mineral density.[7,8] The first step is to determine the usual dietary intake of calcium from a diet record (minimum of 3 days) or from a calcium intake questionnaire. This information will allow the physician to compare the individual patient's intake to the RDA for age and gender and determine if the intake is adequate. It also will provide valuable information about the possibility of increasing the food-based calcium intake and how to prescribe calcium supplementation liquid or tablets, if necessary. The use of dietary calcium, primarily from dairy products, should be encouraged as the first step in increasing calcium intake. Total (food and supplements) calcium intake should be increased to about two times the RDA for the patient. Patients with a history of renal stones may have an increased risk of recurrence of renal stones on a high-calcium diet, and the risks and benefits of calcium supplementation should be carefully considered. In general, patients should not routinely consume more that 4 g of calcium per day, because of increased risks of side effects.

Vitamin D intake and serum vitamin D levels should be evaluated in patients with chronic cholestatic liver disease, chronic pancreatic insufficiency, or chronic malabsorption. Any patient with a low bone mineral density and low or low-normal serum vitamin D levels should be considered for supplementation at about two times the RDA. Serum levels should be checked after supplementation to confirm that the values are normal. Note that most food vitamin D comes from vitamin D fortified dairy products, so a patient who does not consume these products may be at risk. Vitamin D is also acquired from sunlight exposure, so special considerations are needed for patients who are rarely outdoors, live in areas with severe winter conditions limiting outside activities, or have darkly pigmented skin.

Weight-bearing physical activity is also a modifiable determinant of bone mineral density. A component of therapy for low bone mineral density is to encourage weight-bearing activities on a regular basis. Activities that are not fully weight-bearing, such as swimming and bicycling, do not offer as much bone formation stimulation as full weight-bearing activities, such as walking, running, and stair climbing. Patients should be encouraged to include age-appropriate activities in daily routines. This bone-healthy activity will need to be continued throughout the life cycle.

The effect of oral corticosteroid medications in the growing child is not completely understood, although it is well accepted that in adults steroid-induced osteoporosis is a common complication of therapy in a wide variety of diseases. The use of steroid medications is a risk for poor bone mineral density and other complications in children, and in practice, physicians are always alert

k = 1.286   d0 = 146.6(1.000H)

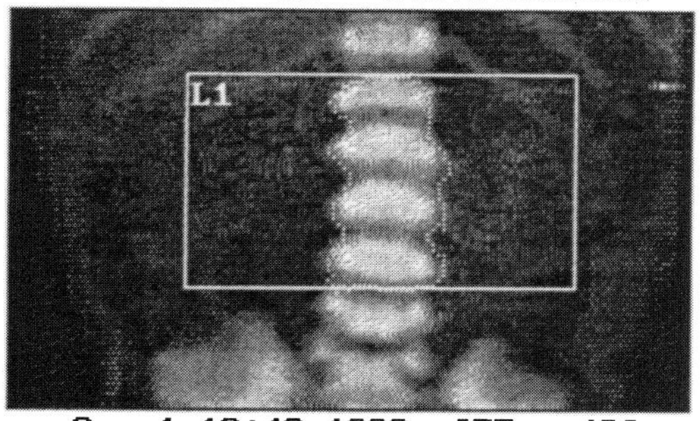

·Sep 1 13:48 1993   [75 x 43]

A   Infant Spine V4.63

```
A11228913    Wed Nov 22 12:42 1989
Name:             Infant Spine - LCM
Comment:
I.D.:                      Sex:    F
S.S.#:          -  -    Ethnic:
ZIPCode: 39SA   Height:  51.00 cm
Scan Code:   J1 Weight:   3.42 kg
BirthDate: 11/21/89       Age:    0
Physician:     PR SALLE
Image not for diagnostic use


   TOTAL BMD CV FOR L1 - L4   1.0%

   C.F.    0.998     1.035     1.000

Region    Area      BMC       BMD
          (cm2)    (grams)  (gms/cm2)
-------  --------  --------  --------
   L1   7.8723    2.7046    0.3436
```

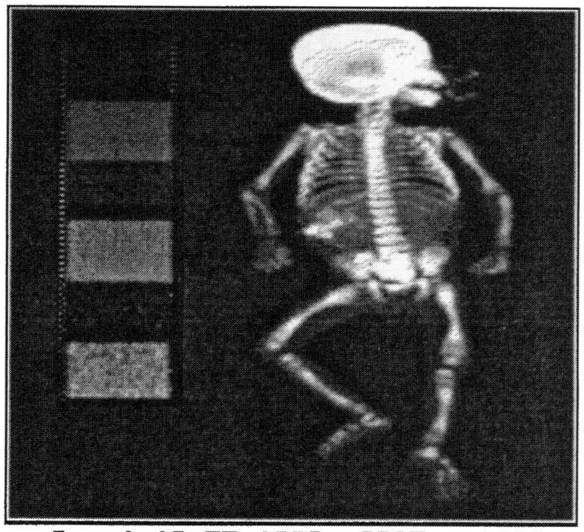

```
V07079203    Tue Jul 7 16:38 1992
Name:               INFANT WB #3
Comment:            CONG OP, PR1
I.D.:          KOO  Sex:      M
S.S.#:          -  -   Ethnic:    C
ZIP Code:           Height:  '   "
Scan Code.          PWB Weight:
BirthDate: 02/02/90      Age:    2
Physician:     WANG/KOO
Image not for diagnostic use

   C.F.    0.997     1.083     1.000

Region    Area      BMC       BMD
          (cm2)    (grams)  (gms/cm2)
-------  --------  --------  --------

GLOBAL  652.95    342.53    0.525
```

·Sep 1 13:57 1993   [267 x 166]

B   Infant Whole Body V5.65

FIGURE 82-1. Example of infant DXA scans evaluating (A) lumbar spine and (B) whole body. BMC, bone mineral content; BMD, bone mineral density.

k = 1.138   d0 =   43.4(1.000H)   7.118

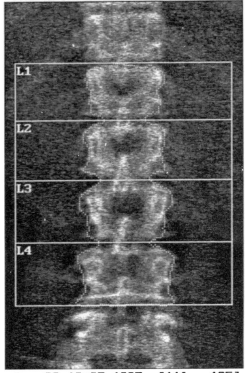

·Aug 22 12:35 1995   [116 x 135]
Hologic QDR (S/N 45018)
Lumbar Spine V8.15a:3

A

R03279506   Mon Mar 27 03:15 1995
Name: COMPARE   SPINE   BJL
Comment: 901
I.D.:   Sex: F
S.S.#:   – –   Ethnic:
ZIPCode: Height: 167.70 cm
Operator: 175 Weight: 68.80 kg
BirthDate: 09/26/42   Age: 52
Physician:
Image not for diagnostic use

TOTAL BMD CV FOR L1 – L4   1.0%

C.F.   1.028   1.006   1.000

Region	Est.Area (cm²)	Est.BMC (grams)	BMD (gms/cm²)
L1	11.55	8.00	0.693
L2	13.06	10.53	0.806
L3	14.54	11.70	0.805
L4	16.75	13.22	0.789
TOTAL	55.90	43.45	0.777

WALTHAM IMAGING CENTER

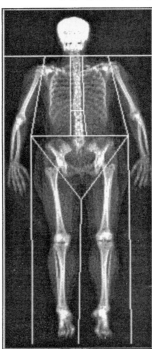

oSep 20 12:18 1995   [318 x 150]
Hologic QDR-4500 (S/N 4500)
Whole Body V8.10a:3

B

W0427950P   Thu Apr 27 16:02 1995
Name: WB #2
Comment:
I.D.:   BCA   Sex: F
S.S.#:   – –   Ethnic: W
ZIP Code: Height:5' 9"
Operator: MEK Weight: 155
BirthDate: 09/08/56   Age: 38
Physician:
Image not for diagnostic use

TOTAL BMC and BMD CV is < 1.0%
C.F.   1.037   1.019   1.000

Region	Area (cm2)	BMC (grams)	BMD (gms/cm2)
L Arm	232.09	192.05	0.827
R Arm	243.72	203.71	0.836
L Ribs	156.94	113.12	0.721
R Ribs	150.30	111.81	0.744
T Spine	144.49	139.39	0.965
L Spine	58.54	78.98	1.349
Pelvis	277.35	296.63	1.070
L Leg	421.01	529.50	1.258
R Leg	410.21	507.11	1.236
SubTot	2094.66	2172.30	1.037
Head	254.52	675.24	2.653
TOTAL	2349.18	2847.54	1.212

to the risks and limit the use of oral steroids as much as possible. Long-term or frequent intermittent use of steroids is an indication for a baseline DXA evaluation. If the medication continues to be clinically required, annual DXA evaluations should be considered as part of monitoring for side effects and response to therapy aimed to improve bone mineral density.

REFERENCES

1. Ponder SW. Clinical uses of bone densitometry in children: are we ready yet? Clin Pediatr 1995;34:237–240

2. Fassler ALC, Bonjour JP. Osteoporosis as a pediatric problem. Pediatr Clin North Am 1995;42:811–824

3. Welten DC, Kemper HCG, Post GB et al. Weight-bearing activity during youth is a more important factor for peak bone mass than calcium intake. J Bone Miner Res 1994;9: 1089–1096

4. National Academy of Sciences. Recommended Dietary Allowances. Washington, DC: National Academy Press, 1989.

5. Semeao E, Stallings V, Peck S. Vertebral compression fractures in pediatric patients with Crohn's disease. Gastroenterology

6. Klein GL, Herndon DN, Langman CB et al. Long-term reduction in bone mass after severe burn injury in children. J Pediatr 1995;126:252–256

7. Johnson CC, Miller JZ, Slemenda CW et al. Calcium supplementation and increases in bone mineral density in children. N Engl J Med 1992;327:82–87

8. Lloyd T, Andon MB, Rollings N et al. Calcium supplementation and bone mineral density in adolescent girls. JAMA 1993;270:841–844

FIGURE 82-2. Example of adult DXA scan evaluating *(A)* lumbar spine and *(B)* whole body. Note that in whole body scans, various body parts may be highlighted.

83

LAPAROSCOPY

ANDREW M. DAVIDOFF
PERRY W. STAFFORD

Laparoscopy represents a new and exciting approach for the performance of "minimally invasive" operative procedures. A laparoscope is passed through a port generally placed in the umbilicus and into the peritoneal cavity, which has been distended by carbon dioxide. This camera is used to observe the performance of an operation that is performed using special instruments passed through additional trocars placed through small stab wounds across the anterior abdominal wall. Vessels can be controlled with electrocautery or endoscopic clips, tissues can be stapled and divided with an endoscopic linear stapler, and specimens can be collected and withdrawn from the peritoneal cavity in an endoscopic sac. Additionally, sutures can be easily placed and knots tied either intra- or extracorporeally.

There has been tremendous enthusiasm in the United States for laparoscopic procedures in adults, and this has now extended to children. Like adult endosurgery, however, pediatric endosurgery is not an innovation. Gans and Berci[1] advocated the use of endoscopy and peritoneoscopy in infants and children for diagnostic and therapeutic purposes in the early 1970s. Several years later, Rodgers and Talbert[2] reported the use of diagnostic thoracoscopy in children for the evaluation of pleural or parenchymal disease, mediastinal lesions, and cancer staging. Widespread acceptance of laparoscopic cholecystectomy for adults occurred following the Southern Surgeons Club report of 1991.[3] Since then the indications for laparoscopic and thoracoscopic approaches for surgical procedures performed in adult patients have expanded dramatically. Acceptance of endosurgical ap-

proaches by pediatric surgeons has followed by about a year. There is now an explosion of papers in the pediatric literature describing successful endosurgical approaches to nearly all of the operations performed by pediatric surgeons.

Real and theoretic benefits of the "minimally invasive" surgical approach for pediatric and school-age patients include better visualization of certain areas, less perioperative pain and anxiety, decreased postoperative ileus, shortened hospital stay, faster return to school and full activity, fewer respiratory complications, and improved cosmetic result. In addition, there may be a lower incidence of postoperative adhesive bowel disease. Limitations of the endoscopic approach include the loss of tactile sensation and depth perception, added expense such as for disposable equipment, occasionally longer operative times, and the necessity for additional training and expertise. The limitations are likely to be overcome by new developments such as endosurgical ultrasound, improved video, cheaper and smaller instruments, and appropriate supervision. Already, the development of high-resolution imaging using the newer three-chip cameras has permitted the miniaturization of the laparoscope to a size appropriate for even small infants. Endoscopes as small as 2 mm are currently available; these small instruments maintain an excellent degree of visualization. Also, several companies are now introducing instruments designed specifically for smaller pediatric patients.

The early experience with pediatric laparoscopy suggests that most, if not all, of the operations commonly performed by pediatric surgeons can be performed safely, with comparable results to open approaches, and expediently with experience. This requires appropriate training and experienced assistance for the more advanced endo-surgical procedures during the learning phase. Long-term results are currently being evaluated. There should be a clearly demonstrated benefit of a laparoscopic approach over the conventional, time-tested open technique. The ability simply to do an operation through the laparoscope is not sufficient.

CHOLECYSTECTOMY

The laparoscopic era was ushered in with laparoscopic cholecystectomy. In the short period of time from the late 1980s when the procedure was first performed in the United States, to 1991 when the Southern Surgeons Club report[3] confirmed its safety and efficacy, the laparoscopic approach has become the gold standard for performing cholecystectomy. Painful subcostal or upper midline incisions are replaced by four small stab wounds, and patients typically go home on the first or second postoperative day. The procedure is performed by identifying, isolating, clipping, and then dividing the cystic duct and artery. The gallbladder is then dissected free from the liver bed with electrocautery. The applicability of the laparoscopic approach to cholecystectomy in children has been confirmed in several large series of pediatric patients.[4,5] The procedure has become so routine that many surgeons have noticed a significant increase in patient referral, particularly patients with sickle cell disease and asymptomatic cholelithiasis.

An intraoperative cholangiogram can be easily performed laparoscopically. Various techniques have been described including passing an angiocatheter through the abdominal wall and into the gallbladder under direct vision or passing a variety of catheters including cholangio-catheters or ureteral stents into the common bile duct through a nick made in the cystic duct after it has been clipped proximally. Many surgeons find fluoroscopic evaluation quicker and easier than taking individual radiographs. The most appropriate management of choled-ocholithiasis remains unsettled and depends in large part on local expertise. Some prefer to clear the common duct with either pre- or postoperative endoscopic retrograde cholangiopancreatography. Others are willing to undertake a laparoscopic common bile duct exploration. This can be performed with ductal irrigation, choledochos-copy and pushing stones through the ampulla of Vater, or wire basket extraction, all done through the cystic duct stump. Very experienced laparoscopists may open the common duct in performing the exploration and then sew it closed it over a T tube.

APPENDECTOMY

Appendicitis is the most common intra-abdominal surgical emergency in children. The assessment of the laparoscopic approach to the performance of this procedure has, therefore, received great scrutiny.[6] The performance of an appendectomy laparoscopically is technically straightforward, requiring two trocar sites in addition to an umbilical port for the laparoscope. The base of the appendix and mesoappendix can be stapled and divided with an endoscopic linear stapler, although a loop or clip can be used, and the appendix then placed in an endo-scopic sac prior to its removal from the peritoneal cavity.

The benefits of the laparoscopic approach over a conventional open one are controversial, however. An open appendectomy can often be performed quickly and through an incision smaller than the sum of the length of the trocar sites. The cost of the laparoscopic equipment currently makes this approach more expensive, although several studies have suggested that this may be offset by decreased narcotic use postoperatively, shorter hospitalization, and earlier return to full activity. Clear benefits include better ability to examine the peritoneal cavity and other viscera in the event that a normal appendix is found and a lower incidence of wound infection. Additionally, many authors have suggested that the laparoscopic approach is also better in cases of perforated appendicitis, as the peritoneal cavity can be better visualized and irrigated. A surgical drain can be placed through one of the trocar sites. Longer follow-up of these patients is required to determine whether the theoretic decrease in the incidence of adhesive bowel disease with the laparoscopic approach is in fact realized.

ANTIREFLUX PROCEDURES

Gastroesophageal reflux is extremely common in infants and children, and antireflux procedures represent one of the most common operations performed at most children's hospitals. Fundoplication is likely to be one of the procedures for which patients would most benefit from a laparoscopic approach. This procedure is often performed in debilitated children with significant pulmonary disease. These patients are among those who would potentially benefit most from a minimally invasive approach that avoids a painful, upper abdominal incision, in addition to the other general benefits of a laparoscopic approach previously mentioned. The laparoscopic approach to Nissen fundoplication, first reported in 1991,[7] appears highly successful in adult patients, although long-term follow-up is not yet available. The earliest description of this technique in children was a case report published in 1993 of a laparoscopic Nissen fundoplication performed in a 10-year-old child.[8] Since that time, a few groups have described a small but successful (short-term) experience with laparoscopic Nissen fundoplication in children and even infants.[9,10]

Pediatric surgeons differ on the details and subtleties of performing both open and laparoscopic Nissen fundoplications. Laparoscopic procedures should, however, satisfy the same anatomic and physiologic goals as the open procedure. One method involves the placement of five trocar sheaths: an umbilical port for the laparoscope, a subxiphoid fan retractor for the liver, two right upper quadrant trocars for the operating surgeon, and a left upper quadrant port for stomach traction. The short gastric vessels can be divided after being secured with clips or staples. The retroesophageal dissection is done bluntly, and the diaphragmatic crura can be closed. A 360 degree circumferential wrap is constructed and secured with several nonabsorbable, braided sutures. A fundoplication is frequently performed in conjunction with gastrostomy tube placement. This is performed easily following the fundoplication, either laparoscopically, by percutaneous endoscopic technique, or open, through a trocar site. Patients with poor gastric emptying may require a pyloroplasty in combination with the fundoplication. This can be done through a trocar site, since laparoscopic pyloroplasty in children has yet to be reported, although this is likely to be feasible as instrumentation improves and endoscopic experience increases. It is also possible to perform other antireflux procedures, such as a posterior gastropexy or anterior fundoplication, with a laparoscopic approach.

The laparoscopic approach to performing a fundoplication is clearly an advanced laparoscopic procedure with a significant learning curve and one where the surgeon should have significant laparoscopic experience. Nevertheless, it is technically quite feasible to perform, as documented by several large series, and the benefit of the avoidance of a large upper abdominal incision is significant.

SPLENECTOMY

Splenectomy, as with fundoplication, when performed using a traditional, open technique, involves a significant upper abdominal incision. Therefore, it is not surprising that splenectomy is another attractive procedure to perform laparoscopically, although, again, this is an advanced laparoscopic procedure. Indications for splenectomy have already been discussed in detail and are generally performed in children with hematologic disorders or for cancer staging.

The procedure is usually performed with four trocars, two in the right upper quadrant and two in the left lower quadrant, in addition to the umbilical port for the laparoscope. The short gastric vessels are controlled with clips, while the hilar splenic vessels are stapled and divided

with an endoscopic linear stapler. The spleen can then be placed in an endoscopic sac and morcellated with a finger fracture technique prior to removal, although tissue morcellating devices are commercially available. Either method allows removal of the spleen without having to enlarge a 12-mm trocar site, although the fracture method provides a better specimen for histologic evaluation. Very large spleens, as encountered in patients with sickle cell disease and splenic sequestration, may be difficult to manipulate for hilar visualization and dissection, thereby precluding a laparoscopic approach. The peritoneal cavity can be easily surveyed to determine the presence of accessory spleens, which can then be removed. Also, where clinically indicated, cholecystectomy can be readily performed using the same trocar sites.

Early reports have demonstrated that splenectomy can be safely and successfully accomplished laparoscopically in children.[11,12] Operative time and equipment costs are currently greater for a laparoscopic approach, although with operator experience and equipment refinement these will decrease. Blood loss can be kept to a minimum and postoperative pain and narcotic use diminished. Generally, patients have a shorter hospitalization, although children with certain underlying diseases may be more amenable to early discharge than others.

DIAGNOSTIC LAPAROSCOPY

In addition to being used to perform specific procedures, laparoscopy can be used as a diagnostic tool. It is of particular benefit when the condition diagnosed is a nonsurgical one, thereby avoiding an unnecessary laparotomy incision. It is also useful for inspecting the entire peritoneal cavity, especially when the exact location of intra-abdominal pathology is not known. This ensures that the appropriate incision can be made to avoid awkward operative exposure. Alternatively, once the diagnosis has been made, many surgical conditions can be treated definitively with a laparoscopic approach.

Abdominal Pain

Laparoscopy can be useful in evaluating children with abdominal pain of unclear etiology, many of whom have undergone an extensive radiographic workup. Findings at laparoscopy are varied. In some patients, there may be evidence of chronic inflammation of the appendix. Some authors have reported relief of pain following an appendectomy even when no pathologic diagnosis is documented. Others believe that tethering bands to the cecum and right colon or other bands or adhesions may cause chronic abdominal pain and have found that when these are taken down, patients' symptoms resolve. It is unclear whether relief is due to the elimination of pathology or a placebo effect.

In other patients, unsuspected abdominal wall defects may be visualized, including ventral, inguinal, or femoral hernias. Fascial defects are very well demonstrated with laparoscopy and pneumoperitoneum. This approach is particularly useful in obese patients or those with a question of recurrence or with an unusually located bulge, where the diagnosis of a hernia can be difficult.

Other findings may include the presence of a Meckel's diverticulum or of an unsuspected intestinal volvulus, both of which can be resected laparoscopically using the endoscopic linear stapler. In the case of volvulus, stomas can be created or bowel continuity restored with laparoscopic assistance. Findings at laparoscopy including bowel wall induration, creeping fat, and serositis are suggestive of inflammatory bowel disease. If the disease is limited, a laparoscopically assisted bowel resection can be performed. Alternatively, laparoscopy can be used to document the presence and extent of multiple areas of disease.

Laparoscopy may also identify pathology of the gonads as the etiology for abdominal pain. In males, torsion of undescended, intra-abdominal testes has been diagnosed and treated. In females, ovarian torsion can be diagnosed and either detorsion or oophorectomy performed laparoscopically. The gynecologic differential diagnosis for adolescent females with pain is extensive and includes endometriosis, adhesions (e.g., postoperative or perihepatic), ovarian cysts or tubo-ovarian abscess, or uterine malformations.[13] Many of these conditions can be treated as well as diagnosed laparoscopically.

Abdominal Mass

Laparoscopy may also be useful for the evaluation of abdominal masses in children. A diagnosis may be made by simple visual inspection of a lesion, or a laparoscopically guided biopsy may provide tissue for histologic evaluation. Cystic lesions such as a choledochal cyst, splenic cyst, or gastrointestinal duplication can be identified and occasionally treated laparoscopically. Intra-abdominal lymph nodes can be biopsied to make the diagnosis of cancer, sarcoidosis, or infection, among other things. Finally, tumors can be biopsied where appropriate and occasionally resected.[14]

The Children's Cancer Group and the Pediatric Oncology Group are currently involved in new intergroup studies to evaluate the role of laparoscopy in the diagnosis and management of children with cancer. With advances in adjuvant therapy, the role of surgery as part of multimodal treatment strategies is being evaluated. Although certain tumors are best treated with traditional open approaches, some in which preoperative chemoradiation is employed may benefit from a minimally invasive approach to obtain tissue for diagnosis. This may hasten postoperative recovery, permit earlier initiation of therapy, and minimize

wound complications while maintaining diagnostic accuracy. In addition to diagnosing primary tumors, laparoscopy can be used to document metastatic spread to the liver or peritoneal surfaces, and staging accomplished through lymph node biopsy and even splenectomy can be performed with a minimally invasive approach.

OTHER PROCEDURES

Meckel's Diverticulum

A Meckel's diverticulum, either diagnosed preoperatively or discovered at exploration, can be easily resected laparoscopically.[15] The base can be secured with either the endoscopic linear stapler or an endoloop. Care should be taken to control the arterial supply of the diverticulum and to ensure that all ectopic mucosa has been removed.

Achalasia

Esophagomyotomy is highly effective in relieving symptoms of dysphagia in patients with achalasia, but enthusiasm for this procedure has been limited because of the need for a thoracotomy or laparotomy. Several series of adult patients and case reports in children have reported the successful performance of an esophagomyotomy both laparoscopically and thoracoscopically.[16,17] Concurrent esophagoscopy is performed during the procedure to distend the esophagus during the dissection and to determine if mucosal penetration has occurred.

Hirschsprung's Disease

The successful performance of laparoscopic pull-throughs for infants and children with Hirschsprung's disease is now being reported.[18] The techniques used involve modification of each of the three main approaches to the pull-through operation—Duhamel, Soave, and Swenson. As with the open procedures, these are being performed both as primary procedures in the neonate and as staged procedures in older children. Although the rectosigmoid bowel is inspected and mobilized intraperitoneally under laparoscopic guidance, much of the dissection and the anastomosis is performed transanally. Difficulties can occur when there is no obvious transition zone or in patients with total colonic aganglionosis.

Hypertrophic Pyloric Stenosis

A few surgeons have expressed enthusiasm for and demonstrated success at performing laparoscopic extramucosal pyloromyotomy in infants with hypertrophic pyloric stenosis, using very small instruments.[19] Documentation of the benefit of this approach over the already minimally invasive traditional, open approach may be difficult.

Adhesive Bowel Disease

The small bowel can be inspected and easily "run" laparoscopically to evaluate sites of obstruction, and bands or adhesions divided. Dilated, obstructed bowel may be very thin and friable and should be manipulated with great care. Dense abdominal adhesions and a "socked-in" abdomen may preclude laparoscopic exploration.

Peptic Ulcer Disease

A vagotomy can be preformed either thoracoscopically in the chest or laparoscopically in the abdomen. Generally, a truncal vagotomy is performed, but a modified highly selective vagotomy can be performed. Anteriorly the neurovascular bundles to the fundus can be clipped and divided, but posteriorly a truncal vagotomy must be performed.

Malrotation

Radiographic studies are frequently equivocal when determining the position of the ligament of Treitz; laparoscopy can be used to assess the rotation of the gastrointestinal tract. The ligament is identified by elevating the transverse colon and rolling the patient to the right to displace the bowel. Fixation of the cecum can also be easily assessed. In cases of malrotation, Ladd's bands can be lysed, the duodenum straightened, the mesentery broadened, and an appendectomy performed laparoscopically.[20] One concern with this approach is that desirable postoperative adhesions that form normally after an open procedure may be minimized with a laparoscopic approach.

Cholestasis

In addition to identifying the presence of a choledochal cyst, as already mentioned, laparoscopy can be used for the evaluation of other causes of cholestasis in newborns. The gallbladder can be searched for and extrahepatic bile ducts can be visualized either directly or by cholangiography. If present, these can be irrigated in cases where there is biliary sludge. A liver biopsy can also be obtained.

Nutrition Support

Patients who need enteral access but either cannot have endoscopy performed or require a jejunostomy may have a feeding tube placed laparoscopically. Once a site has been selected, transabdominally placed T fasteners arranged in a diamond configuration can secure the bowel to the anterior abdominal wall. A feeding tube can then be placed percutaneously into the bowel lumen using a Seldinger technique.

REFERENCES

1. Gans SI, Berci G. Advances in endoscopy of infants and children. J Pediatr Surg 1971;6:199–234
2. Rodgers BM, Talbert JL. Thoracoscopy for diagnosis of intrathoracic lesions in children. J Pediatr Surg 1976;11:703–708
3. Southern Surgeons Club. A prospective analysis of 1518 laparoscopic cholecystectomies. N Engl J Med 1991;324:1073–1078
4. Newman KD, Marman LM, Attori R et al. Laparoscopic cholecystectomy in pediatric patients. J Pediatr Surg 1992;26:1184–1185
5. Davidoff AM, Branum GD, Murray EA et al. The technique of laparoscopic cholecystectomy in children. Ann Surg 1992;215:186–191
6. Gilchrist BF, Lobe TE, Schropp KP et al. Is there a role for laparoscopic appendectomy in pediatric surgery. J Pediatr Surg 1992;27:209–214
7. Dallemauge B, Weerts JM, Jehacs et al. Laparoscopic Nissen fundoplication: preliminary report. Surg Laparosc Endosc 1991;1:138–143
8. Lobe TE, Schropp KP, Lunsford K. Laparoscopic Nissen fundoplication in childhood. J Pediatr Surg 1993;28:358–361
9. Lobe TE. Laparoscopic fundoplication. Semin Pediatr Surg 1993;2:178–181
10. Lloyd DM, Robertson GS, Johnstone JM. Laparoscopic Nissen fundoplication in children. Surg Endosc 1995;9:781–785
11. Moores DC, McKee MA, Wang H et al. Pediatric laparoscopic splenectomy. J Pediatr Surg 1995;30:1201–1205
12. Janu PG, Rogers DA, Lobe TE. A comparison of laparoscopic and traditional open splenectomy in childhood. J Pediatr Surg 1996;31:109–114
13. Goldstein DP. Acute and chronic pelvic pain. Pediatr Clin North Am 1989;36:573–580
14. Holcomb GW, Tomita SS, Haase GM et al. Minimally invasive surgery in children with cancer. Cancer 1995;76:121–128
15. Teitelbaum DH, Polley TZ, Obeid F. Laparoscopic diagnosis and excision of Meckel's diverticulum. J Pediatr Surg 1994;29:495–497
16. Pellegrini CA, Leichter R, Patti M et al. Thoracoscopic esophageal myotomy in the treatment of achalasia. Ann Thorac Surg 1993;56:680–682
17. Robertson FM, Jacir NN, Crombleholme TM et al. Thoracoscopic esophagomyotomy for achalasia in a child. J Pediatr Gastroenterol Nutr 1997;24(2):215–217.
18. Smith BM, Steiner RB, Lobe TE. Laparoscopic Duhamel pullthrough procedure for Hirschsprung's disease in childhood. J Laparoendosc Surg 1994;4:273–276
19. Alain JL, Grousseau D, Terrier G. Extramucosal pylorotomy by laparoscopy. J Pediatr Surg 1991;26:1191–1192
20. Waldhausen JHT, Sawin RS. Laparoscopic Ladd's procedure and assessment of malrotation. J Laparoendosc Surg 1996;6(Suppl 1):S103–S105.

84

PERCUTANEOUS ENTERAL ACCESS AND CARE OF GASTROSTOMY TUBES

SUSAN N. PECK

CHRIS A. LIACOURAS

DOUGLAS C. B. REDD

Providing satisfactory enteric nutrition access in the child with a chronic illness, failure to thrive, or neurologic impairment can be a challenge for the pediatric practitioner. Direct enteral access via a catheter placed into the stomach or small bowel offers a greater cost-benefit ratio for these patients than calories delivered via an intravenous (parenteral) route, which may cost $50,000 to $150,000/patient-year.[1,2] Enteral alimentation prevents mucosal atrophy, maintains normal gut flora, decreases bacterial translocation, and enhances enteral immunologic competence. Other unique applications for gastrostomy include gastric access for gastric decompression or to facilitate esophageal bougienage for esophageal strictures and to permit the administration of unpalatable medications or diets. Selecting the correct feeding appliance may be a challenging task, as the variety from which to choose is continually increasing. The goals of this chapter are to review the available options in feeding catheters and the alternative methods for their insertion to permit the pediatric practitioner to make a more informed decision.

Historically, gastrostomy has been achieved by an open surgical procedure in which a catheter is inserted directly into the stomach (Fig. 84-1). Although this procedure is routinely successful and usually uncomplicated, there are well-documented rates of morbidity and mortality.[3] Percutaneous gastrostomy, either by endoscopic,

fluoroscopic, or laparoscopic guidance, makes use of the Seldinger technique, which was first introduced for gastrostomy in the early 1980s. Once the gastric lumen has been accessed by needle and guidewire, feeding catheters can be placed either in an antegrade manner[4] with the catheter introduced through the oropharynx or in a retrograde manner with the catheter inserted through the abdominal and gastric walls. Technical success rates for these percutaneous procedures are comparable; failures of this technique are principally due to an inability to suitably distend the stomach below the costal margin (Fig. 84-2) and away from adjacent organs so access can be safely achieved.

Unlike surgical techniques for gastrostomy, higher rates of infection have been reported for the antegrade technique of gastrostomy,[5] owing to contamination of the catheter by oral flora.[6] Additional problems with the "pull" technique include the requirement for a patent esophagus, cost,[7] repeated insertion of the endoscope, potential esophageal injury during introduction of the feeding catheter, and the possible need for another sedation or endoscopic procedure for catheter removal. The "push" technique represents a modification of percutaneous gastrostomy and requires insertion of either the endoscope or laparoscope to visualize the insertion site.[8] In children requiring only gastric access for feeds or medication, primary insertion of a low profile gastrostomy cathe-

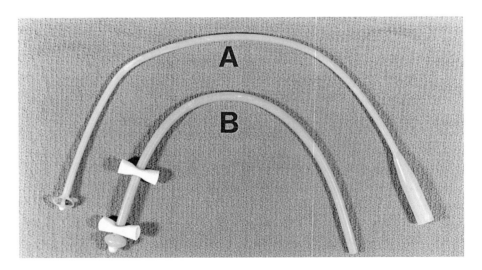

FIGURE 84-1. Surgically placed gastrostomy catheters include the *(A)* Malecot catheter and *(B)* de Pesser catheter.

ter may represent a reasonable option and avoids the need for a future procedure to exchange the surgically or percutaneously placed gastrostomy catheter for a low-profile device.[9] The procedure is no more involved than conventional percutaneous endoscopic gastrostomy (PEG) and has an operative time from needle insertion to button deployment of approximately 12 minutes.[10]

In children with gastroesophageal reflux (GER), anterograde percutaneous gastrojejunostomy may be considered instead of Nissen fundoplication with simultaneous gastrostomy tube placement.[11] This technique has the advantage of avoiding the major complications known to occur following surgery. However, maintenance of chronic transpyloric jejunal feeding catheters is not without problem or cost, with as many as one-third of patients requiring reinsertion because of jejunostomy tube malfunction or malplacement.[11]

Once a candidate for enteral access is identified, an evaluation is performed consisting of a complete history including current medications, past medical history (e.g., GER, failure to thrive, chronic illness, neurologic impairment), previous nutritional interventions (e.g., nasogastric feeds, oral supplementation, tolerance of current feeding regimen), and previous abdominal surgery (e.g., ventriculoperitoneal shunts, pacemakers, splenectomy). A review of prior studies including upper GI, abdominal plain films, pH probe, and endoscopy should be performed to assess the requirements for gastrostomy or gastrojejunostomy access. A physical examination with attention directed to findings that might complicate percutaneous access (e.g., severe scoliosis) is performed. An upper GI examination is indicated prior to percutaneous gastrostomy to exclude unsuspected esophageal stricture, verify satisfactory positioning of the stomach relative to the costal margin and colon, and confirm nor-

mal anatomic positioning of the duodenojejunal junction. Percutaneous gastrostomy can be safely performed in children with ventriculoperitoneal (VP) shunt, immunosuppression including acquired immunodeficiency syndrome (AIDS), and prior operation. In patients with a VP shunt, it is suggested that a minimum of 1 week elapse between shunt tubing insertion and PEG.[12] We believe that relative contraindications for PEG placement include malrotation of the small bowel that has not received operative correction. Patients with these unsuitable findings on upper GI study are referred for evaluation by the pediatric general surgeon for an open or laparoscopic gastrostomy. Other contraindications for percutaneous gastrostomy include uncorrectable coagulopathy, unsatisfactory anatomy including microgastria or partial gastrectomy with either small or inaccessible gastric remnants, massive ascites, portal hypertension with intra-abdominal varices, neutropenia,[1] and inflammatory conditions such as neoplasm or infection that may result in poor wound healing.

PROCEDURE

Percutaneous gastrostomy techniques involve the distention of the stomach with air to position the wall of the stomach against the anterior abdominal wall. In high-risk patients (e.g., neurologically impaired, scoliosis, prior abdominal surgery), a cursory abdominal ultrasound is useful to map out the left lobe of the liver, and the transverse colon should be localized, either by contrast administered on the night prior or by water-soluble contrast enema at the time of gastrostomy tube insertion. Subsequently, upper endoscopy is performed to identify

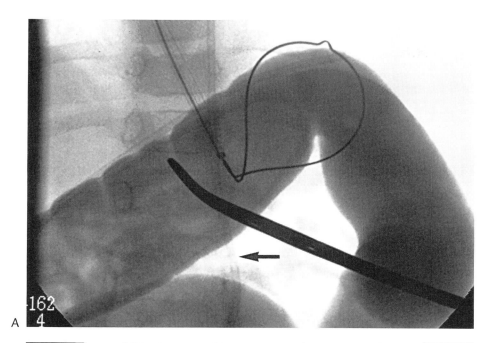

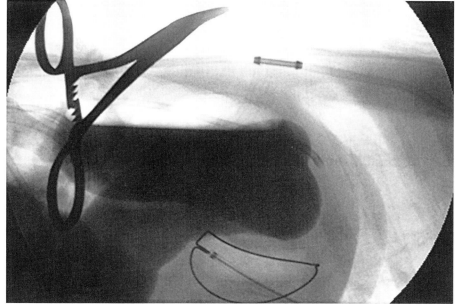

FIGURE 84-2. *(A)* Patient undergoing failed attempt at percutaneous fluoroscopic gastrostomy under conscious sedation. During this procedure, a water-soluble enema was used to opacify the colon, and an orogastric snare catheter was positioned within the stomach to capture the guidewire for antegrade gastrostomy catheter insertion. A hemostat overlies the costal margin. Not shown is the nasogastric catheter used for gastric insufflation, which was unsuccessful in sufficiently distending the stomach to permit safe percutaneous gastrostomy. Also note the presence of a ventriculoperitoneal shunt catheter (arrow) in the left upper quadrant. *(B)* A lateral view in the same patient shows the retrocolic positioning of the stomach. The procedure was successfully completed under general anesthesia using endoscopy, which permitted the stomach to be more completely distended in a better-controlled manner.

any esophageal or gastric mucosal abnormalities and for gastric insufflation. The gastric puncture site is then chosen along the gastric body at the junction of the upper and the middle third of the stomach at some distance from the pylorus. The risk of hemorrhage is diminished if one avoids the inferior epigastric artery that courses at the junction of the medial two-thirds and lateral one-third of the rectus muscle. Lidocaine or bupivacaine is infiltrated into the subcutaneous tissues, a small skin incision (5 mm) is made, and the subcutaneous tissues are bluntly dissected with the tip of a blunt-nosed hemostat. The distance from the skin to the anterior gastric wall is usually 1.5 to 3.0 cm in the child and 4 to 5 cm in the adult.[13] Gastric puncture is made with a brief, forceful thrust so as not to push the anterior gastric wall away from the anterior abdominal wall. However, extreme care is taken to avoid puncturing too deeply, which could compromise the pancreas, left kidney, aorta, or spleen. Once the needle has entered the stomach, the trocar is removed, and a wire loop is passed through the catheter into the gastric lumen. The wire loop is grasped with a forceps by the endoscopist or with a snare catheter and removed from the patient orally. The PEG tube is then attached to the wire loop, and with firm traction applied to the well-lubricated gastrostomy tube, the tube is passed through the patient's mouth, esophagus, and stomach and out through the puncture site on the anterior abdominal wall. Some resistance may be felt as the PEG tube traverses the thoracic inlet and gastroesophageal junction. Care is taken not to cause lacerations in the mouth and esophagus with manipulations of the wire loop and PEG catheter. The endoscope is once again passed into the patient's stomach to inspect for mucosal trauma and to evaluate the PEG tube's position against the anterior abdominal wall of the stomach.

Other percutaneous entry techniques do not require use of the endoscope for gastric insufflation or capture of the wire loop[4] or are performed in a retrograde manner requiring only the placement of a nasogastric tube for distention.[14] The use of gastric anchors has also been described with laparoscopic placement.

POSTPROCEDURE CARE

Postprocedurally, most pediatric series recommend a 1- to 3-day hospitalization for observation, feeding advancement, and the administration of intravenous antibiotics. Early feeding following PEG has been described,[10] but at our institution, the standard of care is a 2-day hospitalization. Patients are seen and evaluated daily in the hospital by the gastroenterologist or pediatric nurse practitioner and the interventional radiologist with whom the procedure is performed. Patients remain NPO for 8 hours immediately after PEG placement.

Feedings are subsequently initiated with the introduction of clear fluids followed by a gradual increase in enteral feeding. We routinely provide 48 hours of intravenous antibiotics (cefazolin sodium) beginning at the time of PEG placement. In PEGs with an external crossbar, the crossbar is turned 45 to 90 degrees every 3 to 4 hours and the PEG site assessed for edema, induration, erythema, and drainage. The external crossbar is manipulated to prevent complications secondary to postoperative edema. Once the edema resolves, the crossbar is repositioned to provide a snug fit against the abdomen. Abdominal radiographs are not routinely obtained, as many patients show some degree of pneumoperitoneum, which usually resolves over 24 to 72 hours without complication. Radiographic workup should be performed in those patients who develop increasing abdominal pain, vomiting, fever, abdominal distention, or abdominal fluid. Intravenous narcotics are avoided for pain, as they induce a pharmacologic ileus; our preference is to use parenteral nonsteroidals for discomfort.

The gastrostomy site is cleaned with soap and water every shift initially. Hydrogen peroxide is avoided because of its association with the formation of granulation tissue. Topical antibiotics are not indicated unless erythema or induration of the gastrostomy site is noted. The site is left uncovered without a dressing. Families often feel more comfortable with a spit gauze against the skin, but this is not typically necessary. Families receive extensive teaching regarding the care of the gastrostomy site and tube prior to discharge home.

COMPLICATIONS

Leakage of gastric contents, intraperitoneally (leading to peritonitis) or out through the skin entry site, resulting in cellulitis, is seen in fewer than 10% of patients. Morbidity associated with aspiration secondary to GER of gastric feedings may be minimized by gastrojejunostomy insertion, which may eliminate the need for surgical fundoplication in some patients.[11] Bleeding following percutaneous gastrostomy or gastrojejunostomy tube insertion has an incidence of 0.7%, slightly lower than seen following surgical gastrostomy.[15] Other potential complications following percutaneous gastrostomy include gastrocolic fistula, which can be seen in 3% to 10% of cases.[16]

CARE OF THE GASTROSTOMY TUBE

Once the gastrostomy tube is placed, daily care is required. Soap and water should be used to clean the area. Agents such as hydrogen peroxide should not be used, as they may cause local irritation. Occasionally, patients develop granulomas. Granulomas are accumulations of vascularized skin and scar tissue that form from the gastrostomy tube site. Granulomas can be controlled by cauterization with silver nitrate applicator sticks; however, surgical removal is sometimes necessary. Finally, the site should continually be monitored for signs of infection including erythema, fever, induration, and tenderness. Often, a yellow-green discharge is noted but without the above signs of infection. This typically represents a foreign body reaction and only requires appropriate cleaning.

TYPES OF CATHETERS FOR GASTROSTOMY FEEDING

The development of the PEG technique has led to the development of many new enteral feeding catheters; however, not all are appropriate for the pediatric population. It is difficult to select one product that will meet the needs of the majority of the patients treated in a pediatric facility. The PEG catheter must accommodate a 3-kg infant yet allow for the nutritional needs of an older child. The diameter of the catheter should be able to allow liquids to pass freely. In some patients, it must also be able to accommodate pureed foods or a jejunostomy tube through the middle to provide jejunal feeding capabilities.

At our facility, we currently use the Corpak PEG system. This system consists of a polyurethane tube with a collapsible internal bumper and an external crossbar. The pediatric system is size 15 Fr and is removable by traction. A jejunostomy tube (6 Fr) can be inserted through the gastrostomy tube to provide jejunal access and gastric decompression (Fig. 84-3). Placement of the jejunal catheter can be performed at the time of PEG placement or later when the need for jejunal feeding is identified.

Some children benefit from the initial placement of a low profile device. Older children prefer this type of tube because of cosmetics, while in younger children, low profile devices offer less chance of accidental removal. In the past, button gastrostomy insertion was a secondary procedure after the initial surgical or PEG placement; however, it can now be placed at time of the PEG. The Surgitek One-Step button (Fig. 84-4) is commonly used for this purpose. Operative time for percutaneous gastrostomy button insertion is short with an average of 12 minutes from needle insertion to button deployment.[18] The tube is made of silicone and is removed easily by traction. It is available in multiple sizes. The shaft length must be sized to the patient. Spacer discs are available, allowing the patient who is between sizes to have an adequate seal and prevent leakage of stomach contents onto the abdomen. The discs are placed between the

FIGURE 84-3. The Corpak gastrojejunostomy system allows for gastric and jejunal access immediately following percutaneous gastrostomy. After placement of the gastrostomy catheter during PEG, it is cut to length, and the gastrojejunostomy hub (large arrow) is attached; a diagnostic catheter is then inserted coaxially through the gastrostomy tube into the gastric lumen. The diagnostic catheter and a guidewire are then advanced across the pylorus and advanced distal to the duodenal-jejunal junction. The catheter is removed, and the jejunostomy catheter (small arrow) is then advanced over the guidewire and passed into the proximal jejunum.

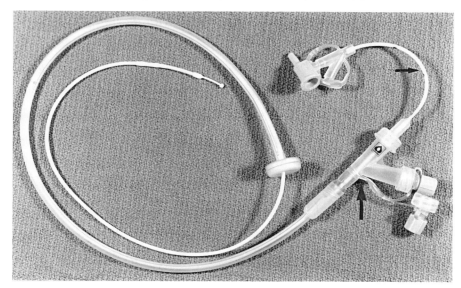

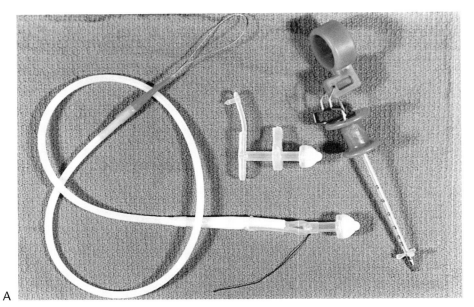

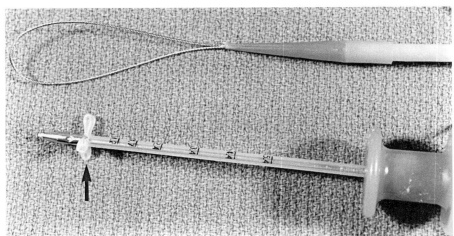

FIGURE 84-4. *(A)* The Surgitek One-Step button gastrostomy catheter system permits percutaneous delivery of a low-profile gastrostomy catheter during the initial percutaneous gastrostomy procedure. By constraining the wings of the gastrostomy tube within a peel-away sheath, the catheter can be safely delivered in the child in an antegrade manner. *(B)* The stomach is punctured using a trocar measuring device, and a wire loop is introduced in a conventional manner for pull-type gastrostomy. The "wings" of the trocar measuring device (arrow) are formed after entering the gastric lumen. The trocar is then gently withdrawn to seat the wings against the anterior gastric wall, and the stoma length is measured directly on the catheter. After the device is drawn through the tissues, the puncture site in the stomach and the tract is progressively dilated as the 18 Fr gastrostomy tube is delivered.

abdominal wall and the outside lip of the button. Gastric decompression is achieved by using a decompression tube that inactivates the antireflux valve in the mushroom tip of the catheter.

A myriad of replacement gastrostomy tubes exist and offer a variety of options for individual patients. "Mushroom-tip" catheters such as the de Pezzer gastrostomy tube and the Malecot gastrostomy tube are available, which are traditionally used in open gastrostomy placement. Both are made of silicone and are available in a variety of sizes (12 Fr to 24 Fr). One disadvantage is that placement of the mushroom-tip catheters requires the use of an obturator. The mushroom tip is extended with the obturator, and then the catheter is pushed through

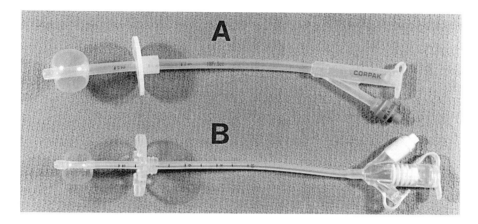

FIGURE 84-5. Replacement gastrostomy catheters include Corpak (A) and MIC (B) appliances, both of which are retained by a fluid-filled retention balloon within the gastric lumen and outer retention disc, which is applied to the abdominal wall.

the gastrostomy tract into the stomach. Placement is verified by aspiration and pH testing of the gastric contents (pH 4 to 6).

Balloon replacement catheters are manufactured by numerous suppliers. Catheters designed as gastrostomy feeding tubes are better suited to meet the needs of the pediatric patient. The external length is decreased, thus minimizing the risk of accidental removal. The internal balloon is designed to be circumferential, providing a tighter internal seal and decreasing leakage of gastric contents around the gastrostomy tube. The internal balloon should also be a low-volume balloon (5 to 10 ml), decreasing the amount of gastric capacity taken up by the gastrostomy balloon. Gastrostomy tube balloons are

FIGURE 84-6. Skin level replacement devices: MIC-KEY skin level jejunostomy (A), MIC-KEY skin level gastrostomy (B), and Bard button gastrostomy catheter (C). When placing these devices, which are available in 14 Fr and 18 Fr diameters, the shaft length must be selected after the tract length of the gastric stoma has been measured.

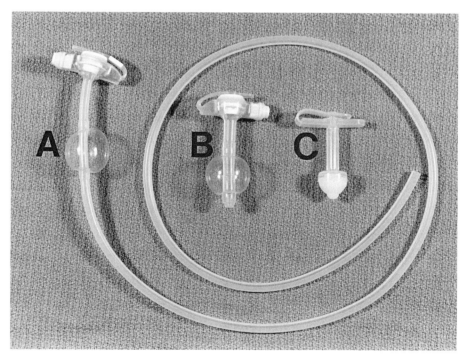

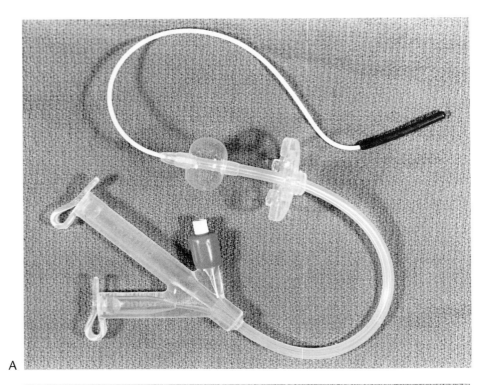

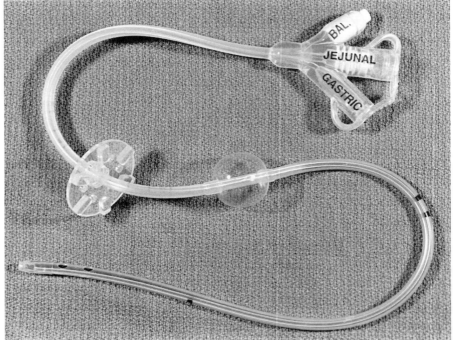

FIGURE 84-7. *(A)* Options in gastrojejunostomy catheters include the MIC gastroenteric catheter, which is retained in a manner similar to the replacement gastrostomy
catheter shown in Figure 84-5. The 16 Fr and 18 Fr diameters are ideally suited for
pediatric use. This appliance may be either placed surgically during open gastrostomy or, more commonly, inserted as a replacement device using fluoroscopic guidance through a mature gastric stoma. A catheter and guidewire are positioned across
the pylorus and advanced distal to the duodenal-jejunal junction. The catheter

inflated with water, not air, to maximize balloon life. Gastrostomy tubes used with children should be made of silicone to decrease the risk of latex sensitivity. External retention discs help minimize the risk of malposition. Many balloon replacement catheters are available as either a triple-port (gastric, medication, and balloon valve) tube or double-port (gastric and balloon valve) tube. The triple-port tube may be converted to a gastrojejunostomy tube by passing a 6 Fr jejunostomy tube through the gastric port. The stomach is then accessed through the medication port, allowing medications to be infused into the stomach and for gastric decompression while feeding through the jejunostomy tube. The size of the gastrostomy tube is printed on the balloon valve. The balloon replacement gastrostomy tubes are available in a variety of sizes (12 Fr to 24 Fr). Insertion of the balloon gastrostomy tube is quite simple and may be performed by trained nursing personnel and families through an established gastrostomy tract. The tube is advanced through the gastrostomy tract approximately 1 to 2 inches. Once in the stomach, the balloon is inflated with 5 to 10 ml of water. After the balloon is inflated, the tube is pulled taut against the abdominal wall, and the retention disc is secured against the abdomen (Fig. 84-5).

Originally, the Foley catheter was used as a gastrostomy feeding tube for many years. The only advantage to using the Foley catheter is its low cost; however, its disadvantages are numerous. The long length of the external catheter allows accidental removal, patient trauma, and malposition internally. Because there is no external retention disc to maintain placement, the catheter is at risk for migration into the small intestine or into the esophagus, resulting in vomiting, diarrhea, and possible perforation.

Surgitek offers a replacement gastrostomy tube without an internal balloon. The tube is secured in the stomach by a crossbar with a feeding port in the middle. It is secured externally by a crossbar as well. It requires an obturator for insertion, which is supplied with the tube. The advantage to this type of replacement tube is that it does not consume gastric space. Thus for children with microgastria or with a history of gastric wall irritation secondary to trauma from gastrostomy tubes, it may offer an alternative option.

Button gastrostomy (skin level or low profile device) is another useful alternative to the traditional gastrostomy tube for the pediatric population. These tubes convert the more cumbersome PEG tubes to low external profile devices and avoid the disadvantages of stoma enlargement and external bulkiness. Skin level and low profile gastrostomy tubes are flush to the abdomen and fit snugly in the stomach to prevent leakage of formula or stomach contents. It is necessary to measure the gastrostomy tract prior to inserting a low profile device to ensure an optimal fit.

The MIC-KEY skin level gastrostomy tube is a balloon skin level device (Figure 84-6 B). It is made of silicone and is easily placed by parents and health care professionals. Sizes range from 14 Fr to 24 Fr diameter with a wide variety of shaft lengths. It is necessary to determine shaft length and diameter prior to insertion. Once the shaft length is determined, the tube is inserted through the well-healed gastrostomy tract into the stomach. The balloon is inflated with 5 to 10 ml of water. It has an antireflux valve in the head of the tube, thus allowing easy gastric access and decompression without a separate apparatus.

The gastrostomy button (Surgitek or Bard) is the original low profile device and has an antireflux valve in the mushroom tip, preventing the backup or leakage of gastric contents should the access port become open between feedings (Figure 84-6C). Gastric decompression is not easily accomplished with the button and requires a separate decompression tube to disable the antireflux valve. The button is removed by traction. The obturator should not be inserted for removal because of the risk of gastric perforation. Spacers may be placed between the abdomen and the outside lip of the button to provide a snug fit for patients whose shaft length is between available sizes.

GASTROENTERIC TUBES (GASTROJEJUNOSTOMY TUBES)

When gastric feeding is not possible, transpyloric feeding may be successful. Many children require gastric access for decompression or medication administration while

---

FIGURE 84-7. *(Continued)* is removed and the guidewire passed through the jejunal lumen of the gastroenteric catheter. The catheter can then be advanced with care over the guidewire to its desired location with the distal tip in the proximal jejunum. *(B)* The MIC transpyloric jejunostomy catheter is available in both 16 Fr and 18 Fr sizes, with jejunal lengths of 30 cm and 45 cm, respectively. The inner diameter of the jejunal lumen is substantially larger than in the MIC gastroenteric catheter, which permits the use of more viscous feeds and allows for longer intervals between device failure secondary to occlusion.

receiving enteral nutrition via a jejunostomy tube. Several manufacturers have recognized the need for a dual-lumen tube providing both gastric and jejunal access. The MIC (Medical Innovations Company/Ballard Medical) gastroenteric tube and the MIC transjejunal feeding tube are dual-lumen tubes that allow gastrojejunal access (Fig. 84-7). They are made of silicone and are placed in interventional radiology under fluoroscopic guidance through an established gastrostomy. They are available in pediatric sizes (16 Fr and 18 Fr) with a 5-ml gastric balloon. They also have an external retention disc to prevent migration of the gastric balloon and tube.

The Corpak Gastrostomy/Jejunostomy System is a two-piece system. The jejunostomy tube (6 Fr) is threaded through the gastric lumen of a Corpak 16 Fr gastrostomy tube. Gastric access for decompression is through the medication port of the gastrostomy tube. This system is available as a percutaneous endoscopic gastrojejunostomy or as a replacement system.

Children who require jejunal feedings but do not need gastric access for decompression or medication administration are candidates for the MIC-KEY skin level jejunostomy tube. This is a skin level device that is similar to the MIC-KEY gastrostomy tube; however, it provides transpyloric jejunal access (Fig. 84-6A) with good cosmetic appearance. The tube is inserted through a traditional gastrostomy and held in place with a gastric balloon. The jejunal limb is placed under fluoroscopic guidance. The jejunal limb may be cut to meet the specific size needs of individual patients. The feeding port is the open end of the jejunal limb.

CONCLUSION

Providing satisfactory enteric nutrition access in children is a challenge. The benefits to the individual are many. By providing adequate nutrition for growth and development, many of the complications encompassed in chronically ill children are avoided. The nutrition industry has started to recognize the special needs of the pediatric population. New devices are being developed that allow for customization to specific patients.

REFERENCES

1. Aquino V, Smyrl C, Hagg R et al. Enteral nutritional support by gastrostomy tube in children with cancer. J Pediatr 1995; 127:58–62

2. Purdum PI, DF K. Short-bowel syndrome: a review of the role of nutritional support. JPEN (J Parent Ent Nutr) 1990; 15:93–101

3. Shellito P, Malt R. Tube gastrostomy: techniques and complications. Ann Surg 1984;201:180–185

4. Towbin R, Ball WJ, Bissett G. Percutaneous gastrostomy and percutaneous gastrojejunostomy in children: antegrade approach. Radiology 1988;1682:473–476

5. Davidson P, Catto-Smith A, Beasley S. Technique and complications of percutaneous endoscopic gastrostomy in children. Aust N Z J Surg 1995;65:194–196

6. Ho CS, Yeung EY. Percutaneous gastrostomy and transgastric jejunostomy, review. AJR 1992;158:251–257

7. Ruge J, Vazquez R. An analysis of the advantages of Stamm and percutaneous endoscopic gastrostomy. Surg Gynecol Obstet 1986;186:13–16

8. Crombleholme TM, Jacir NN. Simplified "push" technique for percutaneous endoscopic gastrostomy in children. J Pediatr Surg 1993;28:1393–1395

9. Treem W, Etienne N, Hyams J. Percutaneous endoscopic placement of the "button" gastrostomy tube as the initial procedure in infants and children. J Pediatr Gastroenterol Nutr 1993;17:382–386

10. Werlin S, Glicklich M, Cohen R. Early feeding after percutaneous endoscopic gastrostomy is safe in children. Gastrointest Endosc 1994;40:692–693

11. Albanese CT, Towbin RB, Ulman I et al. Percutaneous gastrojejunostomy versus Nissen fundoplication for enteral feeding of the neurologically impaired child with gastroesophageal reflux. J Pediatr 1993;123:371–375

12. Graham SM, Flowers JL, Scott TR et al. Safety of percutaneous endoscopic gastrostomy in patients with a ventriculoperitoneal shunt. Neurosurgery 1993;32:932–934

13. Wills J, Oglesby J. Percutaneous gastrostomy. Radiology 1983;149:449–453

14. Malden E, Hicks M, Picus D et al. Fluoroscopically guided percutaneous gastrostomy in children. J Vasc Interv Radiol 1992;3:673–637

15. Rose D, Wolman S, Ho C. Gastric hemorrhage complicating percutaneous transgastric jejunostomy. Radiology 1986;161: 835–836

16. Stefan M, Holcomb G, Ross A. Cologastric fistula as a complication of percutaneous endoscopic gastrostomy. JPEN (J Parent Ent Nutr) 1989;13:554–556

17. Ferguson DR, Harig JM, Kozarek RA et al. Placement of a feeding button ("one-step button") as the initial procedure. Am J Gastroenterol 1993;88:501–504

18. Stylianos S, Flanigan LM. Primary button gastrostomy: a simplified percutaneous, open, laparoscopy-guided technique. J Pediatr Surg 1995;30:219–220

85

PARENTERAL NUTRITION AND CARE OF CENTRAL VENOUS LINES

JULIA A. BILODEAU

CATHY POON

MARIA R. MASCARENHAS

PARENTERAL NUTRITION

Parenteral nutrition (PN) is the intravenous administration of a balanced solution containing all the components of a balanced diet. PN has been used in the United States for the past 25 years. In pediatric patients, the use of PN presents many challenges including changing nutrient requirements with age, specialized needs of children, problems with vascular access, and the sometimes limited ability of children to handle large amounts of fluid, protein, fat, and carbohydrates.[1] In most pediatric tertiary care centers, approximately 5% to 10% of patients receive PN.[2]

Indications

Any patient who cannot receive adequate nutrition via the gastrointestinal (GI) tract for more than 3 to 5 days should receive PN. Some of these patients may have a functioning GI tract but for a variety of reasons may not be able to receive full nutrition. These patients may need supplemental PN. Table 85-1 lists conditions that require PN. Intravenous nutrition may also be used in the malnourished patient to supplement enteral feeds.

Route

PN may be administered via a peripheral vein (peripheral PN) or a central vein (central PN). Peripheral PN is usually used for patients with normal nutritional status, short anticipated period of no or inadequate enteral feedings, and normal nutritional and fluid status. Generally, if the patient will need total PN for less than 2 weeks, a peripheral catheter will suffice. It is often difficult to maintain peripheral access sites for longer than 2 weeks and to deliver adequate calories with the restrictions of a lower (10% to 12.5%) dextrose solution.

Patients who require PN for a long period of time, have abnormal nutritional status, have increased requirements, or require concentrated PN should receive a centrally placed venous catheter. This may be either a peripherally inserted central catheter (PICC) line, a tunneled catheter, or an implantable port. These catheters are considered "central" if the tip of the catheter is at the junction of the superior vena cava and right atrium. It is important to document position of the line by radiologic methods (x-ray) so that malposition of the line can be avoided. Umbilical venous catheters may also be used for the administration of PN. In the case of lines placed in the lower extremities (femoral lines), every attempt is made to have the tip of the catheter in the inferior vena cava above the level of the diaphragm. PN can also be delivered via peritoneal or hemodialysis cath-

TABLE 85-1. Indications for Parenteral Nutrition

Gastrointestinal Disease

Congenital anomalies—atresia

Surgical disease—small bowel resection

Intractable diarrhea

Inflammatory bowel disease

Pseudo-obstruction syndrome

Respiratory Disease

Respiratory failure

Cystic fibrosis

Hypermetabolic Conditions

Sepsis

Burns

Major trauma

Malignancy

Other Conditions

Liver disease

Congenital heart disease

Inborn errors of metabolism

Chronic renal disease

eters. Additional discussion of central venous access devices will be presented later in the chapter.

Components

The usual components of a PN solution are protein, dextrose, fat, electrolytes, minerals, vitamins, and trace elements. In addition, cimetidine, ranitidine, and hydrochloric acid may be added to the PN solution when clinically indicated.

PROTEIN

Current protein solutions consist of synthetic crystalline amino acids. One gram of protein provides 4 calories. It is safe to give most patients their entire daily protein requirements on the first day of PN. The only exceptions are critically ill patients with hepatic and renal insufficiency not on dialysis and patients with disorders of protein metabolism. TrophAmine is a specialized amino acid solution formulated for use in infants (including preterm infants) until 6 months of age. Its composition is based on serum aminograms of healthy 1-month-old breast-fed infants who were born at term. It differs from the adult formulations in that it contains tyrosine, taurine, and histidine, which the preterm infant requires. It also has a higher concentration of branched-chain amino acids and so may be used in patients with chronic liver disease and cholestasis. Novamine is a standard protein

formulation given to patients over 6 months of age. It consists of essential and nonessential amino acids appropriate for the normal growth of children. It is available in 1% to 15% solution. The 15% solution is particularly useful in the fluid-restricted patient. Hepatamine is a specialized amino acid formulation that contains increased amounts of branched-chain amino acids and reduced amounts of methionine and aromatic amino acids. It was designed for use in patients with severe liver failure and hepatic encephalopathy; however, studies have not demonstrated a clear beneficial effect in these patients. Protein needs vary with age and decrease with age when expressed in terms of body weight. Tables 85-2 and 85-3 list guidelines for protein requirements and composition of commonly used protein solutions. Patients with protein calorie malnutrition, protein-losing enteropathy, stress, and increased protein needs will need to be given increased amounts of protein.

CARBOHYDRATES

Carbohydrate is provided in PN as dextrose. Approximately 3.4 calories is obtained from 1 g of dextrose because of its formulation (monohydrate form) for intravenous use. Glucose delivery is usually expressed in milligrams per kilogram per minute (neonates, 5 to 12 mg/kg/min; older children 2 to 5 mg/kg/min). Glucose utilization in neonates has been shown to decrease when glucose delivery is 14 mg/kg/min or greater.[3] Only a 10% dextrose solution should be given via a peripheral vein because more concentrated dextrose solutions can result in osmolalities greater than 900 mOsm and therefore an increased risk of phlebitis.[4] In special circumstances, a 12.5% dextrose solution may be used with caution. Patients with hyperglycemia may require concomitant insulin administration to improve glucose tolerance while meeting the patient's caloric needs. Excessive use of carbohydrates can result in fatty infiltration of the liver and increased carbon dioxide production. Care must be taken

TABLE 85-2. Intravenous Protein Requirements

Age	Protein (g/kg/day)
Infants	
Preterm	2.5–3.5
Full term	
0–6 mo	2.5–3.0
6–12 mo	2.0–2.5
Children	
1–6 yr	1–2
7–10 yr	1–2
11–18 yr	0.8–2.0

TABLE 85-3. Composition of Crystalline and Amino Acid Solutions (milligrams of amino acid per gram of protein)

Amino Acids	Novamine	TrophAmine	Hepatamine	Aminosyn RF
Essential				
L-Isoleucine	50	82	113	88
L-Leucine	69	140	138	139
L-Lysine	79	82	76	102
L-Methionine	50	33	13	139
L-Phenylalanine	69	48	13	139
L-Threonine	50	42	56	63
L-Tryptophan	17	20	8	31
L-Valine	64	82	105	101
Nonessential				
L-Alanine	145	53	96	—
L-Arginine	98	122	75	115
L-Aspartic acid	29	32	—	—
L-Glutamic acid	50	50	—	—
L-Glycine	69	68	113	—
L-Histidine	60	48	30	82
L-Proline	60	38	100	—
L-Serine	39	37	63	—
L-Taurine	—	2.5	—	—
L-Tyrosine	3	23	—	—
% essential amino acids	45%	53%	52%	80%
% nonessential amino acids	55%	47%	48%	20%
% branched-chain amino acids	—	30%	35%	33%

to keep the carbohydrate calories at 50% to 60% of total calories to prevent PN-induced liver disease and balance the regimen.

FAT

Fat is provided to balance out the distribution of calories in PN and provide essential fatty acids, which are required for brain and somatic growth, immune function, skin integrity, and wound healing. Fat provides a concentrated form of calories.

Conventional intravenous fat emulsions contain long-chain triglycerides and are usually made from soybean and safflower oils. Newer intravenous fat formulations consist of structured lipids (medium- and long-chain triglycerides attached to a glycerol backbone), medium-chain triglyceride emulsions, and mixtures of long- and medium-chain triglyceride emulsions.[5–7] Intralipid is a commonly used intravenous fat emulsion that contains soybean oil. It is available as 10%, 20% and 30% emulsions[8] (Table 85-4). The 20% emulsion is used most often. The 10% emulsion is infrequently used because of its high phospholipid-triglyceride ratio, which results in

hyperlipidemia.[9,10] The 30% emulsion can only be used in a total nutrient admixture and cannot be infused alone into a peripheral vein. The total daily dose of intravenous fat should be delivered over 24 hours, except when PN is cycled (see the section *Cycling PN*, below). There is no need to give patients a rest period. Table 85-5 outlines the dosage for intralipid. When a PN regimen is planned, care must be taken to keep the percentage of total calories from fat in the range of 30% to 40% and never more than 60% of total calories, which constitutes a ketogenic diet.

TABLE 85-4. Composition of Intralipids

	10%	20%	30%
Soybean oil (g)	100	200	300
Egg phospholipids (g)	12	12	12
Glycerol (g)	22	22	17
Calories (kcal/ml)	1.1	2	3
Osmolality (mOsm/L)	300	350	310

TABLE 85-5.   Dosage for Intralipid (g/kg/day)

	Preterm & Full Term Infants	Older Infants	Children
Initial dose	1–2	1–2	1–2
Dose increments	0.5–1.0	1	1
Maximum dose[a]	3–4	3–4	3

[a] Percentage of calories from fat should not exceed more than 50% to 60% of total caloric intake.

ELECTROLYTES, MINERALS, AND TRACE ELEMENTS

Electrolytes (sodium, potassium, calcium, phosphorus, and magnesium) are added to the PN solution in maintenance concentrations. These requirements are derived from the recommended dietary allowances (RDA) with allowances made for the efficiency of absorption. Table 85-6 lists dosing guidelines for electrolytes and minerals. It is preferable to obtain a baseline serum electrolyte panel prior to ordering a PN solution and then add electrolytes accordingly. Periodic monitoring of serum electrolytes is required. In neonates and children with high calcium and phosphorus needs, the amounts added to a PN solution may be limited because of solubility issues. Increasing the amount of protein, adding cysteine, thereby lowering the pH of the solution, can allow higher amounts of calcium and phosphorus to be added to the PN solution without precipitation. In instances where the patient's calcium and phosphorus requirements cannot be added to the PN solution, a separate infusion of calcium or phosphorus may need to be given.

In addition, iron, zinc, copper, chromium, manganese,

TABLE 85-6.   Daily Intravenous Requirements for Electrolytes and Minerals

Electrolyte or Mineral (unit)	Preterm	Term	Children > 1 yr
Sodium (mEq/kg)	2–3	2–4	2–3
Potassium (mEq/kg)	2–3	2–3	2–3
Chloride (mEq/kg)	2–3	2–4	2–3
Magnesium (mEq/kg)	0.35–0.6	0.25–0.5	0.2–0.5
Calcium (mEq/kg)	3.0–4.5	3–4	1–2
Phosphorus (mEq/kg)	2.7–4.0	1.5–3.0	0.7–1.4
Zinc (μg/kg)			
Patients < 3 mo	150	250	50–200
Patients > 3 mo	150	100	50–200
Copper (μg/kg)	20	20	20
Chromium (μg/kg)	0.05–0.2	0.2	0.14–0.2
Manganese (μg/kg)	1–5	1–5	1–5
Iron (mg/kg)			
Patients > 2 mo	0.2	0.1	0.1
Selenium (μg/kg)	2	2	2
Molybdenum (μg/kg)	0.2	0.25	0.25

selenium, and molybdenum need to be added to make the PN solution balanced. Adolescent patients who have received 80% or more of their caloric requirements from PN for 3 to 6 months may need to be supplemented with molybdenum. Iodine is not added to PN solutions because patients usually receive enough iodine from unavoidable contamination of PN solutions and from topical administration of iodine-containing antiseptic solutions.

TABLE 85-7.   Daily Intravenous Vitamin Requirements, Recommendations, and Products

	Preterm (per kg)	Term & Children > 1 yr	MVI PED	MVI 12 (5 ml)
Vitamin A (retinol) (IU)	700–1,500	2,300	2,300	3,300
Vitamin D (IU)	40–160	400	400	200
Vitamin E (tocopherol) (IU)	3.5	7	7	10
Vitamin C (mg)	15–25	80	80	100
Folate (μg)	56	140	140	400
Niacin (mg)	4.0–6.8	17	17	40
Riboflavin (mg)	0.15–0.2	1.4	1.4	3.6
Thiamine (mg)	0.2–0.35	1.2	1.2	3
Vitamin B_6 (mg)	0.15–0.2	1	1	4
Vitamin B_{12} (μg)	0.3	1	1	5
Pantothenic acid (mg)	1–2	5	5	15
Biotin (μg)	8	20	20	60
Vitamin K (mg)	0.3	0.2	0.2	—[a]

[a] Patient receiving MVI 12 will get 0.2 mg/day of vitamin K.

TABLE 85-8. Energy Requirements for Infants

Age	Energy (kcal/kg/day)
Preterm	190–110
Full term	
0–6 mo	90–100
6–12 mo	80–100

VITAMINS

The currently used intravenous pediatric multivitamin (MVI) preparation was designed to meet the needs of preterm and term infants and children.[11,12] Table 85-7 lists the vitamin requirements and composition of commonly available preparations. For children older than 10 years, the adult MVI preparation is used with additional vitamin K added. The adult MVI has less vitamin D than pediatric MVI.

Energy Requirements

Basal or resting energy requirements vary widely with age and sex during infancy (Table 85-8), childhood, and adolescence. When determining caloric needs, one must factor in physical activity and severity of illness in addition to age. For children over 1 year of age, a modification of the World Health Organization (WHO) recommendations to calculate resting energy expenditure (REE) may be used[13] (Table 85-9). The equation is based on data from several thousand children and has been found to be accurate in children older than 1 year of age. The REE is then multiplied by a disease activity/stress factor depending on the activity level and severity of illness (Table 85-10). One can also measure REE via indirect calorimetry. Patients in the intensive care setting who have a Swan-Ganz catheter to measure cardiac output can also have their REE calculated based on cardiac output.[14]

Total Nutrient Admixtures

Total nutrient admixtures are solutions in which all the PN components (glucose amino acid solution and fat) are added to one bag and infused through a single IV administration set.[15] Their major advantage is the ease

TABLE 85-10. Disease Activity/Stress Factors[a]

1.3	Well-nourished child at rest with mild to moderate stress (minor surgery)
1.5	Normal active child with mild to moderate stress. Inactive child with severe stress (trauma, cancer, extensive surgery). Malnourished child requiring catch-up growth with minimal activity
1.7	Active child requiring catch-up growth. Active child with severe stress

[a] Multiply REE times disease activity/stress factor for estimated daily energy requirements.

of administration because only one infusion pump is required, and studies have shown fewer infections compared with the traditional methods of PN administration. The egg yolk phospholipids in the intralipid act as the emulsifier and make the solution stable. Other factors affecting solution stability include amino acid, dextrose, calcium, magnesium and iron concentrations, order of addition of PN components, and pH. The disadvantage of total nutrient admixture solutions is that the PN components can precipitate, and because total nutrient admixtures are cloudy, any precipitate needs to be 50 μm or larger to be seen with the naked eye. The use of appropriate (1.2 or 5. μm) in-line filters can help decrease this complication. There have been two reports of calcium-phosphorus precipitates resulting in death.[16]

Formulating a Regimen

Once the decision has been made to give PN to a patient, one must determine the patient's fluid, caloric, protein, electrolyte, vitamin, and trace element requirements. A complete laboratory assessment of the patient's electrolytes, acid-base status, calcium, phosphorus, magnesium, and triglyceride levels should be performed. An assessment of the patient's nutritional status should be made to determine the child's caloric needs based on age, severity of illness, activity level, and degree of catch-up growth required. Next, the route of administration should be decided. If it is anticipated that the patient will need concentrated PN solution for more than 7 to 14 days, a central venous catheter should be placed.

It is usual to start the patient on 75% to 80% of goal

TABLE 85-9. Estimated Resting Energy Expenditure (in kcal) for Children

Gender	1–3 yr	3–10 yr	10–18 yr	18–30 yr
Male	60.9W − 54	22.7W + 495	17.5W + 651	15.3W + 679
Female	61.0W − 51	22.5W + 499	12.2W + 746	14.7W + 496

Abbreviation: W, weight in kilograms.
(Adapted from WHO.[13])

calories and increase this by 10% to 20% every day until the goal of the PN regimen is reached. The total daily protein requirement can begin on the first day unless hepatic or renal insufficiency is present, in which case the amount of protein given is titrated based on clinical parameters. It is customary to start the intravenous lipid dose at 1.0 to 1.5 g/kg/day; if triglyceride levels remain below 300 mg/dl, lipids can be increased. The monitoring of weight gain/loss, electrolytes, and fluid balance initially needs to be performed daily to assess the adequacy and appropriateness of the regimen, and adjustments will need to be made.

Monitoring

The key to the safe administration of PN is close monitoring. Daily measurements of weight, vital sign checks every 4 hours, strict intake and output recording, and monitoring of blood and urine (specific gravity and glucose) tests to determine tolerance of the regimen are essential. Table 85-11 outlines a monitoring schedule. Once the goal regimen has been reached and the patient is demonstrating tolerance, the monitoring frequency can be decreased.

Cycling PN

Stable patients on central or peripheral PN may benefit from decreasing the PN administration time from 24 hours to 8 to 18 hours a day. While this permits more time for daily activity, it also allows for the establishment of oral feedings in some patients. There is also evidence that cycling may help decrease hepatic steatosis and allow for mobilization of hepatic fat stores. In adults receiving a total nutrient admixture PN solution, PN can be stopped abruptly without a tapering schedule, with plasma glucose showing little change after the first 60 minutes.[17] However, in children less than 3 years of age, hypoglycemia is noted after abrupt discontinuation as well as after tapering the PN solution.[18] Therefore, patients receiving more than 10% dextrose should have their PN rate decreased by 50% for the last hour to prevent rebound hypoglycemia. There is no need to give the patient 50% of the PN rate for the first hour of PN administration before increasing to the usual rate. Almost all home PN patients are on cyclic PN for improved lifestyle. Cyclic PN has been shown to be safe in infants less than 6 months of age.[19]

PN Complications and Management

With appropriate use of PN, complications should occur infrequently. Complications related to PN can be categorized as follows: metabolic, infectious, and mechanical (Table 85-12). Metabolic complications are not necessarily unique to PN and can also occur in patients receiving enteral nutrition. Metabolic complications may be further divided into electrolyte abnormalities, glucose

TABLE 85-11. Parenteral Nutrition Monitoring Schedule

Measurement	Frequency
Laboratory studies	
Complete blood count	Baseline & every month
Reticulocyte count	Every month
Serum electrolytes	Baseline, after every change, & every week thereafter
Triglycerides	Baseline, after every change, & every week thereafter
Cholesterol	Baseline & every week
Minerals (Ca, Mg, PO$_4$)	Baseline, after every change, & every week thereafter
Total protein	Baseline & every week
Albumin	Baseline & every week
Liver function tests (ALT, GGTP, ALPH)	Baseline & every week
Iron studies (TIBC, ferritin, % saturation)	Baseline & every month
Vitamins (A, E, 25-HYDROXY D, PT/PTT)	Every 3–6 mo
Trace elements (Se, Zn, Cu, Mn)	Every 3–6 mo
Growth	
Weight	Baseline & then daily for patients < 2 yr & every other day for patients > 2 yr
Height/length	Baseline & every month
Head circumference	Baseline & every month (patients < 3 yr)
Arm anthropometrics	Baseline & every month

Abbreviations: ALT, alanine transaminase; GGTP, gamma-glutamyltranspeptidase; ALP, alkaline phosphatase; TIBC, total iron binding capacity; PT, prothrombin time; PTT, partial thromboplastin time.

TABLE 85-12. Complizations of Parenteral Nutrition

Metabolic

Electrolyte abnormalities

Glucose disturbances

Acid-base disorders

Liver disease

Metabolic bone disease

Refeeding syndrome

Mechanical (central venous access device–related)

Air embolism

Pneumothorax

Hemothorax

Hydrothorax

Perforation of an organ

Malposition—arrhythmias, cardiac tamponade, brachial nerve injury, twiddler's syndrome

Thrombosis

Extravasation

Infectious

Infections—systemic or local

Sepsis

disturbances, acid-base disorders, hepatic dysfunction, metabolic bone disease, and refeeding syndrome. The severity of metabolic disturbances can vary tremendously, and management may sometimes be difficult. Table 85-13 provides a summary of the etiology, clinical manifestations, and management of some common electrolyte and mineral disturbances.

ELECTROLYTES

Electrolyte and mineral disturbances may result from giving too much or too little of a particular PN component (particularly true in neonates and premature infants). Additionally, concurrent disease states and altered end organ functions may contribute to these abnormalities. Complications are easily managed or prevented with appropriate monitoring and early intervention. The most important approach to the management or prevention of imbalances of individual nutrients is to recognize the potential predisposing risk factors and signs and symptoms associated with the various abnormalities and to institute the appropriate therapy quickly.

HEPATOBILIARY

Hepatobiliary complications can also occur.[20–27] The incidence tends to increase with duration of therapy. Risk factors include prematurity, low birth weight, GI surgery, sepsis, bacterial overgrowth, disturbed enterohepatic circulation and absence of enteral intake. Abnormal serum bile acids and elevations in gamma-glutamyltranspeptidase can be observed as early as 2 weeks after beginning PN therapy. Infants and children tend to develop cholestasis, while adults tend to develop more fatty infiltration of the liver. The exact etiology of PN-associated hepatobiliary complications is not known. Various factors implicated are excessive caloric intake, carbohydrate-rich PN regimen, relative carbohydrate-to-nitrogen imbalance, excessive lipid administration, excessive protein intake, PN protein solutions deficient in specific amino acids, bacterial overgrowth, aluminum in PN solutions, and duration of PN. The histologic hepatic changes described include fatty liver, cholestasis, hepatitis, periportal fibrosis, cirrhosis, and hepatocellular carcinoma. Biliary abnormalities include acalculous cholecystitis, biliary sludge, enlarged gallbladders, and gallstones. Measures to decrease the occurrence of hepatobiliary complications of PN include avoidance of excess calories, balancing the components of the PN solution, cycling PN, starting some enteral feeds, and removing the copper from PN solutions in patients with cholestasis.

BONE

Bone disease (osteopenia, osteomalacia, rickets, fractures) can be seen in patients receiving chronic PN,[28–31] especially premature infants, who have high calcium needs. While the exact etiology for PN-related bone disease is unknown, the following factors have been implicated: aluminum contamination of PN protein solutions, decreased calcium and phosphorus intake, altered vitamin D metabolism, and concomitant use of diuretics, which increase calcium losses. Patients with underlying GI disease are at increased risk due to malabsorption.

REFEEDING SYNDROME

The refeeding syndrome refers to metabolic, cardiopulmonary, and neurologic complications (hypophosphatemia, hypokalemia, hypoglycemia, hypomagnesemia, and hypocalcemia) seen in severely malnourished patients after receiving PN.[32–35] These changes are not specific to PN and can occur with enteral refeeding. During starvation, the catabolism of fat and muscle occurs, resulting in loss of lean body mass, minerals, and water with preservation of serum levels. During the reinstitution of nutrition, especially with a carbohydrate-rich regimen, insulin is released, causing increased intracellular uptake of glucose, phosphorus, and other nutrients. A severe hypophosphatemia may occur, which results in cardiac decompensation, neurologic dysfunction, and red cell and white cell dysfunction. At-risk patients include those with anorexia nervosa, kwashiorkor, marasmus, morbid obesity with massive weight loss, prolonged fasting, and chronic malnutrition. The most important measure in the prevention of refeeding syndrome is the recognition of at-risk patients. These patients should have their electrolytes checked prior to the initiation of nutri-

TABLE 85-13. Electrolyte and Mineral Abnormalities during Parenteral Nutrition

Electrolyte/Mineral Abnormalities	Etiology	Manifestations	Treatment/Management
Hypocalcemia	Inadequate calcium intake Increased losses Hypoparathyroidism Pharmacotherapy (e.g., diuretics) Excessive phosphate intake Vitamin D deficiency Magnesium deficiency Hypoalbuminemia	Serum calcium < 11 mg/dl Rickets of prematurity Bone demineralization Carpopedal spasm Positive Chvostek's sign Prolonged QT interval	Exogenous calcium replacement, i.e., separate infusion Maximize calcium supplementation in PN solution (based on calcium and phosphate solubility)
Hyperkalemia	Excessive potassium intake Renal insufficiency Metabolic acidosis Pharmacotherapy (e.g., potassium sparing diuretics, amphotericin B)	Serum potassium > 7 mEq/L Cardiac arrhythmias	Decrease potassium in PN Treat symptomatic patients (e.g., glucose and insulin infusion)
Hypokalemia	Increased GI losses Diarrhea Pharmacotherapy (e.g., diuretics, amphotericin B) Alkalosis Excessive renal losses Refeeding syndrome Insulin therapy High dextrose infusion	Serum potassium < 3.5 mEq/L Lethargy Muscle weakness or paralysis Cardiac arrhythmias	Increase potassium in PN Treat with separate potassium infusion
Hypermagnesemia	Excessive magnesium intake Renal insufficiency	Serum magnesium > 3 mg/dl Hypotension Respiratory depression	Restrict or decrease magnesium in PN
Hypomagnesemia	Excessive losses (i.e., GI) Chronic diarrhea Fistulas Prolonged nasogastric suction Pharmacotherapy (e.g., amphotericin B, aminoglycosides, chemotherapeutic agents)	Serum magnesium < 1.5 mg/dl Numbness Muscle weakness Positive Chvostek's sign Tachycardia Seizure Tremors	Increase magnesium in PN
Hypernatremia	Excessive sodium intake Dehydration Inadequate fluid intake Diabetes insipidus	Serum sodium >145 mEq/L	Restrict sodium in PN Increase fluid intake Diuretic therapy (e.g., furosemide) to increase urinary sodium losses

tional rehabilitation. Caloric intake is started at either 75% of the REE or at the patient's current caloric intake. While fluid, electrolyte, and cardiovascular intake is carefully monitored, caloric intake is increased by 10% to 15% daily, provided the patient's clinical condition is stable. Serum phosphorus, potassium, magnesium, and glucose should be monitored after every change and caloric intake increased only if serum levels of these nutrients are normal.

MECHANICAL COMPLICATIONS

Mechanical complications may be seen during and immediately after insertion of a central venous access device.[36,37] These complications are discussed in the sec-

tion *Catheter Complications and Management* and are listed in Table 85-12.

CARE OF CENTRAL VENOUS CATHETERS

The development of the Silastic catheter[38] has prolonged the use of individual catheters and in essence has made PN a possibility. Today, the practitioner has a larger selection than ever before when it comes to choosing venous access devices. The decision on which type of device to choose is dependent on patient preference, anticipated length of therapy, availability of venous access sites, and institutional availability of products with appropriately trained practitioners. The four types of venous access devices available today include temporary peripheral and central venous catheters, tunneled central venous catheters, and implantable ports.

Once the decision is made to utilize a central venous access device, the physician can choose a PICC or a tunneled Silastic catheter. Many hospitals have specially trained nurses who will insert the PICCs, which has obvious scheduling and cost benefits. In addition, interventional radiologists are trained to insert PICC lines and other tunneled catheters, which previously had been exclusively within the domain of the surgeon.

Types of Central Venous Catheters

PERIPHERALLY INSERTED CENTRAL CATHETERS

PICCs are inserted at or above the antecubital space of the arm with the tip located, ideally, at the lower one-third of the superior vena cava (SVC), 3 to 4 cm above the superior vena cava–right atrial junction[37] (Fig. 85-1c). PICC use started gaining popularity in the 1980s and is now quite popular as there are no known limitations regarding their use related to age, gender, or diagnosis.[37] PICCs are generally indicated in patients when the need for intravenous access is expected to be longer than 7 days or when peripheral access is difficult. PICCs can remain in place as long as needed without complications.

Contraindications include dermatitis, cellulitis, burns at or near the insertion site, and previous ipsilateral venous thrombosis.[37]

PICCs are made of either polyurethane, Silastic, or Aquavene material and come in single and double lumens. They are radiopaque and should be readily visualized via radiograph. PICCs should be placed in an area where aseptic technique can be maintained. It is prudent practice to confirm the placement of the catheter tip prior to initiating therapy, particularly if a hypertonic dextrose solution is to be used through the catheter, to minimize the risk of thrombosis. The incidence of complications with PICCs is very low for infection, central vein thrombosis, and catheter malposition.[37] In addition, there are cost savings with this type of catheter. Management of PICC complications is discussed in the section *Catheter Complications and Management,* below.

TUNNELED SILASTIC CATHETERS

Hickman,[39] Broviac,[38] Leonard (Davol), and Groshong[36] catheters and subcutaneous ports are tunneled Silastic catheters often used to infuse PN (Fig. 85-1a & b). These catheters are generally placed by a surgeon or an interventional radiologist using general anesthesia or conscious sedation. Tunneled catheters are indicated when the intravenous need is expected to be longer than 4 to 6 weeks. Tunneled catheters can be placed either via cutdown or percutaneously. As with PICCs, ideal

FIGURE 85-1. Silastic catheters and peripherally inserted central catheter. (a) Double-lumen Silastic catheter. (From Bard Access Systems, Salt Lake City, UT, with permission.) (b) Single-lumen Silastic catheter. (From Bard Access Systems, Salt Lake City, UT, with permission.) (c) Peripherally inserted central catheter (size 4 Fr). (From Cook, Bloomington, IN, with permission.)

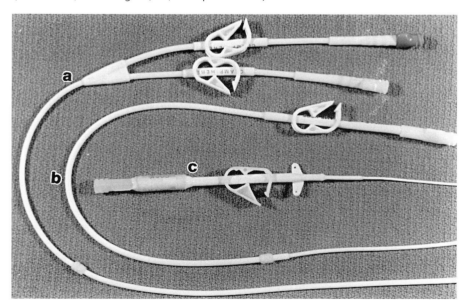

placement is with the tip of the catheter terminating in the superior vena cava.[37,39]

Hickman, Broviac, and Leonard (Davol) catheters are nonvalved catheters that differ primarily in the number of lumens and internal diameter. The catheters are available as either single-, double-, or triple-lumen catheters in various lumen sizes, ranging from 2.7 Fr to 12 Fr. Groshong catheters are catheters that have a two-way valve at the tip of the catheter, which permits aspiration of blood and infusion of fluids, but prevents blood from entering when the catheter is not in use. This two-way valve should decrease the risk of thrombosis and obviate the need for heparin flushes. However, there have been reports of a higher incidence of catheter malfunction with these catheters.[36]

Tunneled catheters have a Dacron cuff located on the midportion of the catheter. This cuff stimulates the formation of dense fibrous adhesions, which anchor the catheter subcutaneously to prevent dislodgement of the catheter, and act as a barrier to potentially ascending bacteria. Sutures are needed at the exit site for several weeks after insertion to allow time for the formation of fibrous adhesions to the Dacron cuff.

PORTS

Implantable ports are available as either single- or double-lumen styles, ranging in size from 5 Fr to 13 Fr catheters, are composed of either Silastic or polyurethane material, and have the option of a Groshong valve. The ports are generally made of plastic or titanium with a compressed silicon disc. The disc is designed for 1,000 to 2,000 insertions with a noncoring needle. Ports are inserted either percutaneously or by cutdown into the jugular, subclavian, or cephalic vein and placed in a subcutaneous pocket over the upper chest wall. There are smaller ports available, which are primarily used for arm placement and for children[36,40] (Fig. 85-2).

Catheter Complications and Management

INFECTIOUS COMPLICATIONS

The use of central venous catheters may be complicated by either local or systemic infections. The most commonly seen life-threatening complication of central venous access devices is septicemia.[41] A patient with a central venous line who develops a fever of 38.5°C should be immediately evaluated for the possibility of an infection. Table 85-14 reviews features of catheter-related sepsis. The work-up for suspected catheter-related sepsis should include the following: a thorough physical examination (looking for other possible sources) and complete blood count with differential, electrolytes, and central and peripheral blood cultures. In addition, a disseminated intravascular coagulation screen (prothrombin and partial thromboplastin times, fibrin split products, and fibrinogen) should be considered in a particularly ill-appearing child. Initiate broad-spectrum antibiotics until culture and sensitivities are available. Catheter-related infec-

FIGURE 85-2. Implanted vascular access devices. (a) Double-lumen chest port. (From Bard Access Systems, Salt Lake City, UT, with permission.) (b) Single-lumen chest port. (From Bard Access Systems, Salt Lake City, UT, with permission.) (c) Peripherally accessed system port (P.A.S. PORT). (From SIMS Deltec, Inc., St. Paul, MN, with permission.)

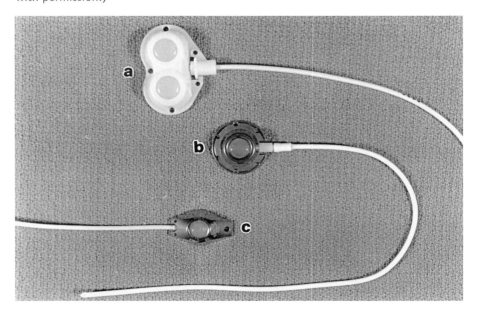

TABLE 85-14. Clinical, Epidemiologic, and Microbiologic Features of Venous Access Device–Related Sepsis

Patient is unlikely candidate for other sepsis event

No apparent source of sepsis

No identifiable local infection

Presence of a venous access device

Inflammation or purulence at insertion site

Abrupt onset associated with shock

Sepsis refractory to antimicrobial therapy or dramatic improvement with catheter removal or infusate

Septicemia caused by staphylococci

(Adapted from Bennett and Brachman,[56] with permission.)

tions are often successfully treated with antibiotics without the need to remove the catheter, and this approach should be tried prior to catheter removal.[42]

The majority of catheter-related sepsis begins with a local infection of the catheter wound. The patient's own cutaneous flora invades the intracutaneous tract at the time that the catheter is placed or sometime thereafter. There is ample evidence that demonstrates the correlation between the organisms colonizing the skin of the infection site and the causative microorganism in catheter-related septicemia.[41,43,44] Gram-positive cocci are the most frequent offenders for line-related sepsis; however, gram-negative rod and fungal infections can also occur.[41] The risk of infection associated with central lines increases with the use of PN. Christenson[45] et al studied 310 oncology patients who had either a Hickman/Broviac catheter or an implantable subcutaneous port before and after being given PN. The mean duration of each central line was 363 days, with an overall infection rate of 0.06/100 days. The infection rate increased to 0.5/100 days when PN was administered.

The Centers for Disease Control and Prevention have developed standard catheter-related infection definitions (Table 85-15).[46] It is important to understand these definitions to properly prevent, recognize, and treat potential infections.

CATHETER SITE CARE

Since the major and most frequent complications of central venous lines are infections, it is reasonable that appropriate care of the catheter site is critical to minimizing these complications. Site care can be divided into three areas: care of the site on initial insertion, care of the site with routine dressing changes, and care of the site with a specific dressing. Recent data[47] support the use of maximal barrier precautions including mask, sterile surgical gown, gloves, and a large drape to reduce the risk of bloodstream infection on catheter insertion. Barrier pro-

tection was found to be more critical than the setting (operating room, intensive care unit,) of the insertion. Skin cleansing around the catheter site is also considered important in reducing the risk of catheter-related infection. The most widely used solution in the United States is 10% povidone-iodine. Maki et al[48] in a prospective randomized trial, assessed the efficacy of three antiseptics used for cutaneous disinfection for central venous and arterial catheters (povidone-iodine, 70% alcohol, or 2% chlorhexidine). The catheters were randomized to one of these three antiseptics prior to catheter insertion and then every other day thereafter during routine site care. Chlorhexidine had the lowest incidence for both local catheter-related infection and for catheter-related bacteremia. Povidone-iodine and alcohol provided comparable protection. Chlorhexidine has the clear advantage of residual antibacterial activity with repeated application, which povidone-iodine and alcohol do not. Unfortunately, the 2% chlorhexidine solution used in Maki's trial is not available in the United States. The current sustained-release chlorhexidine patch (250 μg/g dressing) has been shown to reduce the incidence of catheter colonization in epidural catheters.[49] Some institutions still practice defatting the skin with alcohol-acetone as part of the regimen in disinfecting the catheter insertion site. Acetone is of no benefit in reducing cutaneous colonization.[50] Rather, acetone has the deleterious effect of increasing skin inflammation and patient discomfort.

TABLE 85-15. Definitions of Catheter-Related Infections

Colonized catheter: growth of > 15 colony-forming units from a proximal or distal catheter segment in the absence of accompanying symptoms.

Exit-site infection: erythema, tenderness, induration, and/or purulence within 2 cm of the skin at the exit site of the catheter.

Pocket infection: erythema and necrosis of the skin over the reservoir of a totally implantable device and/or purulent exudate in the subcutaneous pocket containing the reservoir.

Tunnel infection: erythema, tenderness, and induration in the tissues overlying the catheter and > 2 cm from the exit site.

Catheter-related bloodstream infection (CR-BSI): Isolation of the same organism (i.e., identical species, antibiogram) from a semiquantitative or quantitative culture of a catheter segment and from the blood (preferably drawn from a peripheral vein) of a patient with accompanying clinical symptoms of BSI and no other apparent source of infection. In the absence of laboratory confirmation, defervescence after removal of an implicated catheter from a patient with BSI may be considered indirect evidence of CR-BSI.

Infusate-related bloodstream infection: isolation of the same organism from infusate and from separate percutaneous blood cultures, with no other identifiable source of infection.

(Adapted from Centers for Disease Control and Prevention.[46])

TABLE 85-16.   Recommended Procedures for Maintenance of Intravenous Catheters, Administration Sets, and Parenteral Fluids

Frequency of Catheter/Device Change	Frequency of Dressing Change	Frequency of Administration Set Change	"Hang Time" for Parenteral Fluids
Hickmans, Groshongs, Ports NO RECOMMENDATION for frequency of change of tunneled catheters, totally implantable devices (i.e., ports), or the needles used to access them.	NO RECOMMENDATION for the frequency of routine changes of dressing used on catheter site.	NO RECOMMENDATION for intravenous tubing changes beyond 72-h intervals. Change tubing used to administer blood, blood products, or lipid emulsions within 24 h of completing the infusion.	Do not leave parenteral nutrition fluids hanging > 24 h.
Peripherally Inserted Central Venous Catheters Change at least every 6 wk. NO RECOMMENDATION for frequency of change when the duration of therapy is expected to exceed 6 wk.	Leave dressing in place until the catheter is removed or changed or until the dressing becomes damp, loosened, or soiled. NO RECOMMENDATION for the frequency of routine changes of dressing used on catheter site.	Change intravenous tubing, including "piggyback" tubing no more frequently than at 72-h intervals. NO RECOMMENDATION for intravenous tubing changes beyond 72-h intervals. Change tubing used to administer blood, blood products, or lipid emulsions within 14 h of completing the infusion.	Do not leave parenteral nutrition fluids hanging > 24 h. NO RECOMMENDATION for "hang time" of intravenous fluids other than parenteral nutrition fluids.

(Adapted from Centers for Disease Control and Prevention.[46])

TYPES OF DRESSINGS

The use of a transparent, semipermeable polyurethane dressing has become a very common method of covering the catheter insertion site. This type of dressing provides a reliable method for securing the catheter, assessing the catheter site, and allowing the patient to bathe without saturating the site.[51] A substantial area of concern with transparent dressings has been the moisture vapor transmission rate (MVTR), oxygen transmission, and cutaneous adherence. These variables are thought to affect the cutaneous colonization and thus increase the risk of sepsis. This concern has led to the development of a new transparent dressing that has an MVTR five to eight times greater than the other available transparent dressings.[52] The length of time that a transparent dressing should be left in place is still not clear. The Centers for Disease Control and Prevention has recently published recommendations for intravenous catheter care (Table 85-16).[16]

MECHANICAL COMPLICATIONS

Mechanical complications can be divided into those that occur during initial insertion and, later, those that are either nonocclusive or occlusive.

Nonocclusive Complications

Introduction of an air embolus can occur at the time of central venous catheter insertion, with defective catheters (e.g., cracks in the catheter hub, catheter rupture), and with catheters with faulty connections. Symptomatology is directly related to the severity of the air emboli and includes shortness of breath, hypoxia, tachycardia, hypotension, and neurologic changes. Other complications following central line placement include pneumothorax, hemothorax, hydrothorax, intravascular and extravascular malpositioning, and branchial plexus injury. Hydrothorax, like hemothorax, can occur at the time of catheter placement. Additionally, it may occur as a result of delayed catheter perforation due to erosion of the blood vessel after placement. In either case, intravenous fluids being administered through the catheter will empty into the pleural space or mediastinum.

Intravascular malpositioning is more common than extravascular malpositioning and may be the result of a catheter coiling in a vessel, advancing into the right atrium or ventricle, or being located in a peripheral vessel. If the catheter tip terminates in the right atrium, the sinoatrial node can be stimulated, leading to cardiac arrhythmias.

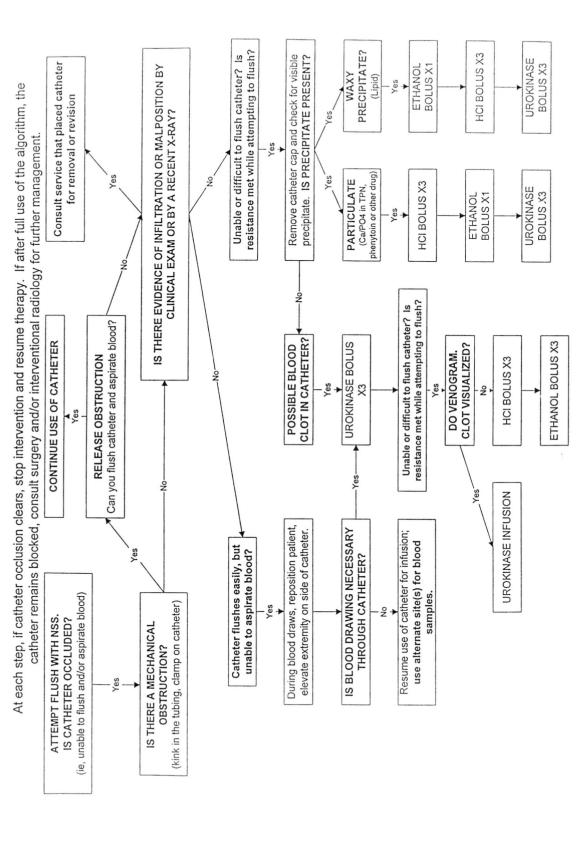

FIGURE 85-3. Algorithm for management of occluded central venous catheters. (From The Children's Hospital of Philadelphia,[55] with permission.)

Furthermore, if the inner wall of a heart chamber is punctured by the catheter, cardiac tamponade may result. Extravascular malpositioning often results when the introducer is accidentally placed outside the vein and thus the catheter becomes lodged into the pleural space or the mediastinum. Lastly, brachial nerve injury may occur during catheter insertion or with malpositioning. Such an injury is manifested as tingling sensation of the fingers and pain and paralysis of the arm.[36,37]

Mechanical complications seen with long-term catheter use are generally related to catheter breakage of the venous access device either in the patient or externally. Small tears, pinholes, or breakage may occur in the Silastic material of the catheter. There are commercially available kits made by each catheter manufacturer that are used to repair the fractured catheter. Damage to the septum of implantable ports may occur if a noncoring needle is not used. This will result in leakage of fluid from the rupture of the self-sealing rubber catheter and then into the surrounding tissue. It may be difficult to aspirate blood from a port whose septum has been damaged.[40]

Catheter fracture and embolization occur infrequently when the catheter becomes pinched closed by the patient as a result of the patient's position, by the catheter's being either caught between the clavicle and the first rib or obstructed, with the catheter tip lodged against the vein wall. The distal segment of the catheter may then embolize and recoil into the pulmonary artery or the right ventricle. This complication requires removal of the fractured segment and the proximal catheter.[36]

Needle dislodgement from an infusaport may occur when the needle slips from the port septum and fluid infuses into the surrounding tissue. The port will not have a blood return, and the patient may complain of localized pain or burning. It is prudent practice to assess the needle position during continuous infusions. Extravasation can occur with tunneled catheters, with fluid also leaking into the surrounding tissue with resultant edema.

Occlusive (Thrombotic) Complications

Catheter occlusion may occur as a result of an intramural thrombus, extraluminal fibrin sleeve, mural thrombosis, or buildup of precipitate from drugs.[53] The occlusion can range from a withdrawal problem, when there is an inability to aspirate blood but fluids infuse without difficulty (the ball-valve effect), to a complete occlusion where nothing can be infused through the catheter. Solutions used to flush the catheter are intended to maintain catheter patency. The most commonly used solutions are anticoagulants (e.g., heparin) and 0.9% saline. Outcome of prophylactic heparin therapy such as inclusion of heparin in PN solutions remains questionable. The risk of potential adverse effects and the optimal dosage regimen remain undefined. Currently, doses of 0.5 U/ml of PN and 1 U/ml of PN solution are recommended for neonates and infants/children, respectively.

The development of a thrombosis may occur as a result of a vascular injury during the catheter placement or from contact with the tip of the catheter. Platelets adhere to the catheter from platelet aggregation, and fibrin is formed from plasma fibrinogen via the clotting cascade. As a consequence, a thrombus develops. These thrombi can develop either within the catheter (intramural thrombi) or at the site of the vascular injury (mural thrombi). Over time, these mural thrombi can become large veno-occlusive thrombi. Fibrin sleeves develop from the catheter's contact with blood. As with the development of a thrombus, platelets and fibrin adhere to the catheter, and a "sleeve" is formed that encapsulates the catheter.

The incidence of catheter-related venous thrombosis is 4% to 68%, and 55% to 100% for fibrin sleeve development, although the clinical presentation is much lower. In addition to the inability to infuse fluids or aspirate blood, other symptoms of an upper extremity thrombosis are pain with infusion, swelling of the arm near the catheter, and observable collateral circulation on the chest. In superior vena cava syndrome, there will be neck and facial swelling. Many patients will have no symptoms.[37] Treatment is aimed at determining the cause for the occlusion and the appropriate intervention. With intraluminal blockages, urokinase, ethanol, hydrochloric acid, and sodium bicarbonate may be instilled in the catheter. Occasionally, a combination of fibrinolytic agents and guidewire manipulation is needed to restore patency.[36]

A radiologic assessment is necessary with extraluminal occlusions.[37] An upper limb venography is a much more sensitive test than a dye study through the catheter as this does not detect extensive obstruction in the deep venous system. Andrew et al[54] evaluated the incidence of catheter-related thrombosis in 12 pediatric patients receiving home PN. The 12 children had had a total of 49 central venous lines placed, 39 of which were removed, with 27 (66%) being removed for occlusion. On venography, 8 of the 12 children had evidence of deep venous thrombosis. The authors conclude that the risk of deep venous thrombosis is a concern and must be considered in patients with catheter occlusion. Venography is warranted in these patients.

A thorough understanding of occlusive problems is critical in responding to occluded catheters. It is imperative to use a stepwise approach to have the best possible outcome. At the Children's Hospital of Philadelphia, an algorithm is utilized to manage occluded catheters in a stepwise approach[55] (Fig. 85-3).

REFERENCES

1. Ament ME, Reylor L, Guss WJ: Parenteral nutrition in infants and children. In: Wyllie R, Hyams JS, Eds. Pediatric Gastrointestinal Disease: Pathophysiology, Diagnosis, Management. Philadelphia: WB Saunders, 1993:1140–1156

2. Heird WC: Parenteral nutrition. In: Grand RJ, Sutphen JL, Dietz WH, Eds. Pediatric Nutrition: Theory and Practice. Stoneham, MA: Butterworth, 1987:747–761

3. Jones MO, Pierro A, Hammond P et al. Glucose utilization in the surgical newborn receiving TPN. J Pediatr Surg 1993; 8:1121–1125

4. Everitt NJ, McMahon MJ. Peripheral intravenous nutrition. Nutrition 1994;10:49–57

5. Bell SJ, Mascioli EA, Bistrian BR et al. Alternative lipid sources for enteral and parenteral nutrition: long- and medium-chain triglycerides, structured triglycerides, and fish oils. Perspect Practice 1991;91:74–78

6. Hyltander A, Sandstrom R, Lundholm K. Metabolic effects of structured triglycerides in humans. Nutr Clin Practice 1995;10:91–97

7. Dahn MS. Structured lipids: an alternative energy source. Nutr Clin Practice 1995;10:89–90

8. Nordenstrom J, Thorne A. Comparative studies on a new concentrated fat emulsion: intralipid 30% vs. 20%. Clin Nutr 1993;12:160–167

9. Haumont D, Deckelbaum RJ, Richelle M et al. Plasma lipid and plasma lipoprotein concentrations in low birth weight infants given parenteral nutrition with twenty or ten percent lipid emulsion. J Pediatr 1989;115:787–793

10. Haumont D, Richelle M, Deckelbaum RJ et al. Effect of liposomal content of lipid emulsions on plasma lipid concentrations in low birth weight infants receiving parenteral nutrition. J Pediatr 1992;121:759–763

11. Greene HL, Hambidge M, Schanler R, Tsang RC. Guidelines for the use of vitamins, trace elements, calcium, magnesium, and phosphorus in infants and children receiving total parenteral nutrition: report of the Subcommittee on Pediatric Parenteral Nutrient Requirements from the Committee on Clinical Practice Issues of the American Society for Clinical Nutrition. Am J Clin Nutr 1988;48:1324–1342

12. Multivitamin preparations for parenteral use: a statement by the nutrition advisory group. JPEN (J Parent Ent Nutr) 1975; 3:258–262

13. WHO. Energy and Protein Requirements. Technical Report Series #724. Geneva: World Health Organization, 1985

14. Liggett SB, St. John RE, Lefrak SS. Determination of resting energy expenditure utilizing the thermodilution pulmonary artery catheter. Chest 1987;91:562–566

15. Driscoll DF. Total nutrient admixtures: theory and practice. Nutr Clin Practice 1995;10:114–119

16. Hill SE, Heldman LS, Goo EDH et al. Fatal microvascular pulmonary emboli from precipitation of total nutrient admixture solution. JPEN (J Parent Ent Nutr) 1996;20:81–87

17. Krzywda EA, Andris DA, Whipple JK et al. Glucose response to abrupt initiation and discontinuation of total parenteral nutrition. JPEN (J Parent Ent Nutr) 1992;17:64–67

18. Bendorf K, Friesen CA, Roberts CC. Glucose response to discontinuation of parenteral nutrition in pediatrics less than 3 years of age. J Parent Ent Nutr 1996;20:120–122

19. Collier S, Crouch J, Hendricks K, Cacallero B. Use of cyclic parenteral nutrition in infants less than 6 months of age. Nutrition in Clinical Practice 1994;9:65–68

20. Baker AL, Rosenberg IH. Hepatic complications of total parenteral nutrition. Am J Med 1987;82:489–497

21. Sax HC, Bower RH. Hepatic complications of total parenteral nutrition. J Parent Ent Nutr 1988;12:615–618

22. Benjamin DR. Hepatobiliary dysfunction in infants and children associated with long-term total parenteral nutrition: a clinico-pathologic study. Am J Clin Pathol 1981;76:276–283

23. Pereira GR, Sherman MS, DiGiacomo J et al. Intrahepatic cholestasis associated with parenteral nutrition in premature infants. Pediatrics 1979;64:342–347

24. Merritt RJ. Cholestasis associated with total parenteral nutrition. J Pediatr Gastroenterol Nutr 1986;5:9–22

25. Drongowski RA, Coran AG. An analysis of factors contributing to the development of total parenteral nutrition induced cholestasis. J Parent Ent Nutr 1989;13:586–589

26. Kubota A, Okada A, Nezu R et al. Hyperbilirubinemia in neonates associated with total parenteral nutrition. JPEN (J Parent Ent Nutr) 1988;12:602–606

27. Quigely EMM, Marsh MN, Shaffer JL, Markin RS. Hepatobiliary complications of total parenteral nutrition. Gastroenterology 1993;104:286–301

28. Verhage AH, Cheong WK, Allard JP, Jeejeebhoy KN. Increase in lumbar spine bone mineral content in patients on long-term parenteral nutrition without vitamin D supplementation. J Parent Ent Nutr 1995;19:431–436

29. Koo WWK. Parenteral nutrition-related bone disease. J Parent Ent Nutr 1992;16:386–394

30. Hurley DL, McMahon MM: Long-term parenteral nutrition and metabolic bone disease. Endocrinol Metab Clin North Am 1990;19:113–131

31. Klein GL, Ament ME, Bluestone R et al. Bone disease associated with total parenteral nutrition. Lancet 1980;8203:1041–1044

32. Weinsier RL, Krumdieck CL. Death resulting from overzealous total parenteral nutrition: the refeeding syndrome revisited. Am J Clin Nutr 1981;34:393–399

33. Solomon SM, Kirby DF. The refeeding syndrome: a review. J Parent Ent Nutr 1990;14:90–97

34. Knochel JP. The pathophysiology and clinical characteristics of severe hypophosphatemia. Arch Intern Med 1977;137:203–220

35. Rudman D, Millikan WJ, Richardson TJ et al. Elemental balances during intravenous hyperalimentation of underweight adult subjects. J Clin Invest 1975;55:94–104

36. Denny DF. Placement and management of long-term central venous access catheters and ports. Am J Radiol 1993;161:385–393

37. Ryder M. Peripherally inserted central venous catheters. Nurs Clin North Am 1993;28:937–971

38. Broviac JW, Cole JJ, Scribner BH. A silicone rubber atrial catheter for prolonged parenteral alimentation. Surg Gynecol Obstet 1973;136:602–606

39. Hickman RO, Buchner CD, Clift RA et al. A modified right atrial catheter for access to the venous system in marrow transplant recipients. Surg Gynecol Obstet 1979;166:295–301

40. Gullo SM. Implanted ports: technological advances and nursing care issues. Nurs Clin North Am 1993;28:859–871

41. Maki DG: Infections due to infusion therapy. In: Bennett JV, Brachman PS, Eds. Hospital Infections. 3rd Ed. Boston: Little, Brown, 1992

42. Nahata HC, King DR, Powell DA et al: Management of catheter-related infections in pediatric patients. J Parent Ent Nutr 1988;12:58–59

43. Snydman DR, Pober BR, Murray SA et al. Predictive value of surveillance skin cultures in total parenteral nutrition-related infection. Lancet 1982;2:1385–1388

44. Bjornson HS, Colley R, Bower RH et al. Association between microorganism growth at the catheter insertion site and colonization of the catheter in patients receiving total parenteral nutrition. Surgery 1982;92:720–727

45. Christenson ML, Hancock ML, Gattuso J et al. Parenteral nutrition associated with increased infection rate in children with cancer. Cancer 1993;72:2732–2738

46. Centers for Disease Control and Prevention. Draft Guidelines for Prevention of Intravascular Device-Related Infections: Part 1. Intravascular Device Related Infections: An Overview; Part 2. Recommendations for Prevention of Intravascular Device-Related Infections. Centers for Disease Control and Prevention, Public Health Service, Department of Health and Human Services, 1995

47. Mermel LA, McCormick RD, Springman SR, Maki DG. The pathogenesis and epidemiology of catheter-related infection with pulmonary artery Swan-Ganz catheters: a prospective study utilizing molecular subtyping. Am J Med 1991;91:197–295

48. Maki DG, Ringer M, Alvarado CJ. Prospective randomized trial of povidone-iodine, alcohol, and chlorhexidene for prevention of infection associated with central venous catheters. Lancet 1991;338:339–343

49. Shapiro JM, Bond EL, Garman JK. Use of chlorhexidene dressing to reduce microbial colonization of epidural catheters. Anesthesiology 1990;73:625–631

50. Maki DG, McCormack KN. Defatting catheter insertion sites in total parenteral nutrition is of no value as an infection control measure. Am J Med 1987;83:833–840

51. Hoffman KK, Weber DJ, Samsa GP, Rutala WA. Transparent polyurethane film as an intravenous catheter dressing: a meta-analysis of the infection risks. JAMA 1992;267:2072–2076

52. Maki DG, Stolz S, Wheeler S. A prospective, randomized, three-way clinical comparison of a novel, highly permeable, polyurethane dressing with 206 Swan-Ganz pulmonary artery catheters: Opsite IV3000 vs Tegaderm vs gauze and tape. Cutaneous colonization under the dressing, catheter-related infection. In: Maki DG, Ed. Improving Catheter Site Care. London: Royal Society of Medicine Services, 1991

53. Cunningham RS, Bonham-Crawford D. The role of fibrinolytic agents in the management of thrombotic complications associated with vascular access devices. Nurs Clin North Am 1993;28:899–909

54. Andrew M, Marzinotto V, Pencharz P et al. A cross-sectional study of catheter-related thrombosis in children receiving total parenteral nutrition at home. J Pediat 1995;126:358–363

55. Children's Hospital of Philadelphia, Medication Protocol Subcommittee of the Therapeutic Standards Committee. Central Venous Catheter Occlusion, 1996

86

MANAGEMENT OF OSTOMIES

LOUISE SCHNAUFER
DIANE S. JAKOBOWSKI

Enterostomies are required in the pediatric population for decompression of the bowel or relief of an obstruction. Fortunately for most children, the stoma is temporary and can be reversed when surgically indicated. In this chapter, we will discuss the indications for an ostomy, briefly review the surgical procedures, and then discuss the management of an ostomy in the hospital as well as at home with anticipatory guidelines for parents.

INDICATIONS FOR AN OSTOMY

Surgical intervention is frequently required for the formation of enterostomies (jejunostomy, ileostomy, colostomy) in the management of certain congenital anomalies and acquired diseases such as inflammatory bowel disease and in the management of abdominal trauma.

CONGENITAL ANOMALIES

HIRSCHSPRUNG'S DISEASE

Almost all infants with Hirschsprung's disease require a diverting colostomy. Many infants have bowel obstruction at birth and are at great risk for developing enterocolitis because of bowel distention and bacterial translocation. Once the diagnosis has been confirmed, generally by contrast studies and suction rectal biopsies, a diverting colostomy should be done at the transitional zone between the proximal normally ganglionated bowel and the distal aganglionic segment. A small left lower quadrant laparotomy is done, the aganglionic segment and transitional

zone are identified, and a biopsy is done of the bowel wall in an extramucosal fashion. The absence of ganglion cells is confirmed by frozen section evaluation, and then the colostomy is done in the ganglionated portion of bowel. A simple loop colostomy is performed, but some surgeons prefer to use a double-barrel colostomy in which both stomas are separated for a short distance. If total colonic aganglionosis is found, then an ileostomy must be done after proving ganglion cells are present in the terminal ileum. Usually an end ileostomy is constructed in which the proximal end of the ileum is brought out as the stoma, and the distal end is closed and dropped back into the abdominal cavity to be resected at a future time. The definitive pull-through procedure is performed when the baby weighs about 16 pounds. However, many surgeons are now doing the pull-through procedure shortly after birth by means of an endorectal Soave procedure without the use of a colostomy. Older children who have just been diagnosed with having Hirschsprung's disease will require a colostomy because of the usually massively dilated colon due to chronic partial obstruction. After several months of decompression, a pull-through procedure is done.

IMPERFORATE ANUS

Newborns with high imperforate anus will require a temporary colostomy. These infants may have either an intermediate type, where the rectum ends blindly at or below the levator sling, or the high type, where there is usually a fistula from the colon to either the urethra or the bladder. This anomaly cannot be reconstructed in the newborn period because of the technical difficulties in such a small child. A completely diverting colostomy must be done because there can be no spillover of stool into the distal colon where it communicates with the urinary tract. Both the proximal and distal stomas are separated for a short distance on the abdominal wall. When the baby weighs 16 to 18 pounds, the definitive pull-through procedure is done.

MECONIUM ILEUS

Approximately 15% of infants with cystic fibrosis have bowel obstruction at birth due to inspissated meconium in the distal ileum. The absence of pancreatic enzymes causes the meconium to be very tenacious and thick, and it often accumulates in the distal ileum, resulting in obstruction. In the past, the large, dilated, meconium-filled ileal segment was resected, and an end-to-end anastomosis was done to reconstitute the gastrointestinal tract. This often resulted in continued obstruction because of the remaining inspissated meconium that could not be passed. Gastrografin enemas are now the method of choice for removing the meconium; however, about 30% of the infants do not respond to the enemas, and a diverting ileostomy must be done. The segment of ileum containing the inspissated meconium is resected, and then the proximal end of the ileum is anastomosed to the side of the distal end, which is then exteriorized as a stoma in the right lower quadrant. This allows irrigation of the distal ileum and colon with pancreatic enzymes or Mucomyst to liquefy the remaining meconium so it can be evacuated. Once intestinal contents pass through the bowel, the ileal stoma becomes defunctional. It may then atrophy and close, or it may need to be closed surgically.

Acquired Diseases

NECROTIZING ENTEROCOLITIS

Bowel perforation and necrosis are often a serious complication in infants with necrotizing enterocolitis. A common site for perforation is the terminal ileum and cecum. Resection of all necrotic segments must be done and the proximal viable bowel exteriorized as an end stoma. In some children, it is necessary to perform multiple stomas if several segments of bowel are resected to preserve as much bowel length as possible. Eventually, if the child survives, intestinal continuity can be restored.

INFLAMMATORY BOWEL DISEASE

Children with Crohn's disease or ulcerative colitis often require a diverting ileostomy because of abscess formation, enteric fistulas, or intractable bleeding. Patients with ulcerative colitis will usually have an endorectal pull-through of the terminal ileum to the rectum. Those with Crohn's disease usually do well after resection of the in-

volved bowel and an end-to-end anastomosis to restore continuity.

MANAGEMENT

Preparation

Parents are devastated that their child is sick, but an enterostomy is a constant reminder that their child is different. Families need to grieve and mourn the loss of their perfect child. With the help of educated health care providers, families can move forward and begin to cope with the situation.

The first step is for the family to realize that a stoma diverts the fecal stream but does not make the child "abnormal." Stooling is a normal function, and their child stools but in a different manner. For a newborn, parental bonding is critical. Parents should be encouraged to hold the baby, make eye contact, and focus on all the wonderful attributes of their child. With an older child, developmental issues must be considered such as change in body image and peer issues.

Parent-to-parent or child-to-child support can be extremely helpful. If the ostomy surgery is being done on an elective basis, talking to a family who has been through the surgery can provide a different focus. Questions can be asked and answered very directly, and issues about lifestyle, friends, sleep-overs, and so on can be addressed. Support groups for parents and those specifically for children are available. The simplest means to contact these groups is through the local United Ostomy Association. Networks and support groups are listed in Table 86-1.

Ostomy site selection is very important. In most situations, except for critically ill infants, the position of the stoma on the abdomen is preselected with input from the child and family. Criteria for site include placement within the rectus muscle and avoidance of any bony prominences, skin folds, old scars, and the belt line. The left and right lower quadrants of the abdomen are the usual sites. This task is especially difficult with adolescent boys, who have a tendency to wear their pants very low on their

TABLE 86-1. Support Organizations for Ostomy Patients

United Ostomy Association (UOA) 800-826-0826

The American Pseudo-Obstruction and Hirschsprung's Disease Society, Inc. (APHS) 617-395-4255

The Pull-Thru Network 201-891-5977

A newsletter for children with ostomies:
"Ostomy Kidzette"
8527 Ridgefield Place
San Diego, California 92129

TABLE 86-2. Teaching Ostomy Care Based on Psychosocial and Cognitive Stages of Children

Age Group	Psychosocial Stage	Cognitive Level	Teaching: Primary Caregiver	Teaching: Child
Infant—newborn to 12 mo	Trust vs. mistrust	Sensorimotor period	Provides total ostomy care. Positive approach can include nuclear and extended family.	Learns by touching, exploring his/her body. Will begin to notice expressions of caregivers.
Toddler—12 mo to 3 yr	Autonomy vs. shame	Sensorimotor period Preoperational period (begins about age 2 yr)	Same as for infant. Positive approach; process that is done with, not to, the child. Encourage child's successes, minimize failures.	Encourage child to "help," e.g., hold measuring guide, peel off paper backing from appliance, play with teaching aid. Give simple "here and now" explanations.
Preschooler—3 to 5 yr	Initiative vs. guilt	Preoperational period concept formation (begins about age 7 yr)	Performs work with scissors. Completes cleansing of peristomal skin. Oversees emptying of pouch/application and removal of clamp. Applies ostomy system. Channels child's curiosity in a positive manner.	Peels off papers. Helps clean peristomal skin. Begins to learn emptying of pouch/manipulation of clamp. Lessons should be of short duration.
Schoolchild—6 to 12 yr	Industry vs. inferiority	Concrete operations	Early (6–9 yr). Same as later preschooler period. Offers child patient, positive encouragement.	Early (6–9 yr). Same as later preschooler period. More adept at manipulating clamp and emptying pouch independently. May begin to help apply ostomy system. Uses scissors with supervision. Avid interest in teaching aids.
			Preadolescence (9–12 yr). Joint effort with child. Offers psychological support and encourages efforts at self-care.	Preadolescence (9–12 yr). Child begins to assume self-care. Uses teaching aids as tools for learning, not toys.
Adolescent—12 yr to late teens, early 20s	Identity formation vs. identity diffusion	Formal operations period	Early to middle (12–18 yr). Instructed along with adolescent. Monitors care, makes appointments, orders equipment. Offers psychological support.	Early to middle (12–18 yr). Client generally assumes self-care.
			Late (18 yr to early 20s). Offers psychological support and encouragement.	Late (18 yr to early 20s). Manages self-care. Generally responsible for obtaining own supplies and making appointments.

(From Edwin-Toth P, with permission.)

TABLE 86-3. Goals of Ostomy Management

Ensure adequate outflow of stool

Protect the peristomal skin from breakdown

Prevent odor

Protect the clothing

hips. It is a challenge to find a location for a stoma below the belt line, not close to the trochanter, and within the rectus musculature.

Once the site is selected, it will be helpful to have the older child or adolescent wear a pouch for several hours prior to the surgery. A small amount of warm water is placed in the pouch to mimic stool and to give the child an idea of what to expect postoperatively. Most children are resistant to this step, but in the long run it has proved very helpful.

Preparation and ongoing professional support are invaluable to a child with an ostomy and to the family. Table 86-2 reviews the psychosocial and cognitive stages children go through and uses those stages as a basis for teaching ostomy care.

Nonappliance Method

The goals of ostomy management are presented in Table 86-3. For infants with a distal colostomy, it is not always necessary to pouch the stoma if the effluent is pasty or semi-formed. The peristomal skin is protected in the same manner as the perineal area if the baby were stooling through the anus. Petroleum- or zinc-based products are applied liberally to the skin around the stoma. A water-soluble product such as K-Y jelly is placed over the stoma to prevent the stoma from sticking to the diaper, which could cause bleeding. This is done by applying the jelly to the inside of the diaper, on gauze squares, or on reusable cotton squares such as cut pieces of cloth diapers. The use of a diaper one size larger than normal is recommended to prevent the stool from getting on the clothing.

Appliance Method

An infant or child with a jejunostomy, ileostomy, or proximal colostomy needs to wear a pouch, since the effluent is liquid and contains proteolytic enzymes that would irritate exposed skin. There are now a variety of pouches (appliances) available to meet the needs of infants and children. They are usually catalogued as one-piece or two-piece appliances (Table 86-4), and each can be purchased as closed-ended or drainable. Appliances are usually constructed of a pectin- or Karaya-based surface that sits on the skin and protects the peristomal area and may come with a "picture framed" hypoallergenic tape for extra adhesive. This skin barrier is usually referred to as a wafer or flange. The pouch is affixed to the barrier in a one-piece system and separate in the two-piece system. The pouch can be clear or opaque, and many come with a soft, cotton-type backing to decrease the problem of skin irritation when the plastic touches the skin and causes increased perspiration. Pouch covers are also available. These muffle noise and also decrease the problem with perspiration.

The one-piece type is flexible, which is important for babies with round bellies or in a situation where part of the appliance rests on the iliac crest, an old scar, or a skin fold. They can be molded onto unusual surfaces. The one-piece appliances are usually thinner than other pouches and are therefore less noticeable under clothing. They come in precut sizes for round stomas or "cut-to-fit" for the usual nonround pediatric stoma. The major disadvantage of the one piece is that emptying the drainage from the appliance requires complete removal of a closed-ended device, which with frequent changes can irritate the peristomal skin.

The two-piece systems are more versatile than the one piece but are not as flexible. This is due to the Tupperware-like ring that holds the two pieces together. With this system, however, the pouch can be changed as the needs of the child change. For example, an adolescent with an ileostomy may wear a small "mini pouch" for swimming, a larger closed-ended pouch for school, and then a urostomy (spout type) pouch at night to allow for continual bedside drainage with a larger collecting system.

TABLE 86-4. Ostomy Appliance Selection

	One Piece	Two Piece	Drainable	Closed-Ended
Advantages	Flexible, does not protrude significantly.	Pouch can easily be changed without changing skin barrier.	Reusable; therefore, less costly.	Ease of use. No need to empty. Place in trash, and apply new system.
Disadvantages	If pouch needs to be changed, entire system must be removed.	May be more noticeable. Not flexible; seal is difficult to achieve on round or scarred abdomen.	If clamp is not secure, pouch could leak. Complete cleaning may be difficult.	Expensive due to need for frequent changing.

Note: One-piece or two-piece appliances come with drainable or closed-ended systems.

TABLE 86-5. Procedure for Changing Ostomy Appliance

1. Carefully remove old appliance with moistened cloth or an adhesive remover packet.
2. Assess integrity of peristomal skin.
3. Clean skin with mild soap and water. Rinse with clear water, and dry skin thoroughly.
4. If needed, apply a pectin-based paste or powder.
   a. Apply a thin coating of powder to peristomal skin if denuded. Brush off excess.
   b. Squeeze paste directly from tube, or place paste in syringe. Apply to irregular areas of peristomal skin or stoma edge.
5. Measure stoma, and cut appropriate opening in flange. Round off internal edge of flange.
6. Remove paper backing from flange. Apply to skin. Firmly press flange around the stoma, working from the inner to the outer edge.
7. If two-piece appliance is used, snap pouch onto flange.
8. Close the end of an open-ended pouch with the appropriate clamp.

Changing the appliance can be a fairly simple task for the child or caregiver if proper discharge instructions and preparations are complete. It is almost always advisable to have a visiting nurse go to the home within the first few days after discharge to assess the parents' skills, answer any questions, and anticipate any problems.

The appliance should be changed approximately every 2 to 5 days. Any less "wearing time" should be investigated to see if the pouching system needs to be altered. If the appliance is intact, it may remain in place for as long as 7 days and then needs to be changed to assess the peristomal skin. It is best to change the appliance right before eating, when the stoma is putting out the least amount of drainage. The procedure for appliance change is outlined in Table 86-5.

ANTICIPATORY GUIDELINES

1. The stoma may decrease in size by as much as one-third following surgery, especially if the child had obstruction preoperatively.
2. The stoma is beefy red and will look like the tissue inside the mouth.
3. Changing the appliance while taking a bath or shower works well. The adhesive is easily removed, and the peristomal skin can be cleaned thoroughly.
4. Cutting several flanges ahead of time will decrease the amount of time needed to change the appliance.

5. Empty the pouch when it is one-third to one-half full.
6. Denuded skin should be covered with the appliance. There is a tendency to leave this area "open to air," but this will make the irritation worse. Apply stoma powder to the denuded skin, brush off the excess, and then apply the flange.
7. The use of any ointments or creams that leave a residue on the peristomal skin will interfere with the adherence of the device.
8. Use of an appliance belt can be helpful if security and wearing time are issues.
9. Infants and toddlers should be dressed in one-piece outfits to prevent them from "exploring" the pouch.
10. Extra appliance systems should be brought with the child for trips or overnight stays.
11. An extra appliance should be left at school, and the school nurse should be familiar with the child's medical needs.
12. If odor is a concern, a few drops of mouthwash or a product called Banish can be put into the pouch.

DISCHARGE PLANNING

A child with uncomplicated ostomy surgery may be discharged from the hospital in 2 to 3 days. In general, this usually does not provide adequate time for the child or family to adjust. Teaching, counseling, and mobilization of community resources must occur quickly. A thorough understanding of the anatomy, characteristics of the stoma, and general concepts of care will need to be reviewed prior to discharge. Ostomy supplies for the home need to be ordered. In addition, arranging for several home care nursing visits can help the child and family adapt to this new situation, review the teaching, and assist with the appliance change.

SUGGESTED READINGS

Bishop HC. Ileostomy and colostomy. In: *Pediatric Surgery*. Chicago: Year Book Medical Publishers, 1986

Davies A. Children with ostomies: parents helping parents. Journal of Enterostomal Therapy 1992;19:207–212

Edwin-Toth P. Teaching ostomy care to the pediatric client: a developmental approach. JET 1988;15:126–130

Garvin G. Discharge preparation of the pediatric patient with an ostomy. Progressions 1990;202: 12–19

Jeter K. *Those Special Children*. Palo Alto, CA: Bull Publishing, 1982

Smith DB. Peristomal skin problems: a nursing challenge. Progressions 1980;112:3–8

Wilkins S, Pena A. The role of colostomy in the management of anorectal malformations. Pediatr Surg Int 1988;3:105–109

INDEX

ISBN 0-443-05542-4